Textbook of ORTHOPEDICS

A Thought from the Student

God created the doctor and his patient. Together they created many hospitals and medical institutions. A happy world is what it would have been, had it not been the emergencies in between.

Let this book come in 'handy' when it matters the most.

— **K Sarawana**

Textbook of
ORTHOPEDICS
Includes Clinical Examination Methods in Orthopedics

Fifth Edition

John Ebnezar
(A "Padma Shri Awardee"-2016)
("Dr BC Roy National Awardee"-2015)
Honorary Doctorate in Medicine-Orthopedics (2016)
PhD (Yoga) MD (Ortho-Hons) MBBS D'Ortho DNB (Ortho) MNAMS Sports Medicine (Australia) IOA-INOR Fellow (UK)
Consulting Orthopedic, Sports Specialist, Spine Surgeon and Holistic Orthopedic Expert
Geriatric Orthopedic Surgeon
Formerly, Vice-President, Indian Orthopedic Association
Founder President, Geriatric Orthopedic Society of India (GOSI)
Founder Director, Geriatric Orthopedic Association of India (GOAI)
Founder President, Orthopedic Author's Association, and All India Medical Author's Association (AIMAA)
President, Neuro-Spinal Surgeons Association of India (Karnataka)
Chairman, Swaasthya Health Foundation®
Chairman, Karnataka Orthopedic Academy®
President, Bangalore WHOlistic Academy
Chairman, Rakesh Cultural Academy
President, Vaidya Kala Ranga, Bengaluru, Karnataka, India
Medical Superintendant, CV Raman General Hospital, Bengaluru, Karnataka, India
CEO, Parimala Health Care Services (AN ISO 9001:2008 Hospital), Bengaluru, Karnataka, India
Chief Orthopedic and Spine Surgeon, Dr John's Orthopedic Center, Bengaluru, Karnataka, India
Chairman, Ebnezar Medical Institute, Bengaluru, Karnataka, India
Author of Over 200 Books in Orthopedics
Editor-in-Chief, Journal of the Geriatric Orthopedic Association of India
Editor, Journal of Yoga and Physiotherapy
District Chairman for Health, Rotary District 3190
Guinness World Record Achiever in Book Writing – 2010, 2nd World Record in Book Writing (103 Books) – 2012
Guinness World Record Achiever in Social Service – 2015, Guinness World Record in Social Service – 2016
Winner of 177 International, National and State Awards/Felicitations
A "Karnataka Rajyotsava Awardee – 2010" (Highest Karnataka Civilian Award)

Co-author
Rakesh John
MBBS MS (Ortho) DNB (Ortho) MNAMS MRCS (England) Diploma SICOT
Senior Resident
Department of Orthopedics
Postgraduate Institute of Medical Education and Research
Chandigarh, India

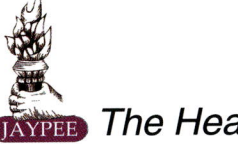

The Health Sciences Publisher
New Delhi | London | Panama

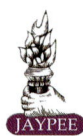 **Jaypee Brothers Medical Publishers (P) Ltd**

Headquarters
Jaypee Brothers Medical Publishers (P) Ltd
4838/24, Ansari Road, Daryaganj
New Delhi 110 002, India
Phone: +91-11-43574357
Fax: +91-11-43574314
Email: jaypee@jaypeebrothers.com

Overseas Offices

J.P. Medical Ltd
83 Victoria Street, London
SW1H 0HW (UK)
Phone: +44 20 3170 8910
Fax: +44 (0)20 3008 6180
Email: info@jpmedpub.com

Jaypee-Highlights Medical Publishers Inc
City of Knowledge, Bld. 235, 2nd Floor, Clayton
Panama City, Panama
Phone: +1 507-301-0496
Fax: +1 507-301-0499
Email: cservice@jphmedical.com

Jaypee Brothers Medical Publishers (P) Ltd
17/1-B Babar Road, Block-B, Shaymali
Mohammadpur, Dhaka-1207
Bangladesh
Mobile: +08801912003485
Email: jaypeedhaka@gmail.com

Jaypee Brothers Medical Publishers (P) Ltd
Bhotahity, Kathmandu
Nepal
Phone: +977-9741283608
Email: kathmandu@jaypeebrothers.com

Website: www.jaypeebrothers.com
Website: www.jaypeedigital.com

© 2017, Jaypee Brothers Medical Publishers

The views and opinions expressed in this book are solely those of the original contributor(s)/author(s) and do not necessarily represent those of editor(s) of the book.

All rights reserved. No part of this publication may be reproduced, stored or transmitted in any form or by any means, electronic, mechanical, photocopying, recording or otherwise, without the prior permission in writing of the publishers and author.

All brand names and product names used in this book are trade names, service marks, trademarks or registered trademarks of their respective owners. The publisher is not associated with any product or vendor mentioned in this book.

Medical knowledge and practice change constantly. This book is designed to provide accurate, authoritative information about the subject matter in question. However, readers are advised to check the most current information available on procedures included and check information from the manufacturer of each product to be administered, to verify the recommended dose, formula, method and duration of administration, adverse effects and contraindications. It is the responsibility of the practitioner to take all appropriate safety precautions. Neither the publisher nor the author(s)/editor(s) assume any liability for any injury and/or damage to persons or property arising from or related to use of material in this book.

This book is sold on the understanding that the publisher is not engaged in providing professional medical services. If such advice or services are required, the services of a competent medical professional should be sought.

Every effort has been made where necessary to contact holders of copyright to obtain permission to reproduce copyright material. If any have been inadvertently overlooked, the publisher will be pleased to make the necessary arrangements at the first opportunity.

Inquiries for bulk sales may be solicited at: jaypee@jaypeebrothers.com

Textbook of Orthopedics

First Edition: 1996
Second Edition: 2000
Third Edition: 2006
Fourth Edition: 2010
Fifth Edition: **2017**

ISBN: 978-93-86056-68-9

Printed at: Samrat Offset Pvt. Ltd.

Dedicated to

My mother (Late) Sampath Kumari
who taught me that life is more than self and there
is more joy in giving and sharing than taking,
My wife Dr Parimala, my lovely children Rakesh and Priyanka
who are an epitome of love, sacrifice, encouragement and inspiration,
All my teachers
who made me what I am today
&
All my students past and present

Comments

I have gone through your book. It is very good for undergraduate students in orthopedics. Please accept my heartiest congratulations.

PS Ramani
Professor Emeritus
World Renowned Spine Surgeon
Formerly, Professor and Head
Department of Neurosurgery
LTMG Medical College
Sion, Mumbai, Maharashtra, India

Presentation is excellent, language is lucid, clarity of subject matter, very nice, illustrations and diagrams very good and sufficient. The author is definitely a good teacher.

Bhaskaranand Kumar
Formerly, Professor and Head
Department of Orthopedics
Kasturba Medical College
Manipal, Karnataka, India

Let me congratulate you on publishing such useful books for the benefit of postgraduate students and orthopedicians.

As it stands today, in my opinion these books are of more value than the Campbells Operative books which contain 900+ techniques and we do not even practise even 50 or 60 of them. Also, the textbooks contain topics which have no relevance to this part of the world. Congratulations once again for the excellent efforts. I will definitely recommend your books to the post-graduates when I meet with them.

NS Laud
(A "Padmabhushan Awardee")
Formerly, Professor and Head
Department of Orthopedics
LTMG Medical College
Sion, Mumbai, Maharashtra, India
Formerly, President
Indian Orthopedic Association

Foreword

I sincerely admire the efforts of Dr John Ebnezar. It is an excellent book for the undergraduate and postgraduate students (their teachers too!). I like the style of his writing.

My heartiest congratulations on his solo herculean effort.

With best wishes.

GS Kulkarni
MS MS (Ortho) FICS
Professor
Department of Orthopedics and Director
Orthopedics Hospital and Post Graduate Institute of Orthopedics
Swasthiyog Pratishthan
Miraj, Maharashtra, India
(Recognised for MS (Ortho), D (Ortho), Courses by
Shivaji University and Medical Council of India,
Delhi and Recognised for Dip NB (Ortho), MNAMS
by National Board of Examinations, Delhi
Editor, Clinical Orthopedics India
Secretary, ASAMI, India (Ilizarov Association)
Chief Research Director, Sandhata Medical Research Society
Miraj, Maharashtra, India

Foreword

I am very glad that Dr John Ebnezar has written an excellent book on orthopedics.

The book is extremely informative and is most up-to-date. It is very stylishly written and is neatly designed. It has so many unique features which is hitherto unprecedented in the history of textbook writing.

What makes this book stand out from the rest is that, it never provides the reader with a single dull moment and makes the reading very interesting and thought provoking. It keeps the reader engrossed and the students will find it very gripping and absorbing.

I am sure students will enjoy reading this book and will find it very useful in their preparation for the examination.

I wish him all the success.

N Ramesh
Formerly, Professor and Head
Department of Orthopedics
Bowring and Lady Curzon Hospital
Bangalore Medical College
Bengaluru, Karnataka, India

Foreword

Dr John Ebnezar has been my assistant and has worked with me for over two years. Knowing him it is hardly surprising that he has written a textbook of orthopedics for such is his keeness and interest in teaching the students. He enjoys teaching and is tremendously popular among the students.

The book is very comprehensive, simple and is neatly written. Never before any book on orthopedics has come out with so many innovations and this kindles and sustains the interest in the readers. A good book is one which apart from evincing interest in the readers about the subject, makes them desirous to know more and more about it. This book does that and I am sure students will enjoy reading it and the roller coaster experience it provides. The practical approach and suggestions will help the students in their preparations for the examination.

This is the first ever textbook written by an Orthopedic Surgeon from Karnataka and I am happy that it comes from my assistant. It is indeed befitting that I write a foreword for his book.

I wish him all the best.

YA Somasundara
Formerly, Senior Professor and Head
Department of Orthopedics
Bangalore Medical College
Bengaluru, Karnataka, India

Preface to the Fifth Edition

It is almost 2 decades when my *Textbook of Orthopedics* hit the market. Ever since I have been deluged with an unprecedented love, support and encouragement from teachers and students from all over the country. More than my effort, it is this universal liking that has made this book what it is today. It has broken all the conventional barriers and is galloping triumphantly into the fifth edition. With each passing year, this book has grown from strength to strength. It is both heartening and humbling to hear encomiums from senior professors to undergraduates. Postgraduate students in orthopedics find this book invaluable. In short, this book has catered to the needs of all and sundry in orthopedics. In this edition, I have made sincere attempts to live up to the expectations bestowed upon me by scores of people. I am placing the fifth edition of this book in your hands with the following changes:

Highlights

- The book has been thoroughly overhauled
- Each and every chapter has been thoroughly updated
- I have inserted about 1,350 mind-boggling color diagrams in this edition
- I have inserted a number of color clinical photographs wherever required
- New X-rays have been added
- Breaking away from the conventional practice, I have introduced lots of innovative and thought-provoking diagrams, which is an idea of my own. Hope students will like it
- Even the appendices have been thoroughly revised
- Due to the sheer number of diagrams, the book has slightly overgrown its size. However, it is an apparent bulk and not the real bulk as diagrams add to the quality of the book.

My book has been widely appreciated for columns like quick facts, vital facts, flowcharts, points to ponder, mnemonics, etc. and many students have told me that they just read these just before the examinations. These columns give them the gist of the entire chapters in a jiffy and it is a great boon to them. Copying is the best complement and I now see so many new books coming out in the market in orthopedics are copying this method of mine thereby stamping their approval of my beliefs and thoughts.

Section on *Clinical Examination Methods in Orthopedics* continues to be offered as a free supplement with this edition.

Nobody is infallible. I am grateful to all those who wrote to me pinpointing certain mistakes in the previous edition. I have corrected these and incorporated the meaningful suggestions. I will be glad to have your feedback on this fifth edition too and help me in my endeavor to maintain high standards. Hope my efforts will be well appreciated by the teachers and students community at large. I will be highly obliged if you can send me your comments, criticisms and suggestions. I will be too happy to make the changes if there are any lacunae.

John Ebnezar
(A "Padma Shri Awardee")
("Dr BC Roy National Awardee")

Rakesh John

Preface to the First Edition

While I was a final year MBBS student, I fell in love with orthopedics lock stock and barrel. The subject fascinated me so much that I was drawn towards it like a magnet. I always wanted to do something to the subject I loved most. This book is a small effort on my part in this regard.

Students often questioned me during my undergraduate teaching sessions as to which book they should read for orthopedics. Whenever I suggested the standard books written for them, they said they found them too inadequate and that the bigger books were too much for them. So they were in a situation of either too little or too much. I then asked them as to what sort of book they need? They said that, they wanted a book which is comprehensive and at the same time examination oriented. I learnt that my notes were actively being circulated among the students and after each examination, students came back to me and told that they had done extraordinarily well after reading my notes. This surprised me as I had always taught them more than required. I was a firm believer of the fact that by pruning the subject one cannot do justice to it. Examination should be a part of the learning process and not vice versa. I then decided to write a book for them which was adequate, neither less nor more. Little did I realize then that I was embarking on a journey which was arduous and tumultous. I slogged for three long years to bring out this book. Hope students find my effort informative and useful.

Despite being meticulous, I am sure there will be plenty of mistakes in the book. I request the students to point them out unhesitatingly so that I can improve upon. This book will be a useful handbook for postgraduate students also.

Now about the highlights of this book:
To make the book more educative and also to present an enjoyable reading, I have tried certain innovative methods which hitherto has not been attempted in textbook writing. I am confident that it will be received well.

- Autobiographical anatomy: I have noticed that majority of students skip anatomy for reasons of monotony. To assure that they read anatomy, I planned to make it different. So I decided to let the structures talk about themselves. I hope this self-talking anatomy appeals
- Good illustrative diagrams
- Differential shading of the tables and columns to highlight the facts in their order of importance
- Quick short summaries during each chapter to make the student focus their attention towards the important and salient features of the topic concerned
- Useful mnemonics wherever feasible to enable the students to remember and recall easily
- Diagrams have been put in tabulated columns with suitable description to make it more useful and attractive
- Orthopedics is a part of life and not vice versa. The philosophies of life applies to it also. Hence, an attempt is made to view orthopedics in a philosophical angle
- Anecdotes, jokes and a word of caution wherever found neessary
- Good flowcharts to convey the ideas effectively
- Though examination is not everything, but still it is an inescapable inevitability in any student life. On their request, a list of examination short cases and relevant points have been given at the end of the book. It will be of use if only the subject has been studied properly. It will be complementary and not a substitute for good reading
- X-rays are put in the end of chapters so that students can browse through it, especially during examinations
- The chapter on instruments is prepared with great care to maximally benefit the students
- History of orthopedics is given equal weightage as much as the recent advances. I firmly believe that it is to the solid foundation laid down by our forefathers we owe our present-day success. It is our duty to remember and know their contributions and build upon it
- Chapter on low backache is written to educate the students about their back. It is a common problem which every student needs to know irrespective of the subject of interest in future. Hence, an attempt is made to present it more realistically
- More importantly, I have used the services of my students rather than professionals and I hope they have done a commendable job, as they know the requirements and pulse of the students better.

John Ebnezar

Acknowledgments

Bringing out the fifth edition of the *Textbook of Orthopedics* turned out to be a marathon effort. My belief that it would be a smooth sailing considering the experience of the previous four editions went topsy-turvy. I ended working harder for this venture. A mammoth effort like this cannot be stage managed by a single person hence I would like to recall with gratitude the role played by these good samararitans in making my dream a reality.

First and foremost, I would like to offer my reverence to my beloved mother *Late* Smt Sampath Kumari, who unfortunately could not live to see the book getting completed. A disciplinarian and idealistic mother to the core. I owe my very existence and success to her. I thank my wife Dr Parimala, my son Rakesh, who is now a Senior Resident in the Department of Orthopedics at Postgraduate Institute of Medical Education and Research, Chandigarh, India, who also has co-authored this book, and my beautiful and lovely daughter Dr Priyanka, for the unstinted and unflappable love, warmth, encouragement and support.

I thank all my teachers who shaped my personality and career right from primary school to my postgraduation in orthopedics. I thank all the colleagues of Victoria Hospital, Bangalore Medical College, for their cooperation. I thank my artist friend Mr Linus, for creating such beautiful diagrams as desired by me. His creativity in imagining and translating my thoughts into pictures and producing the right impressions are worthy of praise. But for his skill, the book would not have been what it is today. I thankfully acknowledge with fond memories the role played by students Dr KR Raghavi, Dr Raghvendra, Dr Santosh and Dr Roopa in this endeavor of mine. I also thank my Junior Reasearch Assistant Dr Yogita in lending me a helping hand. I also thank all the staff of my hospital, for helping me.

A lot of credit should go to Shri Jitendar P Vij (Group Chairman), Mr Ankit Vij (Group President) and Mr Tarun Duneja (Director–Publishing) of M/s Jaypee Brothers Medical Publishers (P) Ltd, New Delhi, India, for kindly agreeing to publish this book and accomplishing the task in a splendid manner.

I thank all the teachers and students for patronizing and supporting my book. Finally, I thank God Almighty, for all the blessings and the gift of life.

Contents

Section 1: Traumatology

1. Trauma—A Modern International Epidemic 3
- ❑ Epidemiology 3
- ❑ Prehospital Care 5

2. Know Your Skeletal System 7
- ❑ Brief Anatomy 7
- ❑ Organization of the Bones 8
- ❑ Types of Bones 10
- ❑ About Joints 11
  - Fibrous Joint or Synarthrosis 11
  - Cartilaginous Joints or Amphiarthrosis 11
  - Synovial Joints or Diarthrosis 11

3. General Principles of Fractures and Dislocations 13
- ❑ Definitions 13
- ❑ Types of Fractures 13
  - Displacement of Fractures 15
- ❑ Approach to Orthopedic Injury 16
- ❑ Investigations in Orthotrauma 19
- ❑ Management of Fractures 20
- ❑ Open Fractures 21
  - Classification (Gustilo and Anderson's) 22
- ❑ Approach in Compound Fractures 22
  - Other Forms of Fracture Immobilization 24
- ❑ Approach to a Polytrauma Case 26
- ❑ Dislocations 26

4. Complications of Fractures 29
- ❑ Acute Respiratory Distress Syndrome (Syn: Fat Embolism) 29
- ❑ Volkmann's Ischemia or Compartmental Syndromes 31
  - Compartmental Syndrome of Forearm 31
- ❑ Nonunion 35
- ❑ Avascular Necrosis 38
- ❑ Traumatic Myositis Ossificans 39
  - Classification (Based on its Location) 40
- ❑ Malunion 40
- ❑ Other Important Complications of Fractures 42
  - Deep Vein Thrombosis and Pulmonary Embolism 42
  - Injury to Blood Vessels 43
  - Injury to Nerves 44
  - Crush Syndrome 45
  - Joint Stiffness 45
  - Reflex Sympathetic Dystrophy 45
  - Osteomyelitis 45
  - Implant Failure 45
  - Post-traumatic Osteoarthritis 46
  - Growth Alterations 46
  - Shortening 46
- ❑ Complications Peculiar to Open Fractures 46
  - Shock 46
  - Gas Gangrene 46
  - Tetanus 47
  - Crush Syndrome 48

5. Emergency Care of the Injured 49
- ❑ First Aid 49
  - Goals of First Aid Treatment 49
  - Initial Care of the Injured 49
- ❑ Modus Operandi in First aid 49
  - Airway 49
  - Cardia 49
  - Bleeding 50
  - Examine the Vital Structures 50
- ❑ Management at the Hospital 51

6. Fracture Treatment Methods: Then, Now and Future 53
- ❑ History of Fracture Treatment 53
  - The Plaster Bandages 54
  - Thomas Splint 54
  - Traction 54
  - Functional Brace 54
  - Open Fractures 54
  - Early Fracture Surgery 55
  - External Fixation 55
  - Intramedullary Fixation 55
  - AO Group 55
- ❑ Fracture Treatment: Now 56
  - General Principles of the Methods of Fracture Treatment 56
  - Splints 57
- ❑ Conventional Plaster Splints 58
  - All you Wanted to Know About Plaster of Paris Splint 58

xxii Textbook of Orthopedics

- ❏ Functional Cast Brace 59
- ❏ Important Splints in Orthopedics Other than POP 60
  - *Thomas Splint* 60
  - *Böhler-Braun Splint* 61
- ❏ Traction in Orthopedics 62
- ❏ Operative Treatment 66
  - *Implants* 66
  - *Types of Implants* 66
  - *Varieties of Implants* 66
- ❏ Plates 68
  - *Types of Plates* 68
  - *AO Plates* 68
  - *Methods of Providing Compression* 68
  - *Dynamic Compression Plates* 69
  - *Intramedullary Nail* 70
- ❏ Other Important Internal Fixation Methods 71
- ❏ Fixation Techniques by Noncompression Methods 73
- ❏ External Fixation 74

7. Recent Advances in Fracture Treatment 78
- ❏ Advances in the Existing Methods of Fracture Treatment 78
  - *Improvements in Plaster of Paris Splints* 78
  - *Functional Cast Brace* 79
  - *Improvements in AO Technique* 79
  - *Improvements in Intramedullary Nails* 79
  - *Interlocking Nails* 79
- ❏ Improvements in External Fixation 80
  - *Ilizarov's Technique* 80
  - *Newer External Fixators* 83
- ❏ Advances in Hip Surgery 83
- ❏ Recent Advances in Spine Surgery 83
- ❏ Recent Advances in Bone Grafting Method 84
  - *Advantages Over the Conventional ABG* 84
- ❏ Computers in Orthopedics 85

8. Fracture Healing Methods 86
- ❏ Methods of Fracture Healing 86
  - *Indirect Fracture Healing* 86
  - *Primary Bone Healing (Direct Bone Healing, Healing by Primary Intention)* 87
  - *Distraction Histogenesis* 87

9. Soft Tissue Injuries 89
- ❏ Introduction 89
  - *Muscle Injury (Strains)* 90
- ❏ Injuries to the Joints 92
- ❏ Special Types of Muscle Injuries 98
- ❏ Important Soft Tissue Problems 99

10. Fractures in Special Situations 100
- ❏ Fractures in Children 100
- ❏ Epiphyseal Injuries 107
- ❏ Pathological Fractures 107
- ❏ Fatigue or Stress Fractures 109

Section 2: Regional Traumatology

11. Injuries Around the Clavicle 113
- ❏ Fracture Clavicle 113
- ❏ Injuries of the Acromioclavicular Joint 117
- ❏ Injuries of Sternoclavicular Joint 118

12. Injuries of the Shoulder Joint 121
- ❏ Dislocation of Shoulder 121
  - *Anterior Dislocation of Shoulder* 123
  - *Recurrent Anterior Dislocation of the Shoulder* 125
- ❏ Fracture of the Scapula 129

13. Injuries Around the Elbow 131
- ❏ Brief Anatomy 131
  - *Posterior Elbow Geometry* 132
- ❏ Injuries Around the Elbow 132
- ❏ Supracondylar Fracture 133
- ❏ Complications that Produce Cosmetic Abnormalities 138
  - *Cubitus Varus (Gunstock Elbow)* 138
- ❏ Dislocation of Elbow Joint 141
  - *Unreduced Dislocation of the Elbow* 146
- ❏ Radial Head Fracture 147
- ❏ Fracture of the Olecranon 148
- ❏ Coronoid Fractures 150
- ❏ Capitellum Fractures 152
- ❏ Physeal Fractures 152
- ❏ Lateral Condyle of Humerus (Jupiter Fracture) 153
- ❏ Medial Condyle of Humerus 154
- ❏ Sideswipe Injuries (Syn: Traffic Elbow, Car Window Elbow) 155

14. Injuries of the Forearm 157
- ❏ Fracture Both Bones of the Forearm 158
- ❏ Isolated Distal Ulnar Fracture (Also Called Nightstick Fracture) 160
- ❏ Monteggia Fracture 161
- ❏ Distal Radius Fracture 163
  - *Comminuted Distal Radial Fracture* 164
- ❏ Colles Fracture 164
- ❏ Distal Shaft Radius Fracture 164
  - *Galeazzi's Fracture* 164

- Essex-Lopresti Fracture 165
- Radial Styloid Fracture (Chauffeur's Fracture) 166
- Smith's Fracture 166
- Barton's Fracture 167
  - *Dorsal Barton* 167
  - *Volar Barton (Palmar Rim Dislocation)* 168

15. Injuries to the Wrist   170
- Brief Anatomy 170
- Carpal Injuries 170
- Scaphoid Fracture 171
- Injuries of the Carpometacarpal Joints of the Thumb 174
  - *Bennett's Fracture* 174
  - *Rolando's Fracture* 175
- Radiocarpal Injuries 176
  - *Anterior Dislocation of Lunate* 176
- Radiocarpal Dislocation 176
  - *Volar Trans-scaphoid Perilunar Dislocation* 176
  - *Dorsal Trans-scaphoid Perilunar Dislocation* 176
- Lunate Fractures 177
- Triquetral Fractures 177
- Pisiform Fractures 178
- Hamate Fractures 178
- Capitate Fractures 179
- Trapezoid fracture 179
- Trapezium Fracture 179

16. Hand Injuries   180
- General Principles 180
- Injuries to the Phalanx 181
  - *Distal Phalanx Fractures* 181
- Mallet Finger (Syn: Baseball Finger, Drop Finger, Cricket Finger) 182
- Distal Interphalangeal Joint Injuries 183
- Fractures of the Middle Phalanx 184
- Dislocations of the IP Joint 184
- Proximal Phalanx Fractures 185
- Metacarpophalangeal Joint Dislocations 187
- Kaplan's Lesion 188
- Dislocation of the Thumb Metacarpophalangeal Joint (Syn: Gamekeeper's Thumb, Skier's Thumb) 189
- Injuries to Metacarpal Bones 189
- Metacarpal Fractures (II to V) 189
- Metacarpal Fracture of the Little Finger (Boxer's Fracture) 191
- Metacarpal Head Fractures 191
- Metacarpal Fracture of the Thumb 191
- Tendon Injuries 192
- Flexor Tendon Injuries 192
- Extensor Tendon Injuries 194
- Soft Tissue Injuries of the Hand 194
- Crush Injuries of the Hand and Amputations 194

17. Dislocations of the Hip Joint   197
- Introduction 197
  - *Clinical Significance of Vascular Anatomy* 197
- Posterior Dislocation of the Hip 199
- Anterior Dislocation of the Hip 205
- Central Dislocation of the Hip 207

18. Fracture Femur   211
- Introduction 211
  - *Fracture Neck of Femur* 211
- Proximal Femur Fractures 211
  - *Subtrochanteric Fracture* 211
- Fracture Shaft Femur 214
- Fracture Distal Femur 220
  - *Supracondylar Fracture of Femur* 221
- Ipsilateral Fractures of Femoral Shaft and Neck 224

19. Injuries of the Knee   229
- Brief Anatomy 229
- Knee Ligament Injuries 229
  - *General Principles* 229
- Collateral Ligament Injury 230
- Cruciate Ligament Injuries 232
  - *Anterior Cruciate Ligament (ACL) Tear* 232
  - *Posterior Cruciate Ligament (PCL) Tear* 236
  - *Combined Knee Ligament Injuries* 236
- Semilunar Cartilage Injuries 237
  - *Medial Meniscus Injury* 238
- Fracture of Patella 242
- Injury to the Extensor Apparatus of Knee 246
  - *Quadriceps Strain* 246
- Acute Dislocation of Patella 247
- Acute Dislocation of Knee 247

20. Fracture of Tibia and Fibula   249
- Proximal Tibial Fractures 249
- Fracture Shaft of Tibia and Fibula 252
- Distal Tibial Fractures 258
  - *Pilon Fractures (Syn: Tibia Plafond Fractures)* 258
- Open Tibial Fractures 260

21. Injuries of the Ankle   261
- Brief Anatomy 261
- Ankle Injuries 261
- Ankle Sprains 265
- Trimalleolar Fracture (Cotton Fracture) 265

- Lateral Ligament Sprain 265
- Medial Ligament Sprain 267
- Tendo-Achilles Injury 267

22. Injuries of the Foot 270
- Forefoot Injuries 270
  - *Phalangeal Fractures 270*
- Interphalangeal Joint Dislocations 272
- Metatarsophalangeal Joint Injuries 272
- Injuries to the Other MTP Joints 273
- Sesamoid Bone Injuries 273
- Metatarsal Fractures 274
- Fifth Metatarsal Injuries 275
- Jones Fracture 275
  - *March Fracture (Insufficiency Fracture) 276*
- Midfoot Injuries 276
  - *Navicular Bone Fractures 277*
  - *Cuboid Fractures 277*
  - *Cuneiform Injuries 278*
  - *Tarsometatarsal Injuries (Lisfranc Injuries) 278*
- Hindfoot Injuries 279
  - *Fracture Calcaneum 279*
  - *Extra-articular Fractures 281*
  - *Intra-articular Fractures 282*
- Fracture Talus 284
  - *Fracture Neck Talus 284*
  - *Fractures of Body of Talus 286*

23. Pelvic Injuries, Rib and Coccyx Injuries 288
- Brief Anatomy 288
- Fracture Pelvis 288
- Injury to the Coccyx 295
- Rib Fractures 296

24. Injuries of the Spine 298
- Brief anatomy 298
- Injuries of the Cervical Spine 300
- Whiplash Injury (Syn: Acceleration Injury, Cervical Sprain Syndrome, Soft Tissue Neck Injury) 300
- Individual Cervical Vertebra Fracture of Interest 307
- Thoracic and Lumbosacral Spine Injuries 308
- Spinal Cord Injury 313
- Cauda Equina Syndrome 317

25. Peripheral Nerve Injuries 319
- Brief Anatomy 319
  - *Microscopic Anatomy 319*
- General Principles of Nerve Injury 320
  - *Nerve Degeneration 320*
  - *Nerve Regeneration 320*
  - *Classification of Nerve Injuries 320*
- Ulnar Nerve Injury 324
  - *Claw Hand 325*
- Radial Nerve Injury 329
- Injury to Sciatic Nerve 333
  - *Foot-drop 334*
- Meralgia Paresthetica 336
- Brachial Plexus Injuries 337
  - *Types of Lesions 337*
- Erb's Palsy 339
- Klumpke's Paralysis 340
- Axillary Nerve Injury 340
- Injury to the Long Thoracic Nerve (Winging of the Scapula) 340

Section 3: Nontraumatic Orthopedic Disorders

26. Approach to Orthopedic Disorders 345
- History 345
- Examination 346
  - *Step I 347*
  - *Step II 347*
  - *Step III 348*
- Investigations 350

27. Deformities and their Management 351
- Definition 351
- Classification 351
- Deformities Since Birth (Congenital) 351
- Acquired Deformities 351
  - *Bone Causes 351*
  - *Joint Causes 352*
  - *Soft Tissue Causes 352*

28. Treatment of Orthopedic Disorders 354
- Operative Treatment Methods 357

29. Regional Conditions of the Neck 362
- Torticollis (Wryneck) 362
- Thoracic Outlet Syndrome 363
- Cervical Rib 365
- Cervical Disk Syndromes 365

30. Regional Conditions of the Upper Limb 366
- Regional Conditions of the Shoulder 366
  - *Frozen Shoulder (Syn: Periarthritis, Adhesive Capsulitis) 366*
- Rotator Cuff Lesions 368
  - *Supraspinatus Tendinitis 369*
- Rotator Cuff Tears 370
- Deltoid Contracture 372

- ❏ Regional Conditions of the Elbow 373
  - *Tennis Elbow* 373
- ❏ Golfer's Elbow (Syn: Epitrochleitis, Medial Tennis Elbow) 376
- ❏ Olecranon Bursitis (Syn: Student's Elbow, Miner's Elbow or Draughtsman Elbow) 377
- ❏ Regional Conditions of the Wrist and Hand 378
  - *Trigger Fingers and Thumb* 378
  - *Ganglia (Ganglion Cyst)* 379
- ❏ Dupuytren's Contracture 380
- ❏ Carpal Tunnel Syndrome 381
- ❏ Compound Palmar Ganglion 384
- ❏ Keinbock's Disease 384

31. Regional Conditions of the Spine 386

- ❏ Scoliosis 386
- ❏ Spondylolisthesis (Spondylos—Spine; Olisthein—to Slip) 391
- ❏ Kyphosis 394
- ❏ Lumbar Canal Stenosis 395

32. Regional Conditions of the Lower Limb 396

- ❏ Regional Conditions of the Hip 396
  - *Coxa Vara* 396
  - *Legg-Calvé-Perthes Disease (Syn: Osteochondritis Deformans Juvenilis and Coxa Plana)* 397
  - *Slipped Capital Femoral Epiphysis (Syn: Epiphyseal Coxa Vara; Adolescent Coxa Vara)* 403
- ❏ Regional Disorders of the Knee 405
  - *Genu Valgum (Knock-Knee)* 405
  - *Genu Varum (Bow Legs)* 407
  - *Genu Recurvatum* 409
  - *Bursae Around the Knee* 409
  - *Popliteal Cyst (Baker's Cyst)* 411
  - *Recurrent Dislocation of Patella* 412
  - *Chondromalacia Patella* 413
  - *Loose Bodies in the Knee (Joint Mice)* 414
- ❏ Lesser-Known But Important Regional Conditions of the Knee 415
  - *Jumper's Knee* 415
  - *Osgood-Schlatter Disease* 415
  - *Sinding-Larsen-Johansson Syndrome* 415
  - *Iliotibial Band Syndrome* 416
  - *Plica Syndrome* 416
  - *Osteochondritis Dissecans* 416
  - *Hoffa's Syndrome (Syn: Fat Pad Syndrome)* 417
  - *Infantile Quadriceps Contracture* 417
- ❏ Regional Disorders of the Foot 421
  - *Arches of the Foot* 421
  - *Pes Cavus* 422
  - *Pes Planus* 423
  - *Foot Pain* 425
  - *Metatarsalgia* 425
  - *Morton's Neuroma* 426
- ❏ Painful Heel 427
  - *Traumatic Disturbances* 428
- ❏ Developmental and Pathological Disturbances of the Heel 428
  - *Plantar Fasciltis (Subcalcaneal Pain)* 428
  - *Calcaneal Spurs* 430
  - *Fat Pad Insufficiency (Atrophy of Fat Pad)* 431
  - *Calcaneal Stress Fracture* 431
  - *Epiphysitis of the Calcaneum (Sever's Disease)* 431
- ❏ Lesser-Known But Important Foot Conditions 432
  - *Plantar Fibromatosis (Lederham Syndrome)* 432
  - *Pump-Bump* 432
  - *Dancer Tendinitis* 432
  - *Hallux Valgus* 432
  - *Hallux Rigidus* 433
  - *Hammer Toes* 434
  - *Claw Toes* 434
  - *Sesamoiditis* 435

33. Disorders of the Hand 439

- ❏ Congenital Anomalies of the Hand 439
- ❏ Infections of the Hand 440
  - *Paronychia* 440
  - *Apical Subungual Infection* 441
  - *Distal Pulp Space Infection (Syn: Felon)* 441
  - *Middle and Proximal Volar Space Infection* 441
  - *Infection of the Web Spaces* 441
  - *Deep Palmar Abscess* 442
  - *Tenosynovitis* 442
- ❏ Arthritic Hand 444
- ❏ Paralytic Hand 444

Section 4: Common Back Problems

34. Low Backache and Repetitive Stress Injury 447

- ❏ Epidemiology of Backache 447
- ❏ Posture 447
- ❏ Pathological Physiology 447
- ❏ Lumbar Disk Disease and Disk Prolapse 449
  - *Disk Anatomy* 449
  - *Disk Physiology* 449
  - *Natural History of Lumbar Disk Disease* 449
  - *Classification of Prolapsed Intervertebral Disk* 450
  - *Etiology of Disk Herniation* 450
  - *Examination of the Back* 451
  - *Chemonucleolysis* 460

- Approach to a Patient with Low Backache 461
  - Causes of Backache 461
  - Pain 464
- Backache in Special Situations 465
  - Backache in Children (School Bag Syndrome) 465
- Repetitive Stress Injury 466

Section 5: General Orthopedics

35. Congenital Disorders 471
- Congenital Disorders of Upper Limb 471
  - Congenital Torticollis (Wryneck) 471
- Sprengel's Deformity 473
- Cleidocranial Dysostosis 474
- Congenital Radioulnar Synostosis 475
- Madelung's Deformity 476
- Congenital Absence of Radius (Radial Club-Hand) 476
  - Congenital Dislocation of Radius 477
- Congenital Disorders of Lower Limbs 477
  - Developmental Dysplasia of Hip (Earlier Known as Congenital Dislocation of Hip) 477
- Congenital Dislocation of Knee 483
  - Congenital Pseudarthrosis of Tibia 484
- Congenital Talipes Equinovarus 485
  - Ponseti Technique 490
  - Structures Released in Turco's Procedure (Posteromedial Release) 491
  - Retention of CTEV Correction 493
  - Congenital Absence of Fibula 494
  - Congenital Absence of Tibia 494
  - Congenital Vertical Talus (Syn: Rocker-Bottom Flatfoot, Congenital Rigid Flatfoot) 494

36. Developmental Disorders 497
- Introduction 497
  - Classification of Developmental Disorders 498
- Achondroplasia 499
- Osteogenesis Imperfecta 500
- Mucopolysaccharide Disorders 501
  - Morquio-Brailsford Disease 501
- Hurler's (Gargoylism) 502
- Hunter's Disease 502
- Hereditary Multiple Exostosis (Diaphyseal Aclasia) 502
- Dyschondroplasia (Ollier's Disease) 502
- Maffucci's Disease 502
- Osteopetrosis 503
  - Marble Bone Disease, Albers-Schönberg Disease 503
- Epiphyseal Dysplasias 503
  - Epiphyseal Dysplasia Multiplexa 503
  - Epiphyseal Dysplasia Punctata 504
  - Epiphyseal Dysplasia Hemimelia 504
- Metaphyseal Dysplasias 504
  - Metaphyseal Dysplasia (Pyle's Disease) 504
  - Craniometaphyseal Dysplasia 504
  - Metaphyseal Chondrodysplasia 504
- Diaphyseal Dysplasia 504
  - Progressive Diaphyseal Dysplasia (Canuati or Engelmann's Disease) 504
  - Craniodiaphyseal Dysplasia 504
  - Fibrous Dysplasia 504
  - Albright's Syndrome 505
  - Nail-Patella Syndrome (Onycho-osteodysplasia) 505
  - Marfan's Syndrome 505
- Homocystinuria 506
  - Acrocephalosyndactyly (Apert's Syndrome) 506
  - Carpenter's Syndrome 506
- Cleidocranial Dysplasia 506
- Congenital Neurofibromatosis (von Recklinghausen's Disease) 506
- Paget's Disease 507

37. Metabolic Disorders 508
- Rickets 510
  - Types of Rickets 510
- Renal Osteodystrophy 513
- Vitamin D-Resistant Rickets 514
- Celiac Rickets 515
  - Gluten-sensitive Enteropathy 515
- Osteomalacia 516
- Hyperparathyroidism 517
  - Primary Hyperparathyroidism (Osteitis Fibrosa Cystica, von Recklinghausen's Disease) 517
  - Secondary Hyperparathyroidism 518
- Scurvy 519
- Metabolic Disorders Leading to Osteosclerosis 519
  - Fluorosis 519

38. Osteomyelitis 521
- Acute Osteomyelitis 521
- Subacute Osteomyelitis 527
- Chronic Osteomyelitis 527
- Osteomyelitis of Special Importance 531
  - Brodie's Abscess 531
- Sclerotic Osteomyelitis of Garre 531
  - Tubercular Osteomyelitis 531

39. Skeletal Tuberculosis 532
- Tuberculosis Spine 536
- TB Spine with Paraplegia 542

- ❏ Tuberculosis of the Hip Joint 544
- ❏ Tuberculosis of the Knee 550
- ❏ Tuberculosis of the Shoulder 552
- ❏ Tuberculosis of the Ankle 553
- ❏ Tubercular Osteomyelitis 553
  - *Tubercular Osteomyelitis without Joint Involvement 553*
  - *Spina Ventosa Type 554*
  - *Tuberculosis of Tubular Bones 554*

40. Disorders of Joints (Arthritis) 556
- ❏ Infective Arthritis (Syn: Pyogenic Infection of Joint or Septic Arthritis) 556
- ❏ Gonococcal Arthritis 558
- ❏ Syphilis of Joints 559
- ❏ Neuropathic Joints (Charcot's) 559
- ❏ Hemophilic Arthritis (Bleeder's Joints) 560
- ❏ Synovial Chondromatosis 562

41. Rheumatic Diseases 564
- ❏ Classification 564
- ❏ Rheumatoid Arthritis 564
  - *Orthopedic Deformities in Rheumatoid Arthritis 566*
- ❏ Seronegative Spondyloarthropathies 575
- ❏ Ankylosing Spondylitis (Syn: Marie-Strumpell Disease) 576
- ❏ Fibromyalgia 579
- ❏ Crystalline Arthropathies 580
- ❏ Monosodium Urate Arthropathy (Gout) 580
- ❏ Pseudogout 582

42. Neuromuscular Disorders 583
- ❏ Cerebral Palsy (Syn: Static Encephalopathy) 583
- ❏ Poliomyelitis 586
- ❏ Arthrogryposis Multiplex Congenita (Syn: Multiple Congenital Contractures) 589
- ❏ Leprosy in Orthopedics 589
  - *Orthopedic Affections in Leprosy 590*
  - *Foot-drop 591*
  - *Plantar Ulcers 591*
  - *Affections of the Hand in Leprosy 591*
- ❏ Muscular Dystrophies 592
  - *Duchenne Muscular Dystrophy 592*
  - *Facioscapulohumeral Muscular Dystrophy 593*
  - *Limb Girdle Muscular Dystrophy 593*
- ❏ Neural Tube Defects (Dystrophism) 593
  - *Spina Bifida 593*
  - *Spina Bifida Occulta 593*
  - *Spina Bifida Aperta of Manifesta 593*

43. Bone Neoplasias 596
- ❏ General Principles of Tumors 596
- ❏ Classification of Bone Tumors 598
- ❏ Bone Tumors of Cartilaginous Origin 598
  - *Osteochondroma (Exostosis) 598*
- ❏ Chondroma (Enchondroma, Hondromyxoma) 599
  - *Chondroblastoma 601*
  - *Chondrosarcoma 601*
  - *Chondromyxoid Fibroma 603*
- ❏ Osseous Origin Bone Tumors 603
  - *Osteoma 603*
  - *Osteoid Osteoma 603*
- ❏ Osteogenic Sarcoma 604
- ❏ Resorptive Bone Tumors 608
  - *Aneurysmal Bone Cyst 608*
  - *Unicameral Bone Cyst 608*
- ❏ Giant Cell Tumor (GCT) (Syn: Osteoclastoma) 609
  - *Benign Giant Cell Tumor 609*
  - *Malignant Giant Cell Tumor 610*
- ❏ Tumors of Nonosseous Origin 612
  - *Ewing's Sarcoma 612*
- ❏ Multiple Myeloma (Plasmacytoma) 613
- ❏ Metastatic Tumors of Bone 615
- ❏ Inclusion Tumors 616
  - *Synovioma (Synovial Sarcoma) 616*
- ❏ Recent Trends in Limb Salvage Surgery 617

Section 6: Geriatric Orthopedics

44. Distal Forearm Fractures 621
- ❏ Colles' Fracture 621

45. Fracture Neck of Femur 633
- ❏ Brief Anatomy 633
- ❏ Fracture Neck of Femur 633
- ❏ Complications of Femoral Neck Fracture 640
  - *Thromboembolism 640*
  - *Nonunion 640*
  - *Osteotomy 640*
  - *Avascular Necrosis 642*
  - *Trochanteric Fracture 642*

46. Osteoporosis 646
- ❏ Definition 646
- ❏ Anti-resorptive Drugs 653

47. Osteoarthritis 658
- ❏ Osteoarthritis of the Knee 658
  - *Primary Osteoarthritis of the Knee (Also Called Idiopathic) 658*

- *Secondary Osteoarthritis of the Knee* 666
- ❑ Osteoarthritis of the Hip (Familiarly Called as Malum Coxae Senilis) 666
  - *Primary Osteoarthritis of the Hip* 666
  - *Secondary Osteoarthritis of the Hip* 667
- ❑ Osteoarthritis of Other Regions 671

48. Cervical Disk Syndromes 673
- ❑ Neck Exercises 675
- ❑ Cervical Collar 675

49. Degenerative Lumbar Disk Disease and Canal Stenosis 677
- ❑ Canal Stenosis 677

Section 7: Common Surgical Techniques

50. Common Surgeries of the Humerus 683
- ❑ DCP Plating for Fracture Shaft of Humerus 683
- ❑ Interlocking Humerus 686
- ❑ Supracondylar Fracture Humerus—Percutaneous Fixation 691
- ❑ Intercondylar Fracture Humerus—Reconstructions 696

51. Common Forearm Surgeries 702
- ❑ Excision of the Radial Head 702
- ❑ Forearm DCP Plating 702
- ❑ Medullary Fixation for Fracture of Radius and Ulna 705
- ❑ Darrach's Operation 706

52. Common Hip Surgeries 707
- ❑ Hemireplacement Arthroplasty 707
- ❑ Surgical Technique of AMP Prosthesis 714
  - *Dynamic Hip Screw Technique* 714
  - *Internal Fixation of Fracture Neck of Femur* 717

53. Common Surgery of the Femur 719
- ❑ Intramedullary Nailing 719
- ❑ Interlocking Nailing 720
- ❑ DCP Plating 724

54. Common Surgery of the Patella 726
- ❑ Patellectomy 726
- ❑ Tension Band Wiring (Modified) 726

55. Common Surgery of the Tibia 729
- ❑ DCP Plating for Tibia 729
- ❑ Interlocking Nailing of Tibia 733
- ❑ Malleolar Fixations 736

56. Turco's One Stage Posteromedial Release for Congenital Talipes Equinovarus 741

57. Common Surgery of the Spine 742
- ❑ Laminectomy 742
- ❑ Posterior Instrumentation for Vertebral Compression Fractures 745
- ❑ Posterior Decompression and Surgical Stabilization 750

58. Common Finger and Toe Surgery (Percutaneous Fixations) 755
- ❑ Finger Fracture 755
- ❑ Toe Injuries 763
  - *Surgical Technique of Percutaneous Fixation of Toe Fractures* 763

59. External Fixation 766

Section 8: Miscellaneous

60. Amputations 773
- ❑ Types 773
- ❑ Principles 775
  - *Closed Amputations* 775
  - *Open Amputations (Guillotine Operation)* 775
- ❑ After Treatment 775
- ❑ Important Amputations of Lower Extremity 776
- ❑ Complications 777

61. Prosthetics and Orthotics 778
- ❑ Prosthetics 778
  - *Prosthesis for the Above Knee Amputations* 778
  - *Prosthesis for Below Knee Amputations* 779
  - *Prosthesis for Syme's Amputation* 780
  - *SACH Foot* 780
- ❑ Jaipur Foot (India's Pride) 780
- ❑ Orthotics 780
  - *Lower Limb Orthosis* 783
  - *Upper Limb Orthosis* 785

62. Sports Injuries 786
- ❑ Classification of Sports Injuries 787

- Physical Examination of the Shoulder Joint 872
- Tests for Shoulder Joint 874
- Other Examination 874

3. Examination of Elbow Joint — 876
- History 876
- Measurements 879
- Special Tests 880
- Other Examinations 880
- Important Elbow Disorders 880

4. Examination of Wrist Joint — 881
- History 881
- Physical Examination of Wrist Joint 881
- Range of Movements 882
- Special Tests for Important Wrist Disorders 883

5. Examination of Hip Joint — 885
- History 885
- Clinical Examination 886
- Examination in Standing Position 887
- Important Tests in Standing Position 889
- Examination in the Lying Down Position 889
- Tests for Hip Stability 897

6. Examination of Knee Joint — 900
- Problems Related to Knee 900
- Clinical Examinations 901
- History 901
- Physical Examination of the Knee 902
- Q-angle (Quadriceps Angle) 904
- Tests Peculiar to Knee 905
- Tests for Collaterals 905
- Tests for Cruciates 906
- Tests for Menisci 906
- Examination of Movements 907
- Examination of the Popliteal Fossa 909
- Other Examinations 909
- Common Knee Joint Disorders 910

7. Examination of Sacroiliac Joint — 911
- Physical Examination of Sacroiliac Joint 911
- Clinical Tests for Sacroiliac Joint 911
- Tests to Differentiate Pain due to Hip Joint and Spine 912

8. Examination of Spine — 914
- General Examination 914
- Examination of the Spine 914
- Methods of Examination 916
- Other Examinations 917
- Range of Movements 917
- Examination of Spine for Low Back Pain 919
- True Back Pain 919
- Nerve Root Pain 919
- Important Spine Conditions 922

Index — 923

- ❏ Common Sports Injuries 787
- ❏ Treatment of Sports Injury 788

63. Arthroscopy 791
- ❏ What is Arthroscopy? 791
- ❏ Indications for Arthroscopy 792

64. Standard Arthroscopy Portals 794
- ❏ Patient Positioning 794
- ❏ Lateral Port (Visualization Port) 794
- ❏ Superolateral Port (Drainage Port) 794
- ❏ Medial Port (Operating Port) 795
- ❏ Superolateral Port (Patellar Tracking Port) 795
- ❏ My Inferolateral Port "Lateral Release Port" 796
- ❏ Other Ports 796

65. 9-Point Diagnostic Knee Arthroscopy 797
- ❏ First Point: Suprapatellar Pouch 797
- ❏ Second Point: Patella 798
- ❏ Third Point: Trochlea 798
- ❏ Fourth Point: Medial Gutter 798
- ❏ Fifth Point: Medial Compartment 798
- ❏ Sixth Point: Intercondylar Notch and Anterior Cruciate Ligament 798
- ❏ Seventh Point: Lateral Compartment 798
- ❏ Eighth Point: Lateral Gutter 800
- ❏ Ninth Point: Patellar Tracking 800

66. Arthroplasty 801
- ❏ Arthroplasty 801
- ❏ Hip and Knee Arthroplasty 801
- ❏ Surgical Steps of Total Hip Replacement 802
- ❏ Surgical Steps of Total Knee Replacment 813

67. Evidence-based Orthopedics 828
- ❏ Cost Effectiveness Analysis 834
- ❏ Studies Other than RCT 834
- ❏ Decision Analysis Study 835
- ❏ Quality of Reporting 835
- ❏ Developing an Evidence-based Balance Sheet 836
- ❏ Communication to a Patient 837

Appendices

Appendix I: Instruments and Implants in Orthopedics 839
- ❏ General Surgical Instruments 839
- ❏ Regular Orthopedic Instruments 839
  - *Bone Holding, Plate Holding and Rod Holding Instruments 839*
  - *Instruments Used to Cut, Nibble, Curette and Make Holes in the Bones 841*
- ❏ Miscellaneous Orthopedic Instruments 842
  - *Instruments Used for Insertion of Plate and Screws 843*
  - *Instruments Used for Cutting Plaster Casts 845*
  - *Instruments Used for Wire Insertion 845*
- ❏ Implants in Orthopedics 846
  - *Dynamic Hip and Ankle Implants 847*
  - *Some of the Special Plates Used in Orthopedics 848*
  - *Different Conventional Intramedullary Nails 848*
  - *Instruments Used for K-nail Insertion for Femur 848*
  - *Küntscher's Cloverleaf Intramedullary Nail 849*
  - *Prosthesis of the Hip 849*
  - *Different Hip Implants 851*
  - *Instruments Used for Hip Hemireplacement Surgery 852*
  - *Instruments Used for Smith-Peterson Nailing 853*

Appendix II: Guidelines for Practical Examinations 854
- ❏ Guidelines to Fare Better in Clinical Examination in Orthopedics 854
- ❏ Avoid the Following Pitfalls in the Examination Hall 855
  - *Instruments Required for Clinical Examination 855*
  - *Common Examination Cases 855*

Glossary 859
- ❏ Important Classifications in Orthopedics 859
- ❏ Important Radiological Appearances 860
- ❏ Important Fractures with Eponyms 861
- ❏ Important Clinical Tests in Orthopedics 861
- ❏ Important Orthopedic Surgeries by Names 862
- ❏ Terminologies Associated with Fractures 863
- ❏ Important Orthopedic Terminologies 863
- ❏ Important Osteotomies in Orthopedics 864

Clinical Examination Methods in Orthopedics

1. Examination of a Bony Swelling 867
- ❏ History 867
- ❏ Physical Examination of a Bony Lesion 868
- ❏ Other Examinations 869

2. Examination of Shoulder Joint 871
- ❏ History 871

Introduction

Orthopedics has come a long way since the days of Nicholas Andry, a French Physician, who is credited for coining the term, orthopedics from two words, *Ortho = straight* and *Pedics = child in 1741*.

What was a primitive branch then restricted to correcting deformities in children, has developed into a full-fledged specialty with diverse scope ranging from simple treatment, as done by traditional bonesetters to highly advanced joint, spine and hand surgeries.

The development of orthopedics as a specialty was pedestrian till 18th century. The discovery of anesthesia and aseptic surgical techniques opened-up new avenues of treatment like open reduction, debridement, etc. The discovery of X-rays by Roentgen and the introduction of the usage of plaster of Paris by Albert Mathysen in 1852 revolutionized the diagnosis and management of orthopedic disorders. Thus, orthopedics started breaking through the deadlocks of a crude branch to that of a science.

But what really set the ball rolling was the sudden surge of orthopedic cases firstly by the two World Wars and of late by the road traffic accidents which is on the rise, both in the developed and developing countries.

Polytrauma, multiple fractures and high-velocity injuries severely exposed the limitations of the conventional treatment in orthopedics, as the fracture patterns were bizarre and complicated. Thus, newer modalities of treatment like improved methods of internal fixation, the AO systems, the interlocking nail system, Ilizarov's method, etc. were introduced into orthopedic management. Suddenly, orthopedics was being considered a highly specialized branch with vast scope.

Needless to say many pioneers both at the international and national level have contributed enormously for the development of this branch to the present what is today. We salute them for their contribution. A fitting tribute to them is to carry on the good work done by them and to raise the level of this branch to such dizzy heights so that the sufferings of mankind due to orthopedic disorders are mitigated.

There is a strong notion among the students that orthopedics is all about trauma. Nothing can be farther from the truth. Though trauma contributes to a major chunk of orthopedic-related conditions yet it is not the sole contributor. Like any other system in the body, bones and joints are affected by a plethora of disease conditions ranging from congenital disorders, infections, tumors, etc. Degenerative disorders that seem to ravage the musculoskeletal system in old age complete the cup of misery. Needless to say one needs to be equipped both with knowledge and skill to gear up oneself to face the orthopedic challenges being hurled at surgeons in double quick time of late.

Through this book, I endeavor to arm my students with the all important knowledge so essential to understand and unravel the mysteries surrounding orthopedic-related conditions. Based on this knowledge, the necessary skills can be acquired through various stages of practical exposures. It always helps to know the common orthopedic terminologies, tests, surgical procedures, etc. for better and easy understanding. This is presented in the glossary. It is imperative to know about the fundamentals of bones and joints before undertaking the arduous journey of problems afflicting the musculoskeletal system. Thus basics of this systems are talked about in relevant sections. The chapters deal extensively first with the traumatic conditions and related problems, followed by non-traumatic conditions.

The tools required to acquire the all necessary skills are mentioned in the Appendix on instruments and implants. I fervently urge my students to be a stickler for basics and sophistication automatically follows. It pays to know, at the beginning itself, that the reverse is not always true.

SECTION 1

Traumatology

- Trauma—A Modern International Epidemic
- Know Your Skeletal System
- General Principles of Fractures and Dislocations
- Complications of Fractures
- Emergency Care of the Injured
- Fracture Treatment Methods: Then, Now and Future
- Recent Advances in Fracture Treatment
- Fracture Healing Methods
- Soft Tissue Injuries
- Fractures in Special Situations

1 Traumatology

CHAPTER 1

Trauma—A Modern International Epidemic

INTRODUCTION

When man was basking in the glory of conquering killer diseases like tuberculosis, smallpox, polio, typhoid, plague and other infective diseases that threatened to wipe out the human race in the past, cutting short the euphoria are certain modern causes of death and morbidity like injuries, HIV, etc. There is, however, one difference that these modern problems are man made and thus offers a greatest hope of conquering these. It is said that 99 percent of the accidents are man made and only 1 percent is providential.

Injuries due to trauma are on an unprecedented high across the globe more so in developing nations like India. The reasons are not far to seek. Road traffic accidents are on the rise, so are the industrial and agricultural accidents. Intolerance, hatred, and unrest have caused escalation in terrorist activities across the world leading to increased mortality and bizarre injuries that could maim and make one disabled for life. Add to this instances of assaults, falls, train, air and other accidents not to forget natural calamities like floods, quakes, etc. and war, all this lead to a plethora of injuries that could be a burden to the entire mankind. With sports and games gaining worldwide popularity, injuries due to these events are also on the rise. Suddenly injuries have gained the tag of a *modern international epidemic* that is ravaging young lives like never before.

EPIDEMIOLOGY

Injuries due to various causes could be either fatal or nonfatal. A look at the injury epidemiology could help you to understand the enormity of the situation.

Fatal Injuries

- Injuries are the 4th leading cause of death over all ages (6%).
- Between 1-44 years of age, it is the leading cause of death.
- Between 15-24 years, 8 out of every 10 deaths in young are due to injuries.
- Injuries account for more premature deaths than cancer, heart disease, or HIV.
- Fifty percent of deaths occur at the scene within minutes or en route to the hospital.
- Twenty to thirty percent dies of neurological dysfunction within several hours to 2 days post-injury.
- Ten to twenty percent dies of infection or multiple organ failure within days or weeks.
- Every year 1.9 million are hospitalized due to injury.
- Twenty seven million are treated in the emergency department.
- Injuries account for an estimated 8 percent of all hospital discharges, 37 percent of emergency department visits, and 35 percent of all emergency medical services transport.
- Nonfatal injures lead to reduced quality of life and high costs accrued to the health care system, employers and society in general.
- Persons less than 45 years account for 60 percent of all injury fatalities and hospitalization and 78 percent of all causality department visits.
- Persons more than 65 years account for 25 percent of all injury deaths and 30 percent of injury related hospitalization.
- Seventy percent of injury deaths and more than 50 percent of nonfatal injuries occur among males.
- Rate of injury deaths in male and female is 2:1.
- Rate of nonfatal injury in male: female is 1.3:1.
- But over 65 year's male: female is 1:1.3.

The above statistics are frightening and calls for immediate attention to rein the deleterious effects of injuries on the mankind.

SECTION 1: Traumatology

Mechanism of Injury Leading to Death

Various mechanisms of injuries lead to death or nonfatal injuries. Let us try and analyze the figures.
- Twenty nine percent — are due to motor vehicle accidents.
- Eighteen percent — are due to firearm injuries.
- Eleven percent — is due to falls.
- Poisonings lead to 17 percent of all deaths.
- Thirty percent of all injury deaths are intentional.

After having identified various mechanisms of injury deaths, a look at the causes of death shows that CNS injuries and hypovolemic shock are the prime causes of deaths in fatal injuries.

Possible Causes of Death

- CNS injuries account for 40–50 percent deaths.
- Hemorrhage — 30–35 percent.
- Multiple organ failure — 5–10 percent.

Mechanism of Trauma

The three leading mechanisms of trauma are motor vehicle accidents, firearm injuries, and falls. Now let us analyze each one in detail.

Motor Vehicle Accidents (WHO Statistics)

Increased movements, crazy driving, alcohol, technology, and recklessness all have led to an increase in the motor vehicle accidents across the world. People tend to forget that motor vehicles are meant for commuting and are for their convenience and not for adventure and thus end up with increased instances of accidents (Fig. 1.1). Let us have a look at the Global and Indian scenario.

Global Scenario

- Leading cause of injury deaths.
- Second leading cause of nonfatal injury.
- Male:Female ratio in injury deaths is 2:1.
- For males aged 15–44, RTA's rank 2nd (behind HIV and AIDS) as the leading cause of premature death worldwide.
- Causes of accidents include speed, alcohol, and poor vehicle and road conditions.
- More than 1.2 million people are killed every year in accidents.
- Three to four percent of gross national product is lost is RTA's.
- One child is killed every 3 minutes in the world.
- Total worldwide death toll of Tsunami in 2004 is about 2,30,000.

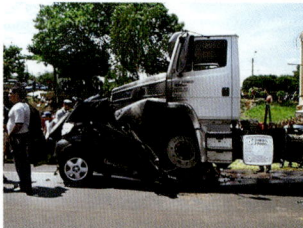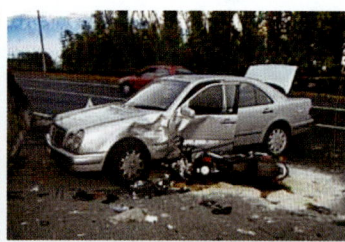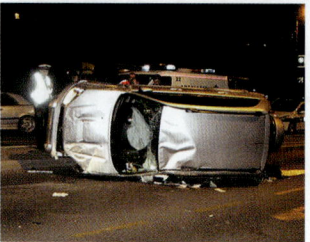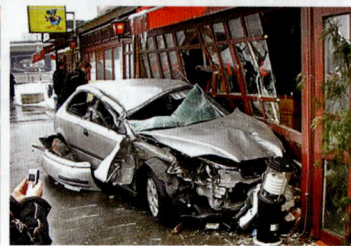

Fig. 1.1: Violent high speed accidents like these can result in fatal injuries and complex polytrauma and multisystem injuries

- So, the annual death toll due to RTA's is 5 times more than Tsunami.
- Three thousand deaths/day.
- Five hundred children/day.
- Fifty million people worldwide are injured in RTA's every year and 15 million seriously.
- Low- and middle-income countries account for more than 85 percent of global deaths.
- Global financial cost of RTA injuries is 518 billion USD/year.

Indian Scenario

- One person dies from injury every 6–10 minutes.
- Presently more than 86,000 people die annually.
- Financial loss due to RTA's is 12,000 crores/year.
- There are 406,730 accidents each year.
- Social cost due to road accidents is 550 crores annually.
- India accounts for 10 percent of the 1.2 million fatal accidents in the world.
- By 2050, India will have the greatest number of automobiles on the planet overtaking USA.

Now let us analyze the other mechanism of injuries.

Firearms

Liberal laws and misuse are leading to increased shoot-out deaths particularly in the Western countries. While most of them are suicides, homicides are also equally high.

Here are a few chilling statistics related to firearm injuries:
- They are responsible for 18 percent of all injury deaths and are the 2nd leading cause.
- Fifty six percent were suicides and 39 percent were homicides.
- Male:Female ratio is 7:1.

Falls

These are mainly accidental and rarely intentional. Increased construction activities, sports, and playful children and fragile elders are all more prone for injuries due to falls.
- Accounts for 11 percent of injury deaths.
- Greater than 1/3 of all injury related hospitalization.
- Under less than 5 years, falls are the leading cause of nonfatal injury, 50 percent at home (less than 4 years) and 50 percent at school (More than 4 years).
- Death from falls is less (0.6–4.7%).
- In the elderly, falls is important cause of death. Thirty four percent in greater than 65 years and 46 percent greater than 85 years.
- It accounts for 80 percent of all injury related hospitalization greater than 65 years.

Overall

Now after analyzing each mechanism of injury in greater detail, the overall global scenario due to injuries is as follows:
- Worldwide injuries account for 1 in every 10 deaths.
- Eleven percent of the global burden of disease.
- By 2020, RTA's will rise from 9th place to 3rd place by 2020.
- Violence will rise from 19th place to the 12th place.
- Self-inflicted injuries from 17th to the 14th place.

Nonfatal Injuries

In injury-related events those who are fortunate to survive deaths or near deaths, may have to face an equally disturbing events in the form of nonfatal injuries. These could range from simple fracture, sprain, strain to major and multisystem injuries. Any possibility of single or combination injuries are possible depending upon the type and severity of accidents. Nonfatal injuries are more morbid and could prove to be an enormous burden in terms of cost and time to the patient, relative, society, country and the world at large.

Among the fatal injuries leading to deaths, motor vehicle accidents rank first. However, a study of nonfatal injuries shows a different scenario.

Mechanism of Injury

- Falls — leading cause and accounts for 1/3 cases.
- RTA's — account for 18 percent of the hospitalizations.
- Firearm injuries — account for less than 1 percent.
- Thirty percent of all injury deaths are intentional.
- Five to fifteen percent injury hospitalizations are intentional.

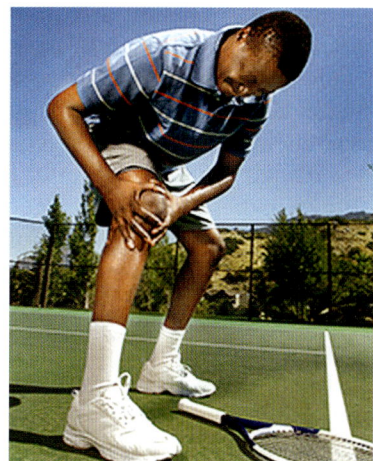

Fig. 1.2: Sports injuries lead to nonfatal injuries most of the times

Interesting Statistics of Nonfatal Injuries

- Upper and lower limb injuries leading cause of hospitalization—50 percent.
- Moderately severe and severe injuries of the extremities account for 33 percent of hospitalization.
- Primary mechanism of injury accounting for hospitalization is falls accounting for 30 percent of all upper extremity injuries and 50–60 percent of all lower limb injuries.
- RTA's are leading to increased hospitalizations due to lower limb injuries.
- Twenty percent of all hospitalizations due to upper limb injuries are due to accidents following machinery and tools.
- Head injury hospitalization accounts for 10–15 percent and is the 2nd leading cause.
- Other leading causes are spinal cord injuries and musculoskeletal injury of the back.
- Work-related back injury accounts for 1/5th to 1/4th of all workers compensation claims.

Sports Injuries

These are the important contributors of nonfatal injuries. Due to increased popularity of major sporting events like football, tennis, cricket, basketball, swimming, etc. injuries following sport activities are on the rise (Fig. 1.2). However, deaths due to sports are far and few and are not of concern.

PREHOSPITAL CARE

To have the best choice of survival, grievously injured victims should receive top quality care from the earliest moments of the accident from the emergency medical services system. Pick and dump attitude by these personnel could spell disaster. Proper first aid, skillful CPR and intelligent handling and shifting of the injured victims by the paramedics or general public can make a world of difference between a certain death and a possible good recovery (Fig. 1.3). Management during the golden hour (first hour post injury) is critical. Thus, prehospital care assumes extreme importance in these backdrops. A good prehospital trauma care system can decrease the mortality due to accidents by 33 percent.

Emergency Management and Research Institute (EMRI): is the first emergency call number and organized trauma care system in India. It has well-equipped ambulances, paramedic training and care on arrival at the hospital. It is responsible for administering proper prehospital care for the injured at the scene of accident and shifting them safely and quickly to the nearest well-equipped center meant for managing these victims (Fig. 1.4).

Once the patient is stabilized by these proper prehospital trauma life support (PHTLS) program effort is made to execute definitive treatment for individual bone and joint injuries.

However, not all well with the prehospital care of the accident or injured victims. The problems being faced by the trauma care systems in India are:
- Lack of human resources
- Lack of physical resources
- Lack of organizational resources
- Lack of trauma care system.

For effective management of the injured, all the above problems need to be tackled in a war footing by the government and the public.

Prevention of Injury

Now that injury is considered a major public health problem, the adage prevention is better than cure applies to it also. However, earlier it was thought that there is no role of prevention in the case of injury-related deaths or morbidities. But now fortunately people have started realizing that preventive measures have a very important role to play in reducing the incidence of injuries due to trauma and needs to be emphasized more. The following preventive steps are suggested:
- Preventive measures should be done like for any other disease.
- Requires an organized and scientific approach.
- It requires a multidisciplinary approach.
- Surgeons need to provide health education to patients (Helmet wear, Alcohol prevention).
- Research into the preventive and treatment aspects of tackling injuries also helps.

CONCLUSION

There is no running away from the fact that injuries have arrived in a big way in terms of deaths and nonfatal injuries across the world. It has all the features of an epidemic and needs to be tackled as such. Here are certain injury related vital issues:
- Trauma is a major public health problem.
- Primary prevention should be emphasized.
- Effective and better treatment plan is required.
- Trauma is called the neglected disease of the modern society.
- It is now the costliest medical problem in the world.

You had a brief overview of the enormity of the problem posed by injuries. Various combinations of nonfatal musculoskeletal injuries could occur. The general principles and individual treatment of these injuries will now be dealt in the ensuing chapters.

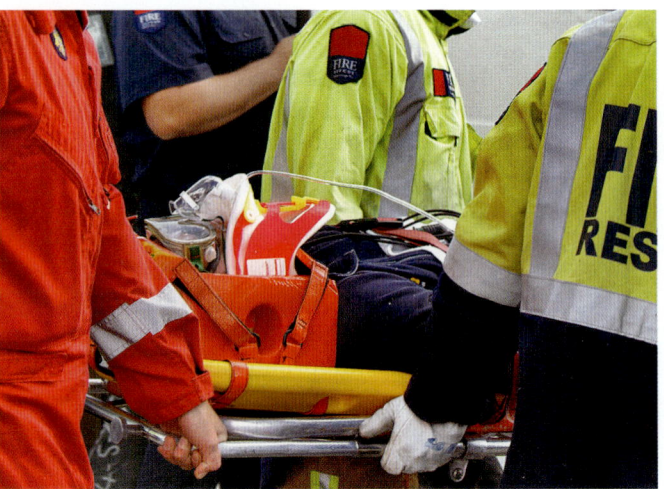

Fig. 1.4: Shifting an injured victim to the nearest well-equipped hospital is the prime responsibility of trauma care systems (EMRI in India)

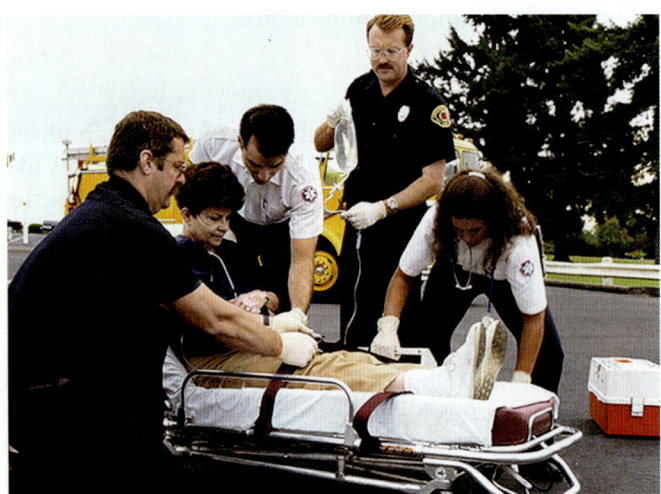

Fig. 1.3: Administering first aid and CPR to an accident victim at the scene of accident

CHAPTER 2

Know Your Skeletal System

BRIEF ANATOMY

Bone Development Speaks
I am a specialized connective tissue. By providing a rigid skeleton, I give the all-important shape to the human beings. I am proud to be entrusted the job of protecting vital structures like brain, lungs, and heart. I am the largest storehouse of the all-important mineral, calcium in the body. I am also concerned with hemopoiesis. I give attachment to the muscles and enable them to act on the joints by acting as a lever for their action. I am made-up of 30 percent organic material (mainly type I collagen) and 70 percent mineral (calcium hydroxyapatite).

Remember the Functions of Bone
- Protection of vital organs
- Support to the body
- Hemopoiesis
- Movement and locomotion
- Mineral storage.

How do I Start Developing?
My development begins with the condensation of the mesenchyme in the embryo. There are certain exceptions like the vault of the skull (membranous ossification), the clavicle (mixed ossification), and the mandible (Meckel's cartilage). From this condensation, I rapidly form a cartilaginous model. Between the cartilaginous bone and plates, I form small clefts for the future joints. During this period of 12 weeks, I am particularly vulnerable to teratogenic influences.

As early as the fifth week of intrauterine life, I develop a primary center of ossification, which gradually replaces this cartilage model to bone by a process of endochondral ossification. During the late fetal stages or early few years of life, I develop secondary centers of ossification.

Growth plate, which keeps the primary and secondary centers of ossification separated from each other until skeletal maturity, helps me grow longitudinally and I increase my width from the growth of the thickened periosteum. In addition, I keep remodeling myself from the fetal stage to the adult stage. Only the rate varies (50% during the first two years of life and 5% per year thereafter until adulthood).

Remember
- Bone development starts as a condensation of mesenchyme
- Later a cartilaginous model develops
- There are two types of ossification—endochondral and membranous
- There are three types of bone cells.

About Osteon

Now let me tell you how exactly I am made-up of internally. I am made-up of many units called "*osteon*." I have three types of cells, osteoblasts that form the bone, osteoclasts which remove the bone and are concerned with remodeling, osteocytes, which are the resting cells. These cells are present in the lamellae, which surround concentrically the Volkmann's canal (which has the nutrient vessel) and each lamellae is interconnected by the canaliculi through which the nutrients pass. Osteoblasts lay down uncalcified matrix, which is subsequently calcified as true bone. These various osteons amalgamate to form large haversian systems, loosely woven in the medullary bone and densely packed in the cortical shell (Fig. 2.1).

Now having known my intrinsic structure, you will be interested to know that I have two major portions, *medulla*, and the *cortex*.

About Medulla

Medulla is my softer counterpart and has the dual role of structure and storage. It stores more than 95 percent of body's calcium and is a storehouse for other minerals too. The other important component of the medulla is the marrow between the medullary bone lattices. This is the source from where the RBCs and WBCs originate. Initially present throughout, it confines itself to the metaphyseal regions of the long bones and in some flat bones like pelvis,

8 SECTION 1: Traumatology

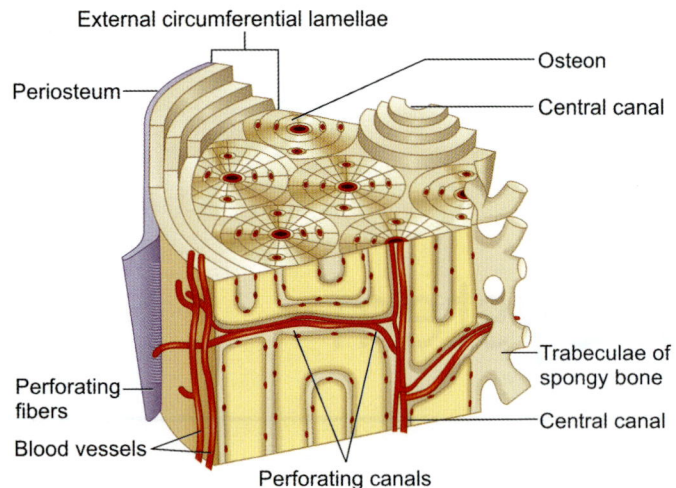

Fig. 2.1: Bone cross-section showing its internal structure

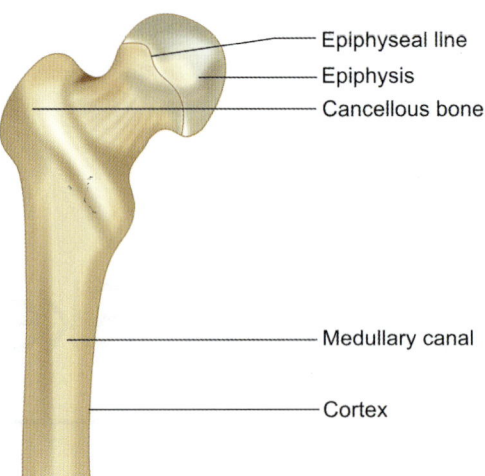

Fig. 2.2: General structure of a long bone

rib, etc. as age advances and is replaced by a *fatty white marrow*.

The medulla plays the structural role by its trabecular organization along maximal lines of stress and clearly identifies itself into *compression* and *traction trabeculae*.

About Cortex

Cortex gives me the remarkable strength, which you all admire particularly during compression. Its periosteal cover allows remodeling throughout life. It also gives attachments to ligaments, tendons, and muscles through the Sharpe's fibers.

> **Remember About Medulla**
> - Softer portion
> - Stores 95 percent of body calcium
> - Marrow is the other important component
> - Also plays a structural role.

About General Structure

Now let me explain to you my general structure. I have an epiphysis and epiphysis plate (which disappears with growth), metaphysis and diaphysis (Fig. 2.2).

Epiphysis is an expanded portion at the end develops usually under pressure and forms a support for the joint surface. It is easily affected by developmental problems like epiphyseal dysplasia, trauma, overuse, degeneration, and damaged blood supply. The result is distorted joints due to avascular necrosis and degenerative changes.

Growth plate (physis) though mechanically weak, it helps longitudinal growth. It responds to growth and sex hormones. It is affected by conditions like osteomyelitis, tumor, slipped epiphysis resulting in short stature or deformed growth or growth arrest.

Metaphysis is concerned with remodeling of bone. It is the cancellous portion and heals readily. It gives attachment to ligament and tendons. It is vulnerable to develop osteomyelitis, dysplasia, and tumors resulting in distorted growth and altered bone shapes.

Diaphysis is a significant compact cortical bone which is strong in compression and which gives origin to muscles. It forms the shafts of the bones. Healing is slow when compared to metaphysis. In remodeling, it can remodel angulations but not rotation. It may develop fractures, dysplasias, infection, and rarely tumors.

> **Remember**
> Parts of a bone
> - Epiphysis
> - Physis (growth plate)
> - Metaphysis
> - Diaphysis.

ORGANIZATION OF THE BONES

We are 206 in numbers and are grouped into two subdivisions namely:
1. Axial skeleton—80 bones.
2. Appendicular skeleton—126 bones.

Axial skeleton forms the upright axis of the body and the *appendicular skeleton* forms the appendages and girdles that attach them to the axial skeleton (Fig. 2.3).

Out of this 206, some of us are short and some are long. We have different shapes. The shape and size depend upon the functions attributed to us.

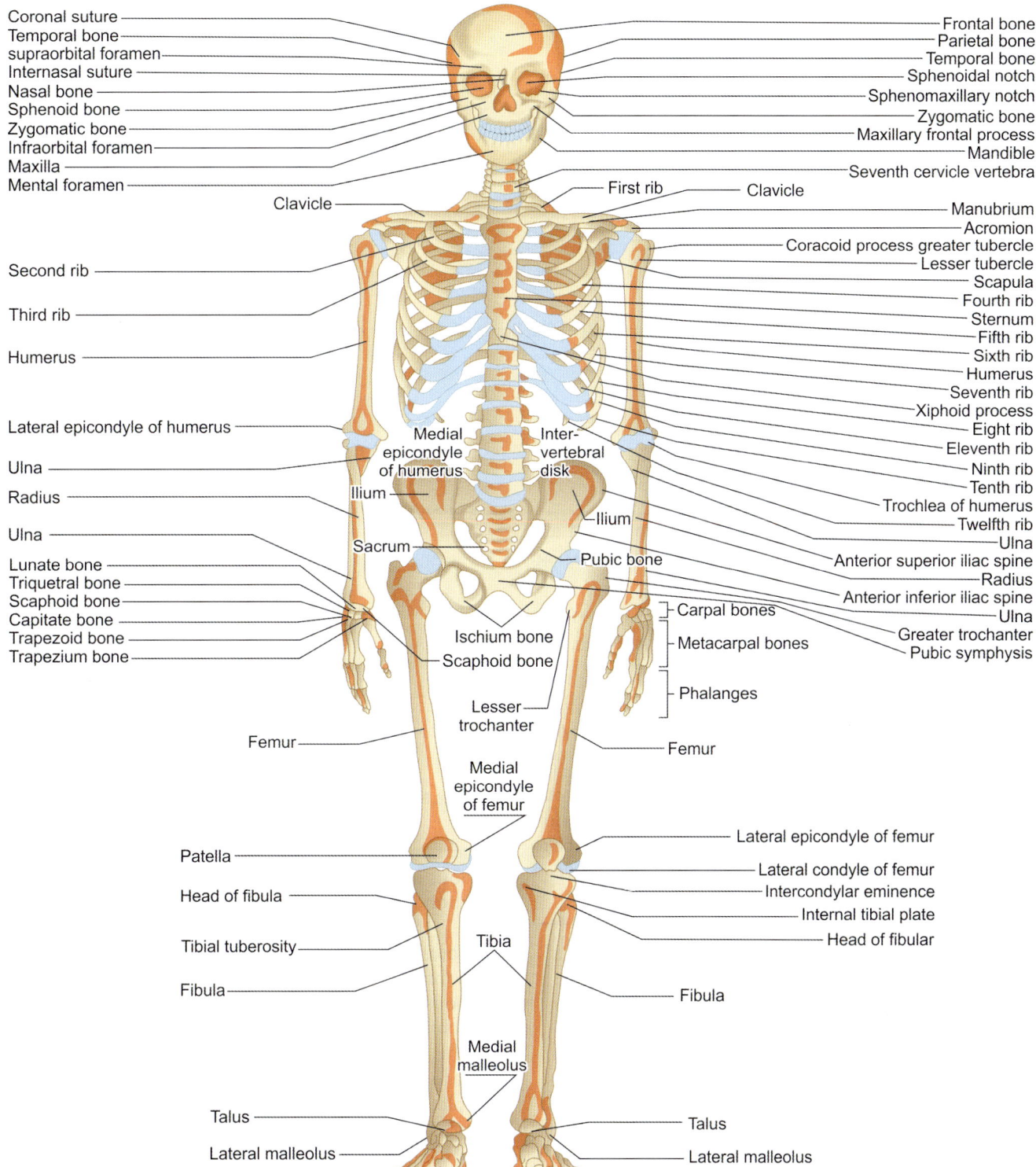

Fig. 2.3: Organization of bones: Axial and appendicular skeleton

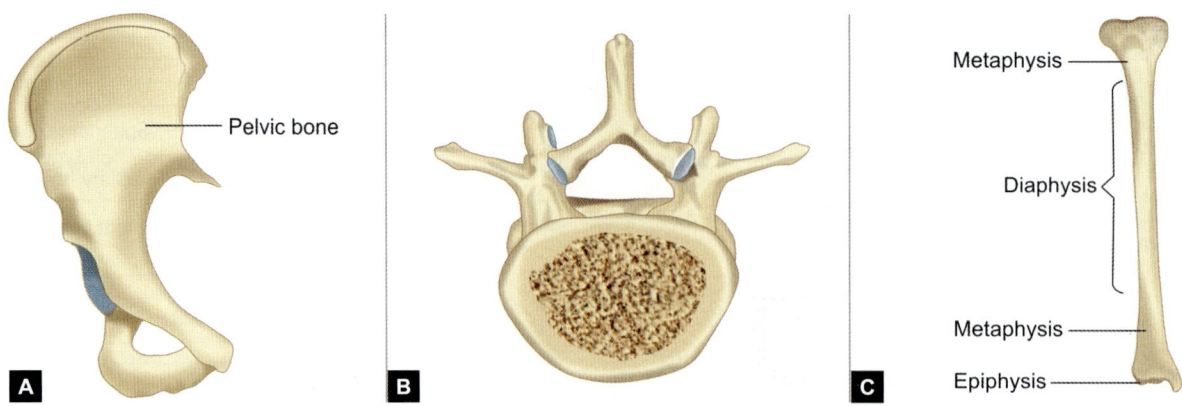

Figs 2.4A to C: Types of bones: (A) Flat bone; (B) Irregular bone; (C) Long bone

TYPES OF BONES (FIGS 2.4A TO C)

Long bones: These serve as levers for the muscle action, e.g. femur, tibia, etc. (Fig. 2.4C).

Short bones: These are generally cube-shaped and are found in areas where limited movements are required (Fig. 2.5). Their primary role is to provide strength.

Flat bones: These consist of parallel layers of compact bone separated by a thin layer of cancellous bone tissue, e.g. scapula, skull, etc. (Fig. 2.4A).

Irregular bones: These have a peculiar and irregular shape and are unique in their appearance and functions, e.g. pelvic bones (Fig. 2.4B).

Sesamoid bones: These are small, rounded, or triangular bones, which develop within the substance of a tendon or fascia. Their name is derived from their resemblance to "sesame seeds," e.g. patella (largest and most definitive of the sesamoid bones).

> **Remember**
> *Types of bones*
> - Long bones
> - Short bones
> - Flat bones
> - Irregular bones
> - Sesamoid bones
>
> *The above bones are arranged in two groups*
> - Axial—80 bones
> - Appendicular—126 bones.

Thus, my duty is to serve you to the best of my ability, so that you lead a healthy skeletal life. Much depends on you in keeping me in a proper shape. You need to take good nutritious diet rich in calcium and vitamins to keep me healthy. Proper exercises, protection against injuries and infection enhance my efficiency in serving you, but there

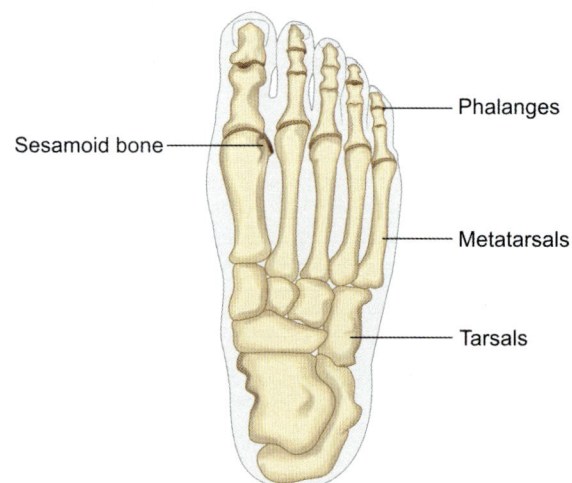

Fig. 2.5: Foot is an assembly of short bones of various sizes

are certain inherent problems in me in which you can do precious little. Congenital problems, hormonal problems, metabolic problems, tumor conditions, etc. are some of these.

However the above problems are troublesome, I develop them infrequently. Nevertheless, the problem that poses a serious threat to my integrity is injuries due to trauma. As a child, you are more playful and more prone to fall and this breaks me quite often. As an adult, you are more prone for road traffic accidents (RTAs) and this subjects me to a plethora of different varieties of forces causing many complexes, grotesque and bizarre breaks. Though you pride in the fast-paced life of yours, I grieve at my misfortune and at my vulnerability to these vast array of incriminating forces, which overcome me putting you out of action for months.

As you age, my faithful friends, proteins and minerals gradually desert me. I cannot provide you the same strength as earlier. In this phase, even trivial forces (pathological fractures) easily overcome me. I am sad that I cannot provide you the same privileges as before but I hope you can realize that I am not being unfaithful to you, but I am made helpless by situations beyond anybody's control.

ABOUT JOINTS

A joint exists where two or more skeletal components—whether bone or cartilage, come together to meet. Without joints in between the bones, your whole body would be rigid and immobile. The existence of these joints makes movement of the body parts possible. Joints are classified into three major groups:

FIBROUS JOINT OR SYNARTHROSIS

These are immovable joints, e.g. sutures of the skull. In these, there are three varieties:

Syndesmosis: This is characterized by a dense fibrous membrane that binds the articular bone surfaces very closely and tightly to each other, e.g. distal tibiofibular joint.

Sutures: True sutures are found in the skull. Here the adjoining bone margins are united into rigid, jagged interlocking processes, e.g. sagittal suture of the skull.

Gomphosis: Here a conical peg or projection that fits into a socket, e.g. teeth and sockets of jawbones.

CARTILAGINOUS JOINTS OR AMPHIARTHROSIS

These are slightly movable joints with either hyaline or fibrocartilage in between. Two varieties are described:

Synchondroses: Here hyaline cartilage is posed in between, e.g. articulations between rib and sternum.

Symphysis: Here the fibrocartilage is interposed in between and is usually found in the midline of the body, e.g. pubic symphysis.

SYNOVIAL JOINTS OR DIARTHROSIS

These form the majority of the joints in the body. They have between the bones, a synovial or joint cavity. They form the most mobile joints in the body and hence are more prone for injuries.

It consists of a fibrous joint capsule that helps to hold the articulating bones together. The synovial membrane lines the joint space and secretes the synovial fluid. This fluid serves to lubricate the joints and provides nourishment for the articular cartilage. The articular cartilage is formed by the hyaline cartilage, which is a unique type of connective tissue formed by specialized cells called chondrocytes.

Types of Synovial Joints

Uniaxial joints: These permit movement in only one plane and one axis (Figs 2.6A to G). In this, there are two types:

Hinge joints: Here movement takes place around a horizontal axis, e.g. elbow joint.

Pivot joints: Here movement takes place around a vertical axis that permits rotation, e.g. atlantoaxial joint.

Biaxial joints: Here movement occurs in two planes and two axes that are at right angles to each other. Two types are described:

Saddle joint: Here the articular surface is concave in one direction and convex in the other while the articular surface of the opposing bone is exactly the opposite, e.g. carpometacarpal joint at the base of the thumb.

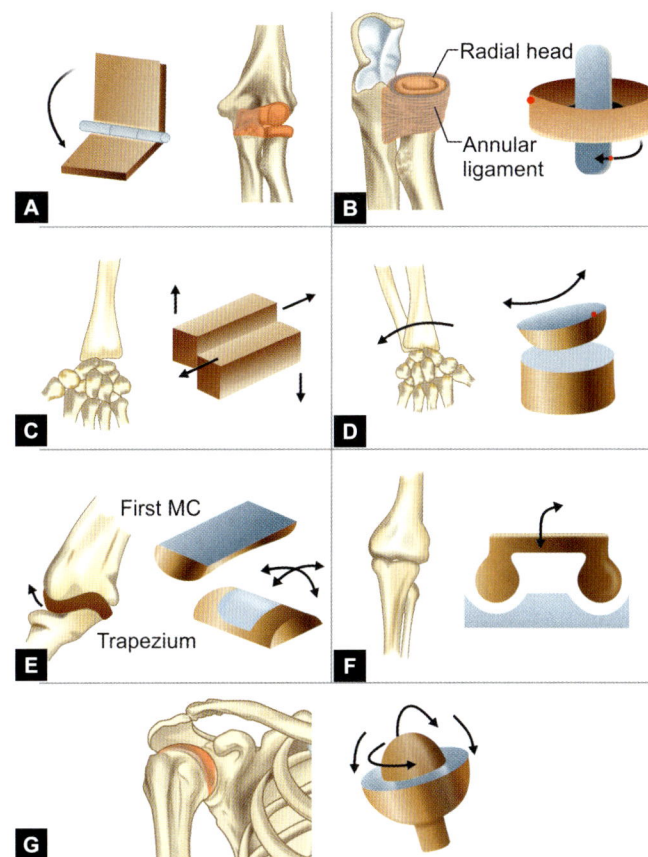

Figs 2.6A to G: Different types of joints: (A) Hinge joint; (B) Pivot joint; (C) Plane joint; (D) Ellipsoid joint; (E) Saddle joint; (F) Bicondylar joint; (G) Ball and socket joint

Condyloid joint: In this, an oval condyle fits into an elliptic socket or cavity, e.g. radiocarpal joints.

Multiaxial joints: Here there are two or more axes of rotation and movement takes place in three or more planes. Two varieties are described:

Ball and socket joint: In this, a ball-shaped head of one fits into a concave socket of another bone. Of all the joints in the body, these provide the widest, most free range of movements in almost any direction or plane, e.g. hip joint, shoulder joint, etc. (Refer Fig 2.6G).

Gliding joints: These are numerous, gliding movements occur in all planes, e.g. joints between the carpal and tarsal bones, and all the joints between the articular processes of the vertebrae (Refer Fig. 2.6C).

3 CHAPTER

General Principles of Fractures and Dislocations

INTRODUCTION

It is not surprising if a bone breaks but what is surprising is the fact that bone does not break more often considering the amount of forces, it is subjected to everyday by the muscle action, load transmission, etc. Bone has devised its own mechanism to ward off the unnatural forces and keep itself intact. But only when the force is too large and occurs suddenly (as in road traffic accidents (RTA), fall, etc.), or when a force is chronic and repetitive (e.g. prolonged standing as in a policeman, nurse, etc.) or when the natural resistance of the bone is eroded by a disease process (e.g. tumor, infection, etc.), that a bone succumbs to the insult and breaks. When it breaks, it is bound to injure the surrounding soft tissues like muscles, ligaments, etc.

DEFINITIONS

Fracture is a break in the surface of a bone, either across its cortex or through its articular surface.

Dislocation is a complete and persistent displacement of a joint.

Subluxation is partial dislocation of a joint.

Sprain is a temporary subluxation of a joint due to ligament injury and the articular surfaces return to normal alignment.

Strain is a tear in the muscle.

The bone can break within its soft tissue envelope and may not communicate to the exterior *(simple* or *closed fractures)* or it may rip through its soft tissues or the soft tissue itself may be damaged by the external forces, exposing the bone to the external atmosphere *(compound or open fractures)*. If the former event is bad, the latter event is catastrophic. In both the situations depending on whether the force is *direct* (as in direct impact in RTA) or *indirect* (e.g. through the muscle action), and depending on the amount of force applied, the direction of force, age and other factors, different fracture patterns are produced and each one poses a problem peculiar to its own.

> **Remember**
> Forces required to break a bone could be:
> - Large and sudden (e.g. RTA)
> - Repetitive (e.g. a stress fracture)
> - Trivial (e.g. pathological fractures).

TYPES OF FRACTURES

- **Simple or compound**—this has been already explained earlier (Figs 3.1A to D).
- **Based on the extent of fracture line:**
  - *Incomplete fractures*—it involves only one surface or cortex of the bone.

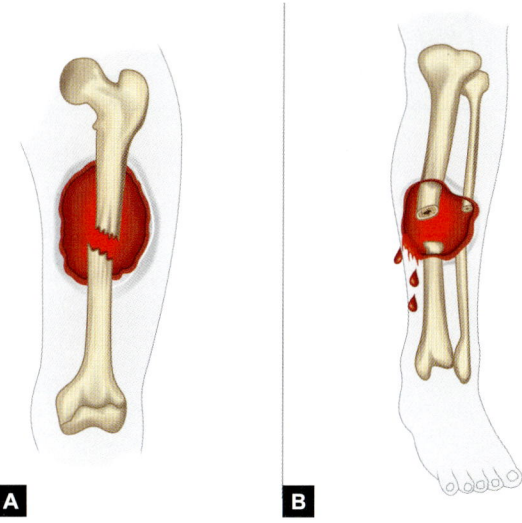

Figs 3.1A and B: Simple and compound fractures

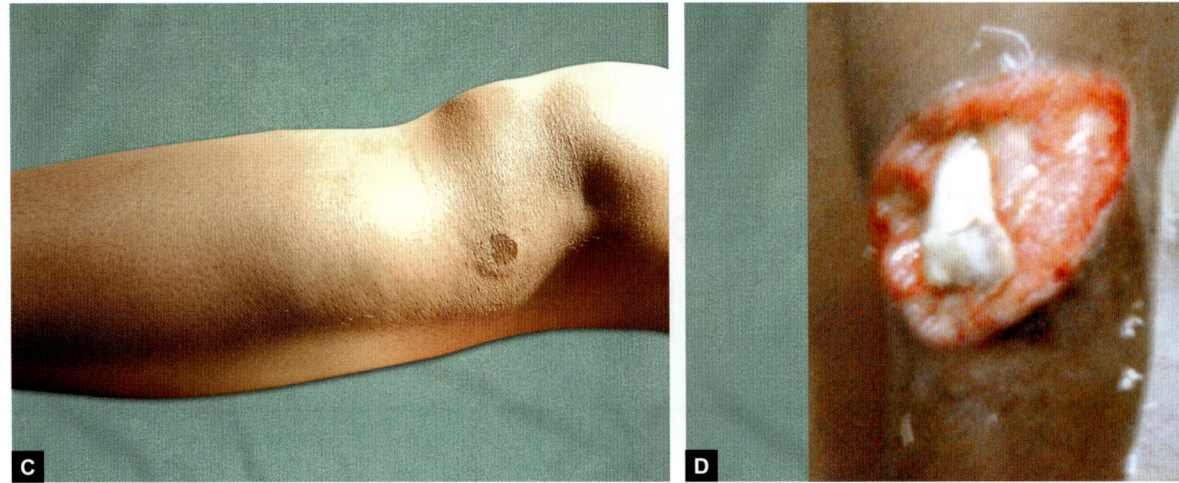

Figs 3.1C and D: Clinical photos showing simple fracture and compound fracture

- *Complete fracture*—here the fracture involves both the cortices and the entire bone. A complete fracture could be *undisplaced* or *displaced*.

Causes for Displacement
- Muscle forces.
- Gravity.
- Obliquity of the fracture line.
- Improper handling of the fracture.

- *Based on fracture patterns* (orthopedic trauma association classification—Figs 3.2A to G)
  - *Linear fractures:* These could be transverse, oblique, or spiral. Any fracture that forms an angle less than 30° with the horizontal line is called transverse. Angle equal to or more than 30° is termed oblique.
  - *Comminuted fractures:* Here the fracture fragments are more than two in number. They are further subclassified into ≥ 50 percent comminution or more than 50 percent comminution. Butterfly-shaped fractures are also included in this group and could be less than 50 percent or equal to or more than 50 percent.
  - *Segmental fractures:* A fracture can break into segments and the segment could be two-level, three-level, and a longitudinal split or comminuted.

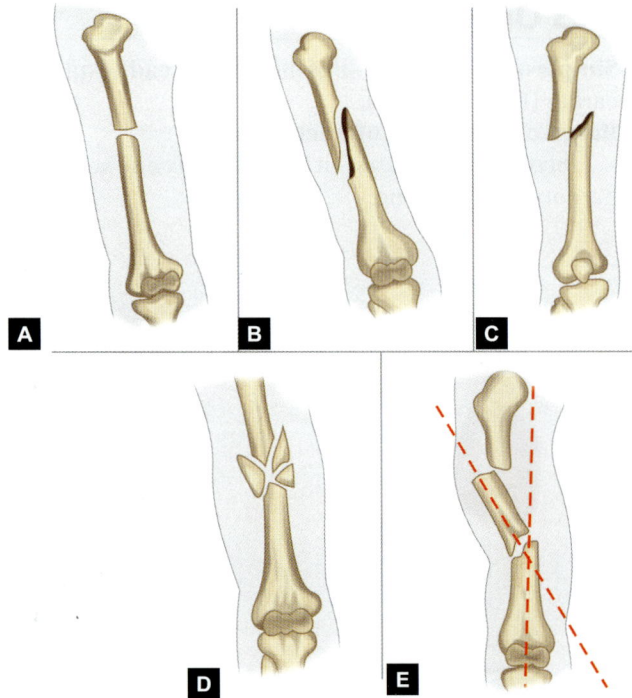

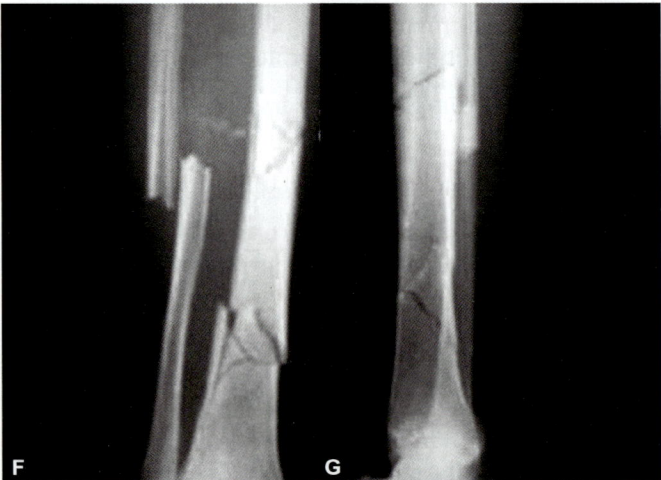

Figs 3.2A to E: Types of fractures based on fracture patterns: (A) Transverse; (B) Spiral; (C) Oblique; (D) Comminuted; (E) Segmental fractures

Figs 3.2F and G: Plain X-rays showing—transverse fracture fibula, short oblique fracture tibia, segmental, comminuted, butterfly fracture tibia

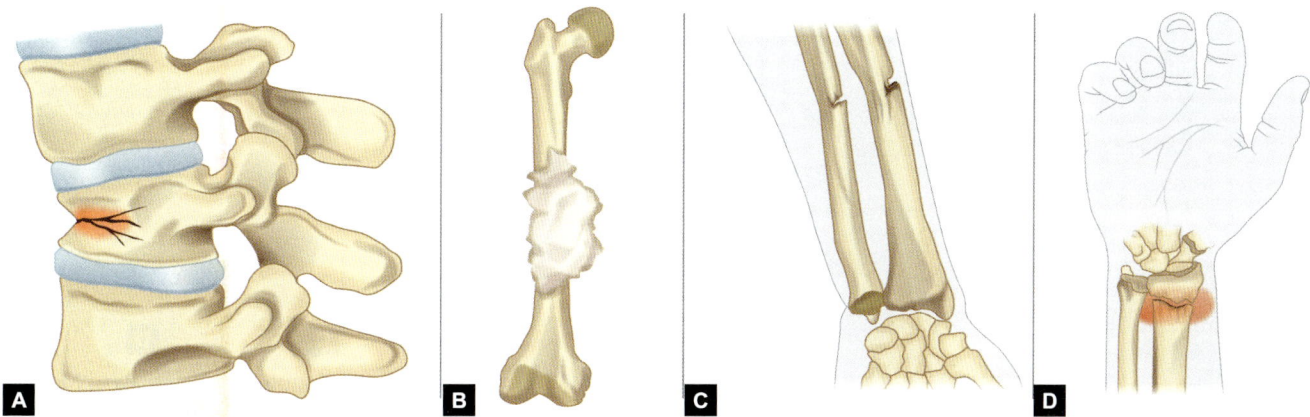

Figs 3.3A to D: Atypical fractures: (A) Compression; (B) Pathological; (C) Greenstick; (D) Torus fractures

- *Bone loss:* This could be a <50 percent bone loss, more than 50 percent bone loss, or a complete bone loss.

Atypical Fractures (Figs 3.3A to E)

a. *Greenstick fractures:* It is seen exclusively in children. Here the bone is elastic and usually bends due to buckling or breaking of one cortex when a force is applied. This is called a greenstick fracture (Fig. 3.3E).
b. *Impacted fractures:* Here the fracture fragments are impacted into each other and are not separated and displaced.
c. *Stress or fatigue fractures:* It is usually an incomplete fracture commonly seen in athletes and in bones subjected to chronic and repetitive stress (e.g. third metatarsal fracture, fracture tibia, etc.).
d. *Pathological fractures:* It occurs in a diseased bone and is usually spontaneous. The force required to bring about a pathological fracture is trivial (Fig. 3.4).
e. *Hairline or crack fracture:* It is a very fine break in the bone that is difficult to diagnose clinically. Radiology usually helps or still better is CT scan.
f. *Torus fracture:* This is just a buckling of the outer cortex (Fig. 3.5).

> **Remember**
> - Greenstick fracture—occurs in children.
> - Stress fracture—common in athletes.
> - Fatigue fractures in occupations like police, nurses, etc.
> - Pathological fractures—usually seen in elderly people.
> - Hairline or crack fracture—is a special variety of incomplete fracture.

DISPLACEMENT OF FRACTURES

A complete fracture usually gets displaced due to various factors already mentioned. Depending on the direction of

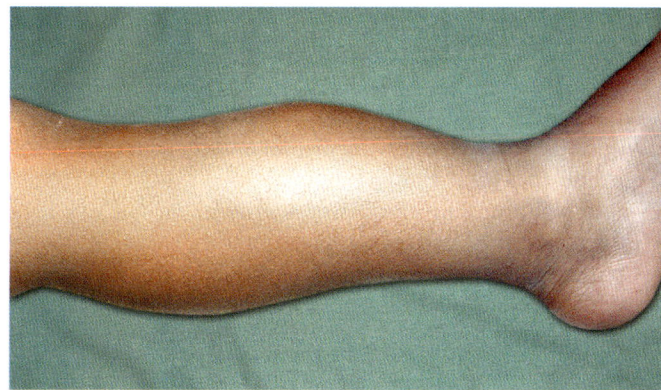

Fig. 3.3E: Clinical photo of a greenstick fracture of tibia

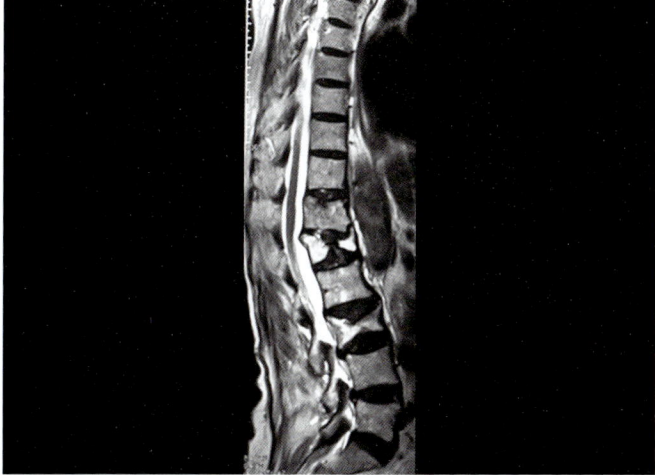

Fig. 3.4: MRI spine showing pathological compression fracture due to osteoporosis

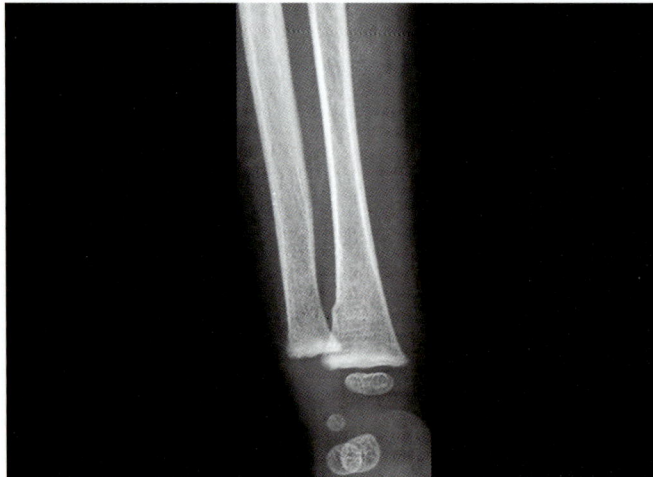

Fig. 3.5: Plain X-ray showing buckling of the outer cortex (Torus fracture)

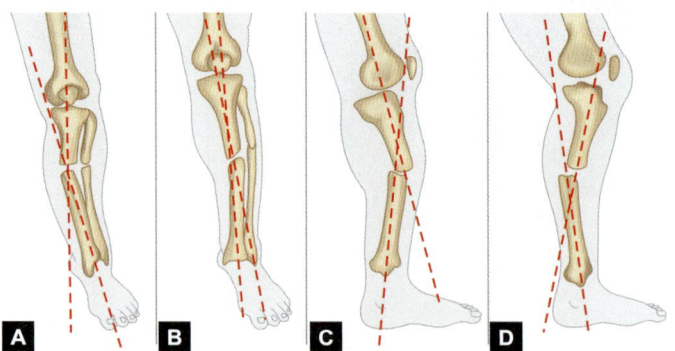

Figs 3.6A to D: Types of angulations in fractures: (A) Medial; (B) Lateral; (C) Anterior; (D) Posterior

force, mode of injury, pull of the muscles, a fracture can show any one of the following displacements or angulations (Figs 3.6A to G):
- Anterior angulations or displacement.
- Posterior angulations or displacement.
- Varus or medial angulations or displacement.
- Valgus or lateral displacement or angulations.
- Shortening.
- Translational.

APPROACH TO ORTHOPEDIC INJURY

Orthopedic injuries encompass a wide range of problems starting from bone and joint injuries, strains, sprains and damage to associated neurovascular structures.

The value of a systematic clinical approach to unravel the myth and mysteries of orthotrauma cannot be less emphasized. Time-honored and time-tested clinical formulae applied so successfully in the diagnosis of various system disorders can be applied for orthotrauma also and consists of the following:

History: Contrary to popular beliefs, a proper history gives vital clues and goes a long way in arriving at a proper diagnosis.

Age: Certain fractures have predilection age groups (Table 3.1). Hence, the practice of first enquiring about the age of the patient is a step in the right direction.

Sex: Colles' fracture is more common in females and supracondylar fracture humerus; posterior dislocations of elbow are more common in males.

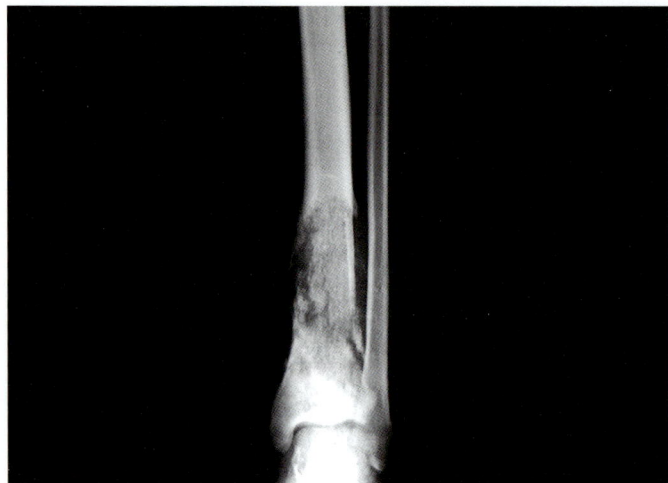

Fig. 3.6E: Pathological fracture

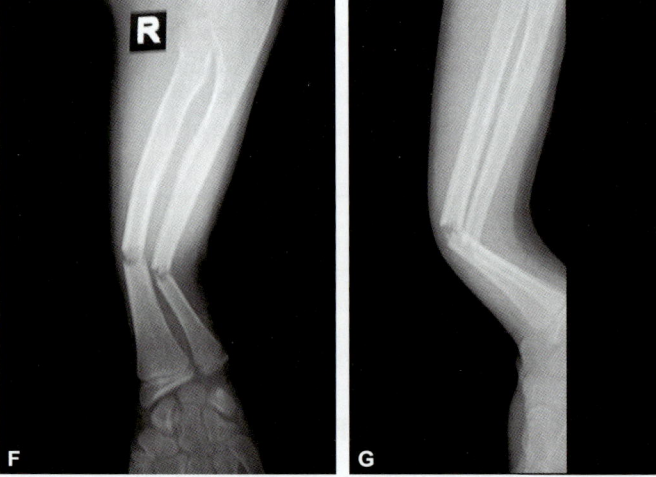

Figs 3.6F and G: Lateral and posterior angulation

TABLE 3.1: Relationship of age and fractures

Age	Fractures and dislocations
• Birth	Brachial plexus injury, fracture, clavicle, fracture humerus, etc
• Early childhood	Supracondylar fracture of humerus. Epiphyseal injuries
• Late childhood	Posterior dislocations of elbow Slipped capital femoral epiphysis Monteggia fractures
• Adult	Fracture of long bones Hip and shoulder dislocations
• Elderly	Colles' fracture Fracture neck femur

Note: In spite of age predilections, any fracture can be seen in any age group as an aberration.

TABLE 3.2: Relationship of age, types of fractures and mode of injuries

Age	Common modes of injury	Examples
Children	Fall on the out-stretched hands usually while on play or from a height	Fracture clavicle, fracture and dislocations of any upper limb bones
Adults	• Fall from height	• Upper limb injuries, spine injuries, etc.
	• Driving injuries	• Cervical spine injuries.
	• RTA	• Any combination of Injuries
		• Whiplash injury
		• Dashboard injuries like fracture patella, posterior hip dislocation, etc.
	• Sports injuries	• Ankle and shoulder, elbow and knee joint injuries
	• Assaults	• Long bone fractures (e.g. nightstick fracture of ulna)
Elderly	Trivial fall	• Colles' fracture
		• Fracture neck femur, etc.

Note: High-velocity trauma due to RTA can produce any combination of bone and joint injuries.

Mechanism of Injury

This could be different in different age groups as mentioned in Table 3.2.

Clinical Features

A patient with limb injuries may present with the following complaints:
- *Pain:* This is a very subjective symptom and is invariably the first and the most important complaint. It may be mild, moderate, and severe and may be due to tearing of periosteum (which contains the nerve endings), soft tissue injury, vascular injury, nerve injury, etc.
- *Swelling:* It is due to soft tissue injury, medullary bleeding, and reactionary hemorrhage. Swelling is usually more in fractures and less in dislocations for obvious reasons.
- *Deformity:* Patients with displaced fractures and dislocations usually present with deformity of varying severity.
- *Inability:* To use the affected part is another frequent complaint.

Having made a note of the history and presenting complaints, effort is now directed towards eliciting the clinical signs, some of which are general and some are injury specific.
- *Tenderness:* This is an important clinical sign in bone and joint injuries and is usually seen after trauma. Importance of tenderness, methods of elicitation and grading is mentioned in the box (refer page 18).
- *Swelling:* The swelling is examined for shape, size (mild, moderate, severe), consistency (cystic, soft, hard), tenderness (see the grades), fluctuation, etc.
- *Deformity:* This is usually seen in displaced fractures and dislocations. Undisplaced fractures, mild strains, and sprains usually show no deformities. Some of the deformities are very characteristic (Figs 3.7A to D) and specific and help in making a spot diagnosis (Table 3.3).
- *Abnormal mobility:* Between fracture fragments is a sure sign of fracture.
- *Loss of transmitted movements:* When one end of the limb is rotated, it automatically is transmitted to the other end. Due to the break in the continuity this is no longer possible in displaced fractures.
- *Crepitus:* This is an abnormal grating sensation produced by the friction between two ragged surfaces of the fracture fragments. Obviously, it is elicitable only in displaced fractures. It should be elicited very gently and at the end of the clinical examination.
- *Shortening:* Limb shortening of various degrees is common in bone and joint injuries.

> **Note:**
> Crepitus, abnormal mobility, deformity, and loss of transmitted movements cannot be elicited in undisplaced fractures, stress fractures, impacted fractures, etc.

> **Remember**
> Clinical manifestations in a fracture are due to:
> - Fracture per se
> - Its complications
> - Or both.

18　SECTION 1: Traumatology

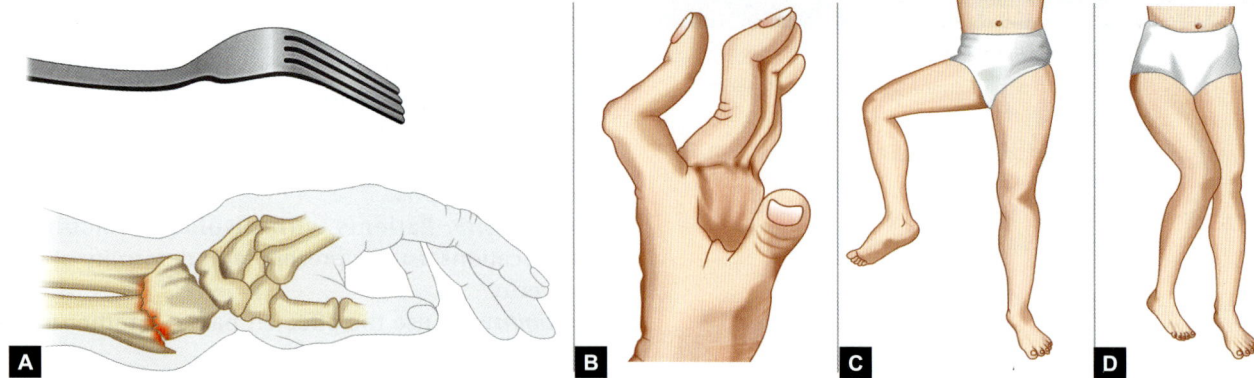

Figs 3.7A to D: Some important deformities in orthopedics: (A) Dinner fork deformity; (B) Swan neck deformity; (C) Anterior dislocation of hip; (D) Posterior dislocation of hip

TABLE 3.3: Deformity facts	
Classical deformities	*Possible diagnosis*
1. Wry neck	Cervical spine injuries
2. Drooping of shoulder	Clavicle fracture
3. Flat shoulder	Anterior dislocation of shoulder
4. S-shaped deformity of humerus	Supracondylar fracture humerus
5. Dinner fork deformity	Colles' fracture
6. Boutonnière deformity	Rupture of central extensor slips of finger
7. Mallet finger	Rupture of distal end of index extensor
8. Jersey finger	Rupture of distal end of flexor digitorum profundus of index finger
9. Flexion, adduction and internal rotation	Posterior dislocation of hip
10. Flexion, abduction and external rotation of lower limb	anterior dislocation of hip
11. Incomplete external rotation of lower limbs	Fracture neck femur (intra-capsular)
12. Complete external rotation of lower limbs	Trochanteric fractures, shaft femur, leg bones fractures
13. S-shaped ankle	Ankle dislocations.

About Tenderness

Remember
Tenderness may be the only evidence of fracture in:
- Crack fracture
- Hairline fracture
- Stress fracture
- Fatigue fracture
- Torus fracture
- Pathological fracture

Method of eliciting: Proceed from normal area to the affected part for better patient compliance.
Grading
- Grade I—just a suspect.
- Grade II—patient winces on pressure.
- Grade III—patient winces and withdraws.
- Grade IV—patient will not allow to touch.

This grading of tenderness is superior to the conventional mild, moderate, and severe grading.

About crepitus, it is defined as an abnormal grating sensation either felt or heard. It could be:
- Fine, e.g. osteoarthritis
- Coarse, e.g. fractures
- Snap, e.g. snapping tendons.

Remember, it is unkind to elicit a crepitus in a fracture for fear of hurting the patient.

About deformity, it is defined as deviation of the normal anatomy of a bone or joint.

Remember
"D" in fracture:
- Deformity is seen often in displaced fractures.
- Displacement could be anterior, posterior, medial, or lateral.
- Distal fragment is the reference point to suggest the type of displacement.
- Dislocation of joints usually presents a deformity.

Interesting Features about the Clinical Signs
Various clinical signs are described in fractures. They can be best represented as follows in order of their importance (Table 3.4).

Clinical manifestations due to neurovascular injuries: Certain fractures are known to cause neurovascular damage quite frequently, e.g. supracondylar fracture of humerus in children. The familiar five Ps detects impending vascular damage and nerve injuries are detected by the classical deformities and screening tests (as described in peripheral nerve injuries).

TABLE 3.4: Relevance of clinical signs

Unfailing signs	• Abnormal mobility • Crepitus
Reliable signs	• Tenderness • Shortening
Important signs	• Bruise • Swelling
Other signs	• Loss of function • Deformity
Late or inconstant signs	• Blisters • Ecchymosis • Swelling due to callus

About Five Ps

In detecting impending vascular damage in musculoskeletal trauma
- **P**ain
- **P**allor
- **P**aresthesia
- **P**ulselessness
- **P**aralysis.

There are certain bones in the body, the fractures of which are usually missed in the initial examination (Box 3.1). These are known to cause diagnostic difficulties and dilemmas.

Box 3.1: Missing Facts

Do you know the fractures, which can give a slip to the clinician?
- Zygoma
- Base of skull
- Odontoid process
- C7 vertebra
- Ribs
- Radial head
- Impacted fracture neck of femur
- Un-displaced pelvic fracture
- Scaphoid fracture
- Carpal dislocations
- Tarsometatarsal joints
- Talus fracture
- March fracture

Note: Among these, scaphoid tops the list.

INVESTIGATIONS IN ORTHOTRAUMA

Radiography

It is an important diagnostic tool for fractures. Minimum two views, anteroposterior, and lateral are required as bone is a cylinder. Sometimes, an oblique view and other special views are required depending upon the clinical situations and bone under study.

Vital Facts: About Plain X-ray

Radiological clues one should look for on plain X-rays for diagnosis of fractures:
- Where is the fracture?
- *Situation:* Whether it is in the diaphysis, metaphysis, epiphysis, and the articular surface.
- *Anatomy:* Look for the fracture line, whether it is transverse, oblique, spiral, segmental, comminuted, etc.
- Also look for the alignment, angulations, displacement, rotation, etc.
- *Number:* How many fragments are seen?
- *Bone condition:* Identify whether the bone is normal or pathological.
- *Joint involvement:* Look for the extension of the fracture line into the joint, joint swelling and for evidence of dislocation.
- *Soft tissue swelling:* The extent of the soft tissue swelling indicates the severity of the injury.

Pitfalls of X-ray
- Presence of a fracture line on an X-ray helps confirm the diagnosis but its absence does not rule out a fracture.
- Hairline fractures tend to be missed (e.g. scaphoid).
- Some dislocations, if associated with fractures could be missed (e.g. Monteggia fracture).
- In comminuted fractures the number of fragments could be misleading.
- Beware of artifacts they could mislead you.
- Be careful in interpreting fracture-like appearances, e.g. apophysis.
- Avoid interpreting a low quality X-ray.

Role of X-ray
- Helps confirm the clinical diagnosis.
- Helps study the fracture anatomy.
- Helps study the fracture displacement.
- Helps to detect crack and stress fractures.
- Helps to plan the treatment.
- Helps to detect fracture dislocation combinations, e.g. Monteggia.
- Helps to ascertain post-reduction status of fractures.
- Helps in medicolegal study.

Remember the Rules in X-rays
- Better no X-ray than one view X-ray.
- X-ray is a shadow. It conceals and distorts. Hence, interpret X-rays with caution.
- A joint above and joint below should be included with the fracture under study.
- The fracture should be in the middle of the film.
- Exposure should be adequate and the soft tissue shadow should be delineated properly.
- X-rays should be read by holding the film in an anatomical position.
- Proper protective measures against radiation should be adopted.
- Avoid unnecessary X-rays.
- Check X-rays are to be taken without disturbing the plaster cast.

CT Scan and MRI

These are the most sophisticated investigative methods available now in orthopedics. Both are noninvasive and are extremely useful in detecting both soft tissue and bony injuries.

> **Note:**
> *CT scan:* This is helpful in detecting fracture of skull, pelvis, spine and identifying loose bodies in the joint.
> *MRI:* This is useful to diagnose any fracture. In addition, it helps to identify soft tissue and ligament injuries. It is certainly the 'Gold Standard' but has its Achilles heel in being expensive.

MANAGEMENT OF FRACTURES

The goal of fracture management is to restore the anatomy back to its normal or as near to normal as possible.

The responsibility of an orthopedic surgeon is to ensure that there is no functional disability to the patient following the treatment of fractures.

Management of fracture can be broadly classified and discussed under the following heads:
- Management of simple fractures.
- Management of open fractures.
- Management of complicated fractures.

Management of Simple Fractures

Simple fractures are managed by conservative and operative methods.

Conservative Methods

1. For un-displaced fractures, incomplete fractures, impacted fractures:
   a. *Cuff and collar sling:* For upper limb fractures.
   b. *Strapping:* For fracture clavicle, fracture ribs, finger, or toe fractures, etc.
   c. *Plaster slabs:* Plaster of Paris slabs can be used to support the injured limb usually as a first aid measure.
   d. *Rest and nonsteroidal anti-inflammatory drugs (NSAIDs):* For pain relief and to reduce the inflammation.
   e. Masterly inactivity in certain cases like impacted fracture neck of femur, etc.
2. For displaced fractures here the aim is to restore back the normal anatomy of the bone by either closed or open reduction.

Management of Fractures by Closed Reduction

This consists of resuscitation, reduction, retention, and rehabilitation (4Rs).

1. *Resuscitation:* Resuscitation is the topmost priority if the patient is in shock following a fracture. A to F management proposed by MacMurthy is to be followed in all situations of emergencies (refer pages 51-52).
2. *Reduction:* Reduction of the fracture fragments if it is displaced. Usually, it is done under general anesthesia after adequate radiographic study.
   Reduction methods are:
   a. *Closed reduction:* It is adopted usually for simple fractures. The technique followed is traction and counter traction method. It is a blind technique and needs considerable skill and expertise. It commonly results in malunion.
   b. *Continuous traction:* Certain examples where continuous traction can be used for reduction of tractions are Gallows traction for fracture shaft femur in children, balanced skeletal traction for adult shaft femur fractures, etc.
   c. *Open reduction:* It is done when the above methods fail or if there are specific, indications (see box).
3. *Retention:* Once the fracture fragments are reduced, it has to be retained in that position till the fracture unites; otherwise it tends to get displaced due to the action of muscles, gravity, and inherent factors.
   Retention methods after closed reduction are:
   a. By plaster of Paris splints this is the most common splint employed. It could be a slab (encircles half the limb) or a cast (encircles the whole limb) or a functional brace (which permits mobility while the fracture is still under the cast) (refer page 59).
   b. By continuous traction to overcome the muscle forces after closed reduction. The traction could be skin or skeletal traction and is employed as fixed; balanced or combined types of tractions (refer page 65).
   c. Use of functional braces this can be used after three weeks, once the fracture becomes sticky (refer page 59).
4. *Rehabilitation* is by way of physiotherapy and exercises (both active and passive).

Fracture Management by Open Reduction (Operative Management)

As mentioned earlier, open method is indicated once, the conservative methods fail and when there are specific indications. These indications could be absolute, relative, or rare as mentioned below:

Indications
Absolute
- Failed closed reduction
- Displaced intra-articular fractures
- Type III and IV epiphyseal injuries
- Major avulsion fractures
- Nonunion
- Replantation of extremities.

Relative
- Multiple fractures
- Delayed union
- Loss of reduction
- Pathological fractures
- For better nursing care
- To avoid prolonged bed rest
- Closed methods ineffective in Galeazzi fracture, Monteggia fracture, femoral neck fracture, etc.

Questionable
- Neurovascular injury
- Open fractures
- Cosmetic reasons
- Economic consideration.

Methods of open reduction: After the exposure, the fracture is reduced by direct methods and in the indirect methods the fracture is reduced without exposing by positioning and traction over the fracture tables, skeletal traction, tensioner, lamina spreader, etc.

Principles of open reduction *(known after Lambotte):* Principles of open reduction as suggested by Lambotte includes:

Exposure: The fracture is adequately exposed through a proper approach.

Reduction of the fracture fragments under direct vision is carried out.

Temporary stabilization of the fracture fragments by K-wire is done first if necessary.

Definitive stabilization of the fracture using plate and screws or intramedullary nail, etc. is done later.

Retention after open reduction: After open reduction, the fracture fragment invariably needs to be fixed internally by various implants (see box).

Choice of Implants
K-wire: For epiphyseal injuries and for fractures of small bones of hand and feet (diameter of the K-wires varies from 1–3 mm).
Screws: For avulsion fractures and butterfly fragments.
Intramedullary nails: For fracture through the narrowest portion of a medullary canal of a long bone.
Plate and screws: For proximal and distal third fractures of long bones.
Interlocking nails: For segmental fractures comminuted fractures, etc. of long bones.
Hip implants: For fracture neck femur. Smith Peterson's nail, Richard's compression screw, multiple cannulated screws, etc. are some of the examples.
Spine implants: Steffi plate and screws (VSP's), Luque's rod, Hart shill frame, Harrington's rods, etc.
Steel Wires No 18–20 gauges: Useful for tension band wiring for fracture of patella, olecranon, etc.

The rehabilitation process is the same as for closed management of fractures.

Contraindications for Open Reduction
- Infection
- Small fragments
- Weak and porotic bone
- Soft tissue damage
- Un-displaced or impacted fractures
- Poor general and medical condition.

Disadvantages of Open Reduction
- Closed fracture converted into an open fracture.
- Fracture hematoma is disturbed.
- Scar tissue.
- Anesthetic problems.
- Foreign body reaction due to metals.

Remember
Success by open reduction depends on:
- Proper indications
- Proper timing
- Proper surgical approach
- Proper technique
- Proper selection of implant
- Proper surgeon.

Quick Facts
About methods of fracture immobilization
- *External:* Plaster of Paris external fixators
- *Internal:* Fixation with plates and screws, rods, K-wire, etc.
- *Traction:* By skin and skeletal traction.

OPEN FRACTURES

Open fracture is a surgical emergency and presents as a problem that is much more difficult than closed fractures.

It is defined as a fracture, which communicates with the external atmosphere due to break in the soft tissue cover. The break in the soft tissues could be from inside to outside or outside to inside.

CLASSIFICATION (GUSTILO AND ANDERSON'S) (FIGS 3.8A TO F)

Type I: Wound is less than 1 cm in size. It is usually due to a low-velocity trauma.

Type II: Wound is more than 1 cm and less than 10 cm, but there is no devitalization of soft tissue and is associated with very little contamination. These are due to high-energy trauma.

Type III: Wounds moderate and severe in size (>10 cm) and the soft tissues are devitalized and contaminated.

Type IIIA: Extensive soft tissue injury but with adequate soft tissue to cover the fractured bone.

Type IIIB: Extensive soft tissue damage and loss. Bone cannot be covered and is exposed to the atmosphere.

Type IIIC: Compound fractures with arterial injuries.

No classification invites so much of debate as for open fractures with only 60 percent of the surgeons across the globe accepting it. Hence, newer modifications are now being suggested like:
a. The modified Gustilo-Anderson's classification.
b. The Trafton classification (this combines the Gustilo-Anderson's and Tscherne classification).
c. AO classification of soft tissue injury with alphanumeric classification of fractures.

APPROACH IN COMPOUND FRACTURES

Compound fractures are usually serious injuries and are due to high-velocity trauma.

They may be associated with multisystem and multi-skeletal injuries. The approach should be more cautious and the following protocol is recommended.

- *General physical examination:* This is of vital importance since the patient is usually in shock. Levels of consciousness, pulse, blood pressure, breathing, etc. should be recorded.
- *Examination of other systems:* Examinations should be carried out for head injury, neck and face injury, chest injury, blunt injury abdomen, pelvic fractures and spine fractures.
- *Examination of the compound injury:* This usually proceeds in the same line as mentioned in examination of closed fractures but here the assessment of the general physical condition of the patient assumes great importance. In addition to the usual clinical features, one should look for soft tissue injury and wound, bone loss, absence of bone pieces, distal neurovascular status of the limb, etc.

> **Note:**
> The term 'open fracture' is more preferable than the old out fashioned term "compound fractures."

Investigations

General investigations: Laboratory tests like Hb%, blood group, bleeding time and clotting time, HIV, HbsAg, routine urine examinations, etc. are carried out.

X-ray of the part as for other fractures and in addition look for missing pieces of bone in open fractures (Figs 3.9A and B).

> **Management Principles**
> Aims of treatment
> - To convert a contaminated wound into a clean wound and thus help to convert an open fracture into a closed one.
> - To establish union in a good position.
> - To prevent pyogenic and clostridial infections.

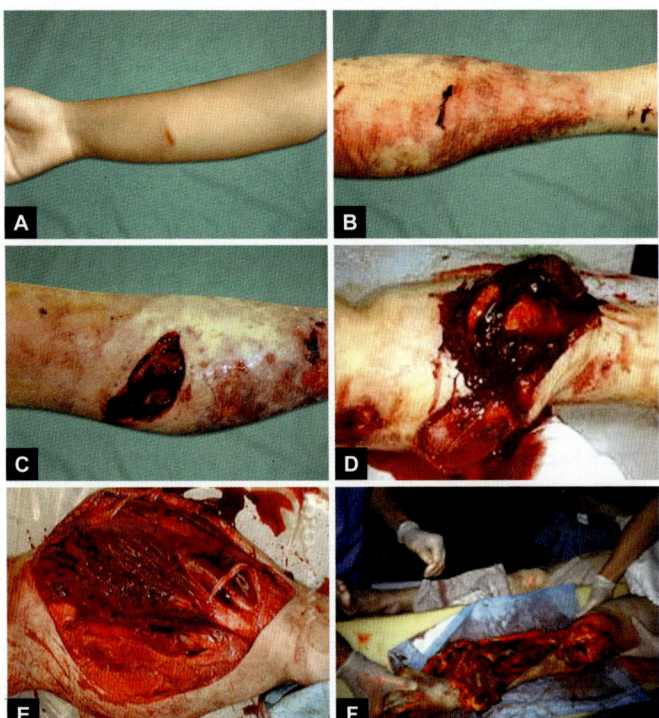

Figs 3.8A to F: Varieties of open fractures: (A) Type I (<1 cm); (B) Type II (>2 cm); (C) Type IIIA; (D) Type IIIB; (E and F) Type IIIC

Considerations

- First to stabilize the general condition of the patient as the patient is usually in shock. This consists of resuscitation, blood transfusion, intravenous fluids, antibiotics, oxygen administration, etc.
- To keep the wound covered with proper sterile bandages until the patient is ready for surgery.
- Open fractures are surgical emergencies and surgery is to be done as soon as the patient is fit.

Treatment Plan

It is a team work and involves a battery of specialists like the vascular surgeon, plastic surgeon, thoracic surgeon, general surgeon, faciomaxillary surgeon, and of course the orthopedic surgeon. Once these specialists manage the injuries to the vital organs and the general condition of the patient is stabilized, the fractures are dealt by the orthopedic surgeon.

After stabilizing the general condition of the patient, surgical debridement is planned under strict aseptic measures in a major operation theater.

Debridement (known as unbridling) this is the most important step in the management of compound fractures. It consists of the following steps (4 Es) (Fig. 3.9C):

- *Exploration of the wound:* The wound should be sufficiently explored proximally and distally to have a proper assessment of the extent of the damage.
- *Excision* of all nonviable structures is important to prevent infection. The recognition of nonviable tissue (see below) before excision is of paramount importance. The tissues are dealt with as follows:
  - *Skin:* Here the plan is to excise all the dead skin and yet be conservative.

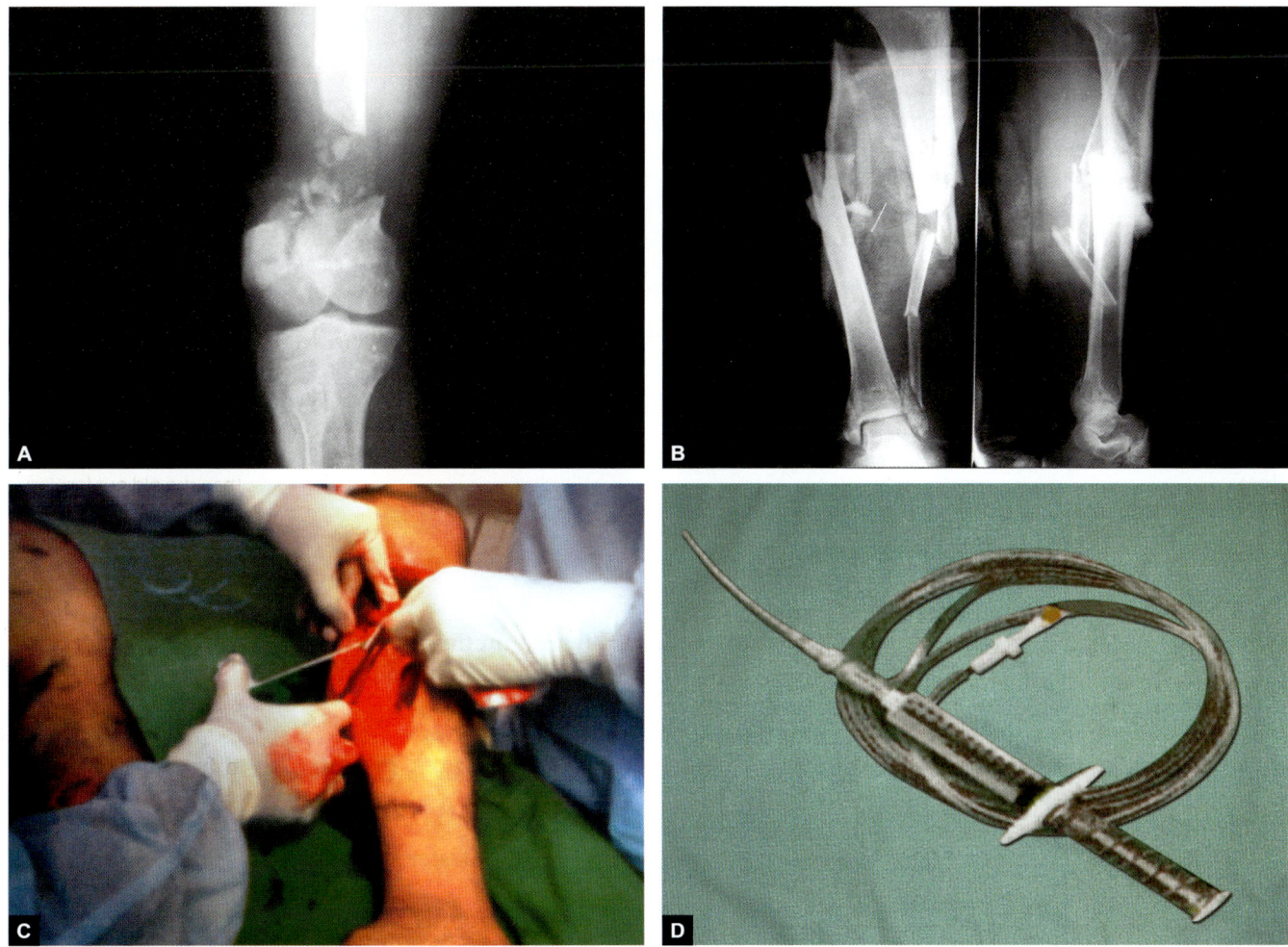

Figs 3.9A to D: (A) Compound fracture of the femur showing bone loss; (B) Compound both bones fractures of the leg; (C) Technique of debridement; (D) Irrigation set used in open fractures

TABLE 3.5: Criteria to evaluate tissue status

Features	Viable	Nonviable
Color	Pink	Pale
Consistency	Firm	Flabby
Capacity to bleed	Preserved	Lost
Circulation	Present	Absent
Contractility	Present	Absent

- *Muscle:* Nonviable muscles should be removed but often it is overlooked hence the axiom, "when in doubt, take it out." 5 Cs help in deciding the muscle viability (Table 3.5).
- *Bones:* Small bits of loose bones devoid of soft tissues are removed. Large fragments with their soft tissue attachments are preserved.
- *Nerves and vessels:* Primary repair is done if the wound is clean. In contaminated wounds, they are dealt with at a later stage.
- *Evacuation* of foreign bodies like dirt, glass, stones, pebbles, etc. These foreign bodies are a source for infection and may invite a foreign body reaction. Hence, they have to be removed by a thorough irrigation (normal saline is used) (Fig. 3.9D).

About Irrigation
- Dilution is the solution of pollution.
- Single most essential step.
- Minimum 10 liters of saline is used.
- Forcible streams are avoided.
- Swirling movements of the irrigation fluid is preferred.
- Irrigation or wound toilet helps to clear the foreign bodies and clots minimizing the chances of contamination.

Note:
- Antiseptic additives kill the bacteria.
- Detergent irrigation aims to remove than kill bacteria.

- *External fixators* are used to fix the fracture fragment after debridement. Plaster of Paris and internal fixation devices have little and controversial role in the fracture management of compound fractures. External fixator's help to stabilize fracture fragments, allow daily wound inspection and dressing, permit procedures like skin grafting to cover the wound, allow soft tissues to heal apart from providing early mobilization. In open tibia fractures, external fixator can be safely exchanged to internal fixation within 3 weeks with only 5 percent incidence of deep infection (Fig. 3.10).

Indications for External Fixation in Open Fractures
- Grossly comminuted fractures
- Grossly contaminated wounds

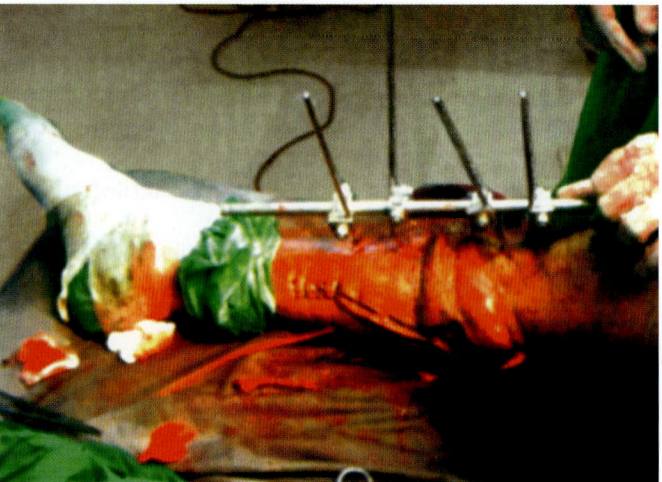

Fig. 3.10: External fixators preferred method of immobilization in open fractures

- Side swipe injuries
- Periarticular fractures
- Pelvic fractures
- Pylon fractures
- Tibial plateau fractures
- Acetabular fractures.

Primary Internal Fixation in Open Fractures
In recent times, this concept is undergoing a 'sea change'. The inhibitions regarding the primary internal fixation is fast disappearing. The reasons for this shift in stance is improved methods of wound care, powerful antibiotics, improvements in the investigations and operative techniques, improvements in the external fixation devices, etc.

Indications for Internal Fixation in Open Fractures
- Intra-articular fractures
- Multisystem injuries
- Multiple fractures
- Elderly patients
- Head injuries
- Vascular injuries
- Tibia shaft fractures.

Preferred method: Interlocking nailing is emerging as a better alternative than plating for internal fixation in open fractures.

OTHER FORMS OF FRACTURE IMMOBILIZATION

- Pins and plasters—limited use, can be tried in type I fractures.
- Limited internal fixation—in grade I and some grade II, grade IIIC fractures
- Skeletal traction—overhead olecranon traction for compound supracondylar fractures. Böhler-Braun

skeletal traction for open femoral shaft fractures is some of the examples.
- Plaster of Paris casts practically have no role.

Open Facts in Open Fractures
About fixation methods in open fractures
- External fixators — liberally used.
- Internal fixates — sparingly used.
- Skeletal traction — rarely used.
- Plaster casts — occasionally used (type I).
- Functional brace — never used.

Poetic Facts
James Learmonth's poem depicts the four major principles of debridement:
 On the edges of the skin take a piece, very thin (1); the tenser the fascia, the more you should slasher (2); of muscles much more, until you see fresh gore (3); and the bundles contract at least the impact; hardly any of bone, only bits quite alone (4).

Remember
Problems peculiar to open fracture:
- In open fractures soft tissue injury is a dreaded problem than the fracture itself.
- It is a surgical emergency.
- *Three problems*:
  – Infection from the environment.
  – Problems of soft tissue loss.
  – Active infection.
- Effective immobilization rendered difficult.
- Bone repair is delayed. Speed is the watchword in treatment.
- Infected nonunion, malunion, chronic osteomyelitis is very common.
- Difficulty in using the standard internal fixation methods renders managing the fractures very difficult.

Some Interesting Treatment Guidelines the World Over for Open Fractures
- Seventeen percent surgeons cultured wounds on admission.
- Ninety eight percent gave antibiotics after initial debridement.
- Ninety seven percent used cephalosporin.
- Except in grade I debridement was done more than once.
- Forteen percent surgeons discharged patients with oral antibiotics.
- Re-operation was done in a few cases.

Definitive wound care: After resuscitation, debridement and application of external fixator's attention is now given to the definitive wound care. This is an extremely important step as the primary objective of treatment in open fracture is to convert an open wound into closed wound. The wound closure could be primary or secondary.

Criteria for Primary Closure
- All necrotic material should be removed.
- Circulation should be normal.
- Nerve supply should be intact.
- The patient's general condition should be stable.
- Wound should be closed without tension.
- No dead space should be left after closure.
- There should be no multisystem injuries.

If all the above criteria are met, primary suturing is preferred to close a wound. The following alternative measures are considered in the event of the above criteria not being met:
- Split skin graft.
- Pedicle or flap graft.
- Secondary suturing after 2 to 3 weeks.
- Relaxing incisions to mobilize the neighboring skin.
- Biological dressings (homologous or heterologous skin).
- To leave it open and to follow by regular dressings, wound inspection and closure later.

Role of antibiotics: It will not replace the wound debridement. Topical antibiotics have very little role. Parenteral administration is recommended. The choice of antibiotics is usually a broad spectrum, bactericidal hypoallergenic agent with adequate serum concentration.

What is New?
Some surgeons have found good results with insertion of antibiotics integrated (2.4 g of Tobramycin powder) PMMA beads into Type III wounds.

Role of AGGS and ATS: The patient has to be protected against tetanus and gas gangrene by effective immunization against them.

Role of primary amputation: In open fractures, this is controversial but can be considered in type IIIC with neural injury and if the warm ischemia is more than 6 hours.

Remember
In open fractures:
- Debridement is the mainstay of treatment
- The procedure is 4 Es:
  – Exploration of the wound.
  – Excision of the devitalized tissues.
  – Evacuation of the foreign bodies.
  – External fixators.
- Devitalized tissue recognized by 5 Cs.
- Wound irrigation is the single most important step.
- Primary aim is to convert an open wound into a closed one.
- Wound closure is to be decided with caution.
- Antibiotics cannot replace wound debridement.
- External fixators have definite role.
- Internal fixators and plasters have limited role.
- Ultimate goal is to restore the patient's limb and function as early as and as full as possible.

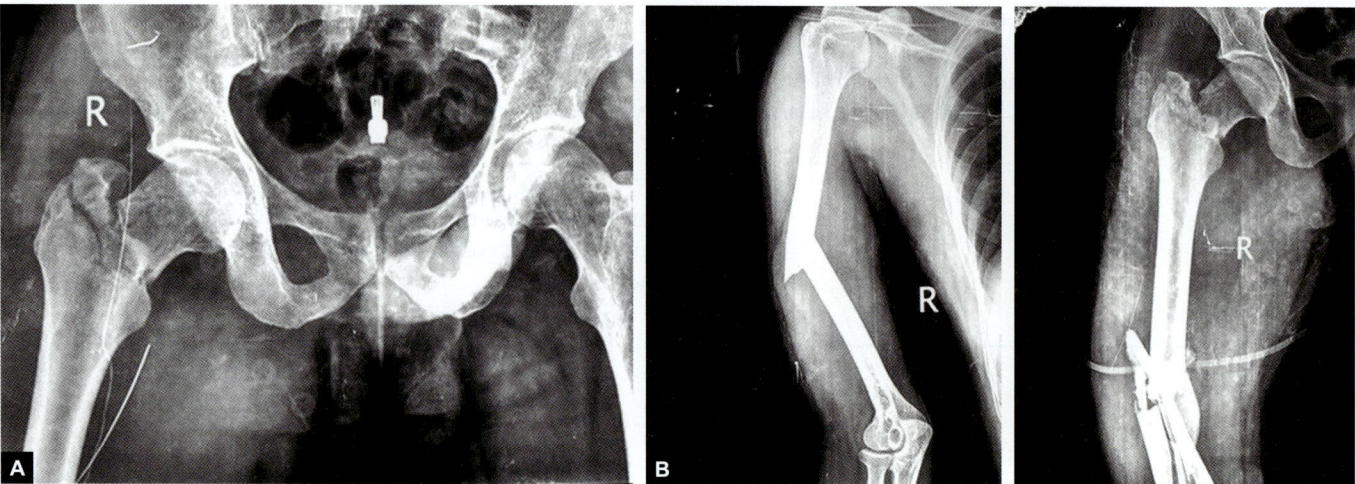

Figs 3.11A and B: Plain X-rays showing a case of polytrauma; (A) Proximal femoral fracture; (B) Humerus and femur fractures

APPROACH TO A POLYTRAUMA CASE

This is as mentioned in the approach to a compound fracture. Speed is the watchword and systematic examination of the injured in the approach towards a multiple trauma case takes a priority and should proceed in the following lines:

- *Initial evaluation:* The ABCDEs of initial examination of a polytrauma case are as follows:
  A—airway, B—breathing, C—circulation, D—disability (neurological examination), E—exposure, F—fracture examination, G—Go back to the beginning for a secondary survey and H—help.
- *Secondary evaluation:* After the initial evaluation and resuscitation, a more systematic and detailed evaluation of the injuries mentioned above are done. Fractures are splinted externally and managed later. Nevertheless, in few cases primary internal fixation is recommended in ipsilateral fractures, multisystem injuries, etc. for faster rehabilitation and better nursing care. Dislocations are promptly reduced.
- *Fracture examination:* This is done systematically as mentioned in the previous discussions.
- *Investigation:* This includes routine blood examinations, radiographs of head, neck, chest, spine and affected parts (Figs 3.11A and B). CT scan and MRI of injured structures are mandatory.

DISLOCATIONS

Dislocation is defined as a total loss of contact between the two ends of bones (Figs 3.12A and B). All dislocations are emergencies unlike fractures, for delay in reduction may damage the articular surface, which are deprived of nutrition by the synovial fluid. Unlike fractures, all dislocations need prompt reduction and early treatment

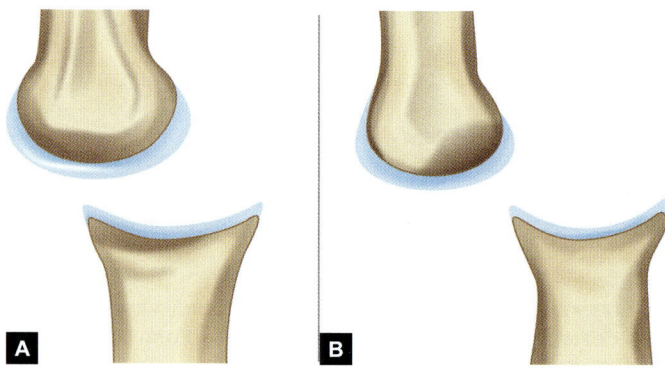

Figs 3.12A and B: (A) Subluxation; (B) Dislocation

because the patient will not be relieved of pain due to the persistent capsular stretch. The capsule contains nerve endings, which give rise to pain.

Pathology

In a dislocation, there could be damage to the capsule, articular cartilage, muscles, and ligaments in varying degrees. There could be osteochondral fractures and avulsion injuries.

Types of Dislocation: Congenital or Acquired

Congenital as in CDH and in acquired the following varieties are seen:
- Traumatic common in young adults due to high-velocity trauma.
- Pathological, e.g. TB hip, septic arthritis, etc.
- Infective, e.g. Tom smith arthritis in infants.
- Paralytic, e.g. poliomyelitis, cerebral palsy, etc.

- Inflammatory disorders, rheumatoid arthritis, etc.
- Here the scope of discussion is about traumatic dislocations.

Clinical Features

Traumatic variety is the most common type of dislocations one encounters in clinical practice (Table 3.6). A patient gives history of trauma usually a road traffic accident (RTA), fall, etc. following which there is pain, swelling deformity and loss of movements. In dislocations of other varieties, clinical symptoms and signs pertaining to that particular disease are seen.

Typical Deformities in Dislocations
- Shoulder—abduction deformity.
- Elbow—flexion deformity.
- Hip: Anterior—flexion abduction and external rotation deformity.
- Posterior—flexion, adduction and internal rotation deformity.
- Knee—flexion deformity.
- Ankle—varus deformity.

TABLE 3.6: Common traumatic dislocations

Area involved	Type of dislocation
1. Spine	Anterior, C5 over C6
2. Upper limb	
– Acromioclavicular joint	Type I/II/III
– Sternoclavicular joint	Anterior/posterior
– Shoulder joint	Anterior/posterior
– Elbow joint	Posterior
– Isolated dislocation of superior radioulnar joint	Anterior
– Fracture dislocation of superior radioulnar joint	Monteggia fracture
– Fracture head of radius and dislocation of inferior radioulnar joint	Essex-Lopresti fracture
– Wrist dislocations	Perilunar, lunar
– Kaplan's injury	Carpometacarpal joint of the thumb
3. Lower limb	
– Hip dislocations	Anterior/posterior/central
– Knee joint	Posterior
– Patella	Lateral dislocations
– Ankle	Anterolateral
– Foot	Intertarsal – Chopart's – Lisfranc's
	Tarsometatarsal

Investigations

Radiograph of the affected part should include anteroposterior and lateral views of the joints (Fig. 3.13).

Treatment

Since dislocation is an orthopedic emergency, early closed reduction under general anesthesia is recommended. The part is immobilized for a period of 3 to 6 weeks to ensure adequate healing. Operative reduction is rarely required and is reserved for compound dislocations or irreducible dislocations.

Complications

Acute: Injury to peripheral nerves and vessels can occur, e.g. sciatic nerve palsy in posterior dislocation of hip.

Chronic

Unreduced dislocation: This is common in Asian countries due to ignorance, delay in seeking treatment, etc.

Recurrent dislocations: Due to inadequate and improper healing of soft tissues following initial trauma, e.g. recurrent dislocation of the shoulder.

Traumatic osteoarthritis: Due to damage to the articular cartilage following impaired nutrition by the synovial fluid.

Joint stiffness: Due to capsular and other soft tissue damage.

Avascular necrosis: Due to injury to the vessels.

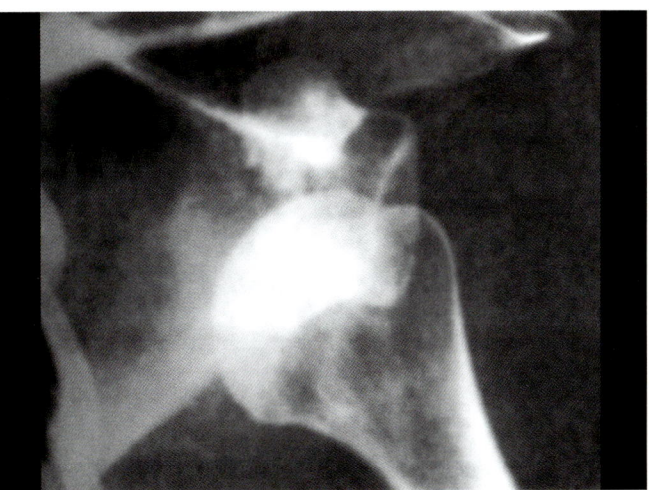

Fig. 3.13: Radiograph showing anterior dislocation of the shoulder

Myositis ossificans: More commonly seen than in fractures due to greater periosteal strip.

> **Remember in Dislocation**
> - It is an orthopedic emergency.
> - Reduction should be quick and prompt.
> - Reduction should always be done under general anesthesia to relax the muscles.
> - Swelling is less when compared to fractures.
> - Movements are more restricted than in fractures.
> - Closed reduction is sufficient most of the times.
> - Open reduction is resorted to if specifically indicated.
> - Reduction technique should always be very gentle.
> - Pain will not subside by splinting unlike fractures.
> - Myositis ossificans is a problem more commonly associated with dislocation.

Subluxation

Subluxation is defined as partial loss of contact between the two ends of the bones. It poses a problem much less serious than dislocation.

Sprain: It is a tear in the ligaments. The severity varies from grade I to grade III. Mild sprains are more common and heal by conservative treatment, whereas grade III sprains cause joint instabilities and need to be repaired surgically. Sprains are commonly encountered in knee joints and ankle joints. They are discussed in detail in appropriate sections.

Strain: It is a tear in the muscles, is more common in young athletes, and usually heals by conservative methods.

These have been dealt in detail in the chapter on Soft Tissue Injuries.

4 CHAPTER

Complications of Fractures

INTRODUCTION

Fracture is a disturbing event more so if it develops complications. The complications could be immediate or delayed. Immediate complications are life-threatening and delayed complications are more morbid. Some complications develop at the time of injury and are beyond the control of the surgeon. They need to be accurately diagnosed and treated. Whenever a surgeon encounters a case of fracture, he should look beyond the fracture and try to detect complications if any. The following are the common complications (Table 4.1).

ACUTE RESPIRATORY DISTRESS SYNDROME (Syn: Fat Embolism)

Acute respiratory distress syndrome (ARDS) is defined as a post-traumatic distress syndrome occurring within 72 hours of skeletal trauma. It indicates the presence of fat globules (palmitin and stearin in children and olein in adults) within the lung parenchyma and peripheral circulation after a long bone fracture. It usually manifests within 24 to 48 hours, but sometimes may be delayed for several days. It is a dreaded complication often associated with multiple fractures, major bone fractures, pelvic fractures, multisystem injuries like chest and abdomen, head injuries, etc. It is seen in 10 to 45 percent cases of multiple fractures and is an important cause of morbidity and mortality (11%) in multiple fracture and multisystem injuries.

> **Historical Facts**
> - Vong Bergman first diagnosed fat embolism syndrome in 1873.

Etiology

Common etiological factor is a long bone fracture in young (usually between 20 and 30 years of age) adult or a pelvic fracture in elderly.

TABLE 4.1: Complications of fractures

Acute open fractures	Chronic	Complications peculiar to

• Shock (Hypovolemic or neurogenic)
• ARDS
• Thromboembolism
• Neurovascular injuries
  1. Radial nerve palsy in fracture shaft humerus
  2. Sciatic nerve palsy in posterior dislocation of hip
  3. Supracondylar fractures causing brachial artery injury
• Acute Volkmann's ischemia
• Crush syndrome
• Deep vein thrombosis
	• Delayed union
	• Nonunion
	• Malunion
	• Shortening
	• Growth disturbances
	• Avascular necrosis
	• Joint stiffness
	• Post-traumatic arthritis
	• VIC
	• Myositis ossificans
		• Infection
		• Chronic osteomyelitis
		• Gas gangrene
		• Tetanus
		• Hypovolemic shock
		• Miscellaneous
		• Implant failure
		• Reflex sympathic dystrophy, etc.

Source of fat: It could be from two sources:
- Mechanical theory
  - From bone marrow (accepted).
- Biochemical theory
  a. *Obstructive theory:* From plasma by agglutination of chylomicrons which later acts as an embolus (less accepted).
  b. *Toxic theory:* The free fatty acid destroys the pneumocytes and causes ARDS.

Pathogenesis

Following injury, the bone marrow fat or the platelet agglutination are sucked into the injured vessels and are transported to various sites as emboli giving rise to varied clinical manifestations.

Classification (Sevitt's)

- *Classical type:* In this variety, the onset is less than 24 hours, *tachycardia* is greater than 140/min, *Pyrexia* is greater than 40°C, *tachypnea, cyanosis, changing cerebral signs* vary from confusion, restlessness and coma. *Petechial rashes* (Fig. 4.1) and in *conjunctiva of lower lids, if present is pathognomonic.* In this type, the blood pressure is maintained throughout.
- *Fulminating type:* Here the sequence of events is very fast and there is no time for the rashes to develop. Patient is comatose within hours and throws repeated seizures. Patient rapidly collapses and death supervenes.
- *Incomplete type:* The manifestation is between the two types. Unexplained tachycardia, fever, and rash are its features.

Features of Rashes in ARDS
- Seen commonly in classical type.
- Presents across the chest, axilla, root of the neck and conjunctiva.
- Fleeting type.
- Fades rapidly.
- Occurs periodically with attacks of coma.
- Can occur in the retina.
- Diagnosed by fundoscopy.
- Retinal rashes are pathognomonic.

Interesting Facts
Do you know the Gurd's major and minor criteria for diagnosis of fat embolism syndrome?
Major criteria
- Axillary and subconjunctival petechiae
- PaO_2 <60 mm Hg
- CNS depression.

Minor criteria
- Pulse >110/min
- Pyrexia >38.5°C
- Retinal embolism
- Fat in urine
- Reduced platelet count
- Increased ESR
- Fat globules in sputum.

Diagnostic criteria: At least one from major criteria and four from minor criteria are required to make a diagnosis of fat embolism syndrome.

Investigations

- *X-ray of the chest:* It may snowstorm appearance and if seen is pathognomonic (Fig. 4.2).

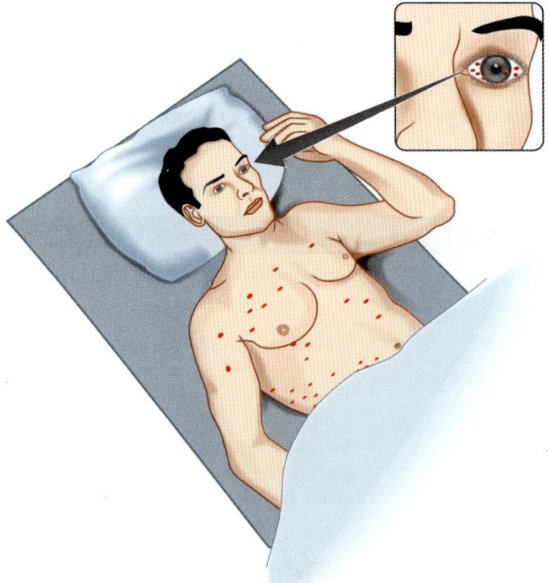

Fig. 4.1: Petechial rashes like these are the hallmark of fat embolism syndrome

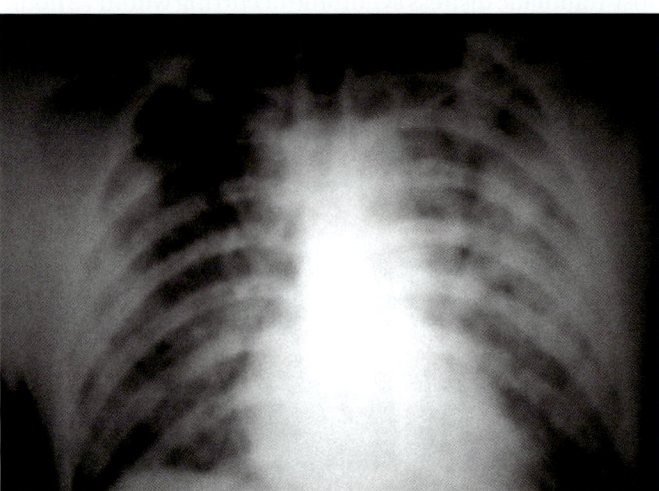

Fig. 4.2: Plain X-ray chest showing snowstorm appearance

- PaO_2 less than 60 mm Hg.
- Platelet counts less than 1.5 lakhs.
- ECG shows prominent S-wave.
- Gurd test: Isolation of fat emboli from the blood.
- There is no pathognomonic laboratory test.
- Anemia, hypocalcemia may also occur.

The Important Diagnostic Triad in ARDS is Represented by the Mnemonic TPR
- Thrombocytopenia.
- PaO_2 <60 mm Hg.
- Rashes.

- CT scan, MRI of the brain helps to grade the severity of fat embolism.

Management

There are two important steps in the management of ARDS:

Nonspecific: It consists of three vital steps:
1. *Keep* (a) airway patent, and (b) fracture immobilized by POP or external fixators.
2. *Restore* (a) blood volume, (b) fluid, and (c) electrolyte balance.
3. *Avoid* (a) careless handling of the injured, and (b) unnecessary transportation.

Specific: Again three vital steps are described:
1. *Respiratory support:* Oxygen administration to restore back PaO_2 or full-fledged ventilator support.
2. *Drug therapy*
   - *Steroids* are given intravenously. These help gas exchange by decreasing inflammation in the lungs.
   - *Heparin:* This acts as a lipolytic and antiplatelet agent.
   - *Low molecular weight dextran:* It acts by increasing plasma volume.
   - *Intravenous alcohol:* It is not universally advocated.
   - *Antibiotics* and other treatment.
3. *Definitive fracture treatment:* It is discussed in appropriate sections. Early fixation of fractures is advocated to prevent worsening of the situation.

Role of Antiplatelets in ARDS
- Should be given early
- Given intravenous every 6 to 8 hours in doses of 2,500 IU.
- It improves microcirculatory flow.
- It increases plasma volume.
- Decreases platelet adhesiveness.

What is Subclinical Fat Embolism Syndrome?
The presence of only laboratory abnormalities with no obvious clinical symptoms. Remember 4T's to diagnose fat embolism syndrome
- T-tachycardia >100/min
- T-tachypnea >25 breaths/min
- T-temperature elevation >37.8°C
- T-thrombocytopenia <2 lakhs.

Interesting Facts
Do you know the common pulmonary problems in orthopedics (Mnemonic PAPA-F)?
- P—**P**ulmonary emboli
- A—**A**telectasis
- P—**P**ostoperative pneumonia
- A—**A**telectasis
- F—**F**at emboli.

VOLKMANN'S ISCHEMIA OR COMPARTMENTAL SYNDROMES

Mubarak defined compartmental syndrome as an *elevation of interstitial pressure in a closed osteofascial compartment that results in microvascular compromise* and may cause irreversible damage to the contents of the space.

Sites
1. Anterior and deep posterior compartments of the legs.
2. Volar compartment of the forearm (Fig. 4.3).
3. Buttocks, shoulder, hand, foot, arm, and lumbar paraspinous muscles are relatively rare sites.

COMPARTMENTAL SYNDROME OF FOREARM

This is one of the most dreaded complications in orthopedics and ranges from mild ischemia to severe gangrene. Early recognition and prompt remedial measures is the key to successful countering of this problem. *This is an orthopedic emergency.*

Definition

It is an ischemic necrosis of structures contained within the volar compartment of the forearm.

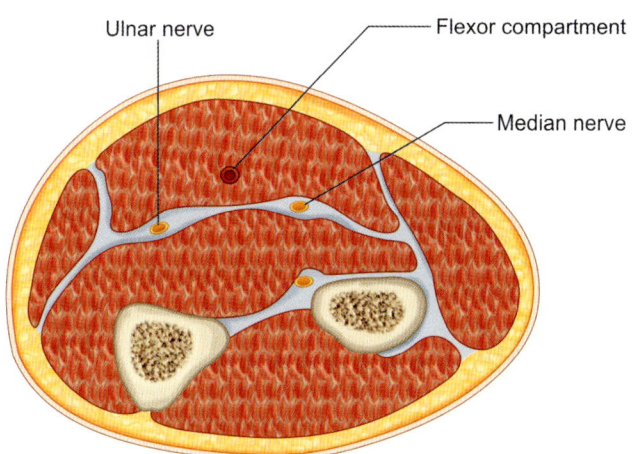

Fig. 4.3: Cross-section of the volar compartment of the forearm

Incidence and Etiology

It is common in children less than 10 years of age.
- Supracondylar fracture is the most common cause in children.
- Crush injuries of the forearm are the most common causes in adults.
- Occasionally fracture of both bones of forearm dislocation of the elbow, vascular injuries and subfascial hematomas may be the cause.
- More recently intra-arterial injections in drug addicts who lie on their forearm for prolonged periods in narcotized conditions are mooted to be a cause (Fig. 4.4).
- Improper application of splints is another important cause.

Usually the flexor muscles of the forearm, especially the flexor digitorum profundus and flexor pollicis longus and rarely flexor digitorum superficialis are involved. Volkmann's ischemic contracture (VIC) is due to the infarction produced by an arterial spasm of the main artery to an extremity with reflex spasm of the collateral circulation. This produces ischemia of the muscle bellies that results in necrosis and is later replaced by fibrous tissue causing contractures.

Pathology

An inelastic and unyielding deep fascia surrounds the forearm muscles. Rise in the intracompartmental pressure due to any cause is not accommodated and the vessels are compressed resulting in muscle ischemia and consequent fibrosis. The picture is one of *central* degeneration in the muscle along the line of anterior interosseous artery. The greatest damage is at the center and the muscles commonly affected are flexor digitorum profundus and flexor pollicis longus (Table 4.2).

Clinical Features

In the acute stages, the patient gives history of trauma and after an interval of few hours; severe, poorly localized pain develops in the forearm. The volar aspect of the forearm is swollen, red, warm, tender, and tense. Fingers are held in flexion and an attempt to extend the fingers increases the pain (stretch pain) (Fig. 4.5). Peripheral pulses, which are present initially, disappear later. Median nerve is more commonly affected than the ulnar nerve.

> **Note:**
> In acute Volkmann's ischemia the patient complains of pain out of proportion to the injury.

TABLE 4.2: Etiopathogenesis of compartment syndrome

Etiology: According to Matson

- ↓ Compartment size
    - Closure of fascial defects
    - Tight dressing
    - Localized external pressure
- ↓ Compartment content
    - Bleeding
    - Vascular injury
    - Bleeding disorders
- ↓ Capillary permeability
    - Burns
    - Trauma
    - Post-exercises
    - Seizures
    - Intra-arterial drugs
    - Exercise
    - Venous obstruction
- ↓ Capillary pressure
    - Exercise
    - Venous obstruction
- Muscle hypertrophy
- Infiltrated infusion
- Nephrotic syndrome

Pathophysiology

External or internal constrictions →↑ Arterial spasm or occlusion → Causes muscle ischemia →↑ Capillary permeability →↑ Intramuscular edema →↑ Intramuscular pressure → Further arterial compromise → Muscle necrosis → Replaced by collagen → Contractures

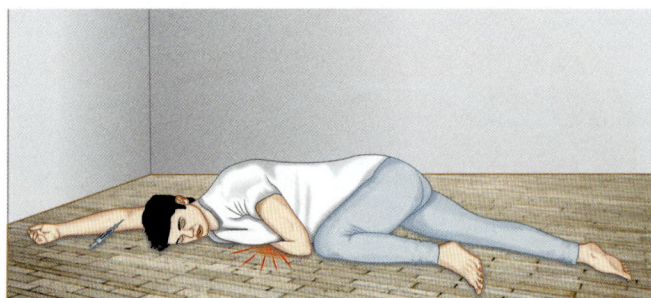

Fig. 4.4: Drug addicts 'beware' lying with your forearm tucked under your body in an inebriated state can lead to compartmental syndrome of the forearm

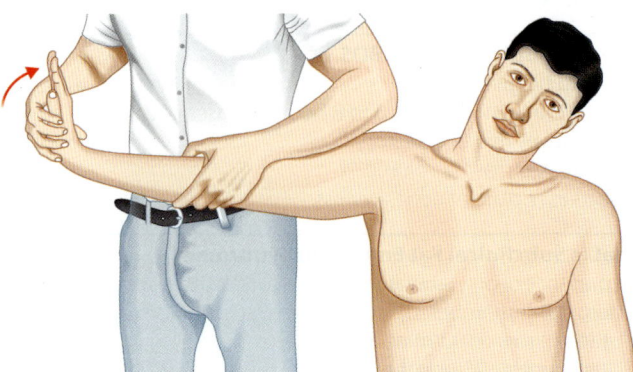

Fig. 4.5: Method of performing the passive stretch test

Impending Volkmann's ischemia is detected by 6Ps
- **P**ain
- **P**allor
- **P**aresthesia
- **P**aralysis
- **P**ulselessness
- **P**ositive passive stretch test.

Investigations

Investigations like routine blood tests, X-ray of the affected part, CT scan and MRI studies, angiograph and Doppler studies needs to be done before planning the treatment (Flowchart 4.1).

Management

Acute stage: It is a surgical emergency. All encircling tight bandages are removed, if present. If there is no improvement, record the pressure within the compartment (Fig. 4.6). If it is more than 30 mm Hg, an emergency surgical decompression is done by fasciotomy (Fig. 4.7). If the pressure is less than 30 mm Hg, continuous monitoring is done.

Methods to Record Intracompartmental Pressure

In any patient with forearm or leg injuries who has a tense compartment and if the patient is unreliable or unresponsive, the intracompartmental pressure should be recorded by using a needle manometer, wick or slick catheter. If the intracompartmental pressure is more than 30 to 40 mmHg or is 10 to 30 mmHg more than the diastolic pressure of the patient, fasciotomy is recommended (Fig. 4.6).

Volkmann's Ischemic Contracture (VIC)

Late cases If mild, flexion contractures of flexor digitorum profundus and flexor pollicis longus develop but in severe cases all the finger flexors, thumb and wrist flexors are affected (Table 4.3). The forearm is thin and fibrotic. Extensive scar tissue may be present. Peripheral nerves may be affected, amongst them median nerve is the most commonly involved. A *classical claw hand* deformity results (Fig. 4.8A) of particular importance is eliciting the *Volkmann's sign* in established VIC. *This test consists of extending the wrist, which exaggerates the deformities, and*

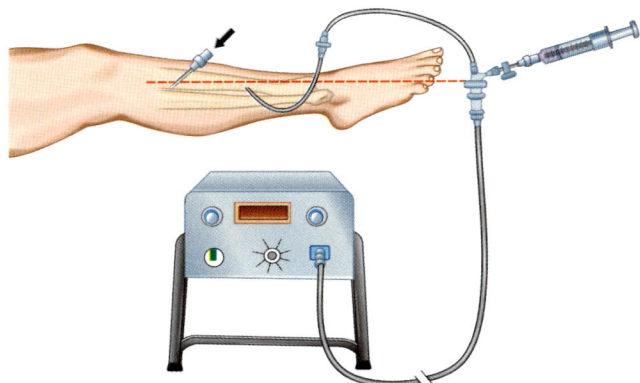

Fig. 4.6: Method of recording the intracompartmental pressure within the leg

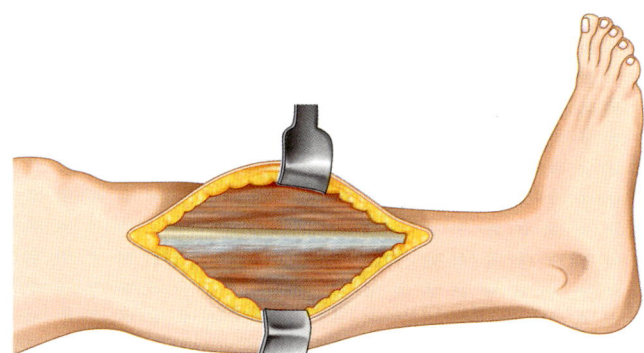

Fig. 4.7: A wide fasciotomy for acute compartmental syndrome

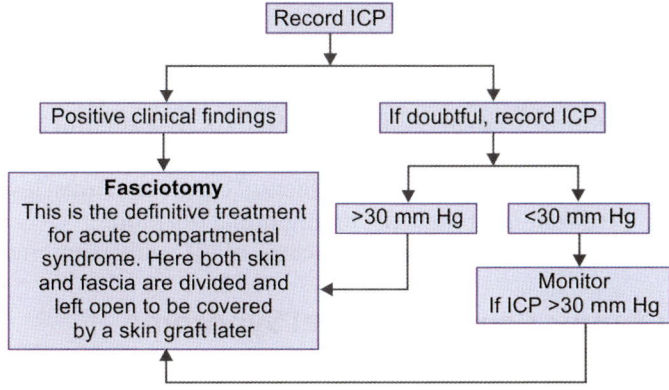

Flowchart 4.1: Treatment plan in VIC

Treatment of choice is early decompression
Ischemia
- More than 4 hours causes' myoglobinuria (crush syndrome)
- More than 12 hours—total ischemia results in contractures

ICP—Intracompartmental pressure

TABLE 4.3: Tsuge's classification of VIC		
Mild	Moderate	Severe
• FDP • FPL involved	• Involvement of FDP + FPL • Superficial finger flexor • Wrist flexors • Thumb flexors	• All flexors. • Few extensors. • Neurological deficit. • Contracture of joint. • Skin scarred.

FDP—flexor digitorum profundus, FPL—flexor pollicis longus.

34 SECTION 1: Traumatology

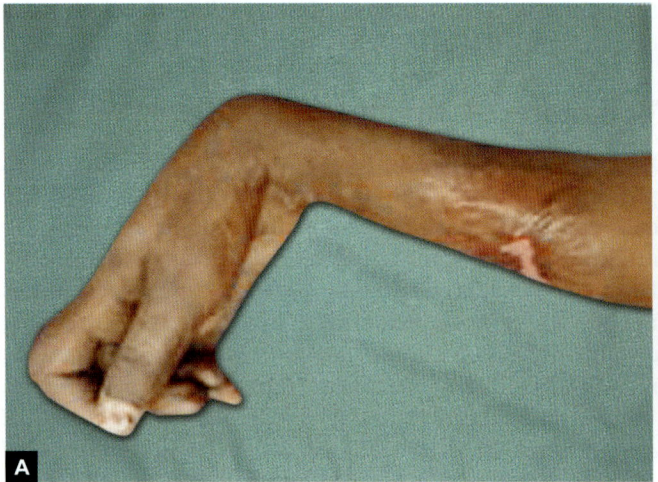
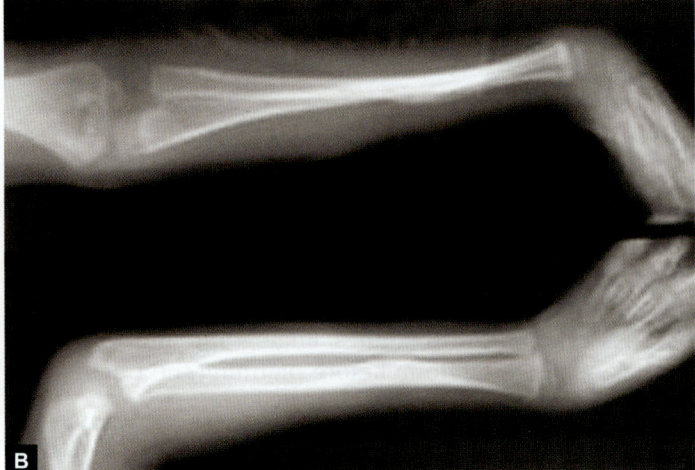

Figs 4.8A and B: (A) VIC of the forearm (Clinical photo); (B) Radiograph of the VIC

on flexion, the deformities appear less prominent (Figs 4.9A and B). Joint contractures and gangrene may also be seen. Plain X-ray of the forearm shows old fracture (Fig. 4.8B).

> **In Established VIC**
> *Look for:*
> - Claw and deformity.
> - Volkmann's sign.
> - Extensive scarring of the forearm.
> - Joint and soft tissue contractures.
> - Neurological deficits.
> - Rarely gangrene.

> **Remember**
> If 5 Ps help in detection of acute cases, 5 Ps also form clue to the management:
> - Pressure to be relieved either external or internal.
> - Pressure to be monitored within the compartment.
> - Pulse to be recorded continuously.
> - Passive stretch test indicates the severity.
> - Putting the fracture back into its position.

Treatment Plan in Established VIC

Here the contractures are well-established and the treatment plan depends upon the severity of VIC.

Mild Type
- Dynamic splinting.
- Physiotherapy.
- Total excision if single muscle is involved.

Moderate Type
- *Max page's muscle sliding operation:* This consists of releasing the common flexor origin from the medial epicondyle and passively stretching the fingers.

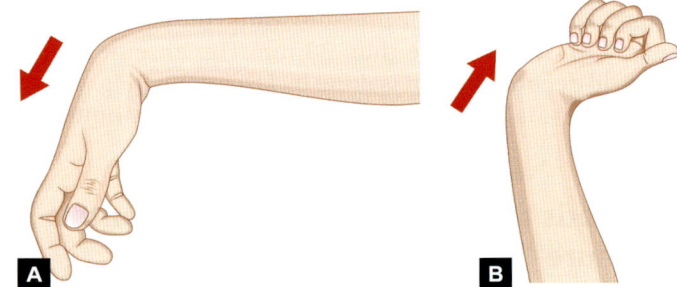

Figs 4.9A and B: Volkmann's sign: Deformity disappears on flexion (A) and appears on extension (B)

This slides the origin of the muscle down and releases the contractures.
- *Excision of cicatrix.*
- *Neurolysis:* It consists of freeing the peripheral nerves from the surrounding fibrous tissue.
- *Tendon transfers:* These are done if criteria's are met.

Severe Type
- *Excision* of the scar.
- *Seddon's carpectomy*—it consists of excising the proximal row of carpal bones thereby shortening the forearm to overcome the effects of contracted muscles.
- *Arthrodesis* of the wrist in functional position.
- *Amputation* for very severe cases of VIC with gangrene.

Chronic Compartmental Syndrome

Chronic compartmental syndrome is a pretibial pain induced by exercise seen in the anterior compartment of the leg in athletes. If the compartmental pressure is more than 15 mm Hg at rest, more than 30 mm Hg during exercise and more than 20 mm Hg for 5 minutes after exercise, chronic compartmental syndrome are suspected. Due to the herniation of fat or muscle through the fascial defect, a soft tissue mass is seen in the anterolateral aspect of the lower third of the leg. The patient is instructed to alter or decrease the level of activity, if no relief is forthcoming, surgical decompression is indicated.

NONUNION

The difference between delayed union and nonunion is of degree. In delayed union healing has *not advanced* at the average rate for location and type of fractures but healing can still take place if the limb is immobilized for a longer period. In nonunion, there is evidence to show clinically and radiologically that healing has *ceased* and union is improbable and needs surgery. Final status of nonunion is pseudarthrosis.

Definition (FDA Panel)

Nonunion is said to be established when a *minimum of nine months* has elapsed since the injury and the fracture shows no radiologically visible progressive signs of healing continuously *for three months*.

Classification

Two classifications are adopted.
[1]**Paley's classification** This classification takes into account the amount of bone loss and includes two varieties:
- Type A less than 1 cm bone loss
- Type B greater than 1 cm bone loss.

Muller and Weber's classification: This classification takes into account the amount of callus at the fracture site (Table 4.4).

Hypervascular Nonunion

In this, the fracture ends are viable and show biological reaction; hence, stable internal fixation is enough, and no bone grafting is required.

Types

Elephant foot nonunion: Exuberant callus is seen in this variety (Fig. 4.10A).

Reasons
- Insecure fixation of fracture fragments.
- Premature weight-bearing.

Horse hoof nonunion: Here poor callus is seen (Fig. 4.10B).

Reasons
- Unstable fixation with plate and screws.

Oligotrophic nonunion: Very poor callus is seen in this variety (Fig. 4.10C).

Reasons
This is usually seen in:
- Major displacements, distraction, etc.
- Poor internal fixation.

Avascular Nonunion

In avascular nonunion (Figs 4.11A to D), the fracture ends are not viable due to poor blood supply. No biological reaction is seen, and this needs rigid internal fixation with bone grafting after decortications of nonviable ends.

Types

Torsion wedge nonunion: Here the intermediate fragment has healed at one end and not at the other. It is seen in segmental fractures.

Comminuted nonunion: It is seen in comminuted fractures.

Defect nonunion: Here there is loss of fragment, seen in compound fractures, osteomyelitis, etc.

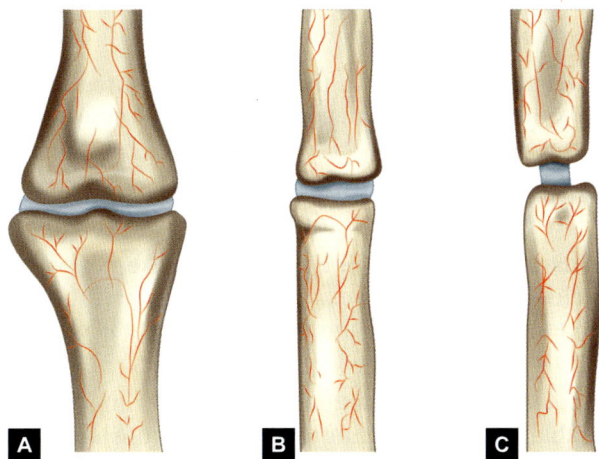

Figs 4.10A to C: Hypervascular nonunion: (A) Elephant foot; (B) Horse hoof; (C) Oligotrophic

TABLE 4.4: Muller and Weber classification	
Hypervascular nonunion	Avascular nonunion
Hypertrophic nonunion (Exuberant callus)	• Torsion wedge nonunion
Horse hoof nonunion	• Comminuted nonunion
Oligotrophic nonunion	• Defect nonunion
	• Atrophic nonunion

---

[1] **Dror Paley**, American Orthopedic Surgeon

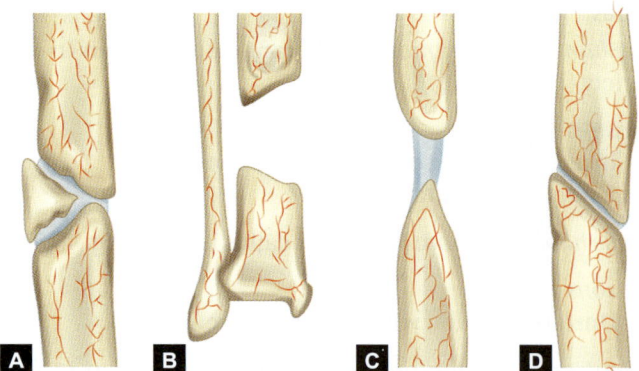

Figs 4.11A to D: Avascular nonunion: (A) Comminuted nonunion; (B) Gap nonunion; (C) Atrophic nonunion; (D) Torsion wedge nonunion

Atrophic nonunion: Here the ends are thin and sclerotic with excessive scar tissue in between and the fracture fragments have tapering ends.

Causes for Nonunion

Nonunion of fractures is a very notorious complication to treat. Infected nonunion challenges the clinical acumen of best of orthosurgeons. There are various causes leading to nonunion and the following are some of those.

Compound fractures: There is extensive damage to the soft tissues in open fractures and there could be even loss of small pieces of bone. The former results in impaired blood supply to the fracture fragments jeopardizing the chances of union.

Infection: This is commonly seen in compound fractures and in postsurgical infections. Hence, infections should be kept at a minimum in treatment of fractures.

Segmental fractures: In this type of fractures there is a maximum risk of damage to the intraosseous vessels resulting in poor union.

Distraction of fracture fragments: This happens when excessive weight is used during skin or skeletal traction.

Soft-tissue interposition: If soft tissues, like periosteum, muscles, tendons, nerves, vessels, etc. are interposed between the fracture fragments, it obstructs the growth of internal callus and thus jeopardizes union.

Ill-advised open reduction: Open reduction damages favorable factors for fracture union like fracture hematoma. Periosteal stripping and intramedullary reaming disturbs the vascular supply. All these are detrimental to fracture healing.

Insecure and inadequate fixation: Insecure and inadequate fixation of fracture fragments by plate and screws or intramedullary fixation allows micro-movements, which prevent union.

Apart from these local factors, the general factors that contribute to poor healing of fractures are anemia, general debility, cachexia, steroid therapy, osteoporosis, malignancy, etc.

Nevertheless, it can be observed that most of the factors, general or local, responsible for poor fracture healing are preventable if one exercises utmost caution and care during the treatment of fractures.

Clinical Features

This can be discussed under three headings.

History: Usually the patient gives history of trauma resulting in fractures, multiple injuries, multisystem or head injuries. There could be history of open fractures, delay, or improper or inadequate treatment. It should be noted that in nonunion the history is of a longer duration.

Symptoms: The acute symptoms seen in fresh fractures are conspicuously absent in nonunion. There is usually history of no pain or minimal pain. There could be presence of a deformity or loss of function.

Signs: The important clinical signs are painless abnormal mobility, no crepitus, shortening, scars, and sinuses, deformity, wasting of limb muscles, etc.

Investigations

Radiograph of the part in AP and lateral views (Fig. 4.12). The following points are looked for:
- Gap between the fracture fragments.
- The fragments are rounded and sclerotic.

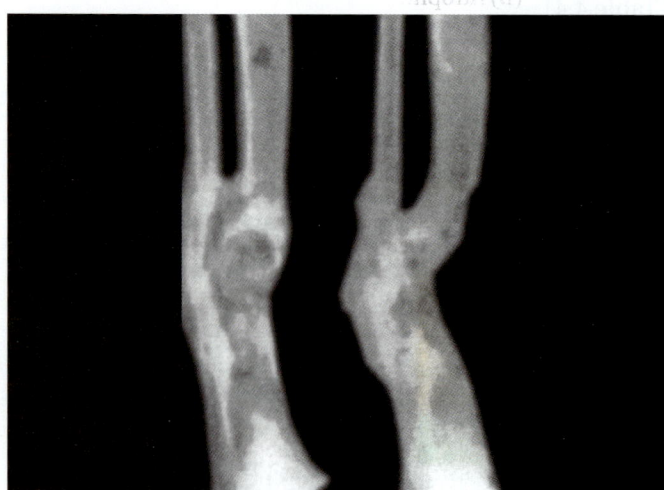

Fig. 4.12: Radiograph showing infected nonunion of tibia and fibula

- The amount of callus formed could be less (avascular nonunion) or more (higher-vascular nonunion).
- Decreased density of bone is due to osteoporosis. Radiology helps classify nonunion depending upon the amount of callus (Figs 4.13 and 4.14).

Management

Principles

- Nonunion is an absolute indication for surgery and it requires open reduction, rigid internal fixation and bone grafting.
- There is no role of conservative treatment.
- Other methods of treatment include electrical stimulation, interlocking nails, and Ilizarov's technique (Table 4.5).

Role of Bone Grafting in Nonunion

Bone grafts help in promoting osteogenesis. They also fill in the gap and provide stability.

TABLE 4.5: Management of nonunion

Uninfected nonunion	Infected nonunion
I. Open reduction and bone grafting	I. Classical method (takes 1 year) stages
1. Onlay grafting	• Wound debridement.
• Single	• One week later split skin graft.
• Dual	• Next week, full-thickness graft.
2. Phemister technique (Subperiosteal bone grafting)	• Bone graft after 6 to 12 months.
3. Cancellous bone grafting	
4. Massive sliding graft	
5. Whole fibular graft	
II. Electrical stimulation	II. Active method (takes less time)
1. Electrical	
• Noninvasive	• Internal fixation of fractures done first.
• Semi-invasive	• Bone grafting next.
• Invasive	• Continuous irrigation with saline and antibiotics.
	• Skin grafting later.
2. Pulsed EMF stimulation	
III. Internal fixation	III. Pulsed electromagnetic field stimulation.
• Interlocking system	
• Rigid compression plating	
IV. Ilizarov's technique	IV. Ilizarov's technique.

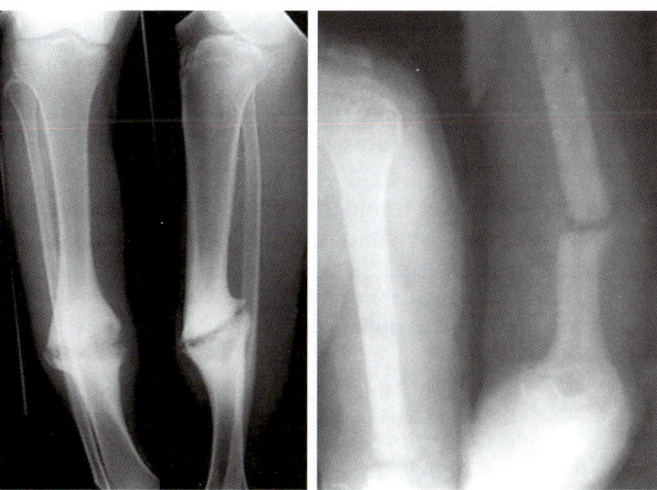

Figs 4.13A and B: (A) Hypertrophic nonunion of tibia; (B) Atrophic nonunion of humerus

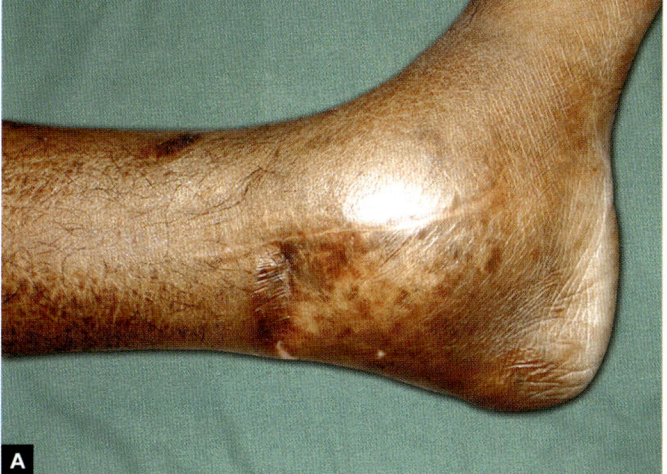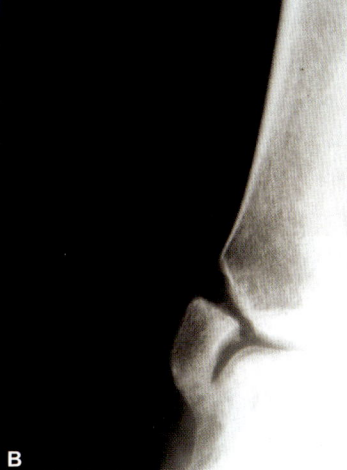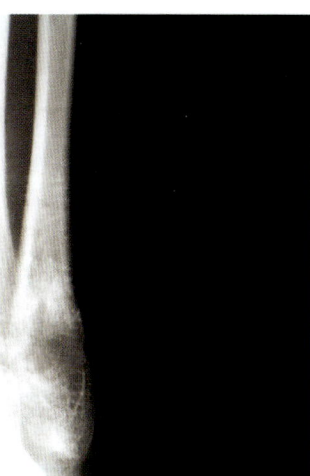

Figs 4.14A and B: Clinical photo of nonunion medial malleolus

Types

Cancellous bone graft: It is useful in defects less than 2.5 cm. It is very commonly used since it is better tolerated and is rapidly revascularized.

Cortical bone graft: It provides sufficient fixation and promotes osteogenesis. It has a stabilizing property and can be used for nonunion of the shafts of any long bone. When placed on one surface, it is called *single only*; when it is placed on both the sides, it is called *the dual only*; and when a piece is sided from above to the fracture site, it is called a *sliding graft* (Fig. 4.15).

Phemister bone graft: Here the graft is placed subperiosteally. It is simple and blood supply is not disturbed. It is placed posterior and is found to be useful in tibia.

Role of Electrical Stimulation in Nonunion

Weak electrical currents of 20 mA delivered to the fracture site by a cathode converts fibrous tissue to fibrocartilage, which is ossified later by endochondral ossification.

Three types: If cathode is placed inside the fracture site, it is called *invasive;* when placed subcutaneously, it is called *semi-invasive;* when incorporated into a plaster cast externally, it is called *noninvasive*.

Pulsed electromagnetic field is the method of delivering the current by electromagnetic field in a pulsed manner. This is also noninvasive.

Union occurs in 85 percent of cases. Large gap greater than half the diameter of the bone will not unite.

Excision of fibrous tissue followed by bone grafting is done first. Immobilization by plaster is done to decrease stress.

Union by electrical means is slow and is not always successful.

Role of Ilizarov's Technique in Nonunion

This allows simultaneous correction of all deformities and bone loss. In hypertrophic nonunion gradual compression helps. In avascular nonunion corticotomy, bone transport and compression helps. *Corticotomy* provides some of the same biological benefits as bone graft. Segmental nonunion is also successful. *Ilizarov's* technique provides dramatic results but is technically very demanding. It is still the best way to treat cases of infected nonunion.

AVASCULAR NECROSIS

Avascular necrosis (AVN) is a rare but severe complication of certain fractures. It occurs when the blood supply to a segment of bone is affected.

Causes

- Extensive stripping of soft tissues, which damage the periosteal blood supply.
- In certain bones where the blood supply is unique and unidirectional, e.g. talus, scaphoid, neck of femur (Figs 4.16A to C).
- Other causes like steroid therapy, Caisson's disease, etc. which may cause an embolic block of the blood vessels.

> **Do you know other causes of AVN other than fractures? Remember the mnemonic 'SCLERA'**
> - S—**S**teroids
> - C—**C**aisson's disease
> - L—**L**upus erythematosus
> - R—**R**adiation therapy
> - A—**A**lcoholism

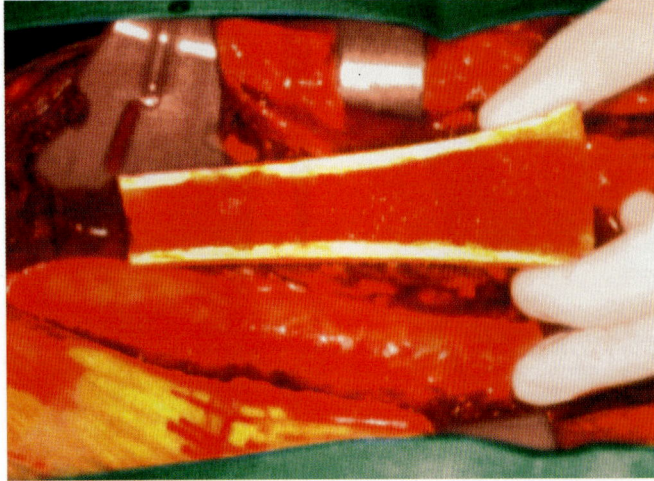

Fig. 4.15: Cortical bone graft

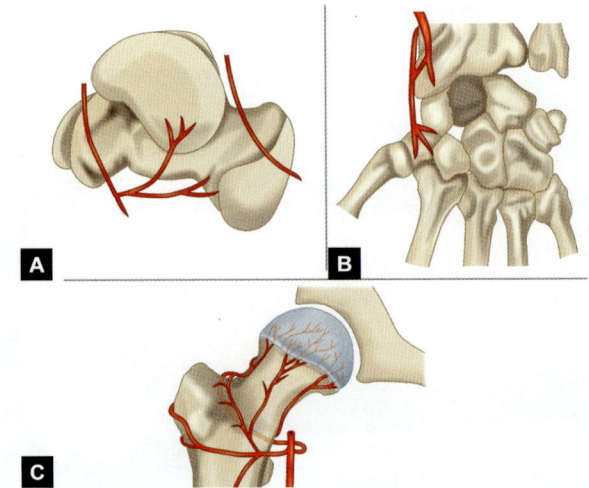

Figs 4.16A to C: Due to the peculiar blood supply, avascular necrosis is common in the above three bones: (A) Talus; (B) Scaphoid; (C) Neck of femur

Common sites of AVN: These are head of femur in fracture neck of femur and dislocations of hip, body of the talus in fracture through the neck of talus, proximal pole of scaphoid in fracture through the waist of the scaphoid.

Problems in avascular necrosis: The loss of blood supply to a major bone segment impairs healing because the avascular segment cannot participate in the reparative process. This defective healing makes the bone weak and susceptible to external forces. This results in collapse of the bone and late osteoarthritis changes.

Clinical Features

Avascular necrosis of a bone is usually asymptomatic in the early stages. In the later stage, the patient may complain of pain, limp and slight loss of movements. In very advanced cases, the patient will show features of osteoarthritis.

Investigations

In the early stages, avascular necrosis can be detected by bone scan, radioisotope study. In the later stages, radiograph shows dense changes in the bone, collapse and osteoarthritis features (Figs 4.17 and 4.18).

Treatment

Early stages require no treatment. Protective braces may be given to prevent bone collapse. Surgical decompression has a doubtful role. In the late stages, total hip replacement is advocated for AVN head of the femur. AVN in scaphoid needs open reduction and bone grafting.

TRAUMATIC MYOSITIS OSSIFICANS

Definition

It is a reactive lesion occurring in the soft tissues and at times in the bone periosteum. It is characterized by fibrous, osseous, and cartilaginous proliferation of the subperiosteal hematoma. This is later followed by metaplastic changes.

Causes

Trauma: This has a definitive role in the causation of myositis ossificans. Injury to the muscles, ligaments, tendons, periosteum, and bones results in bleeding within the soft tissues, which in turn may lead to myositis.

Simple blow or repeated minor trauma: This could also give rise to myositis due to the repeated and constant soft tissue damage.

Dislocations and avulsion injuries: These are more prone to develop myositis than the fractures because of the violent stripping of the periosteum and damage to the muscles.

Ill-advised massage: This is by far the most common cause for myositis. Vigorous and improper massage particularly the elbow joint by quacks, etc. explains the frequent occurrence of this problem in patients treated by traditional bonesetters and osteopaths.

Pathology

Muscles are commonly involved, but fascia, tendon, and periosteum can also be affected. Basically, the process

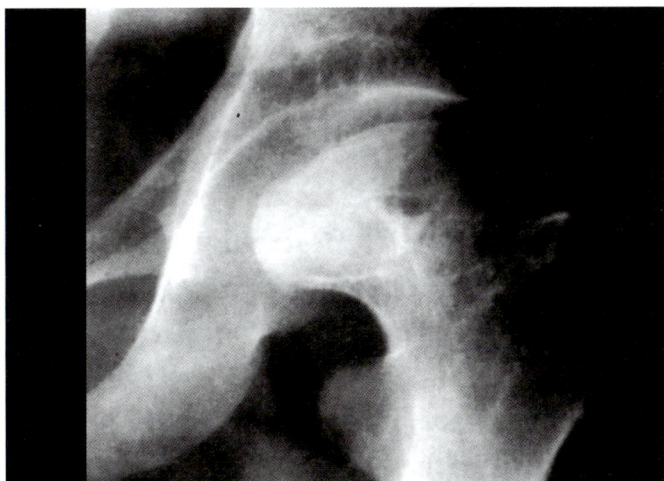

Fig. 4.17: Radiograph showing avascular necrosis of femoral head

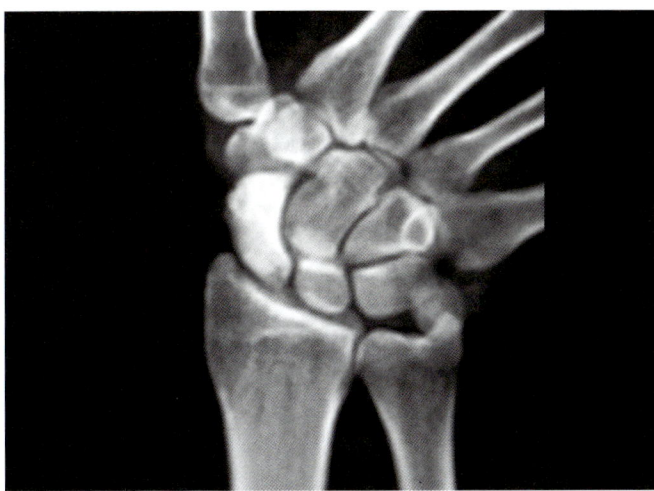

Fig. 4.18: Plain X-ray showing AVN scaphoid

is a peculiar alteration within the ground substance of the connective tissue associated with proliferation of undifferentiated connective tissue.

If the periosteum is involved, the subperiosteal hematoma undergoes proliferation and metaplasia resulting in bone formation. Histological study reveals three zones (Ackermann's zone phenomenon).
- Central highly cellular area.
- Zone of fibroblastic tissue.
- Zone of mature well-oriented bone.

Remember in Myossitis Ossificans
Muscles commonly involved are:
- Brachialis anticus.
- Quadratus femoris.
- Adductor muscles of the thigh.

Note:
All these muscles take origin from a wide area-suggesting role of periosteum in its genesis.

CLASSIFICATION (BASED ON ITS LOCATION)

1. Extra-osseous.
2. Periosteal—beneath the periosteum.
3. Paraosteal.

Hematoma seems to be a prerequisite in all the three situations.

Clinical Features

In the acute stages, the patient may complain of pain, swelling, and loss of movements. On examination, there may be tenderness. In the late stages, there is no pain and a bony hard lump may be palpated. This may act as a mechanical block to the movements.

Remember
Areas commonly affected
- Elbow joint common in young athletes.
- Ankle joint (known as footballer's ankle).
- Knee (known as Pellegrini-Stieda disease).
- Shoulder.
- Hip.
- In head injuries it is more common.

Radiograph

Radiography has little role in the *acute stages* but in the late stages a bony growth may be evidently seen (Fig. 4.19).

Treatment

Acute stages: Conservative treatment is the method of choice and consists of the following:

- *Immobilization of the part by splints, etc.*
- *Drugs*—diphosphonate therapy, calcitonin and nonsteroidal anti-inflammatory drugs (NSAIDs).
- *Physiotherapy:* Active physiotherapy is encouraged and passive stretching is avoided.
- *Manipulation is done under anesthesia*: It is a double-edged sword and has to be done very carefully.

Note:
Adhesions should snap abruptly and should not be broken gradually.

Chronic stages: Surgery is the treatment of choice and consists of soft tissue release and excision of bony spur when it is well formed.

Remember
- The term myossitis ossificans is a *misnomer* because skeletal muscle is often not involved and inflammatory changes are rarely seen.
- Myossitis ossificans progressive. It is a different condition and has nothing to do with the traumatic one. It is a congenital condition affecting all the skeletal muscles.

MALUNION

When fracture fragments heal in an abnormal position, it is called malunion.

Clinical Features

It can pose the following problems:
- It may cause cosmetically unsightly deformity (Fig. 4.20A).
- It may cause alteration in posture and balance in lower limb fractures.
- It may cause shortening (Fig. 4.20B).

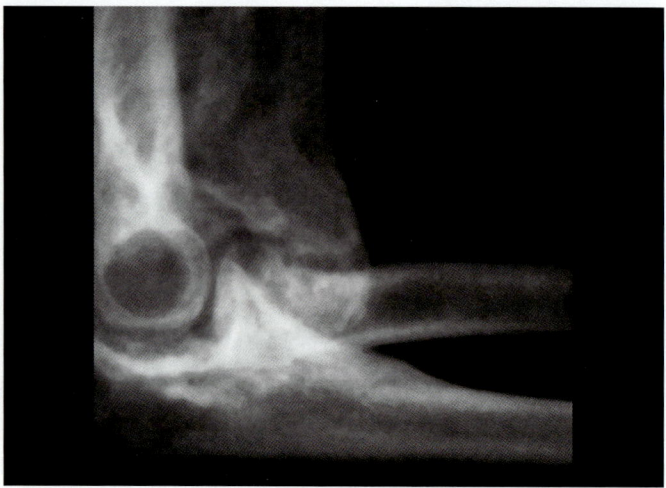

Fig. 4.19: Radiograph showing myossitis ossificans (Elbow joint)

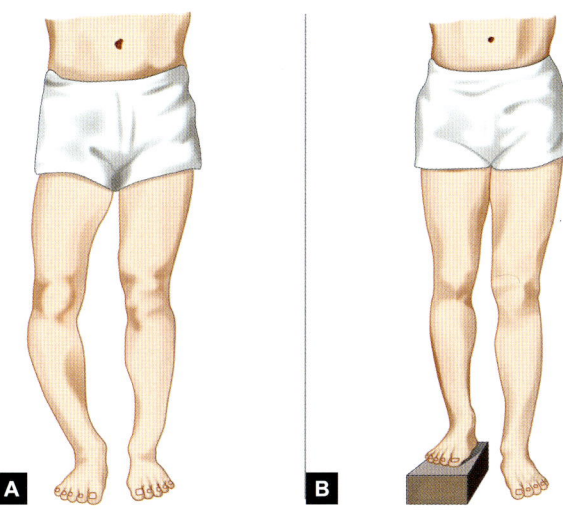

Figs 4.20A and B: Malunion of a long bone like tibia will cause deformity (A) and shortening (B)

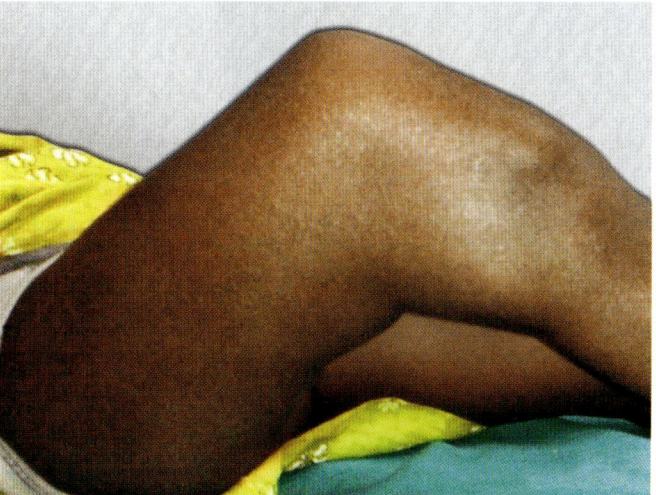

Fig. 4.21: Clinical photo showing malunion of femur

- It may interfere with joint function.
- Altered weight-bearing mechanism may lead to premature osteoarthritis of the hip and knee joints.

Causes

Treatment methods: Malunion is common in fractures treated by closed reduction because it is a blind technique, and it is very difficult to assess the accuracy of the reduction.

Improper immobilization techniques: Following reductions if the fracture is not immobilized properly and if immobilized for inadequate length of time, malunion usually results.

Treatment by quacks: Due to poor knowledge of fracture anatomy, the osteopaths and the traditional bonesetters contribute significantly to the incidence of malunion (Fig. 4.21).

Multiple and multisystem injuries: These are life-threatening and assume more importance during treatment and the fractures may go unnoticed by the treating physicians resulting in malunion.

> **Vital Facts**
> *Postreduction criteria to prevent malunion from developing:*
> In order to prevent the malunion from developing following closed reductions, certain postreduction criteria should be strictly adhered to like (in order of importance):
> - Alignment of fracture fragments to be corrected first.
> - Rotation of the fragments corrected next.
> - Length of the limb is restored.
> - Lastly, position of the fragments is adjusted.

Classification

If there is improper correction of any one of the above-mentioned criteria, the following types of malunion may be encountered:
- *Length malunion:* This commonly results in shortening of the limb and rarely may give rise to lengthening.
- *Rotatory malunion:* This may cause external or internal rotation deformities.
- *Angulatory malunion:* This may cause varus or valgus deformities.

Of all the factors mentioned above the one factor, which is not corrected by remodeling, is rotation, while the other three are successfully overcome over the years by remodeling. Hence, all precautions should be taken to correct the rotation element during the initial treatment of fractures.

Types

Significant malunion: This impairs both the function and causes a major cosmetic problem.

Insignificant malunion: This does not interfere with function but causes only cosmetic problem.

Clinical Features

A patient with malunion of bones may complain of deformity and/or alteration or rarely loss of function of the affected extremities. There may be shortening and wasting of the involved limbs (Fig. 4.22).

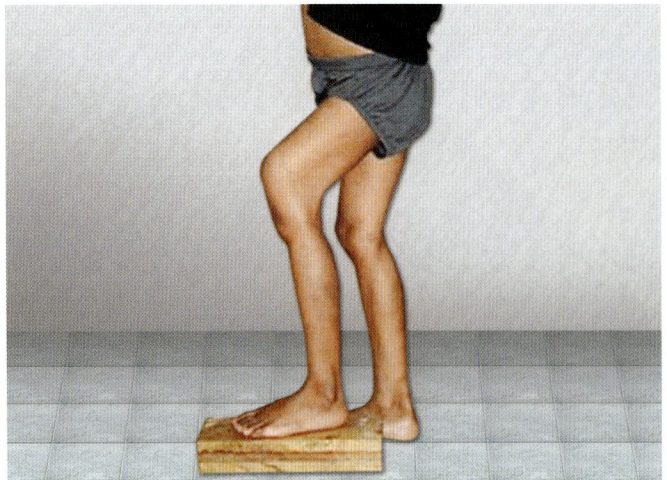

Fig. 4.22: Clinical photo showing shortening in malunion femur

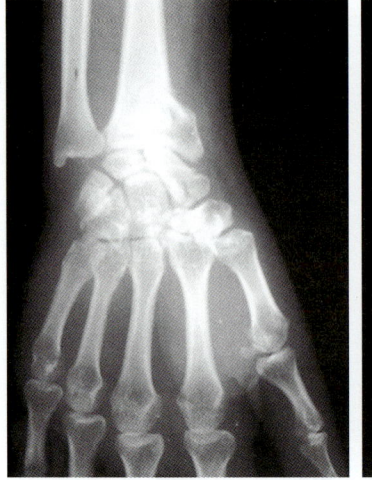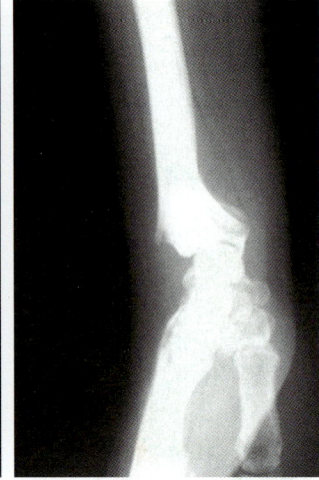

Fig. 4.23: Plain X-ray showing malunion distal radius

Radiograph

Radiograph of the affected part, including the joints above and below are mandatory to assess the malunion (Figs 4.23 and 4.24).

Treatment

Masterly inactivity if the patient has no functional problems. Cosmesis alone does not form a sufficient indication for surgery unless the patient desires so. Nevertheless, operative treatment is highly justified when malunion affects the function. This can be done by a *corrective osteotomy* at the old fracture site or a *compensatory procedure* may be necessary to restore functions (e.g. Darrach's operation in malunited Colles). Sometimes pain may be the only predominant symptom necessitating *fusion of the affected joint*.

The optimum time to carry out surgery for malunion is 6–12 months after the fracture has occurred.

OTHER IMPORTANT COMPLICATIONS OF FRACTURES

DEEP VEIN THROMBOSIS AND PULMONARY EMBOLISM

Introduction

Deep vein thrombosis (DVT) is an important complication seen after fractures of spine, pelvis, femur, tibia, etc. Virchow's triad of venous stasis, vascular damage, and hypercoagulability has described the pathogenesis.

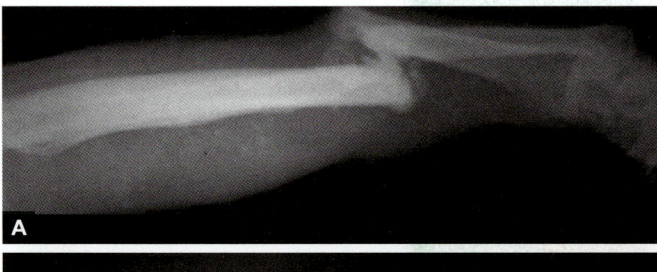
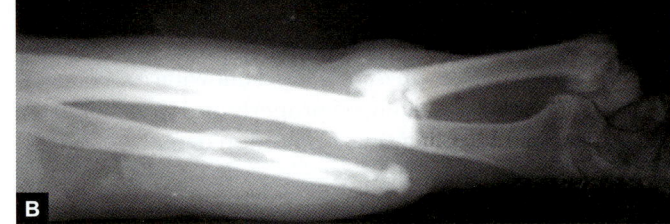

Figs 4.24A and B: Radiographs showing malunited fractures of both bones of the forearm

Clinical Features

The patient complains of mild-to-severe calf pain, swelling, difficulty in standing or walking and cramps in the calf muscles or foot. The clinical signs include unilateral leg swelling, increased temperature, tenderness, enlarged superficial veins, pitting edema, palpable cord along the involved veins, erythema, etc. (Figs 4.25A and B).

Homan's sign: When forced ankle dorsiflexion produces calf pain, Homan's sign is said to be positive and is pathognomonic of DVT (Fig. 4.26).

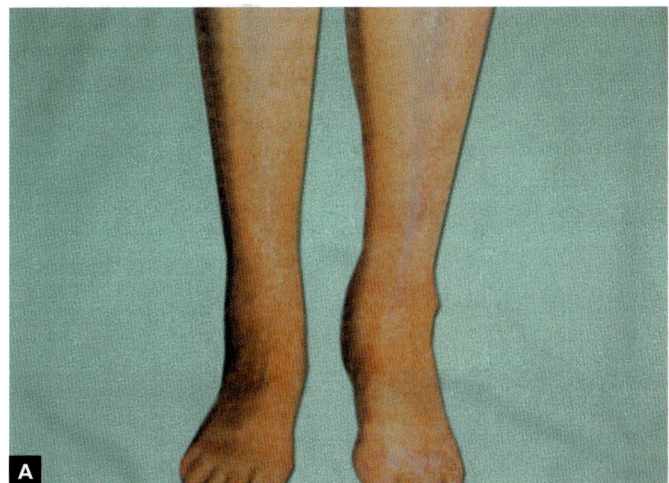

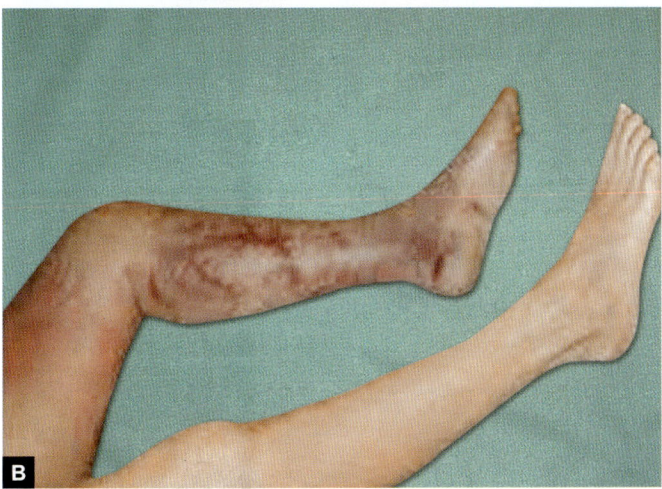

Figs 4.25A and B: Clinical photographs showing deep vein thrombosis

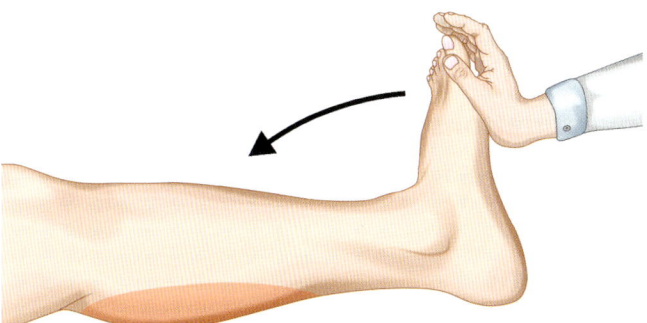

Fig. 4.26: Homan's sign

tachypnea, tachycardia, signs of cor pulmonale, etc. Heparin therapy is the treatment of choice.

Chronic venous insufficiency is the common long-term complication of DVT.

Embolic Facts

Other important predisposing factors for DVT
- Surgery—orthopedic/thoracic/abdominal/GU systems.
- Immobilization due to CCF, MI, stroke, etc.
- Neoplasms
- Estrogen therapy
- Pregnancy
- Obesity
- Age >40 years
- TAO, Behçet's disease, etc.
- Hypercoagulable states.
- Total hip and knee replacement, etc.

INJURY TO BLOOD VESSELS

Blood vessels in close proximity to the bones are injured during fractures and dislocations (Table 4.6).

Causes of Injury

The blood vessels may be injured in one of the following ways: Reflex vasospasm, compression by the fracture fragments or hematoma, incomplete tear, complete tear, partial tear, internal thrombus, tight encircling bandages, etc. (Fig. 4.27).

Effects of Injury

In the initial stages, it may range from mild ischemia to gangrene. In the late stages ischemic contractures may develop.

Clinical Features

Apart from the usual features, the patient may show impending signs of vascular disaster recognized by 5 Ps:

Investigations

Laboratory investigations particularly BT, CT, prothrombin time, blood group, etc. needs to be done.

Treatment

Prophylactic methods consist of early ambulation, foot elevation, elastocrepe bandaging, exercises, etc.

Anticoagulant therapy: This consists of aspirin (600–650 mg), heparin (low dose), low-molecular weight dextran, low-dose warfarin (2.5–16 mg/day daily orally), etc.

Complications

Pulmonary thromboembolism is a serious complication of DVT. The patient with pulmonary embolism complains of unexplained dyspnea, pleuritic chest pain, hypoxia,

Pain, pulselessness, paresthesia, pallor, and paralysis. Cold extremities herald the onset of gangrene (Fig. 4.28).

Investigations

Consists of radiograph of the part, Doppler angiogram studies, etc.

Treatment

This consists of prompt reduction of fractures and dislocations and removal of all tight encircling bandages.

TABLE 4.6: Blood vessel injuries in skeletal trauma	
Injuries	Blood vessel involved
Upper limb trauma	
• Fracture clavicle	Subclavian vessels
• Proximal humeral fractures	Axillary vessels
• Supracondylar fracture of humerus	Brachial vessels
• Posterior dislocation of elbow	Brachial vessels
• Fracture both bones of the forearm	Anterior interosseous artery
Lower limb trauma	
• Dislocation of hip	Femoral vessels
• Fracture femur	Femoral vessels
• Supracondylar fracture femur	Popliteal vessels
• Dislocation of knee	Popliteal vessels
• Proximal tibial fractures	Posterior tibial vessels
• Fracture tibia and fibula	Posterior tibial vessels
• Ankle injuries	Posterior tibial vessels

Thrombectomy, direct end-to-end repair, injection of xylocaine, papaverine, and sympathectomy to relieve the vasospasms are some of the commonly recommended methods of treatment. Amputation is considered in irreversible loss of blood supply.

INJURY TO NERVES

Forty percent of the bone and joint injuries are associated with peripheral nerve lesions (Table 4.7).

TABLE 4.7: Nerve injuries in skeletal trauma	
Trauma	Nerves injured
Upper limb	
• Fracture clavicle	Brachial plexus
• Proximal humeral fracture	Axillary nerve
• Fracture humerus	Radial nerve
• Supracondylar fracture humerus	Radial nerve
• Posterior dislocation of elbow	Median nerve
• Monteggia fracture	Posterior interosseous nerve
• Hook of hamate	Deep branch of ulnar nerve
• Wrist injury	Median nerve
Lower limb	
• Dislocations of hip (posterior)	Sciatic nerve
• Anterior dislocation of hip and shaft femur	Femoral nerve
• Dislocation of knee	Common peroneal nerve
• Proximal tibial fractures and ankle injury	Posterior tibial nerve
• Fracture neck fibula	Lateral popliteal nerve

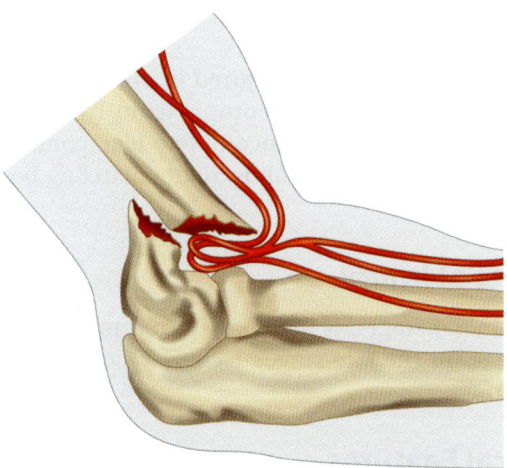

Fig. 4.27: Injury to the brachial vessels can occur in displaced supracondylar fractures of humerus

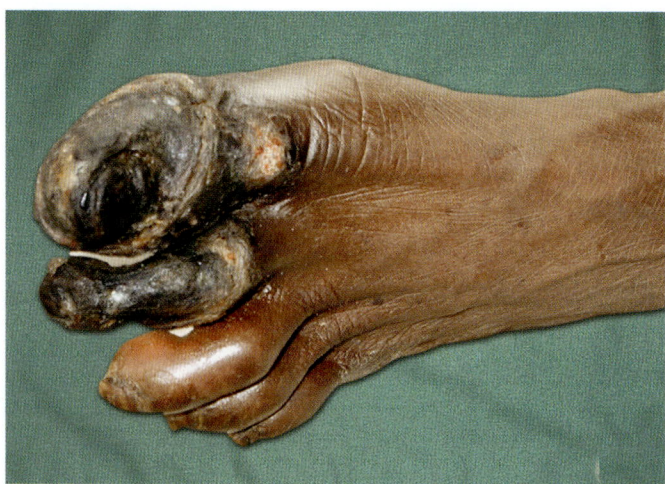

Fig. 4.28: Clinical photograph showing gangrene of the great toe and 2nd toe

Types

Two types are described:
- *Primary:* Here the nerve is injured by the same trauma that resulted in the injury to bone and joint.
- *Secondary:* This is due to involvement of the nerve in infection, scar, callus, etc.

Incidence

Radial nerve is the most commonly injured peripheral nerve (45%), followed by ulnar nerve (30%), median nerve (15%), peroneal nerve, lumbosacral plexus (3%), and tibial nerve.

Mechanism of Injury

The nerve may be damaged by the fracture fragments, entrapment between the fragments during fracture reduction, direct injury by the bullets, sharp cutting weapons, etc. In the late stages, the nerve may be trapped in the callus or fibrous tissue (Figs 4.29 and 4.30).

Types of Nerve Injury

This may be neuropraxia, axonotemesis, or neurotemesis depending upon the severity of injury.

Classification, diagnosis, clinical features, and treatment of individual nerve injuries are discussed in chapter on Peripheral Nerve Injuries.

CRUSH SYNDROME

Crush syndrome is seen in severe crush injuries of the limbs and muscles, which results in massive release of myohemoglobin into the circulation, which blocks the renal tubules and leads to myoglobinuria and acute renal tubular necrosis. Prolonged and improper application of tourniquet, acute compartmental syndromes, gas gangrene is some of the other causes of crush syndrome. Treatment is directed towards managing acute renal failure in case the patient develops oliguria or anuria.

JOINT STIFFNESS

This is due to improper technique of fracture immobilization. This can be fairly a troublesome problem. Intra-articular fractures, periarticular adhesions of soft tissues, capsules, and muscle contractures are some of the other important causes of joint stiffness. Physiotherapy, exercises, manipulation under anesthesia, surgical excision, and lengthening of contractures are some of the important treatment methods.

REFLEX SYMPATHETIC DYSTROPHY

It is an abnormal sympathetic response following fractures. This is commonly encountered in Colles' fracture.

OSTEOMYELITIS

It is common in compound fractures (*see the section on osteomyelitis for details*) (Fig. 4.31).

IMPLANT FAILURE (SEE FIGS 6.39A TO E)

It can occur due to defective manufacturing or biological reactions within the body and due to infection osteoporosis, improper and inadequate fixation, etc.

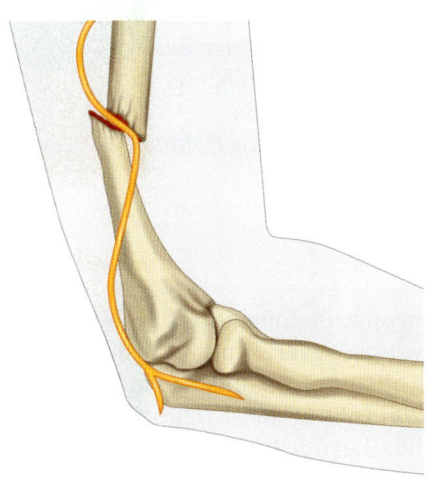

Fig. 4.29: Radial nerve injury can occur in fracture shaft of humerus

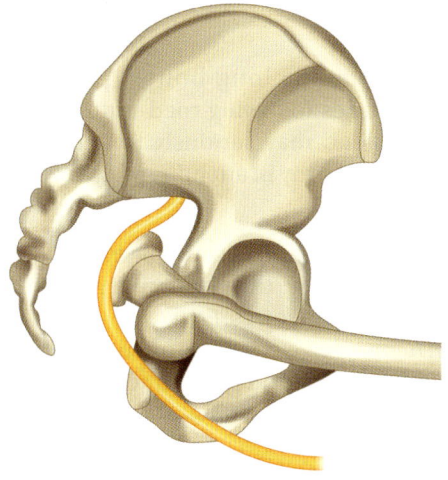

Fig. 4.30: Posterior dislocation of hip joint can damage the sciatic nerve

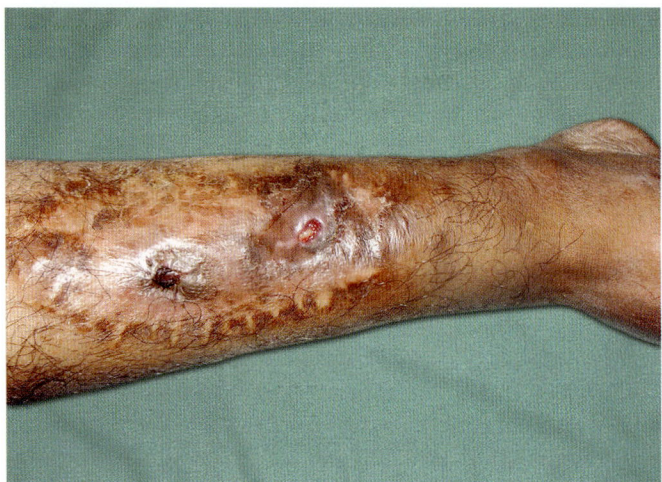

Fig. 4.31: Clinical photo of osteomyelitis tibia

POST-TRAUMATIC OSTEOARTHRITIS

Post-traumatic osteoarthritis is commonly seen in intra-articular fractures, malunion, etc. (see Fig. 47.10).

GROWTH ALTERATIONS

Growth alterations are due to epiphyseal injuries in children.

SHORTENING

Shortening of long bones is the other important complication (see Fig. 4.22).

COMPLICATIONS PECULIAR TO OPEN FRACTURES

SHOCK

In fractures of major long bones, pelvic fractures, multisystem injuries following road traffic accidents, etc. severe loss of blood may seriously threaten the life of a victim. Delay and apathy in attending a hypovolemic shock could prove fatal.

Source of hemorrhage: This could be external or internal.
- *External hemorrhage*: This usually happens in compound fractures, pelvic fractures, etc.
- *Internal hemorrhage*: It is more often seen in blunt injury of abdomen, femur and pelvic fractures, etc.

> **Note:**
> Internal hemorrhage stealthily snuffs out the life of a victim as it largely goes undetected.

> **Bloody Facts: Do You Know the Staggering Blood Loss in Fractures?**
> - Femoral shaft fractures—blood loss could range from 500–2000 mL
> - Pelvic fractures—blood loss could range from 1000–2500 mL. It could be much more in multiple fractures.

Clinical Features

Look for the classical features of shock (see box) apart from the usual features of fractures.

> **Shocking Facts: Look for the Classical Features**
> - Sunken eyeballs
> - Tongue—pale and dry
> - Pale look
> - Low BP
> - Cold clammy skin
> - Cold nose
> - Peripheral pulses feeble or absent
> - Drowsy or unconscious
> - Sweating

Investigations

Laboratory investigations like Hb%, blood group, BT CT, HIV, HBS Ag, etc.
Special investigations like Pain X-ray of the affected limb, MRI, CT scan, etc. can be done once the general condition of the patient is stabilized.

Treatment

Speed is the watchword in the treatment of shock and includes:
- Resuscitation
- Immediate fluid replacement by:
  a. IV fluids like normal saline, Ringer's lactate, etc.
  b. Hemaccel if blood is not available.
  c. Blood is the best alternative.
- Administration of oxygen, etc.
- Splinting of the fractures.
- Controlling the bleeding points.

GAS GANGRENE

Definition

This is an uncommon infection of the superficial and deep fascia following a severe trauma resulting in necrotizing fasciitis. The offending organism in most of these situations is *Clostridium* (about 30%). The presence of gas in the tissues implies that due to anaerobic bacterial metabolism, insoluble gases like hydrogen, nitrogen, and methane are produced.

> **Quick Facts:**
> Organisms, which can cause gas in the tissues
> - *Clostridium welchii* (30%)—Most common
> - *C. perfringes*
> - *Streptococcus pyogenes*
> - Halophilic marine vibrio
> - Fungus of rhizopus and *Mucor* species
> - *Pseudomonas* and Aeromonas

Incidence

It is about 1.76%.

Types of Clinical Presentation

- *Simple contamination*: No clinical signs but clostridia can be cultured from wounds.
- *Local infection only without any systemic features:* Pain and edema seen but no muscle necrosis.
- *Spreading cellulitis and fasciitis with systemic toxicity:* Here there is suppuration, gas in the tissues, toxemia (hemolysis and injury to capillary membrane) without muscle necrosis. Once developed, it spreads rapidly and is fatal within 48 hours.
- *Gas gangrene* sudden onset of pain at the area of the wound heralds the onset of the dreaded gas gangrene. Features of gas gangrene are mentioned in the box.

> **Vital Facts: Gas Gangrene Features**
> - Skin discoloration
> - Skin blebs
> - Drainage of thin, watery, grayish, foul-smelling fluid from the wound.
> - Subcutaneous crepitus
> - Frothy wound exudates
> - Skin is tense, white, and cool
> - Increased pulse rate
> - Temperature more or less normal
> - Profound shock and toxemia and finally
> - Death

Investigations

- Exploration and Gram staining of the exudates.
- Plain X-ray of the part.
- CT scan.
- MRI scans.

Prevention

Early recognition and excision of all necrotizing tissues. The predisposing causes are:
- Penetrating deep wounds of the thigh and buttocks.
- Impaired or loss of blood supply.
- Tight plaster casts.

Treatment Measures

- *Resuscitative measures*: Include fluid and blood transfusion, respiratory support, etc.
- *Surgical excision*: Early surgical excision of all necrotizing soft tissues.
- *Antibiotics*: Penicillin G is the drug of choice (20 lac IU/day in adults is the dose).
- *Antitoxin:* It involves administration of AGGS.
- *Hyperbaric oxygen (HBO):* Here patients are placed in a chamber at three times the atmospheric pressure. HBO inhibits alpha toxin production by clostridia. Its role in non-clostridia infection is not clear.

TETANUS

Definition

Tetanus is a fatal disease caused by *Clostridium tetani* and can occur in a patient with a superficial wound, deep wound or even in no demonstrable wound.

Pathogenesis

Clostridium tetani, usually present in fecal matter of humans and animals, enters the body through breaks in the mucosa or skin following a puncture, laceration, or abrasion. After an incubation period of 7–8 days, it grows and releases two exotoxins, tetanospasmin (acts on the brainstem and spinal cord) and tetanolysin (is cardio toxic and causes hemolysis), with the clinical effects of the latter over-shadowing the former.

Clinical Presentation

A full-blown tetanus patient presents with the following features:
- Restlessness and headache.
- Spasm of the neck and pharyngeal muscles.
- Locked jaw.
- In later stages orthotonus, opisthotonus, etc. occur.
- Generalized toxic convulsions can occur. These are triggered easily by external stimuli like light, sound, breeze, etc. Prone for fractures due to fall, etc.
- Death supervenes after 2 weeks to the hapless victim (mortality rate is 60%).

Investigations

Routine laboratory tests, X-ray of the affected parts needs to be done before treatment is begun.

Treatment

A multidisciplinary approach is recommended:
- Respiratory support by oxygen, ventilators, etc.

- Meticulous management of wound is vital.
- Sedation is very important to prevent or control convulsions. Phenobarbitone, secobarbital thiopental sodium, succinyl choline and magnesium sulphate are some of the commonly used agents.
- Good nursing care is required in a dark isolated room.
- Tracheostomy is required, if the patient develops pharyngospasm or laryngospasm.
- Pharyngospasm is far easier to manage than the troublesome laryngospasm.

Prevention

This is anytime better and easier than the cumbersome curative methods. The measures recommended are as follows:
- *Active immunization:* This is the best and consists of three doses of tetanus-diphtheria booster. The injection needs to be given once in 10 years for the rest of the life.
- *Passive immunization:* This is done by intravascular administration of 250 IU of tetanus immunoglobulin (TIG).

Pearl

This disease proves that, little things are so important than the 'hectic damage control' measures so true of life. What can be prevented by little (simple immunization) cannot be cured by much (the elaborate treatment). A person with a wound who refuses a TT shot is like penny wise and pound-foolish who may unfortunately pay through his life.

After the diagnosis is made, human tetanus immunoglobulin is given in the doses of 500–1000 units until a total dosage of 6,000–10,000 is reached.

CRUSH SYNDROME

This has been discussed on page 45.

5

CHAPTER

Emergency Care of the Injured

FIRST AID

First aid techniques in managing an injured patient should be learnt first and not last. Proper first aid is a skill, which needs to be learnt and developed.

Definition

First aid is the initial care of the injured at the scene of accident.

Anybody can give first aid, but to carry out cardiopulmonary resuscitation measures one should be trained in first aid and should possess a valid certificate issued by a competent body.

First aid executed by a medical person is called *medical aid*.

GOALS OF FIRST AID TREATMENT

Three P's aptly describes goals of first aid treatment:
- **P**reserve life by carrying out appropriate resuscitative measures.
- **P**revent further injuries by careful handling.
- **P**romote recovery.

INITIAL CARE OF THE INJURED

At the Scene of Accident

- Remove the victim from the accident spot.
- Check his or her vital parameters quickly (pulse, BP, consciousness, etc.).
- Seek the help of bystanders if trained in first aid.
- Ensure that police and ambulance have been informed.
- Remember to carry out first aid according to MacMurthy's A to F regimen (refer p. 52).
- Ensure personal safety.

MODUS OPERANDI IN FIRST AID

AIRWAY

First, clear the airway as follows:
- Clear the mouth of clots, dentures, loose teeth, etc. (Fig. 5.1A).
- Extend the neck slightly as this opens up the pharynx (Fig. 5.1B).
- If the patient is not breathing, begin artificial respiration. First keep a thin cloth over the patient's mouth, blow into the patients mouth keeping his or her nostrils closed (Fig. 5.1C). Blow at the rate of 16 per minute and see for the chest raise. Mouth to nose respiration is carried out if there is extensive injury to the mouth. If the patient has suffered extensive facial injuries, put the patient prone, turn the face towards one side and apply pressure over the lower aspect of the chest (Holger-Nelson method).

CARDIA

Examine the radial pulse and the carotid pulse for the function of cardia. If the pulse is absent, initiate cardiac resuscitative measures as follows:
- Ensure that the patient is lying on a hard surface.
- Then pressure is applied with the heel of the palm at the lower end of sternum (Fig. 5.2).
- Optimum pressure should be applied and the depth of each pressure should be 1¼ inch.

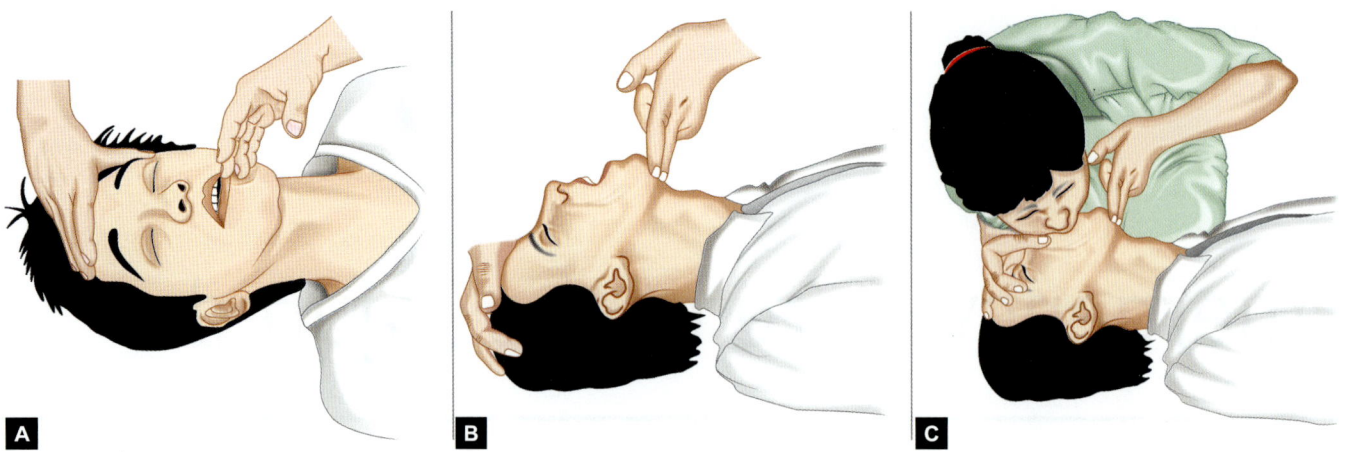

Figs 5.1A to C: (A) Technique of artificial respiration. Clear the mouth of debris first; (B) Extend the neck; (C) Blow into the victim's mouth

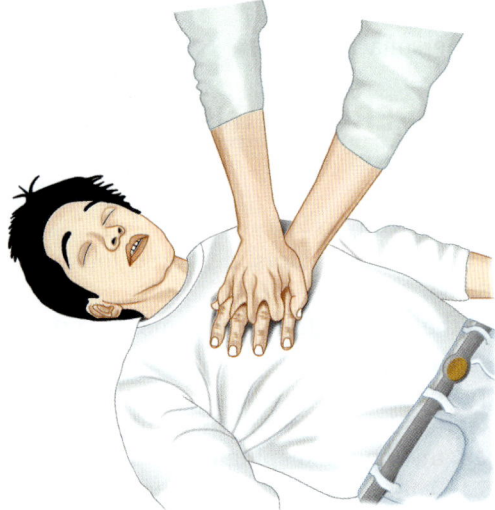

Fig. 5.2: Method of external cardiac massage

- Perform external cardiac massage at the rate of 72 per minute.

  It is preferable to carry out both external cardiac massage and artificial respiration simultaneously by two persons trained in first aid. Nevertheless, if there is no assistance available then cardiopulmonary resuscitation should be carried out by a single person as follows:
  - First artificial respiration is given once and then the same person should quickly change position and carry out external cardiac massage 5 times. So, this 1:5 ratio should be maintained throughout.
  - The cardiopulmonary resuscitation (CPR) should be carried out until the patient recovers or at least for half an hour.

BLEEDING

It is advisable to arrest the bleeding by elevation or direct application of pressure over the bleeding points (Figs 5.3A and B). *Tourniquet should be avoided and used only as a last resort.*

EXAMINE THE VITAL STRUCTURES

Head Injuries

Examine the patient for head injuries, cover the skull injuries with a clean cloth, and examine pupils and the level of consciousness. Look for neurological deficits.

Chest Injuries

Open chest injuries are dangerous as they may cause tension pneumothorax. Application of a clean cloth with firm pressure over the open wounds is all that is required.

Abdominal Injuries

All injured patients should be examined for intra-abdominal injuries, as it is an emergency. Board-like rigid abdomen suggests blunt injury abdomen and there could be damage to the liver, spleen, colon, etc. Arrangement should be made to shift the patient immediately to a hospital. In open wounds of the abdomen, a clean cloth should apply firm pressure.

Pelvic Fractures

Suspect pelvic fracture if the patient complains of pain during compression test or distraction test, which is

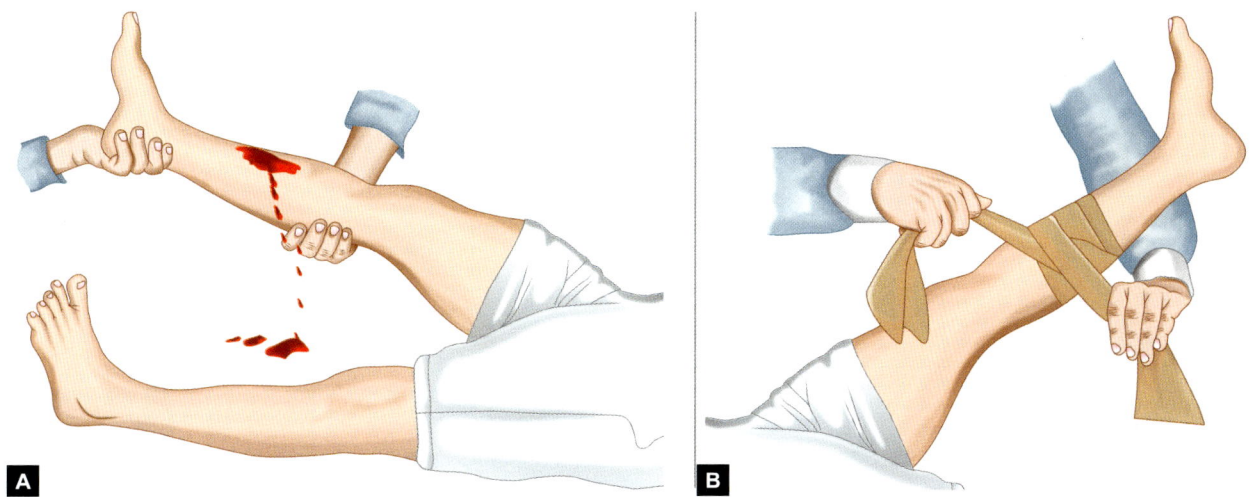

Figs 5.3A and B: Methods to control bleeding: (A) Limb elevation; (B) Firm pressure and bandaging at the bleeding site helps control hemorrhage

performed by applying pressure over the iliac bones. Tenderness over the symphysis pubis is also suggestive.

Injuries to the Genitourinary System

Suprapubic swelling indicates bladder injury, injury to the scrotum or perineal hematoma indicates urethral rupture.

Spine Injuries

Cervical spine injury should be suspected if the patient is lying still and loathes turning the neck. Injuries to the thoracic and lumbar spine should be suspected if the patient has developed paraplegia or complains of pain when individual spinous processes are palpated. *Extreme care should be exercised in managing and shifting a patient with spinal injuries.*

Fractures

Deformity, pain, swelling, loss of function of a limb are suggestive of fracture.

Fracture needs to be splinted with whatever material is available at the scene of accident (Figs 5.4 to 5.6). They can be managed electively after shifting the patient to the hospital.

> **Remember**
> - Fracture is not an emergency.
> - Most of them can be managed electively later.
> - In A to F management of injured fracture treatment comes last.
> - Prepare and improvise splints with available materials at the scene of accident.

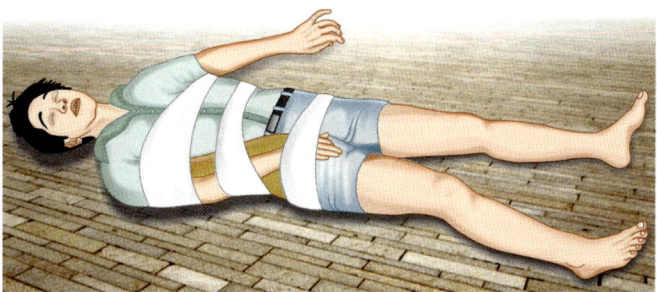

Fig. 5.4: Using victim's own body for splinting of fractures

> **Remember: About Fractures in First Aid**
> *The management of fractures at the scene of accident.*
> **Five Ss**
> - **S**ling for clavicle fractures, shoulder fractures, etc.
> - **S**trap for clavicle and rib fractures.
> - **S**plint, usually improvised. Best would be a Thomas splint or a pneumatic splint.
> - **S**hift the patient with utmost care.
> - **S**eek professional help at the earliest.
>
> **Remember the Priority in First Aid**
> **Three Ss**
> - **S**hock to be corrected first.
> - **S**ystemic injuries to be tackled next.
> - **S**pine injuries call for extreme caution.

MANAGEMENT AT THE HOSPITAL

MacMurthy has laid down the A to F management guidelines to be followed in the institutional care of the injured in the order of importance:
- Airway management

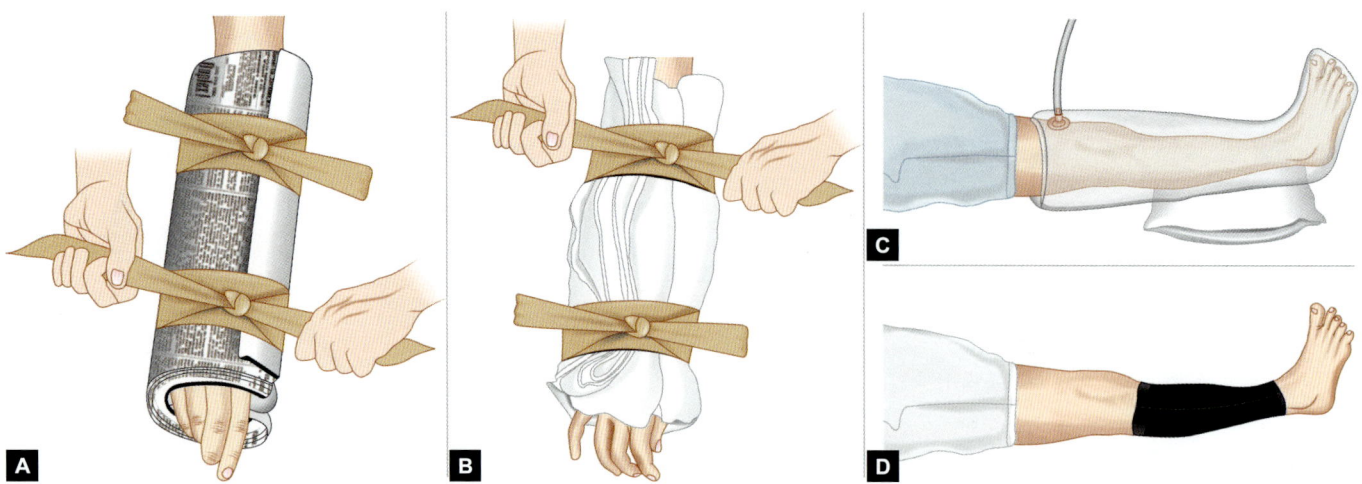

Figs 5.5A to D: (A) Splinting with a newspaper; (B) Splinting with a cloth; (C) Modern pneumatic splint; (D) Splinting with a firm support

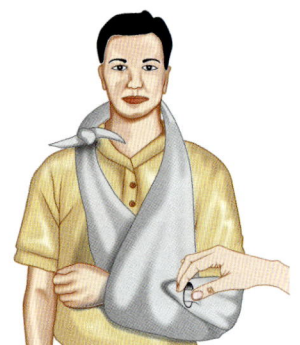

Fig. 5.6: Splinting of the fracture sites with sling and a body bandage

- Blood and fluid replacement
- Central nervous system management
- Digestive system management
- Excretory system management
- Fracture management.

Other emergency measures like administration of antitoxin, antibiotics, anti-gas gangrene serum, and wound debridement should be carried out. Appropriate radiographs should be taken before treating the fractures. The treatment of bone and joint injuries are discussed in detail in the relevant chapters.

> **Remember—The Mnemonic**
> *AID as prerequisites of a good first aider*
> - **A**lertness
> - **I**ntelligence
> - **D**ecisions
>
> *AID as mnemonic of a bad first aider*
> - **A**pathy
> - **I**ndecision
> - **D**elay

> **Remember in First Aid**
> - Delay is dangerous.
> - If improperly executed, first aid will become the last aid!
> - Always aid the patient to recovery and do not send him to mortuary by being apathetic.
> - Shifting the patient to a hospital is extremely important.
> - Terminate first aid measure once medical assistance arrives or after shifting the patient to the hospital.

6
CHAPTER

Fracture Treatment Methods: Then, Now and Future

"They, whose work cannot die, whose influence lives after them, whose disciples perpetuate and multiply their gifts to humanity, are truly immortal." This was how Watson Jones paid tribute to Hugh Oven Thomas.

HISTORY OF FRACTURE TREATMENT

Figure 6.1 represents the historical aspects of orthopedics.

Our ancestors were no less skillful in treating fractures. The Egyptians were known to be skilled at the management of fractures and many healed specimens have been found. Hippocrates and Celsius described in detail the splintage of fractures by using wooden appliances. Nevertheless, Al Zabra, an Arabic surgeon, gave a fascinating account of external splintage. He used clay gum mixtures, flour, and egg white for casting materials. In 1517, Gersdorf described a method of binding wooden splints using ligatures around the assembled splint and tightening it. Chinese described use of willow board splints for the treatment of tibial shaft fractures and Colles' fracture. The Arabians described a technique of pouring a plaster of Paris mixture around an injured limb. Malgaigne was instrumental in popularizing this technique in Europe by the early 19th century. The great disadvantage of all this extensive and heavy forms of immobilization of limb was the possibility of the fracture disease (Fig. 6.2). In 1873, Sir James Paget described about fracture disease. Thus, he advocated the concept of early mobilization to prevent this problem.

> **Remember**
> **Hippocrates (Fig. 6.3) and orthopedics**
> - Hippocrates was born in Greece in 460 BC.
> - He advanced the five concepts of fracture treatment, namely antisepsis, bandaging, reduction, splinting, and traction.
> - He dissociated medicine from religion and philosophy.
> - He wrote three books on skeletal system.

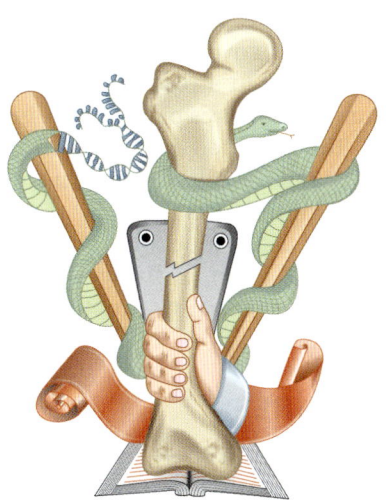

Fig. 6.1: History of orthopedics

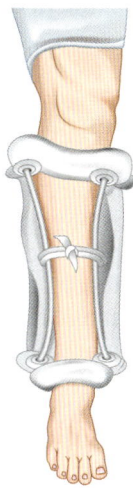

Fig. 6.2: Primitive methods of fracture immobilization

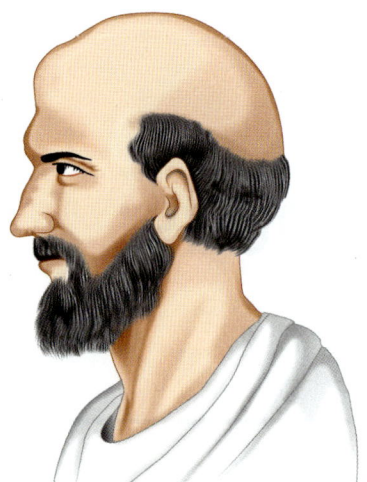

Fig. 6.3: Hippocrates

THE PLASTER BANDAGES

In Holland, in 1852 Antonius Mathysen (1805-1878), a military surgeon, was on the look out of an immobilizing bandage that would permit the safe transport of patients with gunshot injuries to specialized treatment centers. He sought a bandage that could be used at once, would become hard in minutes and be adaptable to the extremity. Thus, he introduced plaster of Paris (POP) in 1876 at the centennial exhibition in Philadelphia. The use of POP bandages as cast and slabs became popular after his death.

THOMAS SPLINT

However, the most brilliant discovery of a splint was by HO Thomas, which came to be known as Thomas splint after his name. It is still used in many centers of the world for treatment of fracture of femur, though it was designed initially to assist in the treatment of TB knee (see box).

TRACTION

Galen (AD 130-200) first described the longitudinal traction to overcome the overriding of fracture fragments. The use of continuous traction in the management of diaphyseal fractures appeared around the middle of the 19th century. In 1800, Albert Hoffa of Wurzburg (the place of Roentgen who discovered X-rays) described the use of tractions for many types of fractures of femur and humerus. Dr Josiah Crosby of New Hampshire gave one of the earliest accounts of the use of continuous skin traction in the treatment of fractures. Professor George Perkins of London described the external splint and advocated a simple straight traction through an upper tibial pin.

Remember
About HO Thomas
- He came from a family of unqualified bonesetters.
- He broke the family tradition by qualifying in medicine in 1857.
- His partnership with his father failed.
- He established his practice individually in the slum of Liverpool.
- He worked there for 32 years taking only six days vacation.
- He died in 1891 at the age of 57.
- He was a great believer of enforced, uninterrupted, and prolonged rest in the treatment of fractures.

Interesting Historical Facts
About HO Thomas
- His brighter side
  - HO Thomas is known as the father of British orthopedic surgery
  - A genius still unparallel in the field of orthopedics.
  - His diagnosis and management in orthopedics was spot on even in those dark days despite the unavailability of X-ray.
  - He said "An inflamed joint, rest it", A truth which is a greater truth even today.
  - He wrote a book on diseases of the hip, knee, and ankle in 1875.
  - He was a master of splints. The ones he invented are:
    a. Cervical collar
    b. Metatarsal bars
    c. Heel wedge
    d. Knee splint
  - He demonstrated the famous 'Thomas Test' to reveal the fixed flexion deformity of the hip joint.
- His darker side
  - Rude
  - Temperamental
  - Critical
  - Unaccomodative

  Nevertheless, a genius who strode the world of orthopedics like a colossus.

FUNCTIONAL BRACE

Gooch in 1767 first described the tibial and femoral functional braces. However, surprisingly, this concept was pushed into oblivion for over two centuries until Sarmiento revived it. He developed a patellar tendon-bearing cast for the treatment of fractures of tibia after initial standard cast treatment. This heralded the renaissance of functional bracing. In 1970, Mooney described hinged casts for the management of femoral casts.

The widespread use of functional bracing has liberated countless patients from prolonged hospitalization and permitted early return to function and to gainful employment.

OPEN FRACTURES

Until 150 years ago, an open fracture was virtually synonymous with death and generally necessitated an immediate amputation. Ambrose Pare, a French surgeon, first described the technique of ligating the bleeding vessels after amputation. Earlier, it was cauterized. Le Petit in 1718 first described the use of tourniquet to control bleeding from amputation. This brought the mortality from amputation of the lower limbs from 75 to 25%. In 1561, it was Pare again who first described the concept of conserving the limb after an open fracture when he himself sustained an open fracture of tibia due to fall from the horse. The discovery of antisepsis by Pasteur, Koch, etc. brought down the rate of infection due to open fractures drastically.

EARLY FRACTURE SURGERY

In 1770, Malgaigne was the first to describe the earliest technique of internal fixation of fractures by a ligation or a wire suture. The use of screws in bone started first around late 1840s by French surgeons Cucuel and Rigaud. Hansmann of Hampburg in 1886 was the first to describe the plate fixation of bone. Lambotte in 1909 designed a diamond-shaped plate and coined the term osteosynthesis by which he meant stable bone fixation. *He is generally regarded as the father of modern internal fixation.* Lane and Scherman devised their own plates. It was Denis in the year 1940 who by forming an association of Swiss surgeons heralded the modern era of internal fixation.

EXTERNAL FIXATION

Malgaigne in 1840 described the first external fixation device. Later, in 1897 Dr Clayton Parkhill of Colorado devised a new and improved apparatus. In 1902, Lambotte devised a more sophisticated type of external fixator in which the protruding screws were bolted to adjustable clamps linked with a heavy external bar. Pitkin for the first time devised transfixion pins with a bilateral frame as the earlier devices relied upon half pins with a single external linkage device. Ilizarov of Russia in 1952 first described the use of circular external fixator frame. He first showed that external fixator device could also be used for limb lengthening and deformity correction.

INTRAMEDULLARY FIXATION

Dieffenbac of Prussia in 1841 performed early intramedullary nailing with ivory pegs. In 1907, Lambotte emerged as a pioneer in intramedullary fixation for trochanteric fractures. Others who advocated intramedullary nails were Hey Groves of England in 1914, and Rush family.

The person who revolutionized the intramedullary nailing technique was the German military surgeon, Gerhardt Küntscher, who devised a cloverleaf nail prior to the World War II. The world was slow to accept Küntscher's design but slowly Sweden in 1943 and America in 1945 absorbed the technique.

In 1958, the Association for the Study of Internal Fixation (ASIF or AO) was born. They suggested many alterations and conducted plenty of educative courses. *They advocated with vigor the concept of rigid fixation and primary bone healing.* Livingston's I beam nail is the earliest example of interlocking nail in the year 1950. At present, interlocking nail has made greater strides.

AO GROUP

Robert Denis of Brussels (1880–1962) is regarded as the father of modern osteosynthesis. He described the interfragmentary compression and the concept of rigid fixation. On 1 March 1950, a young Swiss surgeon, Dr Maurice Muller, was so much influenced by the work of Denis that he started an association in Sweden in 1958 involving a group of young enthusiastic fracture surgeons. Educating young surgeons from all over the world in their technique was their aim. From 1960 to the present day, they conduct regular annual training sessions.

Thus, it is to our ancestors we owe the tremendous achievements we have made of late in fracture treatment. Without their sweat and toil, we would be way behind.

Remember
The pioneers in orthopedics
- Hippocrates—first described splinting of fracture.
- Galen—traction in orthopedics.
- Sarmiento—functional cast brace.
- Malgaigne—technique of internal fixation.
- HO Thomas—Thomas splint.
- Lambotte—external fixator.
- Gerhardt Küntscher—intramedullary nail.
- Robert Denis—father of modern osteosynthesis.
- Ilizarov—circular external fixator.
- Mathysen—plaster of Paris.
- And a score of countless unsung heroes.

Remember
About AO or ASIF technique
- Advocated in 1960 by a group of Swiss surgeons.
- Aims at full and rapid recovery of the injured limb by open anatomic reduction and stable internal fixation.
- Healing is by primary intention.
- Eliminates the problem called the fracture disease.

Our Own Heroes in Orthopedics
Dr BN Sinha and Dr B Mukhopadhya—father of Indian orthopedics. Known as Sir Robert Jones of India.
Dr KT Dholakia—father of modern Indian orthopedics.
Dr SM Tuli—who described the famous middle path regime for TB spine.

Dr TK Shanmugasundaram—known for his outstanding work in skeletal tuberculosis.
Dr BB Joshi—who has described the Joshi's external stabilizing system (JESS) treatment for congenital talipes equinovarus (CTEV).
Dr Singh—Singh's Index.
Dr GS Kulkarni—known for his work on Ilizarov's treatment.
Dr PS Ramani—eminent neuro and spine surgeon known for his work on IDSS, PLIF and bone bank methodology.
Dr Bakshi—pioneering work on muscle pedicle graft for fracture neck femur.
Dr PC Sethi—well-known for his Jaipur foot.
Dr Ashok Johari—known for his pioneering work in pediatric orthopedics.

FRACTURE TREATMENT: NOW

The faithful bones support the entire body until its integrity is broken by fractures. Ironically, what was known to support, now requires to be supported either externally or internally to regain the lost integrity and revert to its original role. Before even the orthopedic surgeons interfere to plan and execute the treatment methodology to restore the bone anatomy, nature has initiated the healing process by immobilizing the fracture fragments by its two important mechanisms, namely:

Pain: The patient loathes moving his or her injured limbs for fear of pain and thus keeps it immobile.

Muscle spasm: The surrounding muscles go into spasm after the injury and prevent mobility between the fracture fragments.

While pain and muscle spasm keep the fracture fragments immobile, SOS signals are sent by the bone induction agents (e.g. bone morphogenic protein, oxygen gradient, etc.) to the bone cells within the periosteum and endosteum to initiate the fracture healing process. The role of orthopedic surgeon is to merely assist nature in its mission of putting back the broken bones to normalcy. The ways and means of how he or she can do it is described as follows.

Remember
- Bones known to support, requires support when broken.
- Pain and muscle spasm are nature's way of immobilizing fracture fragments.
- Role of the physician is to merely assist nature to bring about proper fracture healing.
- Remember the adage *Orthosurgeon merely treats the fracture and God (nature) cures it*.

GENERAL PRINCIPLES OF THE METHODS OF FRACTURE TREATMENT

I. **Conservative or nonoperative methods**
   - **No treatment:** Some fractures needs no treatment. Nonsteroidal anti-inflammatory drugs (NSAIDs) and rest suffices, e.g. rib fractures (because of the efficient splinting action of the intercostals muscles).
   - **Strapping:** Merely strapping certain fractures to the adjacent normal structures like in undisplaced phalanx fracture of fingers (Fig. 6.4) and toes is sufficient (see Fig. 16.15). Other fractures that are treated by strapping are fracture of clavicle, scapula, proximal humeral fractures, etc.
   - **Slings:** These are used to treat undisplaced upper limb fractures or as first aid measures.
   - **Plaster treatment methods:** Two modalities are described.
     a. *Merely support by plaster slabs or splints:* In undisplaced fractures, incomplete fractures, stress fractures, fatigue fractures, support by POP slab often suffices.
     b. *Reduction and support with plaster cast:* Displaced fractures need to be reduced under general anesthesia before splinting with plaster casts. Reduction can be brought about either by manipulative traction and counter traction methods or by skeletal or skin traction. Principles of closed reduction have already been discussed. Plaster of Paris plays a big role in the conservative management of fractures.
     c. *Spica cast:* This is a plaster cast, which encircles a part of the body other than the limb. For example, hip spica, scaphoid cast, etc.
     d. *Traction:* This comparatively plays a less important role and is discussed in detail in a separate section.

Remember
The cardinal rule of reducing any displaced fracture is to reverse the mechanism of injury preferably under general anesthesia.

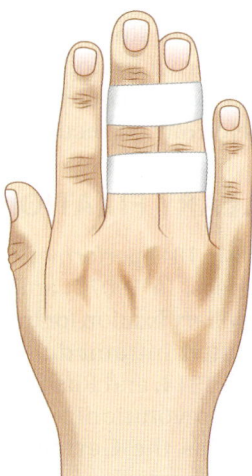

Fig. 6.4: Strapping in a phalanx fracture

Nonoperative Methods

Advantages
- Infection chances are nil.
- Surgical risks are avoided.
- It is less costly.

Disadvantages
- Certain amount of skill is required.
- Fixation is not rigid.
- Prolonged immobilization is required.
- Malunion is more likely.
- Fracture disease is a possibility.

II. **Operative treatment of fractures:** Operative treatment of fractures becomes mandatory once conservative regimen fails or when there are specific indications (see discussions on open reductions). Once fracture is reduced by operative methods, it invariably needs to be fixed internally by implants. Thus, implants act as internal splints. The choice of implants available is as follows:
- *Kirschner's wire (K-wire)*—useful to fix certain fractures in children and small bone fractures, avulsion fractures, distal radial fractures, etc. in adults.

It Pays to Know the Advantages of K-wire:
- Insertion is stress free.
- Less soft tissue damage.
- It allows early exercises after removal.

Certain important technical facts:
- Diameter ranges from 0.6 to 3.2 mm.
- Length ranges from 160 to 310 mm.
- Pointed at both ends for both antegrade and retrograde insertion.

- The shape of the tips could be—trocar, diamond, perforated or threaded.
- *Screws*—used mostly to fasten the plates to the bones and rarely used independently to fix avulsion fractures, butterfly fragments, for interfragmentary compression, etc.
- *Intramedullary (IM) nails*—useful for long bone shaft fractures through the narrowest portion of the medullary canal, which is usually the middle third. Intramedullary nails are not useful when the fractures are outside this ideal situation and in fractures in children.
- *Plates*—are useful in situation where IM nail is not indicated. Proximal and distal third fractures can be treated by this method. It can also be used in children. However, it has its own set of problems and limitations.

Operative Methods

Advantages
- Anatomic reduction.
- Rigid fixation.
- Early mobilization.
- Useful in multiple system injuries.
- Useful in multiple fractures.

Disadvantages
- Infection.
- Biologic process hampered.
- More expensive.
- Failure after removal of plate and screws.

III. **Treatment of fractures by external fixators (Figs 6.5A and B):** Open fractures pose a tough problem in the choice of fixation methods. Loss of soft tissues makes application of plaster casts very difficult. At the same time, the threat of infection discourages the use of internal fixation devices. It is here that the role of external fixators are clearly defined as it provides both stability and immobilization of fractures, so essentially required for both the soft tissues and the fracture to heal. Essentially, all external fixators consist of pins, which are passed through the bones above and below the fracture sites and are fastened to the external metallic frames. From the conventional pin fixator to the more recent Ilizarov's circular fixator, the concept of external fixator has a definite place in the treatment of fractures, especially the compound fractures.

IV. **Functional cast bracing:** It is a new concept developed by Sarmiento wherein the fracture is mobilized once it becomes sticky after a period of 4–6 weeks. Thus, it is a secondary form of treatment and overcomes most of the problems of conventional conservative methods of fracture treatment.

Now let us analyze the fracture treatment methods in detail.

SPLINTS

Any material, which is used to support a fracture, is called a *splint*. From a folded newspaper, wood, cardboard, etc. to the present-day thermoplastics anything can act as a splint.

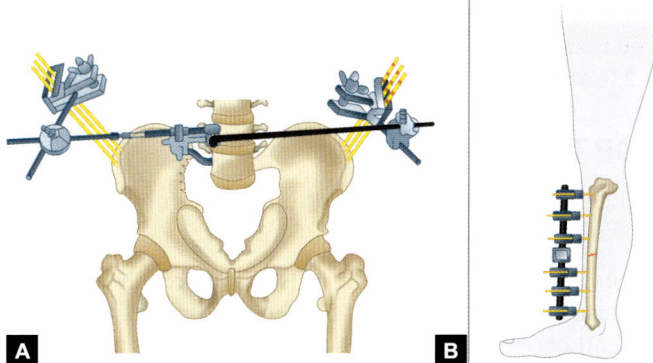

Figs 6.5A and B: Treatment of fractures by external fixators: (A) Pelvic; (B) Tibia fracture

The former is called an "unconventional splint" and is used more as an improvisation splint in carrying out the first aid for fractures in emergency where things are not ideal. The latter can be called "conventional splints" which are more sophisticated and effective. In orthopedic practice, POP splints are the most commonly employed splints.

Remember
- Anything acts as a splint including one's own uninjured part of the body.
- Splint is a material used to support fractures.
- *Unconventional splints* are crude, temporary and are used as a first aid measure, e.g. book, paper, umbrella, board wood, etc.
- *Conventional splints* are refined sophisticated and serve both as first aid and definitive measures, e.g. POP splint, Thomas splint, Böhler-Braun splint, etc.

To attain the goal of fracture treatment of restoring anatomy to normal, splints help a long way. They form the mainstay of conservative treatment of fractures.

CONVENTIONAL PLASTER SPLINTS

ALL YOU WANTED TO KNOW ABOUT PLASTER OF PARIS SPLINT

History

The name plaster of Paris originated from an accident to a house built on deposit of gypsum near the city of Paris. The house was accidentally burnt down. When it rained on the next day, it was noted that the footprints of the people in the mud had set rock hard. Mathysen, a Dutch surgeon, first used plaster of Paris in orthopedics in 1852. It is made from gypsum, which is a naturally occurring mineral. It is commercially available since 1931.

Chemical Formula

It is a hemihydrated calcium sulfate. To make plaster of Paris, gypsum is heated to drive off water. When water is added to the resulting powder, original mineral reforms and is set hard.

$$2(CaSO_4 \cdot 2H_2O) + Heat \leftrightarrow 2(CaSO_4 \cdot \tfrac{1}{2} H_2O) + 3H_2O$$

POP Types

Indigenous Prepared from ordinary cotton bandage role smeared with POP powder.

Commercial: Plaster of Paris rolls commercially prepared consists of rolls of muslin stiffened by starch, POP powder and an accelerator substance like alum. This commercial preparation sets very fast and gives a neat finish unlike the indigenous ones.

Why is Plaster of Paris an Ideal Splint?
- It is cheap.
- It is easily available.
- It is comfortable.
- It is easy to mould.
- It is quick setting.
- It is strong and light.
- It is easy to remove.
- It is permeable to radiography.
- It is permeable to air and hence underlying skin can breathe.
- It is noninflammable.

Its Various Forms

Plaster of Paris is used in four forms as slab, cast, spica, and functional cast brace.

Slab: It is a temporary splint used in the initial stages of fracture treatment and during first aid. It is useful to immobilize the limbs postoperatively and in infections. It is made up of half by POP and half by bandage roll and hence can accommodate the swelling in the initial stages of fractures.

Slab is prepared according to the required length. There are three methods of applying a slab.

Dry method: Here the slab is prepared first and then dipped in water (commonly employed).

Wet method: Here the slab is prepared after dipping the POP roll in water. This is rare and requires experience.

Pattern method: Here the slabs are fashioned in the desired way before dipping it in water.

Casts: Here the POP roll completely encircles the limb (Figs 6.6A to D). It is used as a definitive form of fracture treatment and to correct deformities. There are three methods of applying a POP cast.

Skin tight cast: Here the cast is directly applied over the skin. Dangerous as it may cause pressure sores. It is difficult to remove as hair may be incorporated into the cast and hence it is not recommended.

Bologna cast: Here generous amount of cotton padding is applied to the limb before putting the cast. This is the commonly employed method.

Three-tier cast: Here stockinet is used first over which cotton padding is done before applying the POP cast. It is an ideal method but is expensive.

Spica: This encircles a part of the body, e.g. hip spica for fracture around the hip (Fig. 6.6C), thumb spica for fracture scaphoid.

Functional cast brace: This is used for fracture tibia after initial immobilization (Fig. 6.6D).

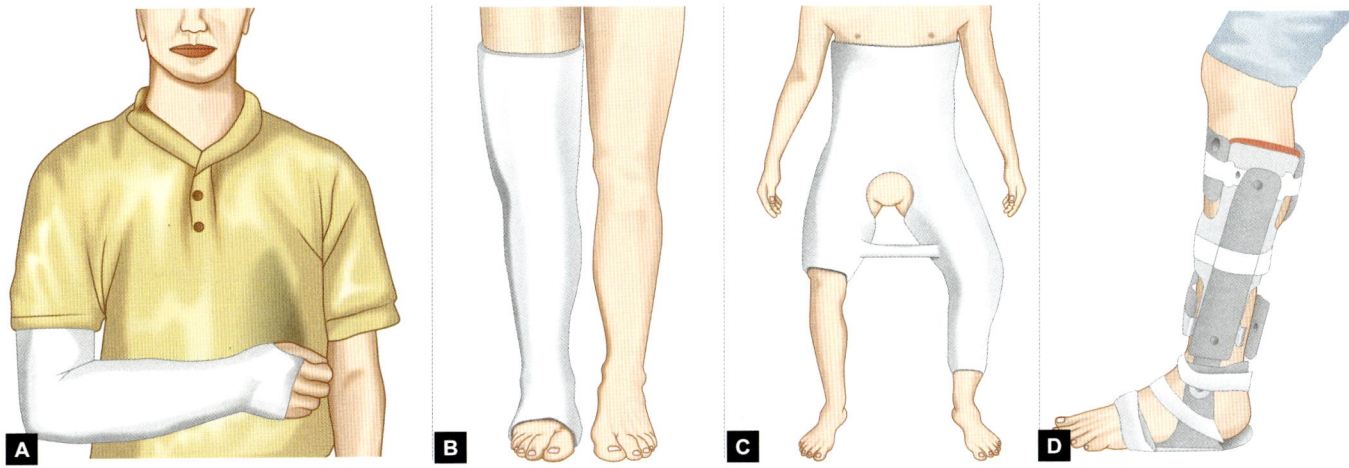

Figs 6.6A to D: Types of plaster applications: (A) Above elbow cast; (B) Above knee cast; (C) Hip spica; (D) Functional cast brace

Rules of Application of POP Casts
- Choose the correct size, 8 inches for the thigh, 6 inches for the leg, and 4 inches for the forearm.
- A joint above and a joint below should be included. Accordingly, we have an above elbow (Fig. 6.6A) or below elbow, POP cast or slab and above knee (Fig. 6.6B) or below knee POP cast or slab. This is done to eliminate movements of the joints on either side of the fractures. However, this is not a hard and fast rule in certain fractures, like a below elbow cast in Colles' fracture, which often suffices.
- It should be moulded with the palm and not the fingers for fear of indentation.
- The joints should be immobilized in functional positions.
- The plaster should just snugly fit and should not be too tight or too loose.
- Uniform thickness of the plaster is preferred.

Stages of Plastering

First stage: Involves application of POP slab or cast (Fig. 6.7).

Second stage or cast setting stage: This is change of POP to gypsum and is defined as the time taken to form a rigid dressing after contact with water.

Third stage or green stage: This is the just set wet cast.

Fourth stage or cast drying: By evaporation of excess water when the cast dries. This results in a mature cast with multiple air pockets through which the skin breathes.

Complications of POP

Due to Tight Fit
- Pain
- Pressure sores
- Compartmental syndromes
- Peripheral nerve injuries
- Cast syndrome (Also called Cast disease).

Due to Improper Application
- Joint stiffness
- Plaster blisters and sores
- Breakage.

Due to Plaster Allergy
- Allergic dermatitis.

Unpleasant Facts about Cast Disease
- Muscle atrophy.
- Osteoporosis.
- Joint stiffness.
- Muscle weakness.
- Skin breakdown.
- Compartmental syndrome.
- Blister formation.

Remember about POP
- Used first in the city of Paris.
- The ideal splint.
- Slab for temporary and initial treatment.
- Casts for definitive treatment.
- Spica for hip fracture, etc.
- Functional cast brace for early mobilization.

FUNCTIONAL CAST BRACE

Introduction

If function is allowed during closed method of fracture treatment, it has been observed that this stimulates

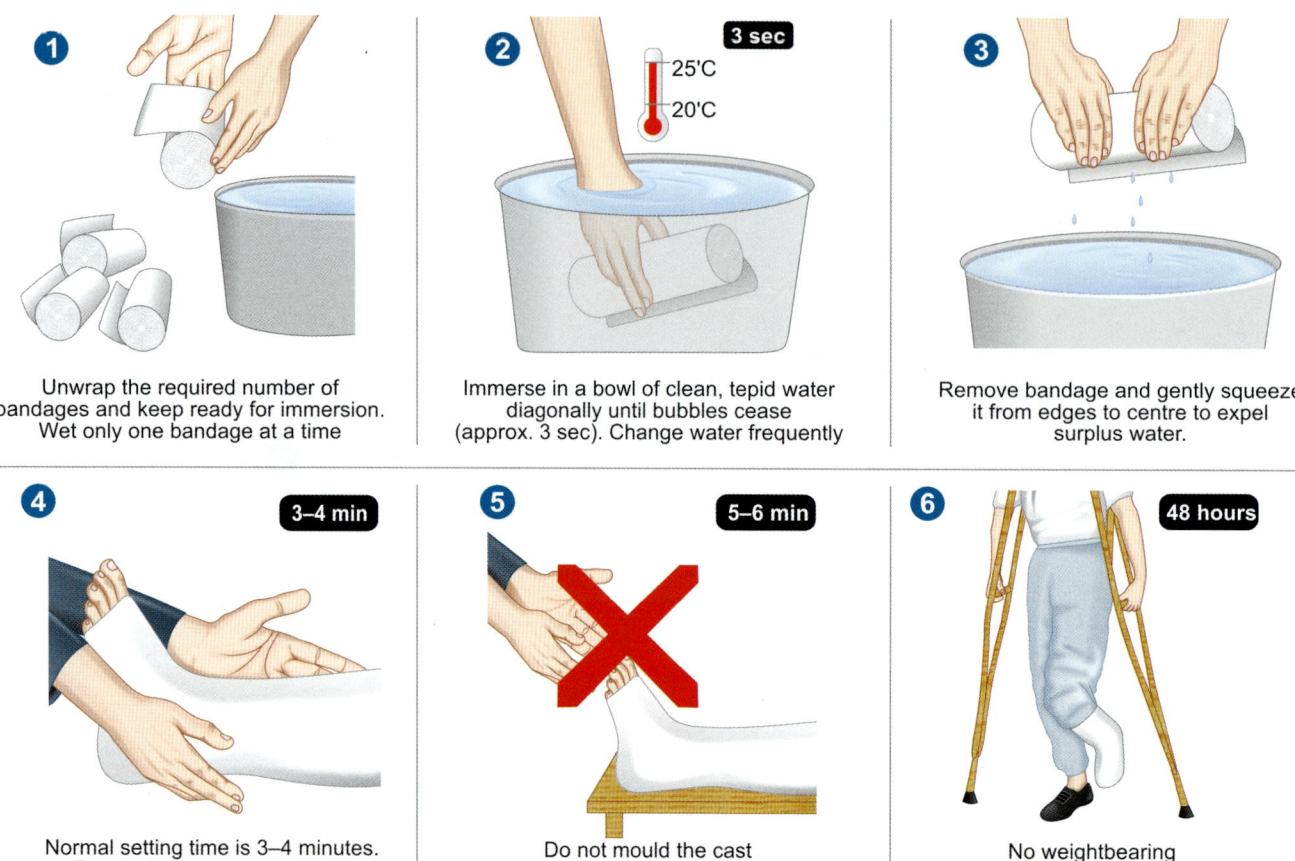

Fig. 6.7: Steps of application of plaster cast

osteogenesis, promotes soft tissue healing, and prevents development of joint stiffness thus hastening rehabilitation. This concept accepts loss of anatomic reduction to rapid healing. It complements rather than replacing other forms of treatment. The observation that fracture ribs still unite in spite of continued movements due to the action of intercostals muscles showed that elimination of movements at fracture site is not mandatory for fracture to unite. It was on this concept that Sarmiento devised functional bracing methods.

The mode of action: Here the hydraulic action of muscles is brought into play. The fracture brace allows movements of the joints and permits the load to be transmitted through the muscles. The muscles, which are surrounded by the inelastic deep fascia if encased in a hard plaster, cannot be stretched beyond the confines of the cast. On movements and bearing weight, the muscle forces are hence driven inwards towards the fracture and not outwards. This helps the fracture to be held firmly. These hydraulic forces control the fragments and resist overlap and angulations until callus forms (Figs 6.8A and B). Rotation is also resisted by the brace and muscle contraction.

In compound fractures, due to severe disruption of soft tissues, this principle will not work until soft tissues have healed.

> **Remember**
> **About functional cast, brace (Fig. 6.9):**
> - Fracture ribs indicate that absolute immobility for fracture healing is not required.
> - It is a secondary form of fracture treatment.
> - Muscle action favors osteogenesis.
> - Hydraulic action of muscles stabilizes the fracture in a closed compartment.
> - Eliminates fracture disease like in AO technique.
> - Not useful in compound fractures.
> - Popularized by Sarmiento.
> - Useful in fracture tibia and fracture femur.

IMPORTANT SPLINTS IN ORTHOPEDICS OTHER THAN POP

THOMAS SPLINT

This is one of the very commonly used splints in orthopedics described by HO Thomas in 1876 to assist for ambulatory

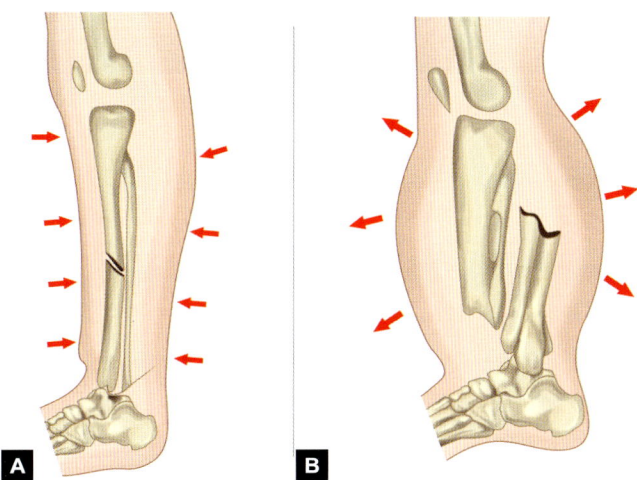

Figs 6.8A and B: Principles of cast bracing: (A) With brace; (B) Without brace

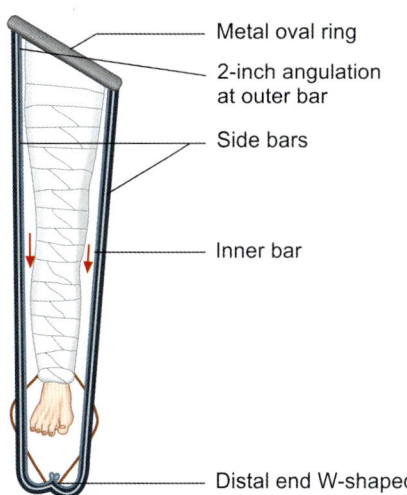

Fig. 6.10: Parts of a Thomas splint and fixed traction method

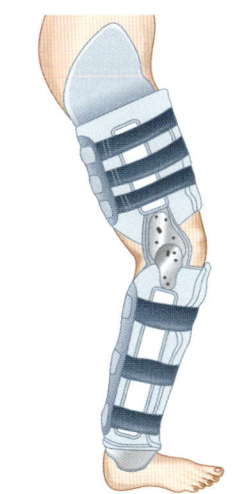

Fig. 6.9: A functional cast braces

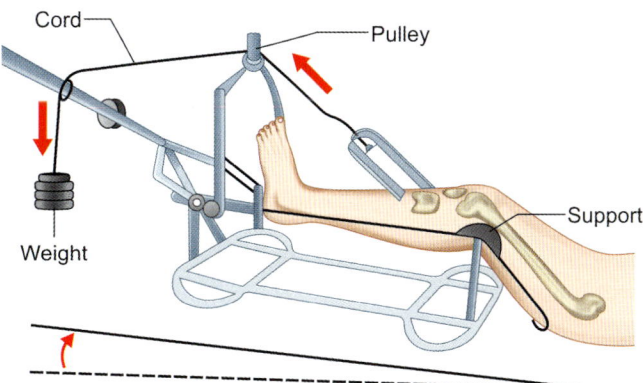

Fig. 6.11: Böhler-Braun splint

treatment of TB knee. It is now widely used for the treatment of shaft fractures of femur.

Parts of a Thomas Splint

A Thomas splint consists of four parts (Fig. 6.10):
1. A padded metal oval ring with soft leather set at an angle of 120° to the inner bar.
2. Two sidebars—one inner and another outer bar of unequal length. They bisect the oval ring. The outer bar is longer than the inner bar.
3. Distal end—where the two sidebars are joined in the form of a 'W'.
4. Outer side bar is angled 2 inches below the padded ring to clear the prominent greater trochanter.

Uses of Thomas Splint

1. To immobilize fracture femur anywhere.
2. As a first aid measure.
3. For transportation of an injured patient.
4. In the treatment of joint diseases like TB knee, etc.

BÖHLER-BRAUN (BB) SPLINT

This is Böhler's modification of Braun splint (Fig. 6.11). It consists of a heavy metallic frame with four pulleys:
1. Proximal pulley prevents foot drop.
2. Second pulley to apply traction in the line of femur.
3. Third pulley to apply traction in the line of supracondylar area of femur.
4. Fourth pulley to apply traction in the line of the legs.

Indications

Skeletal traction is applied through this frame for comminuted trochanteric fractures of the femur. It is also used for the treatment of fracture shaft femur and supracondylar fractures of the femur. Rarely, it can be used for the fracture shaft of tibia and fibula.

One important precaution, which should be taken while using the BB splint, is to provide support at the fracture site and not at the knee joint to prevent angulations, especially in supracondylar fractures of femur.

Problems of BB Splint

1. It makes nursing care difficult.
2. It is a heavy and cumbersome frame.
3. It is associated with recumbent problems like bedsores, hypostatic pneumonia, renal calculi, etc.

Care of the Splints

- *Padding:* The splint should be well padded at the bony prominences and at the injury sites.
- *Bandage:* This should be tied with optimum pressure.
- *Exercises:* Active exercises of the joints and muscles should be permitted within the splints.
- *Checking:* Daily checking and adjustments of the splints are recommended.
- *Neurovascular status:* Distal neurovascular status should be assessed daily.

Table 6.1 shows other common splints used in orthopedics.

TRACTION IN ORTHOPEDICS

Traction plays an important role in the management of fractures in orthopedics (Fig. 6.12).

Uses of Traction

- To reduce a fracture or a dislocation.
- To retain the fracture after reduction.
- To overcome the muscle spasm.
- To control movement of an injured part of the body and to aid in healing.

Methods of Traction

There are four methods of applying traction, namely skin, skeletal, pelvic, and spinal.

Skin Traction

Here traction is applied over a large area of skin. Maximum weight that can be applied through skin traction is 15 lbs or 6.7 kg. If the weight used is more than this, the traction will slide down peeling off the skin. When used in fracture, skin traction is applied to the limb distal to the fracture site.

TABLE 6.1: Practical points—other common splints used in orthopedics

Region	Indications
1. Cervical spine	
– SOMI braces	Cervical spine injury
– 4 post-collar	Neck immobilization
2. Upper limbs	
– Aeroplane splint	Brachial plexus injury
– Cock-up splint	Radial nerve palsy
– Knuckle-bender splint	Ulnar nerve palsy
– Aluminum splints	Finger injuries
– Volkmann's splint	For VIC
3. Spine	
– Milwaukee braces	Scoliosis
– Boston braces	Scoliosis
– Taylor's brace	Dorsolumbar injury
– Anterior spinal hyper-extension braces (ASHE)	Dorsolumbar injury
– Lumbar belts and corsets	Backache
4. Lower limb	
– Thomas splint and BB splints—mentioned already	
– Foot drop splint	Foot drop
5. Miscellaneous	
– Thomas splint	
– Krammer wire splint	For emergencies

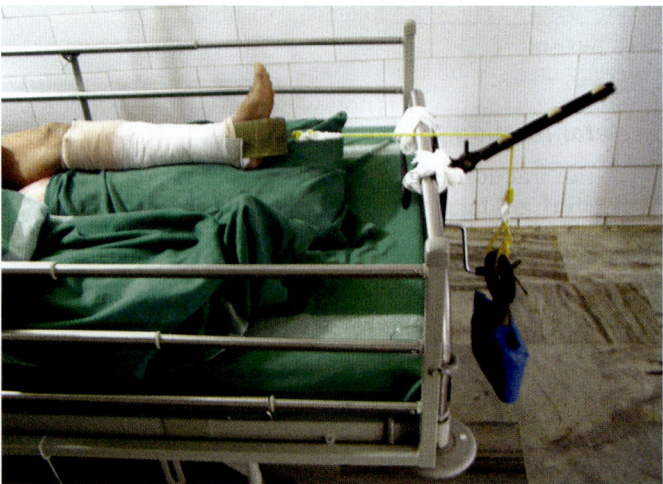

Fig. 6.12: Clinical photograph showing method of skin traction

Types of Skin Traction

Adhesive skin traction: Here adhesive material is used for strapping which is applied anteromedial and posterolateral on either side of the lower limbs.

Nonadhesive skin traction: Useful in thin and atrophic skin and in patients sensitive to adhesive strap. It is less secure than the former.

Contraindications for skin traction: Abrasions, lacerations, impaired circulation, dermatitis, marked shortening, allergy to plaster are some of the important contraindications for skin tractions.

Complications: Allergy, excoriations, pressure sores around the malleoli, common peroneal nerve palsy, etc. are some of the known complications in skin tractions.

> **Remember**
> Rotation of the limb is difficult to control with skin tractions.

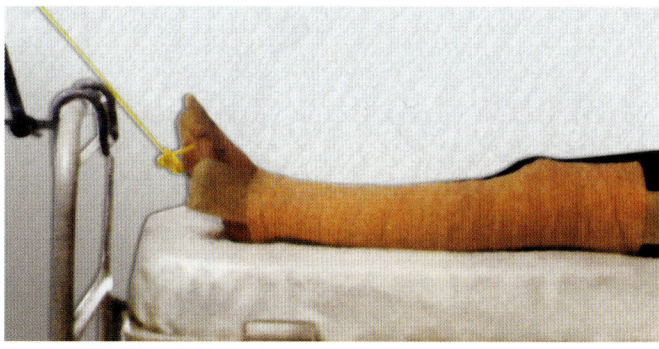

Fig. 6.13: Skin traction (Buck's extension type)

Important Skin Tractions

Buck's extension skin traction: This is the most common type of traction employed for lower limbs. It is used for temporary treatment of fracture neck femur, undisplaced fractures of acetabulum, after reduction of hip dislocation, to correct minor fixed flexion deformity of hip and knee for low backache, etc. (Fig. 6.13).

Dunlop's traction: Used in the upper limbs and is indicated for supracondylar fractures, intercondylar fractures of humerus where elbow flexion causes circulatory embarrassment (Fig. 6.14).

Gallows's traction (Fig. 6.15) or Bryant's traction: Used for fracture shaft femur in children less than 2 years. If used in children above 2 years, it causes vascular complications.

> **Did You Know?**
> Buck first used skin traction in a Cecil war.

Skeletal Traction

Here the traction is given through a metal or pin driven through the bone. It is seldom necessary for upper limb fractures but useful in lower limb fractures for reducing and maintaining the fracture reduction. It is reserved for those cases in which skin traction is contraindicated and where the need to be applied weight is more than 5 kg (Fig. 6.16A and 6.17A).

Steinmann's pin: It is a rigid stainless steel pin 4–6 mm in diameter. Böhler's stirr-up (Fig. 6.16B) allows the direction of the traction to be varied without turning the pin in the bone.

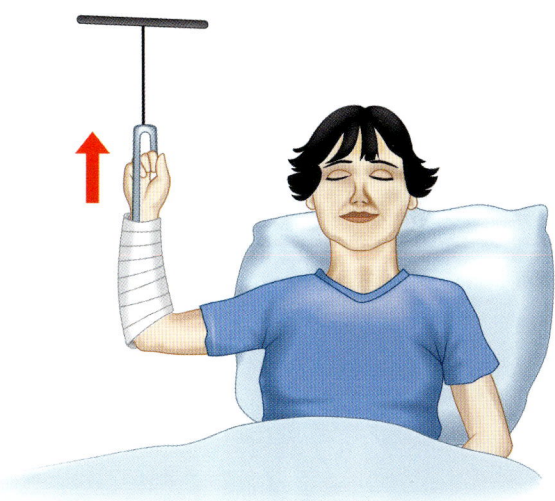

Fig. 6.14: Dunlop's traction

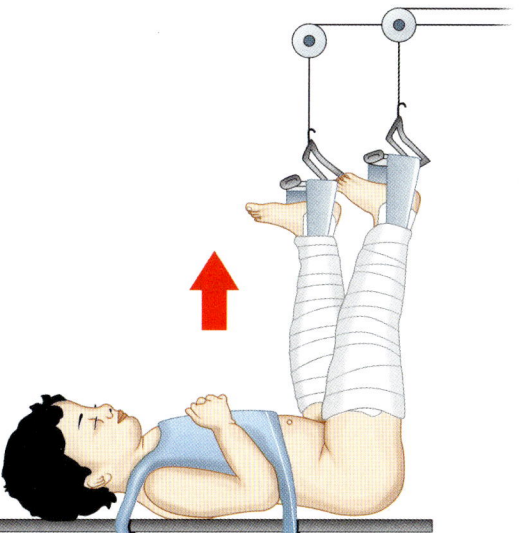

Fig. 6.15: Gallow's traction

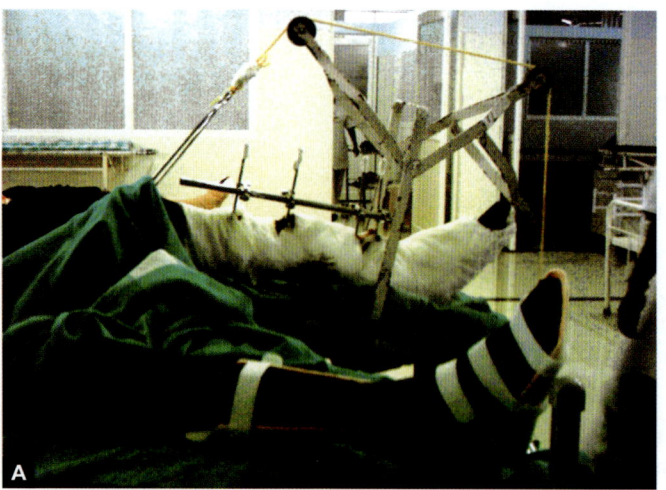
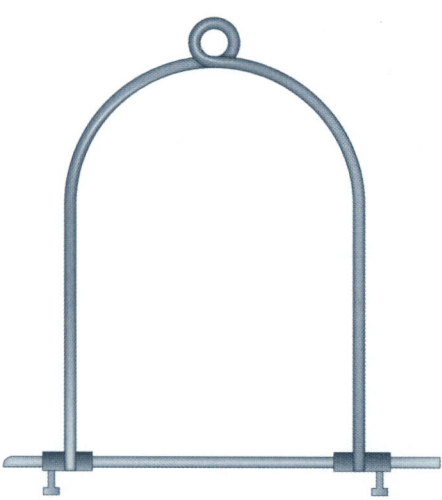

Figs 6.16A and B: (A) Polytrauma case management with skeletal traction and external fixators; (B) Steinmann's pin with Böhler's stirrup

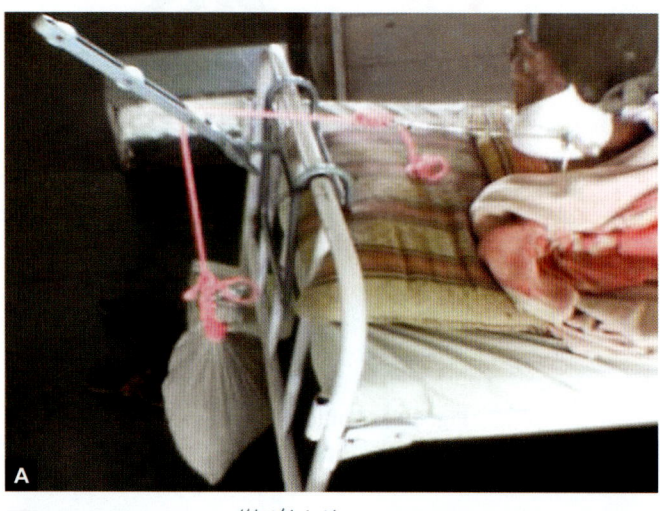

Figs 6.17A and B: (A) Clinical photo showing calcaneal traction; (B) Denham pin

TABLE 6.2: Traction points—well-known traction in orthopedics	
Tractions	Indications
1. Head or cervical tractions	
– Crutchfield or Garden wells	Cervical spine injuries
– Head halter	Cervical spine injuries
– Halo pelvic	Scoliosis
2. Upper limb tractions	
– Dunlop's traction	Supracondylar fracture of humerus
– Metacarpal traction	Compound forearm injuries
3. Lower limb tractions	
– Gallows's or Bryant's	Fracture shaft femur (<2 years)
– Russell's traction	Trochanteric fracture
– Perkins's traction	Fracture shaft femur in adults
– 90–90° traction	Fracture shaft femur in children
– Agnes Hunt traction	Correction of hip deformity
– Well leg traction	To correct abduction and adduction deformity of hip
– Calcaneal traction	Compound fractures of distal leg and ankle
– Buck's traction	Low backache, etc.
– Pelvic traction	Low backache, etc.

Denham pin (Fig. 6.17B): This pin is threaded in the centre and engages the bony cortex. It reduces the risk of pin sliding and is useful in cancellous bone like calcaneum and osteoporotic bones.

Table 6.2 shows well-known traction in orthopedics.

K-wire: It is of small diameter and is often used in upper limbs.

Know the Rules of Application

- Skeletal traction should be applied in a major OT under general or local anesthesia.
- Follow strict aseptic measures.
- Drive the pin from lateral to medial in case of upper tibial traction, to avoid injuring the lateral popliteal nerve.
- Pin should be at right angles to the limb and parallel to the ground.
- Cover the sharp tip on the medial side with a stopper bottle to prevent damage to the normal limb.

Table 6.3 shows the sites and indication for skeletal traction.

Know the Complications of Skeletal Traction

At the time of application
- Anesthetic problems.
- Vasovagal shock.
- Very rarely death due to vasovagal shock.

During application
- Injury to the nerves (lateral popliteal nerve).
- Injury to the vessels.
- Injury to the muscles, ligaments, and tendons.
- Injury to the epiphysis in children (upper tibial epiphysis).
- Pain due to equalization of intraosseus pressure and atmospheric pressure due to the hole made in the bone.

When pin is in situ
- Infection—due to improper aseptic measures.
- Migration—due to loosening.
- Breakage—thin pin or more weight.
- Bending—same reasons as above.
- Loosening—due to osteoporosis, infection, etc.
- Distraction of fracture fragments—due to excessive weight.

Late effects
- Pin tract infection.
- Chronic osteomyelitis with ring sequestra at the site.
- Genu recurvatum due to damage to the anterior epiphysis of tibia in children.
- Depressed scar.

> **How to Take Care of a Patient on Traction?**
> - Patient on traction need to be looked after, as they are unable to take care of themselves.
> - Watch for petechial rashes, confusion, etc. which may suggest onset of fat embolism.
> - Regular monitoring of temperature, pulse, and BP.
> - A balanced mixed diet is recommended.
> - Use of bedpans is advocated.
> - Use of NSAIDs for pain relief.
> - Encourage to keep a healthy mental state.
> - Proper skin care.

Counter traction: Traction force will overcome muscle spasm only if another force is acting in the opposite direction as counter traction.

Types

1. **Fixed traction (see Figs 6.10 and 6.18):** Here counter traction is achieved through an appliance which obtains a firm purchase on a part of the body. *This can maintain but cannot obtain reduction,* e.g. fixed traction on a Thomas splint for a fracture shaft femur.

TABLE 6.3: Know the sites and indications for skeletal traction

Sites of skeletal traction	Exact point	Indications
1. Skull traction	Outer table of parietal bone of the skull with either Crutchfield or Garden wells tongs.	• To reduce dislocation or fracture dislocation of cervical spine. • For postoperative treatment of neck. • For cervical spondylosis with severe nerve root compression.
2. Upper limbs		
Olecranon	1¼ inch distal to the tip of olecranon.	Supracondylar, intercondylar and comminuted fracture lower third of humerus.
Second and third metacarpals	One inch proximal to the distal end of second and third metacarpal.	Fracture both bones forearm.
3. Lower limbs		
Greater trochanter	One inch below the most prominent part of the greater trochanter, midway between anterior and posterior surfaces of femur.	Central fracture dislocation of hip.
Lower end of femur	1¼ inch above the knee joint.	Pelvic fractures, posterior dislocation of hip, trochanteric fractures, shaft fractures, etc.
Upper end of tibia	3/4th inch below and lateral to the tibial tuberosity.	All of the above indications, supracondylar fractures and intercondylar fractures of the femur.
Lower end of tibia	Two inches above the level of ankle joint midway between anterior and posterior border.	• Tibial plateau fractures. • Fracture both bones leg.
Calcaneum	Two centimetres below and behind the lateral malleolus.	Fractures lower one-third of the leg and ankle injuries.
Metatarsal bones	Through the base of the metatarsal.	For calcaneal fractures.

Note: The most common site for skeletal traction is upper end of tibia and common indications for skeletal traction is trochanteric fractures in elderly persons.

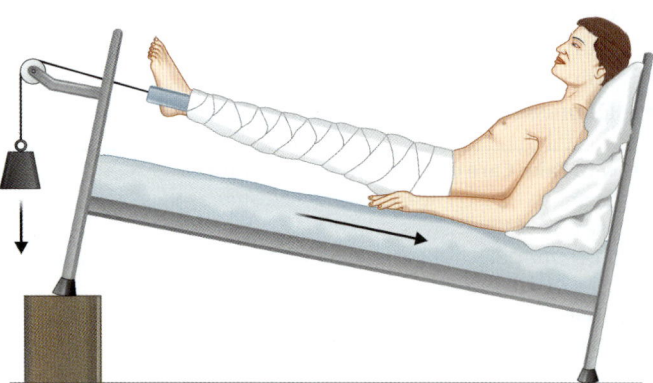

Fig. 6.18: Method of fixed traction for fracture shaft femur (also see Fig. 6.10)

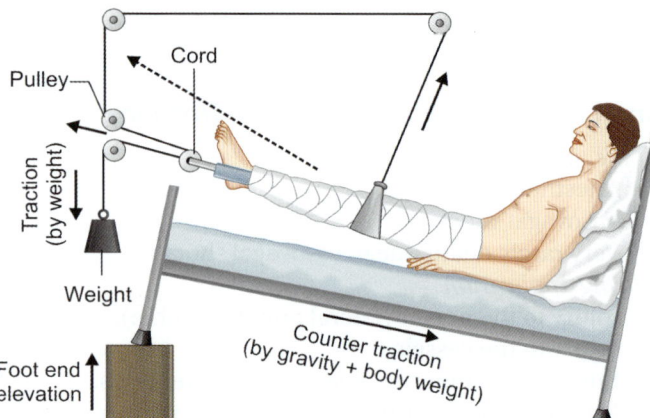

Fig. 6.19: Sliding or balanced traction

2. **Sliding or balanced traction (Fig. 6.19):** Here weight of all or part of the body acting under the influence of gravity is utilized to provide counter traction. This can be achieved by raising the foot end of the bed. *Unlike in a fixed traction, both reduction and maintenance of a fracture can be obtained.*

However, the initial traction weight required to obtain a reduction is greater than the traction weight required to maintain the reduction.

Weight Guidelines
For femoral shaft fracture, initial weight required is 10% of patient body weight. For every 1 lb of weight, the end of the bed should be raised by one inch. A weight of 10–20 kg can be applied through a skeletal traction unlike 6.7 kg in skin traction.

OPERATIVE TREATMENT

IMPLANTS

General Principles

Definition: An implant is defined as a material inserted or grafted into intact tissues or body cavity with some specific purpose.

TYPES OF IMPLANTS

Metallic: Generally, alloys are used. Three varieties are described:

Iron based (stainless steel): Composition of the alloy is, iron 70%, chromium 20%, and nickel 8%, manganese 2%. Commonly used alloy is 18.8S70 stainless steel (18% stands for chromium, 8% for nickel and steel is 70%).

Cobalt based: Here the composition is cobalt 60%, chromium 30%, 5% molybdenum, and 5% nickel.

Titanium based: This consists of 90% titanium, 6% aluminum, and 4% vanadium. Implants made from titanium are very strong and have great corrosion resistance.

Nonmetallic implants usually are made-up of plastic materials. Polyethylene, polymethylmethacrylate (PMMA) and silicones are the commonly used nonmetallic implants.

Remember
Characters of ideal implant
- Should be corrosion resistant.
- Should be biocompatible.
- Should have high tensile strength.
- Should have high fatigue limit.

Three Ps for implant selection
- **P**roper material.
- **P**roper design.
- **P**roper size and fixation.

About polymethylmethacrylate (PMMA)
- Called as bone cement
- It has a polymer and a monomer.
- It is not glue and has no adhesive qualities.
- Called cement because it holds two materials, bone, and metal, together by forming an interlocking network between the irregularities.

Note:
Corrosion is a chronic reaction that weakens the implants. Addition of chromium and nickel makes the implant corrosion resistant.

VARIETIES OF IMPLANTS

Commonly used implants in orthopedics are extramedullary and intramedullary fixations.

Extramedullary fixation: This consists of screws, plates K-wires circlage, transfixion, staples and suture anchors.

Screws

Two types of screws are described.

Machine Screws

These screws are threaded whole length and may or may not be self-tapping (Fig. 6.20). Used widely with standard bone plates. They are not superior to the ASIF screws because the cutting edge of these screws generates heat at the terminal ends of the screw holes resulting in osteonecrosis and consequent loosening of screws at later date. They are not used of late.

Note:
ASIF—Association of the Surgeon of International Fixation (Swiss group).

ASIF Screws or AO Screws

These screws are designed by AO group in which the threads are more horizontal, drill holes are needed as the screws are not self-tapping. Three varieties of ASIF screws are described:
1. *Cortical screws* (Fig. 6.21): These screws are threaded whole length and have a diameter of 2–4.5 mm. This functions as a positional screw or a lag screw for interfragmentary compression.
2. *Cancellous screws* (Fig. 6.22): These have larger threads for more purchase in the soft cancellous bone. It is available as 16 mm, 32 mm length, and 4 mm to 6.5 mm diameter.
3. *Malleolar screws:* These have a sharp-pointed tip and may be inserted without predrilling. Used for internal fixation of malleolar fractures.

Other Screws
- *Cannulated screws:* These are hollow screws modified over the cancellous and cortical screws. It is used widely for fixation of fracture neck of femur.
- *Interference screws:* These are special screws without the usual head and are commonly used for bone ligament bone graft reconstruction for torn ACL.

Parts of a Screw

A screw has a head, neck shaft, and tip. The other important aspects of the screws are:
Pitch: It is the distance between two threads of a screw.
Lead: It is the distance covered by one rotation.
Root diameter: It is the minimum cross-sectional area of a screw.
Outer diameter of the screw.

Methods of Providing Compression by Screws

Lag Effect

To provide compression at the fracture site when cortical screws are used, one has to over drill the proximal cortex so that the screw will slide down through the hole, pulling the far fragment towards the near fragment.

Cancellous Screws

Provide a lag effect (Fig. 6.23) without over drilling of the proximal cortex since it is half-threaded and pulls the far fragment towards the near fragment.

Remember
The uses of screws
- Used mostly to fasten the plates to the bone.
- Used to fix avulsion fractures, butterfly fractures, etc.
- By over drilling the cortex, a cortical screw provides interfragmentary compression by producing the lag effect.
- A cancellous screw can produce compression without over drilling since it is half-threaded.

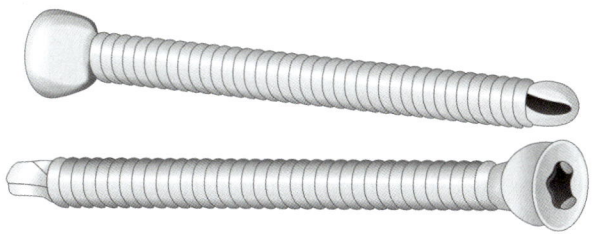

Fig. 6.20: Self-tapping machine screws

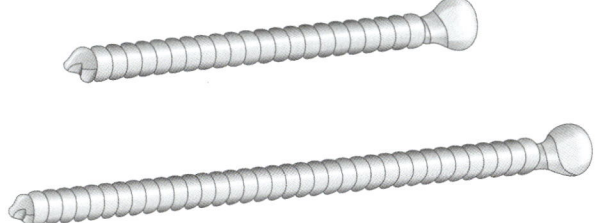

Fig. 6.21: Cortical screws—threaded whole length and not self-tapping

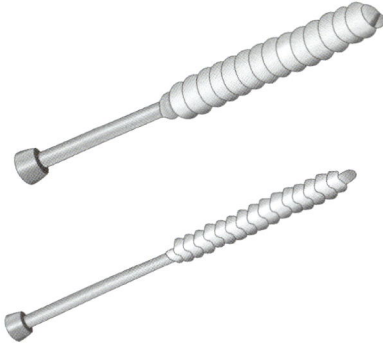

Fig. 6.22: Cancellous screw (above) and malleolar screw (below)

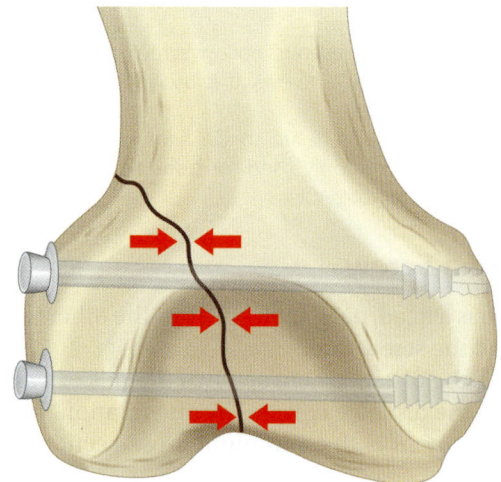

Fig. 6.23: The lag effect produced by cancellous screws

PLATES

Plates are widely used for internal fixation of diaphyseal fractures. Rigidity and strength depend upon the cross-section and the material used. Ranges from very rigid plates to merely positional plates. There is compensating thickness around the holes.

TYPES OF PLATES

Ordinary Plates

These just function as positional plate to hold the fractures but will not bring about any compression between the fracture sites. They are used in subcutaneous locations or where extreme rigidity is not required. The patients need prolonged immobilization once this plate is used, e.g. semi-tubular plate (Fig. 6.24A), Scheurmann's plate, etc. for ulna, clavicle, fibula, etc.

> **Remember about Ordinary Plates**
> - Functions merely as a positional plate.
> - Useful in subcutaneous situations.
> - Needs prolonged immobilization.
> - Hence the role is limited and has given way to compression plating.

AO PLATES

As described earlier, AO techniques aim at early mobilization of the limb by providing a rigid compression at the fracture site and thereby prevent the possibility of fracture disease. Rigid fixation at the fracture site can be obtained by providing compression at the fracture site. The following are the methods to obtain compression.

METHODS OF PROVIDING COMPRESSION

- *Static methods:* This aims to provide compression by causing lag effect, which has been mentioned already.
- *AO plates with external compression device:* Here compression is produced by an external compression device (Müller's device) which is attached to the AO plate. Requires a wider exposure and hence dynamic compression plate (DCP) is preferred.
- *Dynamic compression:* Here, no external compression devices are used; on the contrary, the plate holes are designed in such a way that as the screw is being tightened it pulls the fragment in the same direction and brings about compression at the fracture site. This is by far the best method of providing compression at the fracture site.
- *Tension band principle:* There are two forces acting at the fracture site. One is a distraction force seen over the convex surface of the bone and the other is a compression force seen at the concave inner surface. Now, if the plate is applied on the compression side, the distraction forces will disturb the fixation and cause implant failure. On the other hand, if the plate is applied on the convex border, it will help convert the distraction force into a compression force and will aid in rigid compression at the fracture site, e.g. tension band wiring for fracture of patella and olecranon, DCP plating for tibia, humerus, etc.

Types

- *Static tension band*: If a tension band device produces the compression only at the time of application, it is static tension band.
- *Dynamic tension band*: Here in addition to the above compression effect is produced even during physiologic overloading.

Types of ASIF Plates

- **AO plates:** These are thick plate, with round holes and a slot for the use of compression jig (Fig. 6.24B).
- **DCP** (Fig. 6.24C): These are heavy-duty plates with oval holes.
- **Special plates:** For example, 'T'-plates (Fig. 6.24D), 'L'-plates (Fig. 6.24E), etc. are used for condylar fractures of tibia, proximal humeral fractures, etc.

  Flat buttress plate: This is available in the following shapes:
  a. 'C' or cloverleaf
  b. 'H' plate
  c. 'L' plate
  d. 'T' plate
  e. 'S' or spoon plate.

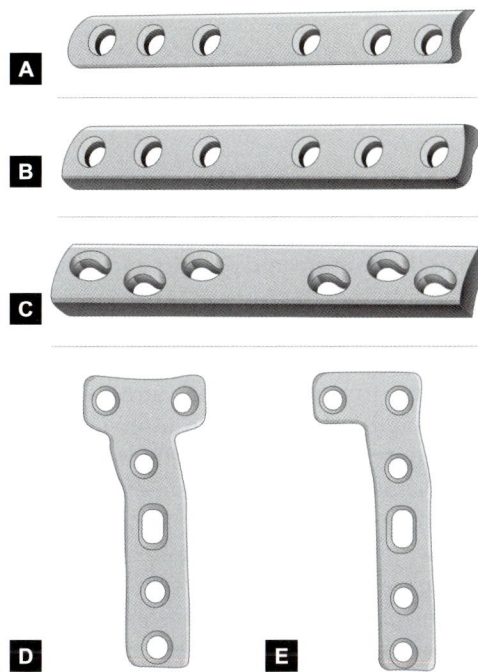

Figs 6.24A to E: (A) Semi-tubular plate; (B) AO plate; (C) A dynamic compression plate (DCP); (D) Special shaped T-plate; (E) L-plate

Indications: It is mainly indicated for buttressing fractures of epiphyseal–metaphyseal junction.

Buttress Plate with an Antiglide Principle

When a lag screw is passed through the buttress plate, it produces both compression and stability and is called the antiglide principle.

- *Wave plate:* Refracture of bone after plate removal is a common pitfall. To prevent this, Weber devised a plate with the cortex not in immediate contact with the plate. Bone graft is used to fill in the gap between the plate and the bone. This is called the wave plate.
- *Reconstruction plate:* These plates are used to fix difficult fractures of pelvis, distal humerus, calcaneum, etc. as they can be contoured in three planes. Their thickness is in between DCP and buttress plate. In between the holes, they have scallop-like notches at the sides.
  Pitfalls: They are less strong than the DCP plates.

Principles of ASIF Plate

The four important principles are as follows:
- *Tension band principle* is already mentioned; here the plate is placed on the convex side of an eccentrically loaded bone. This helps to convert the distraction force into compression force.

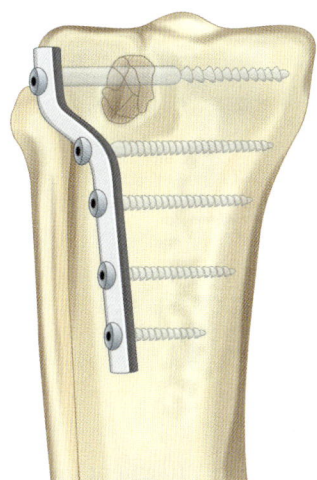

Fig. 6.25: A buttress plate for proximal tibial fractures

- *Neutralization plate* useful in comminuted fracture. Here the plate is attached to two main fragments. Here the force is transmitted from proximal to distal by passing the fracture site and thus the torsional forces are neutralized.
- *Buttress plate (Fig. 6.25)* supports thin bone and functions opposite to tension band. The plate is always under compression and is used in fractures around the joints.
- *Axial compression* for rigid fixation and primary bone healing.

DYNAMIC COMPRESSION PLATES (DCP)

In DC plates screw holes are designed to utilize *spherical gliding principle* with inclined contour of the screw holes and the slope on the under side of the screw head. As the screw is tightened, its head is guided by the contours of the screw whole in such a way that the head glides towards the center of the plate until the deepest portion of the hole is reached. Result is that bone fragment into which screw is being driven is displaced at the same time and in the same direction providing rigid compression. It is called dynamic because the bone fragment moves while the screw is being tightened (Fig. 6.26A).

Advantages of DCP

- Less surgical exposure than the conventional surgery.
- Screw and plate fit congruently in any position (Fig. 6.26B). Plain x-ray of DCP plating is shown in Figure 6.27.
- Screw may be inserted at any angle.
- All other advantages of rigid fixation.

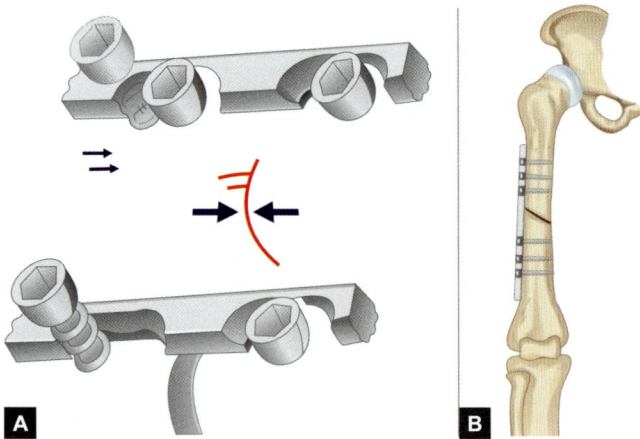

Figs 6.26A and B: In DCP, fragment moves, as the screw is tightened producing compression; (B) Fracture shaft humerus fixed with DCP plate and screws

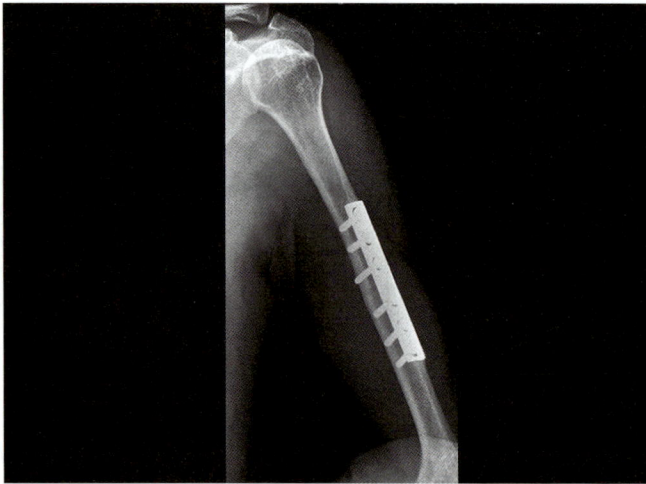

Fig. 6.27: Plain X-ray showing DCP plating

Remember
About rigid fixation plates
- *Compression at fracture site obtained by*
  - Lag effect.
  - By using external compression device as in AO plating.
  - Self-compression as in DCP.
  - Tension band technique.

Advantages
- Early mobilization.
- No fracture disease.

Disadvantages
- Heals by primary intention hence callus is not seen on radiographs.
- Poor fracture welding, as there is no external callus.
- Excessive compression causes osteonecrosis.
- Refracture is common after removal.
- Requires wide exposure.

Irony Rigid fixation no doubt permits early mobilization but this advantage is nullified by the prolonged immobilization required following implant removal to fill up the screw gaps.
Solution. Interlocking nail emerging as an ideal replacement.

INTRAMEDULLARY NAIL

Salient features about intramedullary nail are as follows:
- Firmly fixes the fracture and permits early mobilization.
- Useful in diaphyseal fractures at the narrowest portion of the medullary canal.
- Very suitable in young adults.
- Not indicated for children and adolescents as the epiphysis may be damaged while inserting the nail leading to future growth complications.
- The patient should be able to tolerate major surgery.
- Nails should be of suitable length and diameter.
- Suitable instruments, assistants, and hospital required.
- Closed technique is better than open.
- Union is peripheral and no endosteal healing due to reamed medullary canal.
- Fat embolism is relatively more common.

Types of IM Nails and Indications (Flowchart 6.1)

Broadly speaking, there are three varieties of intramedullary nails, namely:
a. Standard or conventional nails, e.g. Butcher's nail (Fig. 6.28)
b. Interlocking nails (ILN), e.g. GK nail, RT nail, etc. (Fig. 6.29)
c. Flexible medullary nails, e.g. Ender's nails.
Presently, the ILN has largely replaced the conventional IM nails.

Requirements of an IM Nail

- It should be strong and provide a tight fit in the medullary canal.
- It should provide physiologic stimulus to union.
- The ends of the nail must be accessible for easy removal.

Mode of Action of Intramedullary Nails (Fig. 6.30)

- It is a load-sharing device unlike a plate, which is a load-bearing device.
- It fills the medullary cavity.
- It provides three-point fixation (at the ends of nail and at the point where curve of the nail is in contact with the opposite cortex).
- It resists bending movement but is poor against torsional forces.

Flowchart 6.1: Types of intramedullary nails

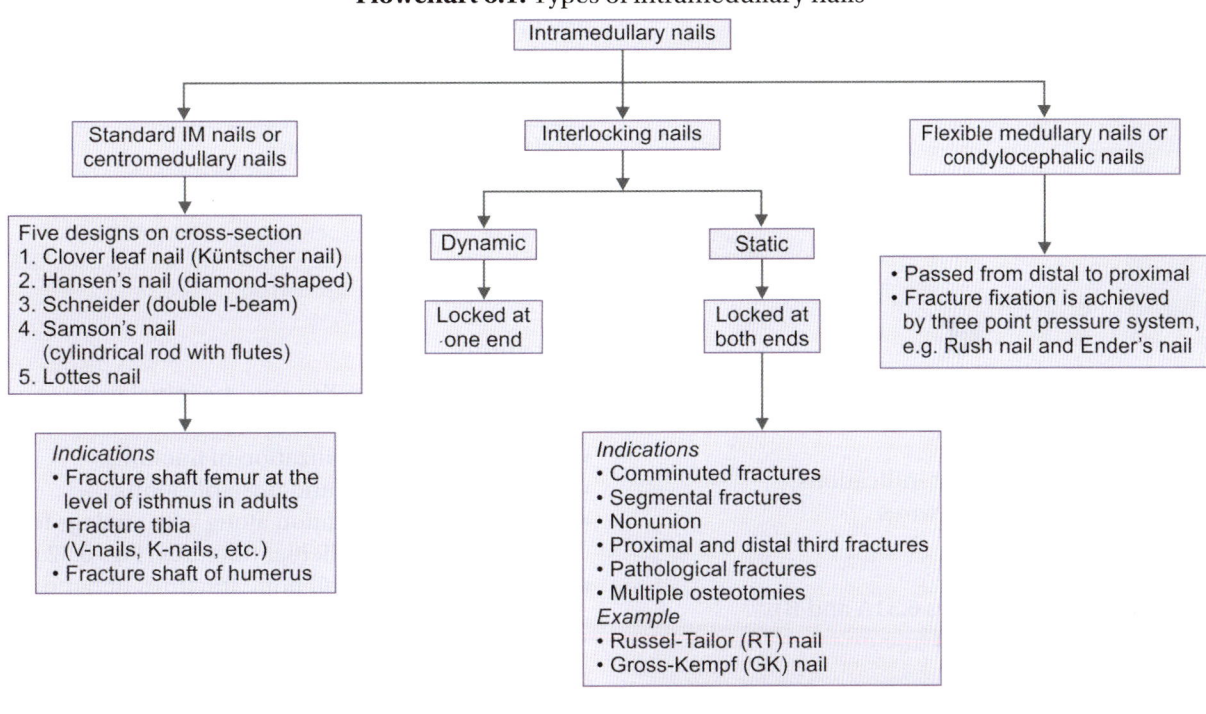

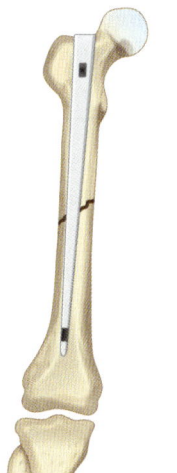

Fig. 6.28: Fracture femur fixed with Küntscher's (IM) nail

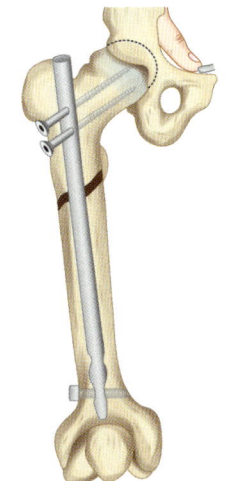

Fig. 6.29: Subtrochanteric fracture fixed with ILN

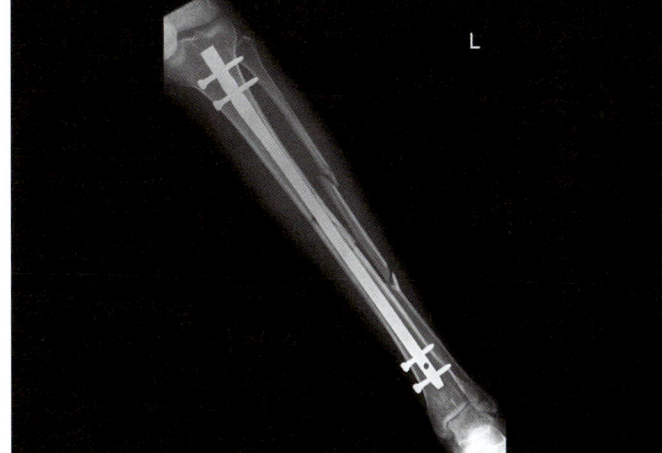

Fig. 6.30: Plain X-ray showing tibia fracture fixation by ILN

Regarding techniques of insertion and complications see chapter on Instruments.

OTHER IMPORTANT INTERNAL FIXATION METHODS

Circlage

This is credited to be the oldest method of internal fixation. It produces an interfragmentary compression effect similar to the interfragmentary screws.

Materials Used as Circlage Wires

- 16-gauge 316 L stainless steel wires
- 18-gauge (1 mm) vitallium
- 24-gauge stainless steel wires woven into three strands.

Indications: Circlage wire like a joker in cards can be combined successfully with various other fixation methods. This creates a number of permutations and combinations for fixations in orthopedics.

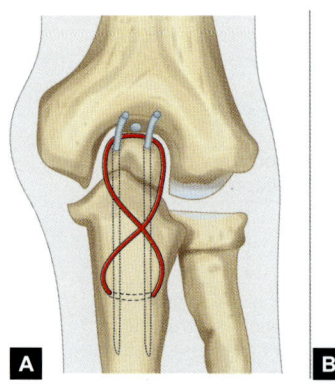 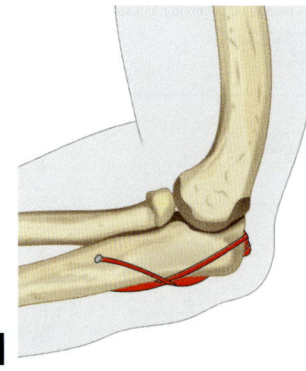

Figs 6.31A and B: Tension band wiring (TBW) in fracture olecranon

Here is a list of some important indications:
- With Steinmann's pin or K-wires
  - Fracture patella.
  - Fracture malleolus.
  - Fracture olecranon (Figs 6.31A and B).
- **With intramedullary nails**
  - Fracture of femur
  - Fracture of tibia, humerus, etc.
- For fixation of avulsion fractures
  - Humerus—greater and lesser tuberosity
  - Femur—greater trochanter
  - Pelvis—symphysis pubis.
  - Tendocalcaneus injury.
  - Acromioclavicular injuries.
- Spine surgeries
  - Sublaminar wiring
  - Posterior segmental stabilization
  - Fixation of grafts.
- It can be used for primary fracture fixations in selected situations too.
- **Miscellaneous**
  - For arthrodesis.
  - For allograft fixation.
  - For tendon and ligament repairs.
  - Periprosthetic fractures

> **Remember**
> **Vital facts about circlage**
> - It helps provide interfragmentary compression.
> - Wires are useful when compression is required and space is limited.
> - Like a joker in cards, it can be suited to various fixation methods.
> - It creates multiple combinations of internal fixation options.
> - This is the oldest method of internal fixation in use since 1775.

Transfixion

Volkmann did the first transfixion surgery in 1875. It literally means fixation of fracture or bone fragment by penetration or piercing. The most famous transfixion surgeries currently in practice are percutaneous fixations of small bone fractures, distal radial fractures, supracondylar fractures of humerus in children, patellar fractures, olecranon fractures, etc.

> **Vital Facts about Transfixion**
> - K-wires or Steinmann's pin is the most common implant used.
> - It is the simplest form of fixation.
> - It can be used both as percutaneous or open fixation.
> - The fixation provided is not stable and needs additional support.
> - Loosening, breakage, backing out can occur.

Indications
- Skeletal fractures: This was the initial use.
- For percutaneous fixation of fractures.
- For temporary stabilization of fractures.
- For stabilizing flail and unstable joints.
- As tension band fixation along with circlage for patella, olecranon, and malleolar fractures (Figs 6.32 and 6.33).
- For fixations of small bone fractures of hand, foot, etc. (Figs 6.34 and 6.35).

Staples

To arrest the growth of the epiphysis, Blount is credited for popularizing the use of staples. They are used in certain special situations.

> **Staple Facts: Indications for Staples**
> - Epiphyseal arrest in children
> - Fixation of valgus tibial osteotomy (Figs 6.36 and 6.37).
> - For arthrodesis of small joints like:
>   - Wrist
>   - Triple arthrodesis.
>   - Subtalar joint.

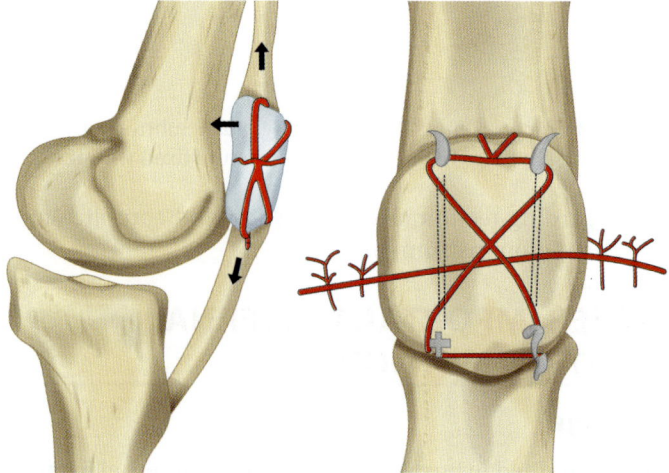

Fig. 6.32: Tension band wiring (TBW) for displaced transverse fracture of patella

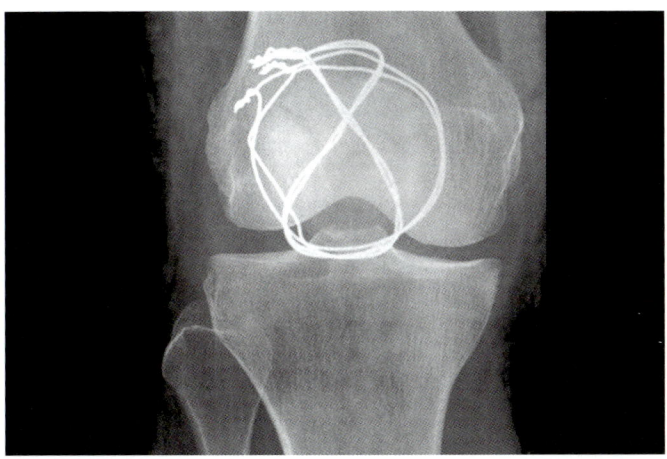

Fig. 6.33: Plain X-ray showing tension band wiring

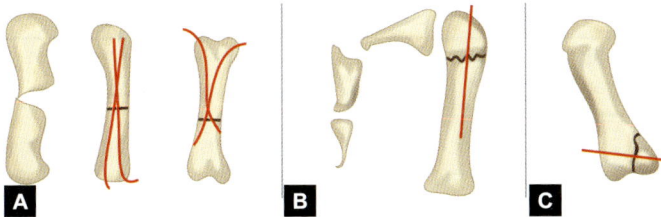

Figs 6.34A to C: Metacarpal fractures treated by closed reduction and percutaneous pinning: (A) Unstable fracture fixed with criss-cross K-wires; (B) Neck fracture fixed by intramedullary fixation; (C) Bennett's fracture fixed with K-wire

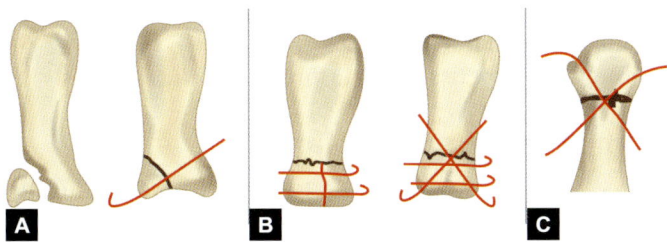

Figs 6.35A to C: Closed reduction and percutaneous fixation of various phalangeal fractures (A) Unstable short oblique fractures; (B) Comminuted fracture; (C) Condylar fracture

- In certain fractures like:
  - Patellar fractures
  - Malleolar fractures
  - Trochanter fractures.

Suture Anchors

Earlier to reattach ligaments or tendons to their insertion points in the bone drill holes were made into them. Of late, this procedure is made easy by attaching a sturdy suture to a

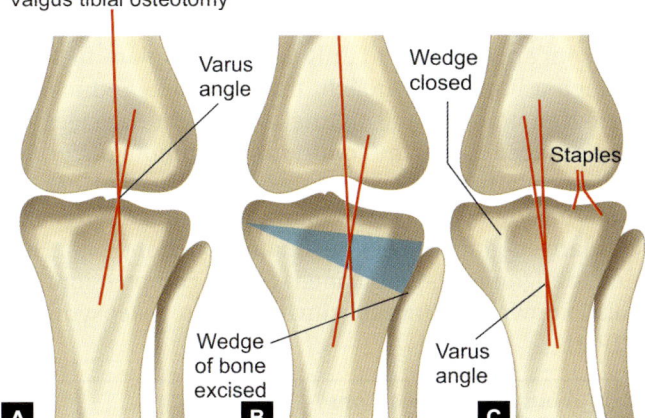

Figs 6.36A to C: Fixation of tibial valgus osteotomy with staples

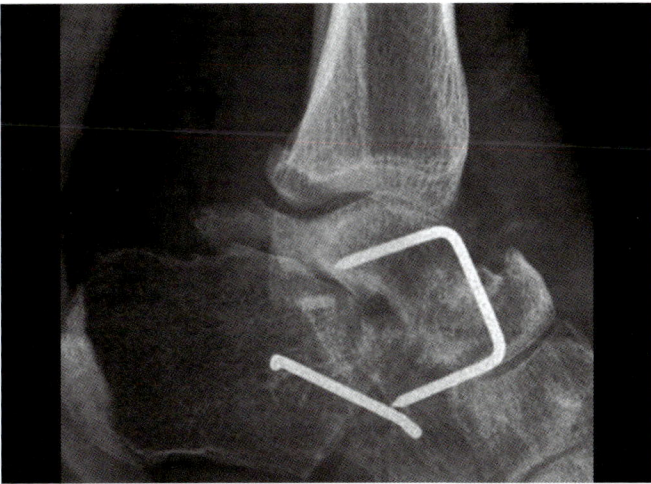

Fig. 6.37: Plain X-ray showing use of staples in fracture

bone with a screw or spring like apparatus. These are called the suture anchors. They have a greater pull out strength.

Indications

- Tendon and ligament surgeries.
- Rotator cuff repairs.
- Shoulder stabilization procedure.

FIXATION TECHNIQUES BY NONCOMPRESSION METHODS

Internal Splints

Intramedullary rods or nails act as internal splints. They do not rigidly fix the fractures but union is most of the times not a problem. The gliding movements that take place between the fracture fragments allow compression. This concept became popular after the discovery by Küntscher.

Biologic Fixation

This concept is being mainly applied to plate fixation. Through a limited approach, the fracture is reduced by indirect methods with minimal soft tissue damage. The plate is placed across the communition without disturbing or manipulating the comminuted fragments. Here, no graft is inserted because the comminuted fragments act as vascularized grafts except in situations of bone loss. Here fracture alignment is maintained without compression. This is also known as minimally invasive plate osteosynthesis (MIPO).

Facts about Biologic Fixations
- Limited exposure.
- Utmost respect for the soft tissue.
- Comminution left undisturbed.
- Limited contact between bone and implant.
- Biocompatible material implants used.

Composite Fixation

This refers to fixation of the metallic implants with bone cement. This concept was developed and popularized by Müller. To qualify the fixation as composite, two different fixation materials are used.

Vital Facts
Composite fixation is useful in filling defects and fixing it in conditions of tumor, crushes injuries, bone loss, etc. Here the gap is filled with cement and the fragments are fixed with nail or plates.

Hybrid Fixation

Here, unlike in composite fixation, only one material is used to provide two different fixation methods. An IM device used with an external fixator is an example of hybrid fixation. This method of fixation helps to attain the advantages of two types of fixation. Some of the most common hybrid fixations in common usages are:
- SP nail and plate.
- Jewett nail and plate.
- DHS screw with wide plate device (most common).

Bioabsorbable Fixation

Reabsorbable internal fixation devices prevent another surgery, and its attendant complications, for removal of implants. These implants slowly disintegrate and get absorbed during the course of fracture union (Fig. 6.38).

Materials used: The rods and screws are made up of:
- Polyglycolic acid
- Polylactic acid.

Mechanism of action: They function as transfixion devices.

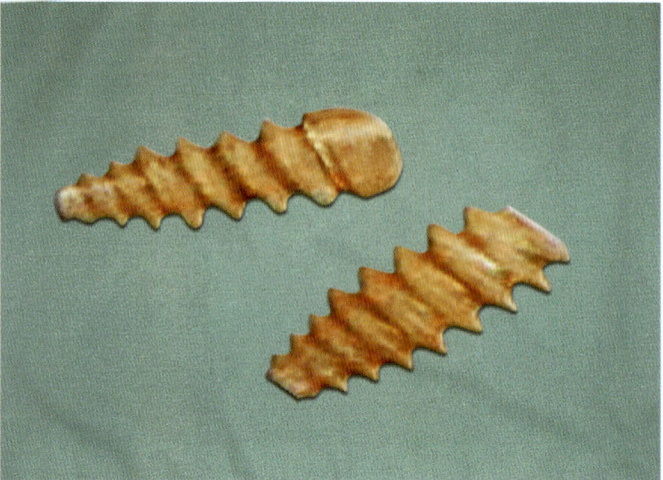

Fig. 6.38: Bioabsorbable screw

Pitfalls
- Fixation attained is not rigid, hence external immobilization is required
- Cannot be used for all fractures and hence has limited applications
- Severe synovial reactions are seen due to polyglycolide when used around the knee
- Sinus track formations are common.

Indications: It has been used in the following situations with varied success:
- Ankle fractures
- Olecranon fractures
- Osteochondral fractures
- Pediatric fractures
- Radial head fractures
- Repair of soft tissues by arthroscopy.

Complications of Implants

There can be a variety of complications with implants like (Fig. 6.39A to E):
- Infection
- Breakage
- Bending
- Migration
- Loosening
- Growth abnormalities

EXTERNAL FIXATION

Definition

An external fixation (EF) is the method of fixing the fractures with a cluster of pins connected to external bars. Lambotte first used it in 1900. From the initial unilateral frames to the subsequent circular frames to the present hybrid fixations, external fixations have come a very long way.

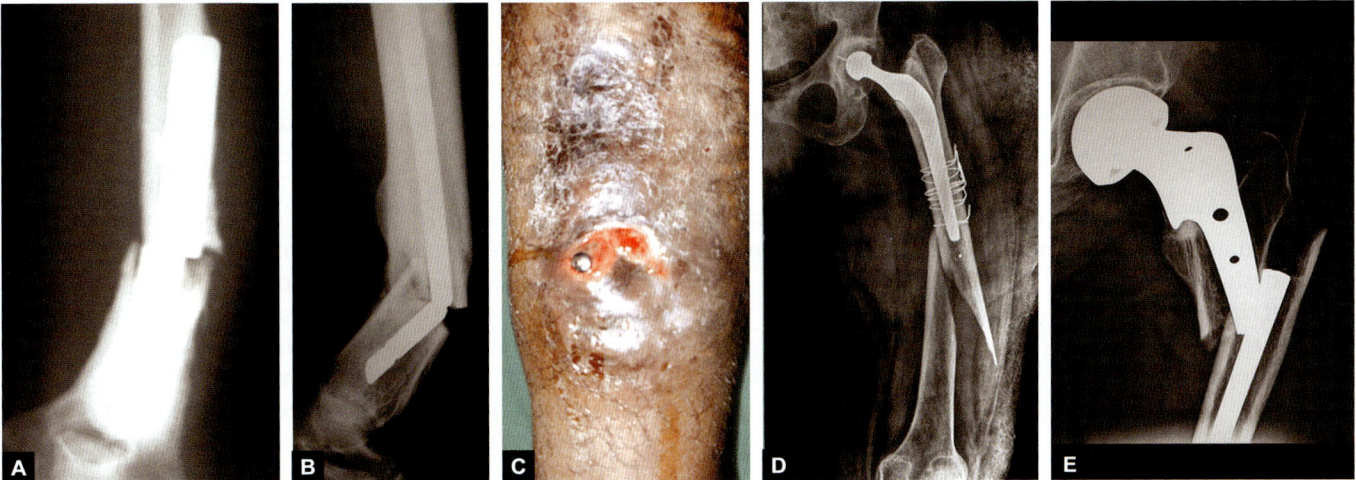

Figs 6.39A to E: Showing implant failures: (A) Plate breakage; (B) Nail breakage; (C) Infection; (D) Periprosthetic fracture; (E) Breakage of prosthetic stem

Highlights of External Fixation

- It provides a stable fixation of fractures and joints.
- Axial, compression, rotation, distraction, translational and angulatory forces can be applied.
- It helps in the wound care and reconstructive surgeries.

Indications: External fixations have specific indications in the following situations:
- Open fractures with severe soft tissue injury.
- To stabilize long bone, periarticular and pelvic injuries in a multiple trauma patient.
- For fixation of pelvic fractures.
- For definitive treatment of some fractures of the long bones and pelvis (Fig. 6.40).
- Circulatory external fixators have its own set of special indications.

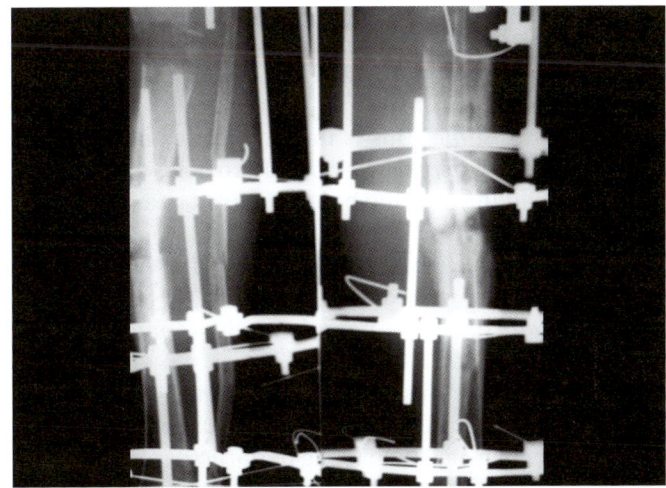

Fig. 6.40: Ilizarov has a definite indication in the treatment of nonunions of long bones

Components of External Fixators

External fixators consist of three basic components, namely the pin, clamps, and external rods.

Pins

The pins are passed through the bones at various levels and fixed to an external frame by the clamps.

Types of Pins

- *Half pins:* These are very commonly used.
- *Full pins*: These are centrally threaded and transfix the entire bone. Diameter—4-5 mm.
- *Thin wires* (1.5-2 mm): These are usually used with circular external fixators and it gains its rigidity by tensioning.
- *Olive wires:* This is a thin wire with a bull protrusion at one end.

Other Varieties

a. *Cortical pins:* Here the thread diameter increases from the tip to the shaft.
b. *Self-drilling pins:* Causes frequent fractures due to osteonecrosis.
c. *Hydroxyapatite coated pins:* These help to prevent pin loosening and migration in porotic bones.

Clamps

These connect the pins to the rods.

Types of Clamps
- *Simple clamps:* This connects single pin or wires to the rod or ring.
- *Modules clamps:* These connect several pins as clusters.

Rings
They are extensively used in Ilizarov's and hybrid fixations. They are made up of stainless steel, aluminum, and carbon. Types of the rings are:
a. Half rings
b. Full rings
c. 5/8 rings.

External Rods
These connect the cluster of pins through various clamps. They are made up of one of the three materials mentioned above and the cross-section varies from circular, square, oval or multiple faced.

Types of External Fixators (Based on Frame Design)
- *Unilateral frame:* This is the simplest external fixator frame. Four pins, two above, and two below the fracture are passed through the bone and fixed to a frame (Figs 6.41A and B).
- *Bilateral frame:* This improves the frame stiffness and helps in better control of bending and torsional forces.
- *Ring fixators:* This has been dealt with separately and is multiplanar (see Figs 7.7A to C).
- *Hybrid fixators:* This helps to combine the advantages of uniplanar and multiplanar external fixator devices. They are especially useful in fixing periarticular fractures.

Mode of Action
- *Compression forces:* These forces help to stabilize certain transverse fractures and for compression arthrodesis.
- *Distraction forces:* These make the ligaments, muscles, capsules and other soft tissues taut by ligamentotaxis. These forces help in reduction and retention of the fracture fragments. This is commonly used in distal radial, tibial plateau and pilon fractures.
- *Neutralization forces:* This provides neutralizing forces across the fracture site. These are frequently used in conjunction with some internal fixation. The common application is seen in distal radial comminuted fractures. Here, distraction forces are provided to reduce the fractures and later are retained by percutaneous fixation and later the distraction forces are released to provide only the neutralizing force across the fractures.
- *Angular forces:* These are used to bend, rotate, and convert the angulations. Used extensively in Ilizarov's technique.

Biotechnical Principles of External Fixation
The following influence the mechanical stability of the external fixator:
- *Pin size:* Greater the pin size, greater is the stability of fixation.
- *Pin number:* More number of pins ensures better stability.
- *Pin placement:* The ideal placement of the pins include very near on either side of the fracture site or farthest away from the fractures. This is known as the "Near Far Construct."
- *Rod placement:* Rods placed closer to the bone gives better stability. Double stacking the rods also increases the stability.
- *Clamps:* The rigidity of fixators decreases considerably if the clamps do not hold the pins firmly. Hence, periodic tightening of the clamp is a useful and effective practice.

> **Vital Facts: Regarding the Case of the External Fixators**
> - Duration of temporary treatment is 4 weeks
> - Duration of definitive treatment is 1 year
> - Conversion of external fixators to internal fixators should be planned once the soft tissues heal well
> - Up to 10% of external fixators end up in pin tract problems
> - Pre-drilling reduces osteosclerosis
> - The tented soft tissues should be released
> - Everyday care of the external fixator and pins is necessary to prevent complications like infections, loosening, etc.

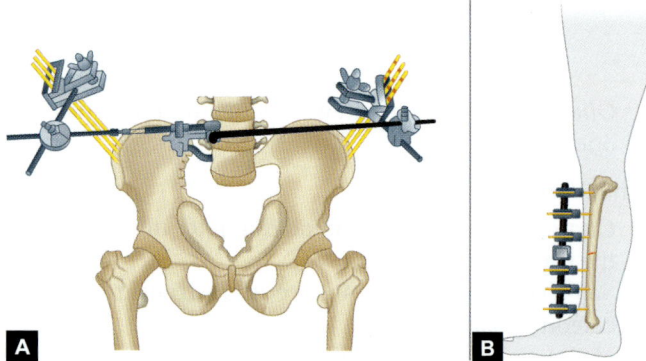

Figs 6.41A and B: Treatment of fractures by external fixators: (A) Pelvic; (B) Tibia fracture

- Resorption of the bone around the pin for more than 1 mm signifies a significant loosening
- Frequent radiograph (once in 2 weeks) is necessary to evaluate the progress of union
- If callus is not seen by 8 weeks, bone grafting should be considered.

Complications

The following are some of the important complications of external fixation:
- Pin loosening
- Pin migration
- Pin breakage
- Pin tract infection (10%)
- Impalement of nerves, muscles, tendons, ligaments, etc.
- Chronic osteomyelitis (0–4% of cases)
- Septic arthritis if pin is placed very close to the joint.
- Soft tissue contractures.

Pin Care Facts
- Inspect the pins everyday
- If there is discharge, dry sterile dressing is advised
- In the event of infections, wash the wound with 50 percent normal saline and 50 percent hydrogen peroxide
- The patient can wash the frame with soap and water for less than five minutes
- Topical antibiotics should be applied if there is infection
- Loose pins should be replaced.

7 CHAPTER

Recent Advances in Fracture Treatment

ADVANCES IN THE EXISTING METHODS OF FRACTURE TREATMENT

Advances are made in the existing methods of fracture treatment. The notable ones are mentioned here.

IMPROVEMENTS IN PLASTER OF PARIS SPLINTS

Now the days are of ultrashort-setting plaster casts or slabs made-up of a material called polyurethane.

What is New in Plasters?

Fiberglass Plasters
The more recent 'polyester cast' is composed of specifically knitted polyester with elasticity, impregnated with polyurethane resin activated by water (Fig. 7.1).

Advantage over Conventional Plasters
- Greater comfort.
- *Strength:* 20 times stronger and is only 1/3rd the thickness of plaster of Paris.
- *Weight:* Much lighter.
- *Shrinkage:* Good shrinkage, hence recasting is avoidable.
- *Durability:* More durable. Water resistant, smooth and soft edges to prevent scratch skin and snatch clothes.
- *Radiolucency:* More radiolucent. Check X-rays are clear.
- *Sanitation:* Moisture resistant porous cast, dries easily, prevents bad odor and other skin complications.
- *Colors:* Available in different colors like white, green, pink, yellow, blue, black, red, purple, etc.
- *Removal:* Easy to remove using conventional cast cutting saw or shear.
- *Dusting:* Significantly less dusting and least harmful.

Indications
- Secondary casting of fractures
- Cast braces
- Reconstruction of joints
- Long-term cast
- For immobilization in injuries
- To reduce arthritic pain
- To stretch the tight muscles
- To protect an area
- For extradurability and strength.

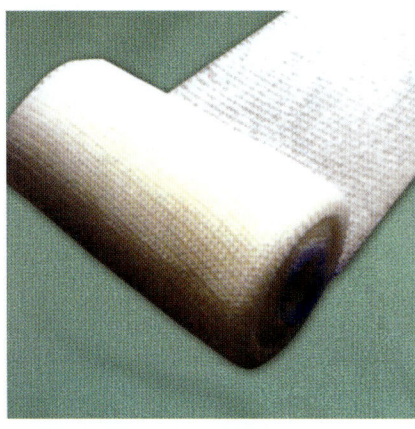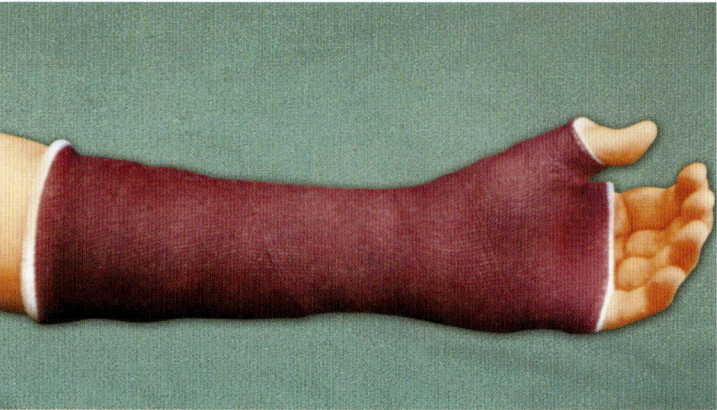

Fig. 7.1: Fiberglass plasters

FUNCTIONAL CAST BRACE

Earlier application of casts or slabs confined the patient to the bed until the fracture united. Now, the concept is to mobilize the patient on the plaster cast by using the functional cast brace, an idea developed by Sarmiento. Discussed at length in the previous section.

IMPROVEMENTS IN AO TECHNIQUE

Introduction of LCDCP (limited contact DCP) is considered as a step in the improvement of rigid fixation by AO technique.

IMPROVEMENTS IN INTRAMEDULLARY NAILS

These are the days of interlocking nails. Earlier intramedullary nails could not be used in proximal and distal third fractures of the long bones because the wider medullary canal in these areas rendered it difficult to control the rotation of the nail. The only alternative left was to use a plate and screw. Nevertheless, the problems associated with plate and screws necessitated the discovery of newer intramedullary nail with the problem of rotation eliminated by locking. Thus, the concept of interlocking nail was born and has made greater strides in the management of difficult fractures of the long bones.

INTERLOCKING NAILS (FIGS 7.2A TO C)

Standard IM nails designed by Küntscher for shaft fractures leave two unresolved problems:
- Rotation of the fracture fragments
- Telescoping at the fracture site.

By locking the nail into the bone by means of self-tapping screw driven through holes located at both the ends, the above two problems are solved. Gross and Kempf locking nail is found to be successful (Figs 7.2A to C).

Advantages

- It can be used for both simple and compound shaft fracture from subtrochanteric to supracondylar area in the femur and from upper third to supramalleolar area in the tibia.
- It can be used in the treatment of segmental fractures, comminuted fractures, bone loss, etc.
- It can be used for the treatment of nonunion.
- For reconstructive surgery following tumor excision.
- Low blood loss, low-risk of infection.
- Short operative time.

Principles

Static Locking

Here screws are placed both proximal and distal on either sides of the fracture. This neutralizes the rotation and restricts telescopy.

Indications

- Comminuted or butterfly fractures
- Spiral fractures
- Comminuted fracture with bone loss
- Lengthening and shortening osteotomies
- Atrophic nonunion
- Pathological fractures.

Dynamic Locking

Here screws are placed either proximal or distal depending on the site of fracture. It neutralizes rotation movements but allows certain movements at the fracture site favoring osteogenesis. It allows immediate mobilization and weight bearing.

Indications

- Proximal and distal fractures where there is good bone contact.
- Proximal and distal nonunion.
- Proximal and distal osteotomies in malunion.

Achieving Dynamization

This consists of removing of either proximal or distal screws of a static locked nail depending on the fracture site. During static locking, the fracture will have healed and become ossified, mobilization of upper and lower joints will not be possible. Dynamization can be performed within third

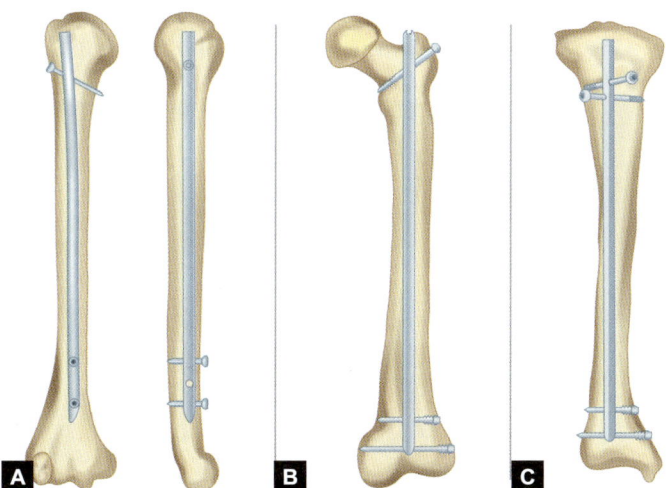

Figs 7.2A to C: Interlocking nails are a gold standard in the treatment of long bone fractures in adults: (A) Interlocking nail of humerus; (B) Interlocking nail of femur; (C) Interlocking nail of tibia

month of treatment. After removal of proximal or distal screws, full weight-bearing is permitted. This hastens the corticalization of the fracture and will lead to a fusiform callus of excellent quality.

What is New in Plate Osteosynthesis?

- *Minimally invasive skeletal stabilization (MISS)*
  a. *For intra-articular fractures* Transarticular joint reconstruction and a retrograde plate osteosynthesis (Mnemonic TARPO).
     Advantages
     - Better visualization.
     - Quicker fracture healing.
     - Better functional outcome.

> **Remember about Interlocking Nail**
> - It is a modification of standard IM nail.
> - It extends the indication of IM nail and can be used for a wide range of shaft fractures.
> - Low blood loss and low rate of infection.
> - Less operative time.
> - Technically demanding.
> - Requires sophisticated equipment like C-arm (Fig. 7.3).

  b. *For extra-articular fractures* (Minimally Invasive Percutaneous Plate Osteosynthesis, to remember use Mnemonic MIPPO).
     This technique consists of percutaneous plate fixation through stab incisions (Fig. 7.4).
- *Less invasive stabilization system (LISS):* This is another alternative, which behaves more like an internal fixator (Fig. 7.5).
- *Locked compression plates (LCP):* This consists of provision of two screw holes, one ordinary and the other to place a locked screw. It can be used in a wide variety of conditions like osteoporosis, pathological fractures, etc. It provides more rigid internal fixation with less bone loss and better union possibilities.

> **Briefly the Newer Techniques of Osteosynthesis are**
> - MISS
> - TARPO
> - MIPPO
> - LISS
> - LCP.

IMPROVEMENTS IN EXTERNAL FIXATION

ILIZAROV'S TECHNIQUE

Dr GA Ilizarov of Kurgan of Russia had developed a research center on the role of external fixators in the management of orthopedic problems. Deviating accidentally from the routine of applying compression, his assistant applied a distraction force much to the discomfiture of Dr Ilizarov. *However, he was surprised to see the bone growth in*

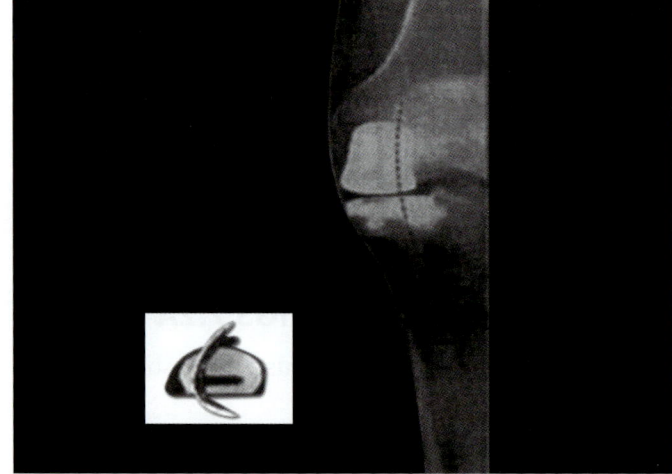

Fig. 7.4: Minimally invasive skeletal stabilization (MISS)

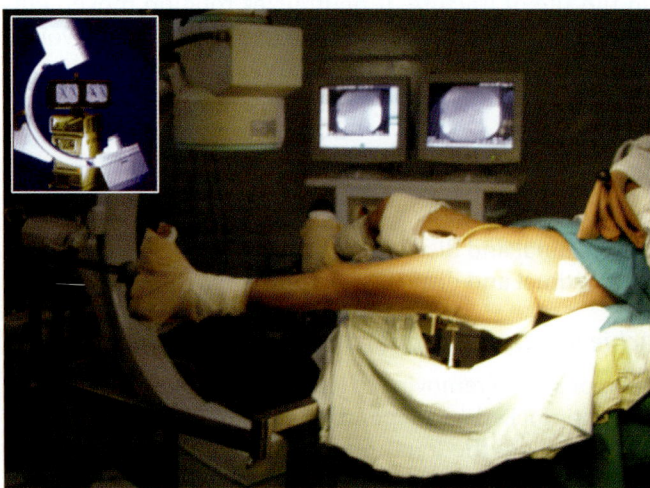

Fig. 7.3: C-arm is a necessary requirement for interlocking nailing and spine surgeries

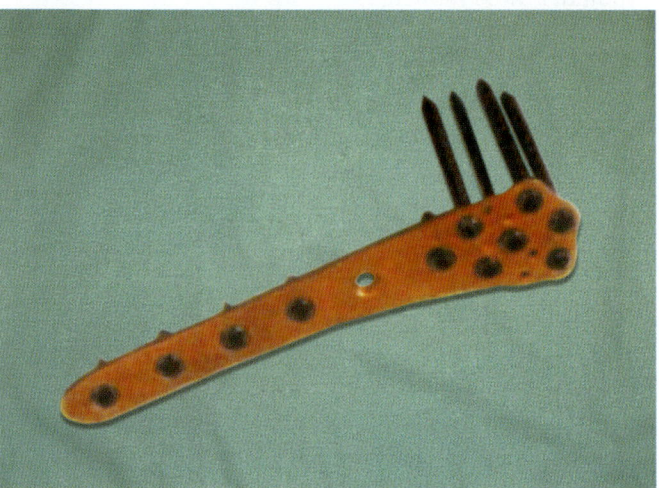

Fig. 7.5: Less invasive stabilization system (LISS)

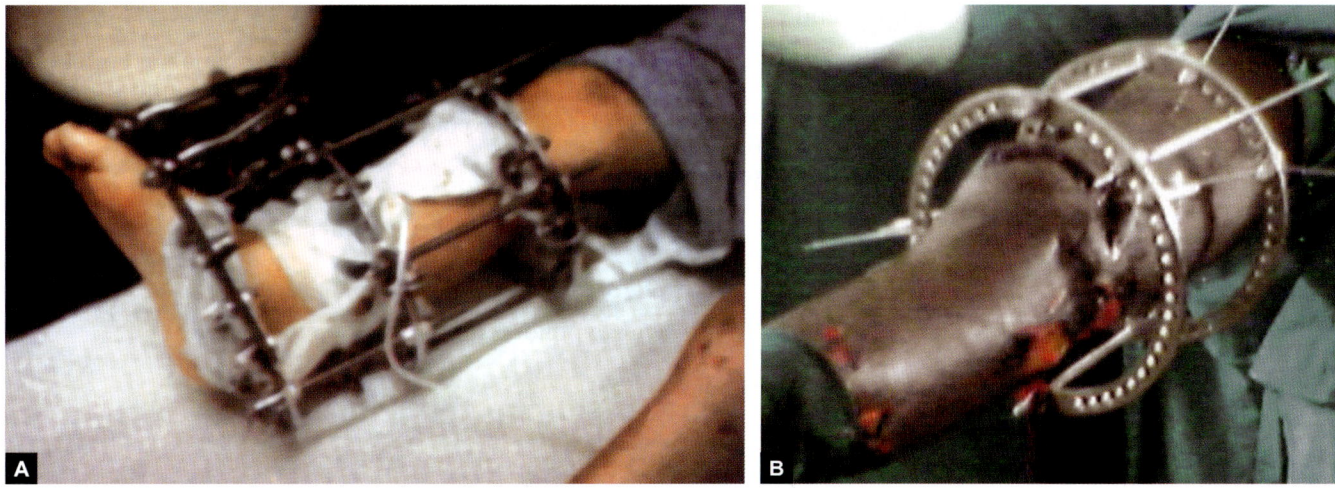

Figs 7.6A and B: (A) Ilizarov's frame; (B) Ilizarov fixator

spite of the distraction force. Little did he realize that he had discovered a new law, which was to revolutionize the management of nearly 65 percent of orthopedic conditions? He had found an answer to complex orthopedic problems hitherto unsolvable by conventional orthopedic procedures.

Hippocrates first described the use of external fixators in the management of fractures 2400 years ago. Conventionally, there are two types of external fixators: Pin fixator and ring fixator. Ilizarov developed the ring fixator in 1951 (Figs 7.6A and B).

Principles of Ilizarov's Method

An important law of nature which was not known to the biologists was "distraction or pulling apart of living tissue creates a new tissue of its own kind". It was the beginning of a new era of successfully treating unsolved orthopedic problems. The following are the principles of his method:

Law of Tension Force

When a living tissue is slowly pulled apart at the rate of 1 mm/day, it creates a new tissue. This is called distraction osteogenesis.

Use of a Unique Ring Fixator

Use of a unique ring fixator which is multilevel, multidirectional, multiplane external fixator and hence it is superior to other external fixators.

Corticotomy

In this procedure, only the cortex of the bone is cut subperiosteally and intramedullary circulation is left intact. Preservation of periosteum and intramedullary circulation produces a better quality of new bone.

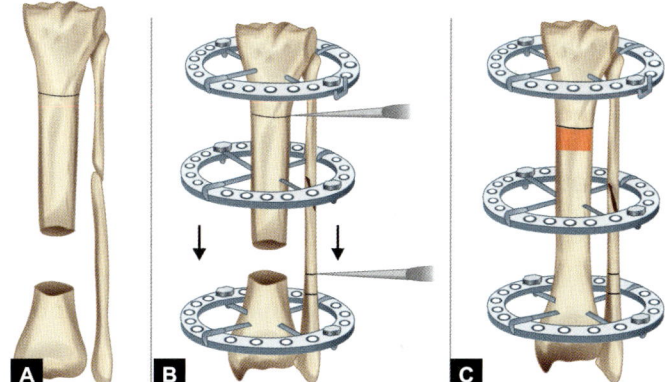

Figs 7.7A to C: Stages of distraction osteogenesis: (A) Bone gap; (B) Corticotomy and distraction; (C) Union

About Ring Fixator

Ring fixator is an exceptionally versatile circular external fixator. The system has good range of hard wires of various sizes and lengths, which can combine to produce a fantastic combination of around 500 types, which allows a precise control of bone segments including angulations, rotation, translation, lengthening and compression.

Stages

Distraction osteogenesis developed by Ilizarov has four stages (Figs 7.7A to C).
1. Stable fixation of low energy corticotomy to preserve the blood supply.
2. A short latency period before distraction for local bridging of the gap by fibrous tissue.
3. Slow gradual distraction to stimulate ossification during elongation at the rate of 1 mm/day.
4. Newly formed bone extends from each end of the osteotomy in full cross-section parallel to the distraction

force. When distraction is discontinued and relative compression is applied, ossification bridges the central gap.

The osteogenic area rapidly remodels to normal macrostructure and microstructure that is indistinguishable from the host bone histologically and roentgenographically.

Benefits of Ring Fixator System

- Simultaneous correction of multiplane deformities.
- Wide variety of indications treatable with one system.
- Thin tensioned wires allow for stable purchase in small fragments and osteoporotic bones.
- Early patient ambulation.
- Single surgical procedure.
- Light weight, high strength, radiolucent, composite half rings.
- Relatively simple method, no major surgery required.
- Ilizarov calls this a bloodless surgery, as no incision is required, if required it is only 1 to 2 cm.
- Removal of the assembly is very easy.

Indications

Complex Fractures

Ilizarov is very useful in treating some of the very complex fractures like open fractures, comminuted fractures, intra-articular fractures, etc.

Compound Fractures

Compound fractures with bone loss. The bone above can be mobilized to cover the gap by gradual distraction (Figs 7.8 and 7.9).

Nonunion

Ilizarov gives excellent result in the management of both infected and uninfected nonunion. It simultaneously attends to all the components of nonunion.

Limb Lengthening

As in achondroplasia and other shortenings.

Deformity Corrections

Due to polio, cerebral palsy, etc.

Other Important Indications

- Congenital pseudoarthrosis of tibia
- Stump-lengthening
- TAO
- Tumor excision and lengthening
- Foot deformities.

Complications

- Poor patient compliance.
- Damage to nerves and vessels during insertion.
- Wire tract infection, loosening or breakage.
- Joint contractures.
- Inadvertent injury to the patient or operating room personnel caused by the K-wire.

> **Remember About Ilizarov**
> - Makes use of the hitherto unknown principle that distraction stimulates osteogenesis
> - A single frame by arranging it in different combinations can be useful to solve 65 percent of orthopedic problems
> - The greatest boon is early ambulation and weight bearing

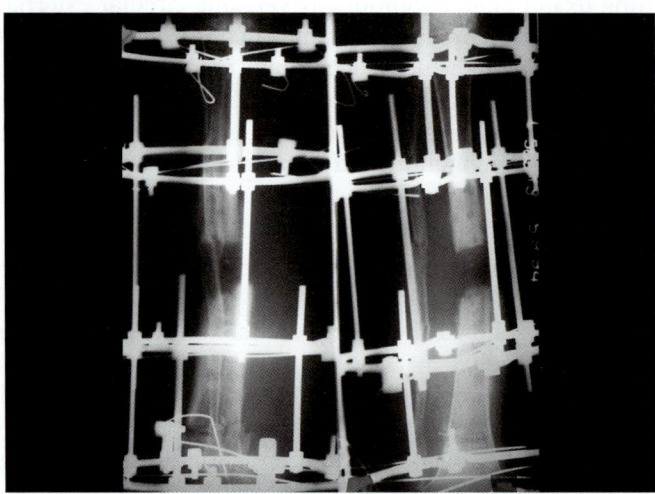

Fig. 7.8: Ilizarov frame indicated in bone loss

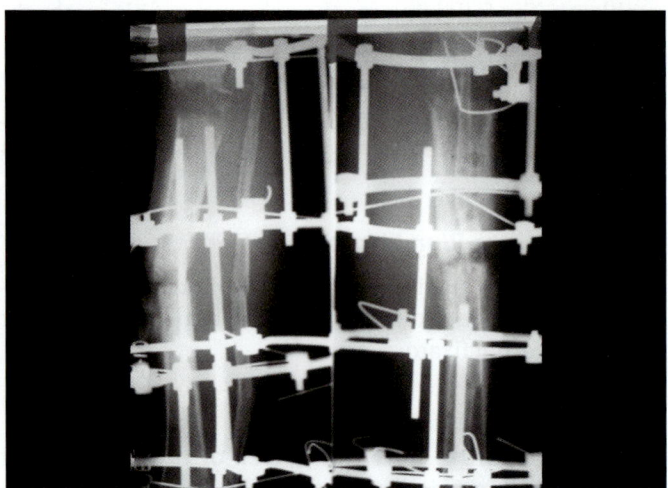

Fig. 7.9: Mobilization and closure of the gap

- Low rates of complications
- Virtually a bloodless surgery
- Very effective in the treatment of nonunion
- Cost-effective.

NEWER EXTERNAL FIXATORS

Umex™—Universal Mini External Fixator

This is an indigenous external fixator frame devised and popularized by our very own Indian pioneers. It has the following advantages over the conventional external fixators:
- It is lightweight
- It is cheap
- It can be applied to any part of the human skeleton unlike conventional fixators. Hence called universal frame
- It can be made indigenously
- Relatively few complications
- Comparatively less learning curve
- It can be customized and modulated according to the needs
- Better patient compliance.

Laser Treatment

Laser treatment for orthopedic problems like disk prolapse, synovitis, etc. is slowly gaining popularity in the West though it is yet to make a huge impact in our country (Fig. 7.10).

ADVANCES IN HIP SURGERY

Like the spine and the knee, the latest to join the bandwagon of minimally invasive procedure is the hip. Dr G Chana of England has devised minimally invasive surgeries for the hip replacement called the minimally invasive hip replacement (MIH) and minimally invasive hip resurfacing (MIHR), for trauma and hip diseases. It has the advantages of minimally invasive procedures like:
- Less blood loss
- Minimal exposure
- Shorter hospital stay
- Reduced hospitalization cost
- Faster mobilization
- Faster ambulation
- Minimal scarring.

Birmingham hip resurfacing arthroplasty: For only the diseased portion of the femoral head like as in AVN, on hip is done. Unlike in JHR where the entire head is removed. This is indicated in more younger patients.

RECENT ADVANCES IN SPINE SURGERY

Recent advances in spinal surgery paradoxically have resulted in less and less exposure for doing more and more inside the spine. Yes, I am talking about the 'keyhole' procedures, which have revolutionized the surgical management of the spine conditions. The notable ones among them are:
- Microscopic lumbar diskectomy: The conventional open method of diskectomy resulted in greater morbidity to the patient. With the advent of powerful operating microscope, C-arm and advanced spinal instrumentation, the same procedure can now be done with minimum exposure. This results in widespread benefits to the patients.

Pearls: Advantages of MLD
- Less exposure (less than 4 cm incision required)
- Minimum blood loss
- Early mobilization (Same day)
- Short hospital stays (2–3 days)
- Relatively inexpensive
- Early return to normal activities and work
- Faster rehabilitation

- Endoscopic lumbar diskectomy (ELD) (Fig. 7.11): This has the same beneficial effects as MLD and is known to further reduce the tissue trauma and blood loss.
- Minimum invasive spinal surgery (MISS): Now through this technique, using an operating endoscope, complex deformities of the spine-like the scoliosis, kyphosis, etc. can be corrected at one stage. Earlier these deformity corrective surgeries involved two-stage procedures with extensive blood loss, tissue trauma and big ugly scars. All these undesirable effects are outdated with the advent of MISS.

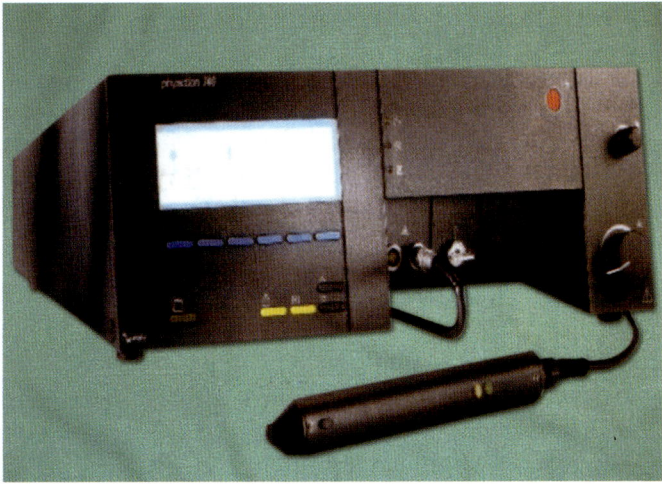

Fig. 7.10: Laser

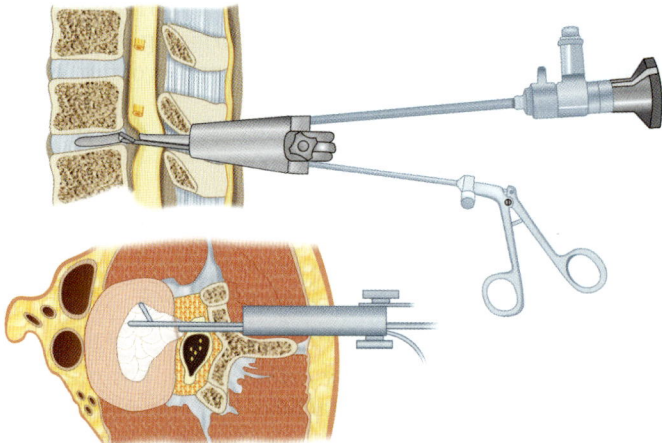

Fig. 7.11: Endoscopic diskectomy

- VATS (video-assisted thoracoscopic spine surgery): This is an endoscope procedure where anterior thoracic spine pathologies like TB, trauma, tumor, thoracic kyphosis and scoliosis can be successfully corrected. Here, the patient gets an opportunity to enjoy all the benefits of a MISS and get the above deformity corrected.

Interesting Facts

Remember 'T': in thoracoscopic spine surgery which is indicated in thoracic spine pathologies like:
- T: Tuberculosis
- T: Trauma
- T: Tumors
- T: Thoracic scoliosis
- T: Thoracic kyphosis

Facts You Need to Now: Get Yourself Familiar with the Following Terminology
- MOSS: Moderately open spine surgery
- MISS: Minimally invasive spine surgery
- MICOSS: Minimally invasive cosmetic spine surgery
- VATS: Video-assisted thoracoscopic surgery
- MLD: Microscopic lumbar diskectomy

- Artificial disk replacement (ADR) (Figs 7.12A and B) of late, damaged disks removed during surgeries is now being replaced by artificial disks. This is known to reduce the postsurgical morbidity and incidences of failed back after surgery.

RECENT ADVANCES IN BONE GRAFTING METHOD

Till recently, autologous bone grafting (ABG) was the 'gold standard' in orthopedic practice. Adaptive periosteal cambiplasty (APC) is fast emerging as an effective

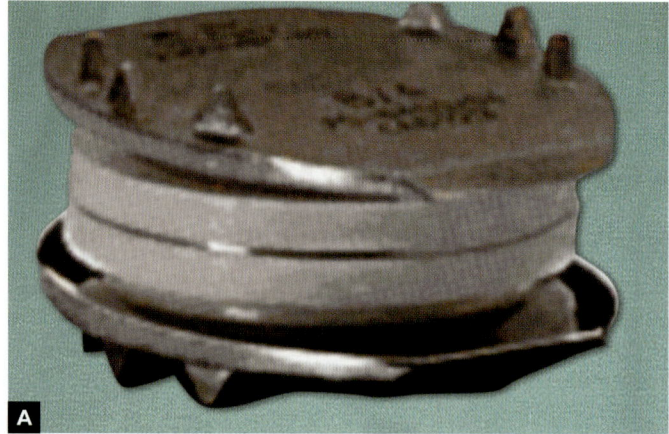

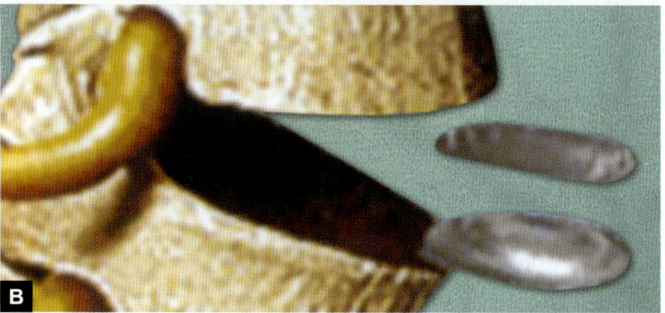

Figs 7.12A and B: Artificial disks

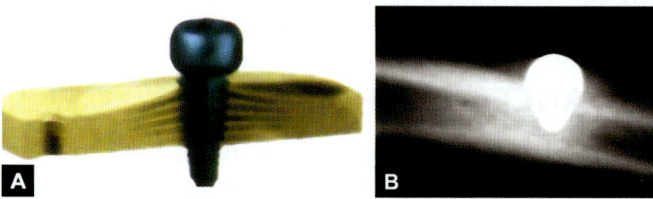

Figs 7.13A and B: Newer techniques of bone grafting by using differential conical screw

alternative for the time-tested ABG. Mechanical stimulation of healthy tibial shaft by percutaneous application of a specially adapted *differential conical screw* yields highly active osteogenic tissue, which can be used for autologous bone grafting (Figs 7.13A and B).

ADVANTAGES OVER THE CONVENTIONAL ABG

- More potent osteoinductor.
- Here the live cells of the cambium layer of the periosteum are activated.
- There is no immune rejection.
- There is minimum artificial injury.
- The healing is faster.

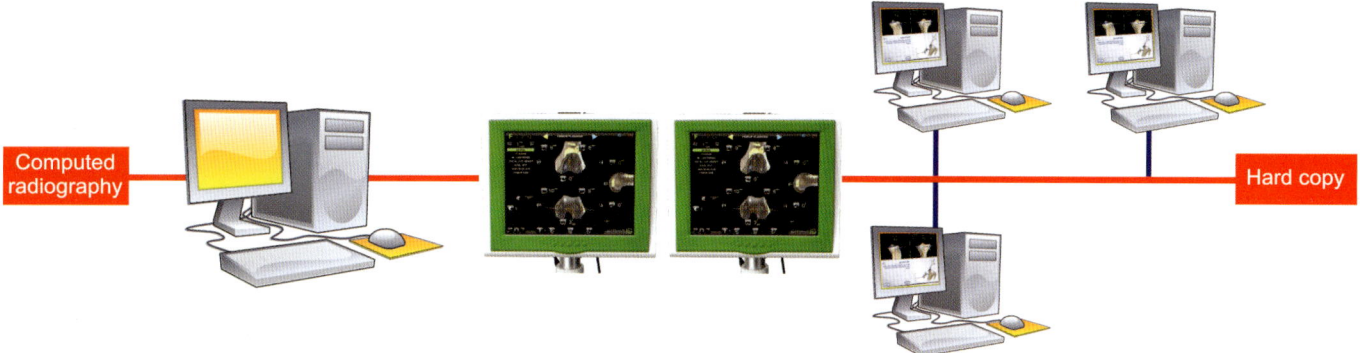

Fig. 7.14: Computers in orthopedics

Indications: It can be used for the same clinical conditions as ABG but with an enhanced healing response.

COMPUTERS IN ORTHOPEDICS

Globally computers have made inroads into almost all spheres of human life, so much so that it is hard to imagine life without them. Hence, it is no wonder that computers have started knocking the doors of orthopedic specialty.

In the West and now in our country surgeons, are relying more and more on computers for investigations, preoperative planning during operative procedures, especially in arthroplasty, better implant design, etc.? Whether all this will improve, the quality of orthopedic services is yet to be ascertained. However, it can be categorically said the future definitely belongs to computer-assisted operations in orthopedics (Fig. 7.14). Computer navigation surgeries for knee replacement, hip replacement and spinal instrumentation is gaining popularity in recent times.

8 CHAPTER

Fracture Healing Methods

INTRODUCTION

Bone makes a valiant attempt to get back to its original shape and form after having suffered humiliating fractures due to a myriad of incriminating forces. *Bone is unique in healing itself completely with a tissue that is indistinguishable from the original tissue hence there is no scar left.* The term *bone regeneration* and not *fracture healing* is more appropriate.

Bone is repaired by *callus*, which is a new tissue that may develop externally or internally. An *external callus* envelops around the outer aspect of the opposing ends of bone fragments. An *internal callus* forms between the bone ends.

During the first two days at the fracture site and away from the fracture site, in the deep layer of the periosteum the *osteogenic cells* proliferate and lift the fibrous layer of the periosteum away from the bone. *Marrow cells* also proliferate but to a lesser degree. These osteogenic cells differentiate into *osteoblasts,* which form the bone trabeculae resembling the embryonic tissue. The osteogenic cells lying away from the fracture site due to *inadequate vascularity* differentiate into chondroblasts and chondrocytes, which form the cartilage. The cartilage is finally converted into bone by endochondral ossification.

The internal callus is formed by the mesenchymal cells that convert into pro-osteoblasts and later to osteoblasts laying down new bone. *Remodeling* is an activity of *osteoclasts,* which slowly remove the necrotic bone and create cavities. Osteoblasts line these cavities and lay new bone.

METHODS OF FRACTURE HEALING

A fracture heals by three ways, indirect, direct and distraction histogenesis as described by Ilizarov.

INDIRECT FRACTURE HEALING

This is the common method of fracture healing where both external and internal callus are formed. Hunter has described six stages in this method of healing (Figs 8.1A to F).

Stage of Impact

This stage extends from the moment of impact until the complete dissipation of energy causing fractures.

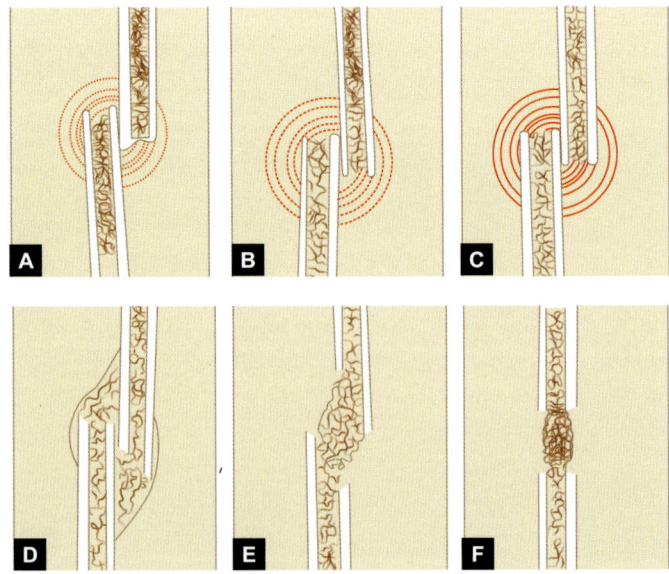

Figs 8.1A to F: Hunter' stages of fracture healing: (A) Stage of induction; (B) Stage of inflammation; (C) Stage of soft callus; (D) Stage of hard callus; (E) Stage of remodeling; (F) Normal

Stage of Induction

Following fractures, cells possessing osteogenic potential are activated. Other inducing factors are BMP (bone morphogenic protein), fall in oxygen tension and bioelectric effects.

Stage of Inflammation

In this stage, the disruption of blood supply results in necrosis of the bone ends. There is hemorrhage, cellular proliferation, and vascular ingrowths.

Stage of Soft Callus

Here the hematoma is organized with fibrous tissue, cartilage and woven bone. Fragments are united with fibrous or cartilaginous tissue or both.

Stage of Hard Callus

Bone fragments are firmly united with bone. If immobilization is complete, membranous bone healing takes place. If incomplete bone heals by endochondral ossification.

Stage of Remodeling

Here fiber bone is converted to lamellar bone. Medullary canal is reconstituted and callus diameter begins to decrease in size that takes a few months to several years. However, there will be no remodeling of rotational misalignment.

This method of fracture healing is seen in fractures treated by plaster immobilization (Fig. 8.2) and other forms of external and some limited internal fixation techniques.

Problems Associated with Indirect Fracture Healing
- Less anatomic union.
- Chances of malunion significant.
- Delayed joint mobilization.
- Possibility of fracture disease.

PRIMARY BONE HEALING (DIRECT BONE HEALING, HEALING BY PRIMARY INTENTION)

This type of bone repair is seen when bone fragments are anatomically reduced and rigidly fixed. This cannot be obtained by closed methods of fracture treatment but can be achieved by operative reduction and fixation with special techniques of plate and screws. Here ideally no external callus forms and there is no interposing fibrous tissue or cartilage tissue between the fracture sites. The fracture site is bridged by direct haversian remodeling which is almost a direct osteon-to-osteon hook-up. The osteoclasts act as cutter heads to remove the bone and are in the forefront promptly followed by osteoblasts behind laying down new bone. This type of bone healing usually occurs in fractures treated by AO techniques developed by Swiss association for osteosynthesis (Figs 8.3 and 8.4).

DISTRACTION HISTOGENESIS

Distraction histogenesis is a recent concept described by Ilizarov (Fig. 8.5). Here bone repair is induced by gradual distraction of osteotomies and fracture after an interval of induction say 5 to 7 days. For osteogenesis to occur

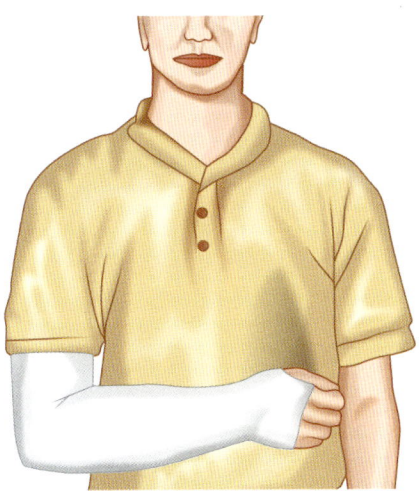

Fig. 8.2: An above elbow cast (Example of indirect fracture healing)

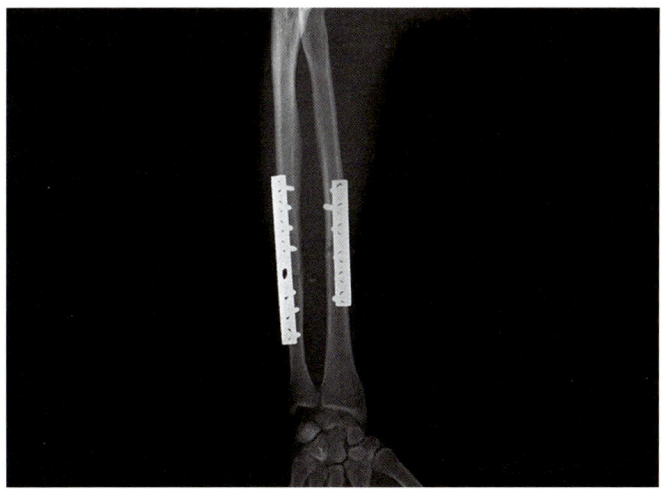

Fig. 8.3: Example of direct fracture healing

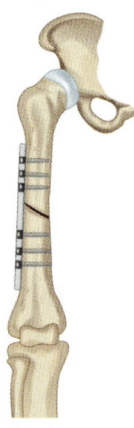

Fig. 8.4: Fracture shaft humerus fixed with DCP plate and screws (Example of direct fracture healing)

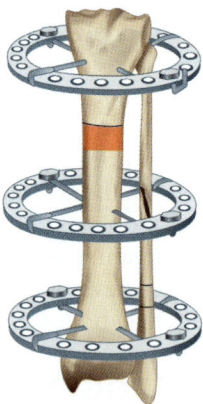

Fig. 8.5: Ilizarov's treatment is an example of healing by distraction histogenesis

the fracture or osteotomy must be stabilized and a slow distraction at the rate of 1 mm per day should be given. For details, see discussion on Ilizarov (refer page 80).

> **Remember**
> **Problems in primary bone healing**
> - Risk of anesthesia
> - Fracture hematoma lost
> - Infection
> - Bone healing is slower
> - Bone healing is inferior to indirect healing
> - Difficult to assess radiological union as no callus is seen
> - Implant failure is a possibility
> - Needs another operation to remove the implants
> - Chances of refracture are high
> - The only advantage seems is good anatomic reduction and chances of early mobilization.
>
> **Factors Affecting Fracture Repair**
> *Factors favoring union*
> - Adequate circulation
> - Hormones like growth hormone, parathormone, thyroxin, etc.
> - Good nutrition and mineral supplements help passively
> - Bioelectric fixation.
>
> *Factors detrimental to union*
> - Poor circulation
> - Infection
> - Distraction
> - Segmental fractures
> - Comminution
> - Osteoporosis
> - Soft tissue interposition
> - Inadequate and improper immobilization, etc.

9
CHAPTER

Soft Tissue Injuries

INTRODUCTION

Soft tissue injuries are not quite 'soft' but 'hard' in terms of management and rehabilitation. The term soft tissue implies skin, subcutaneous tissue, fascia, muscles, ligaments, tendons, synovium, capsules, nerves, etc (Fig. 9.1). Undoubtedly, they are more common than bony injuries. Sportspersons are more prone to suffer from soft tissue injuries than the normal population. Unlike in fractures, the soft tissue injury management is essentially conservative and physiotherapy appears to be the mainstay of treatment.

Mechanism of Injury

Direct Trauma

Due to fall, RTA, assault, etc. Contusion, hematomas, lacerations are some of the examples.

Indirect Trauma

Due to avulsion injuries, muscle pull, ligament sprain, etc. More commonly seen in sportspersons.

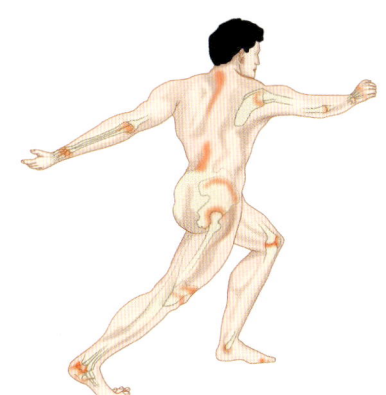

Fig. 9.1: Sites of common soft tissue injuries

Approach to a Patient with Soft Tissue Injury

The Patient's Story

Listen to what the patient has to say about the problem. Do not be swayed by his story. He may be going overboard. Take his complaints with a 'pinch of salt'. This is the subjective assessment.

Your Observation

This is your assessment of the problem based on 'his' story. Make an objective assessment of the injury with regard to site, nature, intensity of pain, etc. of the injury. Your evaluation may or may not correlate with 'his' story. Evaluate carefully the functional problem, interpret it analytically, and individualize the treatment plan.

Goal Setting

A surgeon needs to set-up goals while treating soft tissue injuries. These could be immediate or long-term.

Execution of Your Plan

Having made a careful evaluation of the injury; you have sized up the problem and formulated your modus operandi. Keeping both the short- and long-term goals in mind. Unleash your plan of action now to bottle up this genie.

Treatment Goals of Soft Tissue Injury

Immediate Goals

This aims to 'nip' the problem in the bud and 'prevent' further damages from taking place. A look at the priorities clarifies this:

SECTION 1: Traumatology

- If there is blood loss—arrest it, prevent it, control it.
- If there is swelling—try to minimize it.
- If there is pain—try to alleviate it.
- If there is joint stiffness—try to prevent it.
- In all possibility try to see that there is no further damage whatsoever once you are in charge of the injury!
- In the event of muscle weakness—try to maintain the power.

Thus, immediate goals aim at 'prevention' of further damage and injuries to the soft tissues.

The Distant Goals

Here your efforts are to put the derailed life of the soft tissues back on rails and restore the structures to their pre-injury state. No mean task this and it calls for a sustained and skillful approach. The priorities in this are as under:

- *Movements:* Restore it to as normal as possible.
- *Mobility:* Ensure the affected joints are back to their best.
- *Strength:* The affected muscles need to be given their strength and endurance back.
- *Kinesthetic/proprioception mechanism:* Restore it back to normal.
- *Daily or functional activities:* Restore it back to the original.
- *Confidence:* Boost the patient's morale and that of the affected part.
- *Keep away:* The swelling, edema from raising its ugly head again. Once bitten twice shy, hence no more such injuries.
- *Last but not the least:* Ensure that this problem will not surface again by practicing effective anti-recurrent methods.
- *Inculcate:* A sense of discipline in practicing regular follow-up and valuing the medical advice. Drive home the advantages of 'home care' programs. Instill in them a thought that, "it pays to be your own doctor in the safe confines of their home!"

Classification of Soft Tissue Injury

The four broad classifications for STI are as follows:
- Strains
- Sprains
- Ruptures
- Contusions.

Let us now discuss each one in detail.

MUSCLE INJURY (STRAINS)

Definition

Injury to the muscle and tendons is called *strain* (Fig. 9.2).

Reasons

- Sudden unaccustomed or abrupt action or movements may tear the muscles.
- Direct trauma can also injure the muscles and tendons.
- Overstretching of muscles due to indirect trauma, especially in sportspersons.

Types

Acute strain: This is due to sudden violent force or direct trauma.

Chronic strain: This is due to injury existing since a long period leading to muscle ischemia and fibrosis.

Pathophysiology

Injury to the muscles leads to pain. As a result, the muscle goes into spasm to limit the movements and reduce pain. Nevertheless, paradoxically, this protective muscle spasm causes pain due to stimulation of pain fibers and thus a vicious cycle sets in (Fig. 9.3). The painful stimuli cause muscle spasm through the peripheral nociceptive stimuli (Fig. 9.4).

Severity of Strain

First Degree Strain (Mild Contusion)

This is due to blunt injury and is due to direct trauma of low intensity.

Pathology: Few muscle fibers are torn. Bleeding is minimal and the fascia remains intact.

Clinical Features

- Localized pain and tenderness.
- Pain and spasm prevents muscle stretching.
- Function is not impaired largely.
- Tenderness over the affected muscles.

All the above features are shown in Figure 9.5.

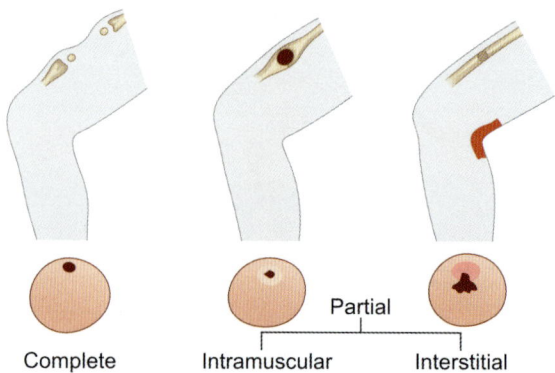

Fig. 9.2: Types of muscle strains

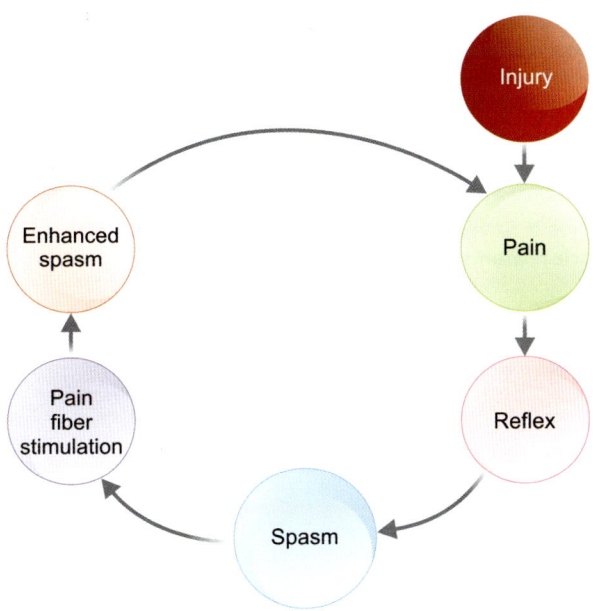

Fig. 9.3: Pain and spasm: The vicious cycle

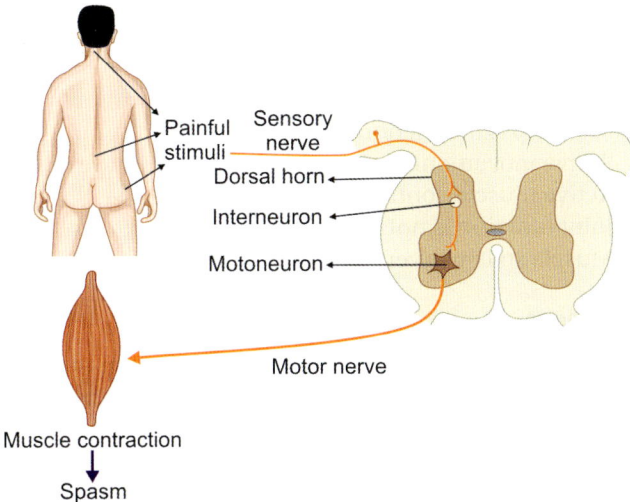

Fig. 9.4: Induction of prolonged muscle contractions (spasm) by peripheral nociceptive stimuli

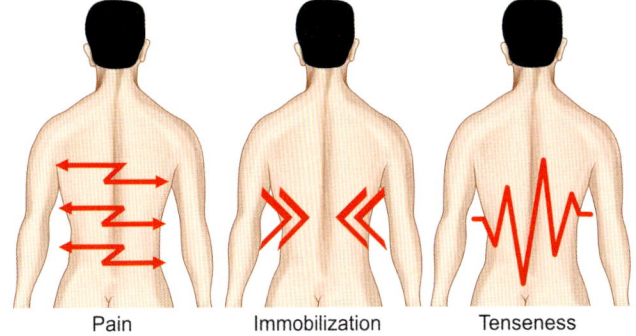

Fig. 9.5: Main symptoms of continuous muscle contractions (muscle spasms) in locomotors system: Pain, immobilization and tenseness-tenderness of muscles

Management
- First aid is by cryotherapy (by application of ice) for a period of 20 minutes.
- Gentle active muscle stretch may be permitted after 20 to 60 minutes.
- Compression bandaging with optimum pressure.
- Low dose and low power ultrasound helps.
- Gentle massaging of the surrounding area helps.
- If pain is minimal, the patient can be allowed to do the light work the next day.

Second Degree Strain

Cause: Here the trauma is more serious.

Pathology
- Greater number of muscle fibers is torn.
- There is bleeding.
- The fascia is still intact.
- Hematoma is still localized.

Clinical Features
- Pain is more severe.
- Tenderness is severe.
- Severe muscle spasm.
- The patient is unable to move the limb.

Third Degree Strain

Cause: Undoubtedly, these injuries are due to trauma of a greater magnitude.

Pathology: Larger area and greater number of muscle fibers are involved. More than one muscle group may be involved. The fascia is partially torn. Bleeding is widespread and more. There could be both intramuscular and intermuscular bleeding. The patient experiences severe pain and loss of function.

Symptoms: Here all the above symptoms are of greater intensity.

Treatment in Grade II and III Strains

For First 24 Hours
- Immediate application of ice.
- Compression bandage.
- Limb elevation.
- Limb immobilized in splints.
- Isometrics to the muscles, which are immobilized.
- Active exercises to the unaffected joints.
- Pulsed electromagnetic field therapy (PEMF) is known to help.
- No active movements to the affected muscles.

During the Next 24 to 48 Hours

- The pressure bandage is removed and active muscle exercises are begun.
- Stretching within the limits of pain is commenced.
- Thermotherapy: Ultrasound, short wave diathermy and TENS help to relieve pain.
- Slow rhythmic massaging helps relieve the muscle spasm.
- Nonweight bearing on crutches is slowly started.
- Rest of the measures is the same as above.

Between 48 and 72 Hours

Apart from all the measures mentioned so far, the additional measures during this phase include:
- More vigorous active movements are encouraged.
- Deep transverse friction massage is added.
- Partial weight bearing can be permitted.

After 72 Hours

- All the above measures are pursued in a more vigorous manner.
- Pressure bandage is totally removed.
- Progressive resisted exercises using the Fowler technique by taking out 10 to 12 repetition maximum (RM), is practiced.
- Full weight bearing should be permitted in injuries of the lower limbs.
- After full movement is regained, the patient is allowed to walk and jog.
- Full functional activity should be regained by 4 to 6 weeks.

The various drugs used in the treatment of muscle strain to relieve pain and muscle stiffness is depicted in Table 9.1.

Grade Four Strain

Cause

This is usually caused by severe trauma.

Pathology

- Complete tear of the muscle (Figs 9.6A and B).
- The fascia is torn.
- Considerable bleeding which is intramuscular and diffuse.
- Gross swelling is present.

Clinical Features

- Excruciating pain
- Severe tenderness is present
- A snapping sound may be heard by the patient

TABLE 9.1: Treatment of muscle strain by conservative methods in a nutshell

Systemic Therapy

Analgesic anti-inflammatory drugs
- Antipyretic analgesics
- Nonsteroidal anti-inflammatory drugs
- Narcotic analgesics

Muscle relaxants
- At muscular level
- At neuromuscular level
- At spinal level
- At supraspinal level

Psychotropic drugs
- Antidepressants
- Neuroleptics
- Minor tranquillizers

Others
- Calcitonin
- Beta-blockers

Local therapy
- Local anesthetics
- Steroids
- Transdermal application of analgesic anti-inflammatory drugs (ointments)

- Palpable gap between the muscles felt
- Severe loss of function
- Active movements produced by the agonist are absent
- Active muscle contraction is absent
- Joint function is not lost
- Muscle spasm is very severe (Fig. 9.7).

Treatment

- Surgery is advised. This involves opening the ruptured site, evacuating the hematoma and suturing the fascial sheath. Direct muscle repair is avoided.
- Compression bandage is applied and the limb is immobilized for 2 to 3 weeks.
- Active exercises to the unaffected joints.
- Slow rhythmic isometric exercises to the affected muscles.
- Non-weight bearing after 48 hours.
- The use of low frequency current (faradism) to obtain passive contraction is very useful.
- Deep heating modalities like ultrasound, etc. help.
- Rest of the measures is same as for Grade II/III injuries.

Note:
Mild muscle strain is also called by lay public as muscle pull.

INJURIES TO THE JOINTS

During an injury to a joint, three things could happen:
- Injury to the ligaments only.

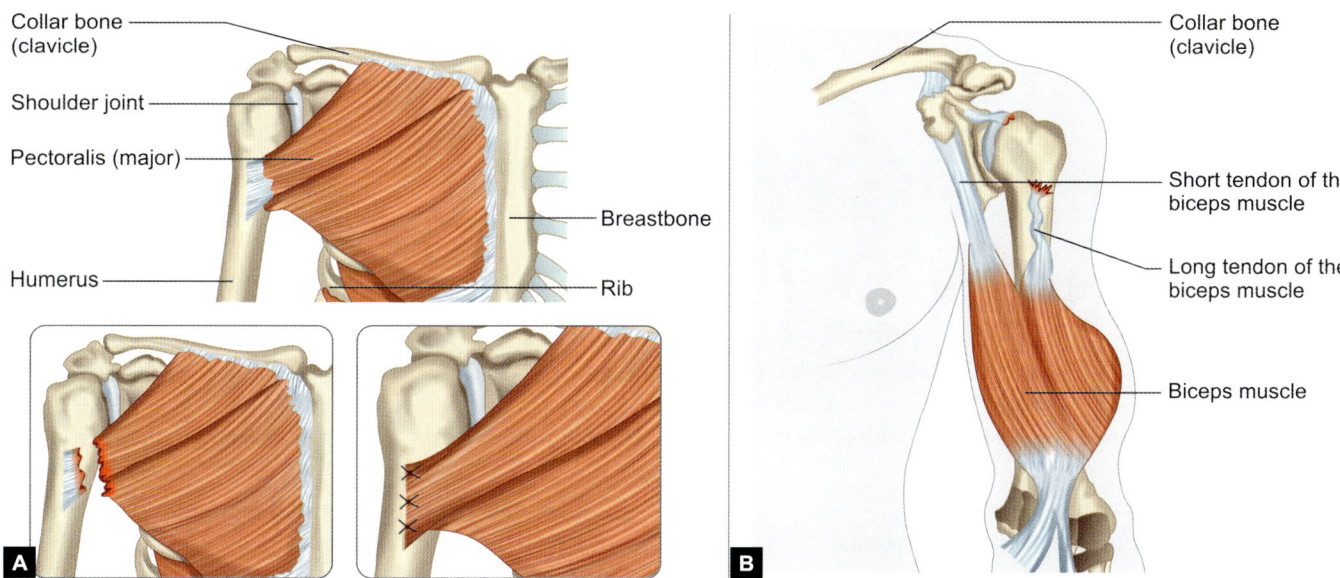

Figs 9.6A and B: Muscle ruptures that are common: (A) Rupture of pectoralis major muscle; (B) Rupture of biceps tendon

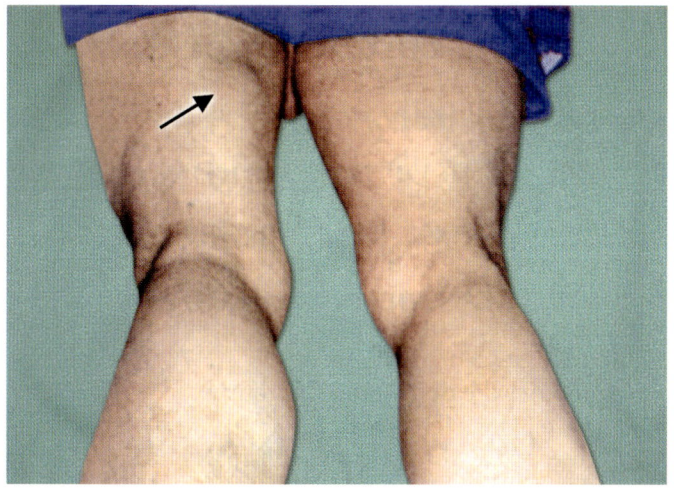

Fig. 9.7: Grade IV muscle strain (Hamstring strain) (Clinical photo)

- Injury to the synovium.
- Both (According to Bass, 1969).

Ligament Injury

A ligament injury is called "Sprain." Depending on the severity, it could be mild (Grade I), moderate (Grade II) or severe (Grade III).

Anatomy

Ligaments are made of fibrous tissues, which are arranged longitudinally. They are tough and elastic. Their vascularity is poor and heals always by scar tissue due to lack of special cells.

Functions

Ligaments serve the following functions:

Support: By reinforcing the capsule, they provide support to the joint.

Stability: By holding the bony ends together, it provides stability.

Protection: The strength of the ligaments offers protection to the joints along with the muscles.

Problems of Healing

- Poor vascularity delays the healing
- Repair is by scar tissue
- Inadequate period of immobilization results in healing with tissue that is more fibrous. This will result in excessive laxity making the joint unstable
- Intermittent stretching strengthens the ligament while continuous stretch leads to adhesions due to periosteal irritation.

Types of Sprain (Fig. 9.8)

Grade I (Minor)

- Slight pain and tenderness at the site of injury
- Slight swelling and loss of function
- Stretch test will be positive clinching the diagnosis.

Treatment

First day
- Cryotherapy to alleviate pain
- Pressure bandage—to prevent swelling

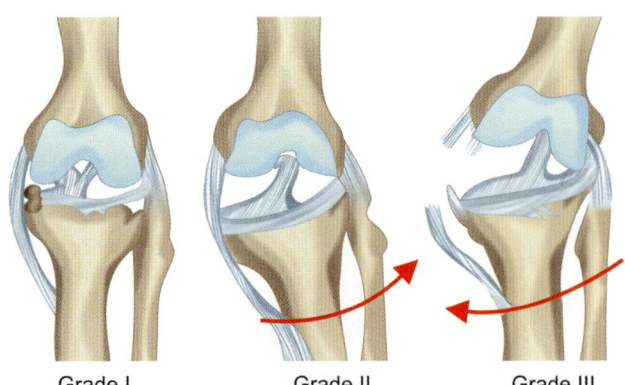

Fig. 9.8: Sprain of medial collateral ligament of the knee

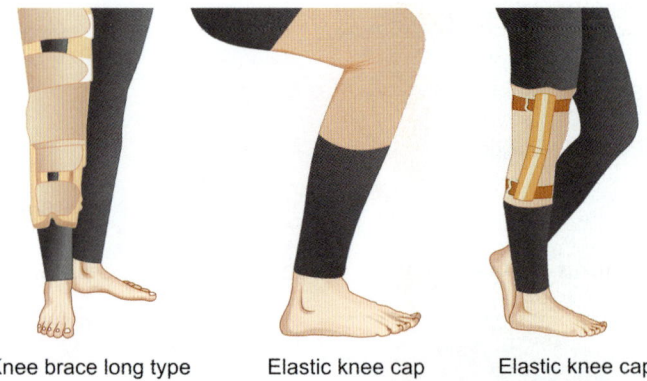

Fig. 9.9: Various elastic knee braces to support the knee joint

- Limb elevation—to prevent swelling
- Active movements of the unaffected joints.

Second day onwards
- Add thermotherapy, stop ice therapy.
- Begin isometric exercises to the affected muscles.
- Weight bearing may be permitted.
- Rest of the measures is same as mentioned above.

Grade II (Severe)
- More force results in this injury
- The ligament may be partially torn or detached from the attachment
- Swelling is more severe
- Pain and tenderness are also more acute
- Movement is grossly restricted
- Weight bearing is difficult
- Function is severely affected.

Treatment
- Cryotherapy
- Compression bandaging or kneecap and braces (Fig. 9.9)
- Elevation
- Rest of the measures same as in Grade I.

Grade III (Complete rupture)
- Severe violence
- Gross swelling
- Pain and tenderness is quite severe
- Joint is unstable
- The patient is unable to bear weight
- Severe loss of function.

Treatment
- *Conservative*
  - Immediate application of ice
  - Compression bandaging
  - Foot end elevation
  - Isometric exercises to the affected limbs
  - Active exercises to affected joints
  - POP cast for 6 to 8 weeks if ligament tear does not cause displacement.
- *Surgical*
  - If the ligament is torn and displaced, it needs surgical repair and immobilization with a POP cast for 6 to 8 weeks.
  - Isometric exercises are started after one week
  - Non-weight-bearing for 3 to 4 weeks

After Removal of the POP Cast

- *Thermotherapy:* Ultrasound, TENS, or SWD helps to relieve pain
- Pressure bandage helps to control the swelling
- Limb elevation to prevent edema
- Transverse friction massage to relieve spasm
- Active exercises to the affected joints are begun slowly and progressed gradually
- Isometrics are done more vigorously
- Passive ROM exercises
- Active, active-resisted, and self-resisted exercises are prescribed
- Weight-bearing is slowly encouraged from partial to full after 6 to 8 weeks
- The patient should be functionally independent by 8 to 12 weeks.

Injury to the Synovium

Relevant Anatomy

Synovium is a lining covering the capsule of the joint, tendon sheaths, etc. It has a rich blood and nerve supply. It is present throughout the body.

Functions

Synovium produces synovial fluid, which serves the following functions:

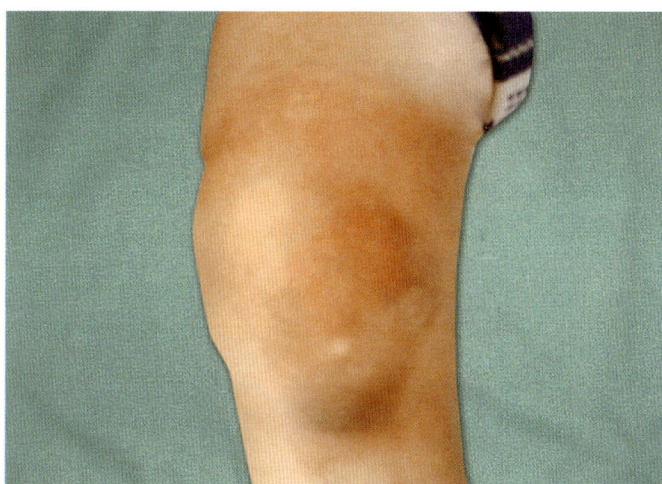

Fig. 9.10: Clinical photo showing traumatic synovitis of the knee joint

- Facilitates frictionless, smooth joint movements.
- Helps in the nourishment of cartilages.

Causes

Inflammation of synovium is called *synovitis*. It could be due to trauma, arthritis, chondromalacia, rheumatoid arthritis, TB, hemophilia, etc. (Fig. 9.10)

Types

- Acute—due to trauma
- Chronic—due to diseases like TB, rheumatoid arthritis, trauma, etc.

Clinical Features

- Swelling of the joint (develops slowly say within 2 to 24 hours)
- The joint is hot and red
- Pain is present over the injured structure
- Feeling of tension or pressure due to swelling
- To accommodate the excess fluid, the joint will assume a flexion attitude (position of ease)
- Muscle atrophy will be quite significant.

In the Event of Synovial Rupture

- The patient feels sudden pain at the back of the knee while getting up from a chair, getting down the stairs, etc.
- The swelling may spread rapidly to the calf muscles. Homan's sign will be positive (see page 42).

Treatment

Aim: To prevent muscle atrophy and joint contractures by a graduated exercise regimen.

Methods

During first 24 hours

- Ice therapy
- Compression bandage
- Limb elevation
- Isometric contraction of the affected limb muscles.
- Active movements of the ankle joint
- Active movements of the unaffected joints
- Splinting of the affected part.

After 48 hours

- Aspiration of the joint if swelling persists even after 48 hours. Aspiration of the knee should be done in major OT under full aseptic conditions by giving local anesthesia. The technique of knee aspiration is shown in Figures 9.11A to E.
- Sustained isometric contraction of the muscles
- Small range gradual active movements with adequate support should now be begun
- Partial weight bearing may be allowed
- Gradually progressive resistive exercises should be started to achieve full function.

Note:
Hemarthrosis vs. synovitis

In hemarthrosis:
- The swelling is rapid in onset (<2 hours).
- Swelling is more generalized.
- Pain on extreme movements.
- Joint instability may be present in cases of complete rupture.

Chronic Synovitis

This is due to various diseases affecting the synovium usually of more than three weeks' duration.

Tuberculosis of the joints, rheumatoid arthritis, etc. is some of the examples.

Problems of Chronic Synovitis

- Firm swelling
- Muscle atrophy may be gross
- Joint stiffness may be considerable
- Lax ligaments create instability
- Mild pain unlike acute synovitis.

Treatment

- Resistive exercises to the affected limbs
- Isometric exercises to the affected parts
- Passive ROM exercises to over come joint stiffness
- Proper gait training

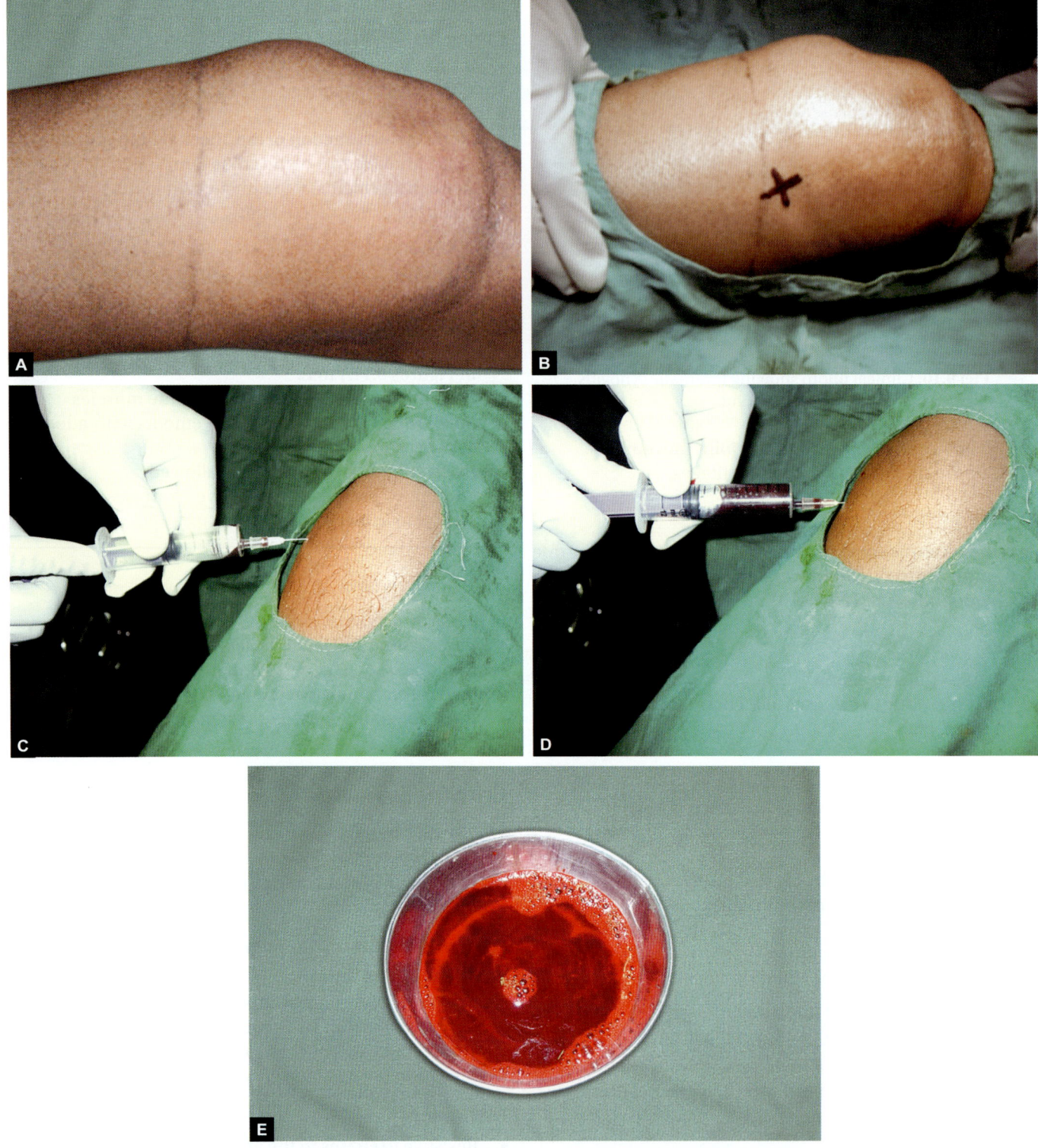

Figs 9.11A to E: Technique of knee aspiration: (A) Gross swelling of the knee (Clinical photo); (B) Mark the point of aspiration; (C) Part prepared and draped, local anesthesia given; (D) Thick blood being drained out; (E) Frank thick blood devoid of fat globules

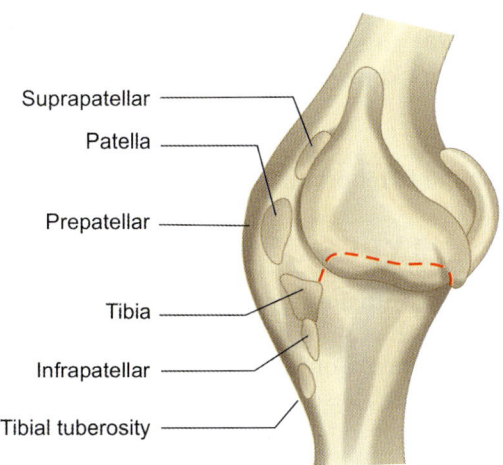

Fig. 9.12: Knee joint has many bursae around it

- Ultrasound, transcutaneous electrical nerve stimulation (TENS), short-wave diathermy (SWD), and other heat modalities to overcome pain and spasm.

Injury to the Bursa

Bursae are thin membranous sac lined with synovial membrane situated at the ends or certain important locations of the bones where tendons, etc. pass over them (Fig. 9.12).

Functions

- To prevent friction between two structures like tendons and bones that is liable to be rubbed against each other.
- To prevent wear and tear of muscles and tendons
- To protect the structures from pressure and injury.

Types

True bursa: They are normally present in the body at certain important situations like beneath the acromion, elbow, knee, heel, etc.

False bursa: They are also called as adventitious bursa. They develop due to external trauma, pressure, etc.

Causes

The causes of bursitis are as follows:
- *Trauma* may be due to a single blow or repetitive trauma.
- *Infection* acute or chronic (e.g. TB)
- *Metabolic disorders,* e.g. gout, etc.
- *Abnormal external pressures,* etc. (e.g. hip ischial tuberosity, etc.).
- *Inflammatory disorders,* e.g. rheumatoid arthritis, etc.
- *Unaccustomed activity,* exercise or ill-fitting shoes, etc.
- *Due to excessive pressure,* friction, etc. (e.g. olecranon bursitis, student's elbow, etc.).

Common Sites

Upper Limbs
a. Subacromion
b. Olecranon

Lower Limbs
a. Prepatellar
b. Tendo-Achilles
c. Medial side of the great toe
d. Lateral side of the little toe.

Clinical Features

- Pain, more so if it ruptures
- Swelling is tender and hot
- Movements of the joint may be painful
- Tenderness may be present
- Limp due to glutei bursitis, etc.

Treatment

In bursitis due to friction

- Rest to the part.
- Thermotherapy: ultrasound, SWD, TENS, etc
- Cryotherapy in initial stages (first 24 to 48 hours)
- Restricted weight bearing
- Isometric exercises to the affected part
- Muscle strengthening exercises
- Joint mobilization if there is restriction
- Injection of hydrocortisone in intractable cases
- Excision of the bursa, if chronic and troublesome.

Infective bursitis

- Appropriate antibiotics
- Rest of the measures is same as above.

Chronic cases

- Appropriate supports like felt pad, footwear modifications, etc.
- Avoiding repeated frictional movements, e.g. shoulder abduction in subdeltoid bursa)
- Relaxed passive movements to avoid friction
- Active limited ROM exercises with strong isometrics
- Progressive resistive exercises
- Deep heating like US, SWD, TENS, etc.
- Deep friction massage
- Active exercises to the unaffected joints
- Isometrics with limb in elevation helps considerably.

Tenosynovitis

This is due to inflammation of the synovial lining of the tendon sheath. The fibrous sheath is, however, not affected.

Types

Irritative: Due to abnormal or excessive friction. There is pain and crepitus on palpation. The movements are not affected and there are no adhesions. There is watery effusion due to sheath inflammation.

Infective: May be due to acute pyogenic infection or chronic infection like TB, etc.

Treatment

Irritative
- Rest to the part by appropriate splints
- Avoid movements at the joints
- Bandaging or POP cast
- Thermotherapy, US, SWD, or TENS
- Deep friction massage
- Difficult cases, hydrocortisone injection
- Intractable cases, surgical excision
- Shoe modifications, etc.

Infective
- Appropriate antibiotics
- Immobilization for 2 to 3 months
- Rest of the measures is the same as mentioned above.

Tenovaginitis

Unlike in tenosynovitis, here the fibrous sheath and not the synovial sheath of the tendon are affected. Though patient may complain of pain, crepitus is conspicuous by its absence, e.g. de Quervain's disease (Fig. 9.13).

Though the exact cause is unknown (Adams 1981), Cyrius (1978) says it may be due to repeated strains. Infection is not known to cause this problem.

Treatment

This is similar to tenosynovitis.

SPECIAL TYPES OF MUSCLE INJURIES

- **Bruise or contusion:** It is nothing but the Grade I muscle strain. This has already been discussed and is called a superficial hematoma.
- **Hematomas:** These are deep in nature and two types are described:

Intramuscular Hematoma

- Here blood is contained within the muscle and is bound by an intact muscle sheath.
- Following an injury, bleeding occurs and stops within two hours.
- There is localized swelling.
- If there is further trauma, more bleeding may occur.

Intermuscular Hematoma

- Here the sheath of the muscle is torn resulting in extravasations of blood between the muscle and fascial planes.
- The hematoma is more diffuse
- Bleeding will be more as the tension does not build-up to stop it.
- Due to gravity, it tracks down and may cause discoloration beneath the skin.
- For the first 48 hours, it is difficult to differentiate between the above hematomas (Fig. 9.14).

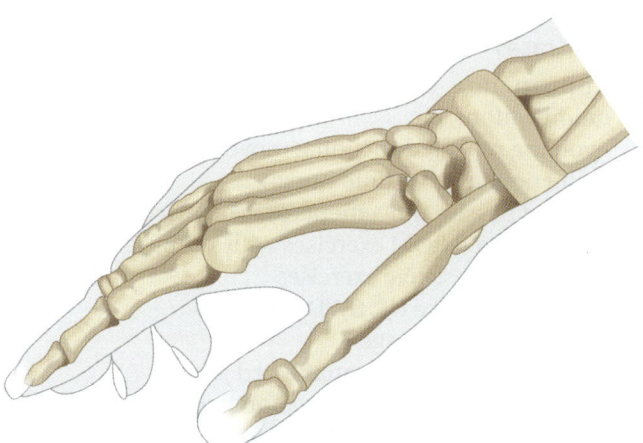

Fig. 9.13: de Quervain's disease, an example of tenovaginitis

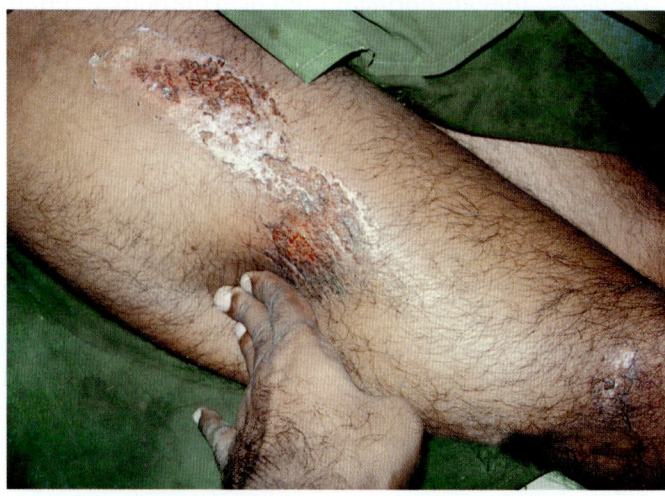

Fig. 9.14: Hematoma of the thigh (Clinical photo)

> **Quick Facts**
> *Features of intermuscular hematomas*
> - Moderate pain
> - Swelling reduces drastically by 48 to 72 hours
> - Muscle contraction is regained first
> - Due to tracking swelling may be seen at a distance away from the site of injury.

Treatment

Aim is to prevent further bleeding.

Methods

- Rest to the part
- Immobilize the affected part with splint
- Cryotherapy to relieve pain and spasm
- Pressure bandage to control the swelling
- Limb elevation to prevent edema.

> **Note:**
> In hematomas, there is no loss of function. If there is loss of function then it may be a Grade II/III muscle strain.

IMPORTANT SOFT TISSUE PROBLEMS

Given below is a list of important soft tissue problems in orthopedics. Please refer the appropriate sections for details.

Upper Limb

Shoulder

- Rotator cuff injuries
- Supraspinatus tendonitis
- Infraspinatus tendonitis
- Subscapularis tendonitis
- Adhesive capsulitis
- Tendonitis of the long head of biceps.

Elbow

- Tennis elbow
- Golfer's elbow
- Student's or Miner's elbow (see page 375).

Wrist

- Ganglion
- de Quervain's disease
- Dupuytren's contracture
- Trigger finger
- Carpal tunnel syndrome
- Mallet finger.

Lower Limbs

Hip and Pelvis

- Piriformis syndrome
- Iliotibial tract syndrome
- Glutei bursitis
- Trochanteric bursitis.

Knee and Leg

- Bursa around the knee
- Collateral ligament injury
- Cruciate ligament injury
- Meniscal injury
- Quadriceps strain
- Hamstrings strain
- Calf muscle strain
- Patellar tendonitis
- Plica syndrome.

Ankle and Foot

- Ankle sprain
- Plantar fasciitis
- Calcaneal spurs
- Morton's neuroma
- Tendo-Achilles injuries
- Tarsal tunnel syndrome.

Tendons and Nerves

- Injuries of flexor and extensor tendons of the hand.
- Injuries to the nerves. Please refer to chapter on Peripheral Nerve Injuries.

10 CHAPTER

Fractures in Special Situations

FRACTURES IN CHILDREN

Fractures in children are different from fractures in adults for the following reasons:
- Complete fractures are rare due to thick periosteal sleeve and greater elasticity
- For the same reasons mentioned above, buckle (Torus fractures) and greenstick fractures are more common
- Fracture displacements are relatively less common
- Fracture bleeding is also less
- Avulsion fractures are more common because bone gives away much earlier than the ligaments
- Disruptions of the epiphyseal plate are relatively more common because they form the weakest portion of the bone in the children and account for nearly one-third of all childhood fractures
- A pediatric fracture unites faster
- Differential periosteal activity causes better remodeling which is more likely in (i) the younger the child, (ii) the nearer the fracture to the epiphyseal plate, and (iii) if the deformity is angulated in the plane of the joint movement
- All tissues in children not only heal well but rapidly too
- Joint stiffness a bugbear in adults, rarely happens in children.

Incidence

- Fracture accounts for 10–25 percent of all injuries in childhood.
- Common between 11 and 14 years of age
- Boys account for 62 percent of all cases
- Fracture distal end of forearm is the most common skeletal injury in children contributing 25 percent of all fractures in them.

Etiology

- Falls are the most predominant cause in children.
- Traffic accidents, especially bicycle accidents account for 12 percent of cases.
- Sporting activities contribute 21 percent.
- *Birth fractures:* The clavicle is the most commonly injured bone during birth (accounts for 40 to 50% of all birth injuries), followed by brachial plexus injury (usually during instrumental rotation of the vertex), the humerus (injured during breech delivery) and the femur in that order.
- *Pathological fractures:* The conditions leading to pathological fractures could be:
  - Generalized, e.g. osteogenesis imperfecta, metabolic disorders, etc.
  - Localized to one limb, e.g. fibrous dysplasia.
  - Localized to the lesion, e.g. benign cystic condition of the bone, infection, benign and malignant neoplasm, etc.

  Pathological fractures usually result from trivial trauma.
- Child abuse (battered baby syndrome)—Eighty percent of child abuse takes place in less than two years of age.
- Stress fractures are not very common. Seen in tibia, neck of femur, etc.

Types of Fractures

Greenstick Fractures

This is a type of incomplete fracture seen exclusively in children. Here one cortex is broken and the other is intact (Fig. 10.1).

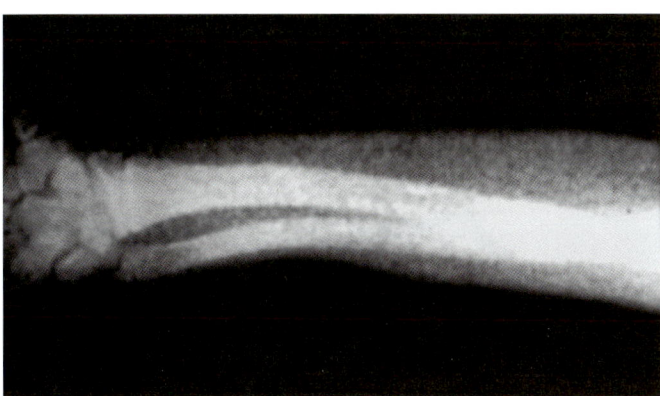

Fig. 10.1: Radiograph showing greenstick fracture of radius and ulna

Buckle Fracture (Torus Fracture)

This is common in metaphyseal region and is due to compressive force. In this fracture, cortex is buckled. Common at distal radius and the treatment is by plaster cast or Futura type of wrist splint.

Plastic Bowing

Here bone deforms but does not break. Seen in paired bones. There is a microfracture on the concave side.

Patterns of Fractures

- It is simple or compound. The latter variety is rare.
- The fracture in either case could be transverse, oblique, spiral, comminuted, or segmental.

Clinical Features

The child complains of pain, swelling, deformity. The child loathes using the affected extremity.

Investigations

AP and lateral views of the plain X-ray of the affected limb is enough to make an accurate diagnosis in children.

Treatment

Problems of Treatment

- The younger child is fretful and difficult to examine fully
- Worried parents and a crying child pose problems
- Many fractures are difficult to see and need X-rays of good quality
- General anesthesia required for manipulation
- Circulatory compromise is relatively common
- Redisplacement after reduction is common during the first week
- Wound care should be the same as in adults
- Overgrowth after long bone fracture is a very common problem and an overlap of 1 cm should be allowed.

> **Remember**
> **The general rules in treatment of fractures in children**
> - Angulations >10° are unacceptable.
> - Rotation will not be compensated and hence is not acceptable.
> - Overlap of the fracture site by 1 to 2 cm is acceptable as there is overgrowth following a long bone fracture.
> - Correction occurs at the average rate of 1° per month.

Conservative Methods

Masterly inactivity NSAIDs, crepe bandage, sling, etc. for undisplaced fractures.

Step by step conservative treatment (closed reduction and casting) green stick bends methods for forearm bone fracture (Figs 10.2A to L).

Closed reduction: If the bones are bent and of one cortex is broken, then closed reduction under general anesthesia and breaking of the other cortex is done. This is followed by plaster cast application. If the other cortex is not broken, then there are chances of malunion due to differential growth of one cortex.

Closed reduction and manipulation: This is preferred if the fracture is displaced and is done under general anesthesia in major OT. Retention is usually by slab, cast and rarely by traction (Figs 10.3 and 10.4).

Closed reduction by traction: This can also be attempted in certain situations, e.g. Gallows's traction, Dunlop's traction, or overhead olecranon skeletal traction in difficult supracondylar fractures of humerus (Figs 10.5 to 10.7).

Surgery

Open reduction and internal fixation: This is rarely done in children. Indications being failed closed reduction, redisplacement, multiple injuries, neurovascular injuries, delayed union and soft tissue interposition.

Closed reduction and percutaneous fixation of late, this method of treatment is gaining popularity due to simplicity of technique and reduced complications rate associated with the open techniques.

The most popular example of this technique is closed reduction and percutaneous K-wire fixation of closed displaced supracondylar fracture of humerus in children (Fig. 10.8).

Corrective osteotomy (Fig. 10.9): This is required in cubitus varus deformity due to malunited supracondylar fracture.

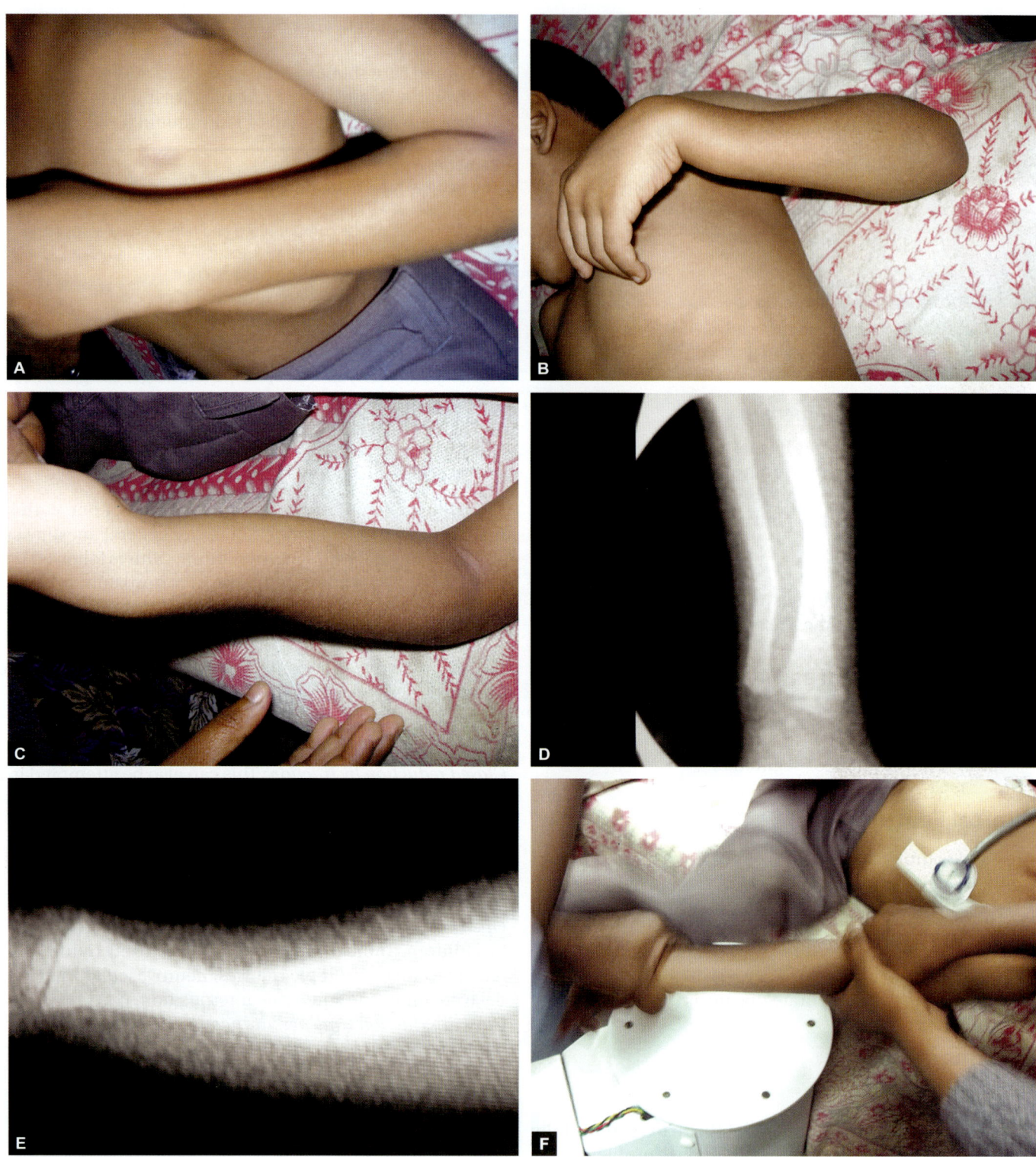

Figs 10.2A to F: Closed reduction of greenstick fracture of forearm: (A) Deformity as viewed from front (Clinical photo); (B) S-shaped deformity from the sides (Clinical photo); (C) Deformity viewed from sides (another view) (Clinical photo); (D) AP view showing both bones fracture; (E) Lateral view showing the dorsal angulations; (F) Reduction by traction and counter traction methods

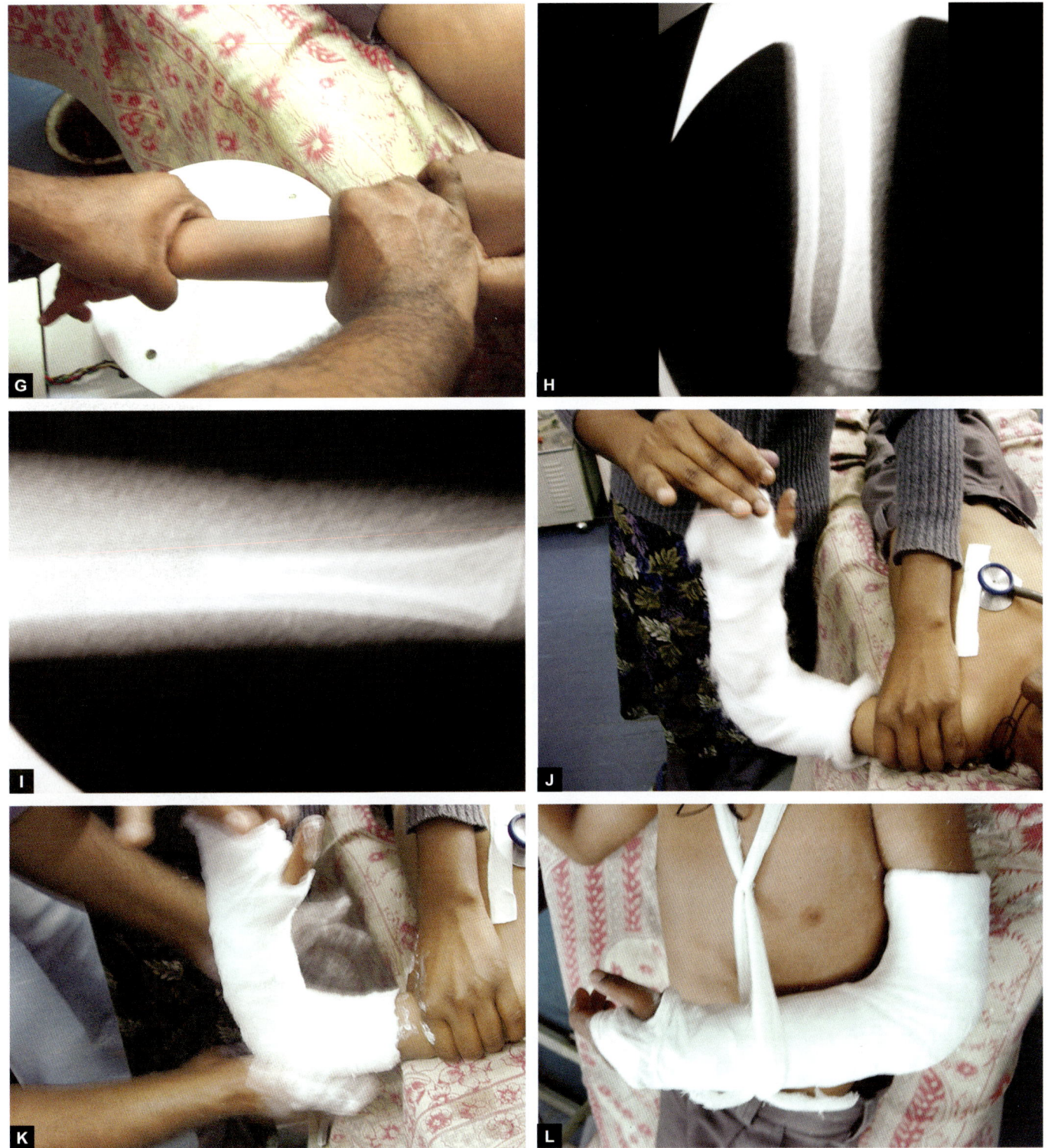

Figs 10.2G to L: (G) Manipulation being carried out; (H) Post-reduction C-arm—AP view; (I) Lateral view showing the reduction; (J) Soff ban being applied; (K) Plaster application continued; (L) Above elbow plaster cast applied

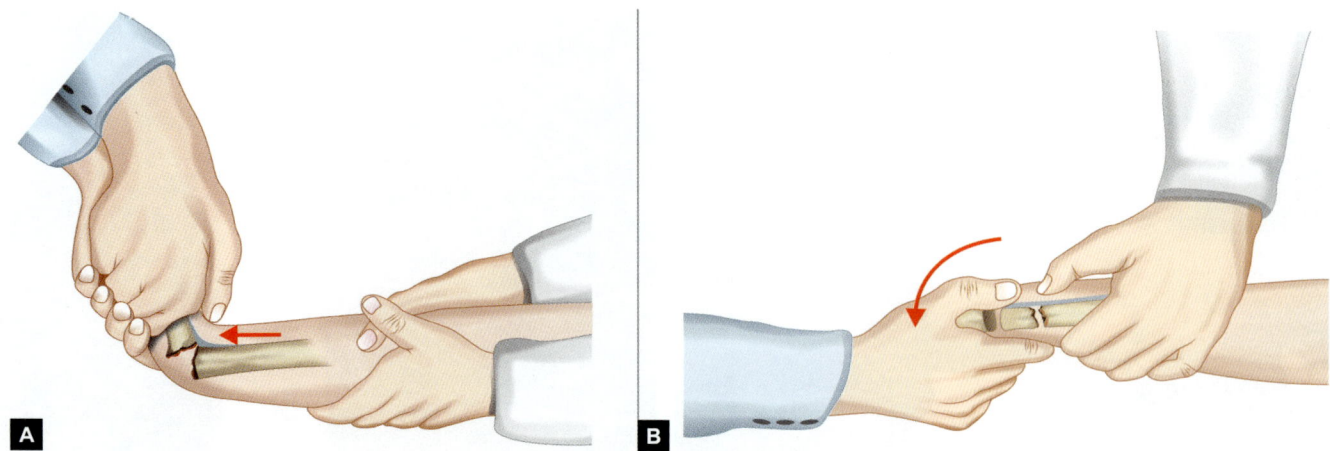

Figs 10.3A and B: Methods of closed reduction of a greenstick fracture in children: (A) The opposite intact cortex is broken; (B) The reduction is done

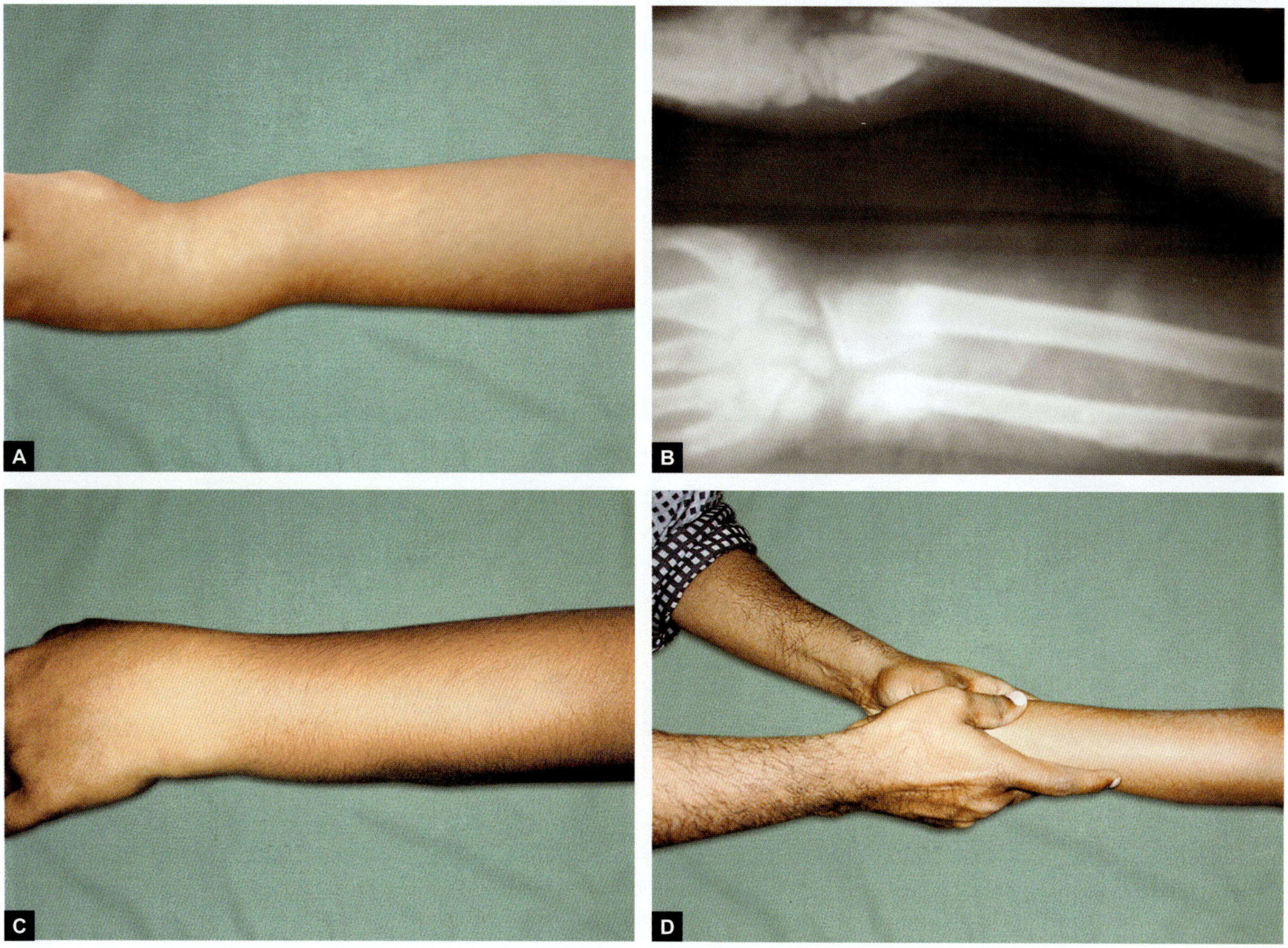

Figs 10.4A to D: Gross S-shaped deformity (Clinical photo); (B) Radiograph showing the displacements; (C) Method of reduction—Step 1 proper positioning; (D) Traction and counter traction

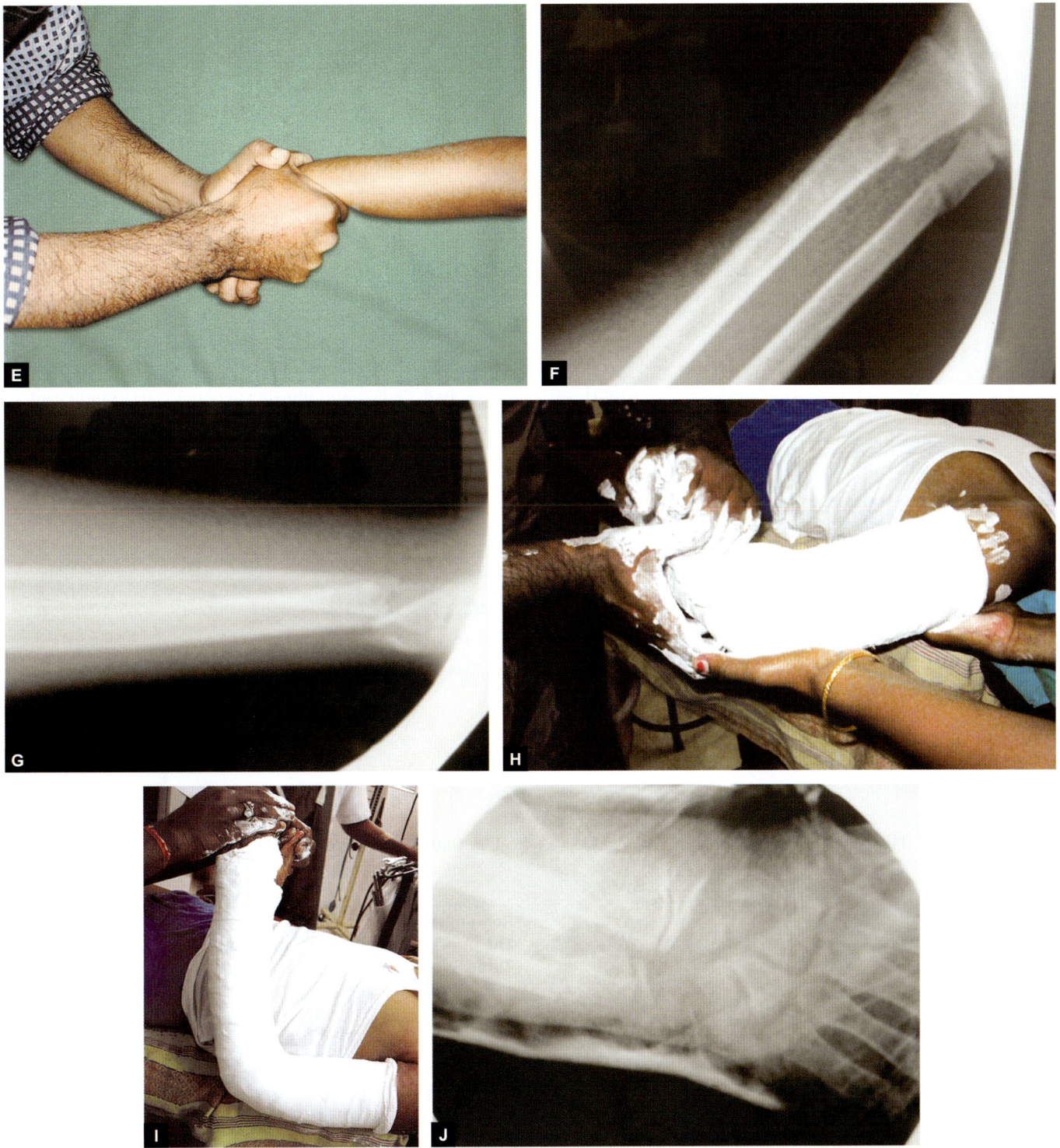

Figs 10.4E to J: (E) Step 3 fracture manipulation; (F) Radiological confirmation—AP view; (G) Radiological confirmation—lateral view; (H) Application of above elbow plaster cast; (I) Completion of the cast; (J) Final view of the corrected displacements

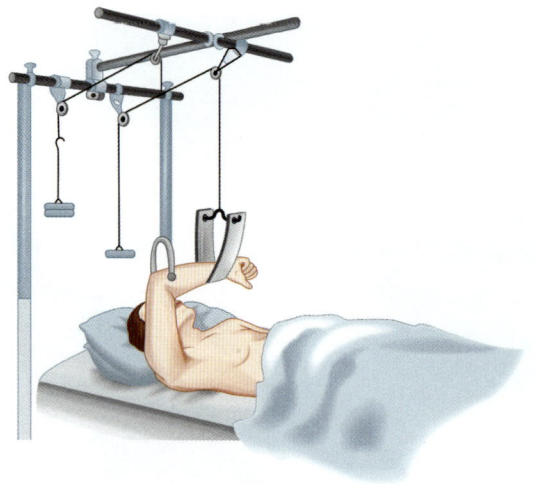

Fig. 10.5: Overhead skeletal traction (Smith's traction)

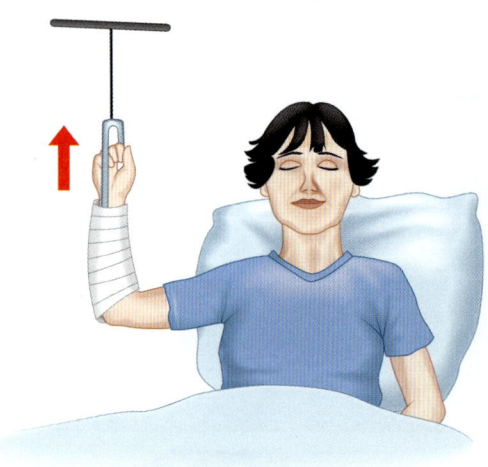

Fig. 10.6: Dunlop's traction

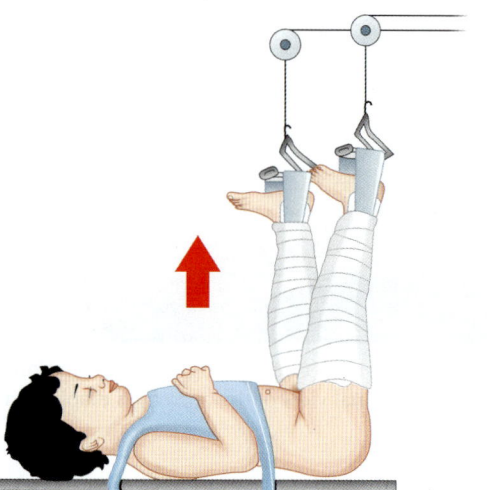

Fig. 10.7: Gallows' traction in children (<2 years of age)

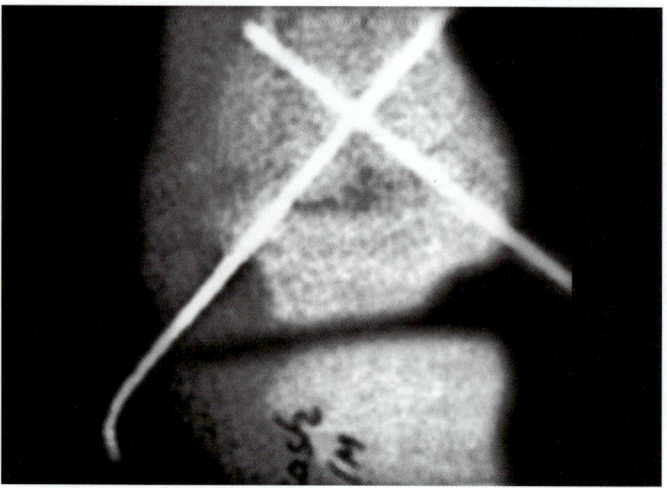

Fig. 10.8: Radiograph showing percutaneous fixation with K-wire of supracondylar fracture of humerus

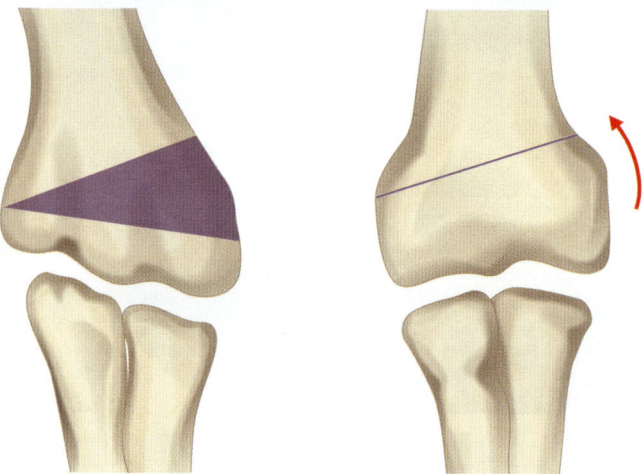

Fig. 10.9: Corrective osteotomy in malunited supracondylar fracture of humerus

> **Remember**
> **The principles of treatment in children**
> **Three Rs**
> - **R**ealign the fracture.
> - **R**espect the soft tissues.
> - **R**emember the child.

Complications

Overgrowth: Due to stimulation and hypervascularity due to epiphyseal injury.

Deformities: Due to unequal damage of the epiphyseal plate.

Growth disturbances: Due to crushing of the growth plate.

Growth arrest: Due to damage of the growth plate.

Shortening: Due to crushing of the growth plate.

Important Fractures in Children
- Monteggia's fracture
- Supracondylar fractures of humerus
- Greenstick fractures and torus fracture
- Radial neck fractures
- Fracture clavicle
- Fracture neck femur
- Epiphyseal injuries of ankle and distal end of radius, etc. Some of these fractures are discussed in detail in appropriate chapters.

Disturbing Facts: Do you know the Problem Fractures in Children?
- *Supracondylar fracture of humerus* because of the fear of VIC.
- *Monteggia's fracture* here radial head dislocation is often missed.
- *Epiphyseal injuries* lead to growth abnormalities in children.

EPIPHYSEAL INJURIES

Definition

The epiphysis is a specialized growth cartilage of long bones and is most likely to be injured after the age of 10 years.

Incidence

It accounts for nearly 17.9 percent of all pediatric fractures. Fifteen percent of these injuries cause growth arrest.

Causes

The junction between the metaphysis and the epiphysis is the weakest point of a long bone in children and is, therefore, most vulnerable to shearing forces.

Types

[1]Salter and Harris have classified epiphyseal injuries into five types (Fig. 10.10). Rang has added the sixth variety.

Type I: Complete separation of epiphysis from the metaphysis without fracture. Common in rickets, scurvy, and osteomyelitis.

Type II: The fracture involves the physis and a triangle of metaphyseal bone (*Thurston Holland sign*). This is the commonest type of epiphyseal injury accounting for 73 percent of cases over 10 years of age.

Type III: The fracture is intra-articular and extends along the physis and then along the growth plate. This injury is relatively uncommon.

Type IV: The fracture is intra-articular and extends through the epiphysis, physis, and metaphysis. Perfect reduction is necessary and open reduction is more often necessary to prevent growth arrest.

Type V: Crushing of epiphysis. Growth arrest usually follows.

Type VI: There is a peripheral physis lesion and is described by Rang.

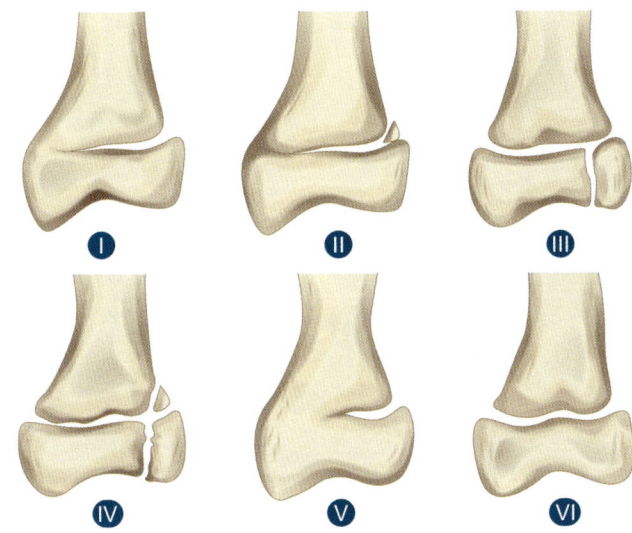

Fig. 10.10: Salter and Harris classification of epiphyseal injuries

Clinical Features

The child complains of pain, swelling, deformity, and loss of neighboring joint functions.

Investigations

A routine AP and lateral views of the plain X-ray of the affected limb is enough to make an accurate diagnosis in children (Fig. 10.11).

Treatment Options

Type I and II injuries can be managed by closed reduction. Type III and IV injuries usually require open reduction. Angular deformity and shortening are the consequences of premature growth arrest.

PATHOLOGICAL FRACTURES

When a fracture occurs through a bone, which has already been weakened by a generalized or localized skeletal disorder, it is called a pathological fracture. Unlike traumatic fractures, these fractures take place either spontaneously or due to trivial trauma (Figs 10.12A to E).

---

[1]Harris WR (Toronto) and Robert Salter (Toronto), 1963. They also described innominate osteotomy for CDH.

108   SECTION 1: Traumatology

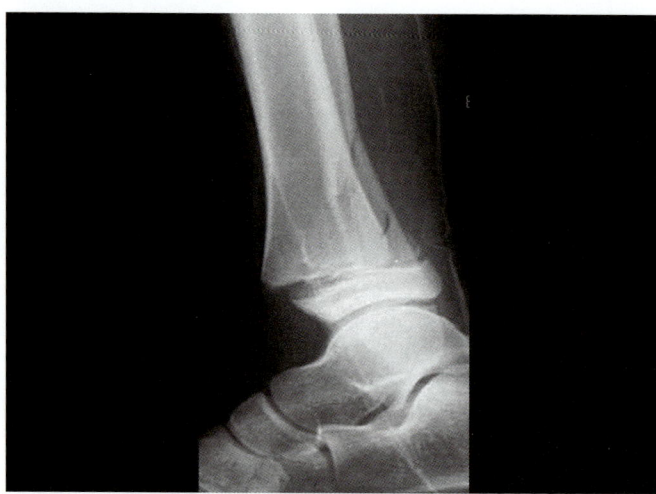

Fig. 10.11: Salter Harris injury

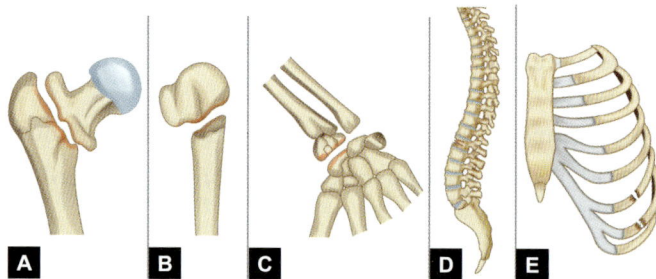

Figs 10.12A to E: Common sites of pathological fractures: (A) Neck of femur; (B) Neck of humerus; (C) Distal end of radius; (D) Compression fracture of vertebra; (E) Fracture of ribs

Quick Glance at the Causes of Pathological Fractures
Localized diseases
a. *Infective disorders*
   - Chronic pyogenic osteomyelitis
   - Tubercular or syphilitic osteomyelitis
b. *Neoplasm*

Benign	Malignant
• Chondroma	• Osteogenic sarcoma
• Giant cell tumor	• Ewing's sarcoma
• Hemangioma spine (Lung, breast prostate, kidney, etc.)	• Solitary myeloma
	• Metastatic carcinoma
• Bone atrophy (e.g. polio, etc.)	• Metastatic sarcoma
• Tabes dorsalis, etc.	

c. *Miscellaneous cause*
   - Simple bone cyst
   - Monostotic fibrous dysplasia
   - Eosinophilic granuloma

General affections of bone
a. *Congenital disorders*
   - Osteogenesis imperfecta.
   - Fibrous dysplasia
   - Gaucher's disease, etc.
b. *Generalized rarefaction of bones*
   - Senile osteoporosis
   - Hyperparathyroidism
   - Osteomalacia
   - Nutritional rickets
   - Scurvy
c. *Miscellaneous*
   - Multiple mycelia
   - Diffuse metastatic carcinoma
d. *Disseminated tumors*
   - Paget's disease
   - Fibroses dysplasia
   - Gaucher's disease, etc.

Clinical Features

The patient usually complains of fracture following a trivial trauma. He/she complains of having suffered pain or discomfort in the region of the affected bone some time before the fracture. The underlying cause for this could be either a generalized disorder or a local skeletal disorder.

Practical Point
Common causes for pathological fractures
Local disorders
a. *Metastatic carcinoma*
   The primary could be in the lungs, breast, prostate, thyroid, or kidney.
   Common sites
   – Vertebral bodies (thoracic/lumbar).
   – Proximal half of femoral shaft.
   – Proximal half of humerus.
b. *Bone cyst* of a long bone.
Generalized disorders
a. *Senile osteoporosis*
   Common sites affected are:
   – Thoracic or lumbar vertebral body.
   – Neck or trochanteric region of femur.
b. *Paget's disease of bone*
   – Shaft of tibia or femur.

Investigations

- *Laboratory investigation:* This includes Hb%, TC, DC, ESR, serum Ca, phosphorous, alkaline and acid phosphatase, etc.
- Plain X-ray of the affected bones including the joint above and below (Figs 10.13 and 10.14).

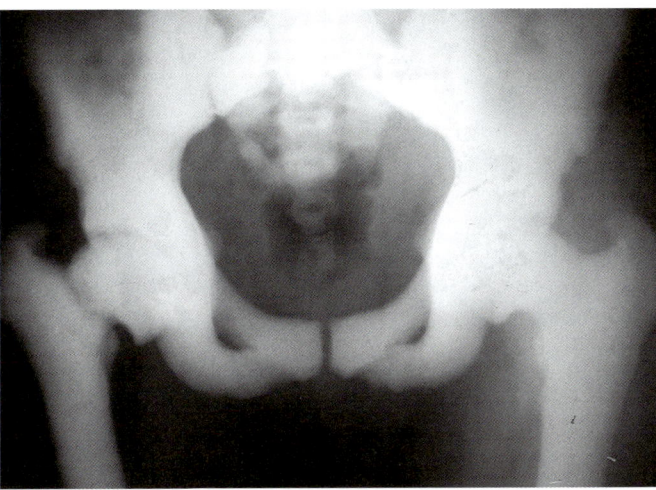

Fig. 10.13: Pathological fracture due to osteopetrosis

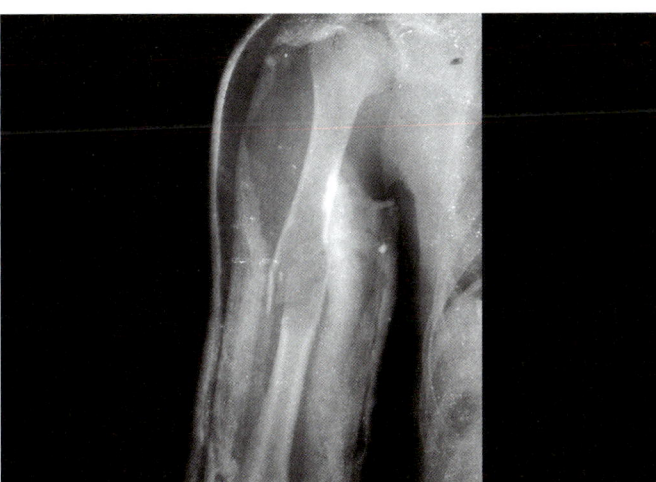

Fig. 10.14: Pathological fracture humerus

- CT scan and MRI are of extreme importance to determine the extent of pathological involvement.
- Bone scan is helpful in determining the spread of disease.

Treatment

Conservative treatment has little role in the treatment of pathological fractures. The treatment recommended is open reduction, rigid internal fixation with or without cement and bone grafting. The aim is to obtain quick union and mobilize the patient early. Pathological fractures due to Paget's disease, osteogenesis imperfecta, etc. unite in the usual time, fractures due to osteomyelitis, bone cyst unite late but fractures due to malignancy, metastasis do not unite at all though union is possible after chemotherapy or radiotherapy.

> **Do You Know the Most Common Causes of Pathologic Fractures?**
> - Osteoporosis first
> - Metastasis into the bones next.

FATIGUE OR STRESS FRACTURES

Definition

Fatigue or stress fractures occur mainly in normal bones due to repeated stress or minor trauma to a particular bone usually of the lower limbs. It is more common in metatarsal bones (Fig. 10.15) and is known as the March fracture.

Clinical Features

Here there is no single specific causative injury as in a traumatic fracture. The onset of pain is gradual or insidious. Activity increases the pain and rest relieves it. On examination, there is significant local tenderness, thickening of bone, local swelling, etc.

> **Vital Facts: Stress Fractures**
> *Who are prone for stress fractures? In alphabetical order*
> - Athletes
> - Dancers
> - Doctors
> - Nurses
> - Policemen
> - Soldiers
> - Sportspersons
> - Surgeons
> - Unknown group

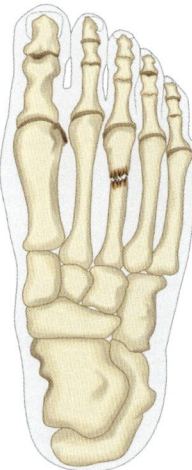

Fig. 10.15: Stress fracture of III metatarsal bone

Radiograph

Radiograph of the part at first may not reveal any fractures but may be seen after 3 to 4 weeks. The fracture itself will be hairline, transverse and undisplaced. More striking than the fracture is a zone of callus that surrounds it (Figs 10.16 and 10.17).

Bone Scan

This is of great help in determining the presence of stress fracture (Fig. 10.18).

MRI and CT scan

There are the other useful investigations but are expensive (Fig. 10.19).

Treatment

Stress fractures usually heal by rest and support to the affected part.

> **Practical Points: Stress Fractures**
> *Common sites*
> - Second and third metatarsal bone—march fracture (due to repeated marching as in soldiers).
> - Tibia or fibula—repeated running or dancing.
> - Femur—occasionally.
>
> *Radiology*
> - 1st week—usually no fracture is detected.
> - 2nd and 3rd week—faint hairline fracture, transverse/undisplaced.
> - Zone of callus that surrounds the fracture is more significant than the fracture itself.
>
> *Treatment is by rest.*

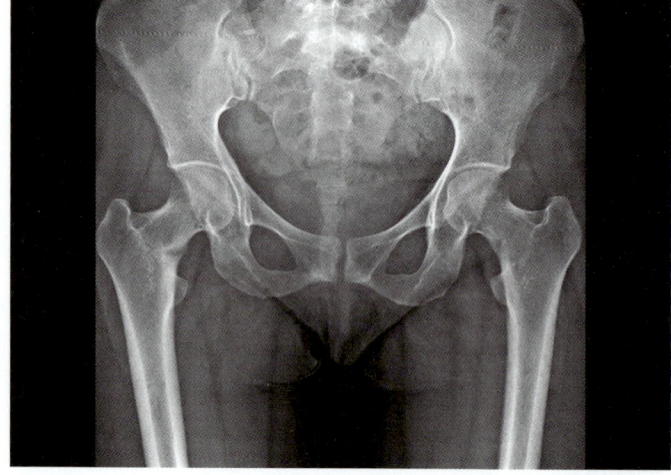

Fig. 10.17: Plain X-ray showing bilateral stress fracture of the femoral neck

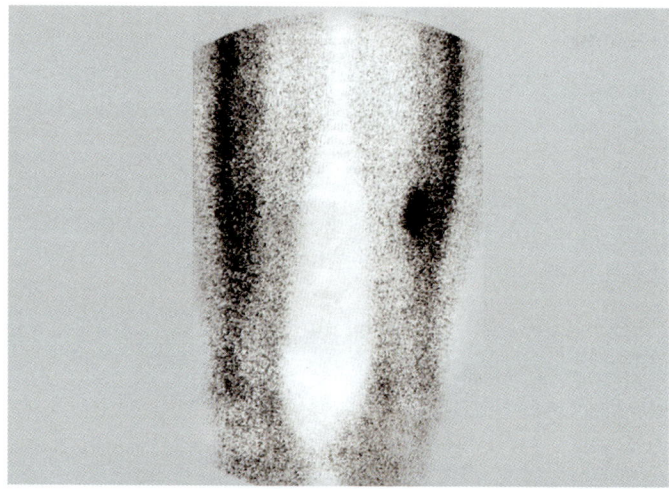

Fig. 10.18: Stress fracture tibia—scintigram

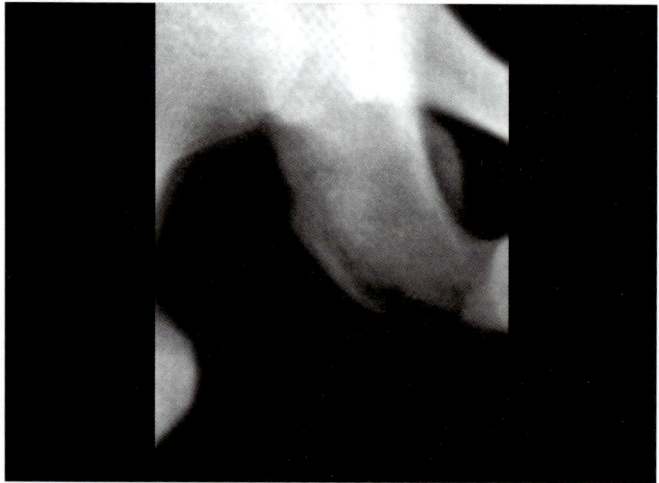

Fig. 10.16: Radiograph showing stress fracture of the ischium

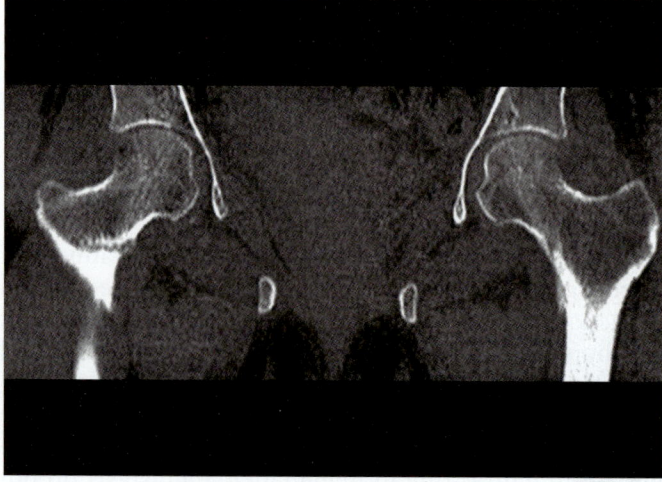

Fig. 10.19: CT Scan gives a better picture of the bilateral stress fracture of the femoral neck

SECTION 2
Regional Traumatology

- Injuries Around the Clavicle
- Injuries of the Shoulder Joint
- Injuries Around the Elbow
- Injuries of the Forearm
- Injuries to the Wrist
- Hand Injuries
- Dislocations of the Hip Joint
- Fracture Femur
- Injuries of the Knee
- Fracture of Tibia and Fibula
- Injuries of the Ankle
- Injuries of the Foot
- Pelvic Injuries, Rib and Coccyx Injuries
- Injuries of the Spine
- Peripheral Nerve Injuries

Section

2

Regional Traumatology

11
CHAPTER

Injuries Around the Clavicle

INTRODUCTION

The shoulder joint complex consists of the glenohumeral joint, the acromioclavicular joint and sternoclavicular joint. The injuries concerning all the three joints and the fractures involving the clavicle, scapula and proximal humerus are discussed in this chapter.

FRACTURE CLAVICLE

The term clavicle (Fig. 11.1) is derived from the Latin root *Clavis* meaning *Key*. Clavicle is 'S' shaped and is linked to the music symbol 'clavicula', hence the name.

The Clavicle Speaks: My Peculiarities
- I am the first bone to ossify in the body.
- I ossify from two primary centers.
- I am the only long bone in the body lying horizontal.
- I am the only long bone ossifying from a membrane.
- I am the only link between the appendicular and the axial skeleton.
- I am the most common bone to be fractured in children.
- I invariably end up maluniting after the fracture.

Functions of Clavicle

- It increases the arm strength mechanism.

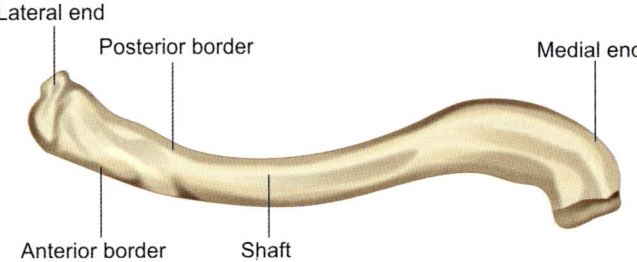

Fig. 11.1: Bony anatomy of the clavicle

- It protects the neurovascular bundle consisting of subclavian vessels and brachial plexus.
- It gives attachments to important muscles around the shoulder.
- It braces the shoulder back during rest and motion (Strut function).

Mechanism of Injury

Direct

Due to fall on the point of the shoulder. This is the most common mode of injury accounting for 91 percent of the cases.

Direct Trauma

Direct trauma over the clavicle due to RTA, direct injury, etc. accounts for 8 percent of the cases (Fig. 11.2).

Indirect fall on the outstretched hands accounts for 1% of the cases.

Sites of Fracture

- Eighty five percent of the fracture clavicle occurs at the junction of middle and outer third (Fig. 11.3).
- One percent at the medial end of the clavicle (5%).
- Lateral end fracture is uncommon (About 10%) (Distal 1/3rd).

Classification of Fracture Clavicle (Allman's)

Group I is fractures involving middle one-third of the shaft.
Group II is fractures involving the lateral third distal to the attachment of the coracoclavicular ligament. This is further subdivided into two subgroups (Proposed by Neer):

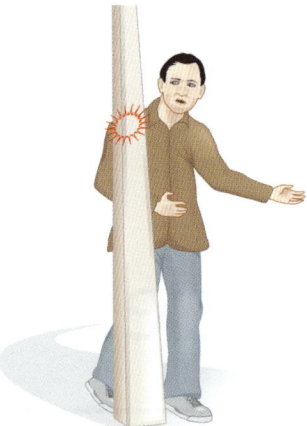

Fig. 11.2: Recklessness like this can break your clavicle bone due to direct injury

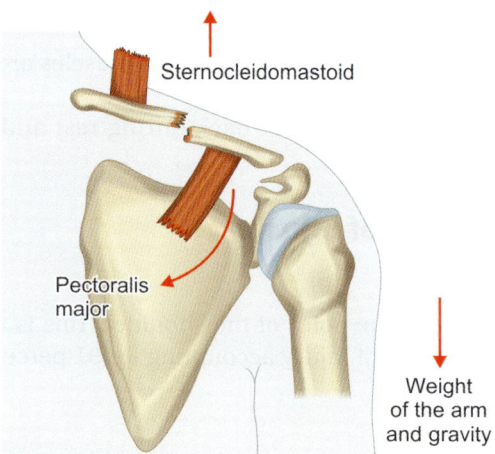

Fig. 11.3: Various displacing forces in fracture clavicle

- *Type A:* Coracoclavicular ligament intact.
- *Type B:* Coracoclavicular ligament ruptured.
- *Type C:* Intra-articular extension into ACM joint.

Group III are medial third fractures.

Clinical Features

The patient presents with pain, swelling, deformity and inability to raise the shoulder. Rarely, the patient may present with pseudoparalysis of the affected arm (Fig. 11.4).

Radiographs

The following views are recommended:
- Routine AP view of the clavicle (Fig. 11.5).
- Lordotic view if the fracture is doubtful.
- Distal clavicle requires special radiography techniques.

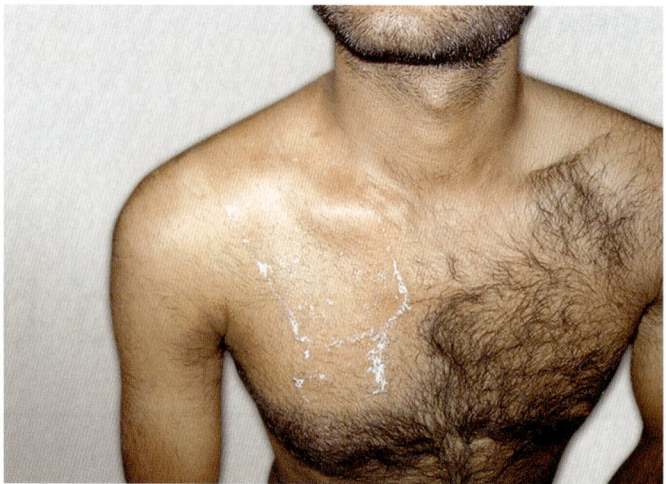

Fig. 11.4: Patient with pseudoparalysis in clavicle fracture

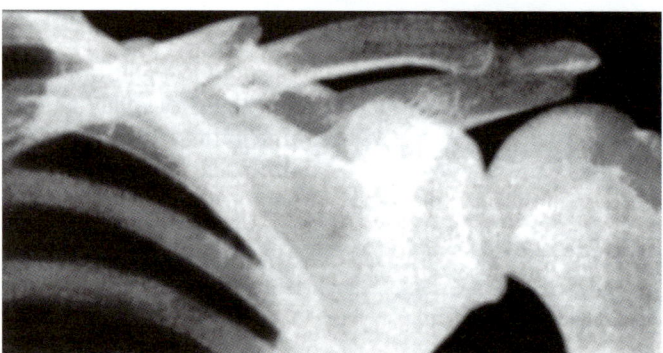

Fig. 11.5: Radiograph showing fracture clavicle of middle third

Principles of Treatment

Before proceeding to the treatment proper one needs to understand the two distracting forces acting on the fracture fragments in clavicle making the treatment difficult. The sternocleidomastoid muscle pulls up the medial end of the clavicle and the pectoralis major muscle and gravity acting through the arm pull down the lateral end (see Fig. 11.2).

To counter the above two detrimental forces, the shoulder should be braced up and back and the arm should be supported while treating fracture clavicle.

Conservative Methods

This was earlier the treatment of choice in fracture clavicle and now is restricted in its usage largely to children and some un-displaced fractures and consists of the following methods:

Cuff and collar sling for undisplaced fractures (Fig. 11.6A).

Strapping of the fracture site after reduction of the fracture by elevating the arm and bracing the shoulder upwards and backwards gives good results in both children and adults (Figs 11.6B and D).

> **Methods in Cold Storage Now:**
> - Sabre method consists of rigid dressing over the fracture. This is no longer used.
> - Billington Yoke method uses a plaster of Paris over a well-padded figure of '8' dressing.

Figure of '8' is popularly used and it acts by retracting the shoulder girdle, minimizes the overlap and allows more anatomical healing. *It does not immobilize the fracture but acts by serving as a reminder to the patient to hold the shoulder up and back neutralizing the forces mentioned above. If they allow the shoulder to slump forward, then the support cuts into the anterior axilla and reminds them to hold the shoulders back* (Fig. 11.6C).

Conservative Treatment Plan

Newborn to perambulatory children: Treated symptomatically, bind arm to the chest.

Ambulatory stage (2–12 years): Figure of '8' bandages, tightened after three days and later one week.

Twelve years to maturity: Commercially available figure of '8' harness.

Operative Methods

Earlier Surgery was rarely indicated, but now it is being done more often and consists of reduction, either closed or open and internal fixation, rigid with plates or biological with K-wires.

Indications

Open fractures, injury to neurovascular bundle, if the fracture is threatening to penetrate the skin, non-union, fracture near acromioclavicular joint, floating shoulder, soft tissue interposition and displaced epiphysis in children.

More Specific Indications for Open Reduction and Internal Fixation of Fracture Clavicle

- Shortening or distraction of fragments for more than 2 cm.
- More than 100 percent displacement or fragmentation.
- Bilateral fractures.

Methods of Internal Fixation

- Intramedullary fixation with K-wires –either retrograde or antegrade, either closed or open techniques (Fig. 11.7)
- Rigid plate and screw fixation with AO semi-tubular or pelvic reconstruction plate (Fig. 11.8).

> **What is New in the Treatment of Fracture Clavicle?**
> - Intramedullary compression clavicular nail
> - Mckeever's threaded IM pin
> - External fixators in open clavicular fractures

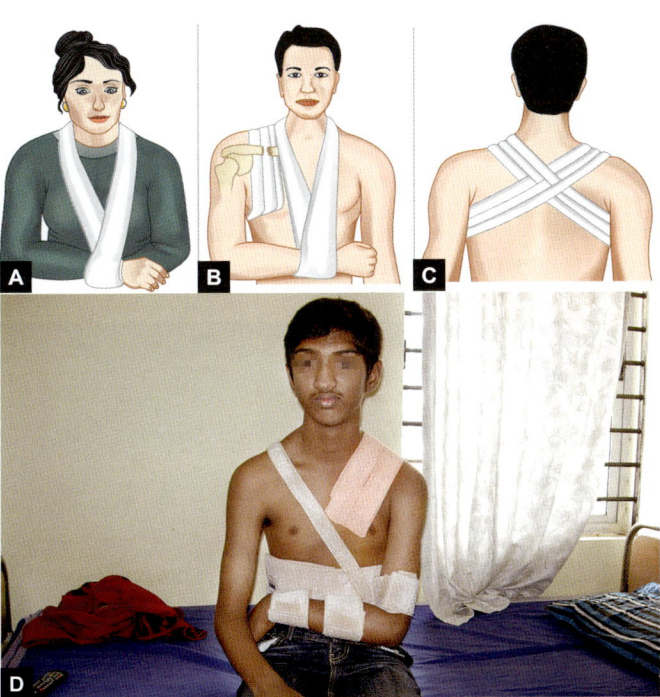

Figs 11.6A to D: Methods of conservative treatment of fractures clavicle: (A) Collar and cuff sling; (B) Strapping and sling suspension; (C) Figure of '8' bandaging; (D) Clinical photo of strapping

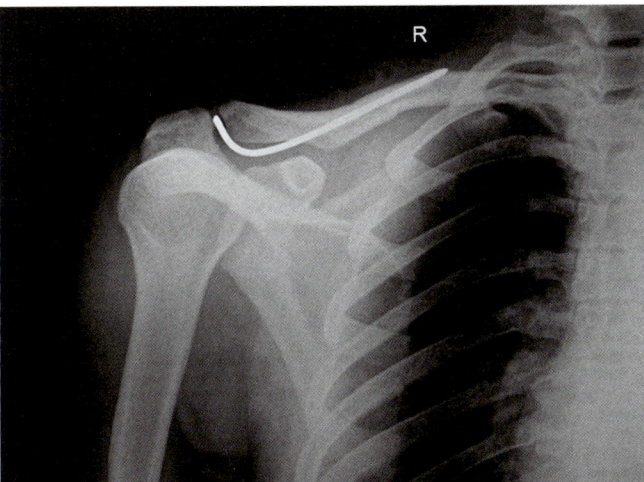

Fig. 11.7: X-ray showing intramedullary fixation with K-wire

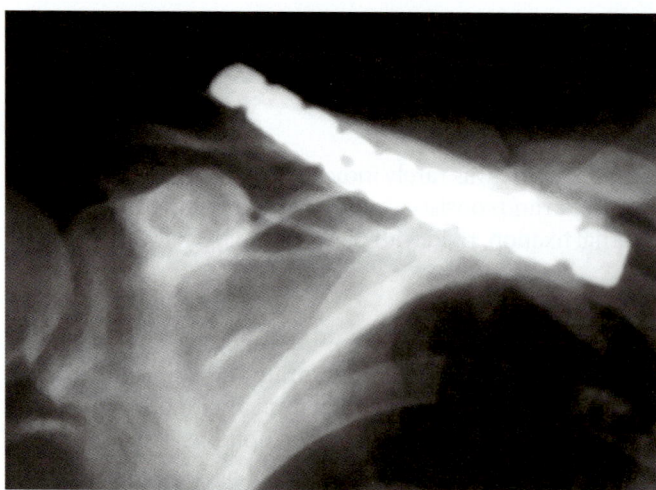

Fig. 11.8: Radiograph showing fracture clavicle plate fixation

Fracture Lateral End of Clavicle

This is less common when compared to the middle shaft fracture and the treatment is essentially surgical fixation (Figs 11.9A and B).

Complications of Fracture Clavicle

Early

Neurovascular injury may be immediate due to direct force or delayed due to a very large callus. The structures commonly injured are subclavian vessels and the medial cord of the brachial plexus through which the ulnar nerve is derived. This occurs in fractures of the middle one-third of the clavicle, which is the most common.

Did You Know?
The ulnar nerve is the commonest nerve to be injured in fracture clavicle due to its compression between it and the first rib.

Late

Malunion is very common due to difficulty in holding the fracture fragments in position because of the distracting forces already explained. It causes only a cosmetic problem and does not usually impair function. Hence, no treatment is required (Fig. 11.10).

Problems Posed by Malunion Clavicle

- Cosmetic complaints—mentioned above.
- Orthopedic complaints—frequent episodes of shoulder fatigue.
- Sleep problems—the patient complains of inability to sleep on the sides.
- Neurological problems—features of thoracic outlet syndrome.

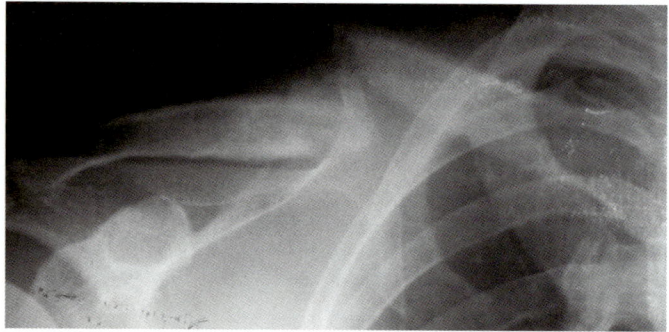

Fig. 11.10: Plain X-ray showing malunion clavicle

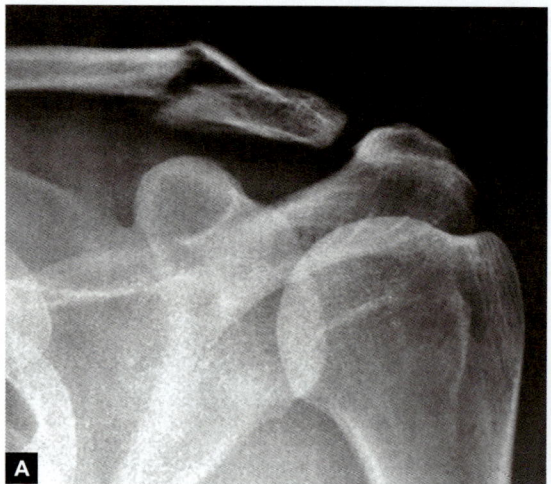
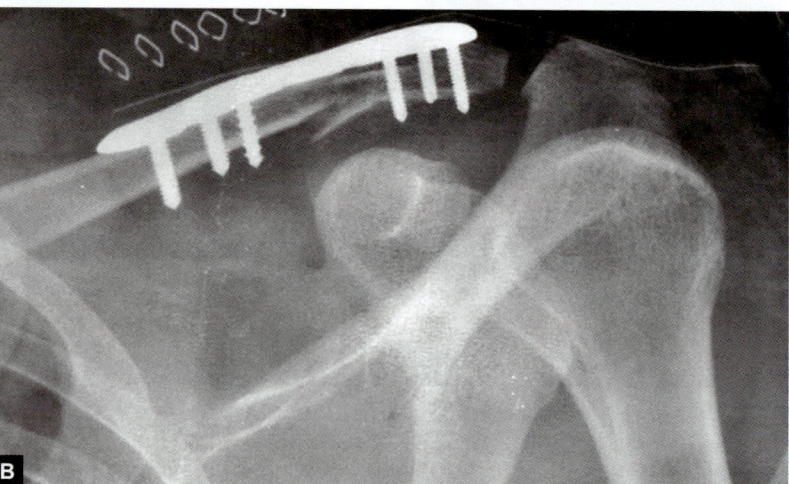

Figs 11.9A and B: Fracture lateral end of clavicle treated with ORIF

Remedy if faced with these situations, the patient requires corrective osteotomy and rigid internal fixation with medullary pins or plate and screws.

Nonunion is rare and requires open reduction, internal fixation and bone grafting.

> **Quick Facts: Fracture Clavicle**
> - Most common fracture in children
> - Common mode of injury is direct
> - Eighty percent break at junction of middle and distal third
> - Nearly all fractures are treated closed
> - Open reduction for specific indications
> - Malunion is a rule, but no functional disability.

INJURIES OF THE ACROMIOCLAVICULAR JOINT

Acromioclavicular (ACM) joint is a diarthrodial joint with a fibrocartilaginous disk between the two bones (similar to a meniscus).

> **The Acromioclavicular Joint Speaks**
> I am essentially a plane joint. I permit gliding rotation between the clavicle and the scapula. My structural integrity depends on the intrinsic capsular element, the superior acromioclavicular ligament and the extrinsic coracoclavicular ligament, which forms a hood over the interval between the coracoid process and the acromion.

Incidence is 12% and is common in the young. Male: Female ratio is 5:1.

> **Do You Know?**
> - The common name for ACL injury is shoulder separation.
> - ACL injuries are 4 to 5 times more common than sternoclavicular injuries.

Mechanism of Injury

Direct force is the most common mechanism (Fig. 11.11) of injury as in RTA, assault, athletic events like the tackling, etc.

Indirect force is due to fall on the outstretched hands.

Downward indirect force through the upper extremity is relatively rare.

Clinical Features

The patient complains of pain, swelling, and difficulty in raising the arm up. The patient supports the affected shoulder by holding the elbow with unaffected hand. On examination, there is tenderness and the lateral end of clavicle is prominently felt (Fig. 11.12).

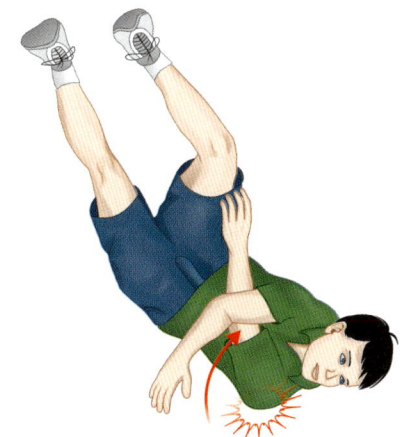

Fig. 11.11: Showing the most common mechanism of injury of ACM joint

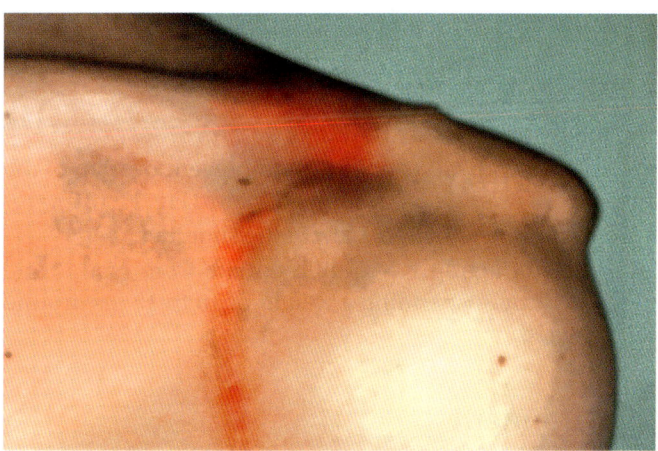

Fig. 11.12: ACM joint injury, the clinical appearance

Classification (Sage and Salvatore's)

Based on injuries to acromioclavicular and coracoclavicular ligaments (Fig. 11.13A):

Type I: Minor sprain to acromioclavicular ligaments.

Type II: Rupture of ACL, sprain of CCL.

Type III: Both ACL and CCL ruptured, clavicle is displaced upwards.

Type IV: Same as type III, but with upward and posterior displacement of clavicle.

Type V: Type III with severe displacement of the clavicle towards base of the neck.

Type VI: Inferior dislocation with clavicle towards base of the neck.

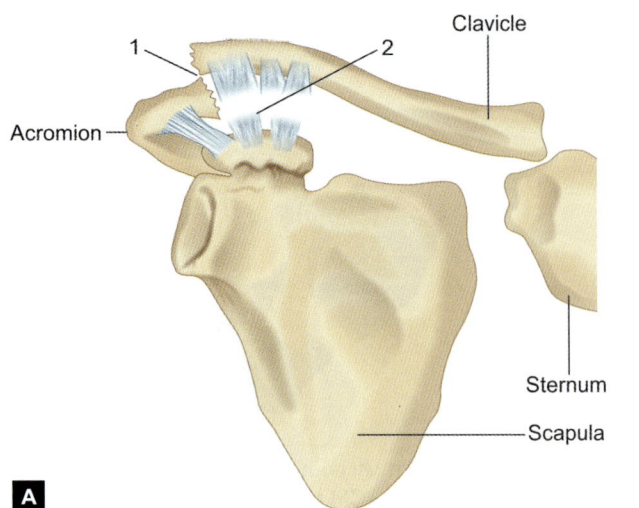 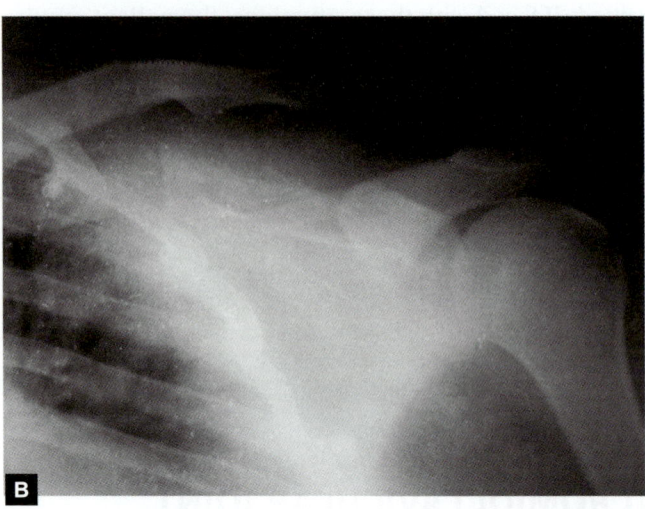

Figs 11.13A and B: (A) Acromioclavicular joint injury shows: (1) Ruptured acromioclavicular ligament (ACL), and (2) Ruptured coracoclavicular ligament (CCL); (B) Radiograph showing ACM joint dislocation

Radiographs

The following views are required:
- AP view with 15° cephalic tilt to prevent overlap of the spine of scapula on routine AP views (Fig. 11.13B).
- Lateral view—axillary view of the shoulder.
- Stress radiographs—to differentiate from type II and type III by suspending a weight of 10 to 15 lbs around the wrist.

Management

Conservative Management

Type I: Rest, ice bags, NSAIDs, etc.

Type II: Sling for 10 to 14 days, adhesive strapping, elastic strapping, cast or harness. Surgery is required for persisting pain.

Type III: Conservative methods like reduction and retention with sling and harness.

Types IV, V and VI: Require open reduction, internal fixation, repair and reconstruction.

Operative Management

Surgical methods include:
- Acromioclavicular repair.
- Coracoclavicular repair.
- Excision of distal end of clavicle for old symptomatic cases.
- Dynamic muscle transfer by transferring the coracoid process.

Complications

Early
- Associated fracture clavicle.
- Complications after surgery like infection, etc.
- Complications after non-operative treatment like joint stiffness, periarthritis, etc.

Delayed
- Step-like deformity
- ACM joint arthritis
- Coracoclavicular ossification
- Osteolysis of distal clavicle
- Pain during weightlifting.

INJURIES OF STERNOCLAVICULAR JOINT

> **The Sternoclavicular Joint Speaks**
> I am a saddle joint and represent the only bone-to-bone connection of the upper limb to the trunk. To absorb the shock transmitted from the arm to the shoulder, I have a fibrocartilaginous disk between clavicle and the manubrii. I derive my structural strength from the interclavicular and costoclavicular ligaments along with the anterior and posterior sternoclavicular ligaments. The intra-articular disk ligaments and the capsular ligaments strengthen me largely.

Mechanism of Injury

This is the least commonly dislocated joint because of the strong ligaments.

Direct force rarely causes this injury. For example, collision of an athlete with another person or a post, etc.

Indirect force is the most common mode of injury. For example, loading the upper shoulder while someone lies on the sides (Fig. 11.14).

Incidence is about three percent and is more common in young males.

Causes

Road traffic accident (RTA) is responsible for 80 percent of the cases, sports-related injuries account for the remaining 20%.

Classifications (Figs 11.15A and B)

Anatomical Classification
- Anterior dislocation (more common)
- Posterior dislocation

Etiological Classification
- Traumatic
  - Sprain
  - Acute dislocation
  - Recurrent dislocation
  - Unreduced dislocation.
- Atraumatic
  - Voluntary
  - Involuntary
  - Congenital
  - Degenerative
  - Infective.

Clinical Features

The patient complains of pain and swelling. Medial end of the clavicle is prominent in anterior dislocation (Fig. 11.16). Affected shoulder is short. Lateral compression test is positive.

Radiographs

- AP view is often difficult to interpret
- Special 90° cephalocaudal views—this helps to see the medial ends of both the clavicles (serendipity view) (Figs 11.17A and B).

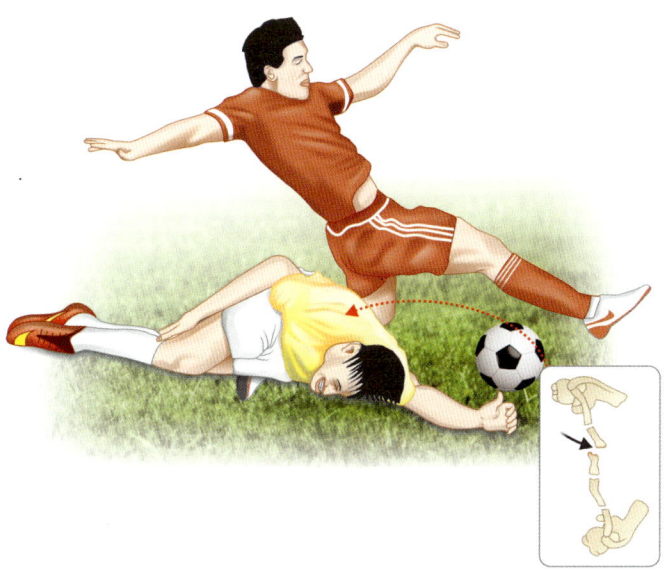

Fig. 11.14: The most common mechanism of injury of the sternoclavicular joint

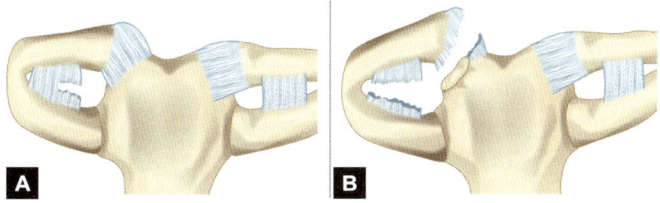

Figs 11.15A and B: Sternoclavicular joint injuries: (A) Partial separation; (B) Total separation

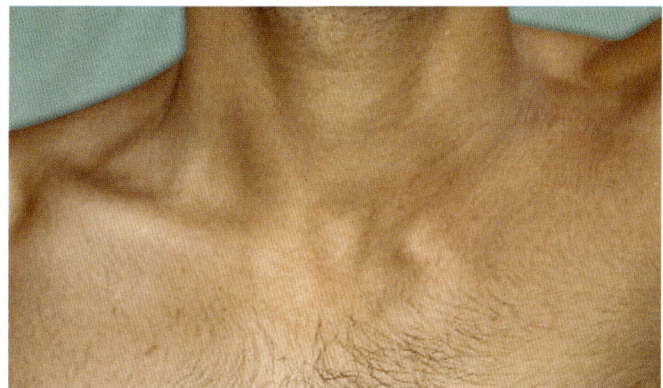

Fig. 11.16: Clinical photo showing sternoclavicular joint dislocation

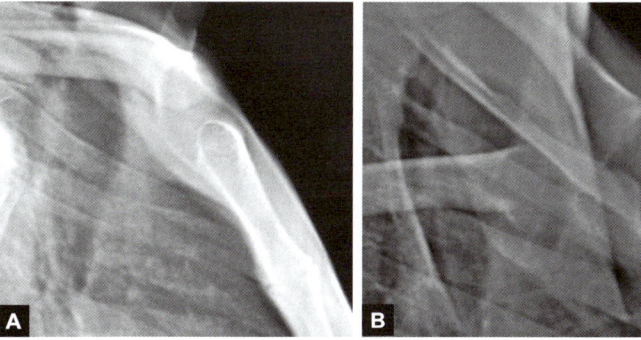

Figs 11.17A and B: Plain X-ray lateral view showing normal position and arm elevated position shows sternocleidojoint dislocation

- Tomograms are useful
- CT scans and MRI help to study the position of clavicle with respect to sternum and soft tissues respectively.

Management

Mild sprain: The treatment consists of ice, sling, painkillers, etc.

Subluxation: The treatment methods are ice (first 12 hours), warmth (24–48 hours), clavicle strap, and figure of '8' and excision of medial end if pain persists.

Dislocation: The treatment of choice is closed reduction by firm digital pressure followed by figure of '8', clavicle strap, sling, etc. If it fails, open reduction and internal fixation using K-wire is done.

12 CHAPTER

Injuries of the Shoulder Joint

Glenohumeral Joint Speaks
I am a multiaxial ball and socket joint. I am proud to be the most mobile joint in the body. Let me introduce my various components (Fig. 12.1) that I am made up of:
- **Humeral head:** It is approximately one-third of a sphere and is oriented at 45° from the long axis of the shaft and retroverted 30°. The indistinct anatomical neck consists two important landmarks, the lesser tuberosity anteromedially and the greater tuberosity superolaterally separated by the bicipital groove.
  The shallow-shaped glenoid cavity is anteverted approximately and inferiorly angulated 5° from the long axis of the scapula.
- **Labrum:** It is a fibrocartilage, which is triangular in cross-section and is attached to the outer perimeter of the glenoid. It increases the contact area by 70% and helps me in my stability.
- **Ligaments:** The fibrous capsule is attached peripherally to the margins of glenoid cavity and anatomic neck. I have three intrinsic capsular ligaments called the glenohumeral ligaments, which reinforce me. The coracohumeral ligament assists the capsule in supporting the arm.
- **Rotator cuff:** This is the name given to four inter-related muscles, infraspinatus, supraspinatus, subscapularis, and teres minor. By their coordinated activity, they provide me help in the finer adjustments of the humeral head within the glenoid cavity.
- **Bursa:** To provide smooth movements, I am aided by numerous bursa of which sub-deltoid or subacromial bursa is the most important. I can carry out various activities like flexion, extension, adduction, abduction, internal and external rotation and circumduction with ease, thanks to the anatomy, which the nature has designed for me.

DISLOCATION OF SHOULDER

Shoulder joint is vulnerable for dislocation more often than any other joint in the body. The extreme mobility it enjoys jeopardizes its stability. The shoulder has an "Achilles point" at the inferior part of the capsule providing the joint with a potential weak spot, so much so that 99% of the anterior

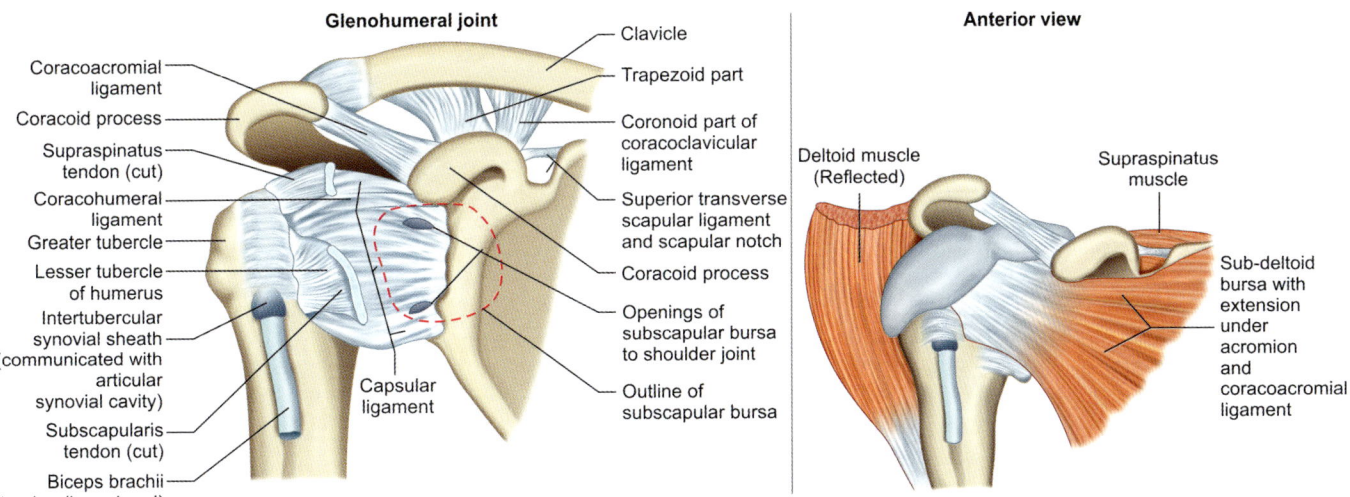

Fig. 12.1: Normal anatomy of shoulder joint

shoulder dislocation occurs here. Ninety-five percent of the shoulder dislocation is anterior and the remaining five % is posterior. An attempt is made here to present a comparative study of both the dislocations for better understanding and easy remembrance (Table 12.1).

Matsen identifies two groups of dislocations with mnemonics TUBS denoting traumatic group, and AMBRI denoting atraumatic group. These are usually applied to anterior dislocation (Fig. 12.2) but can be applied to posterior dislocation also.

TABLE 12.1: Comparative study between anterior and posterior dislocation of shoulder

	Anterior dislocation (95%)	Posterior dislocation (5%)
• Classification – Traumatic injuries	• Sprains • Acute subluxation • Acute dislocation • Recurrent dislocation • Unreduced dislocation	• Sprains • Acute subluxation • Acute dislocation • Recurrent dislocation • Unreduced posterior dislocation
– Atraumatic	• Voluntary or habitual • Involuntary • Congenital	• Voluntary • Involuntary • Congenital
– Based on anatomical location of humeral head	• Subcoracoid • Subglenoid • Subclavicular • Intrathoracic	• Subacromial • Subglenoid • Subspinous
• Mechanism of injury	• *Direct force*—blow from the posterior aspect of the shoulder • *Indirect force*—due to Abduction + External rotation + Extension injury (common)	• *Direct force*—blow from the anterior aspect of the shoulder • *Indirect force*—due to Internal rotation + Adduction + Flexion injury (common)
• Clinical features for diagnosis	• Severe pain • Arm is held in abduction and external rotation • Adduction is restricted • Normal contour of shoulder is lost and there is anterior shoulder fullness	• Severe pain • Arm is in position of adduction and internal rotation (Classical 'sling' position) • Abduction is restricted • Normal contour of shoulder is lost
• Clinical tests for diagnosis	• Posterior aspect is flat • Coracoid process is not identified • Axillary nerve injury may be present	• Posterior shoulder fullness present • Anterior aspect is flat • Coracoid process is more prominent
• X-ray views taken: – Routine X-rays in AP view in internal and external rotations – AP view in plane of scapula. – Axillary lateral view – True scapula lateral view	• *Bankart's lesions* (Lateral defect anterior) • *Hill-Sachs lesion* (Posterolateral defect in the head of the humerus seen in 100% of cases). • *Erosions of rim of glenoid*	• Anterolateral defect • *Vacant glenoid sign* (Fig. 12.8) • *Daylight sign* (complete gap) • *The trough line:* Similar to Hill-Sachs lesion and is found on the anteromedial aspect of the head of the humerus
• Transthoracic lateral X-ray Other investigations – *Arthrography:* It is more helpful to evaluate rotator cuff tears due to previous dislocations. – *CT scan:* It helps to detect the defect in the head more accurately. – *MRI:* It is very useful to evaluate both soft tissues in addition, bony injuries.	C-shaped rolling line (Fig. 12.7)	V-shaped rolling line (Figs 12.9A and B)
• Techniques of reduction	I. *Closed reduction:* Three methods – *Hippocrates's method:* Reduction with foot in the axilla – *Stimson's gravity method:* Patient is in prone position with weight attached to the wrist. Gravity helps in reduction – *Kocher's method:* Most effective and commonly followed method	Reduction under general anesthesia distal traction on the injured limb with lateral rotation on the upper arm

Contd...

Contd...

	II. **Open reduction:** This is indicated in failed closed reduction, soft tissue interposition, greater tuberosity fracture displaced >1 cm after reduction and large glenoid rim fractures	
• Complications	• Recurrent dislocation • Unreduced dislocation • Traumatic osteoarthritis • The risk of developing secondary osteoarthritis following anterior dislocation of shoulder is 10 to 20 times greater than normal people • Axillary nerve damage	• Recurrent dislocation • Unreduced dislocation • Traumatic osteoarthritis

ANTERIOR DISLOCATION OF SHOULDER

As mentioned earlier, this is the most common type of shoulder dislocation.

Mechanism of Injury

It could be due to either direct or indirect forces. The latter is more common.

Varieties

The anterior dislocation of shoulder could be either subcoracoid, subglenoid, subclavicular or intrathoracic. Among these, the most common variety is the subglenoid (Figs 12.3A to E).

Clinical Features

The patient complains of severe pain and inability to use the shoulder joint. Flat shoulder, rounded anterior prominence and the arm held in a position of abduction and external rotation are some of the unmistakable clinical signs. Due to injury to the axillary nerve, there could be loss of sensation on the outer aspect, of the upper arm and is called the 'Regiment Badge' sign (Fig. 12.4). Other clinical tests are denoted in the box (see page 128).

Radiographs

Various views are required to detect the lesions due to the dislocation (Fig. 12.5 and Table 12.1).

Treatment

Anterior dislocation of the shoulder is an emergency and has to be immediately reduced. There are various methods of reduction (Table 12.1 and Figs 12.6 to 12.9), but the most commonly used method is the Kocher's method. The various steps of this method of reduction are under general anesthesia, longitudinal traction is applied along the line of

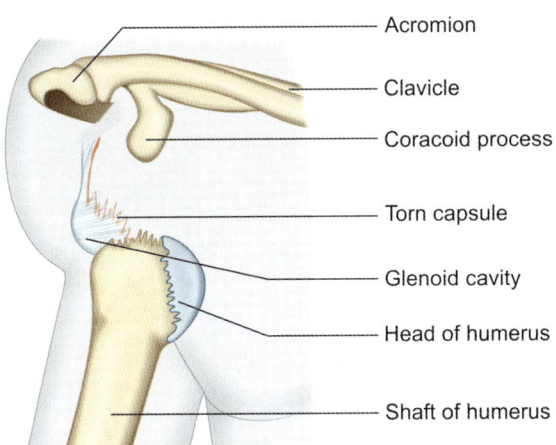

Fig. 12.2: Pathological anatomy: Anterior dislocation of shoulder joint

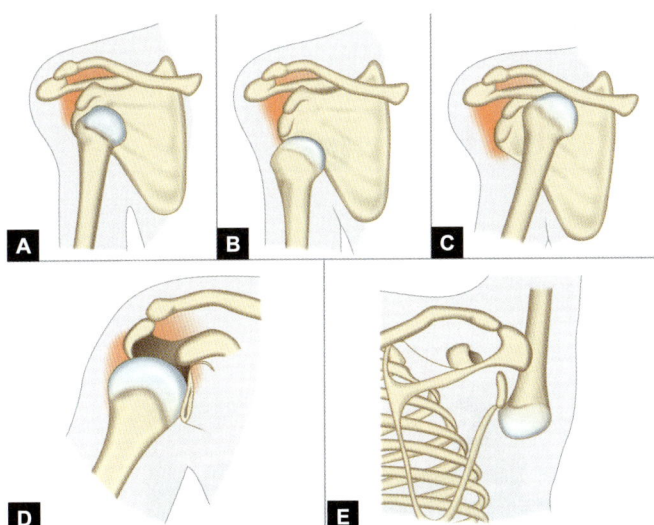

Figs 12.3A to E: Various varieties of shoulder dislocation: (A) Subcoracoid; (B) Subglenoid; (C) Infraclavicular; (D) Posterior; (E) Inferior (luxatio erecta)

124 SECTION 2: Regional Traumatology

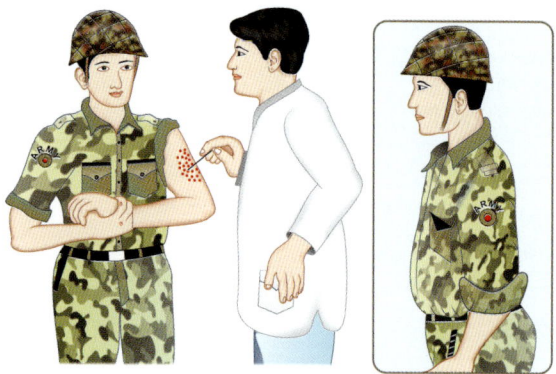

Fig. 12.4: The 'Regiment Badge' sign

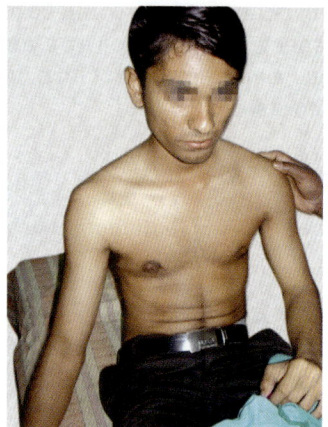

Fig. 12.5: Clinical photo showing anterior dislocation of the shoulder joint

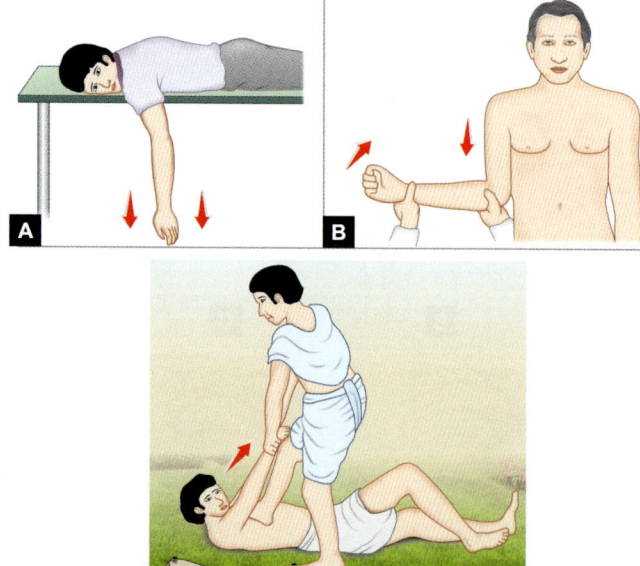

Figs 12.6A to C: Different methods of reduction of shoulder joint dislocation: (A) Stimson's gravity method; (B) Kocher's method (most preferred method); (C) Hippocrates method (outdated)

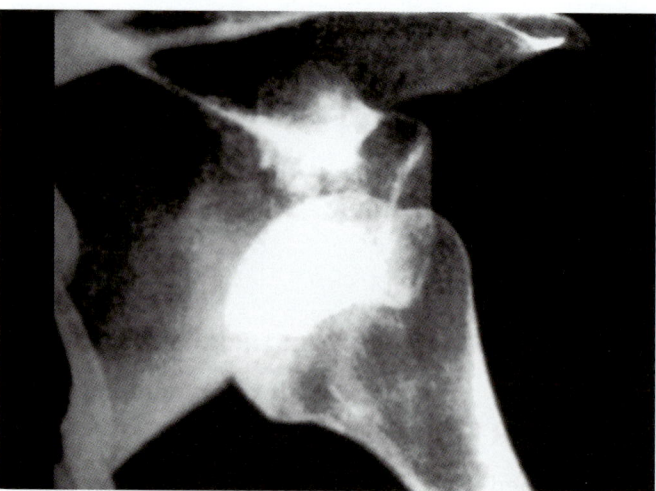

Fig. 12.7: Radiograph showing anterior dislocation of shoulder

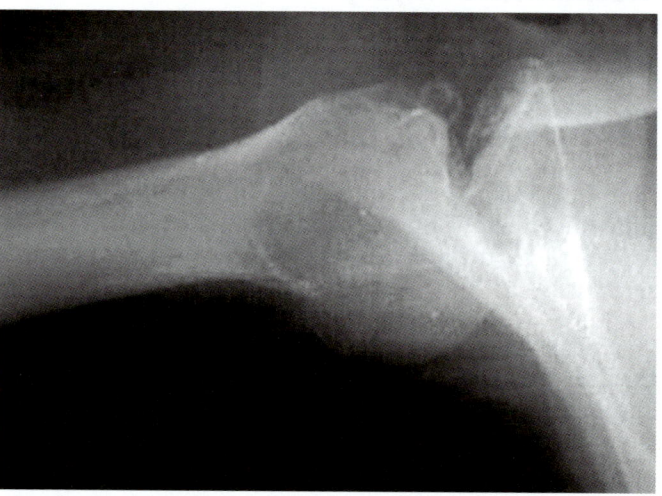

Fig. 12.8: Radiograph showing posterior dislocation of shoulder

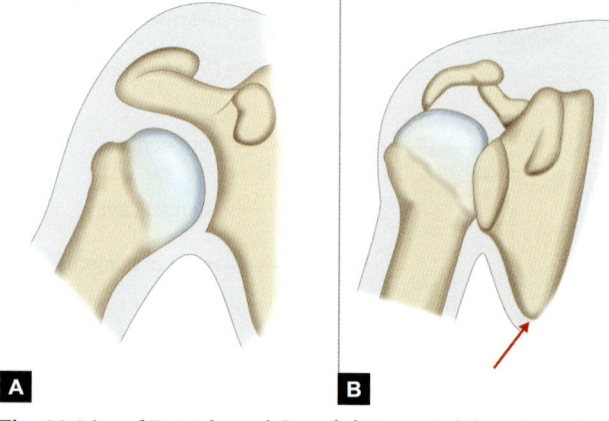

Figs 12.9A and B: Moloney's line: (A) Normal; (B) Moloney's akin to Shenton's line in the hip. Seen in posterior dislocation of shoulder

CHAPTER 12: Injuries of the Shoulder Joint

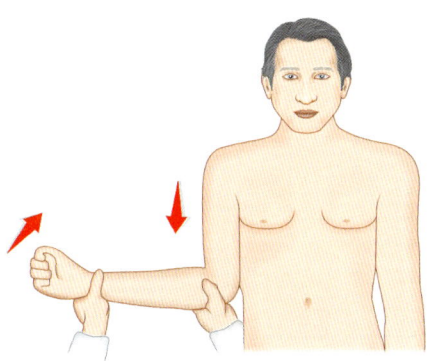

Fig. 12.10: Kocher's method of reduction of anterior dislocation of shoulder. The method consists of four important steps (mnemonic TEAM): T—traction (longitudinal), E—external rotation, A—adduction, M—medial rotation

the humerus, external rotation of the arm, adduction and internal rotation of the arm (Figs 12.10 and 12.11).

> **Note:**
> Reduction should be gentle and should be done preferably under general anesthesia.

After Treatment

After the reduction, the arm should be fastened to the chest with a body bandage for a minimum period of three weeks (Figs 12.12A and B). Failure to do this leads to the development of recurrent dislocation of the shoulder due to the faulty healing of the capsular rent.

> **AMBRI Denotes**
> - A—**A**traumatic
> - M—**M**ultidirectional with
> - B—**B**ilateral shoulder findings responding to
> - R—**R**ehabilitation and
> - I—**I**f surgery, perform an inferior capsular shift.

> **Matsen's Mnemonic TUBS**
> - **T**raumatic etiology
> - **U**nidirectional
> - **B**ankart's lesion present
> - **S**urgery for specific cases.

> **Did you know?**
> Hippocrates was the first person to give a detailed description about the anatomy and dislocation of the shoulder.

> **[1]Kocher's Method of Reduction (Mnemonic TEAM Describes the Various Steps)**
> - **T**raction in line of humerus
> - **E**xternal rotation of the arm
> - **A**dduction of the arm
> - **M**edial rotation of the arm

---
[1]**Theodor Kocher**, Switzerland. Described the method in 1970.

> **Clinical Points**
> Clinical tests of importance in anterior dislocation shoulder
> - *Hamilton's ruler test:* A ruler can be placed between the acromion and the lateral epicondyle. Normally, this is not possible because of the contour of the deltoid muscle.
> - *Callaways test:* The circumference of the axilla is increased.
> - *Bryant's test:* Anterior axillary fold is at a lower level.
> - *Dugas test:* Patient is unable to touch the opposite shoulder.
> - *Regiment badge test:* Area of anesthesia around the deltoid due to injury to the axillary nerve.

> **Quick Facts**
> **Anterior dislocation shoulder**
> - Commonest dislocation.
> - Subcoracoid and subglenoid account for 99% of cases.
> - Capsular injury in 30%: Labral lesion in 60%.
> - Prompt reduction required. Kocher's method is the best.
> - Check for axillary nerve injury before reduction.
> - Immobilize for three weeks and relative immobilization for further three weeks.
> - Prolonged rehabilitation
> - Avoid provocative positions for 6 weeks.

RECURRENT ANTERIOR DISLOCATION OF THE SHOULDER (RDS)

This is a very common complication of anterior dislocation of shoulder and accounts for greater than 80% of dislocations of the upper extremity. Age at the time of initial dislocation is an important prognostic factor, recurrence rate being 55% in patients 12 to 22 years old, 37% in 23 to 29 years old, and 12% in 30 to 40 years old.

> **Did You Know?**
> *One* in every three anterior dislocation of shoulder becomes recurrent dislocation of shoulder.

Causes

- Failure to immobilize the shoulder for 3 to 4 weeks after initial dislocation.
- Size and nature of damage at the time of initial dislocation.
- Greater the trauma, lower the incidence.
- Younger the patient, less is the recurrence.

Mechanism of Dislocation

In some individuals, the dislocation can be predictable and can be avoided. In others, the mechanism is unpredictable and thus makes it a very disabling problem. The usual mechanism of dislocation is external rotation in abducted position (Fig. 12.13).

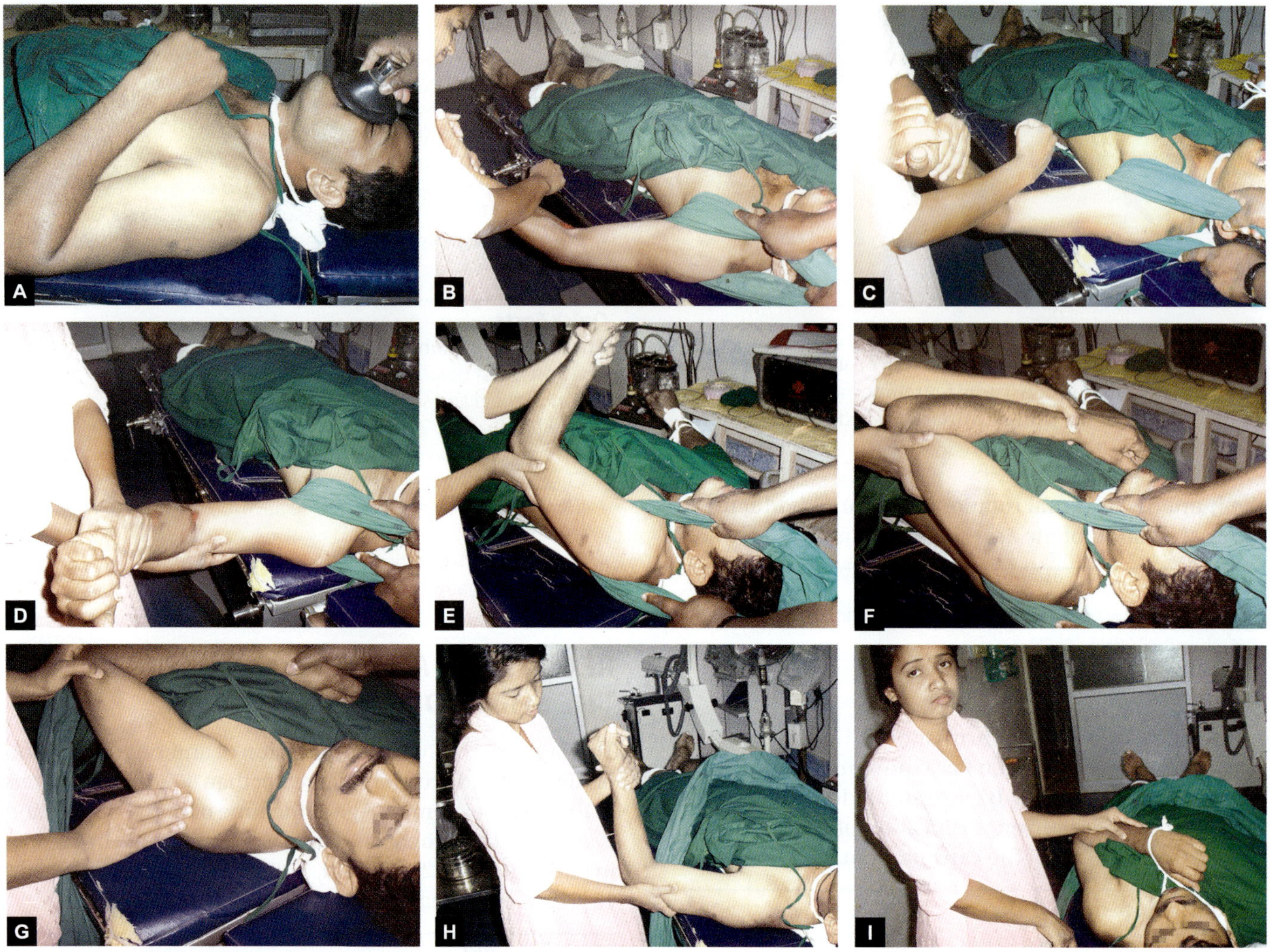

Figs 12.11A to I: (A) Patient is being administered general anesthesia; (B) Kocher's technique—step 1: Longitudinal traction along line of humerus; (C) Traction and counter traction continued; (D) Step 2: External rotation of the arm; (E) Step 3: Adduction of the arm; (F) Step 4: Internal (Medial) rotation of the arm; (G) Shoulder contour restored; (H) Checking for the postreduction stability; (I) Cuff and collar sling being applied

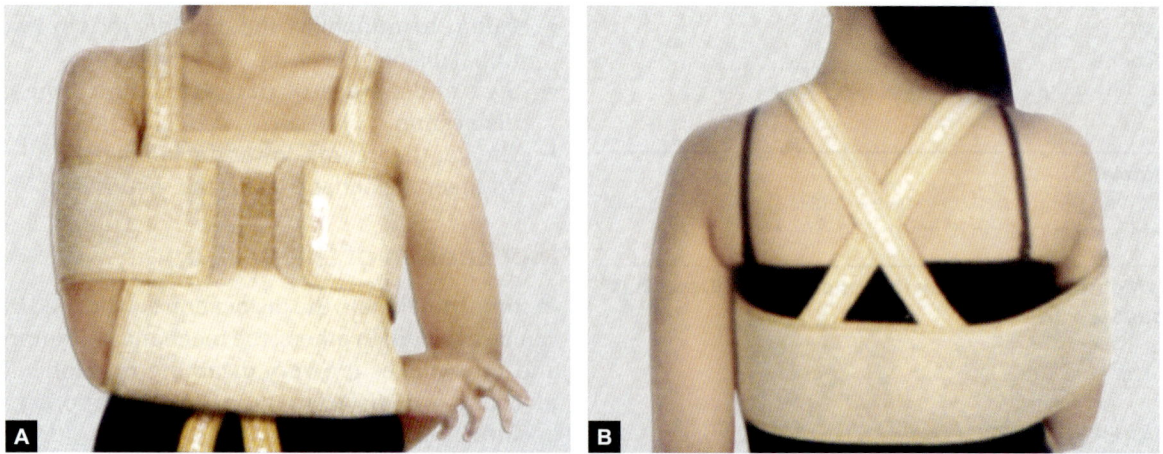

Figs 12.12A and B: Method of shoulder immobilization after reduction of ADS (failure to do this for at least 3 weeks is the prime cause of RDS)

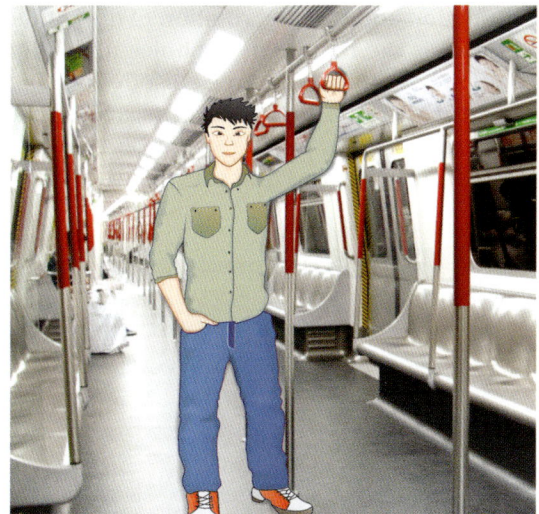
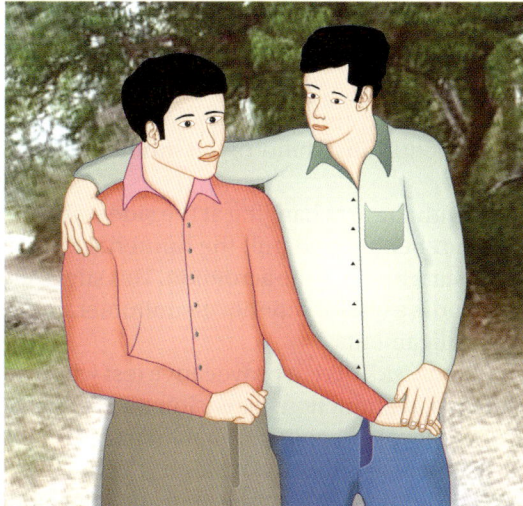
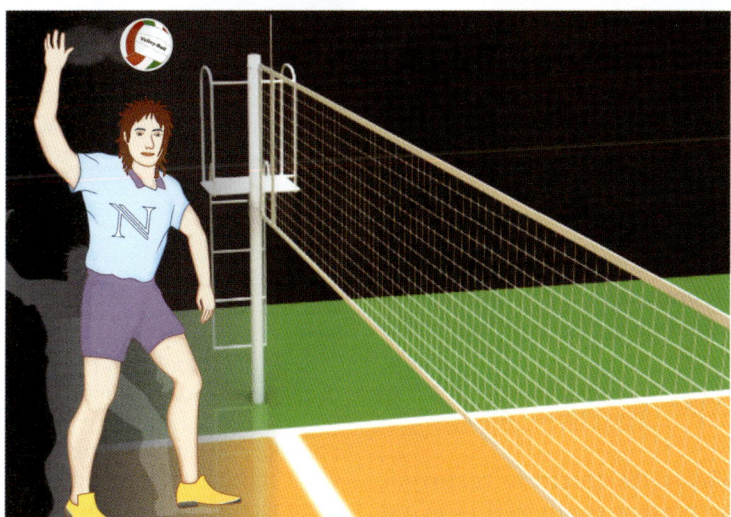

Fig. 12.13: Are you a victim of RDS? If so, beware of routine innocuous activities like these that will knock out your shoulder joint repeatedly

Pathological Anatomy

No single deformity is responsible for recurrent dislocation of shoulder. Three important reasons have been cited and they have been called the essential lesions.

Triad of Essential Lesion

Hill-Sachs lesion: It is a posterolateral defect in the head of the humerus. This is produced due to the impact of the posterolateral part of the head of the humerus against the sharp anterior margin of the glenoid rim.

Bankart's lesion: Perthes first described this as defect in the anterior part of the glenoid labrum and the anterior capsule. If this defect does not heal properly or heals in elongated position, it results in RDS.

Erosion of anterior rim of glenoid cavity: External rotation of the shoulder in abducted position pops out the head of the humerus from the glenoid cavity due to the lax anterior capsular structures. The posterolateral defect now encounters glenoid rim and is levered out of the socket, producing dislocation. Since no single factor is responsible for every recurrent dislocation, no single operative procedure can be applied to every patient.

Clinical Features

Usually, the patient gives history of a previous episode of traumatic dislocation. After that, there could be one or two instances of repeated dislocations during abduction. The clinical features and the presentation will be like in anterior dislocation of shoulder but the far less severity

(Fig. 12.14). There could be wasting of deltoid, supraspinatus and infraspinatus muscles.

Clinical Tests

Three tests help to identify instability of the shoulder prone to develop RDS:
- *The sulcus test* with the arm hanging at the side stabilize the scapula from behind and pull the humerus down. A large gap appears beneath the acromion. This suggests inferior laxity and is a test for superior glenohumeral and coracohumeral ligaments.
- *The apprehension test:* This is a provocative test where if the arm is placed in abduction, extension and external rotation and if a force is applied, the patient becomes apprehensive and resists the provocation (Fig. 12.15).
- *Relocation test:* The joint can be dislocated and relocated back into its position by manual pressure.

Investigations

Radiology: A study of the plain X-ray of the shoulder helps detect the various lesions described above.

CT Scan: Helps to analyze the defects of RDS more clearly.

MRI: This helps to evaluate the entire spectrum of the problem in RDS namely the bony, soft tissue and labral defects that cannot be identified by the X-rays. This helps to plan the treatment better.

Treatment

There is no role of conservative treatment in recurrent dislocation of shoulder. The patient is advised to avoid abduction and external rotation of the shoulder. However, surgery is the treatment of choice and is indicated if the patient has more than three episodes of RDS.

More than 150 operations are devised. Few are mentioned here. All the surgeries aim at correction of the essential lesions and prevent external rotation of the arm.

Name of the surgery	What is done?
[2]Bankart's operation (Fig. 12.16)	Detached anterior structures are attached to the rim of the glenoid cavity with suture
Staple capsulorrhaphy of Destot and Roux	Bankart's lesion attached to labrum with staples
[3]Putti-Platt's operation	Subscapularis tendon and capsule is overlapped and tightened
Magnuson and Stack	Subscapularis tendon and capsule is advanced laterally on the humerus
Eden Hybinette	Bone graft is placed against the anterior aspect of neck of scapula and rim of glenoid cavity
Bristow's	Transplantation of coracoid's process with its attachments to the anterior rim of glenoid
McLaughlin's	Tendon of subscapularis is transplanted into the posterolateral defect

Did You Know?
Bilateral facts about shoulder dislocation. Though anterior dislocation is more common than posterior dislocation, bilateral posterior dislocation is more common than anterior variety. The reason being, the mechanism of injury of adduction and internal rotation of posterior dislocation is common in seizures, which is more prevalent while simultaneous abduction and external rotation for anterior dislocation of shoulder is relatively rare.

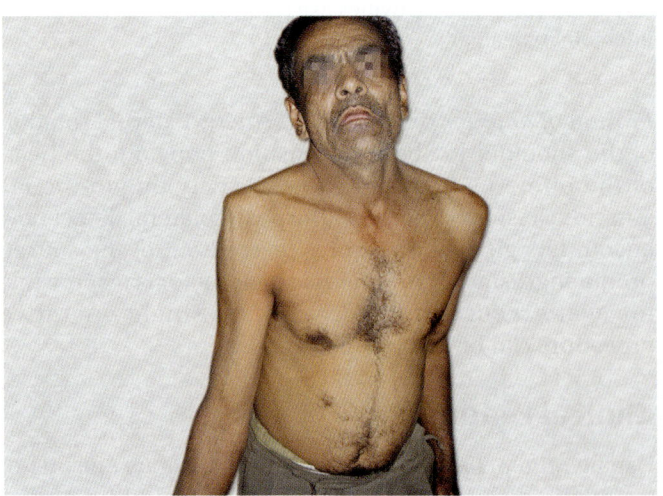

Fig. 12.14: Deformity in RDS (Clinical photo)

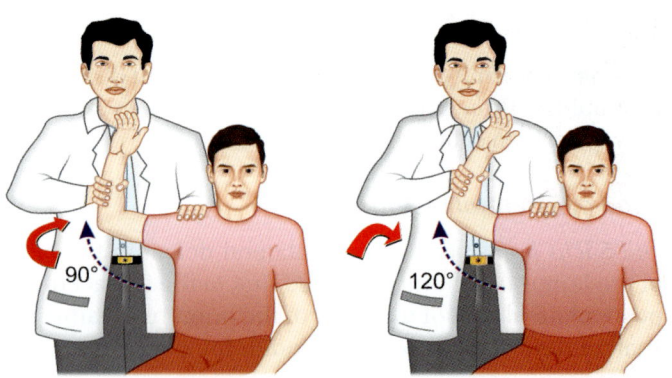

Fig. 12.15: Shoulder apprehension test

---
[2]A and B Bankart (1938). London described pathology and treatment for RDS in 1938.
[3]Putti Vittoria (1880-1940) Bologna, Italy and Harry Platt (1886-1986) Manchester, England.

Inferior Dislocation (Luxatio Erecta)

Here the head of the humerus is below the glenoid cavity and the humeral shaft is pointing overhead. It is due to hyperabduction force and is a rare injury. Here shoulder is locked in 100 to 160° of abduction with the forearm behind the head (see Fig. 12.3E).

Posterior Dislocation of the Shoulder Joint (Fig. 12.17)

Posterior dislocations of the shoulder are seen in a small percentage of patients say about 5% of the cases. They are occasionally due to the violent muscle contractions from *electric shock* or epileptic fits. It is due to the strength imbalance of the rotator cuff muscles. Patients typically presents with a deformity of holding their arm internally rotated and adducted, there is flattening of the anterior shoulder with a prominent coracoid process.

In an *elderly* patient and in some unconscious trauma patient in head injuries it may go unrecognized. An average interval of 1 year is noted in a series by some authors. Plain X-rays may show vacant glenoid sign. Treatment is conservative and if it fails open reduction is done with repair of the labral defects.

FRACTURE OF THE SCAPULA

Scapula is a flat bone thickly covered by muscles (Fig. 12.18).

Incidence

It is a rare injury.
- 3 to 5 percent of all shoulder girdle injuries.
- 0.4 to 1 percent of all fractures.
- Mean age is 35 to 45 years.

Functions

- Stabilizes the upper extremity against the thorax.
- Links the upper extremity to the glenoid.

Mechanism of Injury

- Direct blow—fall of a heavy object on the shoulder blade (Fig. 12.19).
- Axial loading on the outstretched hands.

Classification (Thompson's)

Type I: Coracoid, acromion and small fractures of the body.
Type II: The glenoid and neck fractures.
Type III: Body fractures major (Fig. 12.20).

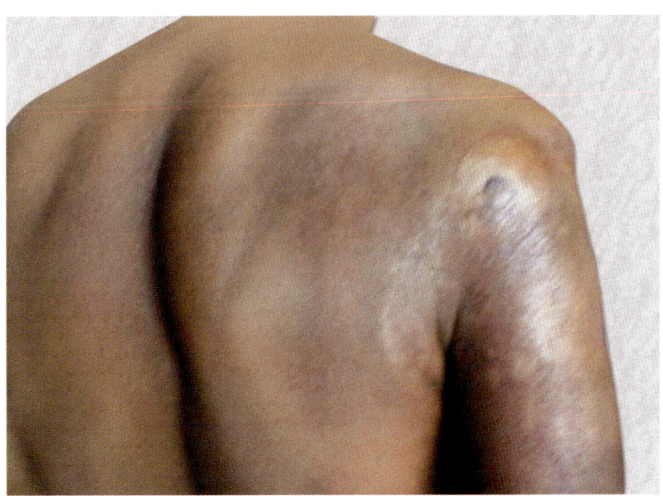

Fig. 12.17: Clinical photo showing unreduced posterior dislocation of the shoulder joint

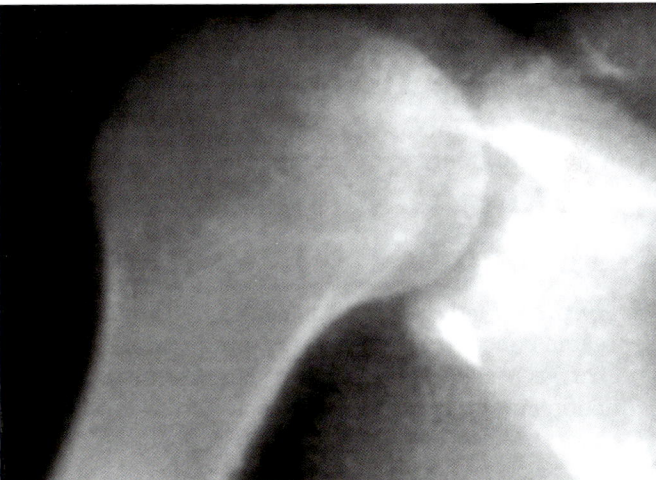

Fig. 12.16: Radiograph showing Bankart's repair

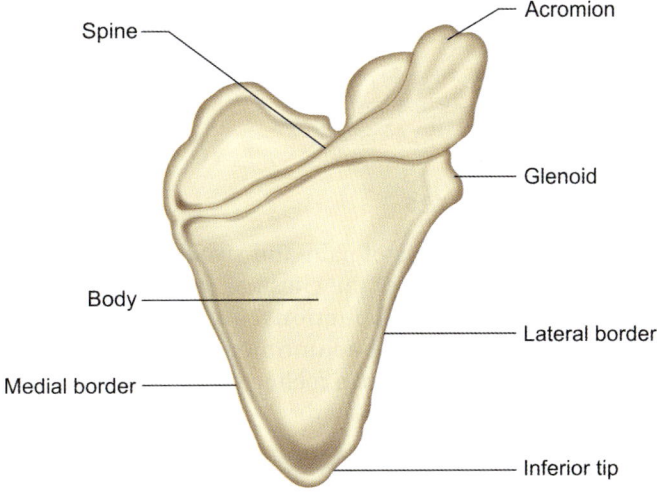

Fig. 12.18: Shows bony anatomical features of scapula

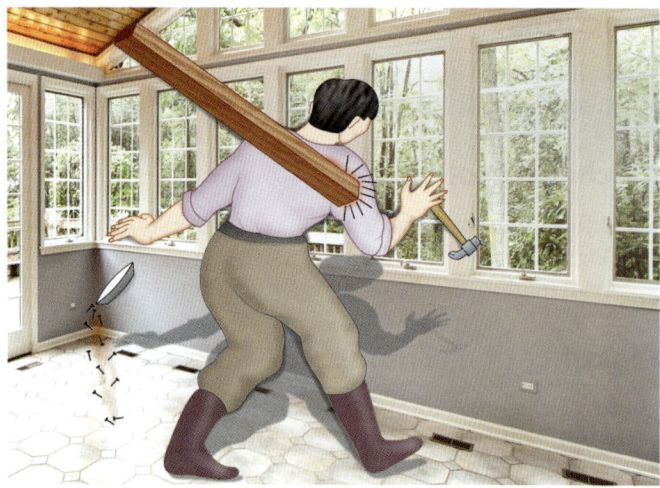

Fig. 12.19: Most common mode of injury causing scapular fracture

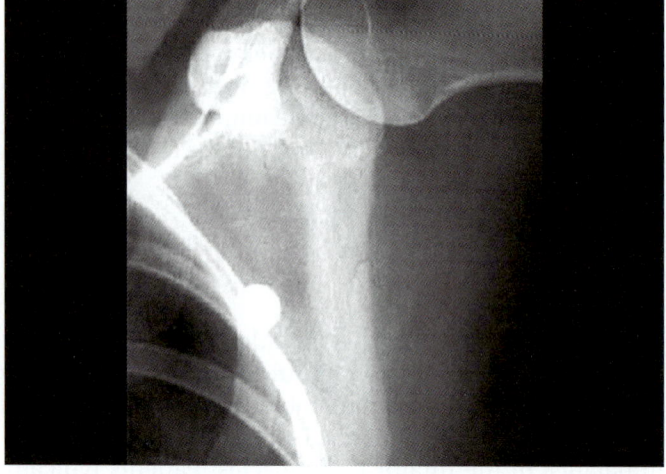

Fig. 12.21: Scapula fracture lateral border

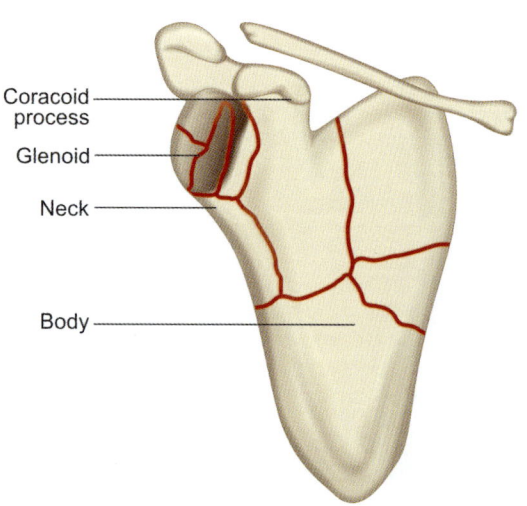

Fig. 12.20: Types of scapular fractures

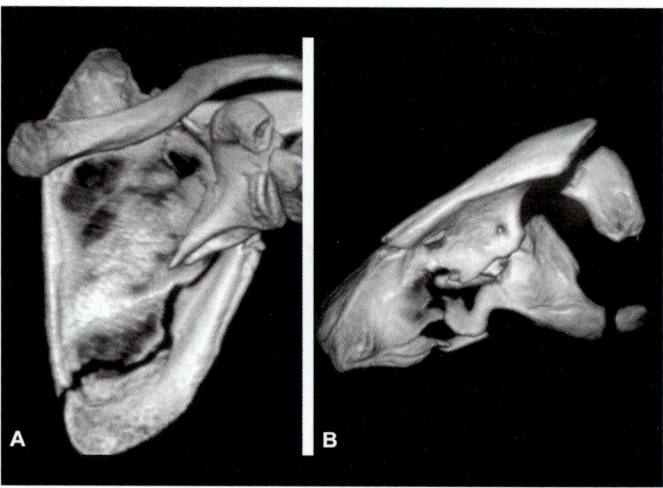

Figs 12.22A and B: CT scan showing Scapula fracture

Note:
- Neck fractures —10 to 60 percent
- Body fractures—49 to 89 percent
- Glenoid fractures—9 percent.

Clinical Features

The patient complains of pain and swelling, arm is held adducted to the sides of the chest, all movements of the shoulder, especially abductions, are painful, may be associated rarely with pneumothorax and inability to elevate the arms may give a feeling of pseudo-rupture of the rotator cuff.

Radiographs

A true scapular AP view and a true lateral view (axillary view) helps to make the diagnosis (Fig. 12.21). CT Scan helps to delineate the fracture better (Figs 12.22A and B).

Treatment

Nonoperative Methods: Undisplaced scapular fractures may be treated conservatively with rest, sling, strap, etc.
Operative Methods: Displaced fractures need open reduction and internal fixation with K-wires, screws, etc.

13 CHAPTER

Injuries Around the Elbow

BRIEF ANATOMY

Elbow joint is the most notorious joint in the body for it is associated with many complications following injury or trauma to the elbow. *It easily becomes stiff and offers stiff resistance to the efforts of treating doctors to make it mobile again.*

Elbow Joint Speaks
- I am a compound paracondylar joint as the lower end of humerus articulates with both radius and ulna. However, I am a hinge joint allowing only flexion, extension through an arc of 150°, more specifically the humeroulnar component of mine is a modified sellar joint, and the humeroradial component is an unmodified ovoid. I have the proximal radioulnar joint, which is a modified ovoid joint. All the three components of mine mentioned so far share the same joint capsule. This makes me respond differently to trauma, exercises, massage, etc. I have a capsule, which is reinforced laterally by the radial collateral ligament and medially by the ulnar collateral ligament. The annular ligament holds the head of the radius in its position (Fig. 13.1).
- I flex mainly due to the action of biceps and brachialis supported by brachioradialis, pronator teres, and common flexors. I extend due to the action of triceps, aided by anconeus and common extensors. Biceps and supinator help me supinate and pronator teres and quadratus help me pronate. Three important nerves of the upper limb pass through me: (i) the radial nerve crosses laterally, (ii) the ulnar nerve passes beneath the medial epicondyle and enters the forearm through the flexor carpi ulnaris, and (iii) the median nerve crosses me in front.

Interesting Facts
What is patella cubitis?
These are accessory bones present in the triceps near its attachment at olecranon.

Vital Facts
- Primary elbow flexor is the brachialis and is called the "workhorse" of elbow flexion.
- Primary elbow extensor triceps.

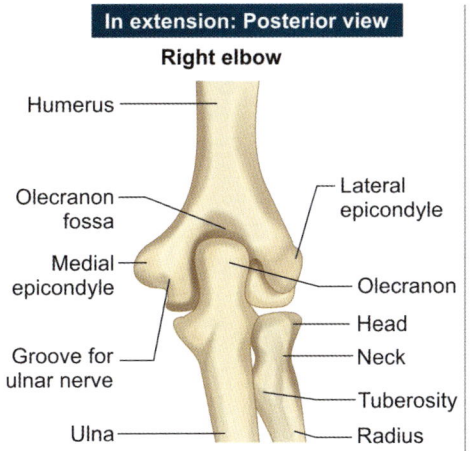
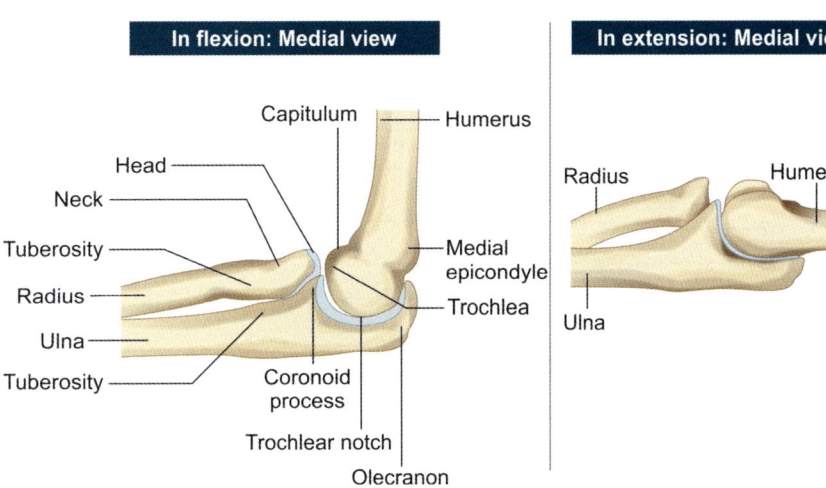

Fig. 13.1: Anatomy of elbow joint

POSTERIOR ELBOW GEOMETRY

Mnemonic CRMTOL: Helps to remember the secondary centers of ossification around the elbow (All are multiples of two) (Fig. 13.2)
- **C**apitulum appears at 2 years (6 months to 2 years)
- **R**adial head (4 years)
- **M**edial epicondyle (6 years)
- **T**rochlea (8 years)
- **O**lecranon (8–10 years)
- **L**ateral epicondyle (12 years)
- Internal epicondyle appears at 6 years
- Trochlea appears at 9 years
- External epicondyle appears at 12 years.

Note:
The importance of these secondary ossification centers is that they are often mistaken as fractures in children.

Triangle Sign

The relation between the three bony points around the elbow namely, lateral epicondyle, medial epicondyle, and olecranon is important to differentiate between fractures around the elbow and dislocations (Figs 13.3A and B). In flexion, these three bony points almost form an equilateral triangle. This is maintained in supracondylar fractures and is disturbed in posterior dislocation of the elbow. In extension, these three bony points lie in the same straight line normally. In posterior dislocation of the elbow, the olecranon process of the ulna lies above the line joining the medial and lateral epicondyle.

Carrying Angle

This varies with elbow flexion and extension. In full flexion, the carrying angle is 0°. In full extension of the elbow, the long axis of the arm and the long axis of the forearm do not lie in the same straight line. The latter forms a valgus angle of 11° with the former. This is slightly more in the females and is called the carrying angle in extension. The carrying angle helps the elbow to clear the pelvis. Increase in this angle results in cubitus valgus deformity (Fig. 13.4) and decrease in the angle forms the cubitus varus deformity. However, the carrying angle disappears with full flexion of the elbow, and it is in this position that the long axis of the forearm and long axis of arm lie parallel to each other.

INJURIES AROUND THE ELBOW

Fall on the outstretched hands is more common in children because they are more playful and hence more prone to fall. Thus, upper extremities are vulnerable to fractures. Sixty five

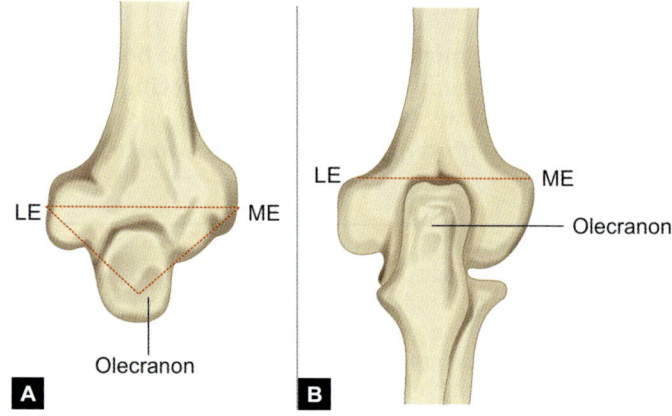

Figs 13.3A and B: Relationship between the three bony points of the elbow in flexion and extension between LE—lateral and olecranon epicondyle, ME—medial epicondyle

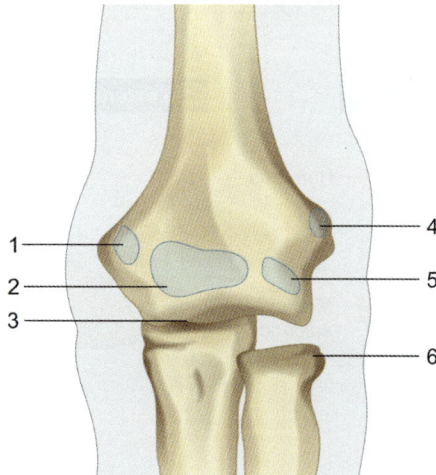

Fig. 13.2: Secondary centers of ossification: (1) Medial epicondyle; (2) trochlea; (3) olecranon; (4) lateral epicondyle; (5) capitulum; (6) radial head

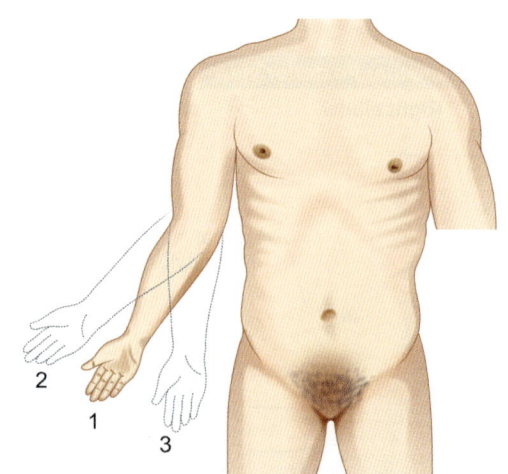

Fig. 13.4: Carrying angle of elbow: (1) Normal; (2) increased (cubitus valgus); (3) decreased (cubitus varus)

TABLE 13.1: Incidence of injuries around elbow	
Injuries	Percentage
• Supracondylar fractures	65.4
• Condylar fractures	25.3
• Fracture neck radius	4.7
• Monteggia's fractures	2.2
• Olecranon fractures	1.6
• T-condylar fractures	0.8
In children, forearm bone fractures rank first followed by fractures around the elbow region. The incidence of distal humeral fractures is as follows:	
• Supracondylar	69
• Lateral condyle	16.8
• Medial condyle	14.1
• T-condylar	1

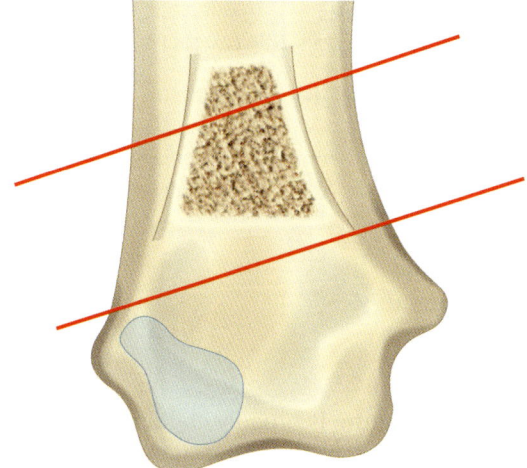

Fig. 13.5: Supracondylar area in children

to seventy five percent of all fractures sustained by children are seen in upper limbs (Table 13.1).

Classification of Fractures of Distal Humerus in Children

A. *Supracondylar:*
   • Flexion type
   • Extension type.
B. *Physeal fracture:*
   • Involving lateral condylar physis
   • Involving medial condylar physis
   • Involving total distal physis
   • Involving medial epicondylar physis
   • Involving lateral epicondylar physis.
C. *T-condylar fracture.*

SUPRACONDYLAR FRACTURE

As mentioned earlier, supracondylar fractures of the humerus is very common in children. The reason lies in the bony architecture of the supracondylar area in children. The mechanism of injury and the predisposing factors exploit this potential weakness in this area and break it more often than any other bone in children (Fig. 13.5).

Do You Know?
Supracondylar fracture of humerus is also called Malgaigne's fracture.

Vital Facts of Pathological Anatomy
Why common in children <10 years?
Bony architecture at the supracondylar region is weak and vulnerable because in this region:
• Bone is remodeling
• It is less cylindrical
• Metaphysis is just distal to 2 fossae, coronoid, and radial

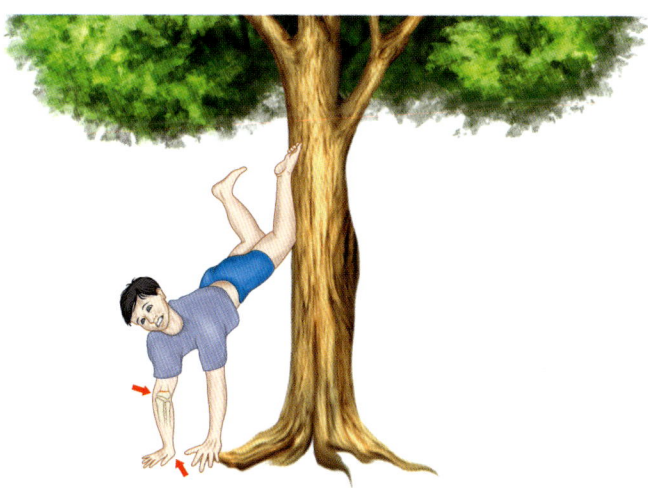

Fig. 13.6: Fall on outstretched hands is a common mechanism of upper limb fractures in children

• Here the cortex is thin
• Anterior cortex has a defect in the area of coronoid fossa
• Laxity of ligaments permits hyperextension at the elbow.

Important Facts
Predisposing factors for juvenile supracondylar fractures are:
• Ligamentous laxity at the elbow leads to hyperextension.
• Hyperextension converts linear force into bending force. Olecranon concentrates this force to the weak supracondylar area.
• Anterior capsule is taut.
• Bony architecture of a supracondylar area.

Mechanism of Injury

Fall on outstretched hands with hyperextension at the elbow with abduction or adduction, with hand dorsiflexed (Fig. 13.6).

134 SECTION 2: Regional Traumatology

> **Quick Review of Statistics**
> - Age—first decade, 5–8 years, 84% cases <10 years
> - Sex—boys 63.6%
> - Sides (L)—58.6%; (R)—42.4%
> - Open fracture—2.3%
> - Nerve injury—7% → Radial nerve—45%
> - VIC—0.5%   Median nerve—32%
> - Fracture of ipsilateral   Ulnar nerve—23%
> - Extremity—1.2%
> - Flexion type—2.3%
> - Extension type—97.7%

Classification

Supracondylar fracture is broadly classified into *extension type* and *flexion type*. In extension type, the fracture line runs *upwards* and *backwards;* and in flexion type, it runs *downwards* and *forwards* (Figs 13.7A and B). Extension type of supracondylar fracture is further classified into the following subtypes (Fig. 13.8).

Gartland's Classification (In Children)

- *Type I:* Undisplaced
- *Type II:* Displaced, but posterior cortex is intact.
- *Type III:* Displaced, but no intact posterior cortex and the distal fragment could be either displaced:
  - Posteromedial or
  - Posterolateral.

Clinical Features

The patient complains of pain and swelling which is gross, S-shaped deformity of the upper arm is obvious and there is loss of both active and passive movements of the elbo (Fig. 13.9). Symptoms relating to vascular and nerve injury may be seen. The patient may also complain of pseudoparalysis. Tests should be carried out for brachial artery and all the three nerves of the upper limb, namely, the radial nerve, the median and ulnar nerves.

The following are the characteristic clinical signs in supracondylar fracture:
- Arm is short, forearm is normal in length
- Gross swelling, and tenderness
- Crepitus is present but should not be elicited for fear of increasing the pain and damaging the neighboring neurovascular structures
- S-shaped deformity
- Dimple sign due to one of the spikes of proximal fragment penetrating the muscle and tethering the skin.
- Relationship between three bony points is maintained.
- "Soft spots" is an effusion beneath anconeus muscle.
- Movements of the elbow both active and passive are decreased.

Radiographs

X-ray of the elbow: A proper study of the radiological signs in both AP and lateral view (Fig. 13.10) of the elbow

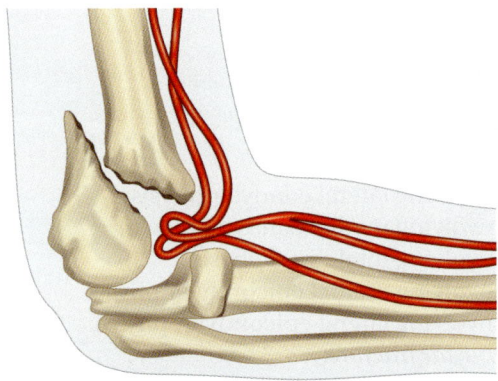

Fig. 13.8: Extension type of supracondylar fracture causing neurovascular injuries

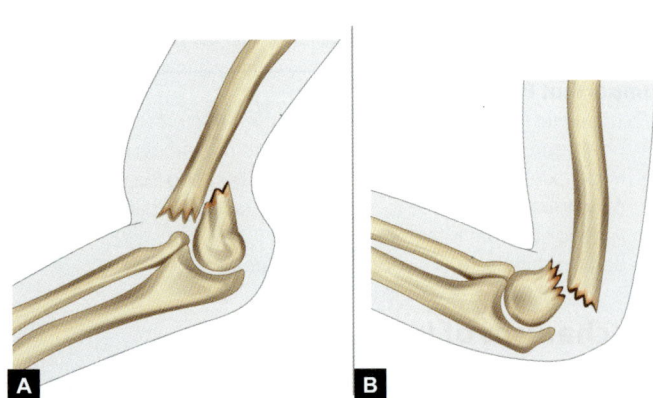

Figs 13.7A and B: Types of supracondylar fracture: (A) Extension type 97.7%; (B) Flexion type 2.3%

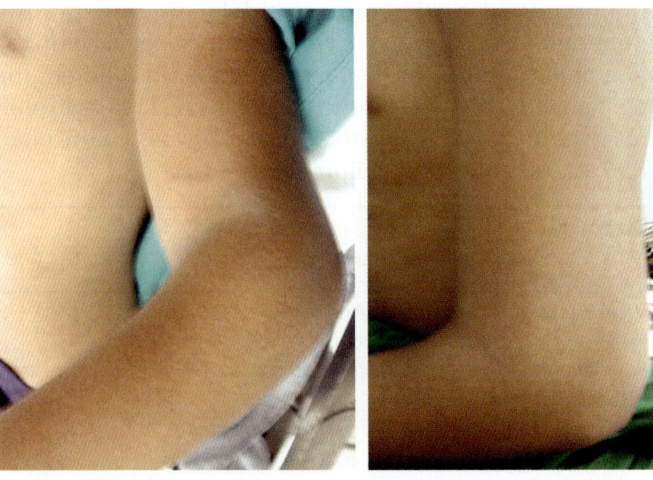

Fig. 13.9: Clinical photo of supracondylar fracture humerus

is extremely important not only to study the fracture anatomy but also to check for the adequacy and accuracy of reduction, a failure of which results in malunion later.

AP view: The following are the radiological parameters of importance in this view (Fig. 13.11A).

- *Baumann's angle:* Angle between the horizontal line of the elbow and the line drawn through the lateral epiphysis and long axis of the arm. Normally, it is less than 5° and should always be compared with the other side.
- Angle between the long axis of humerus and the transverse axis of the elbow is normally 90°.
  - Less than 90° suggests cubitus varus
  - Greater than 90° suggests cubitus valgus.

Lateral view (Figs 13.11B and 13.12A to D)

- *Tear drop sign:* It is disturbed in supracondylar fracture, but it is seen in the normal radiograph.
- Normally, there is an angulation of 40° between the long axis of humerus and long axis of lateral epicondyle.
- *Anterior humeral line:* A line drawn along the anterior border or the distal humeral shaft passes through the middle 1/3rd of capitulum's. If it passes through anterior 1/3rd, it indicates posterior displacement of the distal fragment.
- *The coronoid line*: A line directed proximally along the anterior border of the coronoid process of the ulna should just barely touch the anterior portion of the lateral condyle. Posterior displacement of the lateral condyle will project the ossification center posterior to this line.
- *Fat pad sign:* The olecranon fossa is deep and thus the fat pad here lies totally contained within the fossa. Not seen on the normal lateral radiograph of the elbow at 90°. Distension of the capsule with an effusion due to trauma or infection causes the olecranon pad to be visualized as a radiolucent gap.
- *Fish-tail sign*: Due to rotation of the distal fragment, the anterior border of the proximal fragment looks like a sharp spike (see Fig. 13.11B).

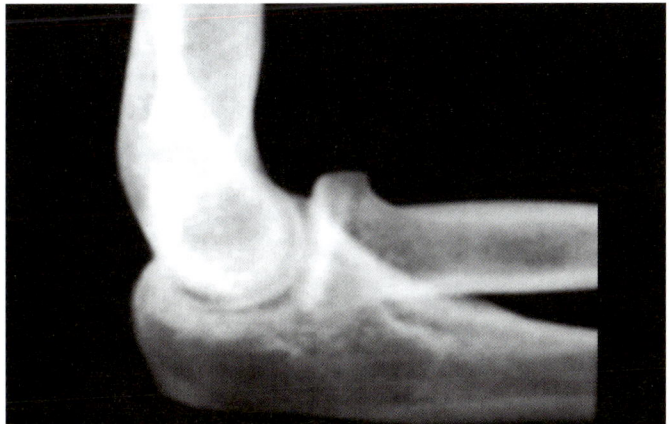

Fig. 13.10: Radiograph showing normal lateral view of elbow

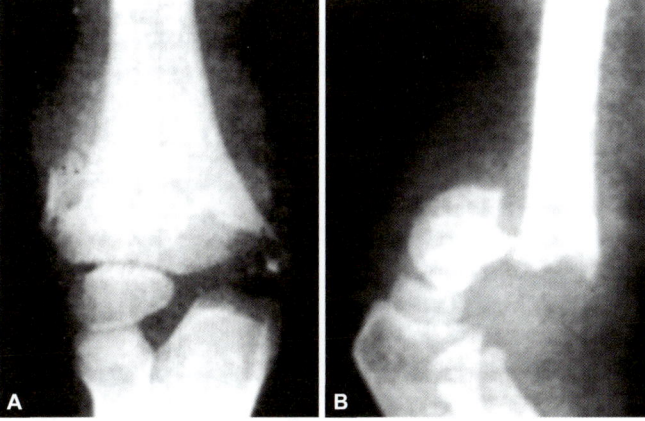

Figs 13.11A and B: (A) Radiograph showing extension type of supracondylar fracture: AP view; (B) Radiograph showing extension type of supracondylar fracture: Lateral view

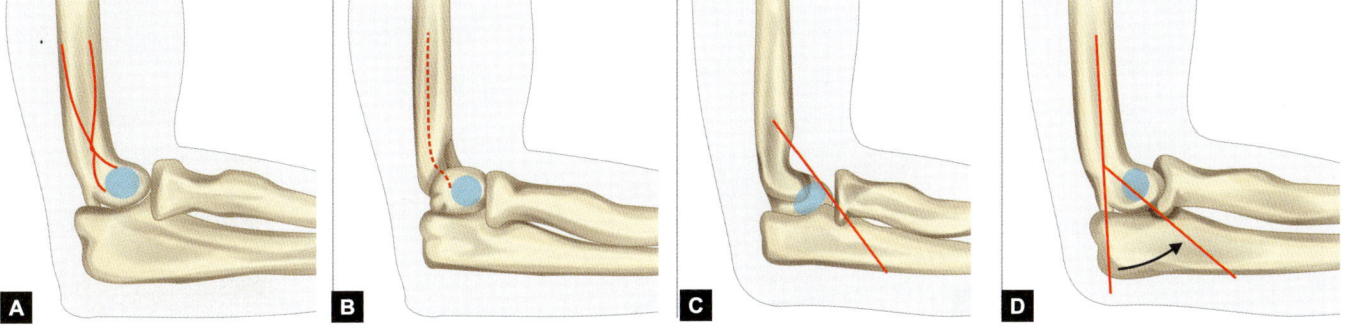

Figs 13.12A to D: Look for these important landmarks on the lateral view of the elbow X-ray: (A) Tear drop sign; (B) Anterior humeral line; (C) Coronoid line; (D) Relationship between axis of humerus and that of lateral epicondyle

- *Crescent sign*: Here the normal radiolucent gap of the elbow joint is missing and a crescent-shaped shadow due to the overlap of the capitulum's over the olecranon is evident and indicates either varus or valgus tilt of the distal fragment.

Quick Facts
Radiological points
Posterior displacement of the distal fragment: Indicated by:
- Loss of tear drop sign
- Coronoid line
- Fat pad sign
- Anterior humeral line.

Coronal tilt of the distal fragment: Usually varus tilt rarely valgus indicated on radiography by:
- Crescent sign
- Baumann's angle.

Horizontal rotation of the distal fragment: Indicated by fish-tail sign.

Management

Conservative management: Initially, closed reduction is tried under general anesthesia by traction and counter traction methods (Figs 13.13A to C). The medial and lateral tilt is corrected first and posterior displacement next. *An immediate check can be made whether the reduction has been successful by noting the long axis of the forearm and arm, which should be parallel.* Any deviation from the normal indicates residual uncorrected deformities. Two to three attempts under the same anesthesia can be made and the elbow is immobilized in hyperflexion, as in this position the triceps acts as an internal splint (Figs 13.14 and 13.15) and the forearm is pronated as in this position the medial periosteal hinge closes the cortex laterally. Check radiograph is taken and all the angles so far discussed should be restored to normalcy, failure of which requires considering alternative methods of treatment like skeletal traction or open reduction and internal fixation. Modified shoulder spica for 3 to 4 weeks has given good results in some.

Traction methods: It is indicated if conservative methods fails (Figs 13.16A to D). Traction methods consist of skin or skeletal traction and are of historical importance of late due to the availability of better and effective treatment methods.

Surgery: This includes closed reduction and percutaneous internal fixation with K-wires or open reduction and internal fixation with wires or plates.

Closed reduction and percutaneous fixation (PCIF): In cases where hyper flexion of the elbow cannot be done due to gross swelling in and around the elbow and in grossly unstable fractures, percutaneous fixation of the

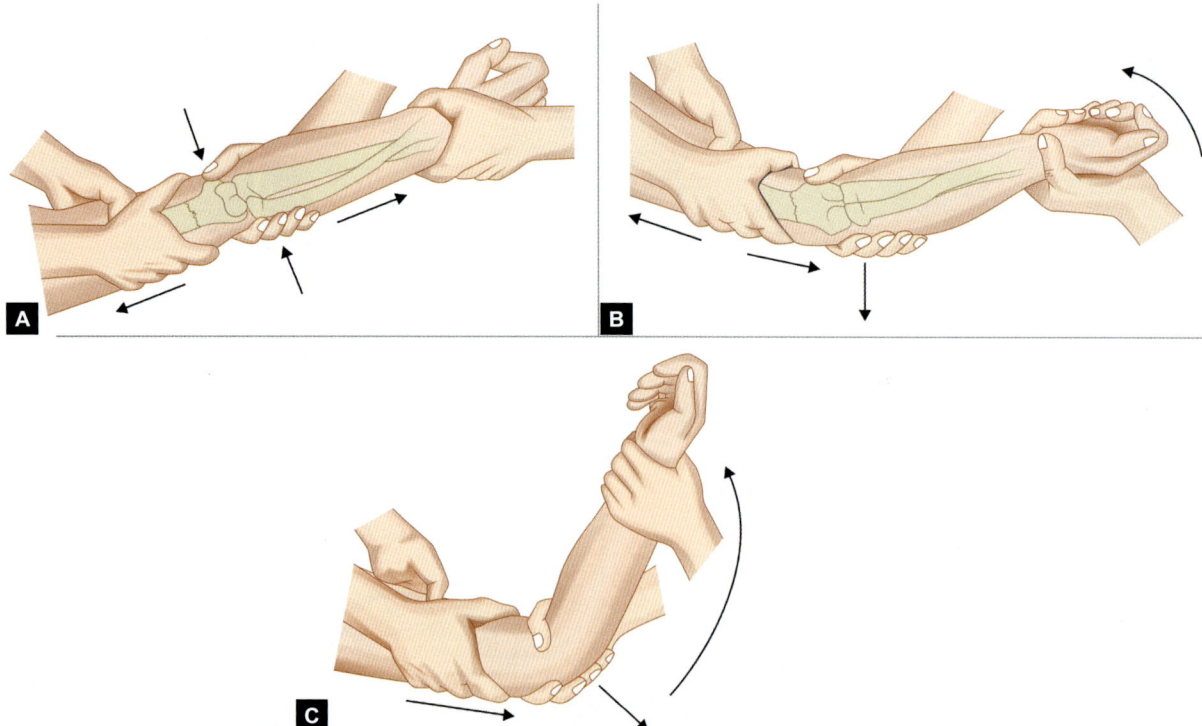

Figs 13.13A to C: Technique of closed reduction of a supracondylar fracture of humerus: (A) Longitudinal traction and correction of medial and lateral tilts; (B) Correction of posterior tilt; (C) Final position

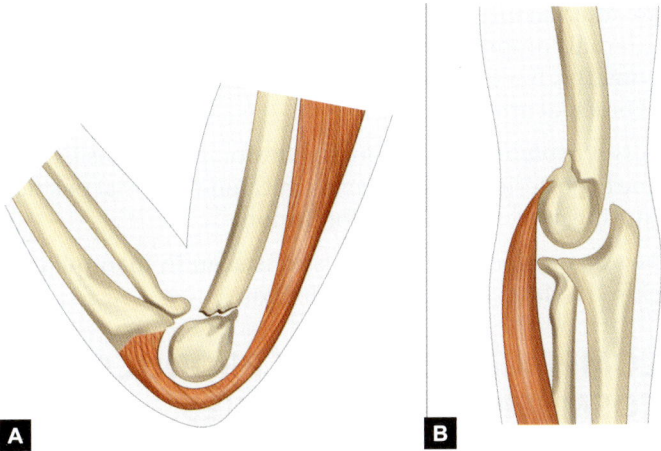

Figs 13.14A and B: Methods of immobilization of supracondylar fracture of humerus: (A) Extension type; (B) Flexion type

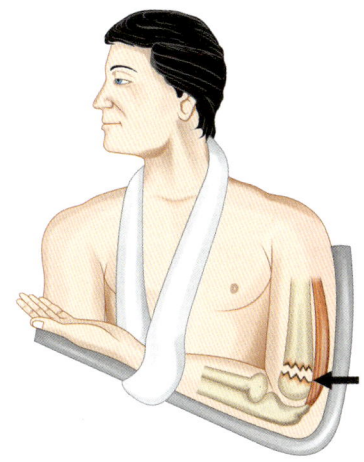

Fig. 13.15: Triceps muscle acts as an internal splint in supracondylar fracture humerus when flexed beyond 90°

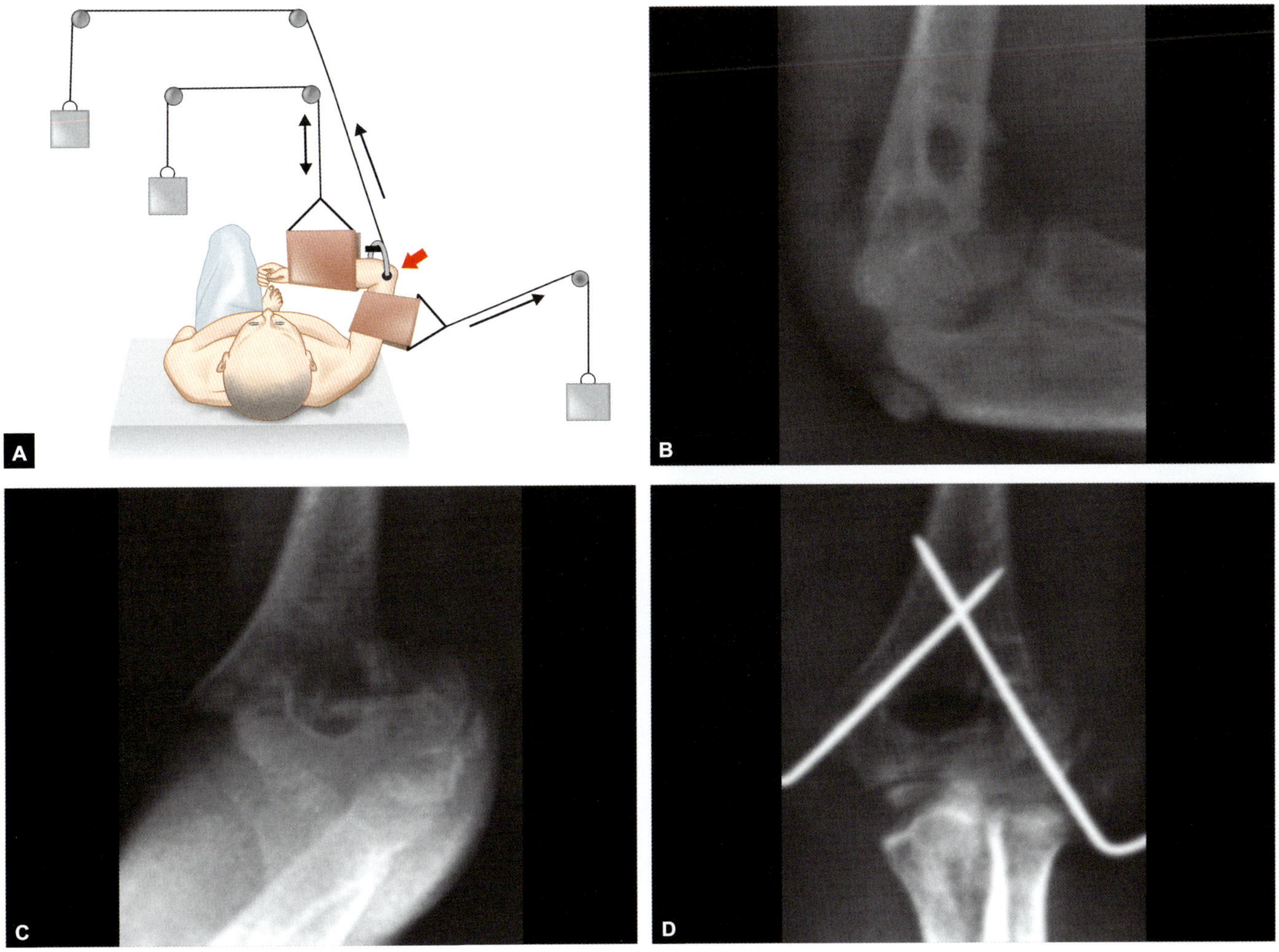

Figs 13.16A to D: (A) Overhead olecranon traction (Smith's traction); (B to D) Radiograph showing percutaneous fixation with K-wire of displaced supracondylar fracture of humerus

fragments with K-wires on either side after closed reduction is an acceptable form of treatment and is widely accepted (Figs 13.16B to D).

Open reduction: This is rarely indicated in certain special indications as depicted in the flow chart. Open reduction is invariably followed by internal fixation with either K-wires or plate and screws (Fig. 13.17). Please see Flowchart 13.1 for the treatment plan of supracondylar fracture of the humerus.

Complications

These are broadly divided into two categories:
1. Those that cause functional impairment of the extremity and is more serious.
2. Those that produce only cosmetic sequel.

Complications Causing Functional Impairment

Neurological involvement: Overall incidence is around 7 percent.

Radial nerve: Most commonly affected and is usually injured in posteromedial displacement.

Median nerve: Injured during posterior displacement.

Anterior interosseous nerve: Injury is seen in posterolateral displacement of the distal fragment.

Ulnar nerve: Injured in overhead skeletal traction and in flexion type of supracondylar fracture.

Vascular injury: The incidence is between 0.5 and 1 percent. Common with extension type and is usually due to direct injury of brachial artery by the fracture. The other causes are internal thrombus, intimal tear, brachial artery spasm, external compression by proximal fracture fragment of the humerus, fracture hematoma, partial or complete rupture of brachial artery.

Loss of mobility: Average loss of flexion is 4° and is usually due to posterior displacement, which unites in that position causing mechanical block for flexion.

Myositis ossificans: It is rare and is seen in manipulative closed reduction and open reduction.

COMPLICATIONS THAT PRODUCE COSMETIC ABNORMALITIES

CUBITUS VARUS (GUNSTOCK ELBOW)

This is so called because the deformity resembles a rifle gunstock (Fig. 13.18) and is the most common complication of supracondylar fracture. Incidence varies from 9 to 58%. The deformity becomes obvious in an extended elbow.

The following are three static deformities of cubitus varus (all with respect to distal fragment):
- Posterior displacement
- Horizontal rotation
- Coronal tilt.

> **Quick Facts**
> Causes of cubitus varus: 4 'I's
> - Improper persons treating
> - Improper reduction
> - Improper interpretation of radiographs
> - Improper follow-up.

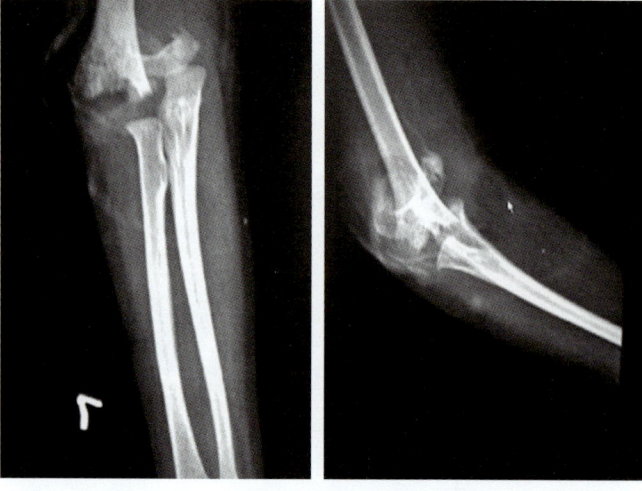

Fig. 13.17: Plain X-rays showing compound supracondylar fracture, needs open reduction

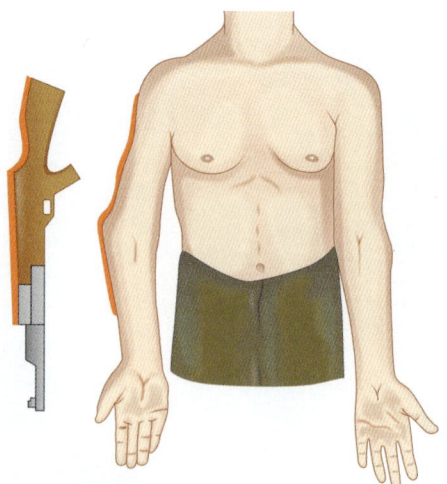

Fig. 13.18: Cubitus varus deformity (also called Gunstock deformity)

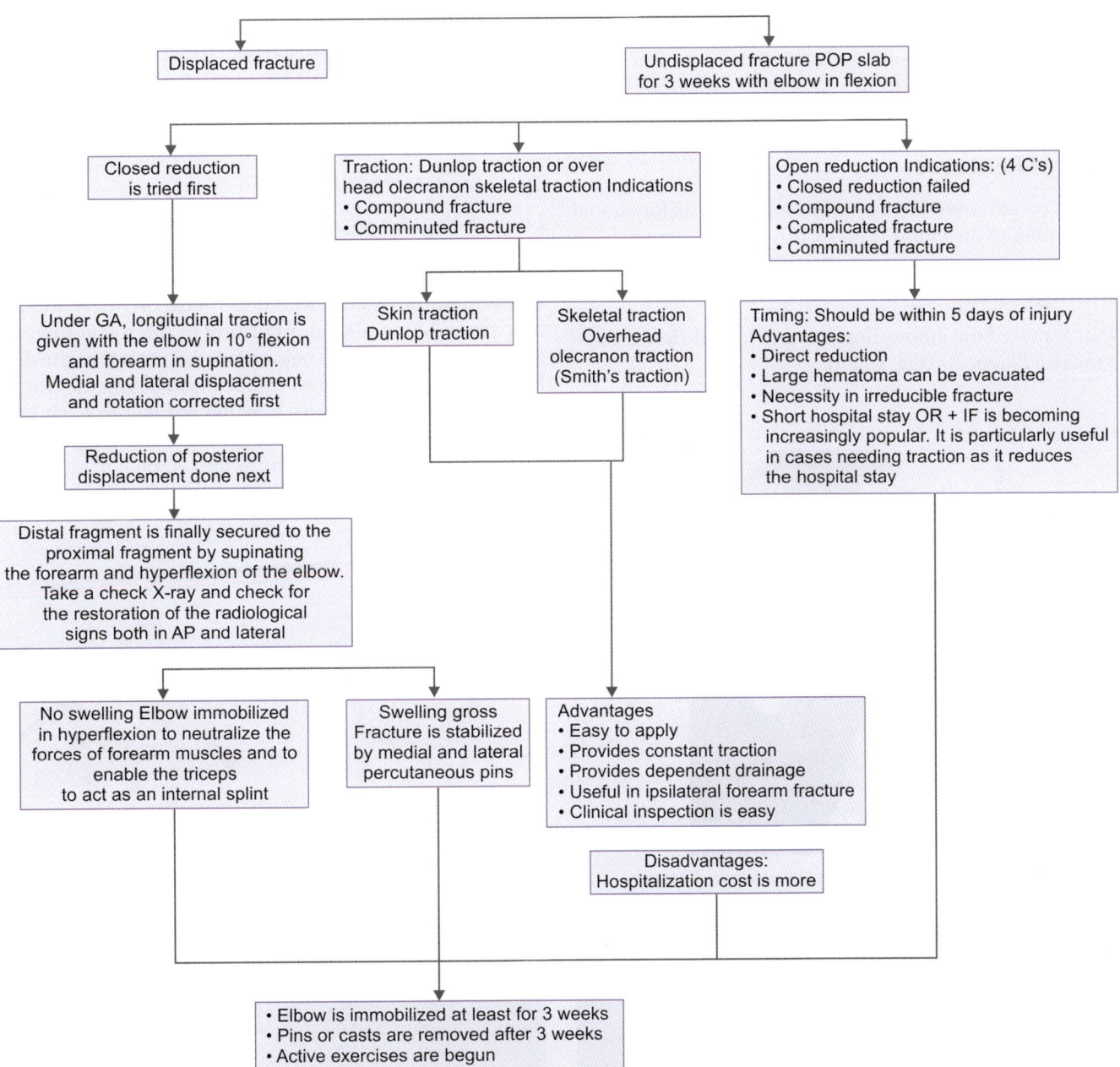

Flowchart 13.1: Management of supracondylar fracture

Pathomechanics

Posterior displacement and horizontal rotation predisposes to coronal tilt. Because the edges of the fracture fragments are thin, there is very little resistance to coronal tilt, if the fragments are horizontally rotated, and contraction of the biceps produce a medial tilting force. All these three components should be corrected during the initial reduction of the fracture otherwise, cubitus varus deformity results. Determination of the quality of fracture reduction after the initial injury can be assessed by the following clinicoradiological tests (Box 13.1).

Box 13.1: Clinical Tests

Long axes of the forearm and humerus should be parallel when elbow is flexed after reduction. This test is done after reduction of an acute fracture to ascertain the alignment has been restored. Ignoring this all important test may lead to Cubitus Varus deformity in future

> **Radiographs**
> *AP view:* Baumann's angle should be less than 5°.
> *Lateral view:* All the normal radiological signs should be restored. If the clinicoradiological criteria are satisfactory, the closed reduction is accepted otherwise re-reduction is attempted. *Ignoring these criteria after closed reduction results in future cubitus varus deformity.*

Clinical Features

Cubitus varus is only a cosmetic disability with no functional impairment of the elbow (Fig. 13.19).

Radiographs

Plain X-rays of the elbow, both AP and lateral views, helps to make a diagnosis (Fig. 13.20).

Treatment

Treatment of choice is corrective osteotomy and is deferred until skeletal maturity as cosmesis gains importance at this age and for the fear of recurrence of deformity, if surgery is done before growth stops since there is still potential for growth left.

Osteotomy Methods

Lateral closed-wedge osteotomy (French and modified French): This operation (Fig. 13.21) is simple and easy to perform and the posterior triceps splitting approach is used. In this method, osteotomy is done between two screws, the first screw being placed anteriorly in the distal fragment and the second screw is being placed posterior in the distal fragment. After the osteotomy, the distal fragment is rotated such that both the screws become parallel to each other indicating correction of rotational deformity (Fig. 13.22). A wedge of bone is removed from the lateral cortex, the gap

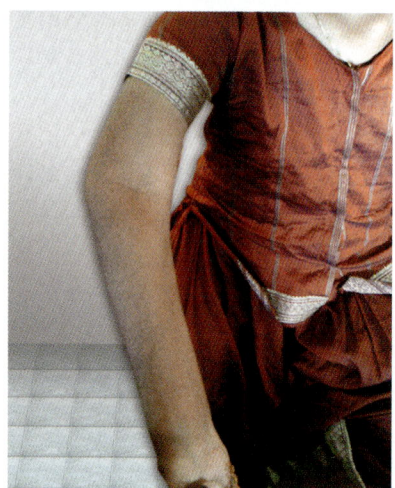

Fig. 13.19: Clinical photo of a cubitus varus deformity

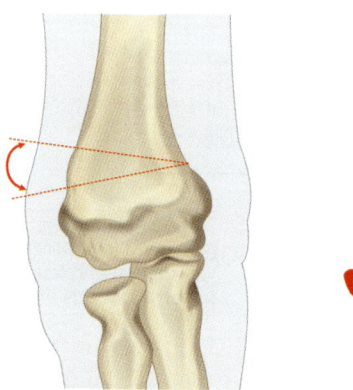 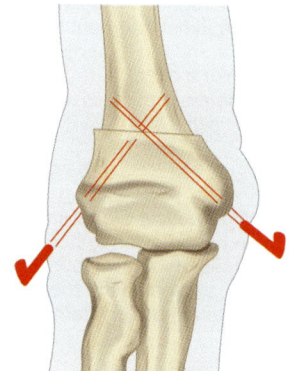

Fig. 13.21: French osteotomy

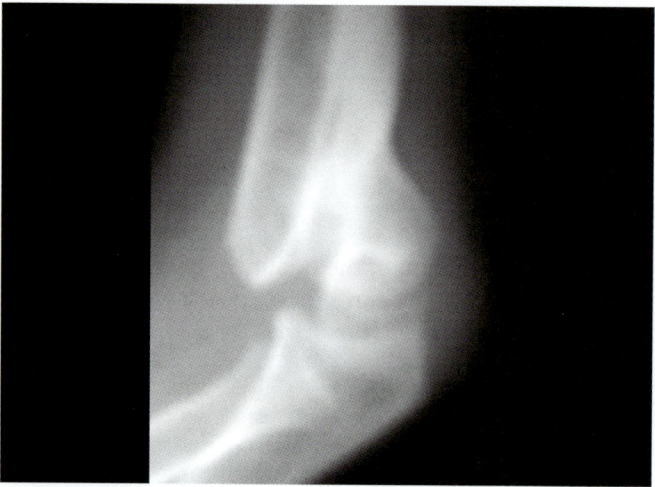

Fig. 13.20: Plain X-rays of the elbow showing cubitus varus (Lateral view)

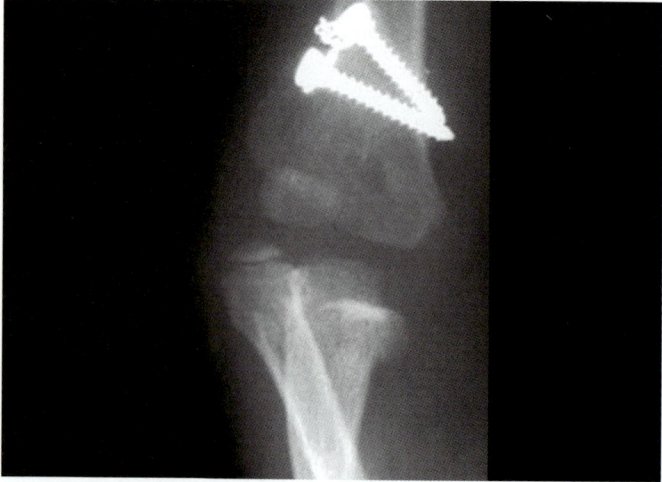

Fig. 13.22: Plain X-ray showing French osteotomy

is closed, and a figure of '8' stainless steel wire secures both the screws against each other. This way the cubitus varus is corrected.

Medial open-wedge osteotomy (King's osteotomy): This is the opposite of lateral closed-wedge osteotomy. In this, a wedge of bone is resected on the medial aspect and the deformity is corrected.

Derotation osteotomy: This technique is not as popular as the lateral closed and medial open-wedge osteotomies mentioned above (see Fig. 13.16B).

> **Treatment Facts of Cubitus Varus**
> **Cubitus varus (see Fig. 13.18) is a cosmetic problem and not functional**
> *Before skeletal maturity*
> - Observation
> - Cosmetic considerations are not very important before 18 years.
> - If surgically corrected, deformity may recur.
> *After skeletal maturity*
> - No further growth left, hence the recurrence chances are nil.
> - Deformity is full blown
> - Girls and boys are more cosmetically concerned at this age and hence corrective osteotomy is performed.

Cubitus valgus: This is rare and may be seen in posterolateral displacement in the extension type of supracondylar fracture. Unlike cubitus varus, it is cosmetically acceptable and the treatment is by medial closed-wedge osteotomy. Tardy ulnar nerve palsy is a distinct possibility in cubitus valgus deformity.

Flexion type of supracondylar fracture: This is extremely rare and has an incidence of only 2.5 percent.

Mechanism of Injury

The common method of injury is direct blow to the posterior aspect of the arm. Angulations seen in lateral radiography are reverse of extension type. This fracture is associated with high incidence of ulnar nerve injury.

Clinical Features

Patient presents with acute pain, swelling, reverse S-deformity, tenderness, loss of elbow movements and functions. Examination for the injury of the ulnar nerve is carried out.

Investigations

Plain X-rays of the elbow both AP and lateral views and CT Scan of the elbow is done to have more clarity in the fracture configurations.

Treatment

Closed reduction and immobilization in above elbow cast in extension is undesirable as it causes elbow stiffness. To overcome this, Sultanpur technique is used. If reduction can be achieved by closed methods, the fracture can be stabilized in flexion with percutaneous pins. If reduction cannot be achieved then open reduction and internal fixation is contemplated.

> **Quick Facts: Sultanpur Technique**
> - Described by Sultanpur of Bahrain
> - A technique, which helps to immobilize flexion supracondylar fracture in flexion rather than the conventional extension (Figs 13.23A and B)
> - Two-stage casting
> - First, cast is put until distal end of the proximal fragment and is allowed to set
> - Next, the distal fragment is pushed back against this cast
> - Cast is then completed with elbow in flexion.

Complications

Injury to ulnar nerve is common in this type of fracture. Loss of elbow flexion is another important complication commonly encountered.

> **Quick Facts: Supracondylar Fracture of Humerus**
> - The second most common injury next to forearm fractures in children.
> - Characteristic pathological anatomy
> - Extension type accounts for 98%
> - Study and restoration of radiological anatomy is very vital
> - Closed reduction difficult
> - Open reduction in specific indications
> - Cubitus varus is the most common complication.

DISLOCATION OF ELBOW JOINT

It is common in adults and rare in children below 10 years of age.
- *Incidence:* 3 to 6%
- *Males:* 71%
- *Non-dominant extremity:* 62%

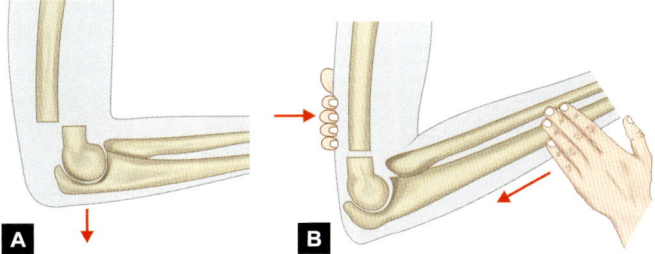

Figs 13.23A and B: Sultanpur technique of reduction

Fifty percent of all elbow dislocations occur in patients less than 20 years of age.

Mechanism of Injury

This is frequently due to fall on the outstretched hands with elbow slightly flexed. A valgus twist is added to the longitudinal force by the projecting trochlea and thus the dislocation is usually posterolateral. Commonly seen in sporting events and in RTA.

Classification (Stimson)

He described elbow dislocation with respect to the position of radioulnar unit to the distal humerus (Table 13.2).

> **Do You Know?**
> What is "terrible triad" of the elbow? (Figs 13.24A and B) Well it is,
> - Posterior dislocation of elbow.
> - Radial head fracture.
> - Fracture coronoid process of ulna.

Clinical Features

Clinical features consist of severe pain, swelling, deformity, severe loss of movements of the elbow (Figs 13.25A and B) and rarely there could be features of neurovascular injuries. It is frequently confused with supracondylar fractures but can easily be differentiated (Table 13.3).

> **Interesting Facts: Associated Fractures in Posterior Dislocation of Elbows**
> - Medial or lateral epicondylar fractures (18–34%)
> - Coronoid process (5–10%)
> - Radial head fracture.

TABLE 13.2: Stimson's classification

Proximal radioulnar joint intact	Proximal radioulnar joint disrupted (divergent dislocation)
A. Posterior (90%) – Posterolateral – Posteromedial	A. Anteroposterior – Radius is anterior – Ulna is posterior
B. Anterior	B. Medial lateral (transverse)
C. Medial	– Radius is lateral
D. Lateral	– Ulna is medial

TABLE 13.3: Comparative features between SC fracture humerus and posterior dislocation of elbow

SC fracture humerus	Posterior dislocation
• Younger children	• Slightly older
• Arm is short	• Forearm is short
• Bony triangle maintained	• Triangle is disrupted
• Swelling is more	• Swelling is less
• Crepitus is present	• Crepitus is absent
• Olecranon is below intercondylar line	• Olecranon is above the intercondylar line
• Step sign is negative	• Step sign is positive
• Movements are restricted	• Movements are grossly
• Radial nerve	• Medial and ulnar commonly affected nerve injured

Radiographs

AP view: Greater superimposition of distal humerus with proximal ulna and olecranon is seen (Fig. 13.26).

Lateral view: Coronoid process lies posterior to the condyles of the humerus.

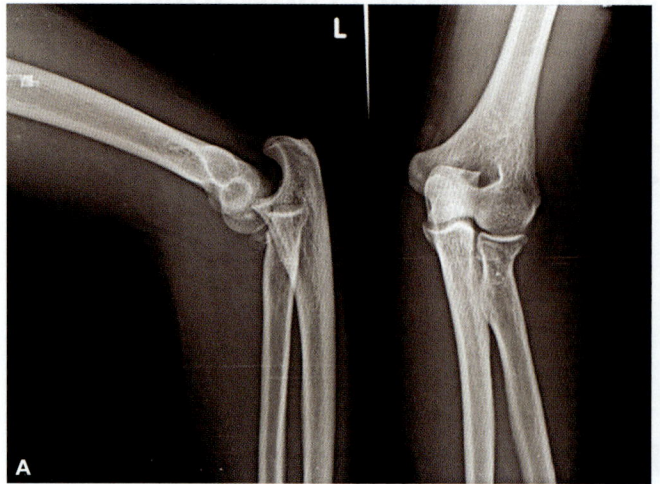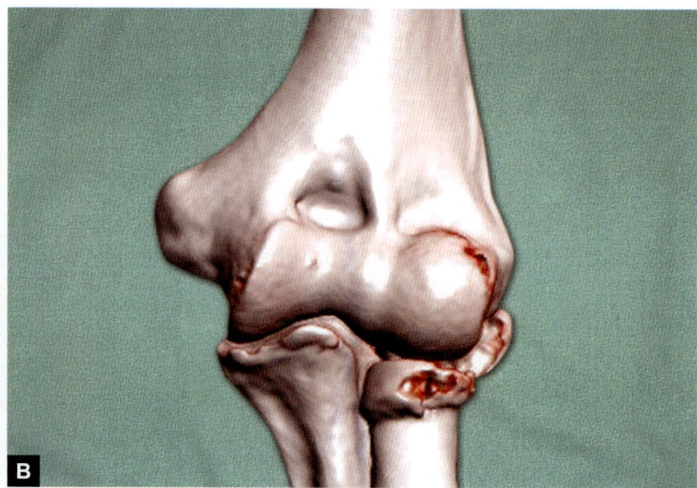

Figs 13.24A and B: Terrible triad of the elbow. Plain X-ray and CT scan showing: (A) Posterior dislocation of elbow; (B) Fracture radial head

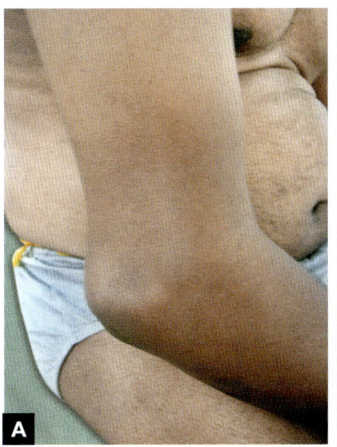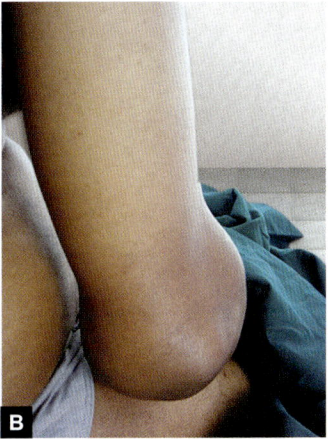

Figs 13.25A and B: Clinical photo showing the posterior dislocation of the elbow from the sides and the back

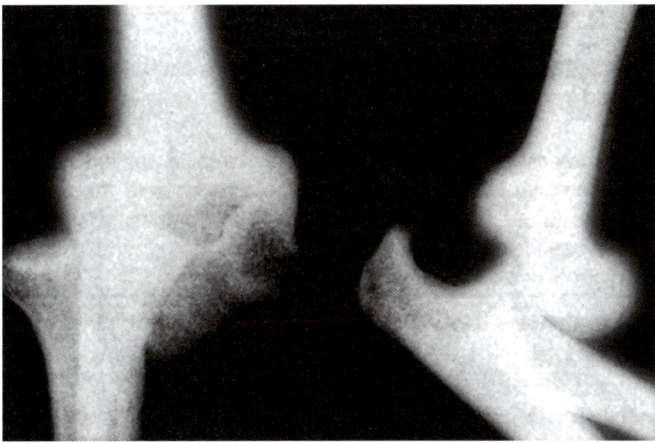

Fig. 13.26: Radiograph showing posterior dislocation of elbow joint: AP and lateral views

Treatment

Conservative Treatment

Elbow dislocation is an emergency and has to be reduced immediately in a Major OT. Closed reduction under general anesthesia is attempted first and reduction by operative methods is reserved for those rare cases of failed closed reduction.

Stimson's principles of closed reduction: According to Stimson, the effective methods of overcoming the muscle forces are:

Step I: Traction along the long axis of the humerus to overcome contraction of biceps, brachialis, and triceps muscles.

Step II: Once these forces are neutralized, second force along the long axis of forearm is employed to pull the proximal radius and ulna back into position.

An above elbow POP slab is applied with 90° elbow flexion and midpronation for a period of 3 weeks after closed reduction under GA (Figs 13.27 to 13.38).

Techniques of Reduction

This could be closed and open. Flowchart 13.2 shows the types of reduction.

Complications

Early

Neurological injuries: In these, the ulnar nerve is very commonly injured, followed by radial and median nerve in that order.

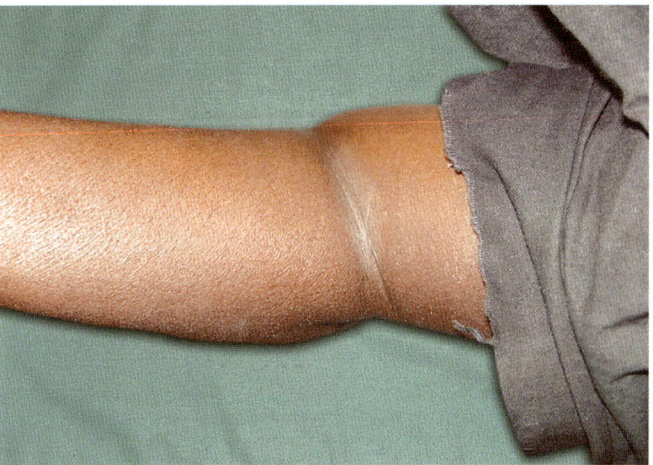

Fig. 13.27: Deformity from the front (Clinical photo)

Flowchart 13.2: Showing techniques of reduction

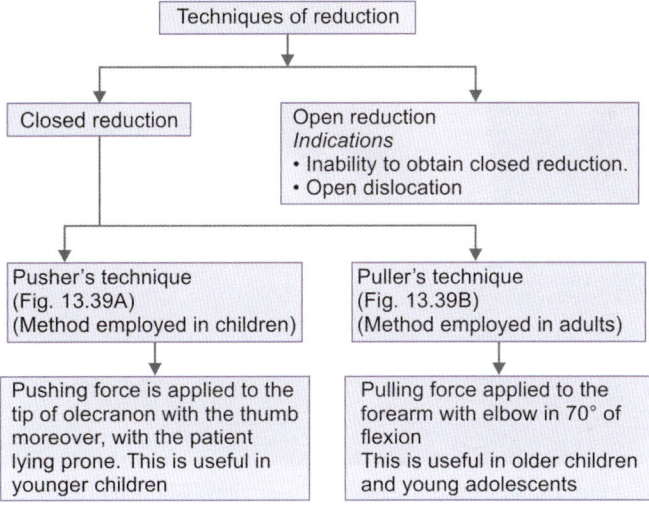

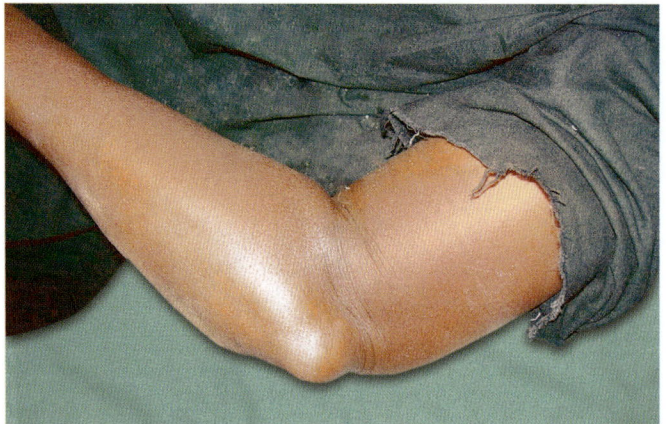

Fig. 13.28: Deformity from the sides (Clinical photo)

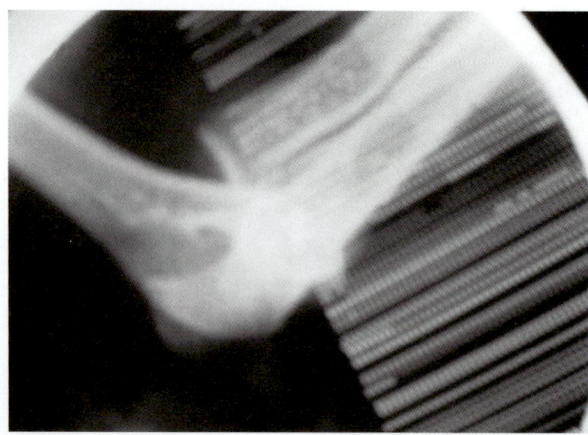

Fig. 13.31: Radiograph lateral view

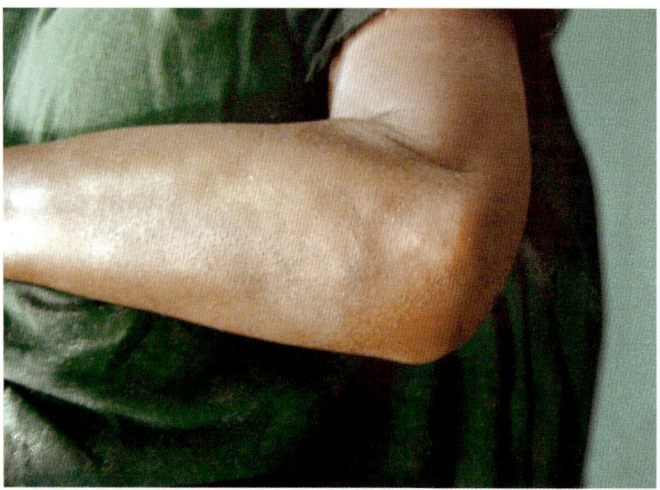

Fig. 13.29: Deformity from the closer view (Clinical photo)

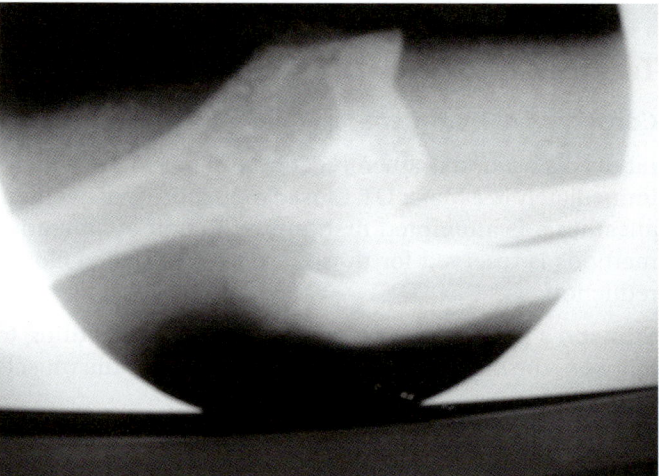

Fig. 13.32: Radiograph lateral view (Another view)

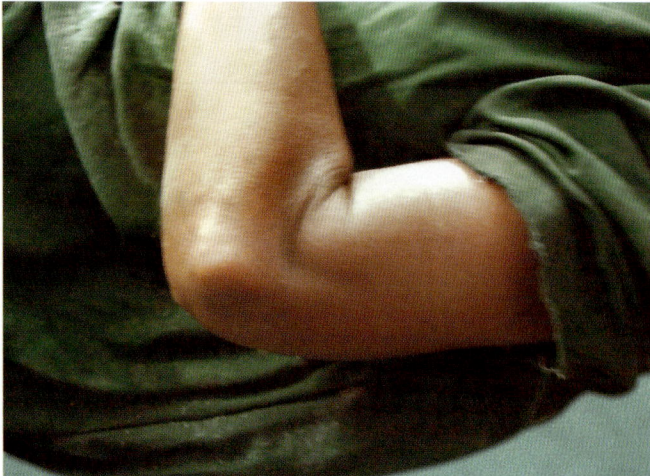

Fig. 13.30: Deformity lateral closer view (Clinical photo)

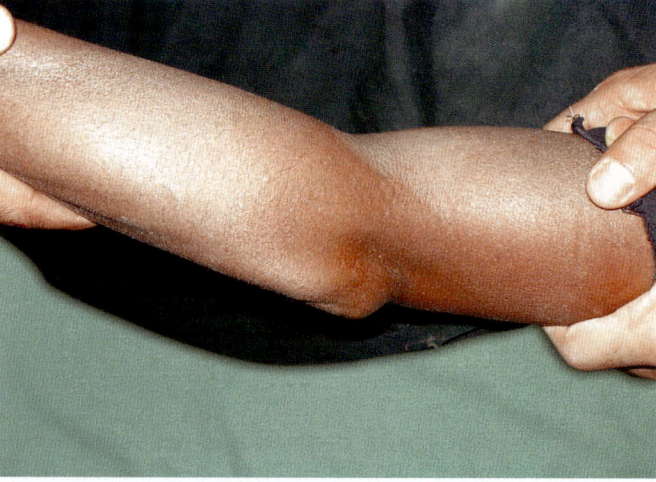

Fig. 13.33: Method of reduction—traction with the elbow slightly flexed

CHAPTER 13: Injuries Around the Elbow

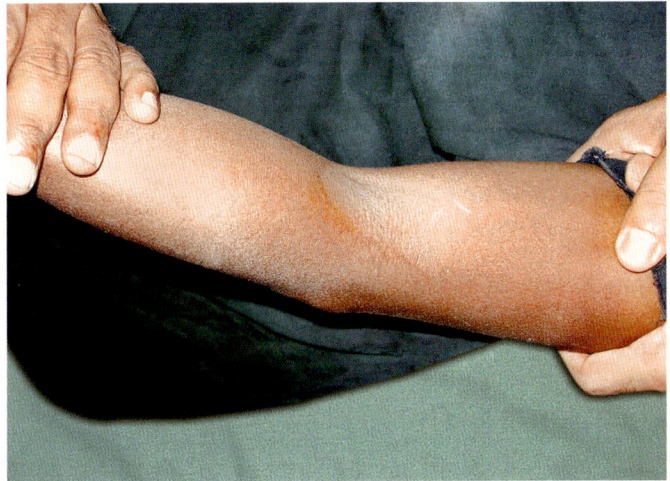

Fig. 13.34: Traction and counter traction continued gently

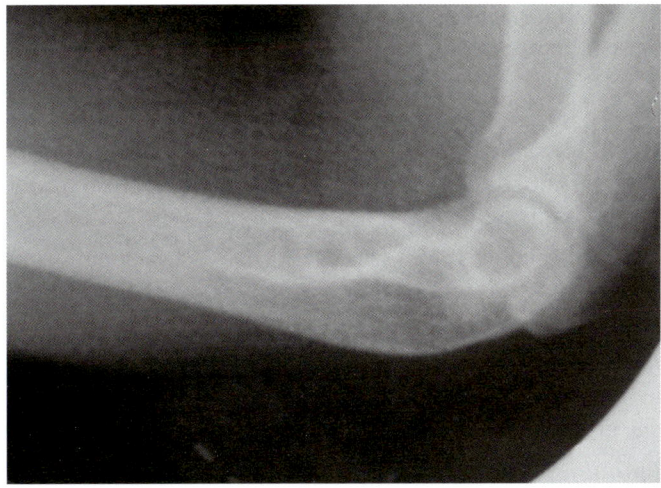

Fig. 13.37: Post-reduction C-arm picture—lateral view

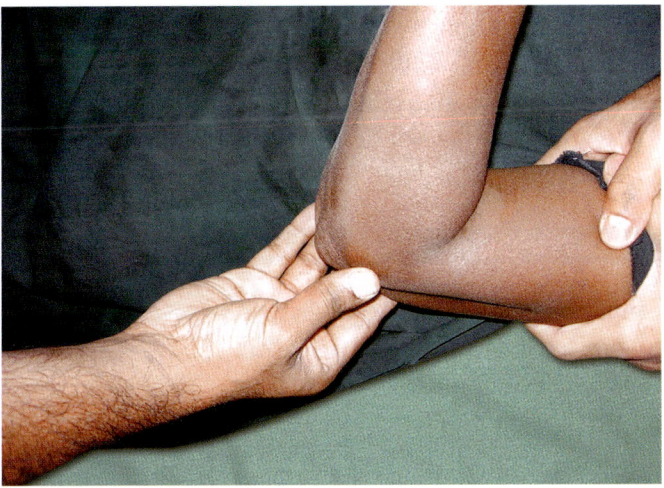

Fig. 13.35: Elbow is gently flexed and reduction is successful

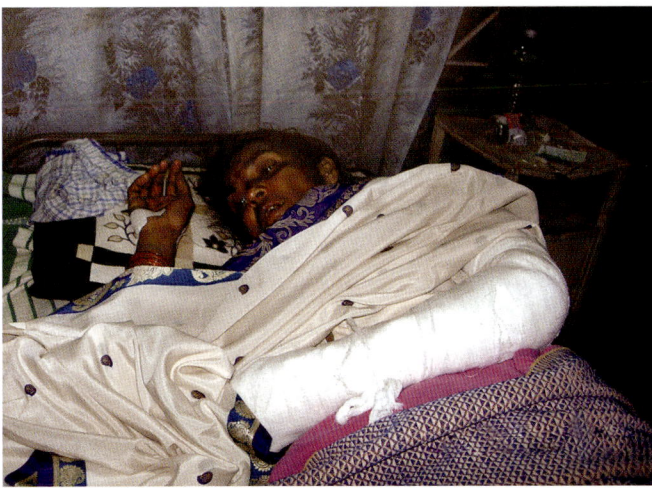

Fig. 13.38: Immobilization in an above elbow slab

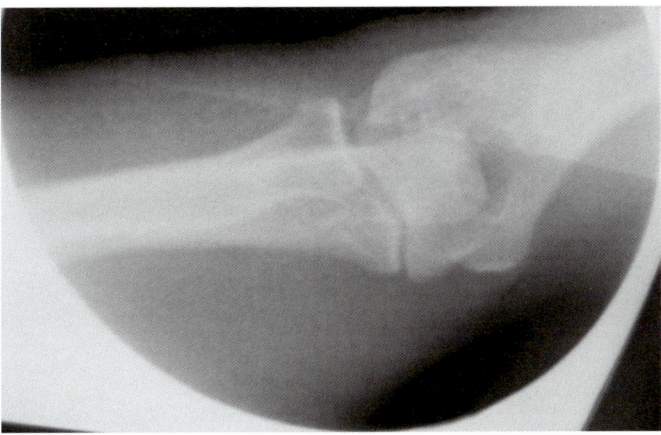

Fig. 13.36: Post-reduction C-arm picture—AP view

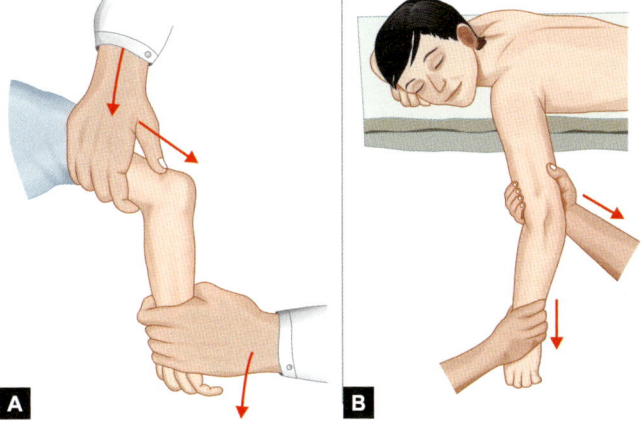

Figs 13.39A and B: Methods of reduction of elbow dislocation: (A) Pusher's technique; (B) Puller's technique

Arterial injuries: They are rare but brachial artery injury may be seen in open fractures.

Late

Myositis ossificans: This has an incidence of 5 to 18% and is generally not due to the injury *per se* but due to the manner in which it is treated.

Causes: Delay in initial treatment; use of hyperextension force during reduction; vigorous active physiotherapy and massage are some of the common causes.

Recurrent dislocation: This is relatively rare but can be seen in males and is usually found to be confined to the pediatric age group.

Pathology: Lax ulnar collateral ligament, pocket in the radial collateral ligament and a defect in the posterolateral aspect of the lateral condyle are the common pathological findings.

Treatment: Surgery is the treatment of choice. Soft tissue procedures consist of tightening the radial collateral ligament. Bony procedures, here a graft is placed to deepen the semi-lunar notch of the ulna.

Proximal radioulnar translation: This is an extremely rare complication and is due to very vigorous force used during reduction methods.

Osteochondral fractures: These are relatively uncommon.

UNREDUCED DISLOCATION OF THE ELBOW

Though rare it is more often seen in Asians due to ignorance, treatment by quacks, etc. Let us know about this complication is more detail.

Clinical Features

The patients with unreduced posterior dislocation of the elbow joint have fixed flexion deformity and gross restriction of elbow movements. There may be wasting of the arm and forearm muscles (Figs 13.40A and B).

Radiographs

Plain X-rays of the elbow helps to make an accurate diagnosis. Some amount of ossification and calcification may be seen.

Treatment Methods

Children: Open reduction and resection of myositis is done in children.

If it is less than 3 months' duration, open reduction alone is done.

If the injury is greater than 3 months, open reduction is combined with arthroplasty if necessary.

Adults: In adults, open reduction is invariably followed with one of the following arthroplasties (Table 13.4).

TABLE 13.4: Different types of elbow arthroplasties

Interpositional (fascial) arthroplasty	Implant arthroplasty	Resection arthroplasty
• Done in mobile joint with minimal pain	• Gives a stable, painless and mobile elbow	Causes instability and is rarely used
• Triceps fascia is used	• Technically difficult and expensive	

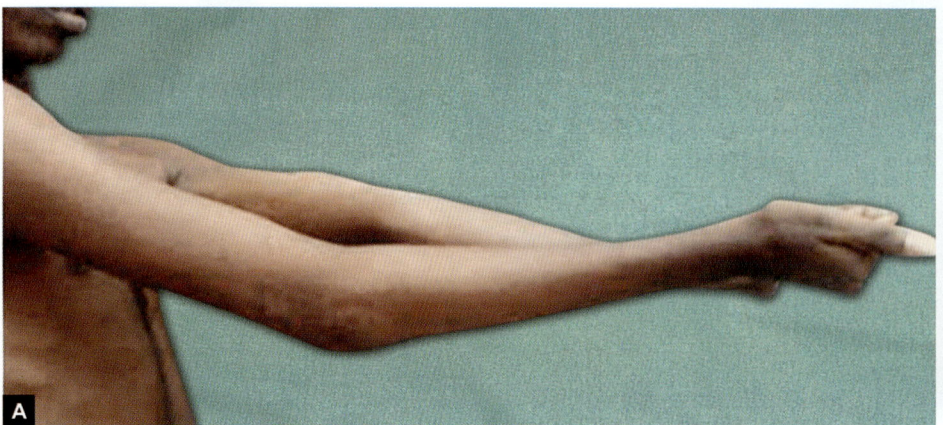 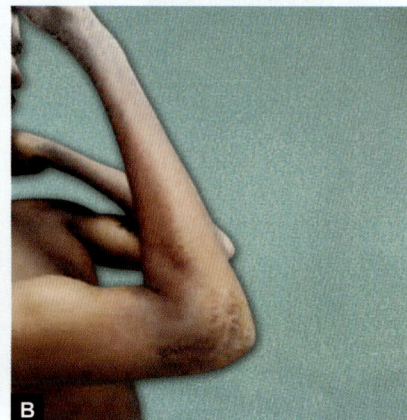

Figs 13.40A and B: Clinical photos showing neglected elbow dislocation

Recurrent Dislocation of the Elbow

If the initial dislocation is not treated or immobilized properly, then there could be development of recurrent dislocation of the elbow which is difficult to treat (Fig. 13.41).

Other Important Complications
- *Loss of motion: About 10 to 15% loss of extension.*
- *Fifteen percent average loss of strength.*
- *Ectopic calcification: Seen in 75% of the cases.*
- *Heterotrophic calcification: Seen in 5% of the cases.*

RADIAL HEAD FRACTURE

Radial head fracture is a common injury in adults and is rare in children.

Mechanism of Injury

- Indirect trauma due to fall on an outstretched hand.
- Direct trauma due to RTA, assault, etc. in adults.

Mason's Classification

Type I: Undisplaced fracture.

Type II: Marginal fracture with displacement.

Type III: Comminuted fractures.

Type IV: Radial head fracture with posterior dislocation of elbow.

Clinical Features

The patient with radial head fracture complains of pain on the lateral side of the elbow, minimal swelling, and restriction of elbow movements and supination, pronation of the forearm. There is tenderness over the radial head and crepitus can be elicited.

Investigations

Plain X-ray of the elbow including the anteroposterior and lateral radiographs of the elbow (Figs 13.42A and B). Additional oblique radiograph delineates the fracture line better. CT scan helps to delineate the fracture pattern better (Fig. 13.43).

Treatment

This varies according to the type of fractures (Table 13.5). In Non-comminuted fractures, reduction and stabilization with K-wires is attempted and in comminuted fractures, radial head excision is the treatment of choice. Of late excision of the head is followed by radial head replacement, and is controversial since excision of the head is usually effective in isolated comminuted radial head fracture that too if the medial collateral ligament is intact (Fig. 13.44A). However, metal radial head replacement is superior to silicone prosthesis (Fig. 13.44B).

Complications

Injury to the posterior interosseous nerve, osteoarthritis, and elbow stiffness is the common complications of radial head fractures.

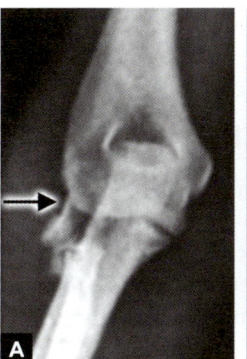
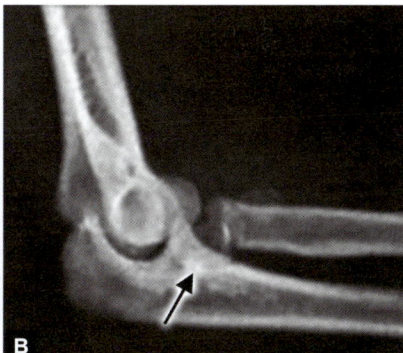

Figs 13.42A and B: Radial head fracture complete

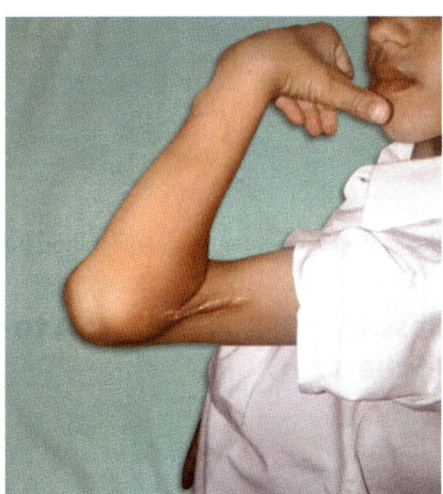

Fig. 13.41: Clinical photo showing RDE

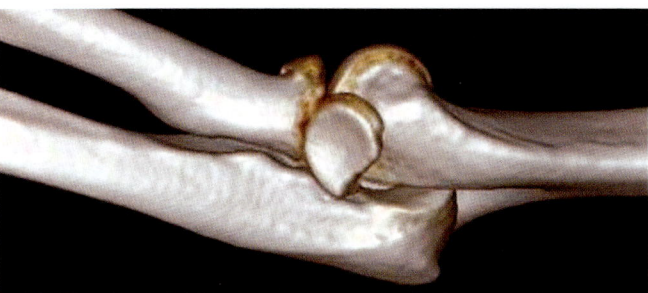

Fig. 13.43: CT scan picture

TABLE 13.5: Methods of treatment for different types of fractures of head of radius

Type I	Type II	Type III	Type IV
Non-operative means • Aspiration of elbow within first 24 hours decreases pain • Early mobilization within 24 hours	Excision head of radius (McLaughlin's criteria for immediate excision) • Angulation >30° • Depression >3 mm • Involvement of >1/3rd of head	• Radial head excision is indicated within first 24 hours • Excised head is replaced with prosthesis	• Prompt reduction of the dislocation is a must • Assess status of the head. If it meets the criteria for excision, do it within 24 hours

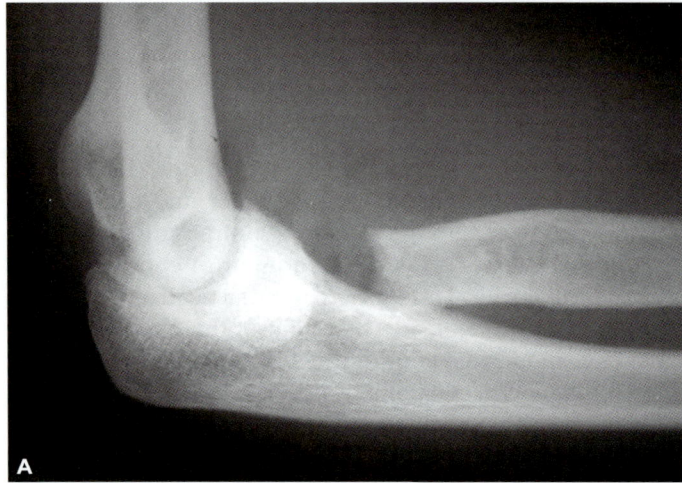 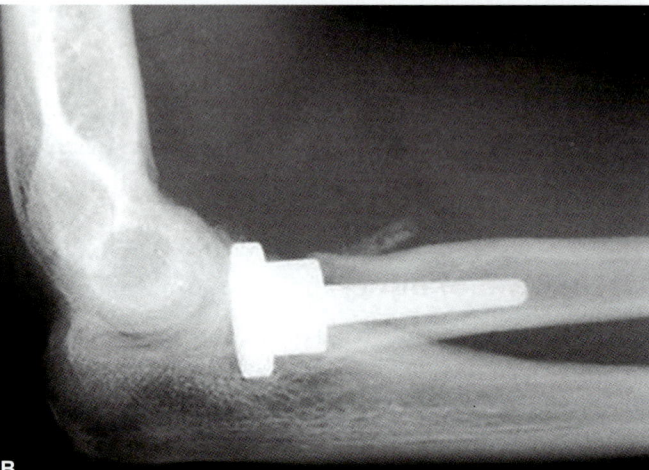

Figs 13.44A and B: (A) Radial head excision; (B) Replacement with prosthesis

Mystifying Facts
Radial head excision does not cause instability (due to the presence of interosseous membrane) or functional impairment (due to the distal radioulnar joint).

FRACTURE OF THE OLECRANON

Fracture olecranon is uncommon in children. Olecranon fracture in adults is comparable to fracture patella. Fracture reduction should be exact since any residual irregularity of the articular surface will cause limited motion, delayed recovery, and traumatic arthritis of the elbow.

The fracture fixation should be strong enough to allow gentle active exercises even before radiographs show evidence of complete union.

As separation of the fracture of the patella causes quadriceps insufficiency so does displaced fracture olecranon causes triceps insufficiency.

Mechanism of Injury

Direct: Trauma due to fall on the point of elbow. This is the frequent cause (Fig. 13.45).

Indirect: Due to forcible triceps contraction.

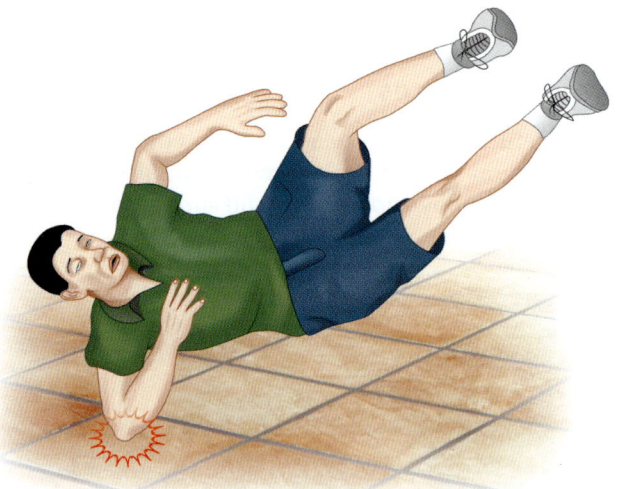

Fig. 13.45: Most common mechanism of olecranon fracture

Colton's Classification (Figs 13.46A to C) (Modified Schatzker)

- Undisplaced fracture
- Displaced fracture
- Avulsion fracture
- Transverse/oblique fracture

- Fracture dislocation (Monteggia group)
- Comminuted fracture.

Clinical Features

The patient complains of pain, swelling, and inability to extend the elbow (Fig. 13.47). Clinically, tenderness and crepitus can be elicited.

Radiographs

Routine anteroposterior and lateral views of the elbow help in confirmation of the diagnosis (Figs 13.48A and B).

> **Note:**
> In olecranon fracture more than 2 mm separation between fracture fragments is called displaced fracture.

Treatment

Conservative Treatment

This is indicated for undisplaced fractures and in fractures with less than 2 mm displacement. In children, closed reduction is done and the limb is immobilized in an above elbow plaster slab or cast for 3 to 4 weeks and this is often successful.

Surgery

In adults, repair of triceps is done for avulsion fractures. There is no place for conservative treatment, because closed reduction needs immobilization in extension for 6 to 8 weeks, which except in children causes permanent stiffness. Hence, surgery is the treatment of choice in adults.

Methods of Operative Treatment

Open reduction and internal fixation with figure of '8' wire loop. This method is used for avulsion and transverse fractures of the olecranon and for fractures which are uncomminuted and proximal to the coronoid fossa (Figs 13.49 to 13.51).

Medullary fixation by a single interfragmentary screw: This is indicated in comminuted fracture of olecranon when

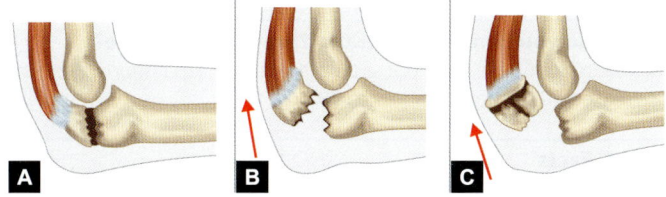

Figs 13.46A to C: Types of olecranon fractures: Undisplaced fractures: (A) Displaced; (B) Comminuted; (C) Fracture of olecranon

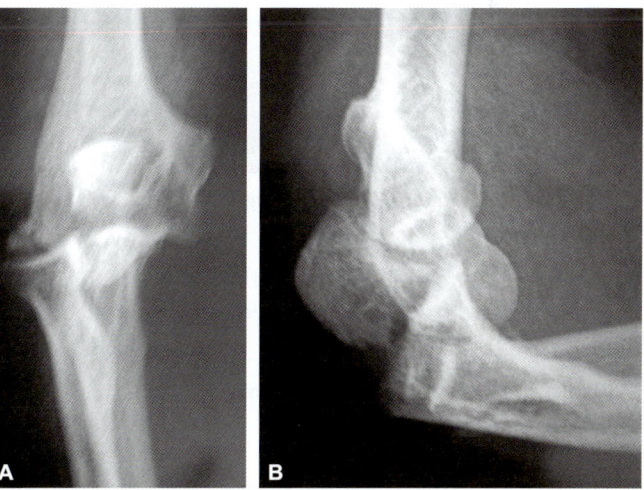

Figs 13.48A and B: Plain X-rays of the elbow showing olecranon fracture

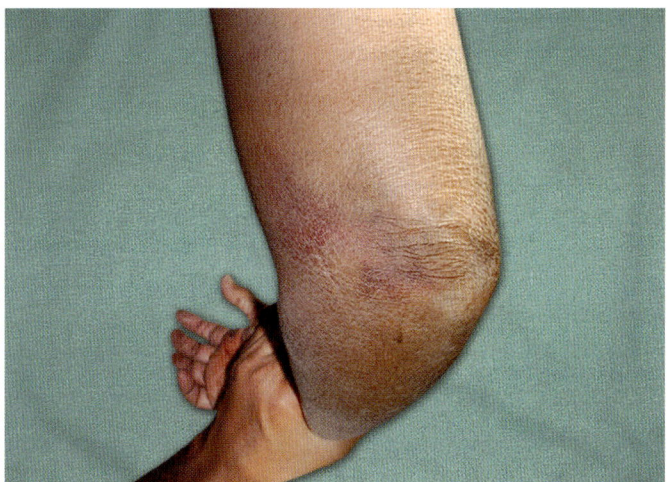

Fig. 13.47: Clinical photo of olecranon fracture

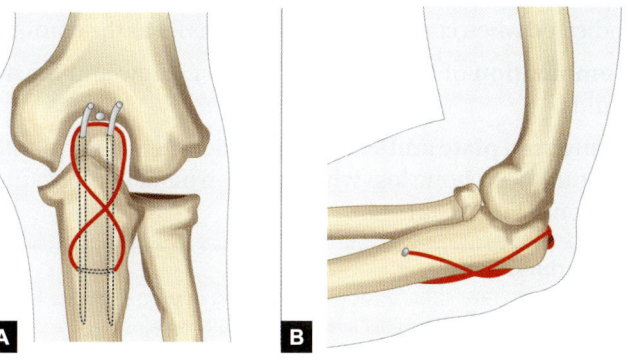

Figs 13.49A and B: Tension band wiring (TWB) in fracture olecranon

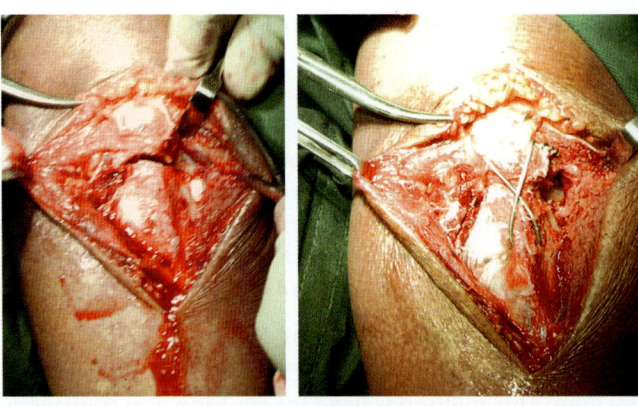

Fig. 13.50: Operative photos showing olecranon fracture and TBW fixation

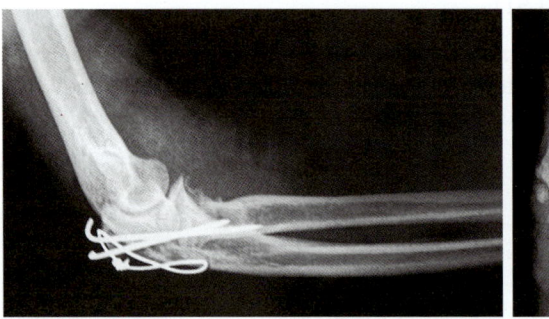 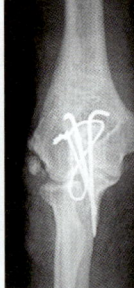

Fig. 13.51: Plain X-rays showing TBW of olecranon

its distal fragment and the head of the radius are dislocated anteriorly. Rigid fixation is required to prevent recurrence of dislocation.

Excision of the Proximal Fragments

Indications
- In comminuted fractures.
- In delayed union or nonunion of fractures in upper half.
- If the patient is greater than 50 years of age and is not involved in heavy work.

This method is useful only if enough of the olecranon is left to form a stable base for the trochlea. Thus, it is not indicated when comminution extends as far as the coronoid.

Combination of intramedullary pin or screw and tension bands.

Contoured plate and screws are indicated in comminuted fractures with bone loss where tension band wiring cannot be done (Fig. 13.52).

Disturbing Facts
Reoperation rate after tension band wiring in olecranon fracture is as high as 71.7% due to backing out of the K-wire.

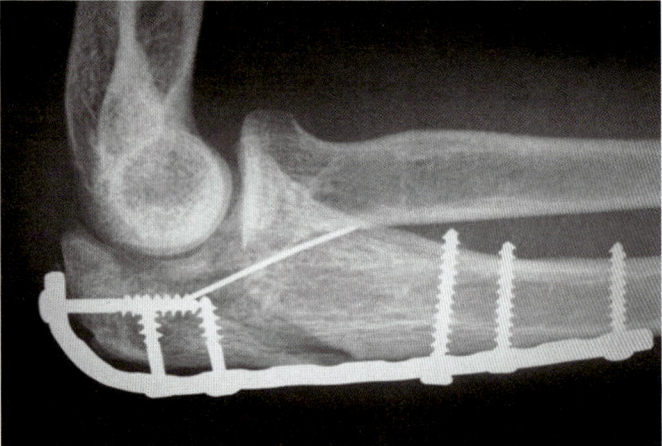

Fig. 13.52: Contoured plating of comminuted olecranon fractures

Complications

Malunion Nonunion of the fracture, osteoarthritis of the elbow, triceps insufficiency and restricted movements of the elbow are the common complications of fracture olecranon (Figs 13.53A and B).

When do you Consider Olecranon Fracture as Stable?
If after reduction it does not separate or if the separation does not increase with flexion of elbow to 90°.

Quick Facts
Treatment of displaced olecranon fractures concisely:
- Avulsion fracture—TBW/LS
- Transverse fractures—TBW/LS
- Transverse fractures with—Plate and screws with bone grafting
- Oblique fractures—LS/Plate
- Comminution—Excision/plate/TBW
- Fracture dislocation—Wire/LS/Plate

TBW—Tension band wiring
LS—Lag screw fixation.

CORONOID FRACTURES

Fractures of the coronoid process of the ulna were earlier thought to be an avulsion fracture involving the brachialis muscle. Of late, this notion has been dispelled as it is found that the insertion of this muscle is more distal.

Interesting Facts about Coronoid Fractures
- Its presence indicates a significant trauma to the elbow.
- It also points towards the possibility of acute recurrent dislocations.

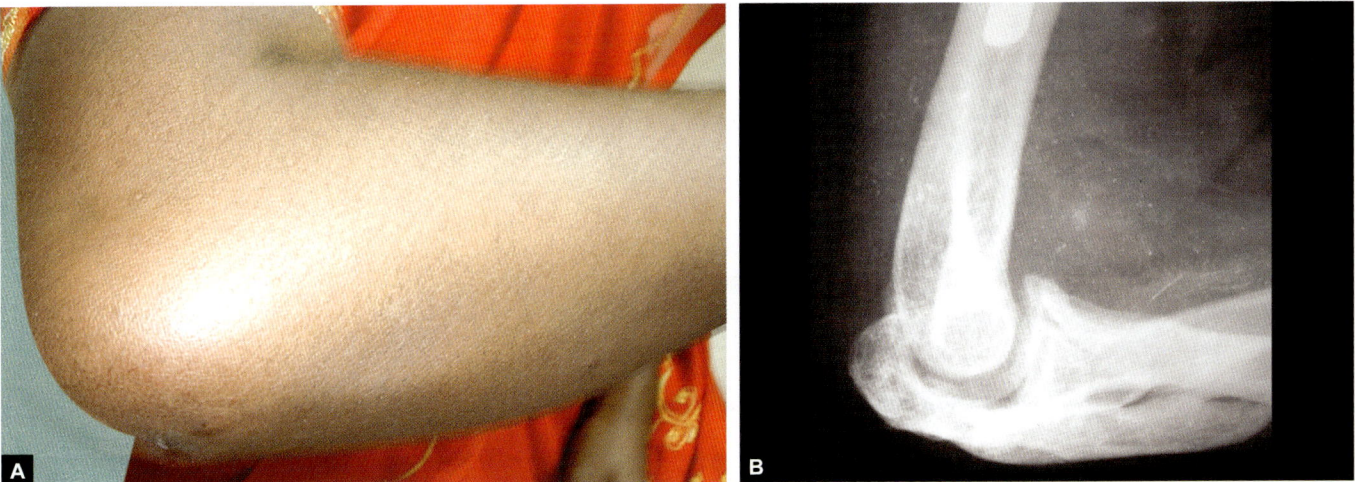

Figs 13.53A and B: Clinical photo and plain X-ray showing malunion olecranon fracture

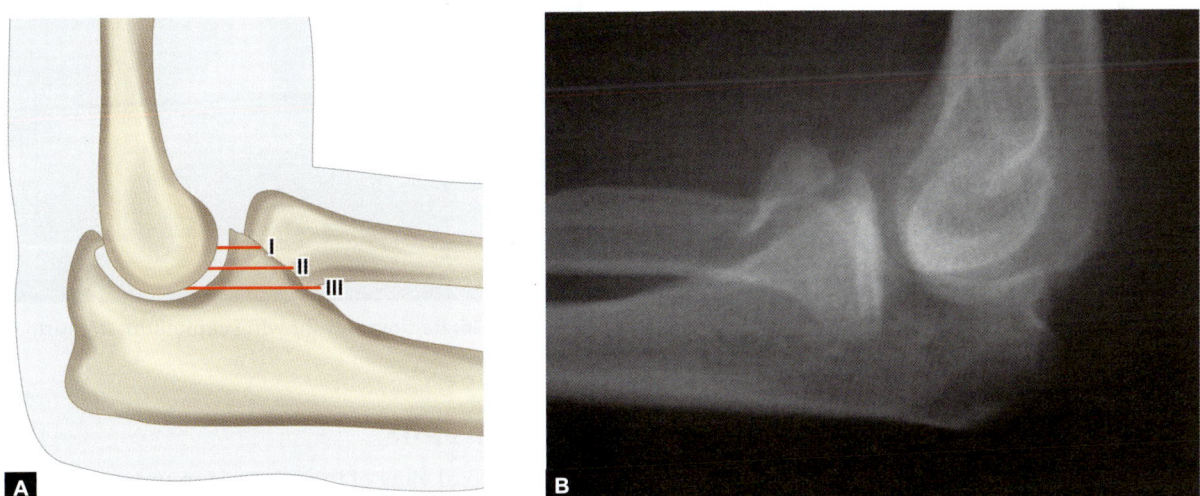

Figs 13.54A and B: (A) Types of coronoid fractures; (B) Radiograph of coronoid fracture

Mechanism of Injury

This fracture occurs due to the impact of the coronoid process against the trochlea following a fall on an outstretched hand.

Classification of Regan and Morrey (Fig. 13.54A)

Type I: Avulsion fracture of the tip of the coronoid.
Type II: Fracture involving greater than 50% of the coronoid.
Type III: Fracture involving the base of the coronoid.

Clinical Features

Isolated fractures of the coronoid process are usually rare and are usually associated with greater elbow trauma. Clinical features like pain, swelling, deformity, movement restriction of the elbow, etc. depends on the extent of damage.

Radiograph

This fracture can be easily identified over a true lateral X-ray of the elbow (Fig. 13.54B).

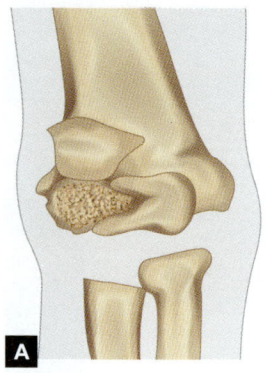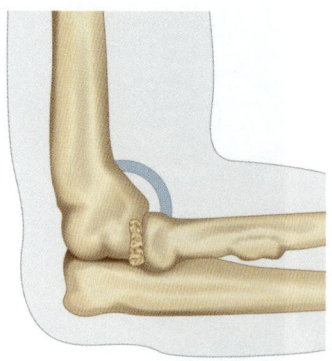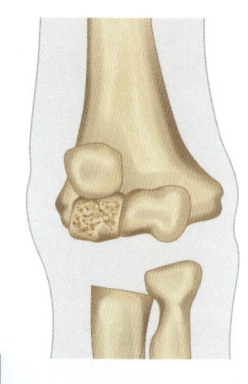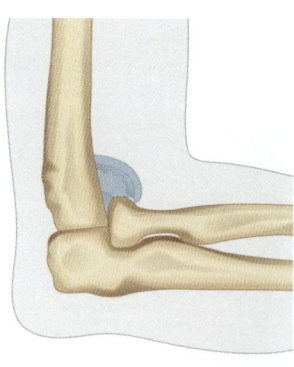

Figs 13.55A and B: Types of capitellum fractures: (A) Type I; (B) Type II

Treatment

Though small-undisplaced fractures can be managed conservatively with an above elbow plaster cast, displaced fractures need open reduction and internal fixation with screw or wires.

CAPITELLUM FRACTURES

Capitellum is the anterior portion of the lateral humeral condyle. This fracture is unique in being intra-articular always.

Mechanism of Injury

Fall on an outstretched hand, with flexion or extension of the elbow and the resulting shear forces through the radial head slices the capitellum.

Classification

Based on the size of the articulating fragment, it is classified into three types (Figs 13.55A and B).

Type I (Hahn-Steinthal variety): This involves a large portion of the capitellum and a small chunk of trochlea with less of subchondral portion.

Type II (Kocher-Lorenz variety): Here only a large portion of the capitellum is involved with a huge chunk of subchondral bone.

Type III: Comminuted fracture.

> **Vital Facts: About Associated Injuries with Capitellar Fractures**
> - Injury to ulnar collateral ligament in 69% of the cases.
> - Fracture of the head of the radius.

Clinical Features

The patient complains of pain and swelling over the lateral aspect of the elbow. Elbow and forearm movements are also restricted.

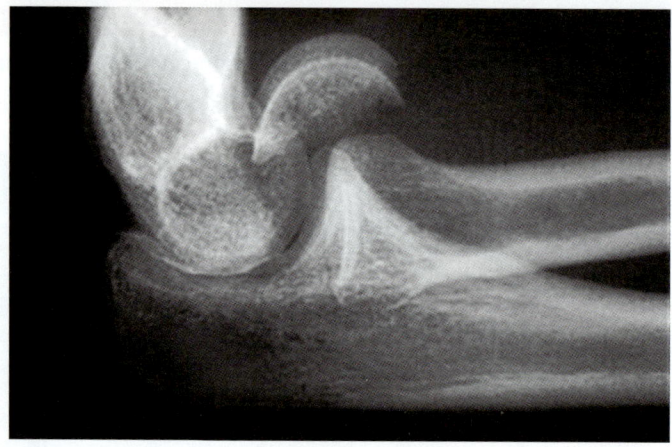

Fig. 13.56: Radiograph showing capitellum fracture—lateral view

Radiographs

A true lateral view of the elbow is mandatory to accurately diagnose this fracture. The characteristic finding of this fracture is the presence of "double arc sign" described by McKay over the X-ray (Fig. 13.56).

Treatment

Undisplaced fractures can be managed conservatively by an above elbow plaster cast or slab for 3 to 4 weeks.

Displaced fractures need open reduction and internal fixation with minifragment screws.

PHYSEAL FRACTURES

These are fractures seen in children. Knowledge of the secondary growth centers around the elbow is important to judge the frequently subtle injuries to the condyles of the humerus. Radiographic comparison with uninjured site is mandatory. Incidence is rare and is less than 5%.

> **Do You Know?**
> Epicondylar fractures in children are also called Granger's fracture.

LATERAL CONDYLE OF HUMERUS (Jupiter Fracture)

Accounts for 16.8% fractures of distal humerus and can be associated with dislocation of elbow and fracture olecranon.

Classification (2 Ways)

Anatomical Location (Figs 13.57A and B)
- Type I: Fracture line lateral to trochlea through the capitulotrochlear groove. Elbow is stable (High Jupiter fracture).
- *Type II:* Fracture line extends into apex of the trochlea; elbow is unstable (Low Jupiter fracture).

Stages of Displacement
- Undisplaced
- Displaced
- Displaced and rotated (Fig. 13.58)

Clinical Features

This consists of little distortion of the elbow and less swelling, tenderness and crepitus is positive over the lateral condyle.

Radiographs

Routine AP and lateral views of the elbow help to make a diagnosis (Fig. 13.59A).

Treatment

In Stages I and II Closed reduction and percutaneous pinning.

For displaced and rotated fracture, open reduction and internal fixation with screws (Figs 13.59 and 13.60).

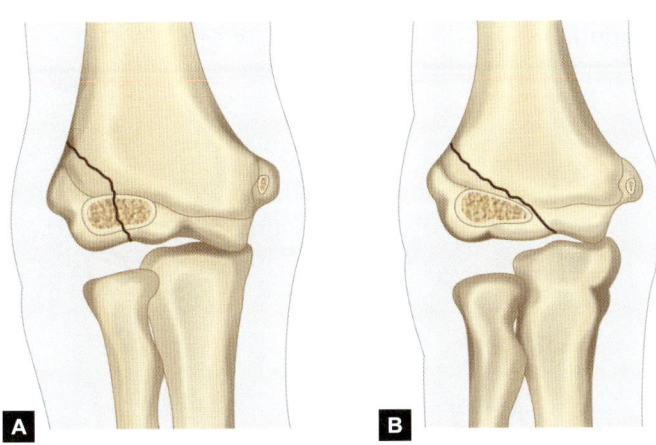

Figs 13.57A and B: Lateral condyle fractures. Undisplaced fractures: (A) Type I; (B) Type II

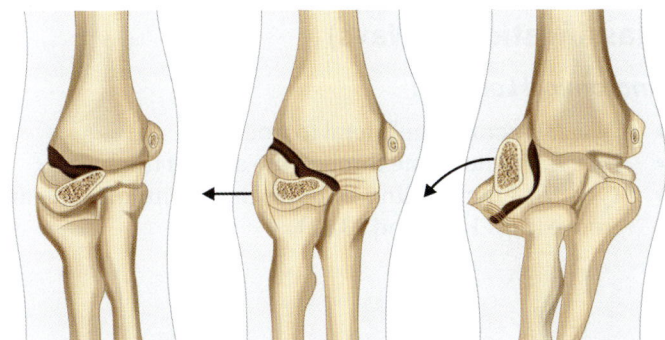

Fig. 13.58: Displaced lateral condyle fractures

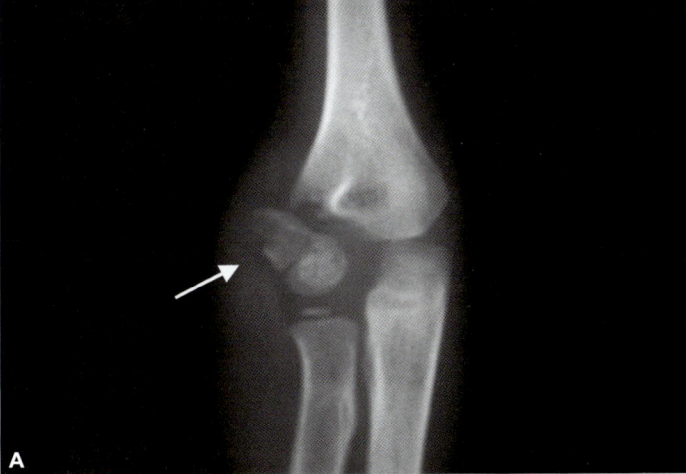

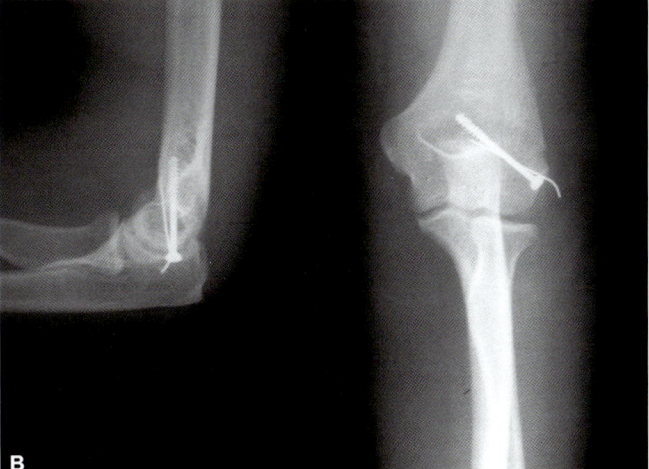

Figs 13.59A and B: (A) Radiograph showing displaced and rotated lateral condyle fracture; (B) Radiograph showing fixation of the lateral condyle fracture

Complications

- Lateral condylar overgrowth
- Delayed union and nonunion can occur if fracture is undetected or left untreated. The cause for nonunion could be due to the constant force exerted by the common extensor tendon. In early stages, it is treated by open reduction and internal fixation and in late stages by osteotomy
- Cubitus valgus: This is a common complication
- Cubitus varus is relatively rare
- Acute injury to posterior interosseous nerve may be seen
- Tardy ulnar nerve palsy—seen after several years
- Physeal growth arrest
- Avascular necrosis—rarely seen
- Myositis ossificans—fairly common.

MEDIAL CONDYLE OF HUMERUS

It is rare in children (1%) and is seen in age group 8 to 14 years.

Classification (2 Ways)

Anatomical Location

- *Type I:* Fracture line lateral to trochlea.
- *Type II:* Fracture line through the apex of trochlea.
- *Type III:* Fracture line through the capitulotrochlear groove (Figs 13.61 and 13.62).

Stages of Displacement (Kilfoyle's)

- Impacted
- Complete
- Displaced and rotated.

Clinical Features

Usual signs and symptoms of fracture, tenderness, and crepitus are positive over the medial condyle.

Radiograph

Routine AP and lateral views help to make an accurate diagnosis (Fig. 13.62B).

Treatment

Stages I and II: Above elbow cast or splint.

Stage III: Open reduction and internal fixation and K-wire fixation.

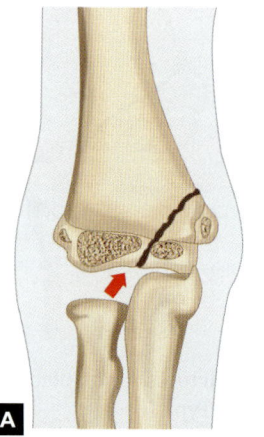
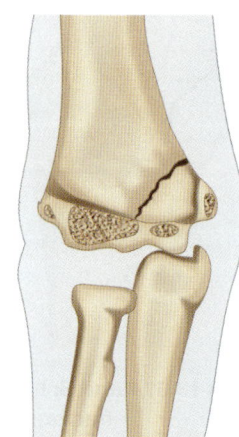

Figs 13.61A and B: Types of medial condyle fractures. Undisplaced (A) Type I; (B) Type II

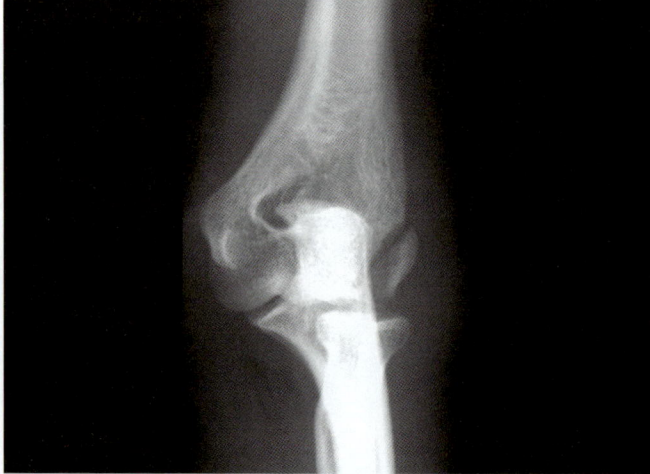

Fig. 13.60: Plain X-ray showing fracture lateral condyle

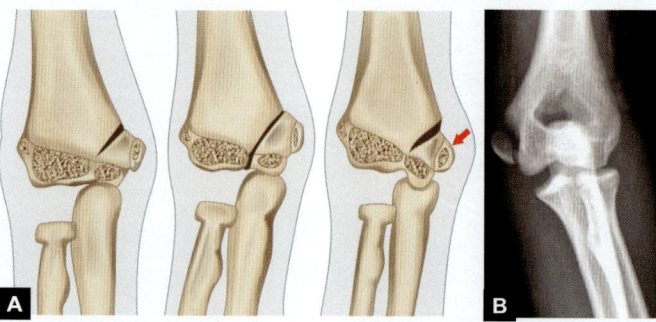

Figs 13.62A and B: (A) Displaced medial condyle fracture; (B) Plain X-ray showing fracture medial condyle

Complications

- Missed diagnosis
- Nonunion with cubitus varus
- Delayed union
- Cubitus valgus due to growth stimulation
- Ulnar neuropathy.

SIDESWIPE INJURIES
(Syn: Traffic Elbow, Car Window Elbow)

Everybody in the metropolis has heard about traffic jam, but have you heard about traffic elbow? Well, it is a shattered elbow syndrome, a consequence of callous neglect while traveling. Traffic jams are police officers' nightmare, while traffic elbow is orthopedicians nightmare!

Mechanism of Injury

It is due to the force applied to an elbow projecting from a car window by a passing vehicle or when it hits a fixed object or when it overturns (Fig. 13.63).

Shorbe's Classification

Group I: Only soft tissue injury.

Group II: Only tip of the elbow is injured and there is fracture olecranon.

Group III: Fracture of both radius and ulna.

Group IV: Variations of comminuted intercondylar fractures of the humerus.

Group V: Severely injured, fracture of all bones around the elbow with considerable soft tissue injury. Extensive open wounds are not unusual.

Clinical Features

This depends on the severity of the fractures. There may be gross swelling, extreme pain, and severe loss of elbow function. Frequently the injuries could be compound. There may be associated distal neurovascular deficits and it could vary from compartment syndrome to gangrene of the forearm and hand (Fig. 13.64).

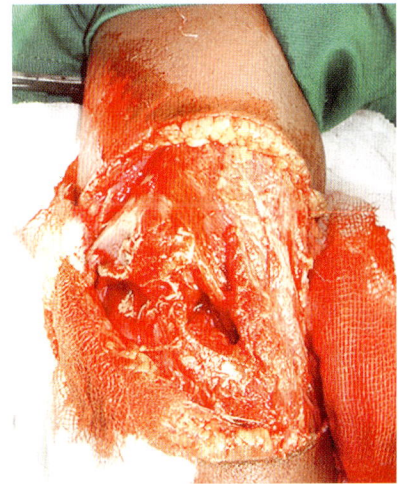

Fig. 13.64: Clinical photo of a traffic elbow (Crushed elbow injury)

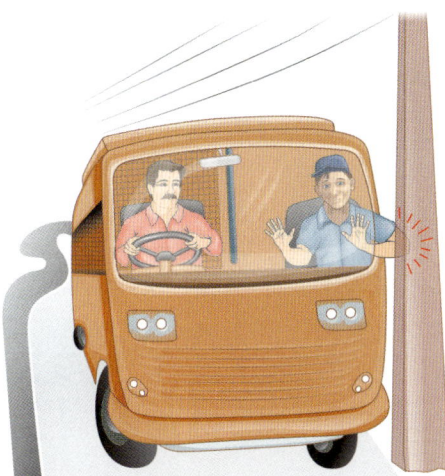

Fig. 13.63: How many times you are guilty of sitting like this while traveling? Thank God, you have not landed up with a "traffic elbow"!

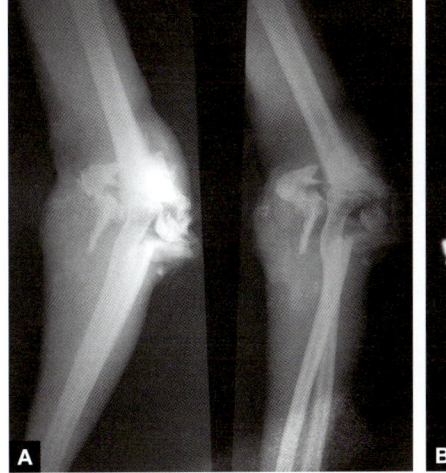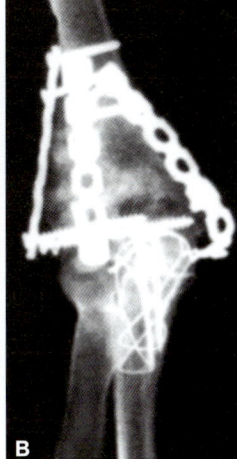

Figs 13.65A and B: (A) Radiograph showing traffic elbow; (B) Radiograph showing reconstruction of fractures due to traffic elbow

Investigations

Plain X-ray (Fig. 13.65A), MRI, CT scan, arteriogram, Doppler study, etc. are some of the important investigation methods.

Methods of Treatment

Treatment must be individualized. Various combinations of internal fixation, external fixation, and traction should be tried (Fig. 13.65B). Initial debridement must be thorough. Primary nerve repair is indicated if the cut is clean. In crushed injuries, nerve should be repaired secondarily.

Primary amputation: This is indicated in the following situations:
- Irreparable vascular damage and a nonviable extremity.
- Segmental disruption of all three nerves around the elbow.

Nevertheless, it should be remembered that a pain-free elbow (either stiff or unstable) is better than amputation.

CHAPTER 14

Injuries of the Forearm

INTRODUCTION

Injuries of the forearm present an interesting combination of injuries like fracture bones of forearm (Fig. 14.1), Monteggia fractures, Galeazzi fractures, Essex-Lopresti fracture, etc. The muscle attachments of the forearm make the treatment of these fractures difficult. The supinator muscle is inserted in the proximal third of the forearm bones and supinates this part of the forearm after the fracture. The middle third gives attachment to the pronator teres muscle and the distal third to the pronator quadratus. When the fracture occurs in the middle third, the forearm is held in the position of midpronation due to the balancing action of supinators and pronator quadratus muscle. In fractures of the distal third, the forearm is pronated due to the action of pronator quadratus. Hence, the treating physician should be aware of the various muscular forces (Fig. 14.2) acting in the forearm to effectively neutralize them and bring about proper union between the fracture fragments. Immobilizing the forearm in *supination* in upper third fractures, *midpronation* in middle third fractures and *pronation* in distal third fracture is found to effectively counter the muscular forces, which threaten to displace the fracture fragments.

Monteggia's fracture along with Galeazzi's fracture forms a rare and interesting combination of injuries where there is fracture of one bone with dislocation of the other. Curiously both are described in the forearm with the former involving the upper and middle forearm, and the latter involving the distal forearm.

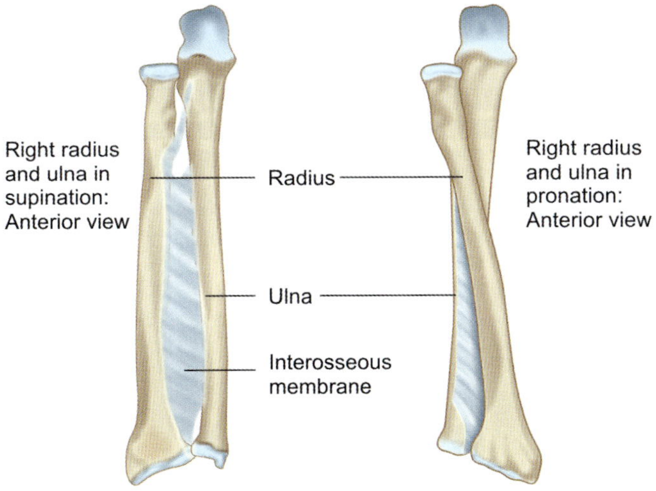

Fig. 14.1: Bones of the forearm

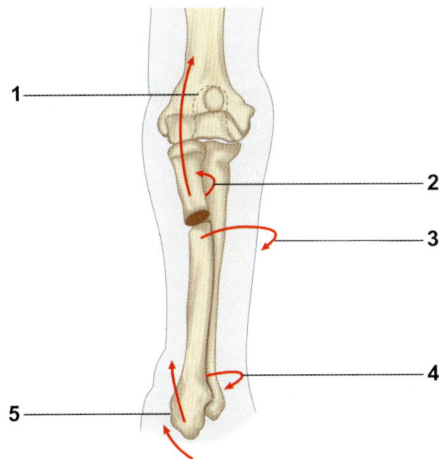

Fig. 14.2: Muscle forces in fracture both bones of forearm: (1) Biceps, (2) Supinator, (3) Pronator teres, (4) Pronator quadratus, (5) Brachioradialis

FRACTURE BOTH BONES OF THE FOREARM

Mechanism of Injury

Fracture both bones of forearm in adults are frequently due to RTA, falls, assault, etc. This is a difficult problem to treat especially in adults. The complex muscle arrangements already described makes retention of the fracture fragments very difficult. The fracture could be due to either direct or indirect trauma (Figs 14.3A and B).

Clinical Features

The patient presents with severe pain, swelling, and deformity of the forearm (Fig. 14.4). Movements of the forearm are severely restricted and all other features of fractures are usually present.

Radiographs

The AP, lateral and oblique views of the forearm help to make an accurate diagnosis (Fig. 14.5A).

Treatment

Conservative Treatment

Undisplaced, incomplete fractures are treated by immobilization with an above elbow plaster slab or cast. The treatment for displaced fractures consists of closed reduction by traction and counter traction methods under general anesthesia followed by an above elbow plaster cast, is usually successful in children.

Surgery

In adults, ORIF is often indicated because it is difficult to regain length, apposition, axial and normal rotational alignment in adults by closed reduction. Open reduction is by two approaches, one for the radius and the other for the ulna (Fig. 14.5A). The choice of implants for ulna is either a medullary nail or plate and screws but for fracture radius, rigid compression plating is usually desired (Figs 14.3C and 14.5B). Cancellous bone grafting is done if the comminution is more than one-third of the circumference of the bone.

The choice of plate osteosynthesis are:
- Dynamic compression plates are still popular.

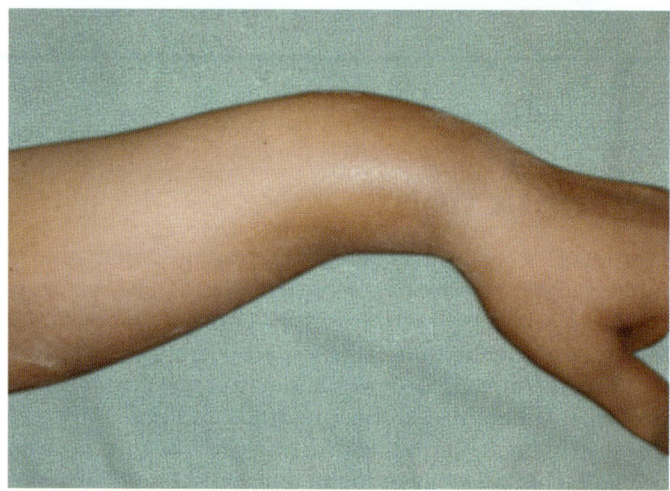

Fig. 14.4: Clinical photo of the deformity in fracture both bones of forearm

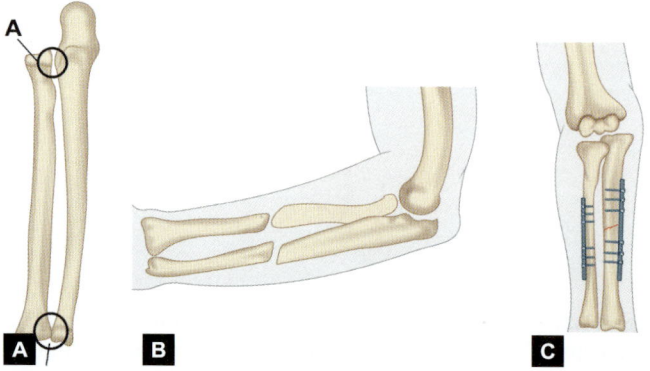

Figs 14.3A to C: (A) Normal both bones of the forearm with superior and inferior radioulnar joints; (B) Fracture both bones of the forearm; (C) Fracture both bones fixed rigidly with plate and screws (Preferred method)

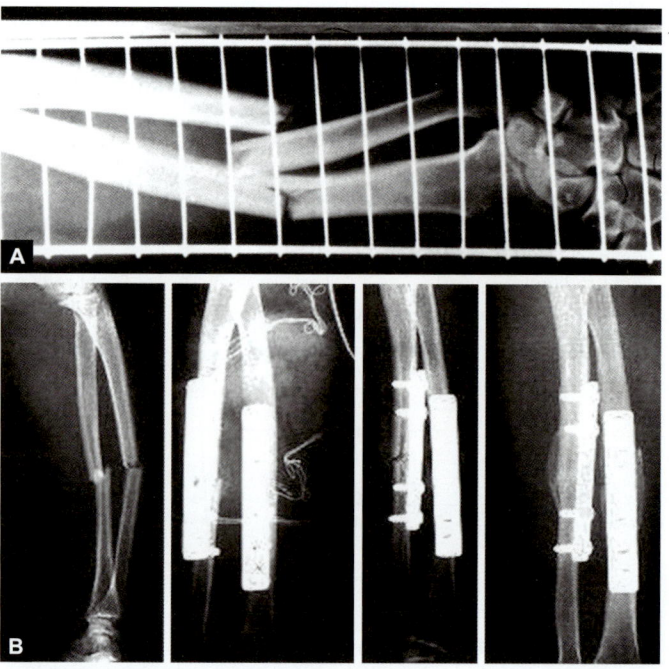

Figs 14.5A and B: (A) Radiograph showing fracture of radius and ulna; (B) Radiograph showing forearms both bones fracture and internal fixation with DCP plates

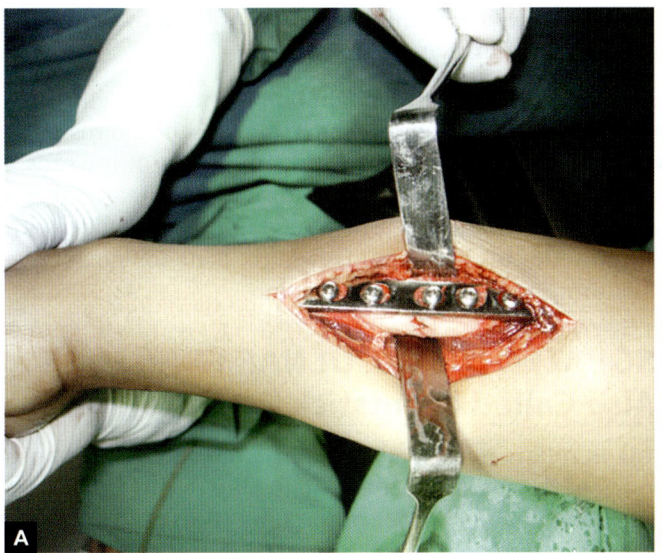
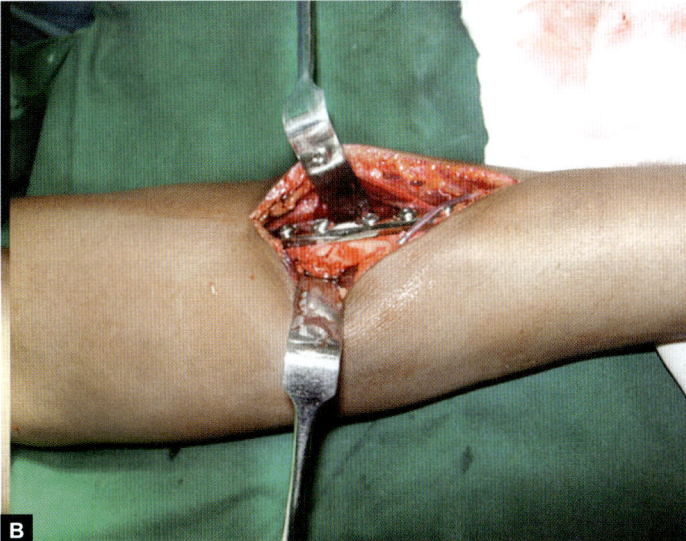

Figs 14.6A and B: Operative photo of plating of fracture both bones forearm (Still the gold standard)

- *Low contact:* DCP have the advantage of less periosteal vascular damage (Figs 14.6A and B).
- DCP plates with preliminary K-wire fixation helps in holding the fracture reduction while the final screws are fixed.
- *Low contact:* Locking dynamic compression plates helps to obtain both rigid fixation and less vascular damage.
- Locked compression plating is the preferred method of late.

Intramedullary fixation: IM nail fixation of both bones fractures with K-wires, Rush nails, etc. was popular in the 1950's and was gradually replaced by plates due to the less rigid fixation it offered. Now they are coming back with a bang thanks to the innovations in the nails technology like the advent of intramedullary interlocking nailing and are being mainly used in the pediatric group than adults.

Indications
- Segmental fracture
- Open fracture with soft tissues injury and/or bone loss
- Multiple injuries
- Failed plating
- Pathological fractures.

Advantages
- Less exposure
- Less periosteal stripping
- Bone grafting is not required.

Choices of IM Nails
- Nonreamed interference fit, prebent star, shaped titanium radial and ulnar nails (Figs 14.7A and B).
- Stainless steel straight distal locking nail system.

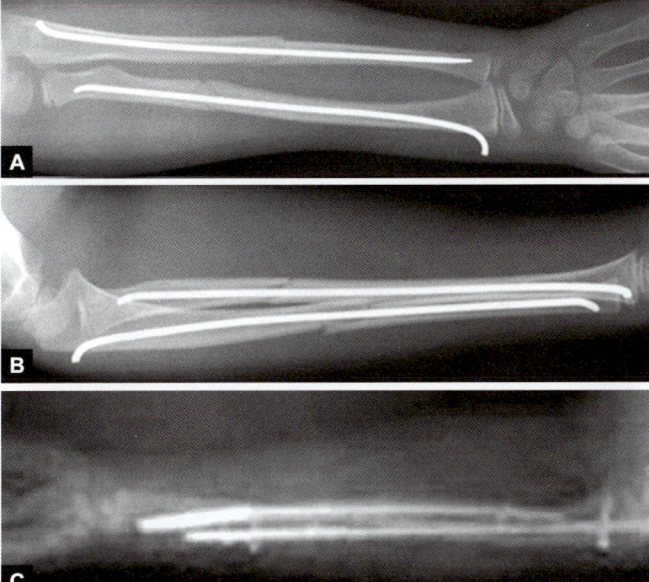

Figs 14.7A to C: Plain X-ray showing intramedullary fixation both bones of forearm, interlocking nailing

- Interlocking nails with both proximal and distal locking (Fig. 14.7C).

Complications of Fracture Both Bones of Forearm

Volkmann's ischemia: Because of the tight fascial compartment, a patient with fracture both bones forearm is more prone to develop acute compartmental syndrome (Fig. 14.8).

Delayed union and nonunion: This can be encountered due to soft tissue interposition, inadequate immobilization, etc. It has to be treated by open reduction, rigid internal fixation, and cancellous bone grafting (Fig. 14.9).

Malunion: Due to the complex muscular forces, it is difficult to retain the position of both bones in perfect alignment after closed reduction (Fig. 14.10). It is in this situation that malunion commonly results. It is treated by corrective osteotomy, plating, and bone grafting.

Cross union: This is due to malunion of a radial fracture in a medially deviated position, which occupies the interosseous space and blocks pronation and supination. If the cross-union takes place in the middle third of the forearm, it can be left alone as the forearm is held in midpronation with less functional damage. Elsewhere, it needs corrective osteotomy and rigid internal fixation.

ISOLATED DISTAL ULNAR FRACTURE (Also Called Nightstick Fracture)

This is relatively rare when compared to fracture both bones of the forearm. It is usually due to direct blow on the subcutaneous border of the ulna (Fig. 14.11A). Three types are described:

Type I: Simple fracture.

Type II: Comminuted fracture without distal radioulnar joint involvement.

Type III: Type II with involvement of the distal radioulnar joint.

> **Interesting Facts**
> Nightstick fracture derives its name from the peculiar incident of a burglar getting caught during his misadventure in the night and trying to ward off the police officer's blow with the stick with his forearm (Fig. 14.5A).

Clinical Features

The patient presents with pain, swelling, and deformity along the subcutaneous border of the forearm. Rotational movements of the forearm are restricted.

Radiograph

The AP, lateral views of the forearm helps to make a diagnosis (Fig. 14.11B).

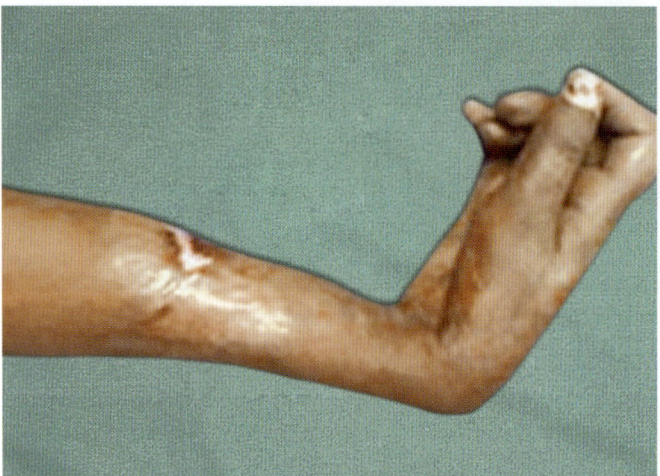

Fig. 14.8: Clinical photo showing VIC

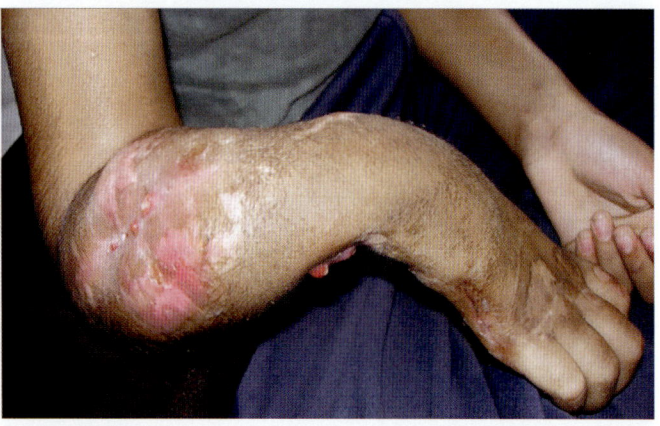

Fig. 14.9: Clinical photo showing nonunion both bones forearm

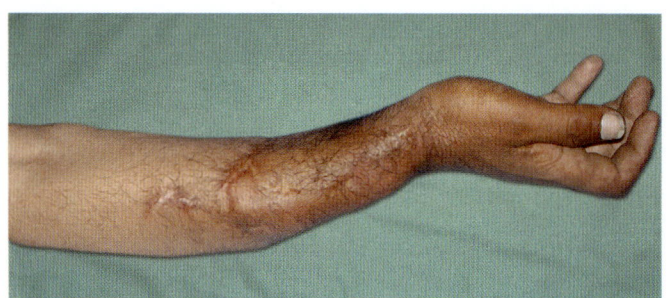

Fig. 14.10: Clinical photo showing malunion both bones forearm

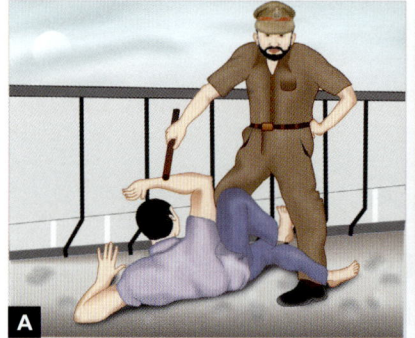 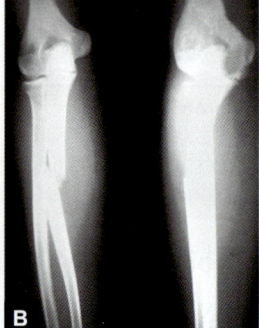

Figs 14.11A and B: Mechanism of nightstick fracture; (B) Radiograph showing nightstick fracture

Treatment

Conservative methods: The type I fractures are treated by immobilization with an above elbow plaster slab or cast for a period of 3–4 weeks.

Surgery: Type II and III varieties are treated by open reduction and rigid internal fixation with plate and screws.

MONTEGGIA FRACTURE

It is a fracture upper third of ulna with dislocation head of the radius. *This is usually called a "treacherous lesion" because the dislocation is often missed (see box for the reasons).* Monteggia first described it in 1881.

> **Monteggia Fractures, why Called as Treacherous.**
> Because dislocation of the head of the radius is often missed.
> *Reasons*
> - *Missed by patient*: As he reflexly pulls the elbow after fall and reduces the dislocation unknowingly
> - Missed by quack due to ignorance
> - *Missed by physician*: Fails to order to include the elbow in radiographs of forearm bone fractures
> - *Missed by radiologist:* If he or she fails to utilize the McLaughlin's line.

Mechanism of Injury

Monteggia's fractures are more common in children and are due to fall on the outstretched hands either in hyperpronation or in hyperextension (Fig. 14.12).

Classification

Bado's classification (Table 14.1) is employed in adults and John Wein's classification (Table 14.2) in children and which takes into consideration the greenstick fractures in them (Figs 14.13A to E).

TABLE 14.1: Bado's classification (adults)	
Type I (60%)	Anterior dislocation of head of the radius with fracture ulna at upper third and with anterior angulations
Type II (5%)	Posterior dislocation head of the radius and fracture proximal ulna with posterior angulations
Type III (20%)	Lateral dislocation head of the radius and fracture proximal ulna with lateral angulations
Type IV (15%)	Fracture radius and ulna in their upper one-third and anterior dislocation of head of the radius with anterior angulations

TABLE 14.2: John Wein's classification (children)
It takes into account greenstick fracture in children.
- Anterior bend
- Anterior greenstick
- Anterior complete
- Posterior
- Lateral

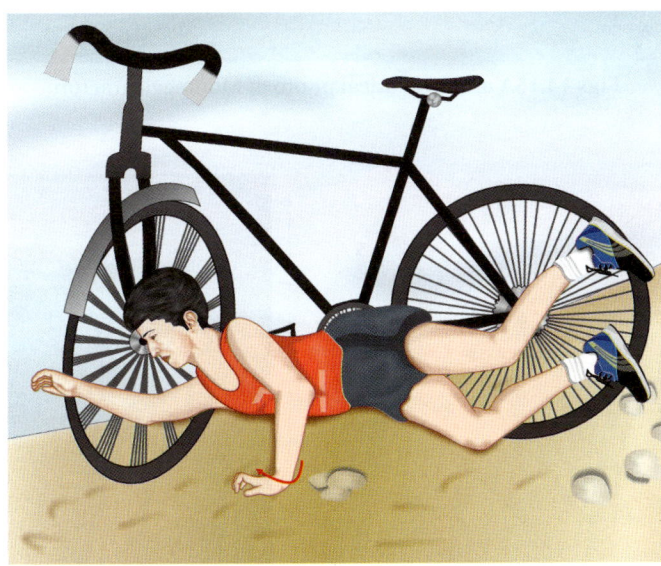

Fig. 14.12: Hyperpronation injury leading to fractures like Monteggia's fracture

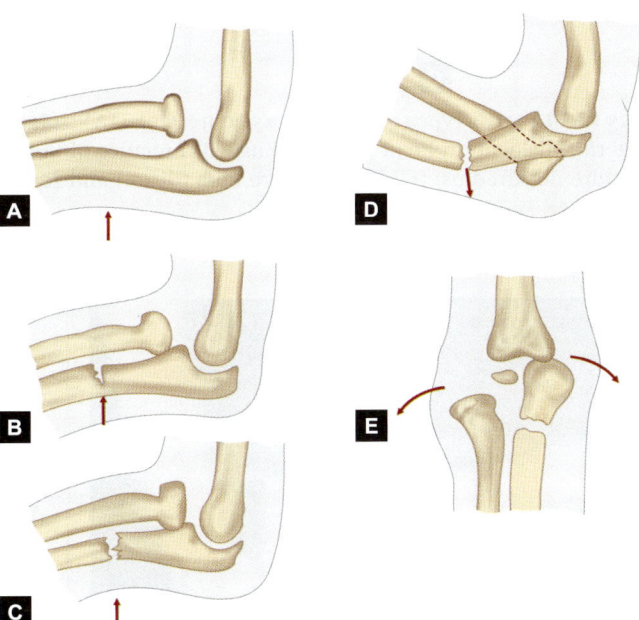

Figs 14.13A to E: Diagrammatic representation of the displacements in Monteggia's fracture; Bado's types (Adults) C-type I, D-type II, E-Type III; John Wein's Types (Children). (A) Anterior bend; (B) Anterior greenstick; (C) Anterior complete

Monteggia's equivalents: These are variants of Monteggia's fracture dislocations and are a result of pronation injuries. The following types are described:
- Isolated dislocation of head of the radius
- Fracture shaft ulna with fracture neck radius
- Fracture shaft ulna with fracture shaft radius (distal)
- Fracture ulna with fracture radial neck, dislocation of shaft of the radius.

In these cases, closed reduction is tried first. If it fails, open reduction and internal fixation is done (Figs 14.14A to C).

Clinical Features

A patient with Monteggia's fracture complains of pain, swelling, deformity, and severe loss of forearm movements. Depending upon the type of Monteggia's fractures, the head of the radius and the ulnar angulation may be felt anteriorly, posteriorly, or laterally (Figs 14.15A and B).

Radiographs

Plain X-ray of the forearm AP, lateral and oblique views including both the elbow and wrist joints needs to be done (Figs 14.16A to C). In order to avoid missing the diagnosis of dislocation of the head of radius, McLaughlin's line is employed as described below (Figs 14.16B). A straight line drawn along the center of the shaft of the radius cuts the capitulum in the center irrespective of the position of the elbow. CT scan image is shown in Figure 14.17.

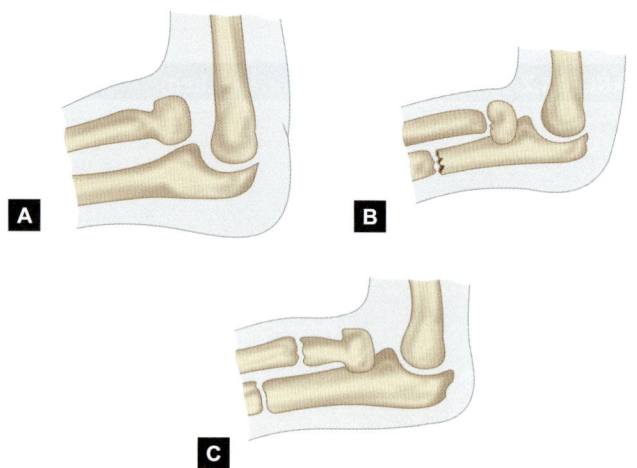

Figs 14.14A to C: Types of Monteggia's equivalents: (A) Isolated anterior dislocation head of the radius; (B) Fracture ulna and fracture neck radius; (C) Both fracture ulna (distal) and radius (proximal)

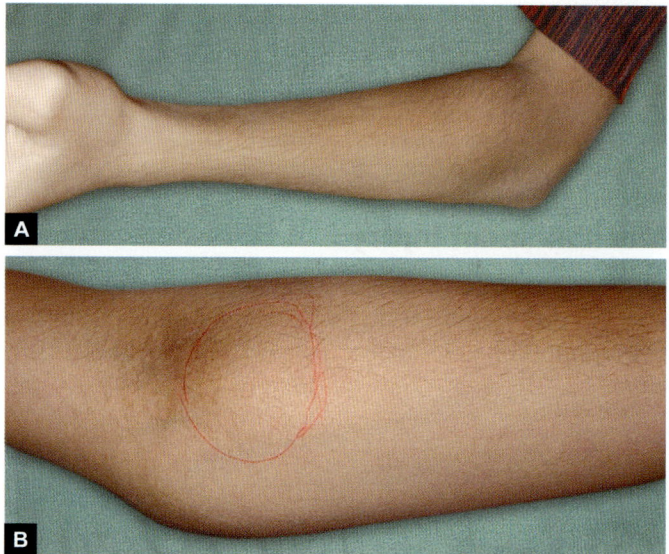

Figs 14.15A and B: Clinical photo of Monteggia fracture

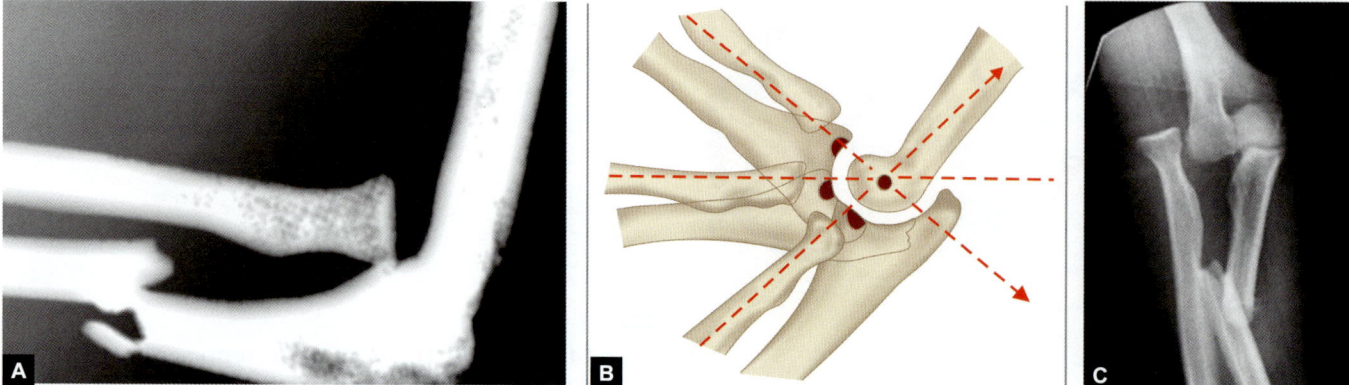

Figs 14.16A to C: (A) Radiograph showing Monteggia's anterior fracture; (B) McLaughlin's line; (C) Radiograph of lateral Monteggia

Treatment

Monteggia's fracture can be managed successfully in children by conservative methods and by operative methods in adults (Table 14.3).

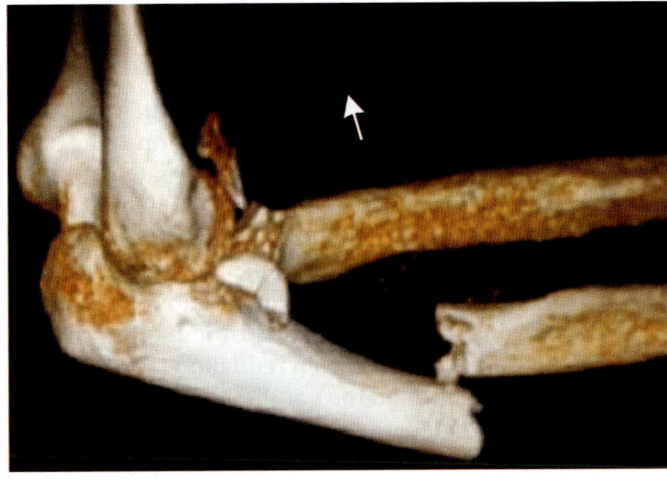

Fig. 14.17: CT image of Monteggia fracture

Complications

- Unreduced dislocation head of radius
- Posterior interosseous nerve palsy
- Malunion of fracture ulna
- Nonunion of fracture ulna
- Myositis ossificans
- Synostosis between radial head and proximal ulna
- Tardy posterior interosseous nerve palsy
- Proximal migration of radius
- Dislocation of inferior radioulnar joint
- Cubitus valgus deformity.

Table 14.3 depicts a comparative study of the various features of different types of Monteggia fractures.

DISTAL RADIUS FRACTURE

These are either extra-articular or intra-articular fractures and are classified based on the mechanism of injury.

Types: They are classified into five types namely:

TABLE 14.3: A comparative study of the various features of Monteggia's fracture

	Type I	Type II	Type III	Type IV
Mechanism of injury Fall on outstretched hands	• Direct blow • Forced pronation • Hyperextension	• Fall with elbow in flexion of 120°	• Forced supination • Forced pronation • Supination with hyperextension	Same as in type I and if force continues
Clinical symptoms: All four types have marked pain and tenderness about the elbow. There will be no flexion/extension/pronation/supination at the elbow. Paralysis of the posterior interosseous nerve may occur.				
Clinical signs	• HOR felt anteriorly • Anterior angulation of ulna	• HOR posterior • Posterior angulation of ulna • Shortening of forearm	HOR is lateral Lateral angulation	HOR is anterior Deformity is at the fracture level
Treatment				
In children	• Closed reduction is tried first • If unsuccessful OR of fracture ulna + CR of HOR is done • If this also fails, OR of fracture ulna with OR of head of the radius with repair or reconstruction of annular ligament using forearm fascia or fascia lata is done	CR tried first OR if it fails	Closed reduction is successful most of the times	CR is tried first if it fails OR + Rigid IF with plate and screws for radius and ulnar fractures is done
In adults	• OR + IF of fracture ulna with plate and screws • CR of HOR • If it fails, OR, HOR + IF fracture ulna is done • If fracture >6 weeks • Excision HOR is done	Same as in type I	Same as in type I	Same as in type I

Note: CR → Closed reduction, OR → Open reduction, IF → Internal fixation, and HOR → Head of radius.

Type I: Extra-articular metaphyseal fractures (e.g. Colles fracture, Smith fracture). These are caused by bending forces.

Type II: Intra-articular fractures and include Barton both dorsal and volar and radial styloid process fractures. They are caused by shearing forces.

Type III: Intra-articular fractures and metaphyseal impaction. Radial Pilon fractures fall in this group. They are caused by compression forces.

Type IV: These are avulsion radiocarpal injuries.

Type V: Multiple comminuted fractures and are due to high velocity forces.

Treatment Plan in a Nutshell

Type I: Colles or Smith fractures can usually managed by closed reduction and plaster casting. Unstable fractures may require percutaneous fixation, plate and screws fixation and comminuted fractures need external fixators.

Type II: Usually, the Barton types require open reduction and rigid internal fixation (Ellis plates).

Type III: Combination of open and closed techniques, wire fixation, open reduction, and bone grafting after plating are some of the options.

Type IV: Avulsion fractures are treated by sutures, K-wire fixation, external fixation, etc.

Type V: Due to severe comminuted open reduction is difficult. Fixation methods may require a combination of K-wire fixation and or external fixations.

> **What is New?**
> *Distraction plate internal fixation:* This is an alternative to external fixation and a distraction plate is used to provide internal distraction forces thereby eliminating the complications of external fixators.

COMMINUTED DISTAL RADIAL FRACTURE

Medoff developed both methods of percutaneous K-wire fixation and plates as when used alone either techniques were found wanting. He described five columns namely:

Radial column: Fixed with radial pin plate consisting of distal K-wire fixation and proximal screws through a radial buttress plate.

Dorsal cortical wall: Treated as dorsal Barton.

Dorsal ulnar split: Fixed with ulnar pin plate as described above. Wire form implants are used to stabilize the dorsal cortical wall.

Volar rim: Treatment as in volar Barton with L-shaped buttress plate.

Central intra-articular fragments: Treatment is with the Trimed system.

COLLES FRACTURE

Discussed in Geriatric Orthopedics. Also called "Piedmont fracture" (after Piedmont Orthopedic Society).

DISTAL SHAFT RADIUS FRACTURE

GALEAZZI'S FRACTURE

This is a fracture of radius at the junction of middle and distal third with associated subluxation or dislocation of the distal radioulnar joint. Subluxation of this joint may be present initially or occur during treatment (Figs 14.18A and B).

French people call this fracture *reverse Monteggia*.

Campbell called it as *fracture of necessity* since it always requires open reduction and internal fixation (ORIF).

The following are the major deforming forces causing loss of reduction and difficulty in reduction (Fig. 14.19).

- Gravity acting through the hand.
- Insertion of pronator quadratus pulls the distal fragment in proximal and volar direction.
- Brachioradialis uses the distal radioulnar joint as a pivot and causes shortening.
- Abductors and extensors of the thumb cause shortening and relaxation of the radiocarpal ligament.

Incidence: It is three times as common as Monteggia's fracture.

Mechanism of Injury

- Fall on an outstretched hand with marked pronation of the forearm.
- Direct blow on the dorsolateral side of the forearm.

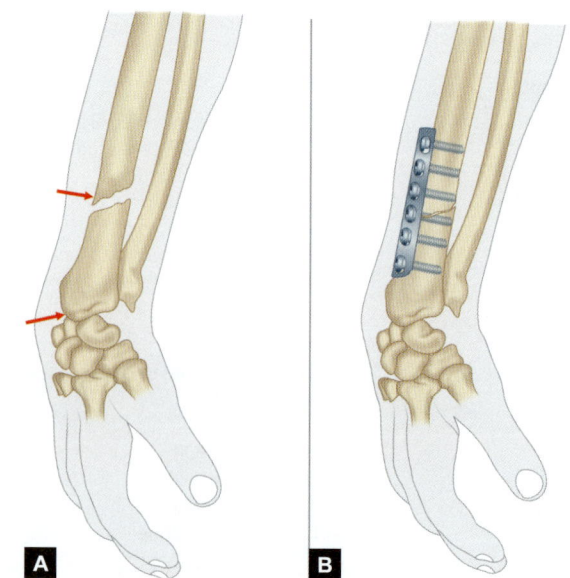

Figs 14.18A and B: (A) Galeazzi fracture; (B) ORIF with DCP plate and screws (Preferred method)

CHAPTER 14: Injuries of the Forearm

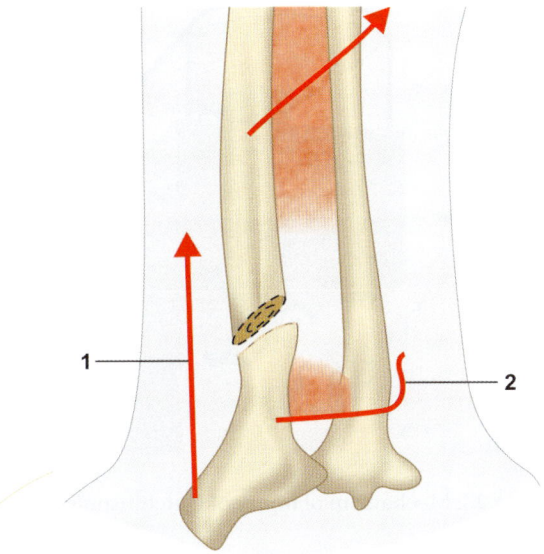

Fig. 14.19: Displacing forces in Galeazzi fractures:
(1) Brachioradialis, (2) Pronator quadratus

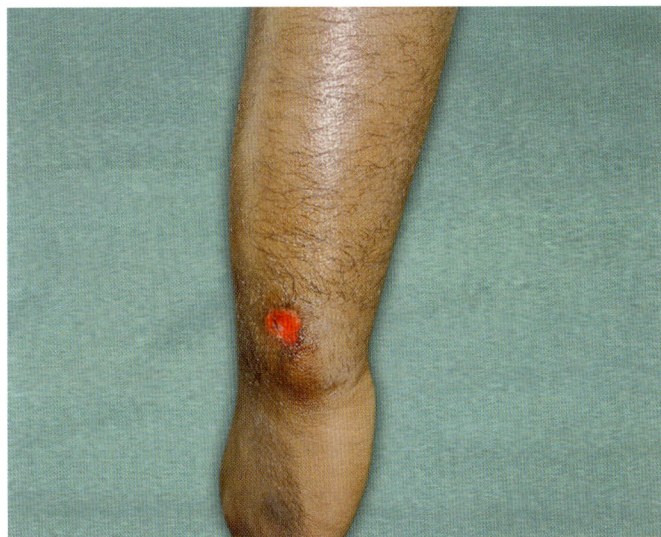

Fig. 14.20: Clinical photo showing Galeazzi fracture

Clinical Features

The patient complains of pain, swelling, and deformity of the lower end of the forearm. Pronation and supination are severely restricted. All other features of fractures are present (Fig. 14.20).

Radiograph

Important radiological features of Galleazzi's fracture are as shown in the box (Fig. 14.21A).

AP view	Lateral view
• Fracture radius, transverse or short oblique • Comminution is less • Distal radioulnar joint is dislocated • Radius appears short	• Radius is angulated dorsally • Head of the ulna is prominent dorsally

Treatment

Closed reduction is usually not successful due to the deforming forces of the muscles. Hence, ORIF is the preferred method of treatment (Fig. 14.21B). Intramedullary nails and small plates do not provide adequate fixation, long plate (LCDCP plate) and screws are thus used and the dislocated distal radioulnar joint may be fixed with K-wire (Fig. 14.22).

Complications

Nonunion and malunion are notorious complications. Angulations of the fracture and subluxation of the distal radioulnar joint can also occur. Rarely entrapment of

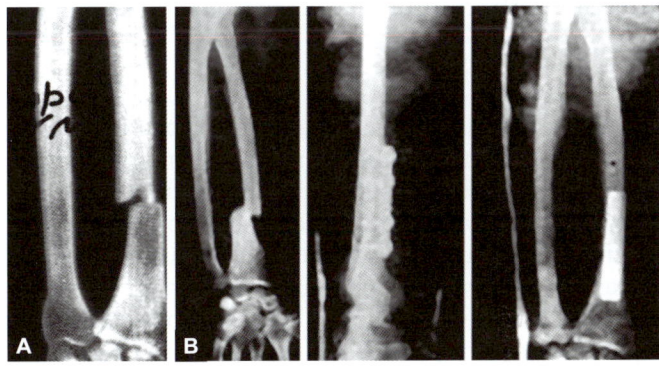

Figs 14.21A and B: (A) Radiograph showing Galeazzi's fracture; (B) Radiograph showing Galeazzi's fracture fixation

extensor carpi ulnaris tendon in distal radioulnar joint is encountered.

ESSEX-LOPRESTI FRACTURE

This is a fracture of the radial head with injury to the distal radioulnar joint and tearing of the interosseous membrane proximally.

Mechanism of Injury

A heavy fall on the outstretched hands.

Clinical Features

Pain and swelling in the radial head region. Pain in the region of the distal radioulnar joint should alert of a possibility. Pain in the wrist could be due to ulnar carpal impingement and pain in the elbow could be due to radiocapitellar impingement.

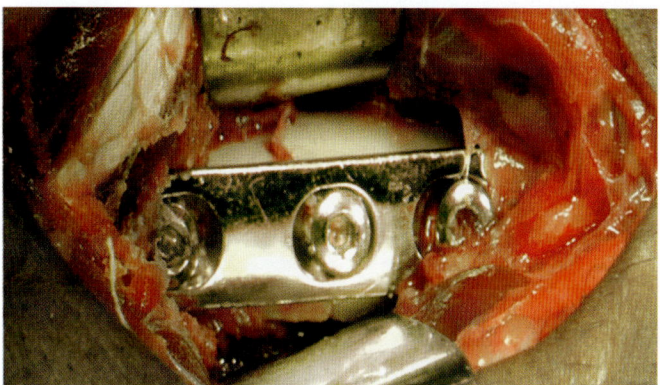

Fig. 14.22: Operative photo showing plating in Galeazzi's fracture (Preferred choice)

Radiograph

It is a relatively rare fracture and in order to avoid missing it, radiograph of the forearm and wrist joint should be taken in all cases of fracture of head of the radius.

Treatment

Open reduction and internal fixation of the proximal radial fracture and pinning of the inferior radioulnar joint is the treatment method of choice. If there is disruption of distal radioulnar joint and if the radial head fracture is grossly comminuted then, excision head of the radius is done. This is likely to aggravate the proximal migration of the radius. Hence, if fracture radial head needs excision, it has to be replaced by silastic prosthesis.

RADIAL STYLOID FRACTURE (CHAUFFEUR'S FRACTURE)

Radial styloid fracture (Hutchinson's fracture) is similar to the posterior marginal fracture of the radius.

Mechanism of Injury

It is usually because of the starting crank of an engine being suddenly reversed by a backfire and striking the wrist with a force. It is common in chauffeurs and is an avulsion fracture of the radiocarpal ligament (Fig. 14.23).

Note:
These are also seen in motorcycle accidents and fall from heights.

Clinical Features

The patient complains of pain, swelling, and tenderness over the radial styloid process. Movement of the wrist, especially radial deviation, is painful.

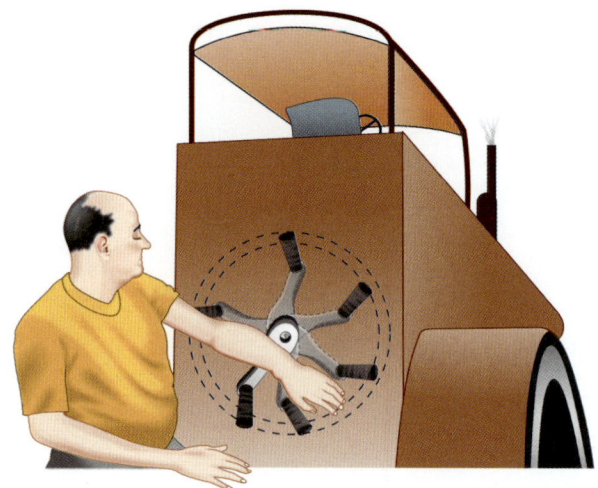

Fig. 14.23: Mechanism of injury of Hutchinson's fracture

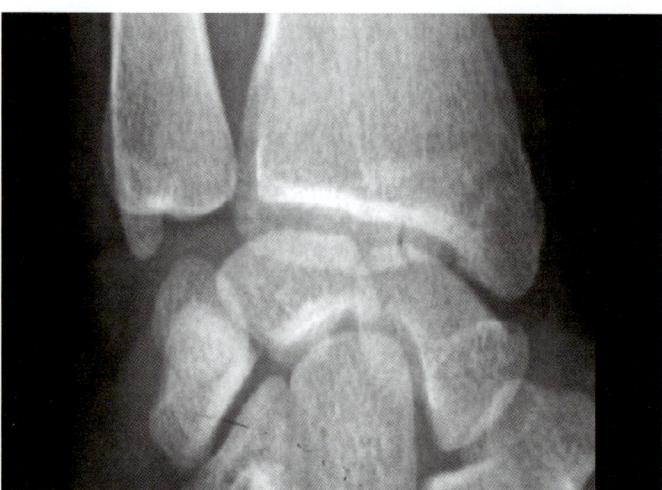

Fig. 14.24: Plain X-ray showing radial styloid process fracture

Radiographs

Radiograph AP view of the wrist shows it as a transverse fracture (Fig. 14.24).

Treatment

This fracture is best treated by an above or below plaster slab or cast in undisplaced fractures and closed reduction and above elbow plaster cast if it is displaced. However, unstable fractures need percutaneous fixation with K-wire.

SMITH'S FRACTURE

It is a fracture of distal one-third of radius with palmar displacement. Hence, it is called as *reverse Colles' fracture*. However, it is less common than Colles' it is readily confused with Colles' fracture. It has a clear fracture dorsally with comminution of the palmar surface (Figs 14.25A and B).

> **Did You Know?**
> Smith's fracture occurs about 1/10 as frequent as Colles' fracture. The greatest problem with this fracture is executing the treatment mistaking it to be a Colles' fracture!

Mechanism of Injury

There are three modes of injury like fall on the back of the dorsum of the hand, fall on the forearm in supination and a direct blow to the flexed hand.

Clinical Features

The patient complains of pain, swelling, deformity, and loss of wrist functions. The deformity is opposite to that of Colles' fracture and is called the 'garden spade' deformity.

Radiograph

Anteroposterior view of the wrist shows the carpus proximally displaced. There will be anterior displacement of the fragment with palmar angulation of distal radial articular surface (Fig. 14.25C). The ulnar styloid process is frequently fractured.

Treatment

The treatment of choice is closed reduction and immobilization in a long arm cast with forearm in supination and wrist in extension. For unstable fractures, fixation with percutaneous K-wire or open reduction and plate fixation may be required (Fig. 14.25B).

Complications

- Misinterpretation of radiographs for Colles'
- Other complication of Colles'.

BARTON'S FRACTURE

Rim fractures of the distal radius are called Barton's fracture. Dorsal or volar rim could be involved and these fractures are invariably intra-articular.

DORSAL BARTON

Dorsal Barton is a dorsal rim fracture of distal radius with dorsal subluxation or dislocation. It is a variant of Colles' (Fig. 14.26).

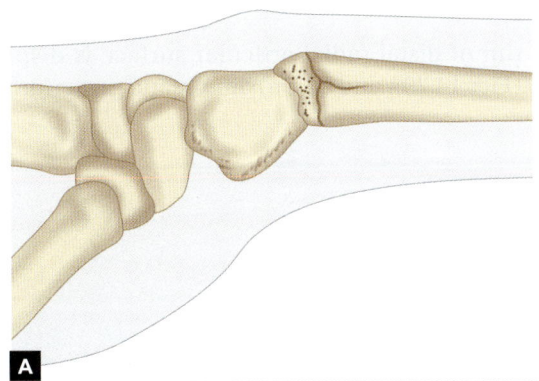
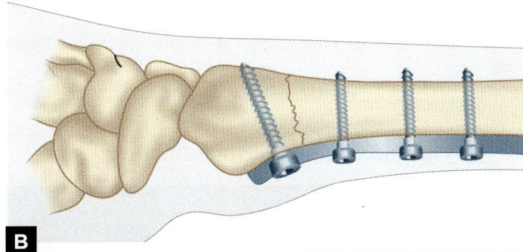
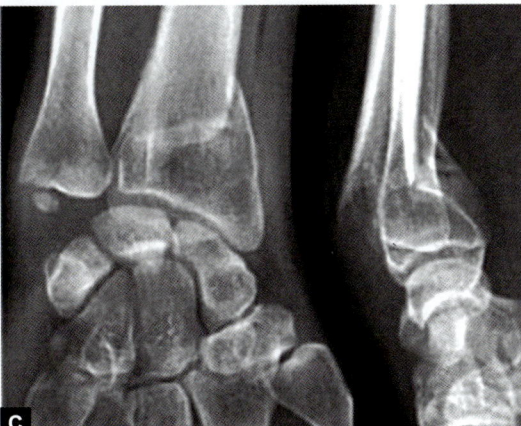

Figs 14.25A to C: (A) Smith's fracture; (B) Method of fixation of Smith's fracture; (C) Radiograph showing Smith's fracture

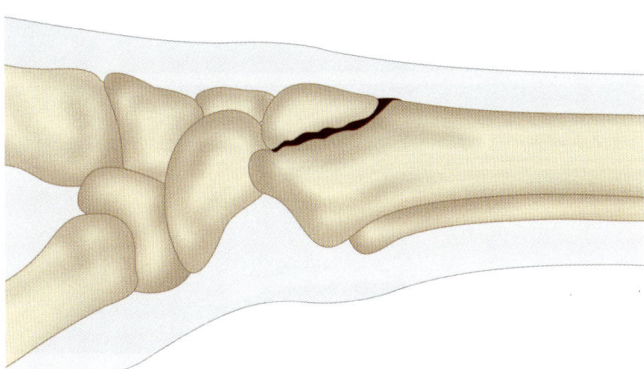

Fig. 14.26: Dorsal Barton's fracture

Mechanism

Fall with dorsiflexion and pronation of the distal forearm on a flexed wrist.

Clinical Features

Patient complains of severe pain, swelling, tenderness over the wrist and restricted wrist movements with painful dorsiflexion.

Radiograph

Best seen on the lateral view. Dorsal lip of distal radial articular surface is displaced proximally and posteriorly and may be associated with dorsal subluxation of the wrist (Figs 14.27A and B).

Treatment

Conservative

Short arm cast with wrist in neutral position.

Surgery

Unstable fracture is fixed by percutaneous pins or small screws. OR + IF with small plate and screws can be done but due to the extensor tendons may be a difficult option.

VOLAR BARTON (PALMAR RIM DISLOCATION)

Volar Barton (Palmar rim dislocation) is a palmar rim fracture of distal radius (Fig. 14.28).

Mechanism

It is due to palmar tensile stress and dorsal shear stress and is usually combined with radial styloid fracture.

Clinical Features

It consists of pain, swelling, tenderness, and loss of wrist movements. Palmar flexion is grossly restricted and painful.

Radiograph

Palmar rim of distal radial articular surface is displaced dorsally (Figs 14.29A and B). Proximally and posteriorly and

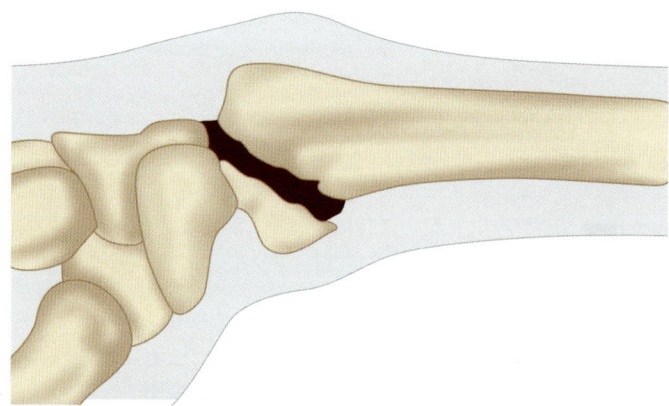

Fig. 14.28: Volar Barton's fracture

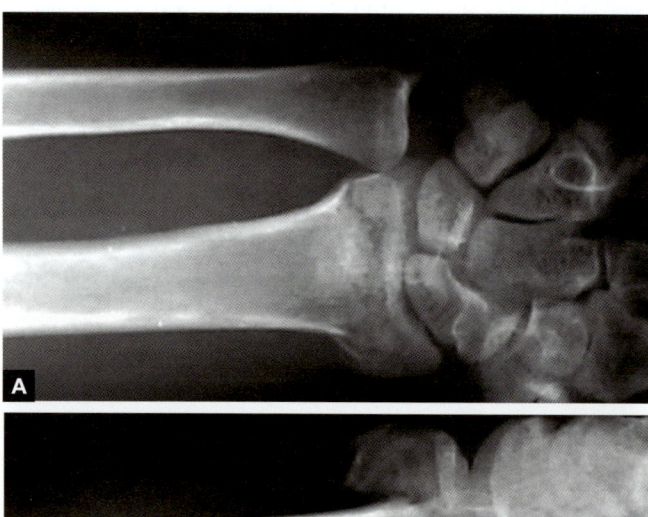

Figs 14.27A and B: Plain X-rays showing dorsal Barton's fracture: (A) AP view; (B) Lateral view

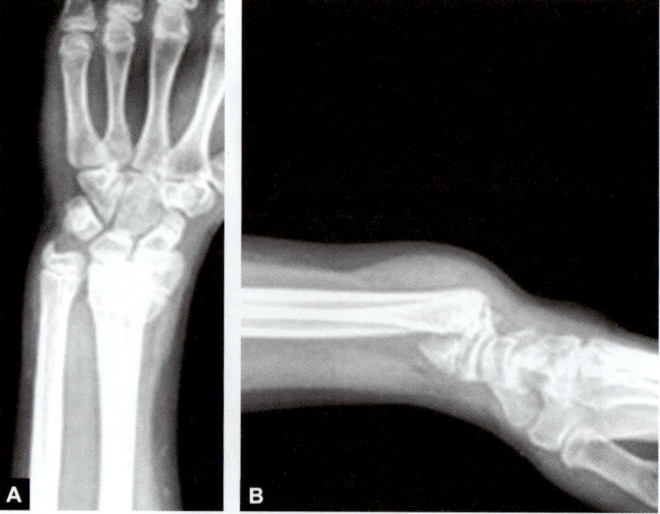

Figs 14.29A and B: Plain X-rays showing Volar Barton fracture: (A) AP view; (B) Lateral view

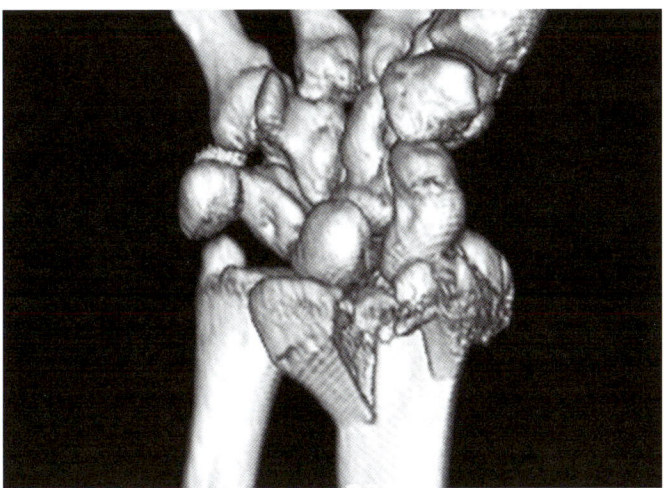

Fig. 14.30: CT images of volar barton fracture

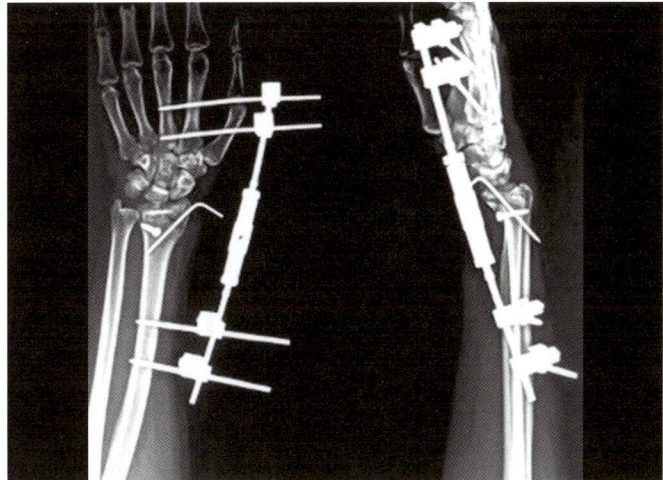

Fig. 14.32: Methods of fixation in volar barton's fracture

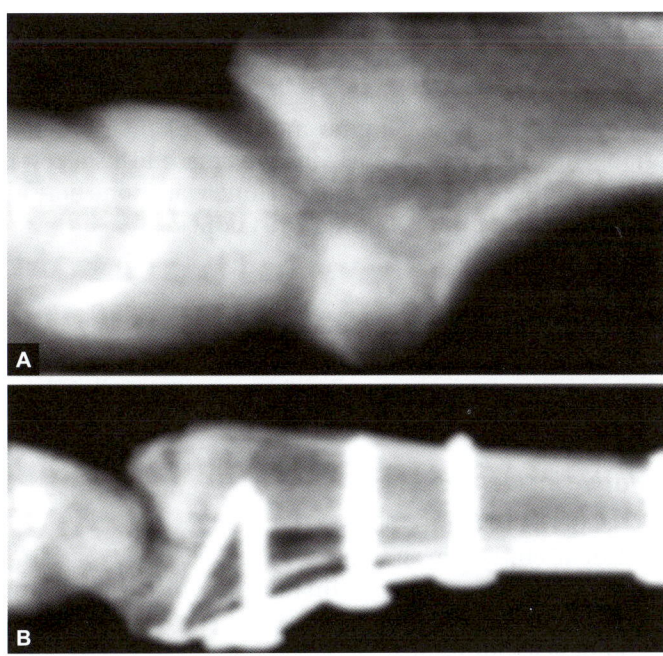

Figs 14.31A and B: Radiographs showing Volar Barton's fracture (A) fixed with plate and screws (B)

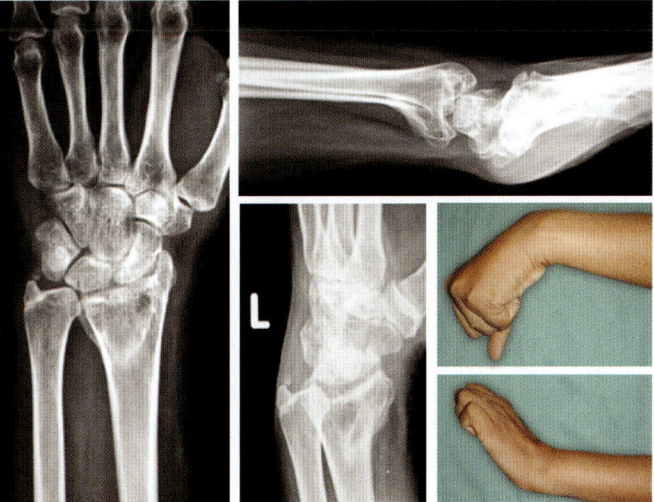

Fig. 14.33: Malunion of volar Barton's fracture

may be associated with dorsal subluxation of the wrist. CT scan gives more accurate picture (Fig. 14.30).

Treatment

Conservative

Reduction is simple, but retention is difficult. Long arm cast is used.

Surgery

If reduction does not remain satisfactorily with wrist in neutral or slight palmar flexion, fixation with K-wire (Fig. 14.32), external fixators and buttress plate, etc. may be done. Ellis T-shaped buttress plate fixation is the preferred method of treatment (Fig. 14.31B).

Complications: Malunion, stiffness, reduced moments of the wrist, pain, osteoarthritis are some of the complications (Fig. 14.33).

15 CHAPTER

Injuries to the Wrist

BRIEF ANATOMY

The Wrist Joint Speaks
I am not a single joint but made up of radiocarpal, midcarpal, and intercarpal joints. The middle finger, the third metacarpal, and the capitate are the axial bones of the hand. The midcarpal component of mine allows flexion and extension as this being a hinge joint (Fig. 15.1). My main flexors are flexor carpi ulnaris and radialis aided by finger flexors. I extend mainly by the action of extensor carpi radialis, longus and brevis supported by extensor digitorum and extensor carpi ulnaris. This movement of mine occurs at radiocarpal joint. I adduct mostly at radiocarpal joint by the action of flexor and extensor carpi ulnaris. I abduct entirely at the radiocarpal joint due to the combined action of extensor carpi radialis longus, extensor pollicis brevis, abductor pollicis longus, and flexor carpi radialis. My normal range of movement includes flexion 80°, extension 70°, radial deviation 20°, and ulnar deviation 30°. My functional position is 30° dorsiflexion.

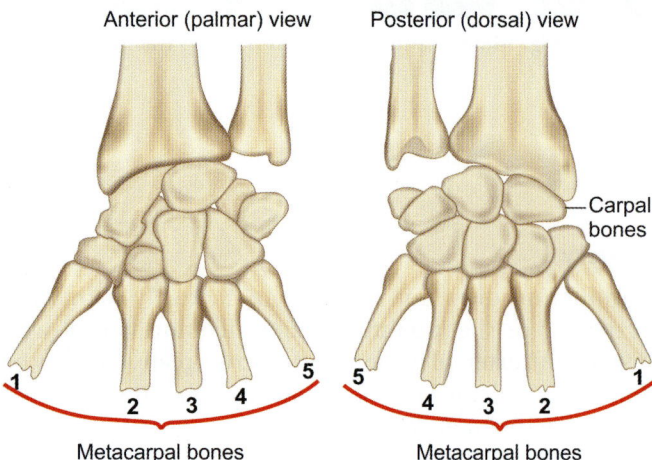

Fig. 15.1: Bony anatomy of the wrist

CARPAL INJURIES

Do you remember the famous mnemonic "She Looks Too Pretty, Try to Catch her" learnt in first MBBS. The starting letter of each word denotes the names of the eight carpal bones (scaphoid, lunate, triquetral, pisiform, trapezoid, trapezium, capitate and hamate), their order of arrangement and placement in the proximal and distal rows. A brief discussion on scaphoid and lunate are done here as they are the commonly injured wrist bones.

General Principles

Incidences
Carpal injuries have an overall incidence of 6% of all skeletal injuries.

Relative Incidences
- Scaphoid fracture—60%
- Dorsal chip radius fracture—10%
- Post-traumatic carpal instability with or without dislocations—10%
- Lunate fracture—3%
- All other carpal bone fractures—7%

Mechanism of Injury

Carpal injuries usually result from fall on the outstretched hands. Frequently misdiagnosed, it is known for complications like early avascular necrosis (in scaphoid), late carpal instability, and arthritis. Hence, prompt and correct treatment is mandatory. Lack of callus in fractures in this region makes judgment about the progress of union difficult.

Clinical Features

Pain, swelling, tenderness, and loss of wrist movements are some of the common complaints of carpal injuries. Careful examination of the entire wrist is mandatory to localize the nature and type of injury.

Investigations

Radiology: Plain X-rays of the wrist preferably the PA view, lateral and oblique views with the wrist in neutral position helps to make an assessment. In the PA view, look for the following:
- The dorsal radioulnar articular surfaces
- The lesser arc at the midcarpal joint (This involves the radial styloid, midcarpal and lunatotriquetral space)
- The greater arc formed by the proximal carpal row and involves the injuries to the scaphoid, capitate and triquetrum
- Radiographs of six views required to make a diagnosis
- AP view
- Lateral view in neutral position
- AP view in maximal radial deviation
- AP view in maximal ulnar deviation
- Lateral view in maximal flexion
- Lateral view in maximal extension.

These views are adequate in 90% of cases. Angular relationship is best visualized in lateral views. Longitudinal axes of long finger metacarpal, capitate, lunate and radius all fall in the same line. The following are the important features on radiographs:
- *Lateral view—scapholunate angle:* It is formed normally between longitudinal axis of lunate and scaphoid and is 30 to 60° (average 47°).
    - Greater than 70° indicates instability.
    - Greater than 80° indicates definite instability of dorsiflexion type.
    - Greater than 20° capitolunate angle (between the long axis of capitulum's and lunate) suggests carpal instability.
- *AP view:* There is constant space between the carpal bones in all the movements of wrist. Joint width between scaphoid and lunate is normally 1 to 2 mm. Space of greater than 3 mm is considered abnormal.

Fluoroscopy: This helps to assess carpal kinematics radiographically.

CT scan: This is a very important investigative tool and it detects features not picked by routine plain X-rays.

MRI: Though less useful, it helps to detect AVN, nonunion, cartilage condition, etc.

Technetium bone scan: It helps to detect carpal bone fractures 6 to 8 hours after injury and those not seen clearly on X-rays.

Arthrography: This helps to detect soft tissue and ligament injury.

Ultrasonography: This helps to detect ganglion, cyst, soft tissue injuries, etc.

Arthroscopy: It has both diagnostic and therapeutic role in wrist fractures.

Treatment

The principles of treatment and the methods of treatment are described below:

Principles
- Most carpal injuries need surgical intervention
- Conservative treatment is reserved for fractures with < 1 mm displacement or <1–2 mm diastases.
- If associated with soft tissue injuries, it needs surgical repair.

Methods

Conservative treatment is by short arm cast immobilization.

Surgery: Operative treatment consists of the following methods:
- Percutaneous fixation for displaced fractures is by fixation with K-wires.
- Open reduction and rigid internal fixation for displaced fractures with K-wires or screws.
- External fixation is indicated for difficult, comminuted and open injuries.

SCAPHOID FRACTURE

This is the most common carpal bone fracture and has several interesting features.

> **Interesting Features**
> - This bone forms the radial part of the carpus
> - Lies obliquely at 45° to longitudinal axes of 2 rows
> - Articulates with 5 bones (radius, lunate, triquetral, trapezium, capitulum)
> - Central indentation is called waist
> - Since it crosses two rows of carpus, it is more susceptible to fracture.

Anatomical Peculiarities
- It articulates with distal radius and with four carpal bones. It moves in all the movements of the wrist.
- It has a precarious blood supply (Fig. 15.2A).

- Sixty seven percent of the scaphoid have arterial foramina throughout its length.
- Thirteen percent have predominant blood supply in the distal one-third.
- In about 20% most of the foramina are in the waist with no foramina in the proximal one-third.

This suggests that one-third of the fractures, occurring in the proximal one-third is without adequate blood supply resulting in avascular necrosis in 35 percent of cases at this level and has poor prognosis.

Etiology

It is common in young adults though it can be seen in patients of 10 to 70 years of age.
- The common mode of injury is fall on an outstretched hand with hyperextension and slight radial deviation at the wrist.
- It is associated with other fractures of the carpus and forearm bones in about 17%.
- It is the commonest fracture among carpal bones.
- Among the wrist fractures, it is second only to the fracture lower end of radius.

Classification

Cooney, Dobyn's, Linscheid's Classification

- *Stable fracture*
- *Unstable fracture:* The following are the criteria to label it as unstable:
  - Scapholunate angle greater than 70°.
  - Capitolunate angle greater than 20°.
  - Separation of scaphoid and lunate greater than 3 to 4 mm.

Anatomical Classification (Fig. 15.2B)

- Proximal pole fracture (20%)
- Waist fracture (70%)
- Distal body fracture (10%)
- Tuberosity fracture
- Osteochondral fracture.

Clinical Features

Patient complains of pain and swelling of the wrist. Tenderness in the anatomical snuffbox is a characteristic finding. The movements of the wrist may be painful.

Investigations

Plain X-rays (Fig. 15.2C): The views of the radiographs are (AP, lateral, oblique and ulnar deviation). These four views can diagnose scaphoid fracture in 97% of the cases.

> **Vital Facts**
> *Signs of instability are:*
> - Displacement of the fracture fragments (>1 mm).
> - Motion between the fracture fragments.
> - Presence of one of the carpal collapse patterns.
> - Angulations or shortening of the scaphoid.

Caution: The X-rays may not show a fracture in the initial stages. Hence, repeat X-ray should be done after 2 to 3 weeks.

CT scan: It is indicated in cases of doubt or if fracture scaphoid is not seen on initial X-ray.

Isotope scan: It shows increased activity in doubtful cases.

MRI: This helps to assess the vascularity, especially of the proximal fragment.

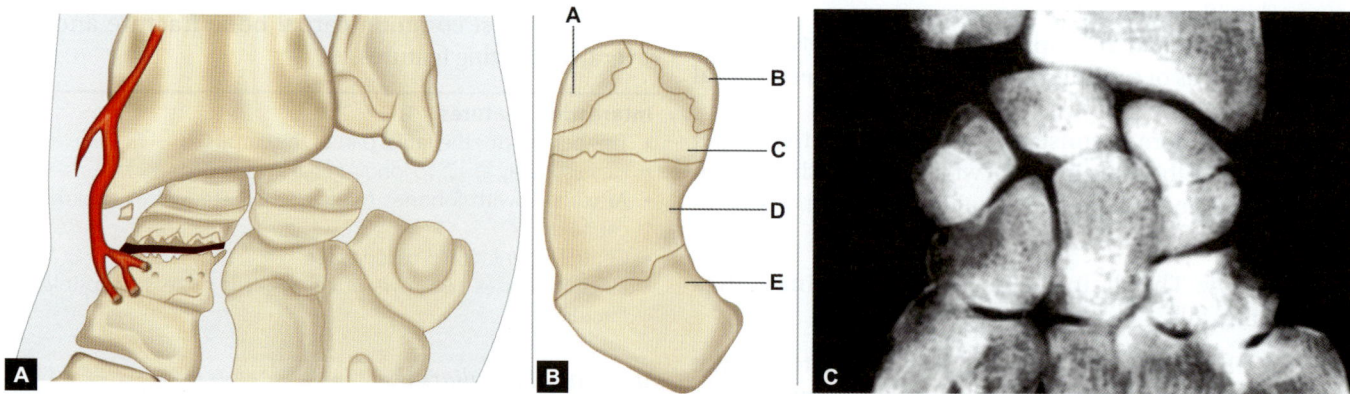

Figs 15.2A to C: (A) Blood supply of scaphoid is peculiar (see text); (B) Different levels of scaphoid fracture: (a) Fracture of the tuberosity, (b) distal articular fracture, (c) distal one-third fracture, (d) waist fracture, (e) fracture of the proximal pole; (C) radiograph showing fracture scaphoid

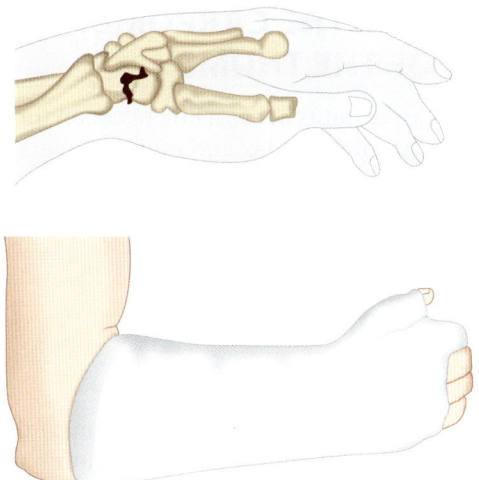

Fig. 15.3: Scaphoid fracture being treated by a "scaphoid cast"

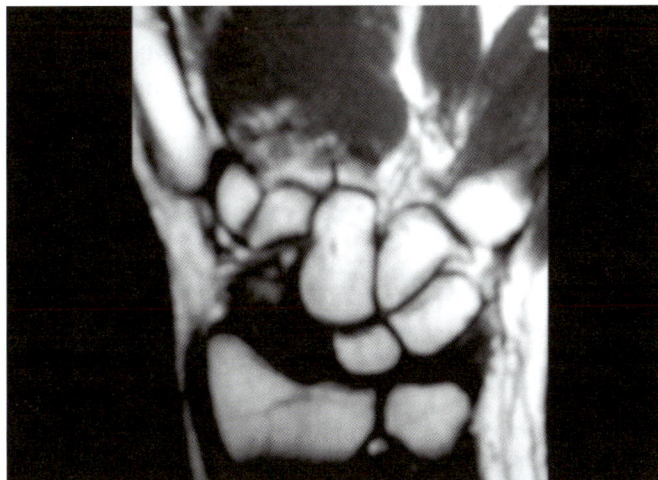

Fig. 15.4: MRI showing AVN scaphoid bone

Principles of Treatment

- Common is transverse fracture of the waist
- Injury to the wrist and tenderness in the region of the scaphoid should be treated as if they had a fracture until the radiographs have disapproved a fracture at 2nd and 4th week.

Conservative Methods

This is indicated in undisplaced, <1 mm displacement or <15° angulations.
- Once a fracture is diagnosed, if undisplaced, Böhler gauntlet type short arm cast from proximal forearm to midpalmar area with proximal phalanx of the thumb is put. Expected rate of union is 95% within 10 weeks of time (Fig. 15.3).
- In displaced fracture treatment is by reduction and casting. Union rate is 54%. Closed percutaneous K-wire fixation is also successful if scaphoid cast cannot retain reduction.

Surgical Management

ORIF is the treatment of choice in displaced fractures.

Indications
- Operative treatment has no place in the management of acute scaphoid fracture except for displaced fractures.
- In delayed union and nonunion (>12–16 weeks)
- Preiser's disease, which is an ischemic necrosis of fracture scaphoid.

Surgical Methods

Closed reduction and percutaneous fixation by three-point pressure.

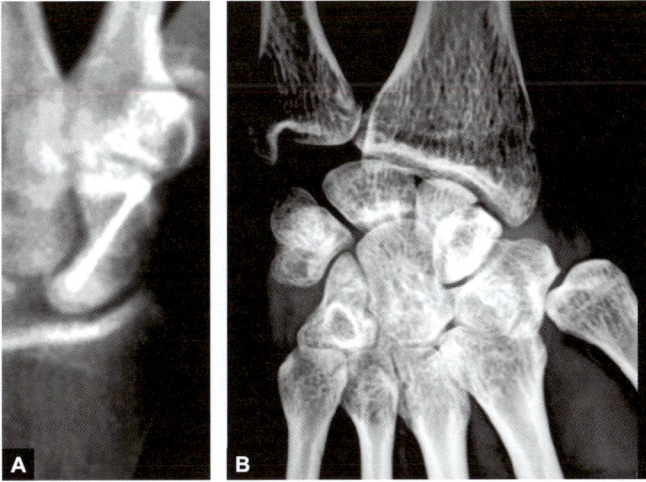

Figs 15.5A and B: (A) Radiograph showing scaphoid fracture treated by ORIF with Herbert screw; (B) Plain X-ray showing nonunion scaphoid fracture

Osteosynthesis: It consists of open reduction and internal fixation or bone grafting or both. K-wire and small corticocancellous screws (Herbert screws, headed or headless and Acutrak screws) along with cancellous bone grafts are used (Fig. 15.5A). *Fusion techniques are used if the patient is young, the opposite hand, wrist are normal, and if much stressful activity is required.*

> **Note:**
> - Open reduction and internal fixation is the most acceptable method.
> - Palmar approach is popular
> - Herbert screw is preferred for internal fixation.

Arthroplasty: This is useful for older patients, with significant osteoarthritis changes in the wrist, e.g. radial styloidectomy, silastic implants, etc.

Arthrodesis: This is less commonly indicated.

Excision of proximal fragments: This is indicated when fragment is less than ¼" in size and when bone grafting has failed.

Flowchart 15.1 depicts the various treatment options in scaphoid fractures.

Complications

- Nonunion due to delayed diagnosis, displacement, and associated carpal injuries (Fig. 15.5B).
- Forty percent cases are undiagnosed in the initial stages of fracture.
- Incidence of avascular necrosis is as high as 40% (Fig. 15.4).

Quick Facts: Scaphoid Fracture
- Accounts for 70 percent of carpal injuries.
- High incidence of AVN.
- Fracture may not be seen on initial radiograph.
- Treat according to symptoms and repeat radiograph at 10 to 14 days.
- If still painful and if still suspicious, cast it.
- If undisplaced, cast it including the thumb.
- If displaced, cast after manipulation.
- Open reduction if gap is more than 2 mm or if a step remains after reduction, if union is slow or if AVN develops open reduction, internal fixation and bone grafting is done.

What is New?
Percutaneous cannulated screw fixation for undisplaced fracture scaphoid bone is found to result in faster radiographic union than the conventional plaster cast immobilization.

INJURIES OF THE CARPOMETACARPAL JOINTS OF THE THUMB

Carpometacarpal joints act as a link between the wrist and hand. The joints of the index and middle fingers are stable while that of the thumb and the little fingers are more mobile. Thumb carpometacarpal dislocations are more common and are dealt here. The two important dislocations are Bennett's fracture dislocation and Rolando fracture dislocation.

BENNETT'S FRACTURE

Bennett's fracture is a fracture dislocation of the palmar base of the first metacarpal bone of the thumb with either subluxation or dislocation of the first carpometacarpal joint. Edward Bennett described it in 1882. It is an intra-articular fracture.

Mechanism of Injury

The common mechanism of injury is an axial blow directed against the partially flexed metacarpal, in most cases during "fist fights."

Characteristics of this Fracture

- Fracture line separates major part of the metacarpal from a small volar lip fragment producing disruption of the carpometacarpal joint.
- It is an avulsion rather than a pure dislocation. It occurs because of strong anterior oblique ligament.

Flowchart 15.1: Depicting the treatment plan in scaphoid fracture

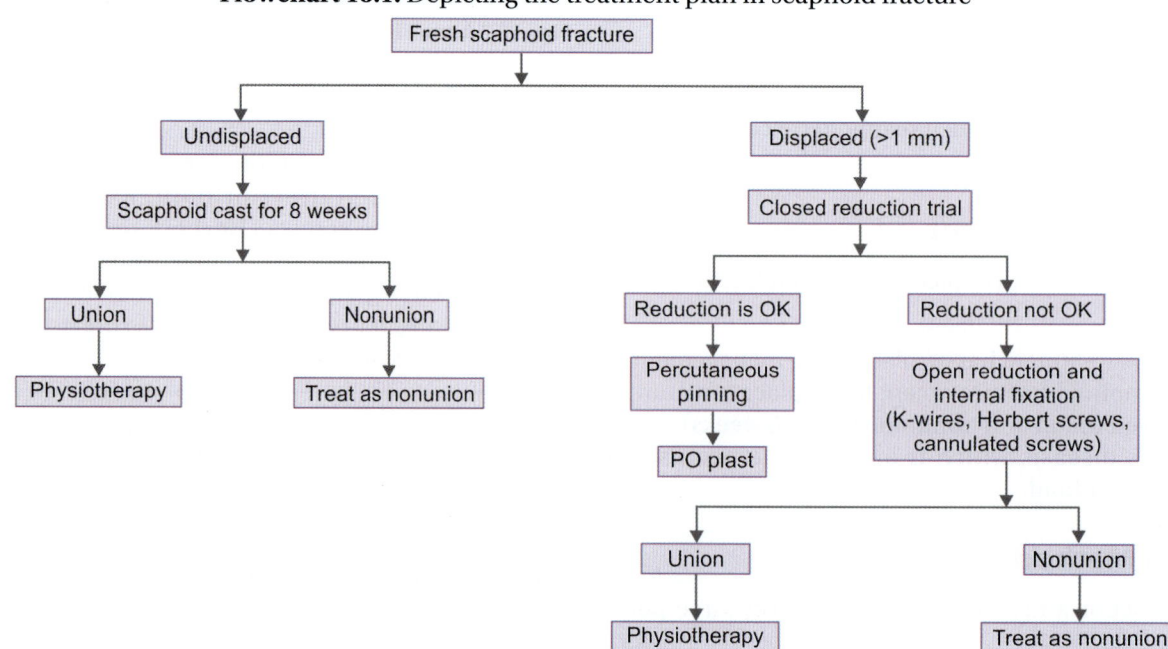

- Size of the volar lip fragment and amount of shaft displacement vary.

Displacing Forces in the Bennett's Fracture
- At the distal fragment, it is the adductor pollicis.
- At the proximal fragment, it is the abductor pollicis longus muscle.

Base of the thumb metacarpal is pulled dorsally and medially by the abductor pollicis longus (Fig. 15.6), while the distal attachment of adductor further levers the base into abduction.

Clinical Features
The patient complains of pain, swelling, and tenderness over the base of the thumb. Movements of the thumb are severely restricted.

Investigations
Radiograph: Plain X-rays help to make the diagnosis accurately (Fig. 15.7).

CT scan: It helps to delineate the fracture pattern better.

Treatment
A single attempt at closed reduction is tried first and a percutaneous fixation with K-wire is usually performed. If it fails, ORIF with K-wire or a small screw is carried out (Fig. 15.8).

ROLANDO'S FRACTURE
Rolando's fractures are comminuted intra-articular fractures of the base of the thumb. Presentation and management are similar to Bennett's fracture.

Clinical Features
Pain, swelling, tenderness over the dorsum of the thumb and loss of the thumb functions are the usual complaints.

Radiograph
Plain X-ray of the thumb AP, lateral and oblique views help to make the diagnosis (Fig. 15.9).

Treatment Methods

Nonoperative Methods
This is indicated in undisplaced fractures and in extra-articular fractures with less than 20° angulation. Closed reduction and external splinting with a thumb spica is the treatment method of choice.

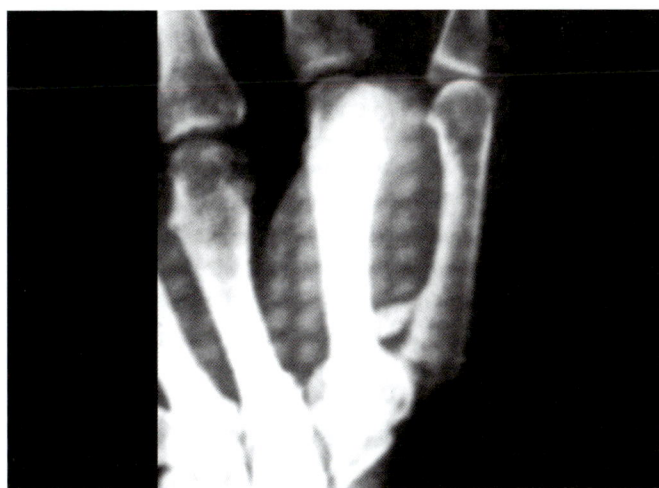

Fig. 15.7: Radiograph showing Bennett's fracture

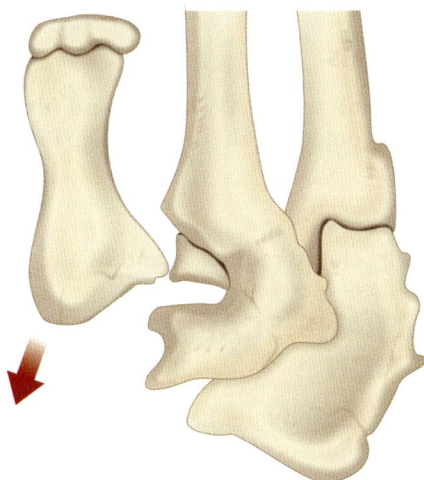

Fig. 15.6: Bennett's fracture. Thick arrow indicates the line of pull of abductor pollicis longus

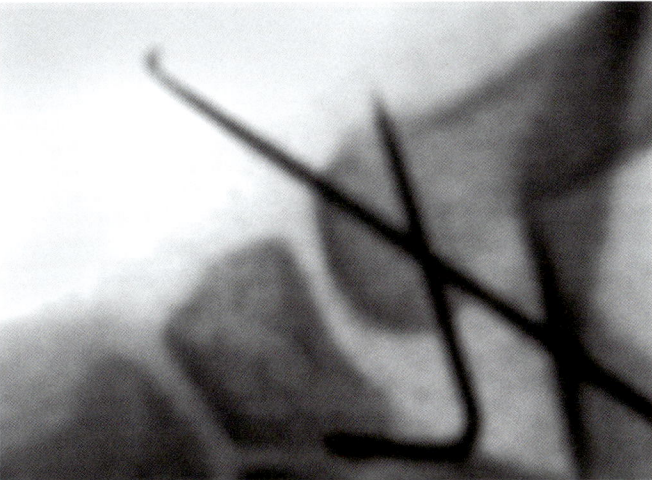

Fig. 15.8: Showing percutaneous K-wire fixation of Bennett's fracture

Closed Reduction and Internal Fixation

This is indicated in:
- Bennett's fracture
- Rolando's fracture
- Oblique extra-articular fracture.

Open Reduction and Internal Fixation

This is indicated in uncomminuted Rolando's fracture and irreducible Bennett's fracture.

External Fixations

This is indicated in highly comminuted Rolando's fracture where internal fixation is contraindicated.

RADIOCARPAL INJURIES

ANTERIOR DISLOCATION OF LUNATE

It is a common carpal dislocation and can lead to severe disability of the wrist function.

Mechanism of Injury

This is due usually due to fall on the outstretched hands. It can cause late carpal instability and arthritis. Hence, prompt and correct treatment is mandatory.

Clinical Features

Patient presents with pain, swelling, tenderness, and loss of wrist movements.

Radiograph

In radiograph of the lateral view, normally lunate forms a half-moon shape, which is lost in this dislocation. Moreover, in the anteroposterior view the normal rectangular profile is lost.

Treatment

Problems
- This may cause compression of the median nerve
- If left untreated it may cause permanent palsy, hence, reduction should be carried out as an emergency procedure.

Methods
- If seen early, reduction is easy and immobilization for 3 weeks with wrist in slight flexion usually gives good results.
- If seen after 3 weeks, open reduction is done.
- If lunate cannot be reduced by open reduction, resection of the proximal carpal bones or arthrodesis of the wrist may be necessary.

RADIOCARPAL DISLOCATION

VOLAR TRANS-SCAPHOID PERILUNAR DISLOCATION

This is a rare injury and is due to fall on dorsum of the flexed wrist.

Mechanism

Mechanism of injury is opposite to the dorsal perilunar dislocation.

Clinical Features

Pain in the wrist, swelling, and loss of wrist function are some of the complaints.

Investigations

Plain X-ray of the wrist (AP, lateral and oblique views) usually helps in detecting this injury (Figs 15.10A and B).

Treatment

Treatment is by closed reduction and casting.

DORSAL TRANS-SCAPHOID PERILUNAR DISLOCATION

It is usually diagnosed late. Early closed reduction is the best treatment. When accurate reduction of the scaphoid is not obtained, open reduction and bone grafting or internal fixation is indicated.

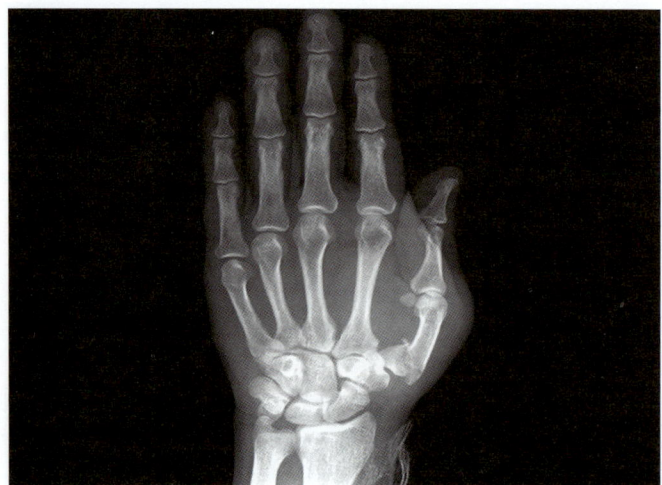

Fig. 15.9: Plain X-ray showing Rolando's fracture

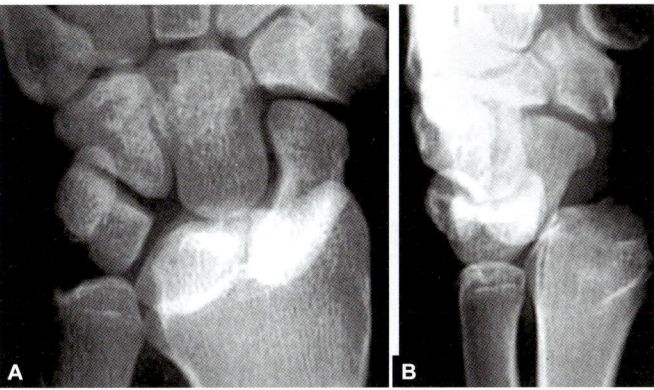

Figs 15.10A and B: (A) Radiocarpal dislocation: AP view; (B) Radiocarpal dislocation: Lateral view

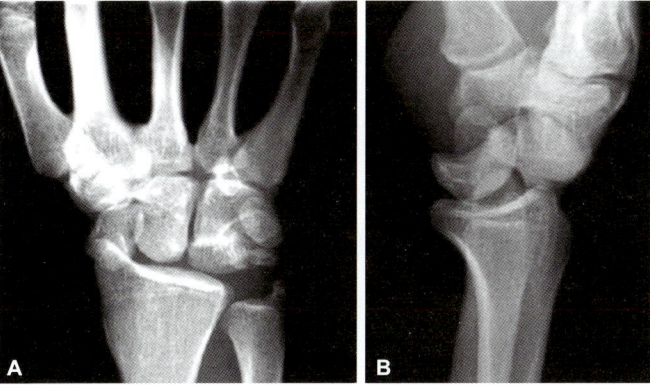

Figs 15.11A and B: Perilunar dislocation: (A) AP view; (B) Lateral view

Clinical Features

Patients may present with pain in the wrist, swelling, deformity, and loss of wrist function.

Investigations

Plain X-ray of the wrist (AP, lateral and oblique views) usually helps in detecting this injury (Figs 15.11A and B).

Treatment

The following are some of the important principles in treating this injury:
- Less than 3 weeks closed reduction can be tried
- More than 3 weeks OR + IF by K-wires
- More than 2 month's arthrodesis or resection of the proximal carpal row is carried out.

LUNATE FRACTURES

These are relatively rare and are due to hyperextension injury of the wrist or may be due to multiple repetitive traumas.

Clinical Presentation

Patients may present with pain, swelling, and tenderness over the dorsum of the wrist, restricted wrist movements, decreased handgrip, and boggy swelling due to synovitis in the late stages.

Investigations

Plain X-rays are inconclusive (Fig. 15.12). MRI is a better option.

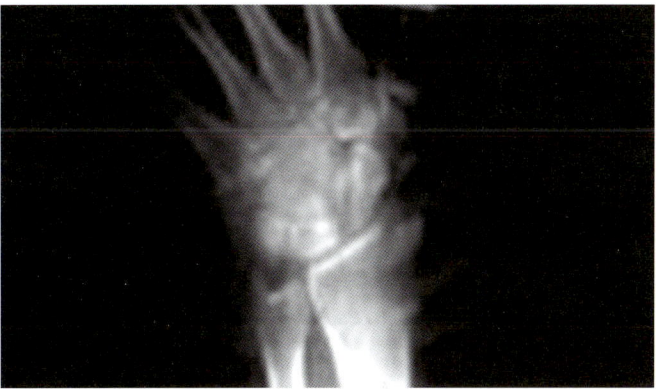

Fig. 15.12: Lunate burst fracture

Treatment

This is essentially conservative and consists of application of a below elbow plaster cast.

Complications

Avascular necrosis of lunate, called the Keinbock's disease is known to occur.

TRIQUETRAL FRACTURES

This is the fourth most common carpal bone fractures (after scaphoid, capitate and lunate). Destot first described it in 1926.

Mechanism of Injury

- Direct blow
- Fall on an outstretched hand
- Avulsion or chip fractures.

Types

These are divided into two types:
- Body fractures
- Peripheral chip or avulsion fractures.

Clinical Features

Pain in the wrist, swelling, and loss of wrist function are some of the complaints.

Investigations

Plain X-ray of the wrist (AP, lateral or oblique views) may reveal the fracture. If still in doubt, CT scan is recommended.

Treatment

Body Fractures

- If undisplaced, it is treated by short arm cast for 4 to 6 weeks.
- If displaced (>1–2 mm), surgery is the treatment of choice namely,
  - Arthroscopic approach and percutaneous pinning
  - Open reduction and internal fixation through K-wires or screws.

Chip or Avulsion Fractures

Symptomatic treatment by orthotics in most of the cases helps and rarely excision may be required in intractable cases.

PISIFORM FRACTURES

There are very rare and account for only 1 to 3 percent of all carpal bone fractures. This fracture is compared to patella fractures.

Mechanism of Injury

- Due to a direct blow resulting is comminuted fractures.
- Due to an indirect force following an avulsion or pull of the flexor carpi ulnaris tendon. This results in transverse fractures.

Clinical Features

Pain in the wrist, swelling, and loss of wrist function are some of the complaints.

Investigations

Pisiform fractures are difficult to visualize on plain X-rays. CT scan is more desirable (Fig. 15.13).

Treatment

Undisplaced fractures are treated by short arm cast for 4 to 6 weeks. Displaced fractures are treated by excision. Open reduction and internal fixation is rarely done in these fractures.

HAMATE FRACTURES

This accounts for 2 to 4 percent of all carpal fractures.

Mechanism of Injury

It could be due to a direct blow or indirect force while trying to grip an object.

Types

Hamate fractures could be either:
- Body fractures
- Hook fractures.

Clinical Features

Pain in the medial side of the palm and comes on with grip is quite typical of hamate fractures. Few patients may present with ulnar nerve (distal) paresthesia or palsy. Ruptures of the ring and little fingers are seen in some severe cases.

Investigations

Plain X-ray of the wrist (AP, lateral and oblique views) usually helps in detecting the fracture. CT scan helps in doubtful cases.

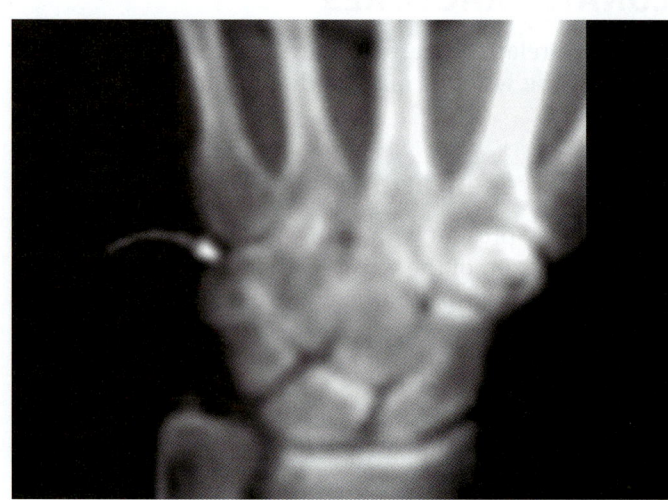

Fig. 15.13: Pisiform bone fracture

Treatment
- Acute fractures are treated by immobilization with short arm cast for 6 to 10 weeks.
- Nonunion of the hook are usually treated by excision.

CAPITATE FRACTURES

These are rare injuries and account for 1 to 2 percent of all carpal fractures. It is often associated with carpal-metacarpal dislocations.

Mechanism of Injury

Isolated capitate fractures are rare and are known to occur due to an axial loading injury to the middle finger to which the capitate is attached below. Direct blow is the other mechanism of injury.

Types

Three types are described:
- Isolated capitate fracture—is rare
- Associated with carpal-metacarpal dislocation
- Scaphocapitate syndrome: This is more common
  This consists of fracture of the waist of the scaphoid and a proximal capitate fracture.

Clinical Features

Pain, swelling and restricted wrist movements are seen.

Investigation

Plain X-ray of the wrist can diagnose capitate fractures. In difficult cases, CT scan is advised.

Treatment

Conservative

Undisplaced fractures are treated by a below elbow cast for 4 to 6 weeks.

Surgery: Displaced fractures and scaphocapitate syndrome are treated by open reduction and rigid internal fixation.

TRAPEZOID FRACTURE

These are very uncommon fractures. Dislocations are more common than isolated fractures.

Mechanism of Injury

- Direct blow
- Axial loading injury to the index metacarpal.

Clinical Features

Pain, swelling, tenderness over the wrist and painful resisted flexion are the usual complaints.

Investigations

Plain X-rays of the wrist are not reliable. CT scan is a better option.

Treatment

- Undisplaced fractures are treated by below elbow cast for 4 to 6 weeks.
- In displaced fractures (>1 mm or diastases >2 mm) open reduction and rigid internal fixation is advised.

TRAPEZIUM FRACTURE

This accounts for 1 to 5% of wrist fractures. It could be isolated fracture or dislocations.

Mechanism of Injury

- Fall on an outstretched hand
- Direct blow over the dorsum of the hand.

Classifications

Trapezium fractures are divided into:
- Body fractures
- Ridge fractures (Palmar)
  - *Type I:* Fracture base of the trapezoid ridge
  - *Type II:* Fracture of the tip of the trapezial ridge.
- *Dislocations:* This could be dorsal, palmar, or radial and may be associated with fracture of the scaphoid and trapezium.

Clinical Features

The patient complains of pain, swelling, and tenderness over the wrist. Resisted flexion produces pain.

Investigations

Plain X-rays though useful are not reliable. CT scan is a better option.

Treatment

- *Undisplaced fracture:* Thumb spica for 4 to 6 weeks.
- *Displaced fracture (>1 mm or >2 mm diastasis):* Open reduction and rigid internal fixation is advised.
- Dislocation is treated by open reduction and K-wire fixation.

16 CHAPTER

Hand Injuries

GENERAL PRINCIPLES

Incidence

Hand fractures account for 17.5% of all fractures.
- *Among the hand fractures:*
  - Phalangeal fractures— 46%
  - Metacarpal fractures—36%
  - V metacarpal bone neck fracture—9.7%
- *Among the phalangeal fractures*
  - Proximal phalanx—57.4%
  - Middle phalanx—30.4%
- Single fracture seen in 98.6% of cases
  Multiple fractures—1.4%
- Male: Female = (1.8 : 1)
- *Mode of injury:*
  - Sports injuries in 3rd decade
  - Workplace injuries in the 5th decade.

Treatment

This includes injuries to the phalanges, metacarpals and carpal bones. The following principles should be followed in treating hand fractures:
- All stable fractures need closed reduction and splinting.
- Burkhalter splint is used universally to immobilize the finger fractures.
- K-wire is the commonly used internal fixation device.
- While using the K-wire, injury to the tendons, ligaments and extension into the joints should be avoided.
- Rotational malalignment of the fingers (Fig. 16.1) should be avoided and this can be done by looking at the alignment of the fingers when the fingers are flexed at metacarpophalangeal and interphalangeal joints. The fingers should point towards the scaphoid bone.
- The safe position for hand immobilization is 70° flexion at MCP joint 15 to 20° flexion at PIP joint, and 5 to 10° flexion at DIP joint. This is called the intrinsic plus position or the James position (Fig. 16.2).

Indications for Open Reduction in Hand Injuries

- Intra-articular fractures with a small fragment
- Severely displaced fractures
- Highly unstable fractures
- Multiple fractures
- Soft tissue (e.g. tendon) interposition.

After open reduction, internal fixation is usually done by K-wires (Figs 16.3A and B). Intraosseous tension band cerclage wiring, intramedullary fixation, small AO plate and screws are the other but less commonly used fixation methods.

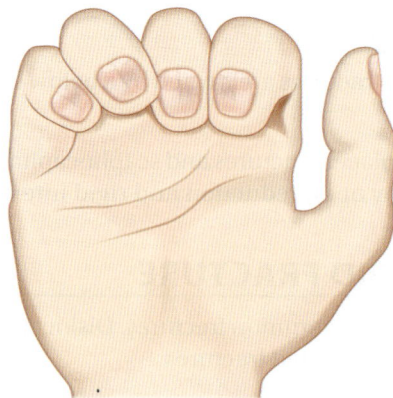

Fig. 16.1: Assessment of rotational malalignment of fingers

CHAPTER 16: Hand Injuries

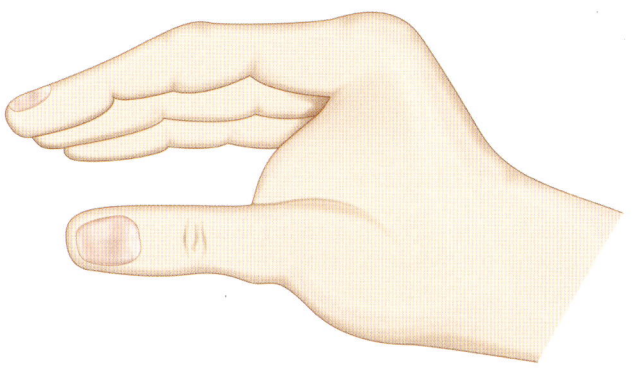

Fig. 16.2: Functional position of the hand (James position)

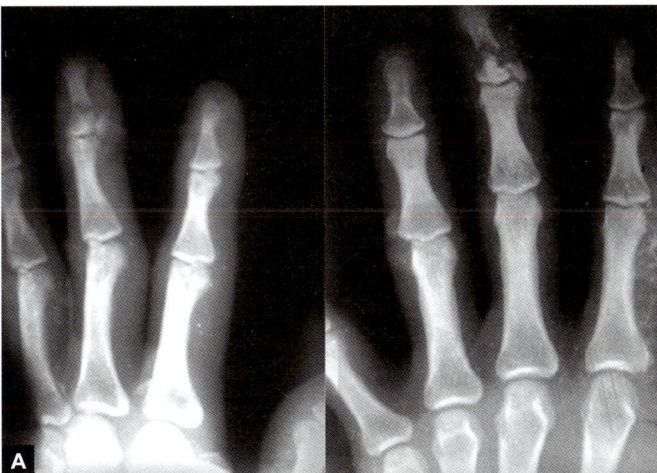

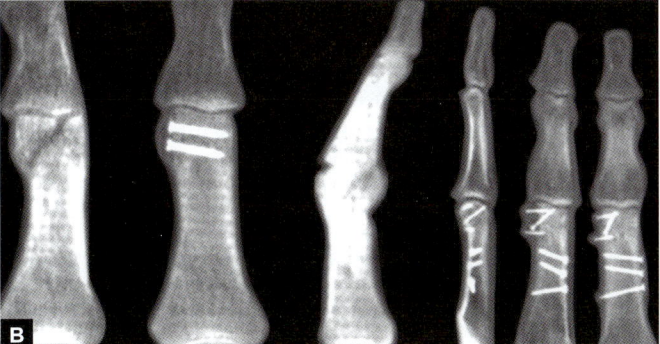

Figs 16.3A and B: Radiograph showing distal phalanx fracture

Steps of Application of the Universal Hand Splint—the Burkhalter Splint

- Fracture reduction of the fingers are done and checked for stability.
- Now the hand and forearm are padded.
- First a volar slab is applied up to the level of the proximal palmar crease with the wrist in extension.
- A second dorsal slab is applied up to the level of the proximal IP joint level with the MP joint in maximum flexion
- This splint neutralizes the intrinsics
- Duration of immobilization: 3 to 4 weeks
- Active movements of the IP joints should be encouraged.

INJURIES TO THE PHALANX

DISTAL PHALANX FRACTURES

These fractures are usually caused by crushing injuries they are frequently comminuted (Fig. 16.3A).

Salient Features

- Very commonly injured
- Soft tissue coverage is less
- In nail bed injuries, hematoma can be seen through the nail bed.

Mechanism of Injury

It is mainly due to direct crush injuries. Indirect forces may result in avulsion injuries.

Classifications

Distal phalangeal fractures are classified into:
- Longitudinal (36%)
- Transverse
- Tuft (63%)
- Basal fractures (18%)
  - Dorsal
  - Volar
- Intra-articular complete fractures.

> **Do You Know the Difference Between Dorsal Base and Mallet Fracture?**
> - *Mallet fingers:* <25% involvement of articular cartilage and hence stable.
> - *Dorsal basal fractures:* > 25% involvement of articular cartilage and hence unstable.

Clinical Features

Pain, swelling, tenderness and deformity of the tip of the finger. Loss of function of the distal IP joints is seen.

Radiograph

Plain X-ray of the finger AP, lateral and oblique views help to make the diagnosis (Fig. 16.3A).

Treatment

Three modalities of treatment are described namely:

Conservative Method: This is reserved mainly for undisplaced, longitudinal and tuft fractures. The method employed is splinting for 3 to 4 weeks (Fig. 16.4).

Closed Reduction and Percutaneous Fixation:

This is reserved for:
- Transverse shaft fractures where external splinting fails to hold the fragments.
- Dorsal base fractures with >25% involvement of articular surfaces. Here the K-wire pinning should be done across the DIP joint (Fig. 16.3B).

Open Reduction and Internal Fixation:

This is indicated in:
- Volar base fractures with disruption of the flexor digitorum profundus (FDP) insertion.
- Dorsal base fractures with 30 to 40% involvement of the articular surface.

MALLET FINGER (Syn: Baseball Finger, Drop Finger, Cricket Finger)

Mallet finger is a common injury usually due to forced flexion of the distal phalanx while the extensor tendons are actively trying to extend the finger. The baseball catcher, football receiver and others are vulnerable to this injury. Depending upon whether the thin extensor tendon is torn in its substance or pulls off a small piece of bone at its insertion, two types are recognized:
- Mallet finger of tendon origin
- Mallet finger of bony origin.

Tendon Origin

This is due to loss of extensor tendon continuity at the distal finger joint.

Mechanism of Injury

Here the end of the finger is forcibly flexed, when extensor tendon is taut, e.g. while tucking the bed, catching a ball, striking an object with extended finger, etc. (Figs 16.5A and B).

Clinical Features

Pain, swelling, tenderness, flexion deformity of the tip of the finger and inability of the patient to actively extend the finger at the distal PIP joint (Fig. 16.6).

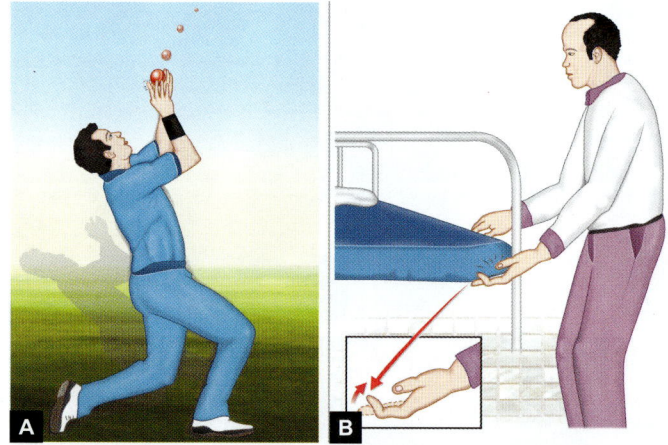

Figs 16.5A and B: Common mechanism of injury pertaining to mallet finger

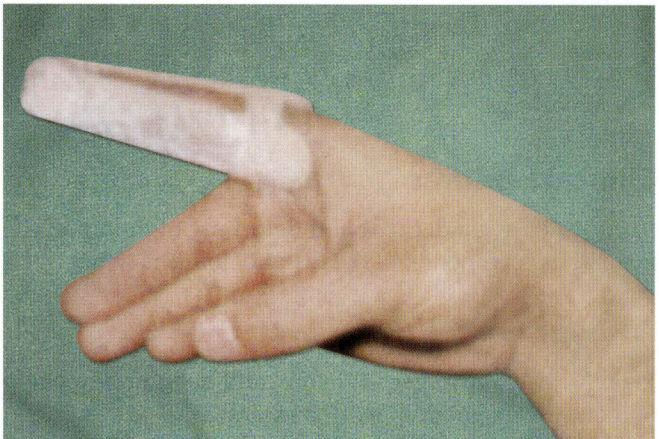

Fig. 16.4: Finger cot splint

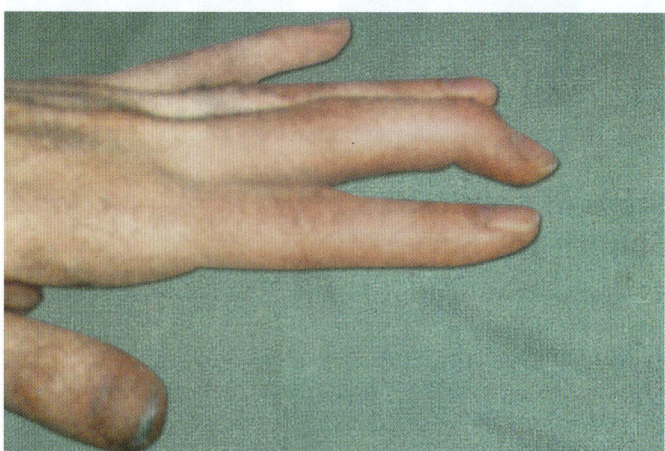

Fig. 16.6: Mallet finger (Clinical photo)

Several Types

The following deformities could be seen based on the types of injuries.
- *Extensor tendon stretched* in this, degree of drop is less. There is loss of 5 to 20° of extension. There is weak active extension.
- *Extensor tendon ruptured* from its insertion into distal phalanx. There is 40 to 45° loss of extension. No active extension.
- *Avulsion fracture.* A small fragment of distal phalanx is avulsed with the extensor tendon. There is no active extension and it should be treated as tendon injuries rather than fractures.

If the flexion deformity is severe, a secondary hyperextension deformity of PIP joint occurs, because of imbalance of the extensor mechanism.

Radiographs

X-ray of the affected finger may show an avulsion fracture of the dorsal lip of the base of the distal phalanx (Fig. 16.7).

Treatment

Nonoperative measures: This is reserved for pure dislocations, collateral ligament injuries and mallet finger. Various custom-made dorsal hyperextension splints (Mallet splints) are used for immobilizing the DIP joints.

Closed reduction and percutaneous fixation: This is reserved for mallet injuries in professionals like dentists, surgeons, sportspersons, etc. who cannot keep their fingers immobilized for long due to professional commitments.

Open reduction and internal fixation: This is indicated in the following situations:
- Avulsion of the profundus tendon and its reinsertion.
- Chronic subluxation of the DIP joint (> 3 weeks).
- Irreducible dislocations.

Mallet Finger of Bony Origin

This is less common. It is usually fixed with K-wire, if more than one-third of the dorsal articular surface is involved and if remainder of the distal phalanx is subluxated volar-wards.

> **Facts about Mallet Splints**
>
> In these cases, proximal interphalangeal joint of the finger is not immobilized but only the distal joint is immobilized by using:
> a. Simple volar unpadded aluminum splint, which provides three-point pressure.
> b. Dorsal padded aluminum splint.
> c. A stack plastic mallet finger splint (Figs 16.8A and B)
>   Distal joint is put in slight hyperextension. The splint may cause pain and the amount of hyperextension should not cause blanching of the skin over DIP joint.
>   Splints are useful in cooperative patients, and in uncooperative patients. Smellie's cast is used. About 6 to 10 weeks of continuous immobilization is required. K-wire fixation is considered in patients like dentist or surgeon who wants to return to work quickly.

> **Lesser-Known but Important Thumb Injuries**
> - *Bowler's Thumb:* It is a traumatic neuropathy of the digital nerve of the thumb due to repeated friction from gripping a ball.
> - *Game Keeper's or Baseball Thumb:* This has been explained earlier.

DISTAL INTERPHALANGEAL JOINT INJURIES

These injuries are usually due to ball catching sports.

Salient Features

- Pure dislocations without tendon ruptures are rare.

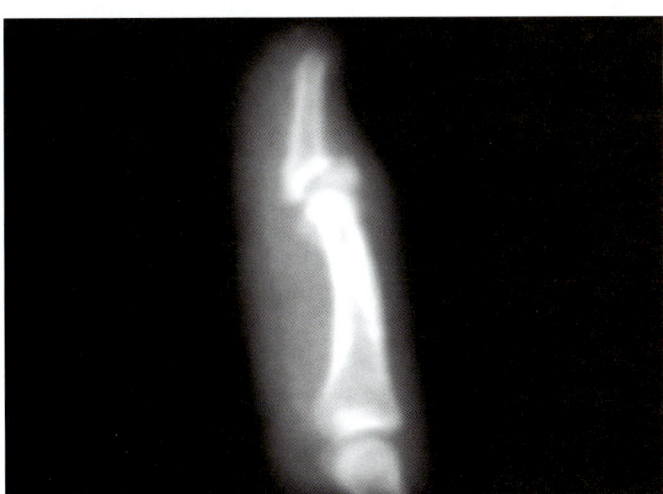

Fig. 16.7: Radiograph showing mallet fracture (Avulsion type)

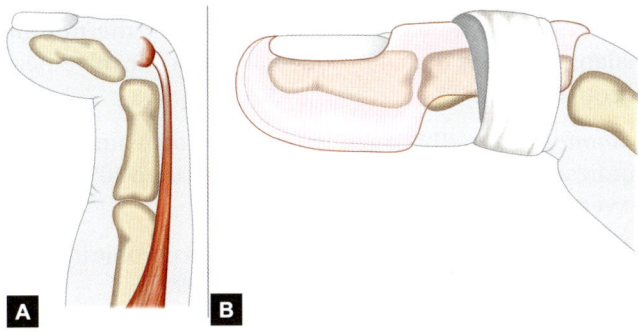

Figs 16.8A and B: (A) Mallet finger; (B) Treatment by a dorsal splint

- Most of the times DIP joint dislocations are missed initially.
- Dislocation is mainly dorsal
- Isolated injury to the collateral ligament and volar plate are rare.

Jersey finger: It is due to avulsion of flexor digitorum profundus from its insertion on distal phalanx. This is the opposite of 'mallet finger' and the patient is unable to flex the distal interphalangeal joint. It is seen in football and rugby players.

FRACTURES OF THE MIDDLE PHALANX

The three important injuries of special interest relating to the middle phalanx are:
- Isolated fracture of the volar base
- Isolated fracture of the dorsal base
- Pilon fractures. This consists of extensive metaphyseal comminution with involvement of the entire articular surfaces and bone loss.

All these injuries can pose problems in the management.

Clinical Features

Pain, swelling, tenderness, deformity of the finger and loss of finger functions are the usual complaints.

Radiographs

Plain X-ray of the finger AP, lateral and oblique views help to make the diagnosis.

Management

Volar Base Fractures

Nonoperative treatment: This consists of extension block splinting of the PIP joint and is indicated in volar base fractures with less than 40% involvement of the articular surface.

Closed reduction and internal fixation: This is indicated for both dorsal and volar base fractures of the middle phalanx with less than 40% articular surface involvement (Figs 16.9A to C).

Dynamic traction: This is a unique method of treatment and is indicated in volar base fractures of more than 40% and in the very difficult Pilon fractures.

Volar plate arthroplasty: This is indicated in chronic injuries and in volar base fractures greater than 40%.

Open reduction and internal fixations: This is indicated in single large fragment and in fixing bone graft to the metaphysis.

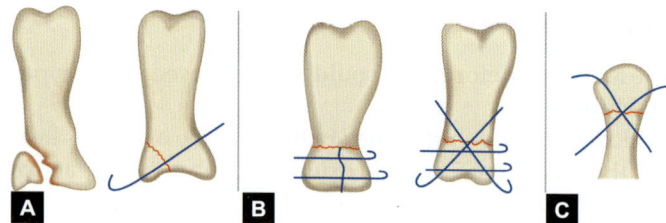

Figs 16.9A to C: Closed reduction and percutaneous fixation of various phalangeal fractures: (A) Unstable short oblique fractures; (B) Comminuted fracture; (C) Condylar fracture

For dorsal base fractures, extension block pinning after closed reduction is the treatment of choice.

DISLOCATIONS OF THE IP JOINT

This could involve the proximal or distal interphalangeal joints.

Salient Features

- These are frequently missed
- Common in ball catching sports
- There is complete disruption of the collateral ligaments and the volar plate
- About 50% cases occur in the middle finger followed by the ring finger
- It is accompanied by gross swelling at the PIP joint.

Clinical Tests

Localized tenderness can be elicited by careful palpation of the PIP joint.

To test the integrity of the central slip: Instruct the patient to actively extend the PIP joint with the MP joint held in hyperextended position.

Tests to identify the development of Boutonnière deformity: Inability to passively flex the DIP joint while the PIP joint is held in extension heralds the onset of the Boutonnière deformity.

Stress tests: Lateral stress testing is performed with the fingers in complete extension and 30° of flexion. Greater than 20° of opening indicates complete tear of collateral ligaments.

Types

- Dorsal dislocation (most common)
- Pure volar dislocation
- Rotatory volar dislocation
- Complete collateral ligament disruption.

Clinical Features

Pain, swelling, tenderness and deformity. Loss of function of the distal IP joints is seen (Fig. 16.10).

Radiographs

Plain X-ray of the finger AP, lateral and oblique views help to make the diagnosis (Figs 16.11A and B).

Treatment

Nonoperative Management

This is indicated for closed injuries and for reducible injuries. After reduction:
- Buddy taping with immediate AROM for rotatory volar dislocation (Fig. 16.12).
- For collateral ligament injuries buddy taping with immediate AROM.
- For central slip disruption and volar dislocation, 4 to 6 weeks of PIP extension, splinting followed by a 2-week daytime dynamic splinting and a static night splinting. Throughout the period of splintage, DIP joint should be actively exercised (Fig. 16.13).
- Extension blocks splinting for 3 to 4 weeks for hyperextension injuries (dorsal dislocation).

Operative Management

Open reduction is indicated for open injuries, irreducible dislocations and injury to the collateral ligament of the index finger.

PROXIMAL PHALANX FRACTURES

These are due to direct blow on the dorsum of fingers.

Salient Features

- Due to the deforming forces of the intrinsic muscles, transverse and short oblique fractures of the proximal phalanx angulate dorsally.

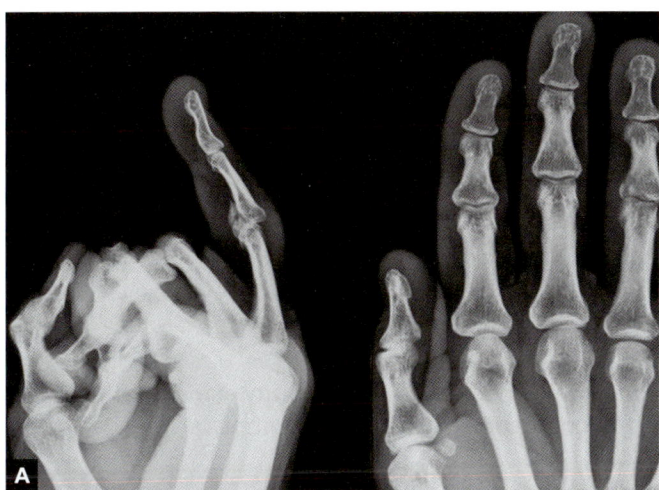
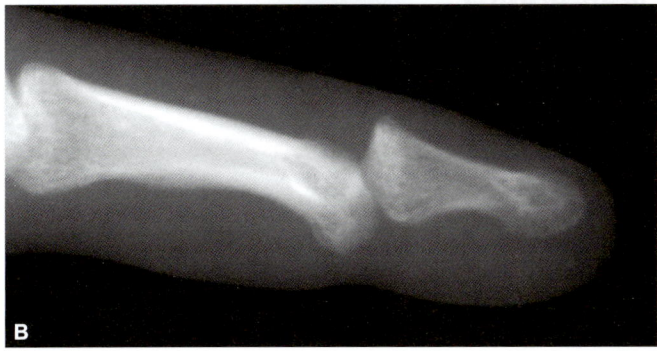

Figs 16.11A and B: (A) Plain X-ray showing proximal PIP joint injury; (B) Dislocation of the distal IP joint

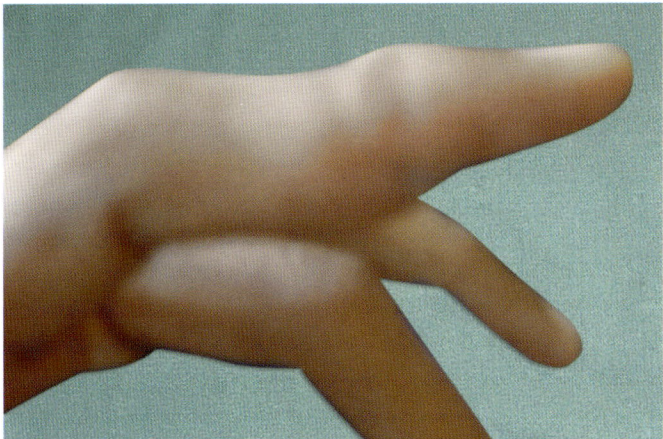

Fig. 16.10: Deformity as viewed from the sides (Clinical photo)

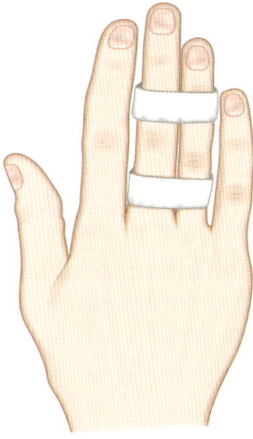

Fig. 16.12: Buddy taping

- The spiral and long oblique fractures shorten and rotate rather than angulate.
- Due to the action of FDS, fractures of the middle phalanx tend to angulate in either direction.

Classifications

- Head fractures—mainly intra-articular.
- Neck and shaft fractures—Extra-articular.
- Base—both extra-articular and intra-articular.

All these fractures could be:
- Minimally displaced but stable
- Reducible but stable
- Reducible but unstable
- Irreducible.

Clinical Features

Pain, swelling, tenderness, deformity of the finger and loss of finger functions are the usual complaints.

Radiographs

Plain X-ray of the finger AP, lateral and oblique views helps to make the diagnosis (Fig. 16.14).

Treatment Methods

Nonoperative Treatment

This is indicated for undisplaced and for reducible but stable extra-articular fractures. The methods employed are Buddy taping (Fig. 16.15) for undisplaced fractures and Burkhalter splint for the rest.

Closed Reduction and Percutaneous Fixation

This is reserved for transverse shaft fractures where external splinting fails to hold the fragments (Figs 16.16A and B).

Closed Reduction and Internal Fixation (IF)

This is indicated in the following situations:
- Oblique neck fracture.
- Reducible and stable intra-articular fracture of the middle phalanx.
- Reducible and unstable extra-articular fractures.

Open Reduction and Internal Fixation

This is indicated in:
- Open fractures
- Multiple fractures
- Soft tissue injury.
- Intra-articular proximal phalanx fractures.

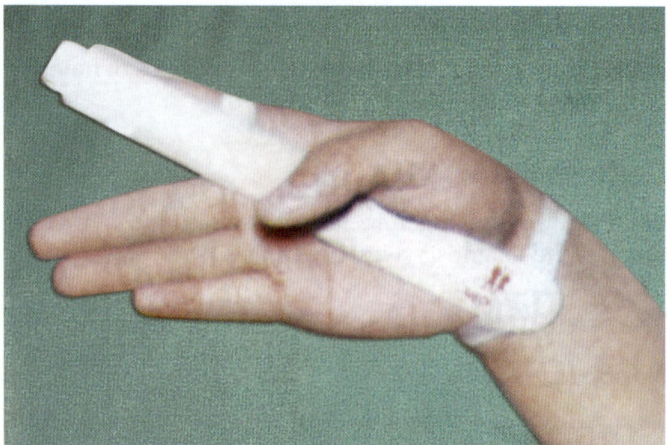

Fig. 16.13: Finger extension splint

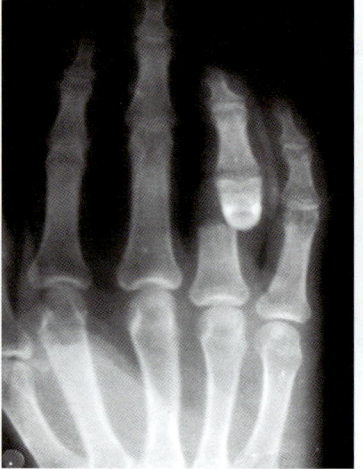
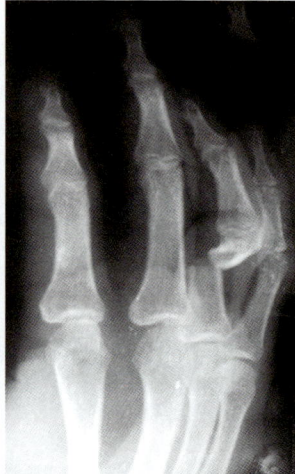

Fig. 16.14: Radiograph showing proximal phalanx fracture (Transverse)

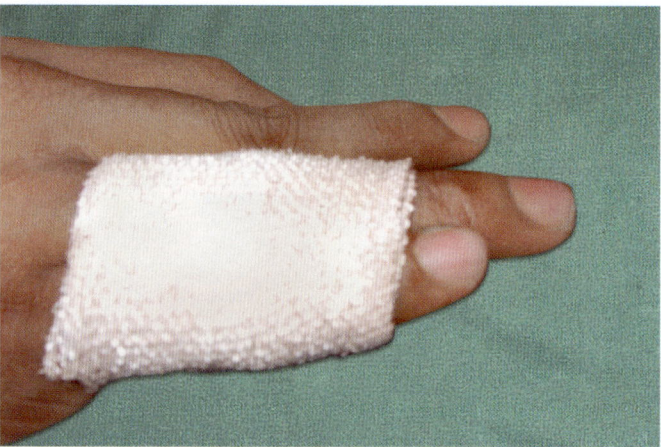

Fig. 16.15: Buddy taping

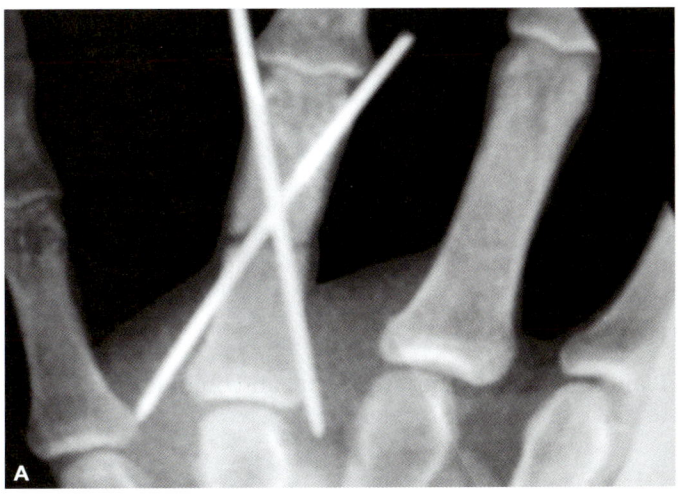
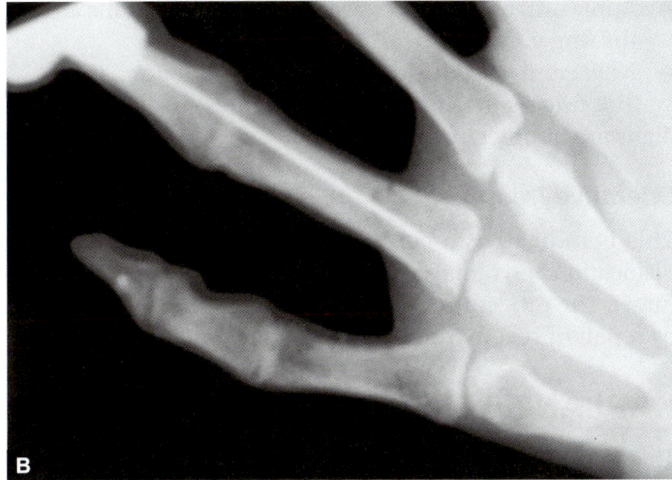

Figs 16.16A and B: (A) Radiograph showing proximal phalanx fracture fixed with criss cross K-wires; (B) Radiograph showing K-wire fixation

The options for internal fixation after open reduction are:
- Intraosseous wiring
- Composite wiring
- Screws only (Fig. 16.17)
- Plate and screw fixation.

The choice of the fixation depends on the experience and familiarity of the technique by the operating surgeon.

Complications of Phalangeal Fractures

Phalangeal fractures are very notorious to develop complications as the PIP joint is very less tolerant joint of the hand:
- Malunion
- Nonunion
- Stiffness
- Extension lags.

METACARPOPHALANGEAL JOINT DISLOCATIONS

Salient Features

- Dorsal dislocations are more common than volar.
- Small finger collateral ligament injuries are more common followed by the index finger.
- Dorsal dislocations are present with hyperextension deformity and are easy to reduce.
- During the dislocations, the volar plate does not get disturbed.
- Irreducible dislocations are called complex dislocations and are due to the volar plate entrapment. This is more common in index finger. Pathognomonic sign is

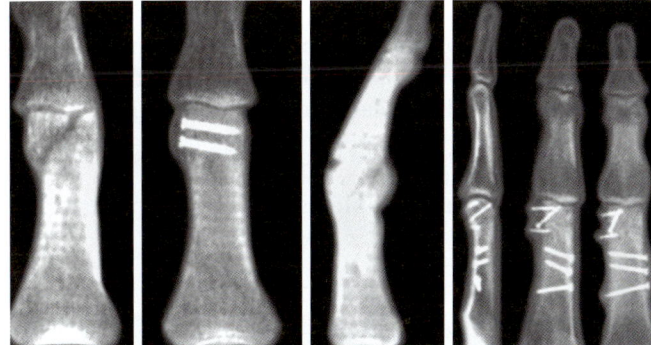

Fig. 16.17: Screw fixation of phalangeal fracture

the presence of sesamoid bones within the joint and puckering of the volar skin.
- Volar dislocations are very unstable but fortunately rare.

Clinical Features

Pain, swelling, tenderness over the MCP joint and loss of the affected finger and hand functions are the usual complaints.

Radiographs

Plain X-ray of the hand AP, lateral and oblique views help to make the diagnosis (Fig. 16.18).

Treatment

Nonoperative Treatment

This is indicated in simple dorsal dislocations and collateral ligament ruptures. Reduction methods include:
- Flex the wrist to relax the flexor tendons.

- Apply firm but not excessive longitudinal tractions along the finger.
- Now gently flex the joint to achieve reduction.

The fingers are immobilized in Jones position as the digits are buddy taped.

Operative Treatment

This is indicated in complex dorsal dislocations, volar dislocation and radial collateral ligament injury of the index finger. The procedure consists of open reduction followed by repair or reconstruction of the collateral ligaments.

KAPLAN'S LESION

This is a complex irreducible dorsal metacarpophalangeal (MCP) dislocation of fingers. Kaplan described buttonholing of the metacarpal head into the palm. Here there is an interposition of volar plate between the base of the proximal phalanx and the head of the metacarpal (Fig. 16.19).

Incidence: This is commonly seen in the index finger next is thumb, little finger. It is rarely seen in long and ring fingers. Two types of dorsal dislocation occur in MP joints:

Simple: This can be reduced by closed methods.

Complex: This is irreducible and usually requires open reduction.

Both results from hyperextension injuries and in both the volar plate are torn at its proximal insertion into the metacarpal neck.

Clinical Features

Pain, swelling, hyperextension deformity at the MCP joint, tenderness over the dorsum of the hand and loss of the hand functions are the usual complaints (Figs 16.20A and B).

Radiographs

Plain X-ray of the hand AP, lateral and oblique views helps to make the diagnosis (Fig. 16.20C).

Diagnostic Clues

There are three clinical and radiographic clues to diagnosis:
- The metacarpophalangeal joint is only slightly hyperextended, and the interphalangeal joint is flexed. In the radiographs, proximal phalanx and metacarpals are nearly parallel.
- A constant finding is puckering of the volar skin, which is more readily seen in thumb than index finger.

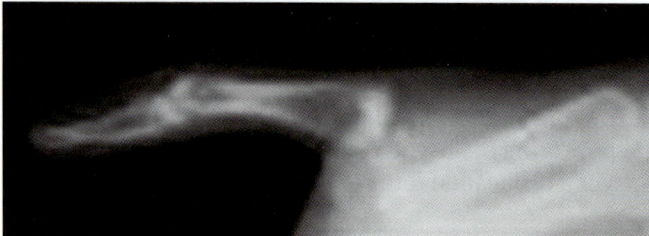

Fig. 16.18: Radiograph showing dislocation of 1st MCP joint

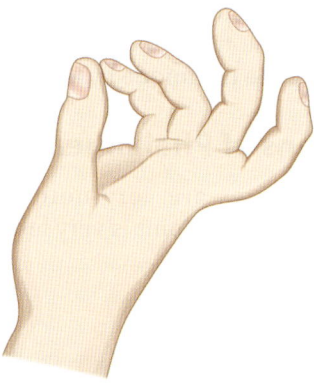

Fig. 16.19: Dislocation of II MP point (Kaplan's lesion)

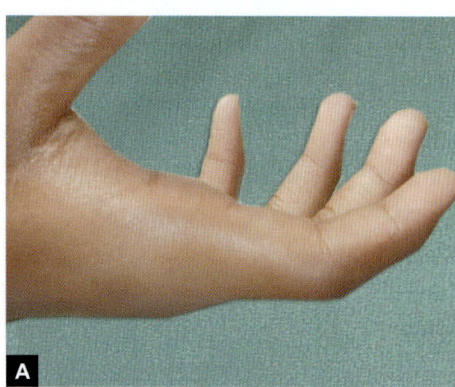
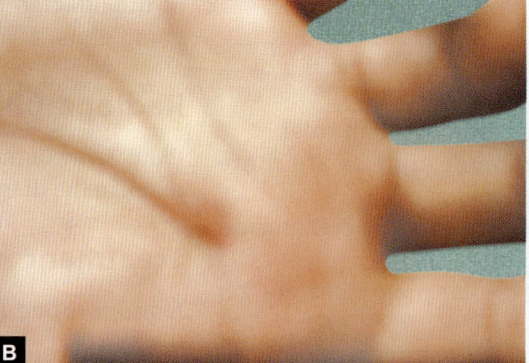
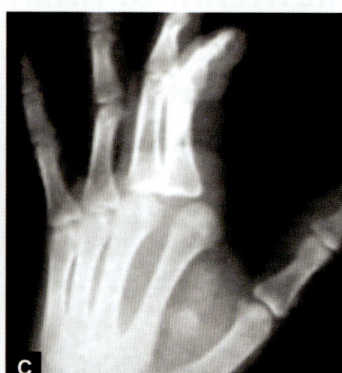

Figs 16.20A to C: (A) Kaplan's lesion (Clinical photo); (B) Volar view showing the puckered skin (Clinical photo); (C) Radiograph of Kaplan's lesion

- Pathognomonic radiographic sign is the presence of a sesamoid bone within a widened joint space. This is normally present with volar plate.

Treatment

A single attempt at closed reduction is made and if this fails, surgical reduction either by the volar (Kaplan's operation) approach or by the dorsal approach is done.

> **Note:**
> The single most important element preventing reduction in a complex metacarpophalangeal dislocation is interposition of volar plate within the joint.

DISLOCATION OF THE THUMB METACARPOPHALANGEAL JOINT (Syn: Gamekeeper's Thumb, Skier's Thumb)

Injury to the ulnar collateral ligament of the first metacarpophalangeal (MCP) joint is very common but a complete dislocation is rare. It heals with some residual instability (Fig. 16.21).

Diagnosis is made by direct palpation and stress tests. Treatment is by operative or nonoperative methods.

INJURIES TO METACARPAL BONES

Metacarpal shaft fracture the common causes for these injuries are direct hit on the dorsum of the hand as in assault, boxing, fall, road traffic accident (RTA), etc. These fractures should be accurately reduced with no rotational malalignment and immobilized with either plaster (common) or percutaneous or open K-wire fixation (less common).

METACARPAL FRACTURES (II TO V)

Salient Features

- The normal neck shaft angle in the metacarpal is 15°.
- A typical apex dorsal angulation is seen in transverse metacarpal neck and shaft fractures.
- This angulation is compensated clinically by a hyperextension deformity.
- Spiral and oblique fractures tend to shorten and rotate than angulate.
- Rotational malalignment is not acceptable more than 10°.
- Due to the overlapping bone shadows, special X-ray views, as the Brewerton view is required (Reverse oblique views and the Skyline views are other special views).
- Metacarpals are responsible for the formation of the following three arches of the hand:
  - Transverse arch at the carpometacarpal joints.
  - Transverse arch at the MP joints.
  - A longitudinal broad convex dorsal arch.

These arches are maintained by:
- The interosseous ligaments at the bases
- Deep transverse intermetacarpal ligaments distally:
  - Volar aspect of the neck of the metacarpal is the weakest point
  - Intrinsic muscles are the primary deforming forces, which can be neutralized by MP joint flexion
  - Reduction can be achieved by longitudinal traction and by flexion of the PIP joint.

Clinical Features

Pain, swelling, tenderness over the dorsum of the hand and loss of the hand functions are the usual complaints (Fig. 16.22).

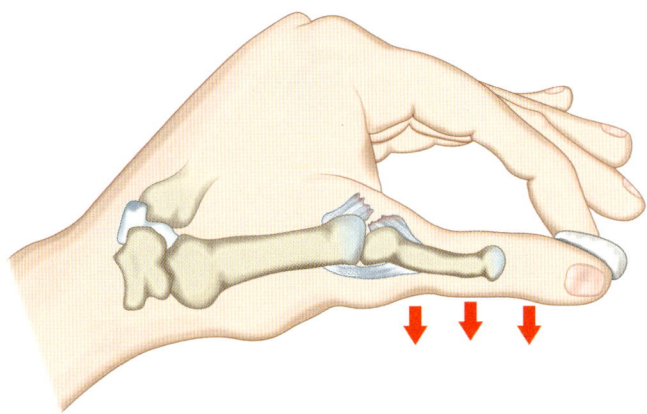

Fig. 16.21: Gamekeeper's thumb

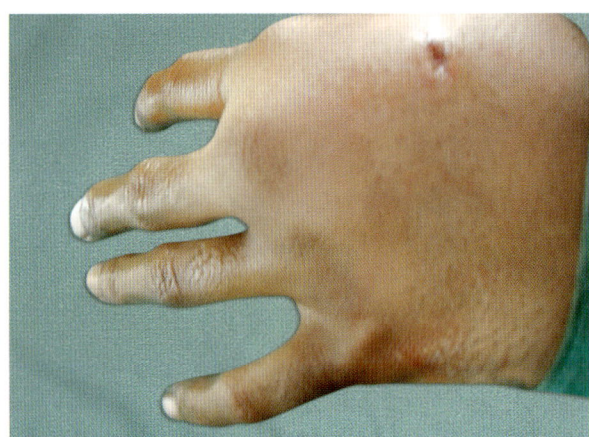

Fig. 16.22: Deformity and pin point compound (Clinical photo)

Radiographs

Plain X-ray of the hand AP, lateral and oblique views helps to make the diagnosis (Figs 16.23A and B).

Treatment Methods

Nonoperative Treatment: This is indicated in the following situations:
- Undisplaced fractures.
- Stable fractures (These have < 50% displacement, <40° angulation and fracture obliquity of <60°).

Methods: The hand can be immobilized by:
- Burk halter splint: This is ideal and is known to give good splints
- Compression glove for 2 weeks
- Hand-based cast is also effective and permits the patient to return to the work early.

Closed Reduction and Internal Fixation

This is indicated for fractures that are unstable after reduction and for base fractures. This is mainly used for extra-articular fractures but can also be used for intra-articular fractures that are stable with K-wire fixation alone after reduction (Fig. 16.24).

Open Reduction and Internal Fixation

This is indicated in the following:
- Multiple fractures
- Open fractures
- Irreducible fractures
- Displaced intra-articular fractures.

The choice of the method of internal fixation devices could be:
- Intramedullary fixation through a Steinmann's pin, multiple prebent K-wires, etc.
- Screws only
- Plate and screws
- Intraosseous wiring
- Composite wiring.

The choice of fixation should be the one with which the surgeon is most familiar with (Figs 16.25A to C).

External Fixations

This is reserved for comminuted intra-articular fractures of the base of the fifth metacarpal bone where internal fixation is not suitable.

Complications

- Nonunion
- Avascular necrosis in periarticular fractures.
- Angular malunion
- Rotational malunion
- Intra-articular malunion
- Stiffness of the fingers.

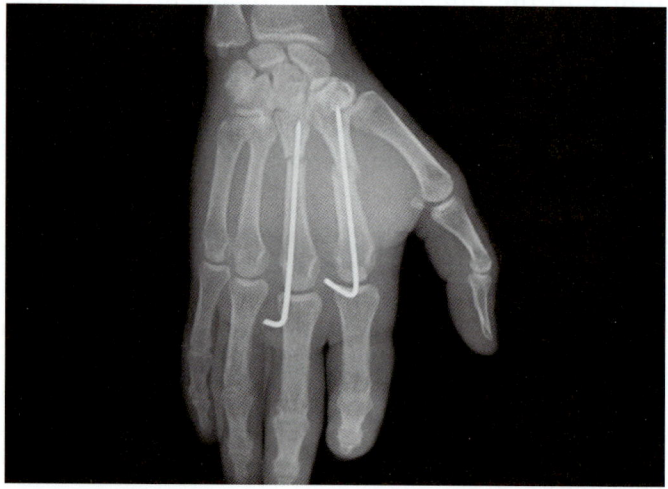

Fig. 16.24: K-wire fixation of metacarpal fracture

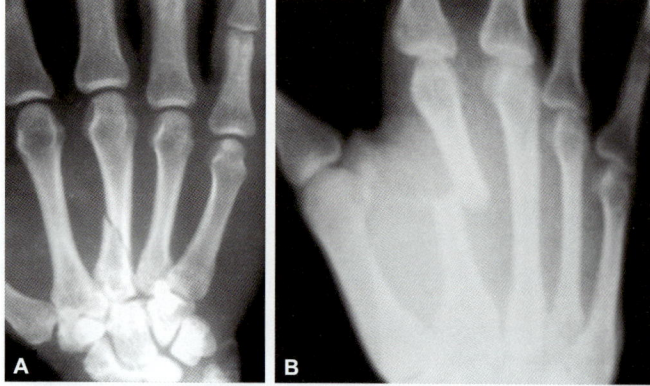

Figs 16.23A and B: (A) Radiograph showing oblique metacarpal fracture; (B) Radiograph showing transverse midshaft fracture

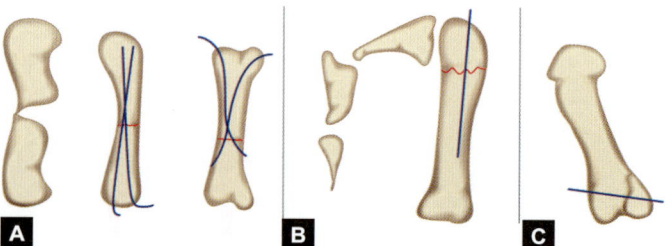

Figs 16.25A to C: Metacarpal fractures treated by closed reduction and percutaneous pinning: (A) Unstable fracture fixed with criss-cross K-wires; (B) Neck fracture fixed by intramedullary fixation; (C) Bennett's fracture fixed with K-wire

METACARPAL FRACTURE OF THE LITTLE FINGER (Boxer's Fracture)

When a boxer punches the jaw of his opponent with his fist and wins the bout, his ecstasy may be short-lived when he finds his little finger is broken, what he has actually broken is the neck of the fifth metacarpal bone and this is due to a direct impact on the dorsum of the hand (Fig. 16.26).

Mechanism of Injury

This injury is also seen in assaults, RTAs, fall, etc.

Clinical Features

Patient may present with pain, swelling, tenderness over the dorsum of the ulnar border of the hand.

Radiographs

Plain X-ray of the hand AP, lateral and oblique views helps to make the diagnosis (Fig. 16.27).

Treatment

These fractures need to be accurately reduced with no rotational malalignment. Closed reduction and fixation with either plaster cast or percutaneous K-wire fixation can do this (Fig. 16.28).

METACARPAL HEAD FRACTURES

These are also known as *'fight bite'* fractures as they occur when the patient strikes an opponent's teeth in a fist fight. The clinical presentation and the investigations are the same as for metacarpal neck fractures. They are frequently intra-articular and need open reduction and internal fixation with K-wire.

METACARPAL FRACTURE OF THE THUMB

Salient Features

- Most of the thumb metacarpal fractures are intra-articular at the carpometacarpal joint.
- The volar beak of basal fracture is not palpable.
- Special X-ray views consisting of true AP and lateral views are required.
- Basal fractures of the thumb are divided into:
  - Extra-articular fractures: Transverse/oblique.
  - Partial articular fracture (Bennett's).
  - Total articular fracture (Rolando's).
  These fractures have been dealt in the previous chapter.

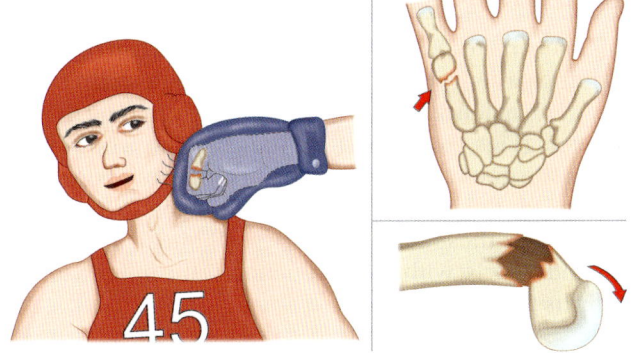

Fig. 16.26: Mechanism of injury in boxer's fracture

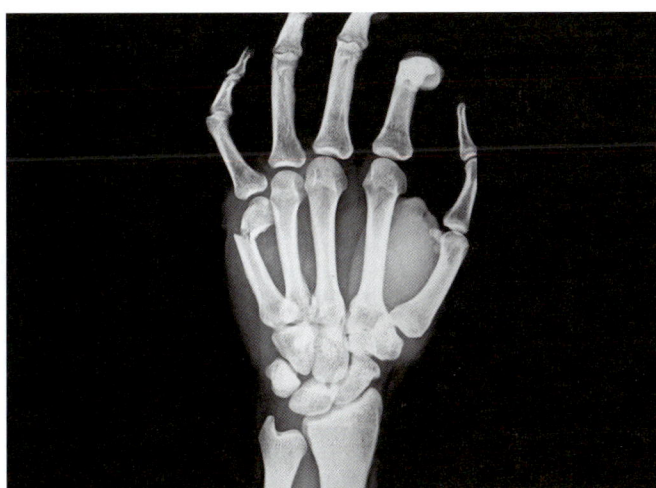

Fig. 16.27: Plain X-ray showing boxer's fracture

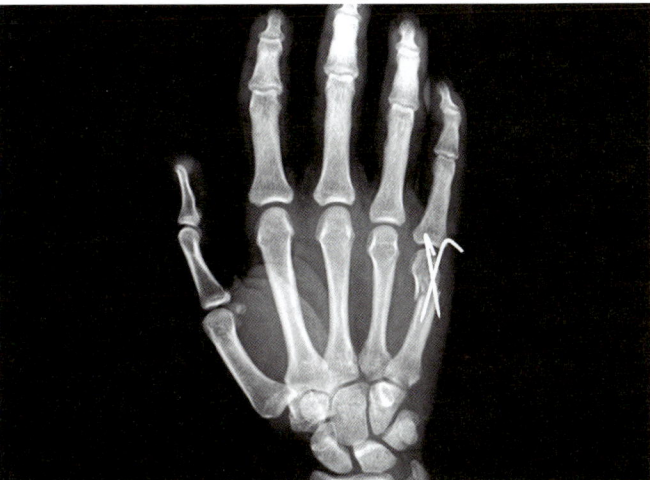

Fig. 16.28: Closed reduction and percutaneous fixation with K-wires

TENDON INJURIES

Either flexor or extensor tendons of the hand can be injured when the patient sustains hand injuries by a sharp cutting object. Flexor tendons are more commonly injured than the extensors (Figs 16.29A and B). The clinician who treats it, if he or she does not explore the hand or the wrist wounds and look for the possibility of tendons being severed more often misses these tendon injuries. Old healed scars over the hand or wrist with loss of function of the injured tendon confirms the diagnosis.

FLEXOR TENDON INJURIES

Flexors of the wrist, fingers and thumb are discussed here.

Wrist Flexors: The main wrist flexors are the flexor carpi radialis and flexor carpi ulnaris. They together bring about palmar flexion of the wrist in the midline. If the flexor carpi radialis is cut, wrist deviates medially towards the intact flexor carpi ulnaris and laterally towards intact flexor carpi radialis if flexor carpi ulnaris is cut.

Finger Flexors: Flexion of the proximal interphalangeal joint of the fingers is brought about mainly by FDS and since FDP crosses this joint, it also aids FDS but FDP is solely responsible for the flexion of distal interphalangeal joint. Both flexor digitorum superficialis (FDS) and flexor digitorum profundus (FDP) could be injured, singly or together. Flexion of the proximal interphalangeal joint of the fingers is brought about mainly by FDS and since FDP crosses this joint, it also aids FDS, but FDP is solely responsible for the flexion of distal interphalangeal joint.

Clinical Features

There could be pain, swelling and deformity of the affected finger (Fig. 16.30A). The patient will be unable to flex the finger. The finger can be moved passively by grasping the torn tendon with a forceps and pulling it (Fig. 16.30B).

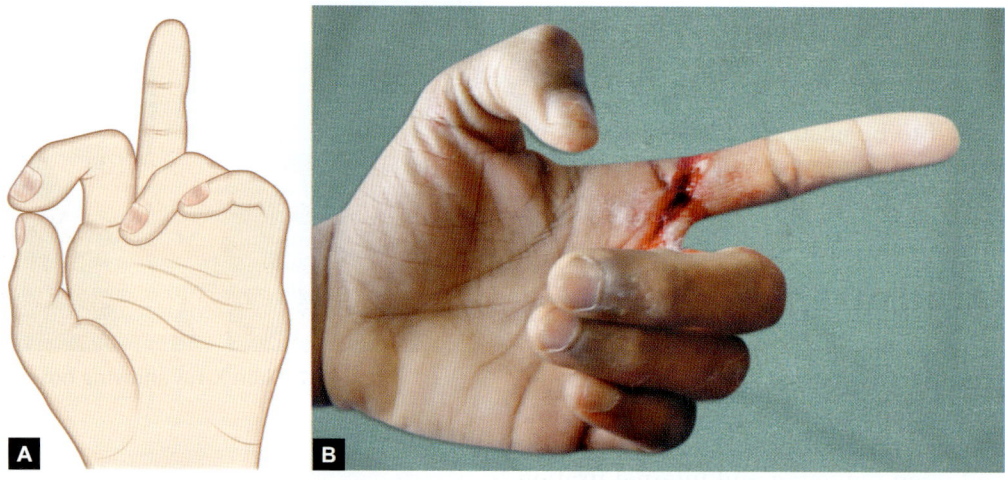

Figs 16.29A and B: (A) If the flexor tendon is injured, the finger does not flex but remains straight; (B) Injury to the finger flexor (Clinical photo)

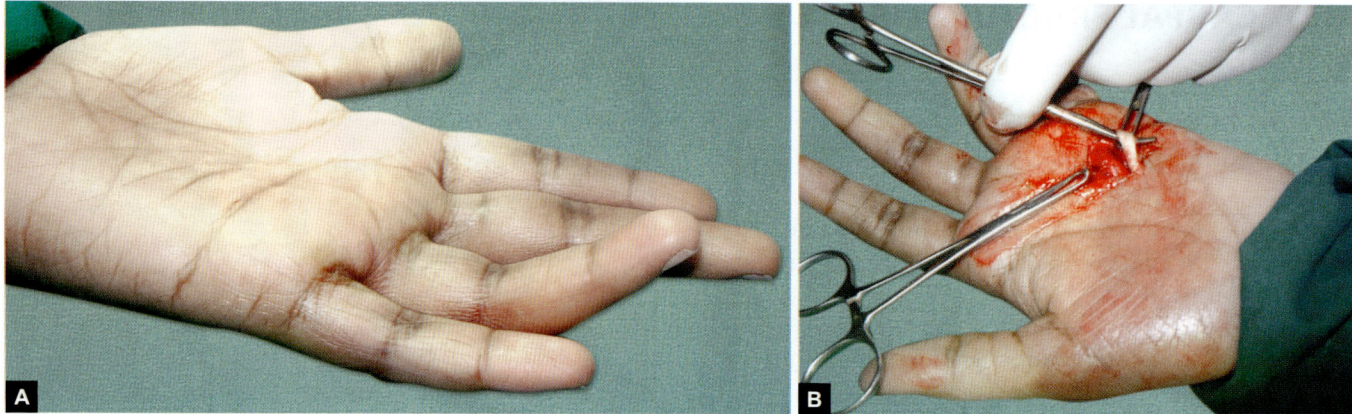

Figs 16.30A and B: Flexor tendon injury: (A) Deformity of the affected finger; (B) Injured tendon

Tests to Diagnose Flexor Tendon Injuries

Test for Profundus

FDP: Instruct the patient to actively flex the DIP joint while you stabilize the PIP joint. If he or she can flex it, there is no injury to FDP tendon (Fig. 16.31).

Test for Superficialis

FDS: Hold the two adjacent fingers in complete extension. This anchors the FDP tendon in the extended position and prevents it from flexing the PIP joint, if he or she can do it, FDS is intact (Fig. 16.32).

Both FDS and FDP: Stabilize the metacarpophalangeal joint and instruct the patient to flex the finger. If he or she cannot flex either the DIP or the PIP joints, both the tendons are cut.

Flexor pollicis longus: Stabilize the MP joint of the thumb and instruct the patient to actively flex the IP joint, if he or she can do it, FPL is intact.

Flexor Zones of the Hand

It is extremely important to know the zones of injury with regard to flexor tendon injuries of the hand and wrist. There are five zones (Fig. 16.33):

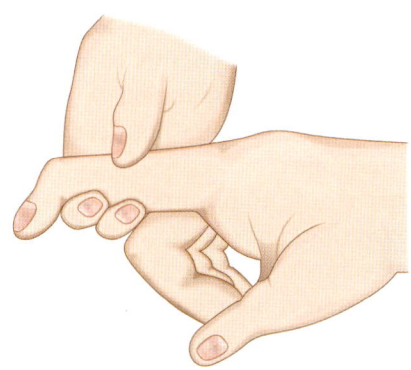

Fig. 16.31: Clinical method of testing FDP

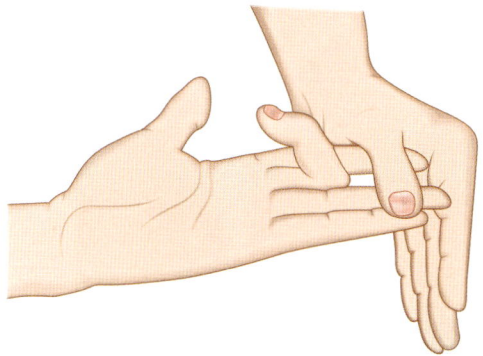

Fig. 16.32: Clinical test to examine FDS

Zone I   : This extends from the tip of the finger to the middle of the middle phalanx.
Zone II   : This extends from the middle of the middle phalanx to the distal palmar crease.
Zone III   : This overlies the palm.
Zone IV   : Overlies the transverse carpal ligament of the wrist.
Zone V   : Extends from the wrist crease to the level of the musculocutaneous junction of the flexor tendons.

Importance of the Zones

Bunnel has labeled Zone II as *no-man's* land and is a critical area of pulleys. These pulleys help in the tendon movements. Primary repairs at this level invariably fail due to the adhesions in the area of pulleys.

Methods of Treatment

Primary repair: This is indicated in fresh, clean-cut wounds. Here the tendons are primarily sutured end-to-end, end-to-side or by various special suturing techniques.

Secondary repair: This may be necessary in severe hand injury, contamination, skin loss, etc. Here after the initial debridement, tendons are secondarily repaired after 2 to 3 weeks.

Tendon transfers: This can be thought of if the patient comes to the treatment late or the previous measures have not been successful. In this, a normal functioning tendon is used to replace the damaged tendon; and for this to happen, all the necessary criteria for tendon transfers should be fulfilled.

Tendon grafting: In the event of loss of tendons due to crush injury, tendon grafting can be considered. Donor tendons

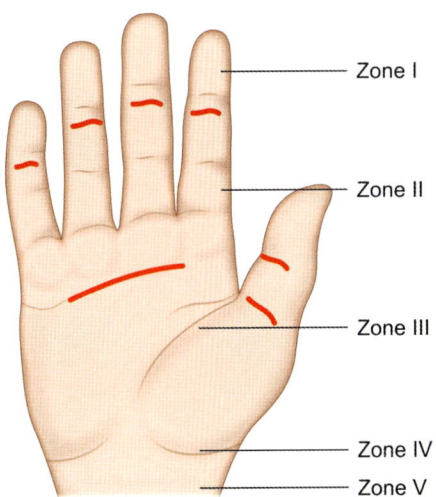

Fig. 16.33: The flexor zones of the hand

for grafting in order of preference are the palmaris longus, the plantaris, the long extensors of the toes, etc.

EXTENSOR TENDON INJURIES

Extensor tendons of the hand are less commonly injured than the flexor tendons.

Clinical Features

There could be pain, swelling and deformity. The patient will be unable to extend the injured finger. Due to the action of the intact flexor tendon, the finger gives auto-flexion deformity (Figs 16.34A and B).

Test

Instruct the patient to extend the metacarpophalangeal joint. If the long extensors are severed, he or she will not be able to do so. However, he or she can extend the IP joints due to the action of the intrinsic muscles of the hand.

Treatment

The extensor surface of the hand is also divided into six zones. Nevertheless, unlike in the flexor tendons, extensor tendons can be primarily repaired at almost any level if the injury is clean-cut. In contaminated or crushed injuries, secondary repair after 2 to 3 weeks can be done with good results.

> **Quick Facts**
> - Flexor tendons are more commonly injured than extensors.
> - Primary flexor tendon injury repair is unsuccessful in Zone II.
> - It is likely that tendon injuries can be missed during the initial evaluation and treatment of hand injuries.
> - Primary repair is done in clean-cut injuries while secondary repair is done in contaminated wounds.
> - Extensor tendons can be successfully sutured in any zone.

SOFT TISSUE INJURIES OF THE HAND

Subungual hematoma: This is due to blunt injury of the fingertips. If it is painful, decompression can be done by puncturing it with a 16-gauge needle.

Nail bed lacerations: Before repairing the wound, distal phalangeal fractures should be reduced if any and the original nail if available should be reinserted back (Fig. 16.35).

Fingertip avulsions: If the soft tissue defect is more than 1 cm, it should be closed by split or full-thickness grafting.

Frostbite injury: In this condition, extreme cold causes vasoconstriction, which may result in thrombosis of the digital vessels. The treatment consists of rapid rewarming in a water bath at 40 to 45°C.

CRUSH INJURIES OF THE HAND AND AMPUTATIONS

Crush injuries of the hand are very serious injuries seen in industrial accidents, RTAs, firecracker injuries, machine tool injuries, etc. (Figs 16.36 and 16.37). Amputation of the fingers or hand is not readily advocated and the following considerations are taken into account before making this painful decision:

- Is the part injured suffering from absolute or irreversible loss of blood supply? If so, this is the only absolute indication for primary amputation.
- Are the other fingers normal? If not, delay the amputation of the affected finger.
- If the finger is left unamputated, will the ultimate function of the hand be good?
- What is the status of the five tissue areas namely, the skin, tendon, nerve, bone and joint? If three or more than three of these five areas require special procedures

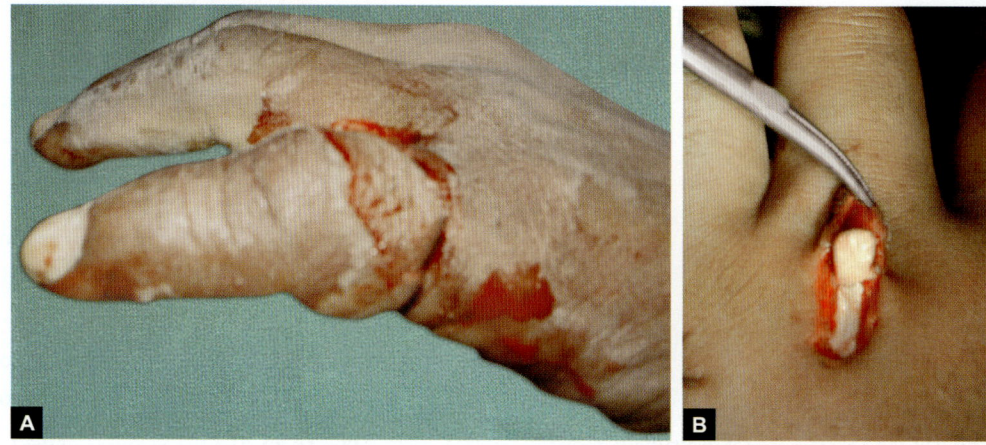

Figs 16.34A and B: (A) Extensor tendon injury (Clinical photo); (B) Clinical photo showing extensor tendon injury

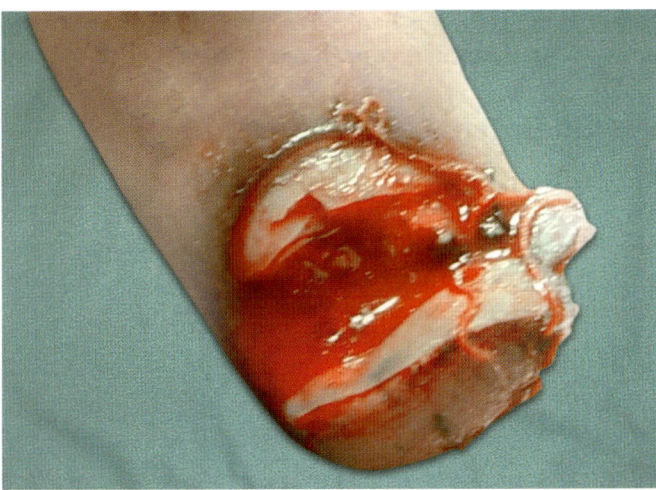

Fig. 16.35: Clinical photo showing nail bed injuries

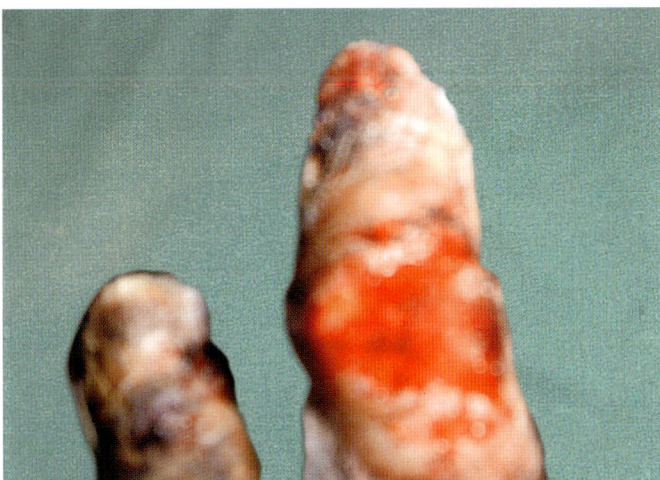

Fig. 16.36: Crush injury of the fingers (Clinical photo)

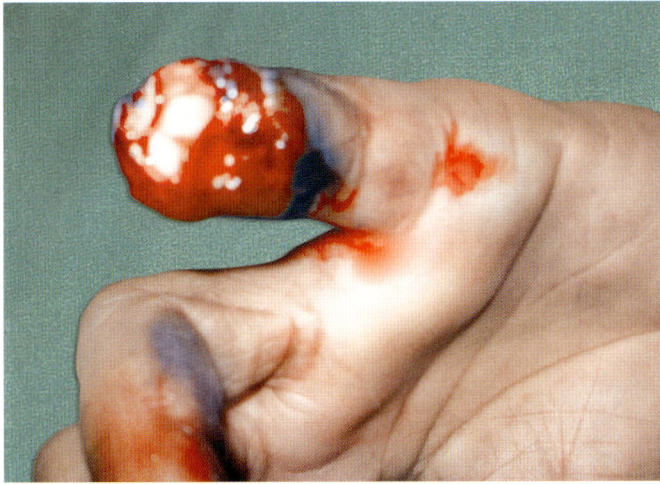

Fig. 16.37: Autoamputation (Clinical photo)

like grafting, etc. give a serious thought about the possibility of amputation.
- Is the victim a child. If so exercise caution.
- If both the flexor tendons and digital nerves are damaged and if the patient is an adult, consider amputation.
- Is the thumb badly injured? Do everything to salvage the thumb.

Thus, in badly crushed hand injuries, it is advisable to avoid radical amputations and to be as conservative as possible in excising the vital parts of the all-important hand.

Principles of Amputation of Fingers

After thorough debridement and removal of all the foreign bodies, amputation is planned keeping the following principles in mind:
- The volar skin flap should be long enough to cover the stump and join the dorsal flap.
- The digital nerves should be resected at least 6 mm proximal to its end and allowed to retract back.
- The digital arteries should be cauterized.
- The flexor and extensor tendons should be pulled distally, cut and allowed to retract.
- If the amputation is through the joint, the flares of the bony condyles are excised.
- No much consideration should be given to the dog-ears.
- Tourniquet should be released before closing the wound and all the bleeders should be cauterized.
- Small interrupted sutures are used to close the flaps.

Treatment Protocol in Crush Injuries

Whatever treatment protocol is followed, it should aim to fulfill the following objectives:
- It should promote primary healing
- The injured parts should be salvaged
- It should aim to prevent infection.

The recommended protocol is as follows:

First aid: These measures include covering the wound with a sterile dressing, hand elevation and judicious application of a tourniquet if required.

First examination: Here status of the skin is assessed in sterile conditions without probing the deeper structures. After the skin, tests are conducted to assess the damages to bones, tendons and nerves. Each of these structures should be considered as damaged until proved otherwise. Radiograph of the hand and general measures like IV fluids, antibiotics, etc. is then done.

Second examination: This is the most important step and is done in a major operation theater under general anesthesia or a regional block. After a thorough debridement, all the structures are very carefully inspected again. Skin is examined for viability, bones, nerves, tendons; vessels are inspected for crushing, loss, viability, etc. All the nonviable structures are excised and loose small pieces of bones are removed.

If the wound is clean, all the structures are primarily repaired and the bone is fixed either by K-wire or Joshi's external fixators. If the wound is contaminated, secondary repair of the tendons, nerves, etc. are planned after 2 to 3 weeks. If the wound is badly crushed and nonviable, then primary amputation is considered as discussed above.

Postoperative Considerations

After the surgical procedures mentioned above, the hand is splinted in functional positions (see Fig. 16.2) as discussed earlier and is kept elevated. Active and passive physiotherapy, wax bath and other rehabilitative measures are planned and appliances given if necessary.

17 CHAPTER

Dislocations of the Hip Joint

INTRODUCTION

When God designed the 65 joints in a human body, he made the hip joint very big and strong to support his weight on a biped stance. Consequently considerable force is required to bring it out of its socket. These forces are provided 70–100% of the times by high-speed motor vehicle accidents. Though hip dislocations were reported earlier to the discovery of the X-rays, it was Funsten in 1938 that first reported a series of 20 hip dislocations and also coined the term "dashboard dislocation." In his series and in subsequent series by other authors, it was found that these dislocations usually happen when the knees of the front seat occupants in a vehicle strike against the dashboard of the vehicle usually in a head on collision. Depending on the position of the limb at the time of impact, there could be either pure dislocation or fracture dislocations. The enormity of the trauma could also cause multisystem injuries of the head, trunk, abdomen, pelvis, etc.

> **Look what could happen in hip dislocations?**
> - Pure hip dislocations.
> - Fracture hip dislocations: Fracture acetabulum, fracture head of femur, fracture neck of femur
> - Other injuries: Knee ligament injuries, fracture patella, supracondylar fracture femur, shaft femur, etc.
> - Other limb fractures
> - Multisystem injuries
> - Pelvic fractures, rib fractures, spine fractures, etc.

Now you know why managing hip dislocations are a gigantic challenge to a treating orthopedic surgeon. Depending upon the presentation it may be a solo or a multimodality and multispecialty approach. Nonetheless hip dislocations are an emergency amidst life-threatening emergencies if any and needs to be treated on a top priority basis. If hi; joint is 'out' pushing it back 'in' should be the mantra lest troublesome delayed complications like AVN, degenerative arthritis, etc. stare in your face.

CLINICAL SIGNIFICANCE OF VASCULAR ANATOMY

Avascular necrosis of femoral head and post-traumatic degenerative hip are the two very important and common complications of hip dislocations. A thorough knowledge of the vascular anatomy is a must to understand the reasons behind (Fig. 17.1). Femoral head circulation is through three sources:
- Intraosseous cervical vessels
- Artery of ligamentum teres
- Retinacular vessels (Man supply).

If there is damage to these vessels during dislocation, or during reduction and also due to the delay in diagnosis and treatment, this could lead to avascular necrosis of the femoral head and later to degenerative arthritis.

"Therefore, the aim of treatment is early anatomical reduction to protect the existing circulation of the head of the femur."

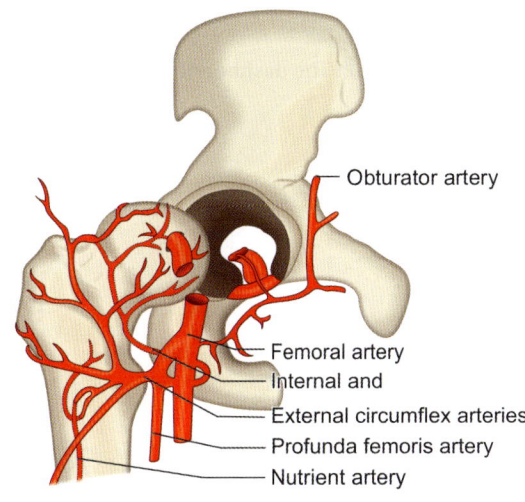

Fig. 17.1: Vascular anatomy of the hip joint
(*Courtesy:* Paul Levin, MD)

Causes

- High speed RTA's
- Violent falls from heights
- Sports related injuries
- Industrial accidents
- Natural calamities, etc.

Note:
Nearly 70–100% of the hip dislocations are due to RTA.

Mechanism of Injury

The notorious incriminating forces that knock the hips out of its safe confines could arise from three sources:
- The front part of the flexed knee striking against an object (dash board events).
- From the sole of feet with the ipsilateral knee extended.
- From the greater trochanter
- Rarely, it could be from the posterior pelvis.
- Look at these interesting developments in a dashboard injury (Fig. 17.2):

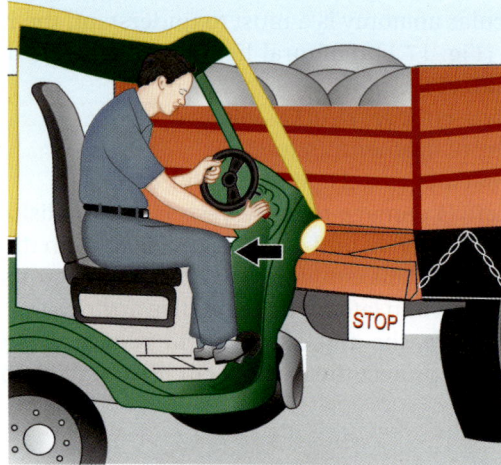

Fig. 17.2: The dashboard injury

- Left hip may develop a pure dislocation of the hip since the left foot is on the clutch with the hip and knee flexed at 90°.
- Right hip may develop a fracture dislocation, because the right foot is either on the brake or accelerator pedal with the hip in 60–70° of flexion and slight abduction.

Classification

Depending upon the position of the head with respect to the acetabulum, hip dislocations are classified as:
- *Posterior dislocations:* Commonest and is seen in 80–90% of the cases.
- *Anterior dislocations:* Seen in 10–15%.
- *Central dislocations:* Relatively rare.

Overall Classification of the Hip Dislocations (Stewart and Milfort, Based on the Hip Stability and Femoral Head Condition, Both Anterior and Posterior)

Type I: Dislocates with either no fracture or an insignificant ace tabular rim fracture.
Type II: Dislocations with either a single or a communized posterior wall fracture but the hip is stable.
Type III: Fracture dislocations with gross instability due to loss of structural support.
Type IV: Dislocations with femoral head fracture.

Comprehensive Classification (Both Anterior and Posterior) (Figs 17.3A to E)

Type I: No significant associated fractures, no clinical instability following concentric reduction.
Type II: Irreducible dislocation without significant femoral hear or acetabular fracture (reduction must be attempted under GA).
Type III: Unstable hip following reduction or incarcerated fragments of cartilage, labrum, or bone.

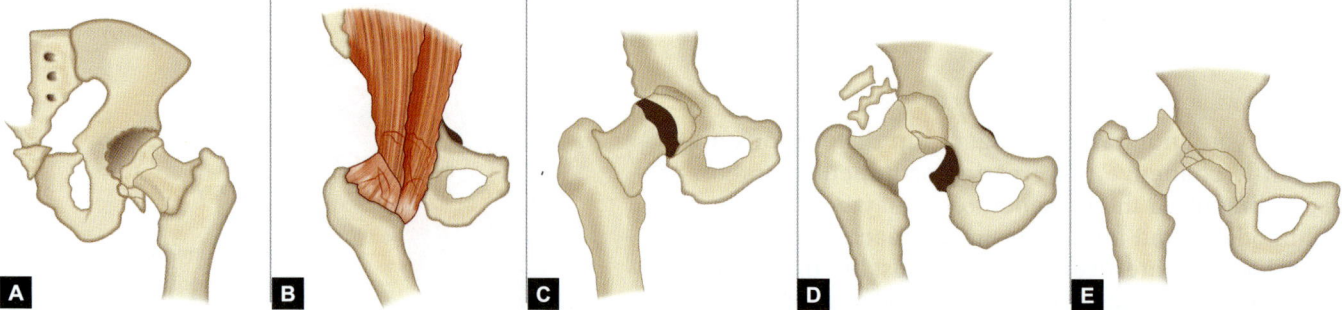

Figs 17.3A to E: The comprehensive classification of posterior dislocation of the hip (*Courtesy:* Paul Levin, MD)

Type IV: Associated acetabular fracture requiring reconstruction to restore hip stability or joint congruity.
Type V: Associated femoral hear or femoral neck injury (Fracture or impactions).

POSTERIOR DISLOCATION OF THE HIP

As mentioned earlier this is the most common variety of hip dislocations. The dislocation could be simple or may be associated with fracture dislocations. Thompson and Epstein have further classified the posterior dislocation of the hip into four types and Pipkin has given four sub-classifications for the femoral head fracture in type IVB fracture of the Thompson and Epstein variety.

Thompson and Epstein Classification (Figs 17.4A to E)

Type I: With or without minor fracture.
Type II: With a large single fracture of the posterior acetabular rim.
Type III: With communition of the rim of the acetabulum with or without a major fragment.
Type IV: With fracture of the acetabular floor.
Type V: With fracture of the femoral head. This has been further classified by Pipkin into four types.

Pipkin Types (Dislocation of the Hip with Fractures of the Femoral Head) (Figs 17.5A to D)

Type I: Femoral dislocation of the hip with fracture of the femoral head caudad to the fovea centralis.
Type II: Posterior dislocation of the hip with fracture of the femoral head cephalad to the fovea centralis.
Type III: Type I and Type II with associated fracture of the femoral neck.
Type IV: Type I, II, or III with associated facture of the acetabulum.

Clinical Features

There is usually history of trauma and the patient has a flexion, adduction, and medial rotation deformity of the affected limb (Figs 17.6A and B). There is marked shortening and gross restriction of all hip movements. Head of the femur is felt as a hard mass in the glutei region and it moves

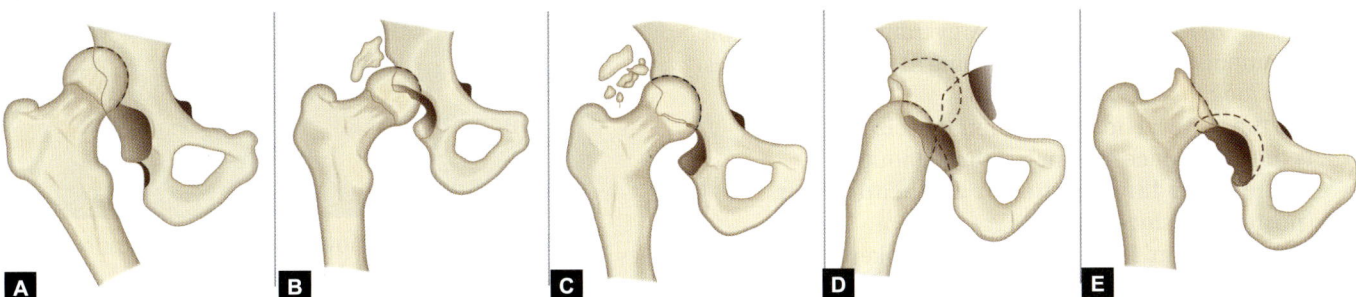

Figs 17.4A to E: Thompson and Epstein's classification of posterior hip dislocations (*Courtesy:* Delee JC. Fractures and dislocations, 2nd Edition, Vol. 2. In: Rockwood CA Jr, Green DP (Eds). Fractures, JB Lippincott, 1985)

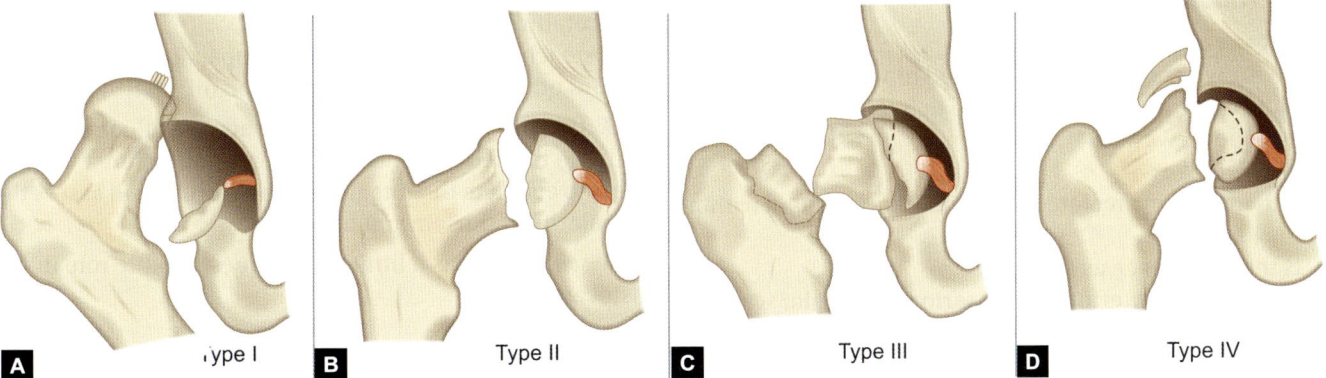

Figs 17.5A to D: Pipkin's classification (*Courtesy:* Delee JC. Fractures and dislocations, 2nd Edition, Vol. 2. In: Rockwood CA Jr, Green DP (Eds). Fractures, JB Lippincott, 1985)

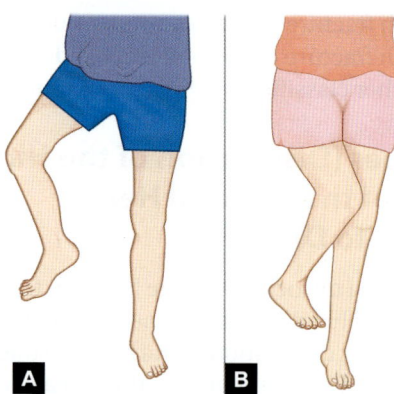

Figs 17.6A and B: Appearance of classical deformities in dislocation hip: (A) Anterior; (B) Posterior

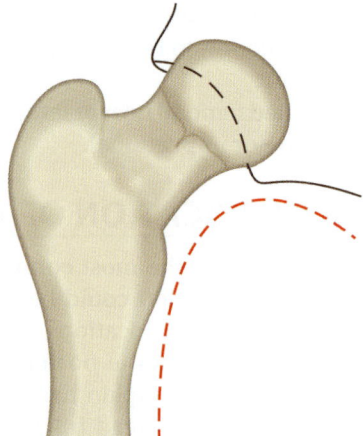

Fig. 17.7: The Shenton's line

along with the femur. There could be features of sciatic nerve palsy. It may be difficult to feel the femoral pulse (Vascular sign of Narath is negative). In fracture posterior hip dislocation, this classical presentation may not be seen.

Investigations

Before Reduction

Laboratory tests: Hb%, BT, CT, blood group, RBS, etc. needs to be done as for any other major surgery.

Plain X-ray of the hip: All high-energy trauma and multiple injury patients should have a screening AP view of the pelvis.

What to look for in the initial X-ray:
- Are the femoral heads symmetric in size?
- Is the joint space symmetric throughout?
- Is the head large (anterior dislocation) or small (posterior dislocation)?
- Is the Shenton' line maintained or broken? (Fig. 17.7)
- Is the greater trochanter prominent (posterior) or inconspicuous (anterior) reverse with lesser trochanter?
- Is the femoral neck normal?

After Reduction

Plain X-ray of the hip
- AP X-ray centered on the affected hip (Fig. 17.8).
- Judet views with the affected hip in internal and external oblique views at 45°.

What to look for?
- Is there any incarcerated osteochondral fragment within the joint?
- Is the joint space asymmetric?
- Look for the anterior and posterior ace tabular wall.
- Look for any indentation on the femoral head.

CT scan: CT scan should be routinely done after a successful or failed closed reduction. The importance of CT lies in:
- Assessing the femoral head (*see* Fig. 17.13).

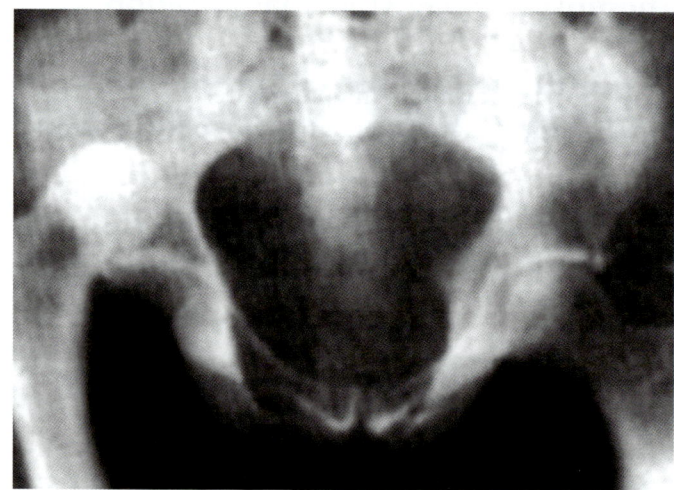

Fig. 17.8: Radiograph showing posterior dislocation of the hip joint

- To demonstrate the presence of small intra-articular fragments.
- To assess the congruence of the femoral head and acetabulum.
- Osteochondral fractures, occult impactions, indentations and other fractures are easily seen on a CT.

MRI: This has its limitations in the acute evaluation of the multiple injured patients. However, as an adjunct to CT it helps to evaluate the integrity of the labrum and assess the vascularity of the femoral head.

Bone scan: This has a limited and questionable role in hip dislocations.

Management

All hip dislocations are emergencies and need to be reduced within 6–12 hours following injury to prevent troublesome late complications like AVN and traumatic degenerative hip. Once reduction is done urgency is reduced and now the diagnostic workup, CT scan, and surgical intervention if necessary can all be done once the general condition of the patient is stabilized.

Goals of Treatment

Immediate goal—Prompt reduction of the femoral head.

Types of reduction: This is either closed or open. Thompson Epstein believed that closed reduction should be reserved for simple hip dislocations and open reduction for hip dislocations, while majority of the authors believe that closed reduction should be tried initially in all cases of simple and fracture dislocation and open reduction shoulder be reserved for the patients in whom;
- Closed reduction fails
- Reduction is unstable
- After reduction, if there are trapped fracture fragments within the joint.

Type I Dislocation

Here prompt closed reduction of the hip is the treatment of choice.

Methods of Closed Reduction

There are various techniques described in the literature. The important methods are the ABC'S.
A – **A**llis method
B – **B**igelow method
C – **C**lassical Watson Jones method
S – **S**timson's gravity method.

Note:
All the reductions should be done under general anesthesia.
Now let us try to know each method of reduction in greater detail.

A. Allis Method (Fig. 17.9)

- Patient is supine
- An assistant stabilizes the pelvis by applying pressure on both the ASIS.
- Traction is applied in the line of the deformity.
- The hip is gently flexed to 90°.
- The hip is now gently rotated, internally and externally, with continued longitudinal traction till reduction is achieved.

Bass's method (Modified Allis method): This is the flexion adduction method. With the patient under general anesthesia, the hip is flexed to 90° in maximum adduction as the longitudinal traction is applied in the axis of the femur while an assistant stabilizes the pelvis.

B. Bigelow's Method (Fig. 17.10)

- Patient is supine
- An assistant applies counter traction on both the ASIS.
- Surgeon applies longitudinal traction in the line of the deformity.

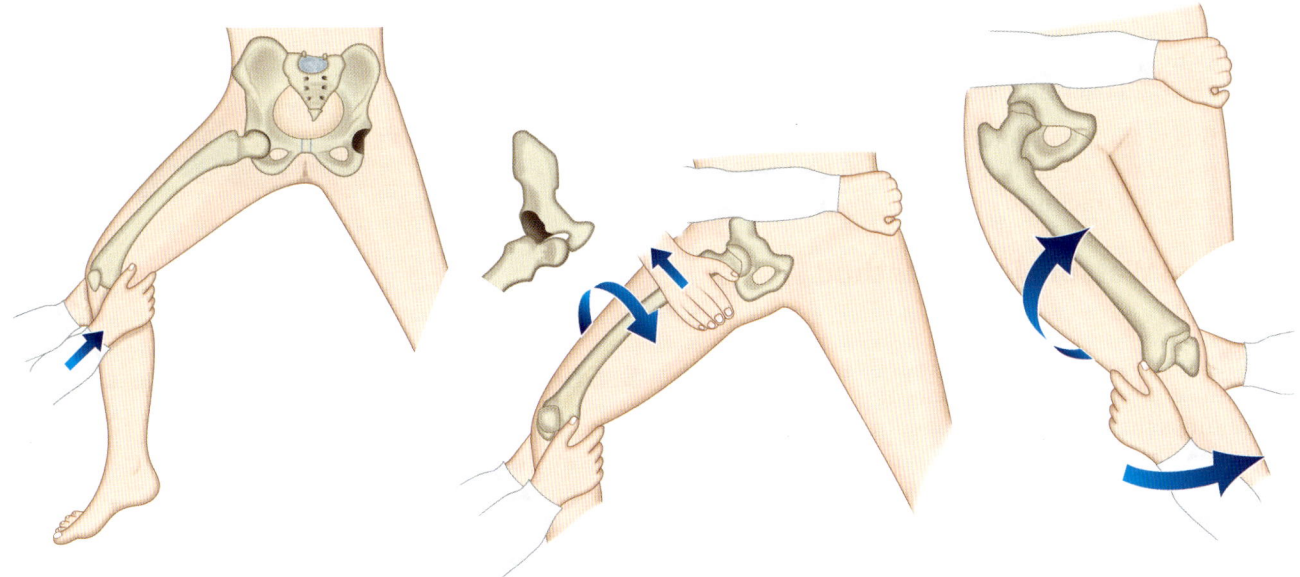

Fig. 17.9: Technique of Allis method of reduction of the hip dislocation (*Courtesy:* Delee JC. Fractures and dislocations, 2nd Edition, Vol. 2. In: Rockwood CA Jr, Green DP (Eds). Fractures, JB Lippincott, 1985)

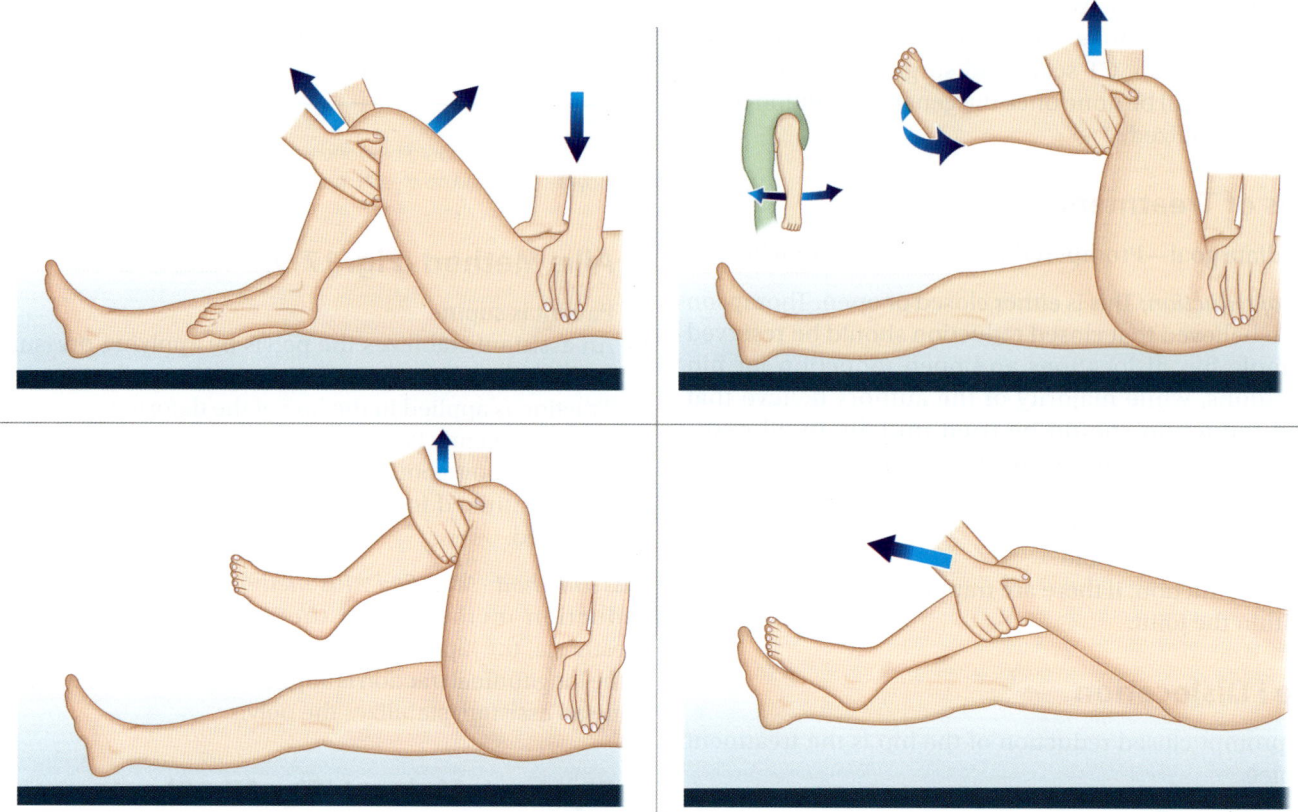

Fig. 17.10: Bigelow's method of reduction (*Courtesy:* Delee JC. Fractures in adults: Rockwood and Green (Eds), 1996)

- The hip is gently adducted, internally rotated, and bent on the abdomen. This relaxes the Y-ligament and brings the femoral head near the poster inferior aspect of the acetabulum.
- By adduction, external rotation, and extension of the hip, head is levered back into the acetabulum.

Caution: This technique should be done with lot of care, as it requires more force and could result in iatrogenic soft tissue damage and fractures.

C. Classical Watson-Jones Method (Fig. 17.11)

This technique is useful in both anterior and posterior dislocation of the hip. Irrespective of the type of dislocation the limb is first brought to the neutral position. In this position, the head of the femur lies posterior to the acetabulum even in anterior dislocation. Now with an assistant steadying the pelvis the head of the femur is reduced into the acetabulum by applying a longitudinal traction in the long axis of the femur. It is simple and effective when compared to Bigelow's method.

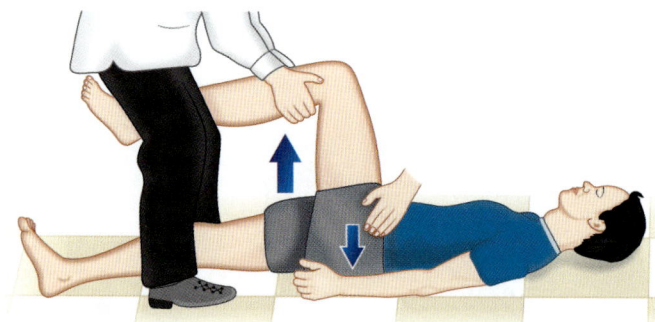

Fig. 17.11: Watson Jones classical method of reduction

S. Stimson's Gravity Method (Fig. 17.12)

In reality, this is the reverse Allis method of reduction. The steps are as follows:
- Patient is prone
- Patient is brought to the edge of the table
- An assistant stabilizes the pelvis by applying downward pressure over the sacrum.
- The affected hip and knees are flexed to 90°.

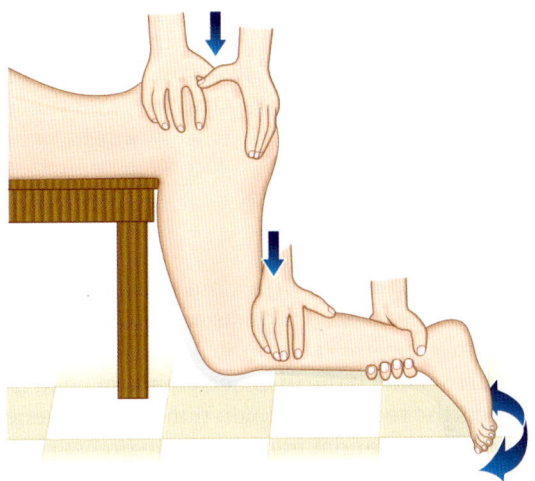

Fig. 17.12: Stimson's Gravity method of reduction (*Courtesy:* Delee JC. Fractures and dislocations, 2nd Edition, Vol. 2. In: Rockwood CA Jr, Green DP (Eds). Fractures, JB Lippincott, 1985)

- Downward pressure is applied on the flexed knee.
- To facilitate the reduction, gentle rotations needs to be done.

Postreduction Protocol

Radiographic verifications: AP and lateral views of the affected hip and pelvis AP views should be taken. The X-ray has to be carefully evaluated for the concentric reduction by looking for the subtle widening of the joint space. If there are any significant acetabular factures, Judet views are recommended.

Evaluation of the postreduction stability: After the radiographic verification of the dislocation, a stability check is carried out as follows:
- Flex the hip to 90-95° in neutral, abduction and adduction and rotation.
- A strong posterior force is thus applied.
- If there is evidence of subluxation, additional diagnostic studies are required and surgical exploration or traction may be required at a later date.

Postreduction CT evaluation: This is very important and the role of CT has already been discussed. Now the final staging of the hip dislocation is carried out.

Postreduction traction: If the hip is stable after reduction, Buck's traction is applied and if the hip is unstable then skeletal traction is applied through the tibia pin.

> **Traction Facts**
> - Permissible weight: 5 to 8 lbs
> - Permissible time: 2–3 weeks (till the hip is pain free and has good range of movements)

> - Traction requirement: It should prevent the hip from flexion, internal rotation, and adduction
> - Weight bearing can be resumed after 2–4 weeks once the pain and spasm disappears.

Bad News for Spica Cast: Spica cast should not be used for postreduction stabilization. Since it prevents early range of movements necessary to promote healing. This damages the articular cartilage and leads to post-traumatic arthritis in future.

Treatment of Type II, III and IV: Here there is an argument over the closed vs. open reduction. Most authors' worldwide feel that hip dislocations with acetabular fractures should be reduced at the earliest. This they claim gives a better long-term outcome than operative reduction. However, Epstein recommends early primary open reduction and he claims better results with this approach. However, theoretically acceptable, practically it has its lacunae as optimum operating conditions for major hip procedure as an emergency procedure is seldom found. If open reduction is warranted it can always be done later, after stabilizing the patient without compromising on the long-term safety of the patients.

Whether the choice is closed or open reduction techniques for posterior fracture dislocations, the following factors are prognostically important:
- Degree of initial trauma
- Reduction either closed or open should be performed within 12-24 hours
- If closed reduction is the choice, it has to be attempted only once failing which open reduction should be attempted.

Indications for Open Reduction

- Failed closed reduction
- Failed stability test
- Big posterior lip fragment
- Bone fragment within the acetabulum
- Fracture of the femoral head
- Sciatic nerve palsy.

Techniques of Open Reduction

- Approach: Posterior approach is favored though some have tried anterior Watson Jones or transtrochanteric approach.
- Debridement: Joint is thoroughly irrigated to remove all pieces of bone and cartilage.
- Reduction of the hip, if it has not been done previously.
- Reposition of the fracture fragments carefully and reconstruct the acetabulum.
- In Type II injury with the large Acetabular chunk can be fixed by single cancellous screws.

- In Type III with several pieces reconstruction is attempted as accurately as possible and fixation is done with cancellous screws or small malleable plate, etc.
- In severe comminution reconstruction is done through a full thickness iliac graft/auto graft.
- In type IV fractures are fixed based on the location and Epstein claims poor results in these cases irrespective of the type of treatment.

Postoperative Treatment

- Skeletal traction (10-15 lbs) with the hip in slight abduction and extension.
- Within 3-5 days, gentle active and passive exercises in traction are begun.
- Traction to be maintained for 6-8 weeks.
- Later protected weight bearing is allowed.

Type V Posterior Fracture Dislocations (Fig. 17.13)

- There is associated femoral head fracture
- First reported by Birkett in 1869
- Incidence is 6-7%
- Incidence is on the rise due to increase in RTA's.

Mechanism of Injury

- In a dashboard injury if the hip is in 60° of flexion or less and is in neutral position it could result in a combined dislocation and fracture of the femoral head.
- Avulsion of the femoral head through an intact ligamentum teres.

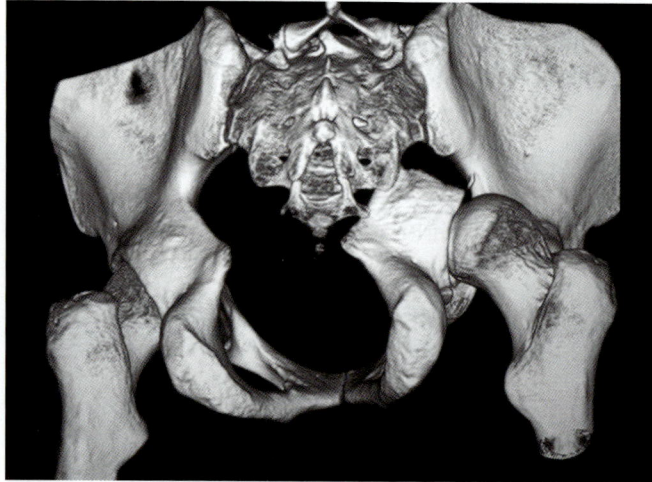

Fig. 17.13: Posterior facture dislocation (Type V)

Classification

Pipkin's types: Here posterior dislocation of hip could be associated with fracture head of the femur and has been discussed earlier.

Management

Type I:
- Closed reduction is often successful. Pipkin has suggested after closed reduction the fragments return back to their normal anatomical position.
- Surgical excision if the displaced femoral head fracture obstructs the reduction Pipkin noted that degenerative changes in the caudal fragment have no bearing in the long-term result.

Type II: According to Swintkwoski in Pipkin I and II, if the displacement of the fracture is less than 2 mm on postreduction CT scan.

Methods of Treatment

- Primary closed reduction
- Excision (Epstein): If the fragment is less than one-third of the articular surface.
- Open reduction and internal fixation in large fragments. This is indicated if the femoral head fracture cannot be reduced by closed means. Internal fixation is done by Herbert Screws.

In this injury since the ligamentum teres is still attached to the head fragment, blood supply to the fragment is still maintained and it heals well.

Type III: Only 13 cases have been reported in the literature and 5 of these were iatrogenic and happened at the time of performing the closed reduction for the hip dislocation. These fractures can be treated as follows:
- Open reduction and internal fixation of the femoral neck fracture. The femoral head fractures were then treated as in Types I and II.
- These can also be treated as primary insertion of endoprosthesis or other types of arthroplasty.

Type IV: Here there is associated fracture of the acetabulum and fracture of the femoral head could be Type I/II/III. The treatment plan is dictated by the degree of ace tabular cartilage damage. Small fragments can be excised and the larger fragment needs to be fixed with screws. Later femoral head fracture is treated as in I and II.

Complications

Myositis ossificans (2%): It is seen commonly in posterior dislocation with head injury and is unknown in simple posterior dislocation. It may be seen after reduction also. It can be prevented by avoiding repeated manipulation, early immobilization and by immobilizing for 6 weeks in hip spica.

Sciatic nerve injury: Incidence of this injury is 10 to 13% and it leads to foot drop (Fig. 17.14). It is 3 times more common in fracture dislocation than simple dislocation. Usually, it is a neuropraxia and the peroneal division is commonly affected. It may be due to stretch of the nerve or may be due to impalement between the fracture fragments. If it is associated with acetabular fracture the nerve should be explored. Prognosis is variable (*see* Fig. 25.28).

Traumatic osteoarthritis due to avascular necrosis (35%): For head of the femur major blood supply enters from the capsule and to a lesser extent through the ligamentum teres. If both these sources are damaged, it gradually leads to AVN followed by osteoarthritis of the hip joint. Incidence is about 10%.

Recurrent dislocation: This is due to fracture acetabulum and sometimes due to rent in the capsule and gluteus minimus. This requires exploration and fixing of the acetabular fragments with screws.

Unreduced dislocation: This is common in Asian patients due to ignorance and illiteracy. Manipulative reduction is tried first. If it is unsuccessful operative reduction is attempted. Arthrodesis if acceptable is the best treatment. Total hip replacement is usually not preferred because the patient is usually young. In hips where there is useful range of painless movements corrective osteotomy is done. In painful stiff joints, girdlestone excision is preferred.

Irreducible dislocation (31%): This may be due to bony (acetabular fragments, femoral head, etc.) or soft tissue (acetabular labrum, etc.) obstruction. It may also be due to coma, ipsilateral fracture femur, or dislocation of opposite hip. It may require exploration and open reduction.

ANTERIOR DISLOCATION OF THE HIP

Incidence: This is rare and is seen in 10–15% of the cases.

Causes

- In RTA's, when the knee strikes the dashboard with the thigh abducted
- Violent fall from the height
- Forceful blow to the back of the patient in a squatted position (Fig. 17.15).

Mechanism of Injury

Due to the above forces, the neck of femur or the greater trochanter impinges on the rim of the acetabulum and through a tear in the anterior hip capsule; the head of the femur is levered out of the acetabulum. If the hip is in simultaneous abduction, external rotation and flexion, an inferior type (obturator) of dislocation results. And on the contrary if the hip is in abduction, external rotation and extension, it results in a pubic or iliac (superior) dislocation. There could be associated fracture of the head of the femur.

Classification

Comprehensive classification: This is same as for the posterior dislocation of the hip discussed earlier (Figs 17.16A to E).

Epstein' Classification

Type I : Superior dislocation (includes pubic and subspinous dislocation).
Type IA : No associated fracture (Simple dislocation).

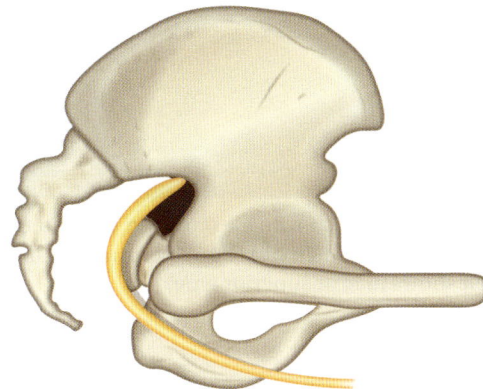

Fig. 17.14: Sciatic nerve injury in posterior dislocation of the hip

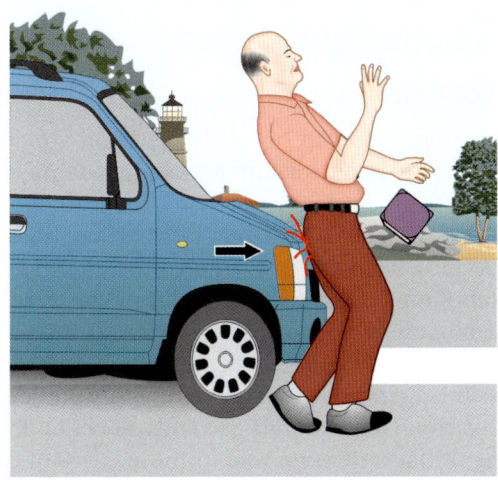

Fig. 17.15: Mechanism of injury in anterior dislocation of the hip

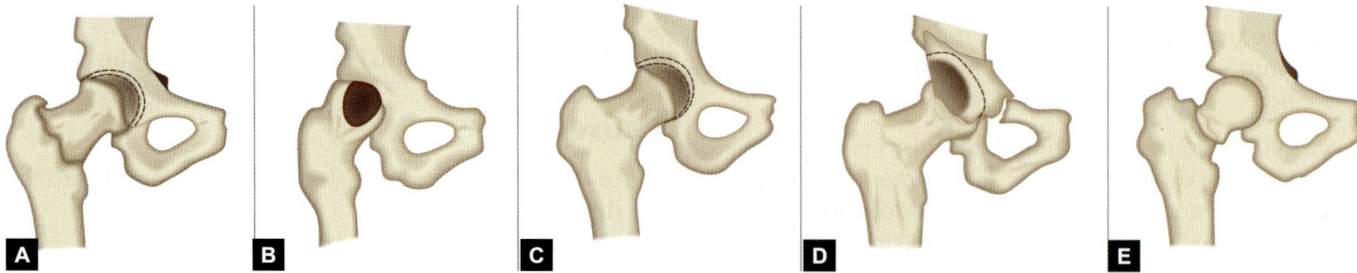

Figs 17.16A to E: Comprehensive classification of the anterior dislocation of the hip (*Courtesy:* Paul Levin, MD)

Type IB : Associated facture of the head (transchondral or indentation type) and/or neck of the femur.
Type IC : Associated fracture of the acetabulum.
Type II : Inferior dislocation (includes obturator, thyroid, and perineal dislocation).
Type IIA : No associated fracture (Simple dislocation).
Type IIB : Associated fracture of the head (transchondral or indentation type) and/or neck of the femur.
Type IIC : Associated fracture of the acetabulum.

Clinical Features

- Multisystem injuries are a possibility and have to be carefully evaluated.
- Position of the limb suggests the diagnosis:
  - *In the superior type (Iliac or Pubic):* The hip is extended and externally rotated and the head is felt near the anterosuperior iliac spine in the iliac type and in the groin in the pubic type.
  - *In the inferior type (Obturator/Thyroid/Perineal):* Here the hip is in abduction, external rotation and in varying degrees of flexion. Head is palpable in the region of the obturator foramen.
- Distal neurovascular status has to be assessed due to the possibility of injuries to the femoral vessels and nerve.

Investigations

- *X-ray:* Diagnosis can be easily made on a plain X-ray (Fig. 17.17). Look for any associated damage to the femoral head, neck, etc.
- *CT Scan:* This helps to detect intra-articular fragments if any and also helps to evaluate the femoral head and acetabulum. CT is also indicated after closed reduction or if closed reduction fails before doing the open reduction (Fig. 17.18).
- *MRI:* This helps to evaluate the integrity of the labrum, vascularity of the femoral head and osteochondral lesion if any. It has a definite role in these cases of unstable hip after dislocation or in widened joint space after reduction.

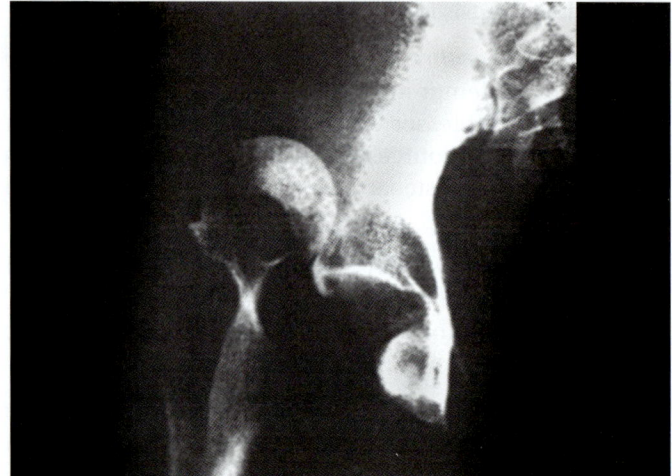

Fig. 17.17: Radiograph showing the iliac type of anterior dislocation of the hip

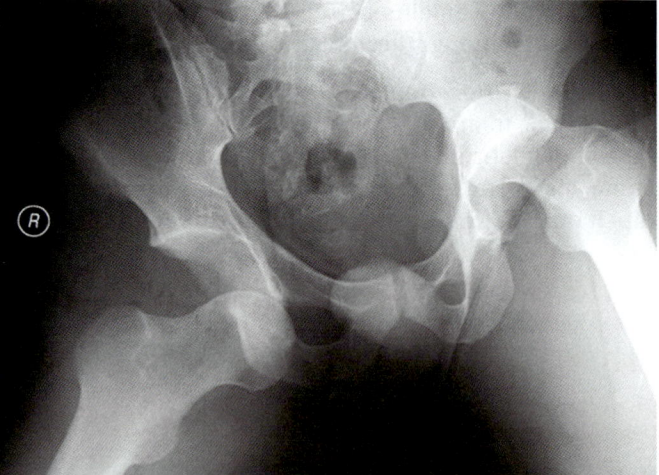

Fig. 17.18: Plain X-ray showing a rare case of bilateral anterior dislocation of the hip. Right hip shows obturator or inferior type and the left shows iliac or superior type

Treatment

Goal: Prompt diagnosis and immediate closed reduction under general anesthesia.

Caution: Single and not multiple attempts are advised, failure warrants open reduction at the earliest.

Methods: ABCDE's Method of Reduction

- *Allis method:* This is the same as for the posterior dislocation
- *Bigelow's method (Actually this is a reverse Bigelow):* Here the hip is in partial flexion and abduction. He has described two methods:
  - *The traction method:* Here the traction is applied in the line of the deformity and the hip is adducted, internally rotated, and extended.
  - *The lifting method:* Here a flexed thigh is lifted with a sudden jerk. However, this method is not successful in pubic dislocations.
- *Classical Watson-Jones' method:* This is the same as described previously in posterior dislocation of the hip.
- *Delee and Epstein method:* This is a modified Allis technique. It consists of continuous traction in the line of the deformity, hip in slight flexion, lateral force to the thigh with slight internal rotation and adduction.
- *Stimson's gravity method:* Same as for posterior dislocation. However, it is not useful in superior dislocation as the hip here is in an extended position. A careful X-ray evaluation is must after closed reduction. Look for any associated transchondral fracture, femoral neck or head fracture. A transchondral fracture needs excision; open reduction an internal fixation for a large fracture of the femoral head and indentation fracture needs to be left alone.

Postreduction Protocol

- Traction for a period of 1–6 weeks.
- Controlled range of movements is instituted during the traction.
- Avoid extremes of abduction and external rotation.
- If there are associated fractures, longer period of immobilization are required.

Complications

Immediate Complications

Neurovascular compromise: In superior and open dislocations, there could be pressure on the femoral artery, vein and nerve leading to distal neurovascular compromise. It warrants immediate reduction of the hip dislocations.

Irreducibility: These could be due to the following reasons:
- Bony block in the obturator foramen.
- Soft tissue interposition could be from rectus femoris, iliopsoas muscle, and anterior hip capsule. This necessitates open reduction.

Delayed Complications

Post-traumatic arthritis: This is reported in more than one-third to one-half of cases and the reasons could be:
- Femoral head fractures
- Acetabular fractures
- AVN
- Transchondral and indentation fractures.

AVN

- Incidence is 8%
- Less common than posterior dislocation
- May appear 2–5 years later
- Reasons could be due to delay or repeated attempts at reduction
- Extent of initial injury has an important role.

Recurrent dislocations: Defective capsular healing due to inadequate immobilization could lead to recurrent dislocations.

Unreduced dislocations: Commonly seen in developing condition than developed condition. The three methods of treatment are:
- *Open reduction:* This could lead to a painful hip at a later stage.
- *Osteotomy of the proximal femur:* This has been tried with varying results.
- THR in late cases.

CENTRAL DISLOCATION OF THE HIP

This is the least common and most difficult of all dislocations of the hip joint.

Table 17.1 gives a comparative study of the various types of dislocations of the hip joint.

Mechanism of Injury

It could be due to direct blow on the greater trochanter as in the case of RTA or fall on the sides (Fig. 17.19). It is invariably associated with the fractures of the acetabulum and this is what makes it a very difficult problem to treat.

Classification: Judet's Types

- Undisplaced fractures (Either single-line or stellate types).
- Inner wall fractures:
  - Femoral head concentrically reduced beneath the dome on initial X-rays.
  - Femoral head not reduced under the acetabular dome but centrally dislocated.
- Superior dome fractures:
  - Gross outline of the acetabular dome intact and congruous with the femoral head.

TABLE 17.1: Comparative features of dislocations of the hip

	Posterior dislocation	Anterior dislocation		Central dislocation	
Incidence	Common (70%)	10–15%		Rare	
Mechanism of injury	• Dashboard injury as in RTA • Flexed knee + neutral adduction results in simple dislocation • Flexed knee + slight abduction results in fracture dislocation	• Dashboard injury with thigh abducted • Fall from height • Blow to the back in squatted position		• Due to direct blow over trochanter • Common in patients with epilepsy, convulsions, etc.	
Classification	Thompson and Epstein • *Type I* with or without minor fracture • *Type II* with a large single fracture of rim acetabulum • *Type III* comminution of acetabular rim with or without major fragment • *Type IV* with fracture of femoral head	*Type I (Superior)* • IA No fracture • IB Associated head fracture • IC Associated fracture acetabulum	*Type II (Inferior)* • IIA No fracture • IIB Associated head fracture • IIC Associated fracture acetabulum	Judet's Dislocation associated with • Undisplaced fracture • Inner wall fracture of acetabulum • Superior rim fracture of acetabulum • Bursting fracture of acetabulum	
Clinical features	• Limb shortening • Flexion/add/IR deformity • Thigh rests on the contralateral limb • Head felt in the gluteal region • Vascular sign negative (Narath) • Movements of hip • Injury to sciatic nerve	Superior type flexion + ABD + external rotation deformity Inferior type hip is extended and externally rotated • Head felt superiorly or inferiorly • Vascular sign (Narath) positive • Injury to femoral nerve artery or vein		• No limb shortening • Limb is neutral in position • Bruising over the greater trochanter • Per rectal examination reveals head of femur	
Treatment	Four methods of closed reduction 1. *Stimson's gravity method*: Least traumatic but associated injuries prevent prone positioning 2. *Allis*: Traction is given in line of deformity 3. *Bigelow's method*: Reduction is done by causing the opposite methods of ext/abd/ER 4. *Classical Watson-Jones method*: Limb is brought to the neutral position first then longitudinal traction in the line of femur is given.	1. *Stimson's gravity method* 2. *Allis method* 3. *Reverse Bigelow's method*: Here position of hip is flexion and adduction 4. *Classical method*: It is as described for posterior dislocation		Reduction is attempted through skeletal traction on greater trochanter in line of the neck of femur. If it fails, open reduction is indicated	
Complications	*Early* • Sciatic nerve palsy • Irreducible fracture dislocation • Missed knee injuries • Recurrent dislocations *Late* • Myositis ossificans • Avascular necrosis of bone • Post-traumatic arthritis • Unreduced posterior dislocation	*Early* • Neurovascular injuries • Femoral artery, vein, nerve injury • Irreducibility *Late* • Post-traumatic osteoarthritis • Aseptic necrosis • Recurrent dislocation		*I Early* • Sciatic nerve palsy • Superior gluteal artery injury • Bowel obstruction • Thrombophlebitis • Infection • Recurrent dislocation	*II Late* • Post-traumatic arthritis • AVN • Nonunion • Myositis ossificans

– Gross outline of the acetabular dome not intact and not congruous with the femoral head.
• Bursting fractures (All elements of the acetabulum are involved):
  – Fractures in which congruity remains between the femoral head and acetabular dome.
  – Fractures in which there is incongruity between the femoral head and acetabular dome.

Clinical Features

Interestingly none of the features as in ADH or PDH is seen. On the other hand, in CDH there is no limb shortening, no external rotation deformity, head is not externally palpable. The limb is in neutral position; there is pain, severe restriction of hip movements and a huge bruise over the greater trochanter. Head is felt easily by a per-rectal examination.

Investigations

X-ray evaluation: Plain X-ray plays a very important role in the diagnosis of these injuries (Fig. 17.20). The recommended views are AP view of the pelvis, internal and external oblique views. The former view helps in the demonstration of the femoral head acetabular relationship

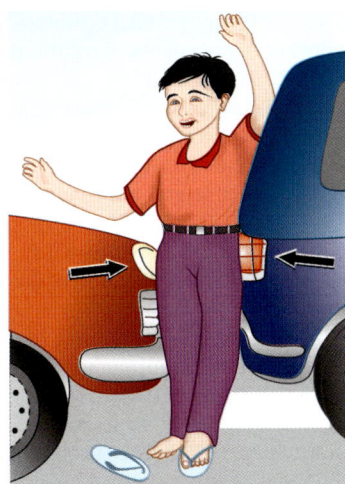

Fig. 17.19: Common mechanism of central dislocation of the hip

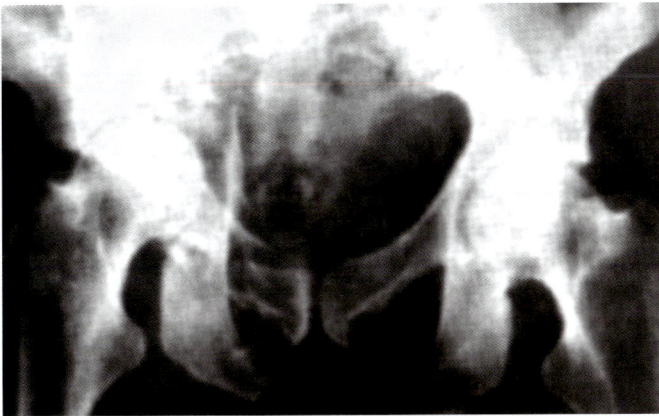

Fig. 17.20: Radiograph showing central fracture dislocation of the hip joint

while the latter views helps in delineating fracture lines and displacement.

CT scan: This helps to delineate the fracture lines better and with far more great accuracy than plain X-rays.

MRI scan: This helps to study the vascularity of the femoral head and the bony and cartilage architecture.

Treatment

Reduction of the dislocation assumes lot of clinical importance, as it is essential to obtain as accurate a reduction as possible to restore the acetabular congruity. This helps prevent post-traumatic osteoarthritis.

- *Skeletal traction:* Reduction is achieved through skeletal traction over the greater trochanter in line of the neck of femur. Open reduction is reserved for cases of failed closed reduction. The skeletal traction is maintained for 10–12 weeks if the acetabulum is reasonably reconstructed.
- *Open reduction and internal fixation:* If the reconstruction of the acetabulum is far from satisfactory, after the mandatory skeletal traction, then open reduction and surgical reconstruction of the acetabulum is recommended.
- *Primary arthroplasty or arthrodesis:* This is recommended in extreme cases where closed reduction fails and open reduction reveals severe articular damage.

Complications

Early complications: This includes sciatic nerve palsy, superior gluteal artery injury, thrombophlebitis, bowel obstruction, aseptic necrosis, pin-tract infection, recurrent central dislocations, etc.

Delayed complications: Post-traumatic osteoarthritis is an escapable complication in central dislocation. Other fearful complications include myositis, avascular necrosis of the femoral head and a stiff and disabling hip.

BIBLIOGRAPHY

1. Allis OH. An enquiry into the difficulties encountered in the Reduction of Dislocations of the Hip, Philadelphia, Dornan Printer; 1986.
2. Armstrong JR. Traumatic dislocation of the hip joint. Review of one hundred and one disorders. J Bone Joint Surg. 1948; 30B:430-45.
3. Bigelow HJ. Luxation of the hip joint. Boston Med Surg J. 1870;5:1-3.
4. Birkett J. Description of a dislocation of the head of the femur complicated with its fractures. Trans Med Chir Soc. 1869;52:133.
5. Brav EA. Traumatic dislocation of the hip. Army experience and results over a twelve-year period. J Bone Joint Surg. 1962; 44A:1115-34.
6. Bromberg E, Weiss AB. Posterior fracture-dislocation of the hip. South Med J. 1977;70:8-11.
7. Bucholz RW, Wheeless G. Irreducible posterior fracture dislocation of the hip. The role of the ilio-femoral ligament and the rectus femoris muscle. Clin Orthop. 1982;167:118-22.
8. Butler JE. Pipkin type II fractures of the femoral head. J Bone Joint Surg. 1981;63A:1292-6.
9. Catkins MS, Zycth G, Latta L, et al. Computed tomography evaluation of stability: Posterior fracture dislocation of the hip. Clin Orthop. 1988;227:152-63.
10. Canale ST, Manugian AH. Irreducible traumatic dislocations of the hip. J Bone Joint Surg. 1979;61A:7-14.
11. Chakraborti S, Miller IM. Dislocation of the hip associated with fracture of the femoral head. Injury. 1975;7:134-42.
12. Crock HV. An atlas of the arterial supply of the head and neck of the femur in man. Clin Orthop. 1980;152:17-27.
13. Delee JC. Dislocations and fracture dislocations of the hip. In: Rockwood CA, Green DP (Eds). Fractures and dislocations, 2nd Edition, Philadelphia, JB Lippincott; 1984.pp.1287-327.

14. DeLee JC, Evans JA, Thomas J. Anterior dislocation of the hip and associated femoral head fractures. J Bone Joint Surg. 1984;62A:960-4.
15. Derian PS, Bibighaus AJ. Sciatic nerve entrapment by ectopic bone after posterior fracture-dislocation of the hip. South Med J. 1974;67:209-10.
16. Epstein HC. Traumatic dislocations of the hip. Clin Orthop. 1973;92:116-42.
17. Epstein HC. Posterior fracture dislocations of the hip: Long-term follow-up. J Bone Joint Surg. 1974;56A:1103-27.
18. Epstein HC. Traumatic anterior dislocations of the hip. Management and Results. An analysis of fifty-five cases. J Bone Joint Surg. 1972;54A:1561-2.
19. Epstein HC, Wiss DA, Coze L. Posterior fracture dislocations of the hip with fractures of the femoral head. Clin Orthop. 1985;201:0-17.
20. Funsten RV, Kinser P, Frankel CJ. Dashboard dislocations of the hip. A report of twenty cases of traumatic dislocations. J Bone Joint Surg. 1938;20:124-32.
21. Garrett JC, Epstein HC, Harris WH, et al. Treatment of unreduced traumatic posterior dislocations of the hip. J Bone Joint Surg. 1979;61A:2-6.
22. Hardinge K. The direct lateral approach to the hip. J Bone Joint Surg. 1982;64B:17-9.
23. Hougard K, Lindenquest S, Nielsen LB. Computerized tomography after posterior dislocation of the hip. J Bone Joint Surg. 1987;69B:556-7.
24. Judet R, Judet J, le Tournel E. Fractures of the acetabulum. Classification and surgical approaches for open reduction. J Bone Joint Surg. 1964;46A:1615-46.
25. Pipkin G. Treatment of grade IV fracture dislocation of the hip. J Bone Joint Surg. 1957;39A:1027-42.

18 CHAPTER

Fracture Femur

This includes proximal femur fractures, fractures of the shaft and distal femoral fractures.

FRACTURE NECK OF FEMUR

This is discussed in geriatric trauma.

PROXIMAL FEMUR FRACTURES

SUBTROCHANTERIC FRACTURE

Subtrochanteric region is defined as an area between the lesser trochanter and a point 5 cm distal to it. Subtrochanteric fracture is a difficult fracture due to problems like malunion, delayed union, nonunion, shortening, angular deformity, rotational malalignment, etc. (Fig. 18.1). Two factors responsible for slow union are:
- Fracture through the cortical bone
- Large biomechanical stress at the fracture site results in implant failure.

Mechanism of Injury

It is usually due to direct trauma due to RTA or fall and is common in young individuals.

It can be broadly considered under two headings:

Stable fracture: Intact or possible to re-establish bone-to-bone contact of the medial and posterior femoral cortex anatomically.

Unstable fracture: Posteromedial cortex apposition is not obtainable.

Classification

Fielding's Classification

This is based on distance at or below the lesser trochanter (Fig. 18.2).

Type I : Fracture at the level of the lesser trochanter.
Type II : Fracture 1" below the lesser trochanter.
Type III : Fracture 2" below the lesser trochanter.

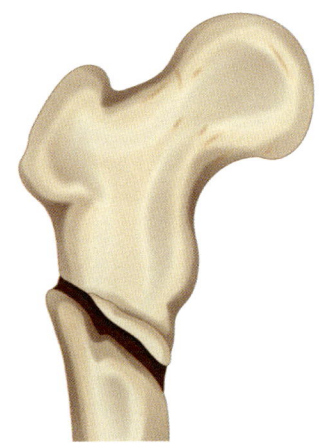

Fig. 18.1: Subtrochanteric fracture

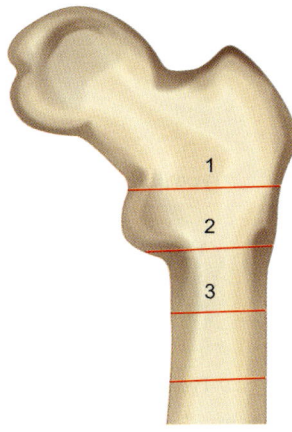

Fig. 18.2: Fielding's classification

Seinsheimer's Classification

This is based on the number of major fragments and the location and shape of fracture lines (Fig. 18.3).

Type I	:	Undisplaced fracture.
Type II	:	Two part fracture.
Type III	:	Three part fracture.
		A—Lesser trochanter is the 3rd fragment
		B—Butterfly fragment is the 3rd part
Type IV	:	Four part fracture.
Type V	:	Subtrochanteric comminuted fracture with intertrochanteric extension.

Russel Taylor Classification

This is based on the involvement of the subtrochanteric fracture with the pyriformis fossa.

Type I	:	Subtrochanteric fracture does not extend into the pyriformis fossa.
Type II	:	The fracture extends proximally into greater trochanter and extends into the pyriformis fossa.

Clinical Features

The patient presents with pain, swelling, shortening, complete external rotation deformity and other usual features of fractures.

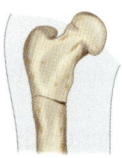 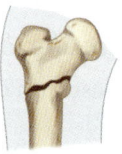

Type I (Below lesser trochanter)   Type II (At the level of lesser trochanter)

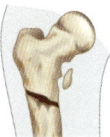 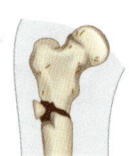 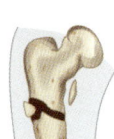

Type III A   Type III B   Type IV

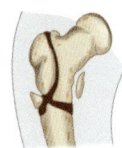

Type V

Fig. 18.3: Seinsheimer's varieties of subtrochanteric fractures of femur

Radiographs

Radiograph helps to study the level and pattern of fracture and thereby plan the treatment (Fig. 18.4).

Treatment

Conservative: Methods are advocated if the patient is young. In severely comminuted fractures, modified cast brace with pelvic band is used.

Surgery: This is the preferred method of treatment in adults and ORIF is chosen for those fractures, which can be made stable by closed or open reduction. The choice of implants in different levels of the fracture is shown in the Box 18.1.

Box 18.1: Fixation Facts

For internal fixation of subtrochanteric fractures, the choice is made from the following:
- Spiral blade plate for pathological or impending pathological subtrochanteric fractures.
- Proximal femoral nail (PFN) (Fig. 18.5A).
- DHS is not ideally suited.
- Dynamic condylar plate, condylar blade plate, and dynamic condylar screw are other useful options (Fig. 18.5B).

Pattern of fracture	Choice of implant
Low transverse fracture and short oblique fracture with 1" intact cortex	IM nailing or a interlocking nail
In fracture above this level without trochanteric extension	Locking nail or Zickel nail
In fracture above this level with trochanteric extension	Sliding compression hip screw *Medial stability is obtained by either compression of interfragment or medial*

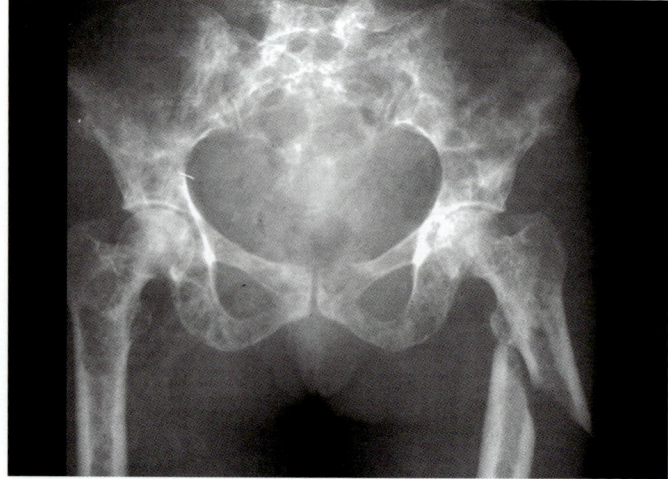

Fig. 18.4: Radiograph showing subtrochanteric fracture femur

displacement or valgus reduction. Fixed nail plate is not recommended. Bone graft is used.

Recent trends in the fixation of pertrochanteric and subtrochanteric fractures: With the gamma nail, stable osteosynthesis of subtrochanteric and pertrochanteric fracture femur is obtained independently of the fracture classification (Fig. 18.6). Patients can be mobilized immediately with this method. However, care must be taken to avoid technical errors.

The Russel Taylor reconstruction nail has greatly improved the fixation methods for subtrochanteric fractures. This has proximal and distal interlocking screw fixation and is a closed nailing technique.

Fixation Methods in a Nutshell
For subtrochanteric fractures (This is based on the Russell Taylor classification)
Type IA: With intact Pyriformis fossa and lesser trochanter: Standard interlocking IM nail.
Type IB: With Piriformis fossa intact, lesser trochanter fractured: Reconstruction IM Nail.
Type IIA: Pyriformis fossa fractures but lesser trochanter is intact: Reconstruction nail or hip screw.
Type IIB: Both Pyriformis fossa and lesser trochanter fractured: Same is in Type IIA but with bone graft along with hip screws.

Complications

- *Malunion:* This is a possibility with conservative treatment (Figs 18.7A to D)
- Shortening.

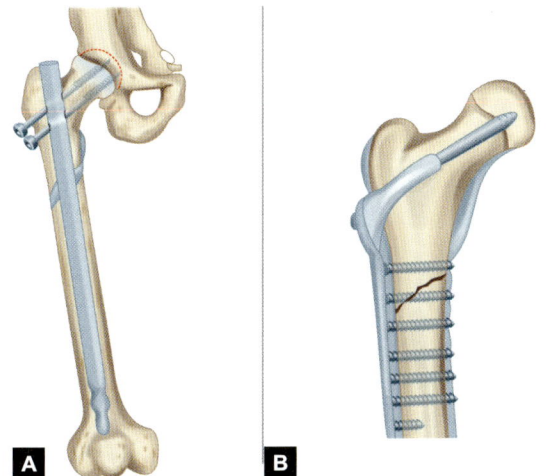

Figs 18.5A and B: Different methods of fixation for subtrochanteric fracture: (A) Interlocking nail; (B) Fixation with DCS

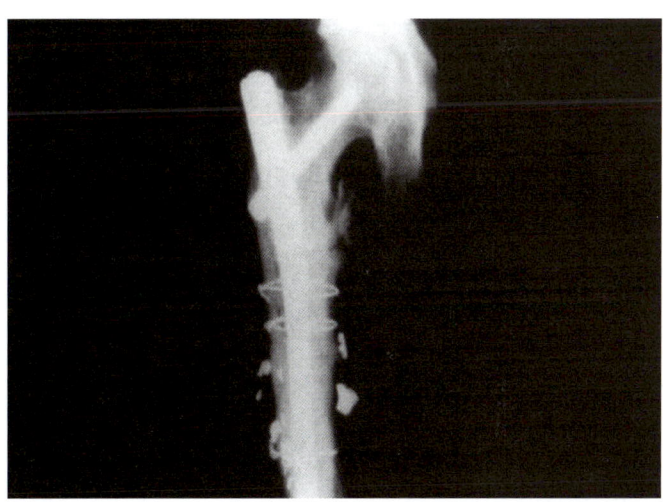

Fig. 18.6: Radiograph showing subtrochanteric fracture fixed with gamma nail (PFN)

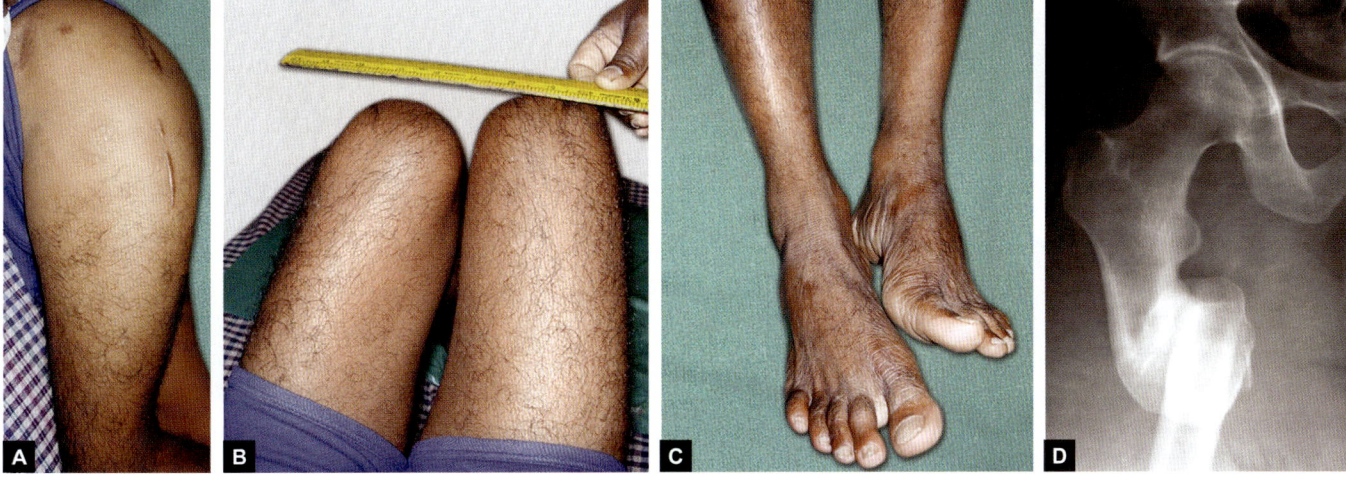

Figs 18.7A to D: Clinical photos and plain X-ray showing malunion subtrochanteric fracture

- Nonunion due to soft tissue interposition and is relatively rare.
- Secondary osteoarthritis of the hip
- Contralateral hip and knee pain due to limp and altered weight bearing mechanism.

Salient Features about Femur
Femur: A Must Know Facts
- It is the longest and the strongest bone in the body
- It is the heaviest bone
- A person's height is four times the length of femur.
- It has three parts: Proximal end, distal end, and shaft.
- The shaft extends from the level of the lesser trochanter to the flare of the condyles.
- The shaft is slightly bowed anteriorly and is narrowest at the mid-shaft.
- The cross-section is circular
- Linea aspera is the thick ridge of bone-situated mid-posterior.
- Muscle forces acting on the femur at different sites (Fig. 18.8).
  Proximal third: Iliopsoas flex, abductors abduct, and external rotators cause abduction and external rotation of proximal fragment, while adductors adduct the distal fragment.
  Middle third: There is shortening and adduction.
  Distal third: This is flexed due to the action of gastrocnemius muscle (Fig. 18.9).
  The blood supply to the shaft of femur is rich and adequate and thus the fracture in this area usually unites well.
  The above muscular forces should be taken into consideration while planning the treatment for fracture shaft femur.

FRACTURE SHAFT FEMUR

Fracture shaft femur is a serious injury and is usually due to severe violence. It may be associated with severe blood loss (up to 1,500 mL), multiple fractures, and multisystem injuries, but heavy musculature, however, provides unlimited blood supply and thus the fracture heals well.

Mechanism of Injury

Usually, it is due to major violence, and is common in young adults because the strong metaphyseal areas transmit the forces to the shaft causing fracture (Fig. 18.10). In old age, the metaphyseal areas are brittle and hence the shaft fracture is rare, but fracture of metaphyseal region is common (Box 18.2).

Box 18.2: Quick Facts: Mechanism of Injury
In Adults
- RTA commonest cause
- Industrial accidents
- Fall from height
- Gunshot injuries

In Children
- Fall
- Birth injuries
  Male-female ratio = 3: 1
  Average age of occurrence = 25-35 years

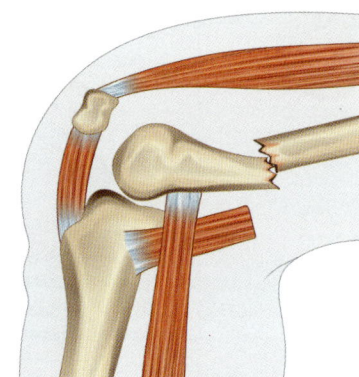

Fig. 18.9: In the distal third, the gastrocnemius flexes the distal end of femur

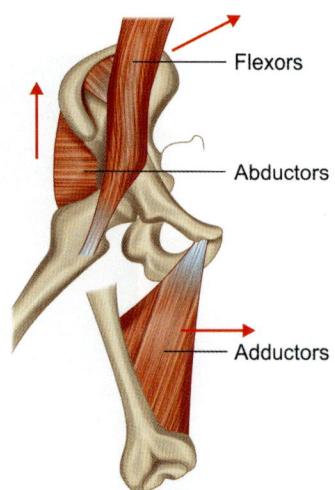

Fig. 18.8: Muscle forces acting across the shaft of femur

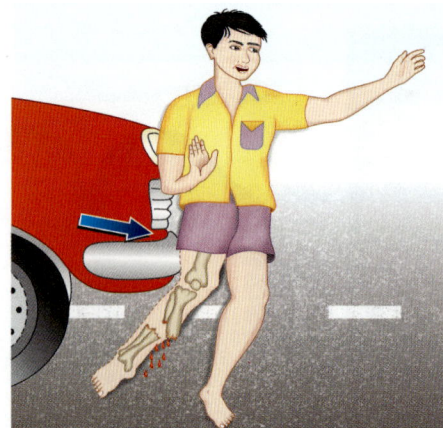

Fig. 18.10: Bumper injuries in RTA commonly cause fracture femur and tibia

Classification of Femur Fractures (Figs 18.11A to E)

- Femoral fractures could be in the proximal, midshaft, or distal fragments.
- Each of the above fractures could be transverse, oblique, spiral, segmental, or comminuted.
- Based on the degree of comminution, Winquist and Hansen have described four types:
    - Type I: None or significant comminution.
    - Type II: <50% comminution.
    - Type III: 50–100% comminution of the cortex.
    - Type IV: No contact between major fragments.
- AO/ASIF classification.
    - Type A: Simple fracture (transverse/oblique/spiral/minimal comminution).
    - Type B: Wedge fractures and greater than one fracture line.
    - Type C: Extensive comminution.

Clinical Features

Apart from all the features of fractures, there could be shortening of the lower limb and complete external rotation deformity such that the lateral border of the foot touches the bed (Fig. 18.12). Since the fracture femur is usually due to major violence, the patient may also present with features of shock, like unconsciousness, pallor, cold nose, tachycardia, cold and clammy skin, hypotension, etc.

Radiographs

Routine anteroposterior and lateral views (Figs 18.13 and 18.14) of the femur suffice, but care should be taken to include the neighboring joints (hip and knee) to rule out the possibilities of injuries to these joints.

Management

General Principles

- Almost 100% union occurs whether fracture is treated by closed or open reduction methods.
- By internal fixation, hospital stay is reduced.
- Simpler the fracture, more likely to be treated by open reduction and internal fixation (ORIF).
- More comminuted the fracture, less likely is the internal fixation attempted. For severely comminuted fracture and extensive soft tissue damage, traction is the safest. Interlocking nailing is the other popular alternative.

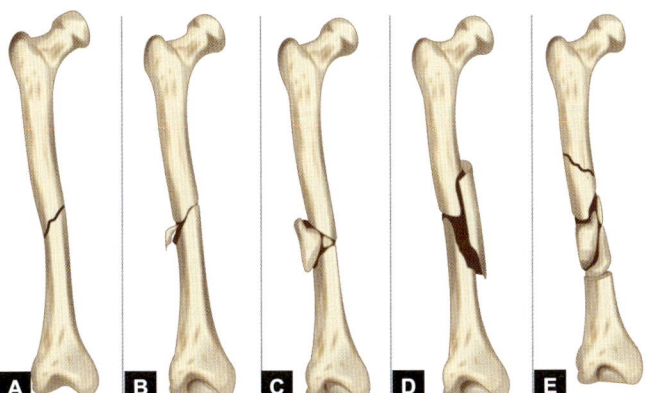

Figs 18.11A to E: Varieties of femoral shaft fractures: (A and B) Simple fracture; (C) Wedge fracture; (D) Butterfly fracture; (E) Comminution

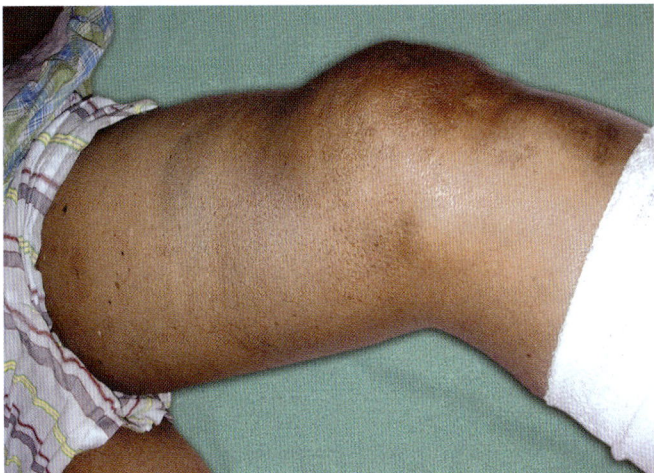

Fig. 18.12: Deformity in fracture femur (Clinical photo)

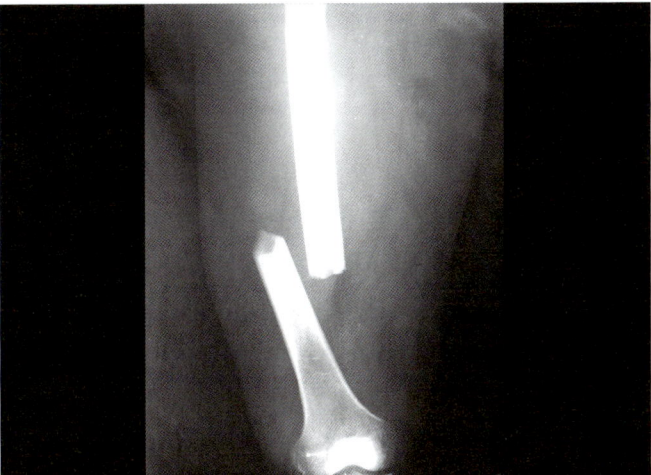

Fig. 18.13: Radiograph showing fracture shaft femur

216 SECTION 2: Regional Traumatology

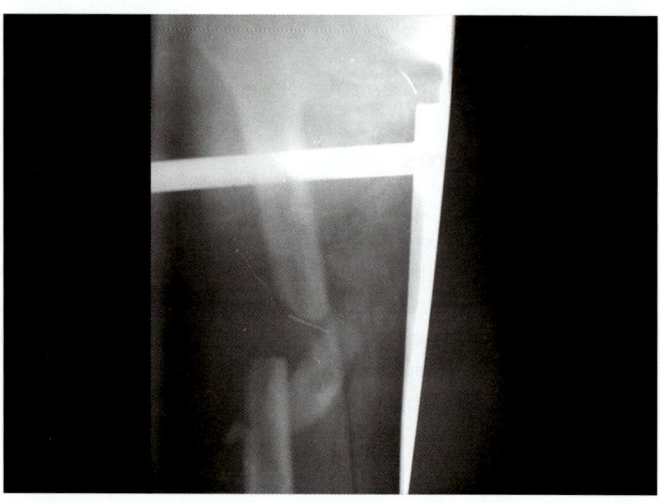

Fig. 18.14: Radiograph showing comminuted fracture shaft femur under Thomas splint

Treatment Methods (Flowchart 18.1)

Conservative Methods

Children: It is mainly conservative in children more than 15 years of age.

0 to 2 years	— Plaster spica in human position[1] or modified Bryant or Gallows's traction (Fig. 18.15).
2 to 10 years	— Most femoral fractures are seen in this age group. Here split Russell traction (Fig. 18.16) is more useful.
10 to 15 years	— 90 to 90° femoral skeletal traction or hip spica or both (Fig. 18.17).
More than 15 years	— Treatment is as in adults.

Flowchart 18.1: Depicting the treatment plan in fracture shaft of femur

```
Treatment plan in fracture shaft of femure
├── Closed fractures (common)
│   ├── Conservative
│   │   ├── Children
│   │   │   • Gallow's traction
│   │   │   • Hip spica
│   │   │   • Russel traction
│   │   │   • TEN (Titanium elastic nailing)
│   │   └── Adults
│   │       • Skin traction
│   │       • Skeletal traction
│   │       • Russel traction (Only as first aid measure)
│   └── Surgical methods
│       ├── Open methods
│       │   ├── K-nail (For fracture at isthmus level)
│       │   └── Plating
│       │       ├── DCP
│       │       │   Problems are
│       │       │   • Infection
│       │       │   • Fracture hematoma lost
│       │       │   • Quadriceps scarring
│       │       │   • Refracture
│       │       └── MIPO
│       │           Bridge plating (Biological fixation)
│       │           Here plate is fixed proximally and distally and the central fracture area is rendered untouched. Here fracture hematoma and soft tissue damage is minimized
│       └── Closed methods (ILN) (Gold standard)
│           For fractures other than isthmus like proximal, distal, comminuted and segmental fractures
│           ├── Dynamic
│           │   Advantages
│           │   • Early mobilization and weight bearing
│           │   • Biological fixation
│           │   • Less infection rate
│           │   • Less blood loss, etc.
│           └── Static
└── Open fractures (rare)
    └── Debridement
        ├── Closed interlocking nailing (A better option)
        └── External fixator
            Problems
            • Shortening
            • Pintract infection
            • Quadriceps scarring
            • Malunion
            • Knee stiffness
```

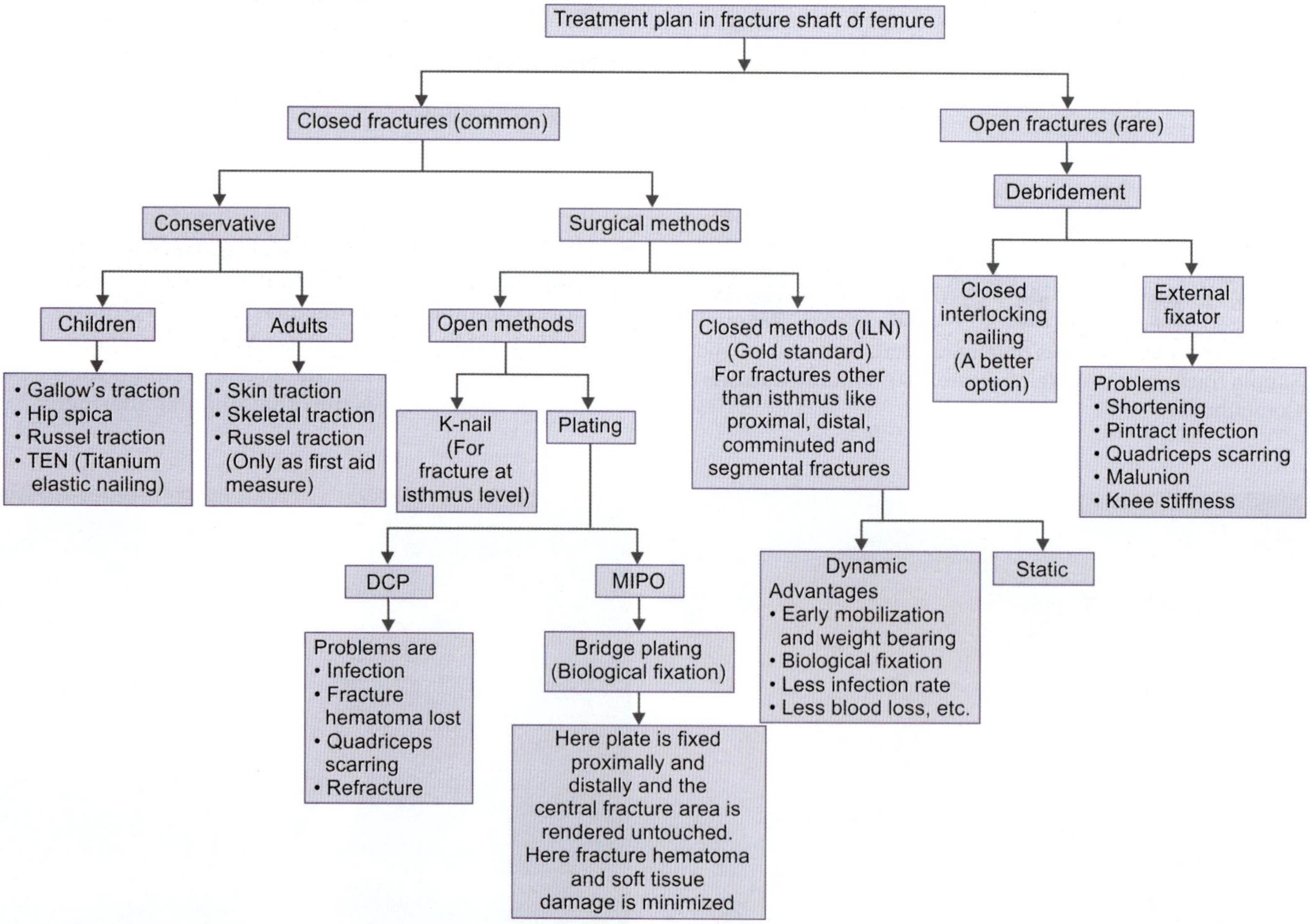

Note:
• Metaphyseal fractures are the only indication for primary plating.
• Minimally invasive plate osteosynthesis (MIPO).

---

[1]Human position is 90° of flexion and 45° of external rotation at the hip.

What is New?
Of late, femur fractures in children are increasingly being treated by operative methods. A special IM nail is being used for this purpose in children [titanium elastic nail (TEN)] (Fig. 18.18).

Adults: Three modalities of conservative treatment are described.
- *Traction:* This could be:
  - *Skin traction:* It is useful only during transportation as a first aid measure.
  - *Skeletal traction:* It is useful only in early stages and hence its role is limited. However, the patient treated in traction shows 100% union, but it causes shortening, and hence is not acceptable. The average time of traction required is 12 weeks and this gives rise to recumbency complications like bedsores, pneumonia, renal calculus, etc.
- *Cast bracing:* This method causes an unacceptable varus of more than 8° and hence is not recommended (Fig. 18.19).

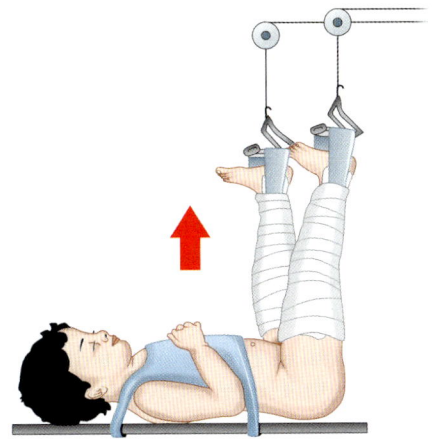

Fig. 18.15: Gallows' traction in children (<2 years of age)

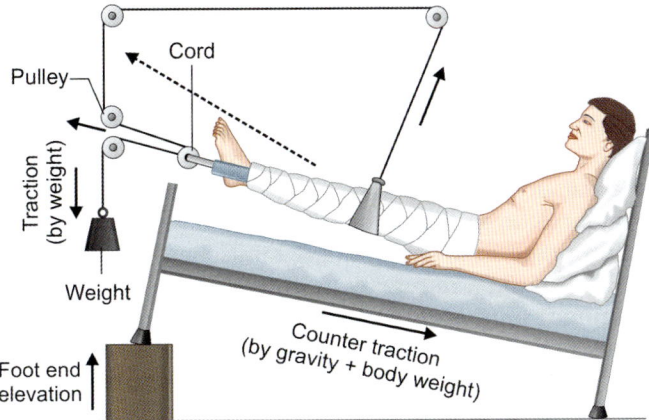

Fig. 18.16: Russell traction

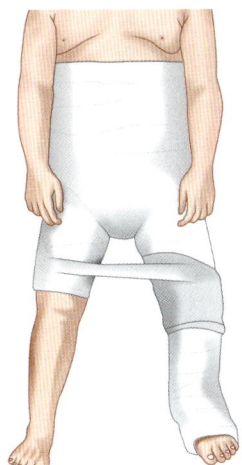

Fig. 18.17: Treatment of fracture shaft femur in children by hip spica

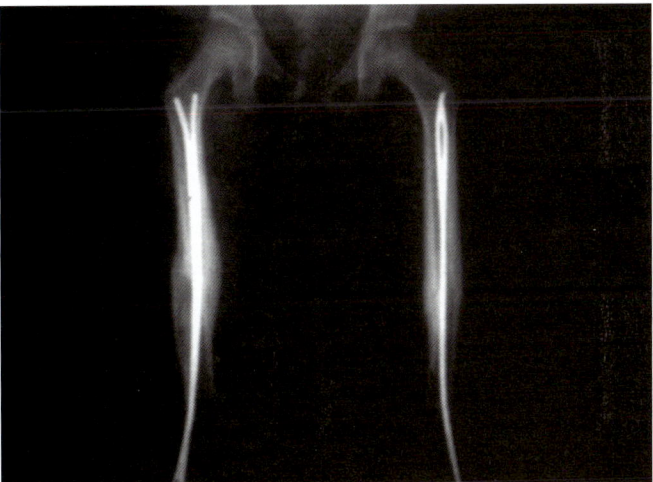

Fig. 18.18: Radiograph showing femur fracture in children treated with titanium elastic nails (TENs)

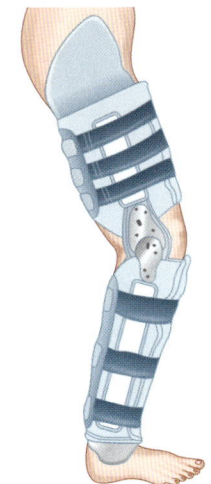

Fig. 18.19: Functional cast brace

Surgery

The best method of managing a fracture shaft femur in adults is by ORIF. The choice of the implants could be from a standard intramedullary nail (K-nail), interlocking nail, or plating (Figs 18.20A to C). Now let us try to know about these in detail:

Intramedullary (IM) nails can be used for fractures 2.5 cm below the lesser trochanter to that 8–10 cm above the knee joint. It can be used in simple or comminuted fractures (Fig. 18.21). It can be done immediately or delayed. Infection and nonunion is rare (0.8%).

Types of Nails in Common Usage for Fixing Fracture Shaft Femur
- *Standard IM nails (Küntscher's nail):* The ideal indication for this nail is the fracture shaft femur in adults at the level of isthmus. Isthmus is the portion of the femoral shaft. It is the junction between the upper and middle one-third and is the narrowest portion of the shaft.
- *Interlocking nails (Gross-Kempf nail):* These extend the indications of standard IM nail and can be used in the following situations where IM nail is less successful:
  - Comminuted fractures
  - Segmental fractures
  - Proximal and distal fractures
  - Nonunion, etc.
- *Flexible medullary nails* like Ender's nail, which is usually passed from below upwards through the distal femur.

What is New in Femoral Nails?
- UFN: Unreamed femoral nail
- CFN: Cannulated femoral nail
- PFN: Proximal femoral nail
- DEN: Distal femoral nail
- TEN: Titanium elastic nail used in children.

Cardinal Points in IM Nailing Technique
- Full set of nail size and length should be available before surgery.
- K-nails are available in 8 diameters from 8 to 15 mm. Average diameter is 11 to 12 mm.
- Ream the canal by reamers with progressively increasing size.
- Select the nail diameter equal or 1 size more of the reamer to provide a snug fit.
- The open slot of the K-nail is placed anterolaterally on the convex (tension) side of the femur. This helps convert the tensile force into compressive force at the fracture site.
- The eye of the nail should face posteromedially, so that extraction can easily be made later.
- The upper end of the nail should be less than 2.5 cm above the trochanter and the distal end should extend to the level of the proximal pole of the patella.
- The clover shape of the K-nail helps prevent rotation in the canal.

Intramedullary nail can be inserted either through the open or closed techniques. A comparative study is presented in Table 18.1.

Technique of Intramedullary Nailing (Küntscher's Nail)

After anesthesia (preferably spinal), strong traction is exerted on the affected limb to reduce the fracture and the patient is firmly fastened to the operating table. The limb is painted and draped. Through a lateral or posterolateral approach, the fracture is exposed. By using suitable sized medullary reamers, the proximal and distal fragments are reamed. Appropriate sized snugly fitting Küntscher's nail is chosen and driven in a retrograde fashion through the proximal fragment until it emerges into the subcutaneous tissue through the greater trochanter. The fracture is now reduced under direct vision and the nail is driven down into the distal fragment. The wound is closed in layers over a drain.

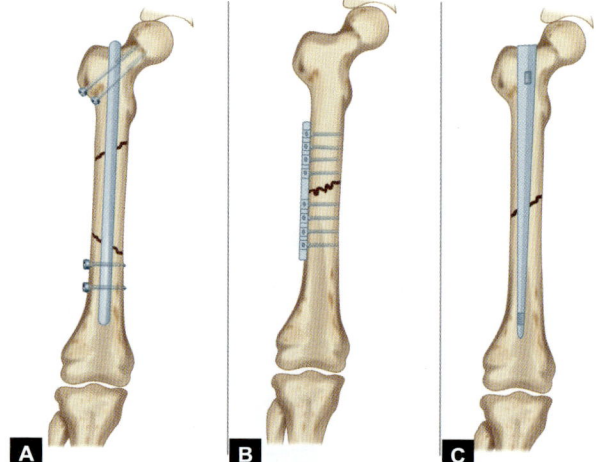

Figs 18.20A to C: Methods of internal fixation for fracture shaft femur: (A) Interlocking nail; (B) DCP plate and screws; (C) Küntscher's intermedullary nails

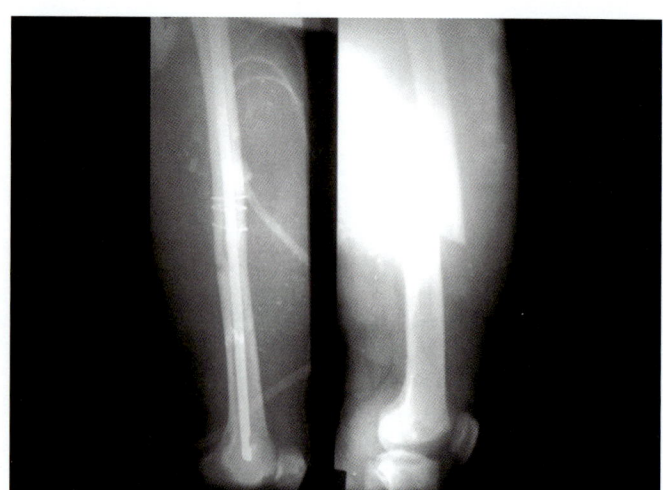

Fig. 18.21: Radiograph showing IM nailing femur

TABLE 18.1: Open and closed techniques compared

Sl.No.	Features	Open technique	Closed technique
1.	Equipment required	Less expensive	More expensive
2.	Fracture table	Not a must	Always required
3.	C-arm	Not required	Required
4.	Anatomic reduction	Easier to obtain	Difficult to obtain
5.	Method of nailing	Retrograde	Antegrade
6.	Blood loss	More	Less
7.	Direct visualization of fracture site	Possible	Not possible
8.	Fracture hematoma	Lost	Preserved
9.	Exposure time	More	Nil
10.	Skin scar	More	Less
11.	Infection rate	High	Less
12.	Tissue trauma	More	Less
13.	Technique	Simple	Demanding
14.	Morbidity	More	Less

Complications of K-nail

The following are some of the well-known complications of K-nail:
- If the nail size is small—it may bend, break or migrate in the proximal or distal direction.
- If the nail size is large—it may splinter the bone or the nail gets jammed in the medullary canal.
- If the nail is projecting more than 2–5 cm in the upper end, it may lead to the development of an adventitious bursa in the glutei region which if inflamed causes pain and limp.
- If the nail is extending more into the distal fragment, it may cause a reactionary effusion in the knee joint.
- Faulty asepsis during insertion leads to infection.

Note:
- Standard IM nailing has given way to interlocking nails in a very big way.
- Open method allows direct visualization of fracture site and hence fracture can be anatomically fixed. Nevertheless, the chances of infection are quite high with this technique.

Interlocking Nailing Technique (Gold Standard)

In this, the patient is securely fixed to a fracture table (Fig. 18.22). Under C-arm control, a suitable sized IM nail is passed through the trochanter into the proximal fragment and driven down into the distal fragment after reducing the fracture and reaming it. The interlocking nail has two holes in the upper and lower ends unlike the standard IM nails. Transverse screws are passed through the upper and lower holes and the nail is locked into position (Fig. 18.23).

Note:
Interlocking is the best method of internal fixation for fracture shaft femur, but technically difficult as it requires sophisticated equipment like C-arm, instrumentation, etc.

Plates

Dynamic compression plating is used for proximal and distal one-third fractures. However, it is less commonly used nowadays. However in the management of non-union femur, open reduction and rigid internal fixation with bone grafting, it still has a place (Fig. 18.24).

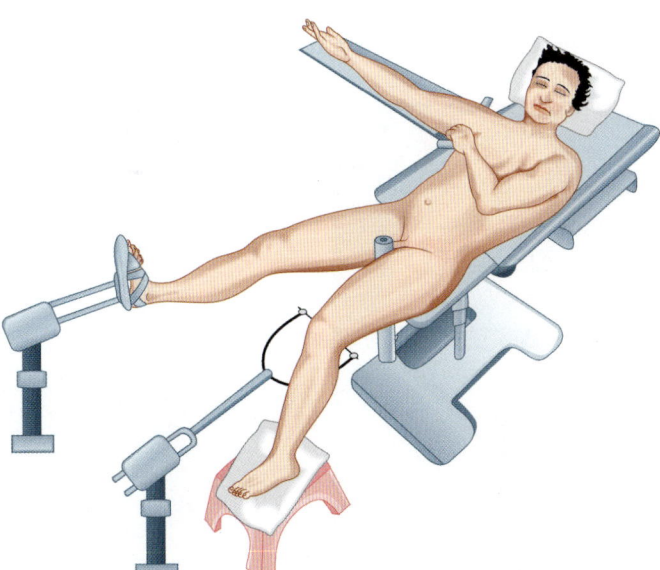

Fig. 18.22: Positioning for ILN femur

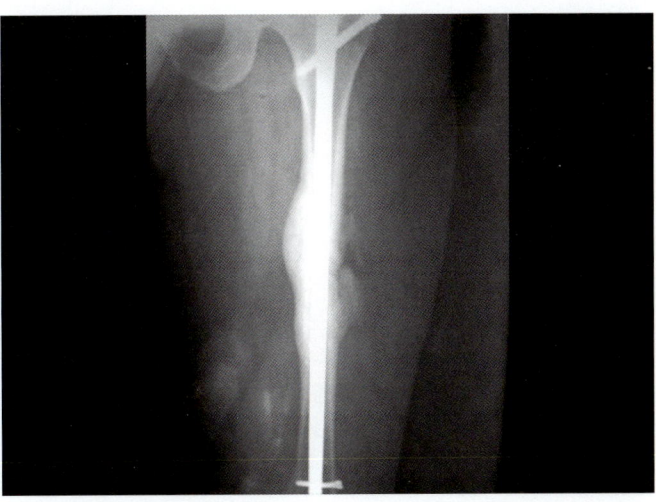

Fig. 18.23: Radiograph showing interlocking femur

Vital Facts

Standard IM nailing and plating have fallen into disrepute. Interlocking nail has emerged as the gold standard in treating most of the shaft femur fractures in adults.

Future trends: What does the future hold for fracture femur treatment?
- Titanium metal
- Bioabsorbable polyesters (Polyglycolide or polylactide). This eliminates need for extraction.

Complications

- *Immediate complications:* These are life, threatening and the common ones are shock, fat embolism neurovascular injury to the femoral artery, sciatic nerve, etc.
- *Delayed complications:* These are more common and include:

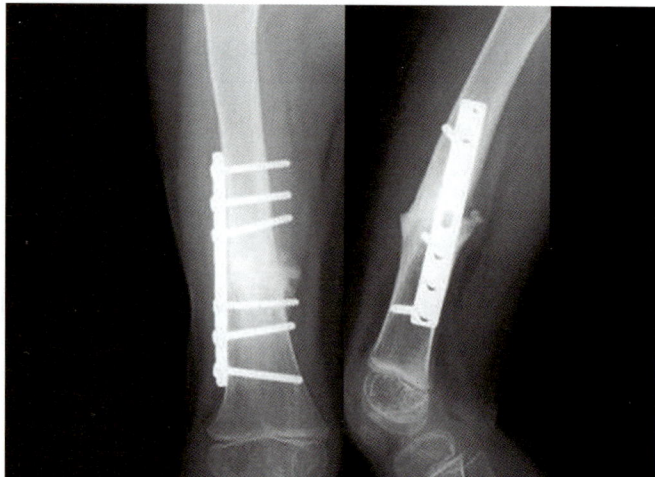

Fig. 18.24: Plain X-rays showing DCP plating for nonunion fracture femur

  – *Refracture:* This is the most embarrassing complication and is commonly seen in simpler fractures due to poor welding of the fracture site by the callus and after plate removal due to the holes left over by the removal of screws which takes time to fill up leaving a potential weak spot for refracture. The incidence of this complication is around 9–15 percent.
  – *Complications of fixation devices:* The problems usually encountered with intramedullary nails are breaking, loosening, proximal or distal migration, jamming, bending, infection, etc. These may be due to faulty implants, techniques, or choice.
  – *Nerve injury:* Injury to the common peroneal nerve is more often seen in these fractures. However, it is not a very common occurrence.
  – *Malunion:* This is one of the most common complications seen in fracture shaft femur and is due to the strong and variable muscular forces already described. Malunion is more often seen following conservative treatment and traction than in operative treatment (Figs 18.25A to D).
  – *Nonunion:* It is not that common as, fracture shaft femur is known to unite well. If it happens all the features of nonunion can be seen (Figs 18.26A to C).
  – *Joint stiffness:* In fracture shaft femur knee joint may become stiff due to quadriceps atrophy following prolonged immobilization and due to intra-articular or extra-articular adhesions.

FRACTURE DISTAL FEMUR

The distal part of the femur encompasses the lower one-third. It varies between 7.6 cm and 15 cm of distal femur. The supracondylar area is a transition zone between the

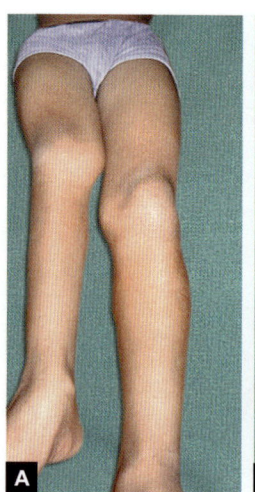
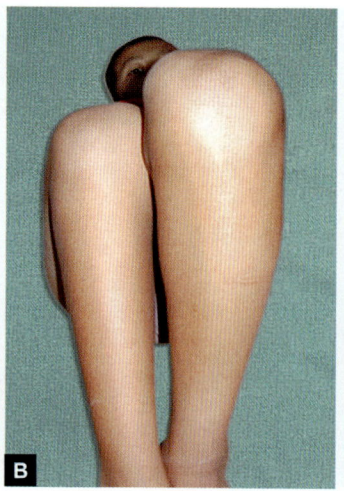
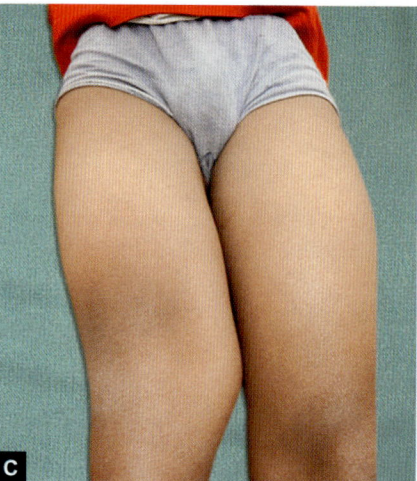
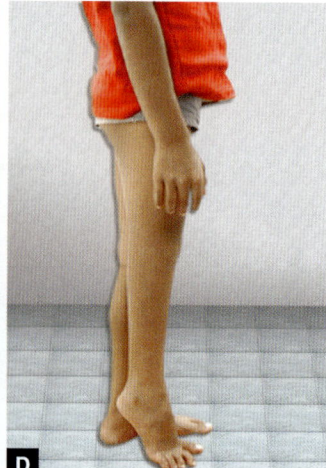

Figs 18.25A to D: Clinical photos in malunion fracture femur

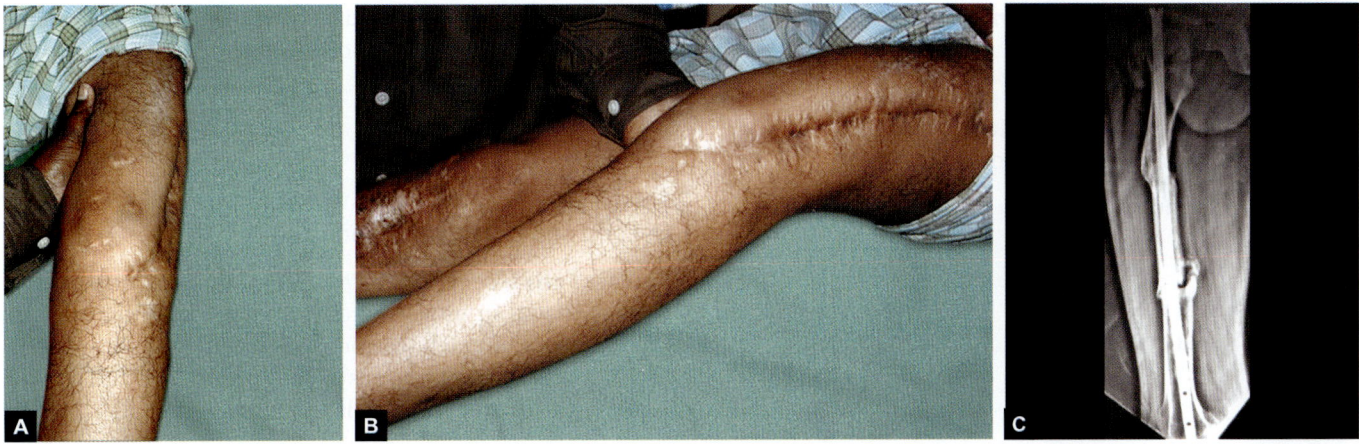

Figs 18.26A to C: Clinical photos and X-ray showing nonunion fracture shaft femur

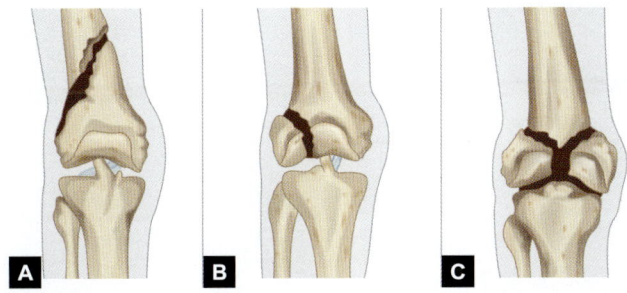

Figs 18.27A to C: Fractures of distal femur: (A) Supracondylar fracture; (B) Unicondylar fracture; (C) Comminuted fractures (Bicondylar)

distal diaphysis and the femoral articular surface. The distal femur is subjected to the quadriceps force anteriorly and the flexion force of the gastrocnemius posteriorly (see Fig. 18.8). The fractures of the distal femur could be classified into supracondylar, intercondylar, unicondylar and comminuted fractures (Figs 18.27A to C). The distal femur fracture accounts for 7% of all femoral fractures and consists of supracondylar fractures and intercondylar fractures.

SUPRACONDYLAR FRACTURE OF FEMUR

Supracondylar region extends from the femoral condyles to the junction of metaphysis with femoral shaft. The distal fragment is displaced and angulated posteriorly due to the pull of gastrocnemius muscle.

Mechanism of Injury

It is due to severe valgus or varus forces with axial loading and rotation due to RTA, fall, etc.

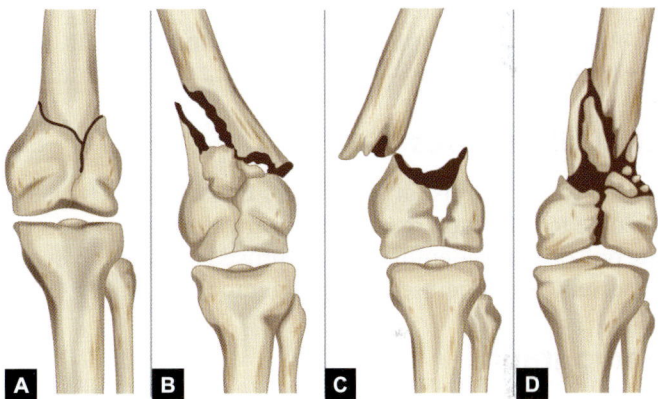

Figs 18.28A to D: Neer's classification for supracondylar fractures: (A) Undisplaced; (B) Displaced and medial; (C) Displaced and lateral; (D) Comminuted

Classification

Neer's Classification (Figs 18.28A to D)

- Undisplaced fracture
- Displaced fracture:
  - Medial displacement
  - Lateral displacement
- Comminuted fractures.

Müller's AO Classification

- Type A: Extra-articular fractures
- Type B: Unicondylar fractures
- Type C: Bicondylar fractures.

Each is further subdivided into 1–3 depending on the severity of comminution.

OTA Classification of Supracondylar Fractures of Femur

- Type A: Extra-articular.
- Type B: Partial articular (Unicondylar).
- Type C: Total articular (Bicondylar).

Further Subdivisions

Type A
- Simple.
- Metaphyseal wedge.
- Metaphyseal comminution.

Type B
- Fracture lateral condyle.
- Fracture medial condyle.
- Frontal fracture.

Type C
- Articular and metaphyseal simple.
- Articular simple and metaphyseal comminution.
- Total comminution.

Clinical Features

It consists of the usual features of fractures, but what is specific to this fracture is the flexion deformity caused by the pull of gastrocnemius. Hemarthrosis is commonly seen, especially with fractures extending into the joint.

Radiographs

Radiograph helps to study the fracture pattern more accurately. Routine AP, lateral and oblique (45°) views are required (Figs 18.29 and 18.30).

Arteriography: This should be performed in suspected vascular damage or in associated dislocation of the knee joint.

Treatment

The treatment usually consists of conservative methods, traction and operative methods.

Conservative methods: This has a limited role and is usually useful in impacted and undisplaced fractures. In the former, a long leg or spica cast is sufficient and in the latter, a long above knee cast after an initial period of skin or skeletal traction is all that is required (Figs 18.31A and B).

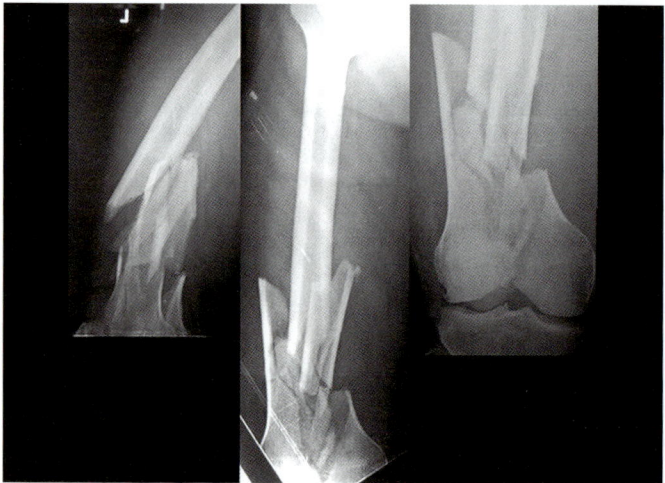

Fig. 18.30: Plain X-ray showing comminuted supracondylar fracture femur

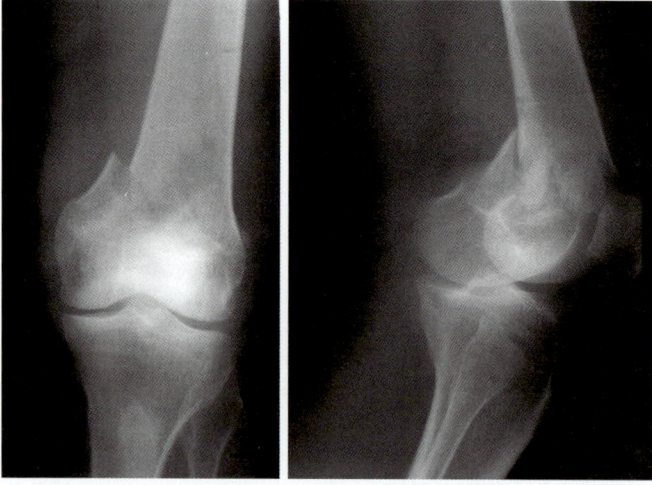

Fig. 18.29: Radiograph showing supracondylar fracture

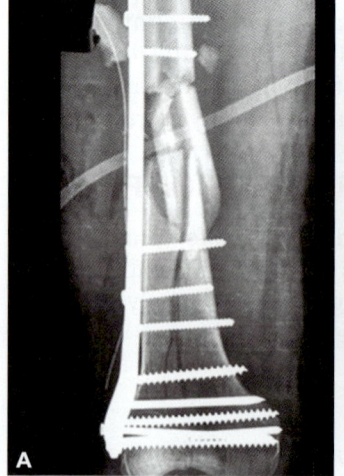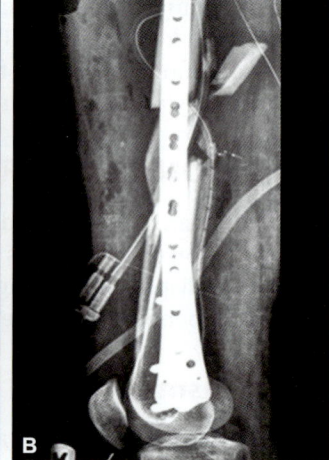

Figs 18.31A and B: Fixation techniques for fractures of distal femur

Traction methods: The choice is mainly skeletal traction and two methods are described:
- *Upper tibial traction:* Here the skeletal traction is applied through the upper end of tibia (Fig. 18.32). Initial weight used is around 15–20 lbs and is subsequently reduced. The traction is given for a period of 8–12 weeks and the patient is put on cast braces. To prevent the knee stiffness from developing, the patient is encouraged to carry out the knee movements during the traction itself.
- *Two-pin traction method:* In this method, traction is added through the distal femur apart from the traction given through the upper end of tibia. This helps in accurate reduction of the fracture and maintains the reduction so obtained. The disadvantage of this technique is that it is cumbersome and may cause neurovascular compressions in and around the knee.

Operative methods: This consists of ORIF (Fig. 18.33) and is preferred as the closed reduction is associated with troublesome complications like limited knee motion, residual varus, and internal rotation deformities. The advantages of open reduction are early mobilization of the knee joint and an accurate reduction and rigid fixation.

Fixation methods: The choice is between medullary fixation and blade plate fixation (Fig. 18.34).

Intramedullary fixations: Rush pins, Ender's nail, medullary nails, split nails, static locking nails, etc. are some of the commonly used medullary fixation methods. They offer biological fixation but the fixation offered is less stable.

Blade plate fixations: AO plates, Elliott or Jewett plates comprise the blade fixation methods, but they are technically demanding (Fig. 18.35).

Dynamic condylar screw (DCS) also gives good fixation and is a better option. But it requires a minimum of 4 cm of uncomminuted bone over the intercondylar notch for effective fixation.

Buttress plate is recommended in highly comminuted fractures.

Condylar locking plates with special screws that help the plates to be locked to the bone are now being increasingly used and are giving good results. The offer good fixation and prevents varus angulations.

External fixation is being used either for temporary or permanent fixation of these fractures in open distal femoral fractures and if associated with vascular injuries.

LISS (Less invasive stabilization system) has a learning curve and gives good results in trained hands. This has less morbidity and offers all the advantages of a minimally invasive procedure.

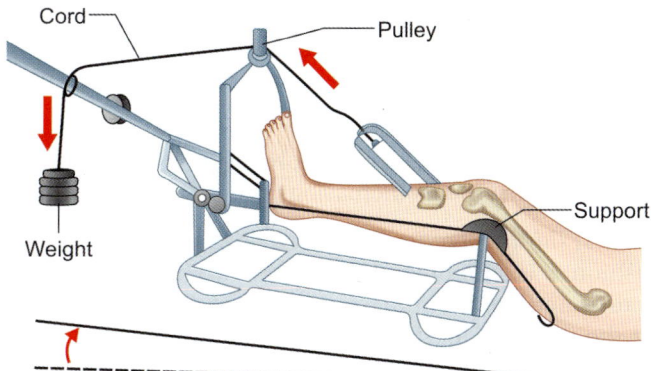

Fig. 18.32: Skeletal traction through Böhler-Braun frame for supracondylar fracture. Note the support is given at the fracture site and not the knee to prevent angulations

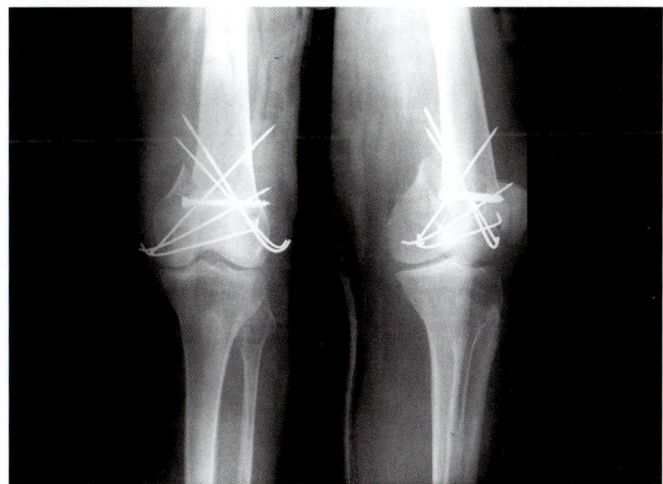

Fig. 18.33: Radiograph showing one of the fixation method in supracondylar fracture femur

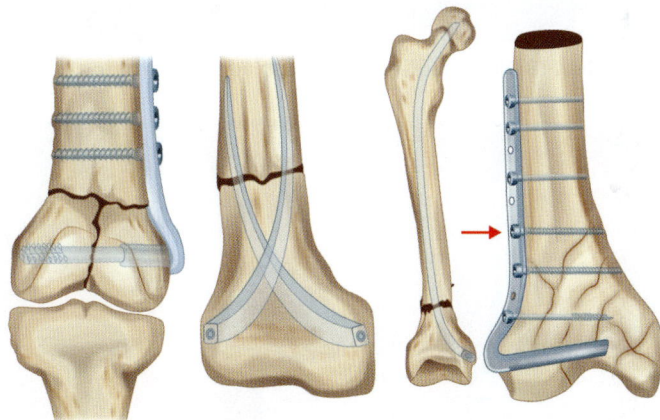

Fig. 18.34: Different methods of internal fixation of supracondylar fracture of femur

Double plate fixation: This is preferred in very low comminuted distal femoral fractures. Here lateral plating alone may not provide the necessary fixation and a medial plate needs to be applied.

Minimally invasive surgeries involving the DCS or condylar blade fixation is being increasing tried for obvious benefits.

Trigen (Third generation) Knee Nail: Inserted in a retrograde fashion. It is a titanium nail and has two holes for oblique screws and one for transverse screw at the insertion end. At the opposite locking end two holes are present in the anteroposterior plane and 2 holes in the lateral plane. The results are encouraging.

Complications

The complications commonly encountered in supracondylar fractures are delayed union, malunion (Fig. 18.36), nonunion, injury to the popliteal vessels and common peroneal nerves, knee stiffness, deep vein thrombosis, infection, implant failure, etc.

> **Do you Know Why Fractures of the Distal Femur are Difficult to Manage?**
> - They are frequently comminuted
> - Due to distractive muscle forces
> - Due to its proximity to the knee
> - Due to associated trauma in the young and due to medical problems in the old.

IPSILATERAL FRACTURES OF FEMORAL SHAFT AND NECK

INTRODUCTION

It is not for nothing that femoral neck fractures are infamously called the unsolved fractures. The statement from Watson Jones that we come into the world under the brim of the pelvis but go out through the fracture neck of femur aptly sums up the enormity of the challenge posed by these fractures both to the patients and the orthopedic surgeons alike. What sends the surgeons scurrying out for cover is the twin threat of nonunion and AVN associated with fracture neck of femur.

Femoral shaft fractures on the other hand pose different sets of problem different from the ones encountered in neck fractures. Nonetheless they are no less challenging than the neck fractures but the saving grace is that we the orthopedic surgeons are spared the ignominy of encountering union problems and this spares us the blushes.

Now imagine the gravity of the problem when both these injuries co-exist in the same bone thanks to those injury forces that rattle both the shaft and neck simultaneously. However, the impact of these enormous loads is first taken by the relatively sturdy shaft thus blunting the forces to a great extent by the time they reach the neck. This is no doubt strong enough to cause a neck fracture but fortunately is weak enough to cause significant displacements that are the bone of the isolated neck factures. What a combination of these two injuries does is it provides a double trouble to the surgeons, who first have to detect it and then pull

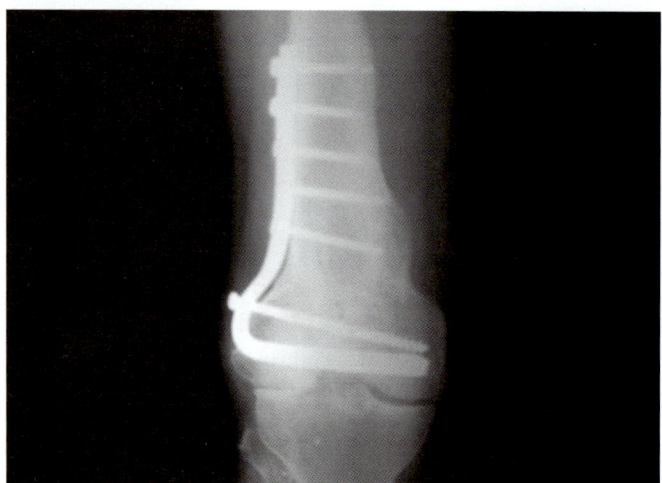

Fig. 18.35: Plain X-ray showing blade plate fixation

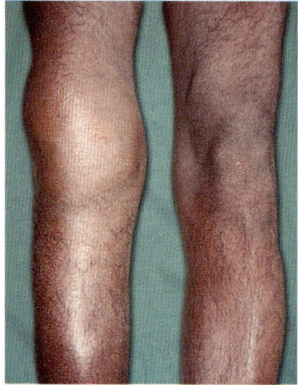 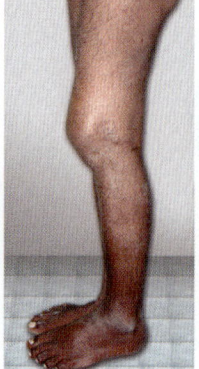 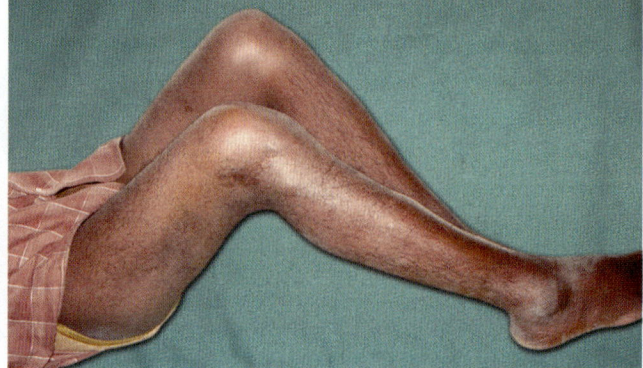 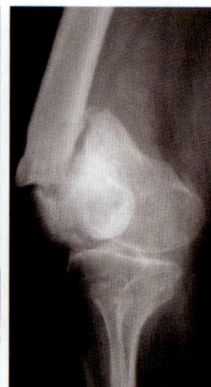

Fig. 18.36: Clinical photos and plain X-ray showing malunited supracondylar fracture femur

out a right combination of treatment plan. A missed neck fracture causes considerable embarrassment to a surgeon and places him on a very sticky wicket. This is what makes these injuries unique and fearsome!

Incidence

First the good news: These are relatively rare injuries and the overall incidence reported in the world literature is around 2.5%. This has been quoted in few studies, first by Winquest et al. in a study of 520 cases and Winquest et al. in a study of 300 cases. Ipsilateral trochanteric fractures are still rare and only 50 cases have been reported so far in the literature.

Now the bad news: In about 20-30% of cases at the time of initial presentation the detection of the fracture neck of femur is often missed. Over attention to the fracture of the shaft of femur lulls the treating orthopedic surgeons into a state of complacency and the fact that there could be an associated fracture above slips his notice. He fails to order for an X-ray of the hip that could have helped him detect this fracture on the X-rays ordered may be taken improperly with no proper internal rotation of the hip. The only way to overcome this iatrogenic slip is to have a high degree of suspicion of the presence of this twin fractures especially in patients with high velocity accidents. Missing fracture neck of femur at the initial diagnosis is a big deal simply because of the development of the notorious complications like nonunion and AVN due to delay in the diagnosis and management. Nonetheless, these twin threats are comparatively less (about 10%) when compared to isolated events of fracture neck of femur (10-30%), thanks to the less displacement encountered in these fractures.

Causes

- Needless to say, high velocity road traffic accidents due to car or motorcycle usually head on injuries.
- Violent falls from great heights
- Catastrophic industrial and agricultural accidents.
- Natural calamities like the earthquakes, floods, etc.

Other Vital Statistics

- *Age:* Average age is 34 years, with a range of 3-76 years. It is rare in children.
- *Sex:* 78% of the cases are male and 22% are female.
- Associated multiple and multisystem injuries: 44%.
- Associated hip fractures: Seen in 0.8-8.6% (Average is 2.5%).
- Diagnosis is missed in 20-30%.

> **Quick Recap**
> - Incidence: 2.5-6%.
> - Missed in: 20-30%. Reasons being failure to have a high degree of suspicion about the possibility of these injuries and failure to order for a proper X-ray of the hip
> - AVN and nonunion could be a distinct possibility due to the missed diagnosis
> - Average age: 34 years
> - Sex: 78% male
> - Multiple and multisystem injuries: 0.8-8.6%.

Mechanism of Injury

High velocity injuries causing axial loading of an abducted femur could lead to fracture shaft of femur and neck fracture (Fig. 18.37). Due to the weakening of these forces as they travel proximally the fracture neck of femur is either undisplaced or minimally displaced. If there is trochanteric fracture it tends to be transverse. The distribution of these hip fractures is as follows:
- Subcapital: 2%
- Midcervical: 21%
- Basicervical: 39%
- Pertrochanteric: 14%
- Intertrochanteric: 24%.

Clinical Features

- Patient could present in shock
- There could be multisystem injuries of the head, spine, trunk, abdomen, and pelvis. Look out for these.
- Pain, swelling, gross external rotation deformity and other sings of fracture are extensively present.

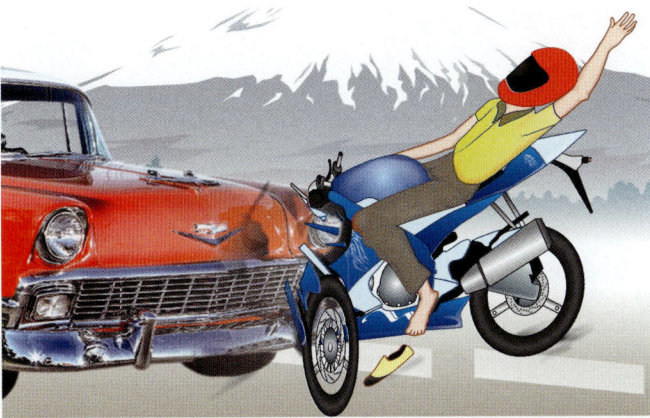

Fig. 18.37: High speed motor vehicle accidents like these can result in ipsilateral fractures of the femoral shaft and fracture neck of femur

Investigations

- *Hemogram:* Like HB%, BT, CT, blood group, random sugar, etc. just like as for any other major surgery.
- *X-ray (Fig. 18.38):* To be done before the surgery in the causality and again in the OT after stabilizing the femoral shaft fracture. These include:
  - *X-ray of the shaft of femur:* The recommended views are AP and lateral views of the shaft.
  - *X-ray of the hip:* If the pelvis X-ray does not show a fracture, try to do an X-ray of the hip in internal rotation as an external rotated limb due to the shaft and neck fracture may cause the fracture to be missed initially.

Other Special Investigations

- Bone scan in people who complain of hip and groin pain following stabilization of the femoral shaft fracture.
- CT scan to detect occult hip fractures in poly-trauma patients.

Methods of Treatment

Conservative treatment: This is mentioned here only for the sake of completion. There is very little role of conservative treatment in these fractures as prolonged hospitalization may lead to fatal pulmonary complications.

Surgery: This is the treatment method of choice in these fractures. There is no dispute over the fact that both these fractures need to be fixed surgically. But there is a fierce debate over which fracture to be fixed first and what should be the choice of the hardware in fixing these fractures. Now let us consider the first debate:

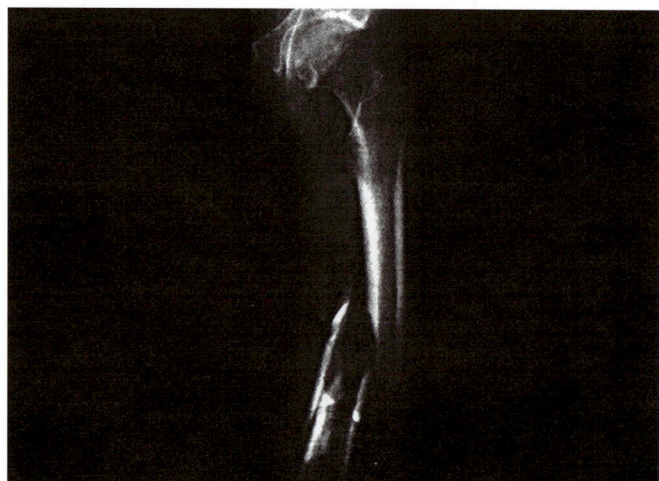

Fig. 18.38: Radiograph showing ipsilateral fractures of the neck of femur and shaft

Which fracture to fix first? Shaft first or neck first? This has led to animated discussion and has clearly divided the surgeons into two groups, one favoring early shaft fixation and neck fixation later while the second group is equally vociferous in advocating neck fixation first and shaft fixation next!

The first group argues that stabilization of the femoral shaft fracture first helps in the better reduction and fixation of the neck fracture. The second group feels that fixing the neck fracture should be the top priority to keep the troublesome AVN and nonunion at an arm's distance. But ironically the incidence of AVN and NU in these combination fractures is rare when compared to isolated neck fractures due to reasons mentioned earlier. But still the advocates of this method vociferously argue that one needs to fix the neck first to prevent these very complications, which are seldom reported.

Choice of Fixation

For the neck: Here there is no much argument and the choice seems to be two cannulated screws.

For the shaft: Here the choice is in between plate fixation and intramedullary fixation. Though plate fixation makes the technique of screw fixation for fracture neck of femur easier, it has not found universal favor due to higher rate of complication like infection, nonunion, etc. when compared to the intramedullary fixation. Hence, it is the intramedullary fixation that has found universal favor.

Methods of Fixation

In the world literature more than 60 methods of fixation have been documented. Since these are complex injuries the methods of fixation are also complex. Surgeons are divided over the choice of the method of fixation simply because nobody seems to know the perfect choice. Not let us know explore the options of fixations:

- Open reduction and internal fixation with lag screws for fracture neck of femur and a cephalomedullary nail for shaft fracture (According to Swiontkwoski, Hansen and Kellam) (Fig. 18.38).
- Femoral neck fixation with screws and retrograde nailing through the intercondylar route.
- Conventional interlocking nailing and cannulated screw fixation for neck fracture (according to Buchlog and others).
- Russell-Taylor reconstruction Nail has been specifically designed for this combination of injuries. This nail allows the fixation of the neck fracture with two self-compressing lag screws and cephalomedully nail to fix the shaft fracture. Here again the priority is to fix the neck fracture first after obtaining its anatomical reduction. Various authors like Russell and Ayan, Koldenhoven et al.

Henry and Seligxon have all reported successful results with very few complications like nonunion or AVN.
- Retrograde femoral nailing through the intercondylar notch of the distal femur has also been reported.
- Antegrade intramedullary femoral nailing with placement of cancellous lag screws around the nail is another technique described by Bennet and associates. They reported 100% union after a 26-month follow-up.
- Chaturvedi and Sahu fixed the femoral neck fracture first with multiple screws and then did antegrade nailing for femoral shaft fracture. They reported very good results with all the fractures uniting by 6 months and there was no incidence of AVN.
- DCP plating of the femoral shaft with a lag screw fixation of the neck is another method of treatment (Fig. 18.39). This method is easy and reliable and can be done in centers that do not have the facilities. It does not disturb the proximal femur to implant the neck. But the disadvantages being increased blood loss increased periosteal stripping, leading to union problems and also the potential need for bone grafts.
- Reconstruction nail that can be locked distally and proximally placement of two compression screws anterior and posterior to the nail seems to be a better option (Fig. 18.40).

Complications

This can be discussed under two heads:

Those Related to Fracture Neck of Femur

The complications related to fracture neck of femur in this combination of injuries is the one that is more troublesome and requires utmost skill on the part of the surgeon to prevent it from happening in the first place. The twin devastating complications are:
- *AVN:* In a young adult there can never be a more devastating complication than this. Not that this happens only where there is this combination fractures. It is as much seen even in isolated neck fractures to the tune of 5–8% for undisplaced fractures and 9–35% for displaced fractures. In contrast, ironically though, AVN happens less often in ipsilateral fractures with a rate of just 0–2%. This is because with these injuries the displacement of neck fracture is considerably less and most of the forces that cause femoral shaft fracture weaken by the time they reach the neck. Philosophically, I feel God compensates for the tragedy of twin fractures by toning down its complications.

Consider this in one series by Casey and Chapman; there was no single case of AVN in those patients treated with traction! However, in studies by Wiss et al and Swiontkowski et al. it ranged between 6–22% respectively over a 3 year follow-up through they had addressed the fracture neck of femur first. This categorically proves that it is not the subsequent treatment but the initial injury that decides the development of osteonecrosis. And moreover gleaning the available literature does not establish a relationship between the development of AVN and the delay in the diagnosis of these injuries. Despite this we keep emphasizing that detecting these fractures early and fixing it securely is the mantra to avoid the troublesome AVN and the next to be discussed nonunion.
- *Nonunion:* Majority of the authors, hold your breath, have reported a 100% union rate for both these fractures.

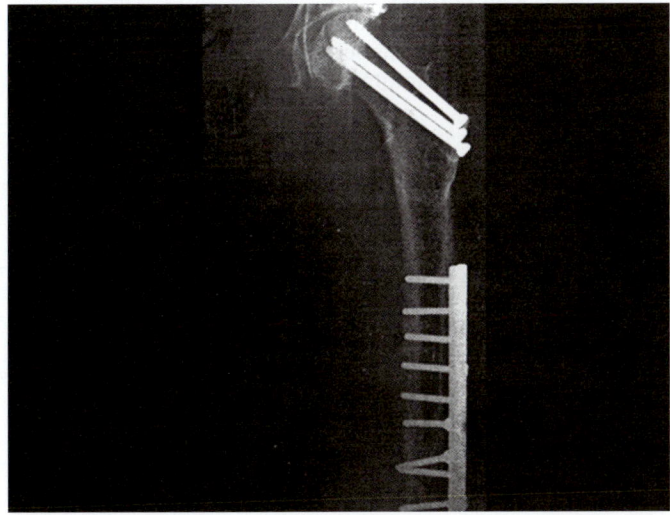

Fig. 18.39: Radiograph showing the fixation of neck fracture with cannulated screws and shaft of femur with DCP plate and screws

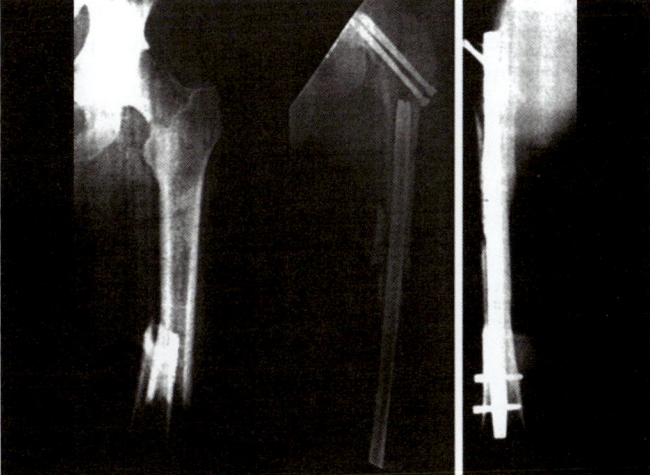

Fig. 18.40: Radiograph showing methods of fixation of these fractures: Cannulated screws and intramedullary fixation (left) and second generation reconstruction nail (right)

But however not all are that successful. Now consider these statistics:
- Wiss et al. reported an 18% (6/33) incidence of nonunion in those patients treated with interlocking nailing.
- Shaheen and Badr reported a 25% incidence of nonunion (4/16) in patients treated with fixed angle nail plate. This throws up the question is the nonunion device related?
- Bennett et al reported a nonunion incidence of 3% in displaced fractures.

Related to fracture shaft of femur: These are fortunately and mercifully rare and include:
- Femoral shaft malunion and shortening.
- Femoral shaft nonunion: In a study reported by WU and Shih, 15 percent (5 cases) developed non-union of the femoral shaft and all these cases had open reduction and internal fixation lading to excessive soft tissue and bony devitalization due to periosteal stripping, loss of blood, etc.

Conclusion

Ipsilateral fracture shaft of the femur and nonunion are relatively rare injuries and are due to high speed RTA's. Neck fractures are frequently missed leading to a possibility of complications like AVN and nonunion. Hence, a high degree of suspicion is required for the presence of these fractures and a hip X-ray is mandatory in all femoral shaft fracture cases. Both these fractures need to be surgically fixed and it is now more or less settled that fracture neck of femur should be fixed first to avoid the above said complications from developing. Cannulated screw fixation for the fracture neck of femur and intramedullary fixations for fracture shaft of femur seems to be the ideal combination. Good fixation is achieved recently by the second generation Russell Taylor interlocking nail.

BIBLIOGRAPHY

1. Alho A. Concurrent ipsilateral fractures of the hip and shaft of the femur. A systematic review of 722 cases. Ann Chir Gynaecol. 1997;326-36.
2. Alho A, Ekeland A, Groggard B, et al. A locked hip screw-intramedullary nail (cephalomedullary nail) for the treatment of fractures of the proximal part of the femur combined with fractures of the femoral shaft. J Trauma. 1996;40:10-6.
3. Barei DP, Schildhauer TA, Nork SE. Noncontiguous fractures of the femoral neck, femoral shaft, and distal femur. J Trauma. 2003;80-6.
4. Bennett FS, Zinar DM, Kilgus DJ. Ipsilateral hip and femoral shaft fractures. Clin Orthop. 1993;296:168-77.
5. Bernsrein SM. Fracture of the femoral shaft and associated ipsilateral fractures of the hip. Orthop Clin. 1974;5:799-818.
6. Bose WJ, Corces A, Anderson LD. A preliminary experience with the Russell-Taylor reconstruction nail for complex femoral fractures. J Trauma. 1992;32:71-6.
7. Chaturvedi S, Sahu SC. Ipsilateral concomitant fractures of the femoral neck and shaft. Injury. 1993;24:243-6.
8. Chen CH, et al. Ipsilateral fractures of the femoral neck and shaft. Injury. 2000;719-22.
9. Daffner RH, Reimer BL, Butterfield SL. Ipsilateral femoral neck, and shaft fracture: An overlooked association. Skeletal Radiol. 1991;20:251-4.
10. Johnson KD. The reconstruction locked nail for complex fractures of the proximal femur. J Orthop Trauma. 1995; 9:453-63.
11. Kates SL. The role of computerized tomography in the diagnosis of an occult femoral neck fracture associated with an ipsilateral femoral shaft fracture: a case report. J Trauma. 1991;31:296-8.
12. Peljovich AE, Patterson BM. Ipsilateral femoral neck and shaft fractures. J AM Acazd Orthop Surg. 1998;106-13.
13. Reimer BL, Fogelsong ME, Miranda MA. Femoral plating. Orthop Clin. 1994;25:625-33.
14. Swiontkowski MF. Ipsilateral femoral shaft and hip fractures, Orthop Clin. 1987;18:73-84.
15. Swiontkowski MF, Winquist RA, Hansen ST. Fractures of the femoral neck in patients between the ages of twelve and forty-nine years. J Bone Joint Surg Am. 1984;66:837-46.

19 CHAPTER

Injuries of the Knee

BRIEF ANATOMY

Knee joint is a complex joint in the body. The problems relating to it are also complex. Here dislocation is not common but injuries to its various ligaments pose severe problems to the patient. An unstable knee can spell doom to the well-being of a person. Meniscal injuries and fracture patella can further compound problems. It is imperative to know how your knee joint is structured before attempting to know about the injuries related to it.

The Knee Joint Speaks

You will have to agree with me that I am the most remarkable joint in the body by any engineering standards. Being the most heavily stressed joint in the body, I have amalgamated two apparently incompatible properties of stability and mobility. During complete extension, I am very stable, and during flexion, I am very mobile. I have a hinge joint between the lower end of femur and upper end of tibia and a saddle joint between the patella and the femur. Hence, I am rightly called a *compound synovial joint*.

I am heavily dependent for stability on the following ligaments (Fig. 19.1):

Medial side: Here in the anterior third I am supported by the anterior capsule and extensor retinaculum, in the middle third by the superficial and deep layers of tibial collateral ligament, in the posterior third the capsule is reinforced by posterior oblique ligament, expansions from semitendinosus, etc.

Lateral side: In the anterior third, capsule and the lateral extensor retinaculum; in the middle third, the iliotibial band; in the posterior third by the arcuate complex formed by fibular collateral ligament, and a slip from the popliteus, biceps femoris, etc.

Anteroposterior stability: For this, I have two cruciate ligaments: One anterior and the other posterior who are the primary stabilizers in the anteroposterior plane.

Anterior cruciate ligament (ACL) restrains me during anterior glide. It has two main functional components, the smaller anteromedial bundle supports me best in flexion and the larger poster lateral bundle supports me best in extension. Both are taut at full extension. Posterior cruciate ligament (PCL) is thicker and is approximately twice as strong as anterior either cruciate or medial collateral ligaments. It restrains me mainly during the posterior glide and is under tension throughout the whole range of movements.

I have two wonderful structures in the form of menisci whose structure and function are discussed in the section on menisci injury.

Knee Stability Depends Upon
- Mechanical axes of the joint
- The bony contours
- Extra-articular stabilizers (synovium, capsules, collaterals, muscles, and tendons)
- Intra-articular stabilizers (menisci and cruciates).

KNEE LIGAMENT INJURIES

GENERAL PRINCIPLES

Etiology

- *Athletes:* Knee ligament injuries are very common in athletes who are involved both in contact and non-contact sports. The injury could be either direct due

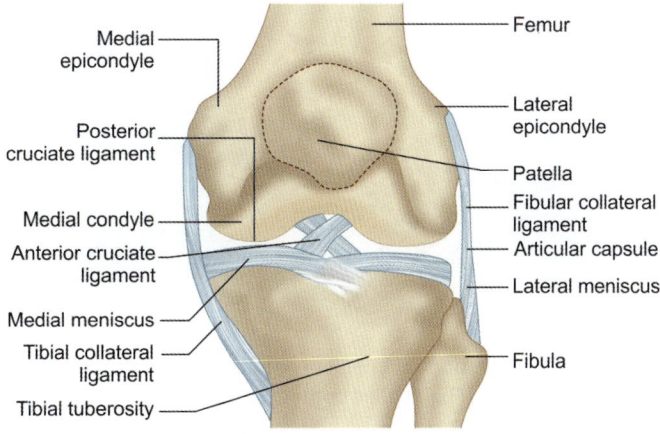

Fig. 19.1: Anatomy of knee joint

to the collision with another athlete or indirect due to rotation and twisting injuries.
- *Road traffic accident (RTA):* Here the mechanism is usually direct and could be due to a dashboard injury.
- *Fall* from a height with twisting force.

Mechanism of Injury (Palmar)

The following are the common mechanism of knee ligament injuries (Fig. 19.2):
- Direct valgus force.
- Rotational or twisting forces.
  - *Abduction, flexion, and internal rotation of femur on tibia (Ab FIR):* This causes damage to medial structures, like tibial collateral, medial capsule and if more force is applied ACL and medial meniscus may also tear.
  - *"O' Donohue's unhappy triad" (Fig. 19.3):* Indicate injuries to medial structures + ACL tear + medial meniscus injury.
  - *Adduction, flexion and external rotation of femur on tibia (Ad FER):* Causes damage to fibular collateral, lateral capsule, arcuate complex, popliteus, iliotibial band, biceps, common peroneal nerve, anterior, posterior or both cruciates.
- *Hyperextension force* may cause either anterior or posterior cruciate ligament injury.
- *Anteroposterior displacement* either anterior (dashboard injury) or posterior cruciates may be injured due to a direct force in RTA.

Goals of Treatment

The goals of treatment in knee ligament injuries are restoration of anatomy and stability to normal or near to normal.

COLLATERAL LIGAMENT INJURY

Collateral ligament injury is due to direct or indirect violence as described earlier. Medial collateral ligament injury is more common due to the valgus stress caused by striking the lateral aspect of the knee joint during collision in sports. The varus force on the medial side required to cause the lateral collateral ligament injury is less common because of the protection offered by the other leg.

However, a severe varus force may cause avulsion of the lateral collateral ligament from the head of the fibula (Fig. 19.4A).

Do You Know?
About Pellegrini-Stieda disease: It is a calcification seen at the adductor tubercle visualized on AP X-ray of the knee in MCL injury of greater than 6 weeks.

Mechanism of Injury

This has already been described.

Types

Depending upon on the degree of tear collateral ligament injuries are graded into three types (Flowchart 19.1 and Fig. 19.4B)

Clinical Features

The patient gives history of valgus and external rotation force in mild sprains. In severe sprains, the patient gives

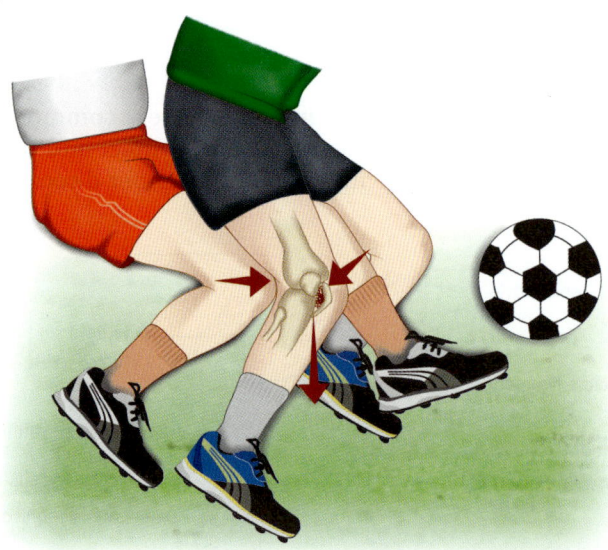

Fig. 19.2: Common mechanism of knee ligament injuries (High speed contact sports)

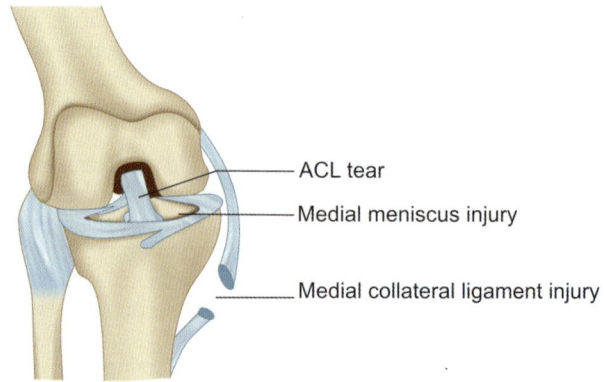

Fig. 19.3: Unhappy triad of O'donoghue

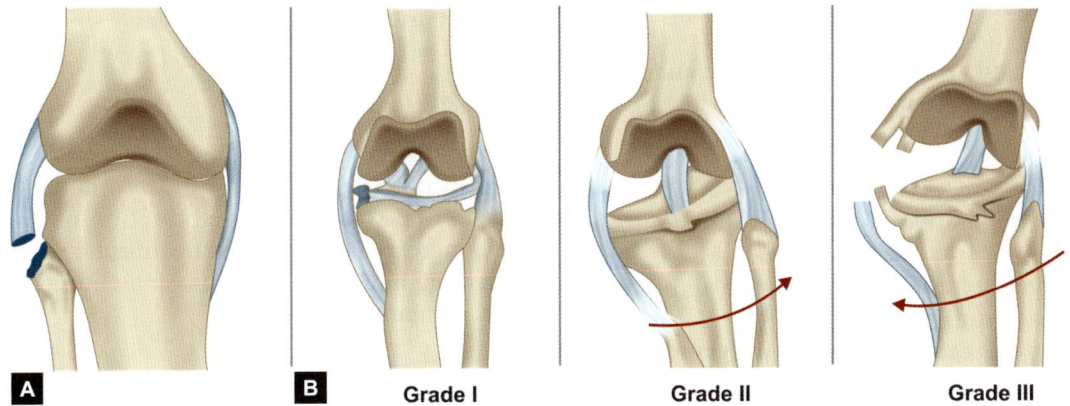

Figs 19.4A and B: (A) Avulsion of lateral collateral ligament from the head of the fibula;
(B) Sprain of medial collateral ligament of the knee

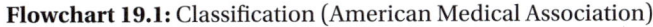

Flowchart 19.1: Classification (American Medical Association)

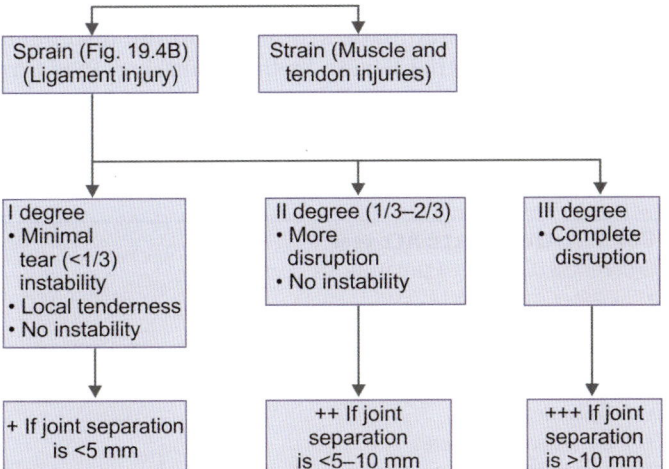

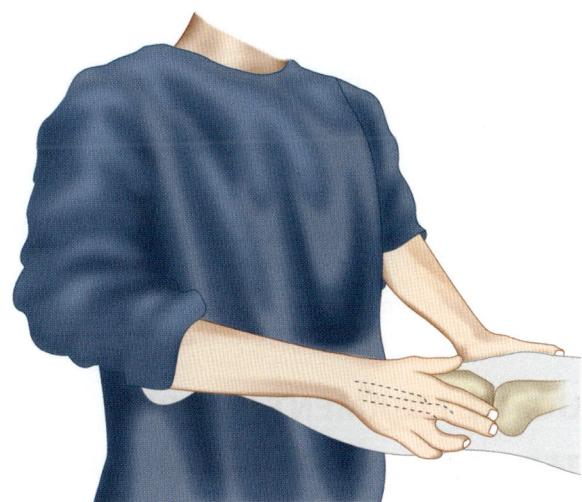

Fig. 19.5: Method of eliciting joint line tenderness

history of valgus stress force due to the direct blow on the lower thigh or upper leg seen commonly in contact sports like football, rugby, etc. It may be associated with ACL tear or meniscal injury and then the patient may present with pain, swelling, hemarthrosis, etc.

On examination, the point of local tenderness could be at adductor tubercle, joint line or at the insertion of tibial collateral ligament (Fig. 19.5). About 10–20% of patients have damage to the extensor mechanism of the knee.

Clinical Tests

These are abduction stress in 30° knee flexion and extension. The amount of opening on the medial side should be assessed (Figs 19.6A and B). To rule out the associated injuries, do the anterior drawer test and Lachman's test.

Investigations

- Stress radiographs at 15–20° of valgus

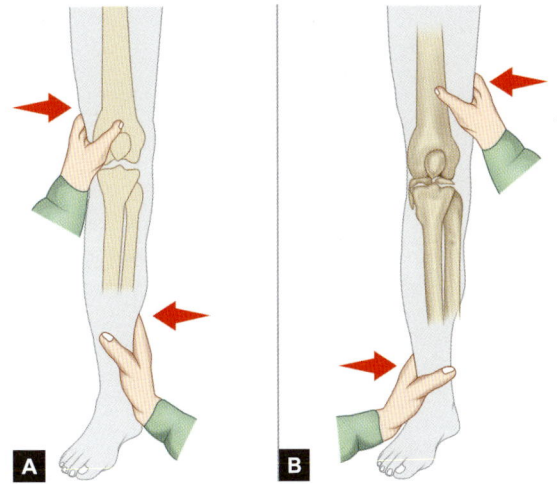

Figs 19.6A and B: Stress tests: (A) Abduction or valgus stress test; (B) Adduction or varus stress test

- MRI helps to localize the MCL tears, ACL, meniscal injuries, etc.
- Arthrograms and arthroscopy to evaluate and rule out meniscal and cruciate pathology.

Treatment

Fresh injury nonoperative treatment is the mainstay of treatment.
- I° Sprain → symptomatic treatment, nonsteroidal anti-inflammatory drugs (NSAIDs), etc.
- II° Sprain → long leg cast for 4–6 weeks with knee in 30–40° of flexion.
- III° Sprain → surgical repair in isolated tears. Repair and reconstruction in old tears or in associated injuries (Fig. 19.7). Brace is required for 4–7 months.

Old Cases

Here surgery is the main stay of treatment and consists of mainly reconstruction.

Tibial collateral ligament (TCL) injury: If TCL is intact but lax, and then distal transfer is done. If ligament is destroyed, reconstruction using hamstrings or semitendinosus is done.

Fibular collateral ligament injury: If adequate and thick, distal transfer is recommended. If destroyed, reconstruction using fascia lata, biceps tendon, etc. is done.

CRUCIATE LIGAMENT INJURIES

ANTERIOR CRUCIATE LIGAMENT (ACL) TEAR

Of all the knee ligament injuries, ACL tear is the most common (Fig. 19.8).

Know the Role of ACL in Your Knees
- AP stability
- Proprioception
- Mechanical function.

Mechanism of anterior cruciate ligament (ACL) tear has already been discussed. The most common mode of injury is external rotation with abduction of the flexed knee or hyperextension of knee in internal rotation. This is a disabling injury and the knee may immediately collapse and is painful.

Clinical Features

Popping sensation felt or heard at the time of injury signifies ligamentous injury (ACL tear). The patient also tells that the knee "gave away" or buckled at the time of injury. Swelling of the knee could be either due to hemarthroses or traumatic synovitis and the distended knee is held in partial flexion by the hamstrings (see Box 19.1 for differential diagnosis).

Note:
Sixty seven percent of ACL tear is sports related.

Box 19.1: Quick facts: ACL tear
Differential diagnosis: Hemarthrosis
- Ligamentous tears (ACL, PCL, etc.)
- Osteochondral fracture
- Peripheral menisci tear
- Capsular tear
- Patellar dislocation
- Intra-articular fractures

Note: Commonest cause is ACL tear.

Did You Know?
Galen first described ACL tear in AD 170.

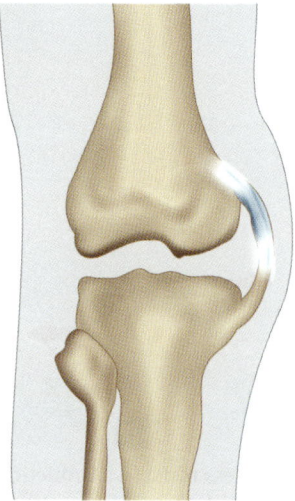

Fig. 19.7: Direct ligament repair in fresh tears

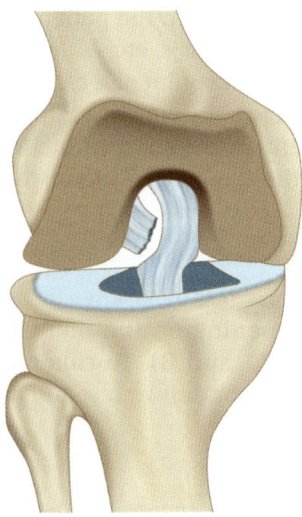

Fig. 19.8: ACL tear

TABLE 19.1: Clinical tests to diagnose various knee ligament injuries

	Tests	How to perform	Inference
I.	Adduction or varus: Abduction or valgus stress test (Fig. 19.9A) 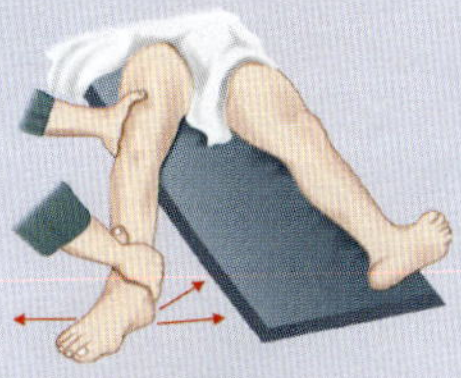 ![Fig. 19.9A]	Patient is supine, knee is flexed to 30° **For abduction test:** One hand is on the lateral aspect of the knee and the other at the ankle, force is applied outwards **For adduction test:** Change hand to the medial side of the knee and give an adduction force	Positive in injury to the medial structures of the knee like tibial collateral ligament. Positive in injuries to lateral structures of knee like fibular collateral ligament
II.	Lachman's* test (Fig. 19.9B) 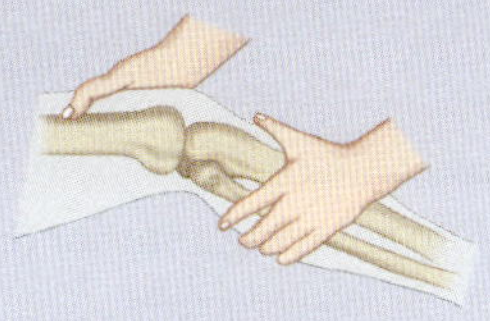	This is an anterior drawer's test done at 20–30° of knee flexion with patient in supine position	Indicates ACL tear. This test is used in acute injuries of knee to test ACL tear where knee cannot be flexed to 90°
III.	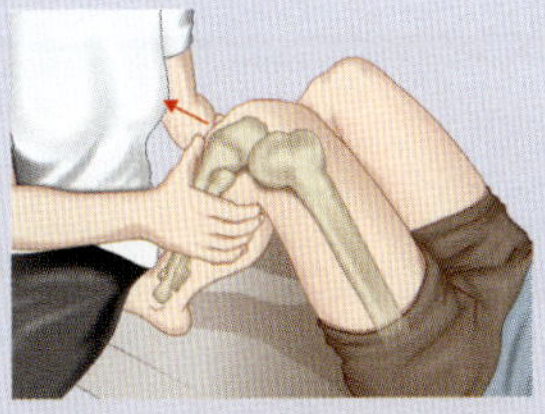 Anterior Drawer's test (Fig. 19.9C)	Patient is in supine position. Hip is flexed to 45° and knee to 90°. Examiner sits on the dorsum of the foot and pulls the tibia forwards. The anterior drawer's test is done in 3 positions a. Foot in neutral position—if positive, it indicates ACL tear, etc b. Foot in 15° internal rotation—if positive, indicates damage to anterolateral structures c. Foot in 15° external rotation—if positive, indicates damage to anteromedial structures	If the tibia shifts anteriorly more than 6-8 mm, then it indicates torn ACL and the test is considered as positive This should always be compared with the normal knee
IV.	Posterior Drawer's test (Fig. 19.9D) Fig. 19.9D 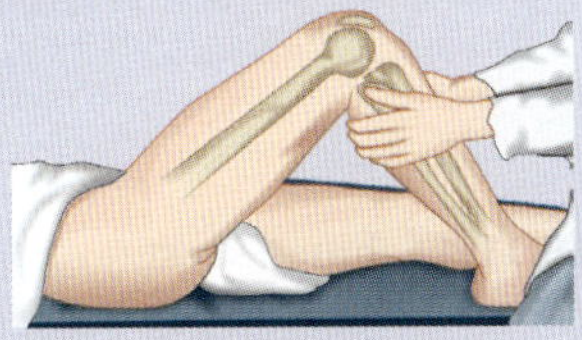	Same as above but tibia is pushed backwards Positive test is indicated by the movement of the tibia backwards.	Indicates posterior cruciate ligament tear.
V.	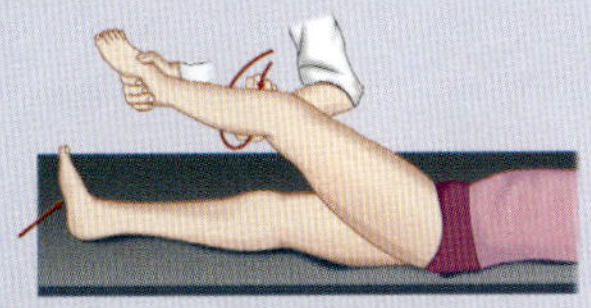 Jerk test of Hughston (Fig. 19.9E)	Patient is supine, knee is flexed to 90°. Tibia is internally rotated with a valgus force applied at the knee, it is slowly extended. *Lateral tibial condyle subluxates at 30° and spontaneous relocation occurs as knee extends*	*Inference* indicates anterior cruciate ligament tear and is more specific than Drawer's test in detecting ACL tear
VI.	Pivot shift test (Fig. 19.9F) 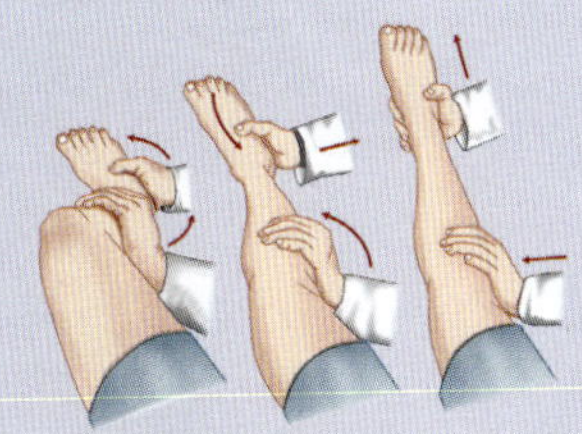	Patient is supine. The knee is extended, with a valgus stress applied on the knee and the tibia is internally rotated. The knee is slowly flexed. Subluxation occurs at 30–40°	A positive test indicates anterior cruciate ligament tear

Clinical Examination

Always examine the normal knee first and form a basis for "comparison." Clinical findings depend on associated ligamentous injury or meniscal injury or bone damage. Depending on the combination, there will be specific instabilities (see Table 19.2) that will allow anterior displacement of tibia on the uninvolved side. Anterior subluxation of more than 5° suggests lax or disrupted ACL. Isolated injury is rare. Anterior drawer test and Lachman's test are specific to ACL tear and various other clinical tests to detect ACL tear are depicted in Table 19.1 and Figures 19.9 and 19.10.

> **Disturbing Facts: About ACL Tear**
> ACL tear → Knee instability → Repeated episodes of instability leads to damage to menisci, cartilage and other ligaments → This ultimately leads to secondary OA knee.

Clinical Tests

- *Slocum test:* It is an anterior drawer's test (rotary test) performed with 15° of internal rotation and 30° of external rotation. The former is positive in anterolateral instability and the latter in anteromedial instability.
- *External rotation recurvatum test (posterior sag sign):* When the leg is passively lifted by holding the toes, the knee sags posteriorly indicating injury to PCL and poster lateral structures.
- *Lachman's test* (Fig. 19.11) as already described, this is an anterior drawer's test done at 20–30° of flexion. It has several advantages over 90° flexion anterior drawer's test. The following are some of them:
  - It can be done in the presence of effusion and hence is useful in acute cases when knee cannot be flexed up to 90°.
  - Evokes less pain as full flexion is not required.
  - Hamstrings and torn menisci will not block forward glide easily.
  - More specific for posterolateral fibers of ACL tear.

> **Grading of Lachman's Test**
> - Grade I: End feel appreciation (0–5 mm displacement).
> - Grade II: Visible anterior movement of tibia (5–10 mm displacement).
> - Grade III: Gross anterior tibial translation (more than 10 mm displacement).

Investigations in ACL Tear

Radiograph of the knee: The views recommended are anteroposterior (AP) view, lateral view, intercondylar notch view, sunrise views, etc. Radiographs are usually normal in ACL tear. Avulsion fracture of tibial spine if present indicates ACL tear (Fig. 19.12).

> **Did You Know What a Segond Fracture is?**
> It is an avulsion fracture of the inferior lateral capsule adjacent to the tibia. If present, it suggests ACL tear.

MRI: This is the best diagnostic tool. It is noninvasive and demonstrates the ACL tear with remarkable accuracy. This

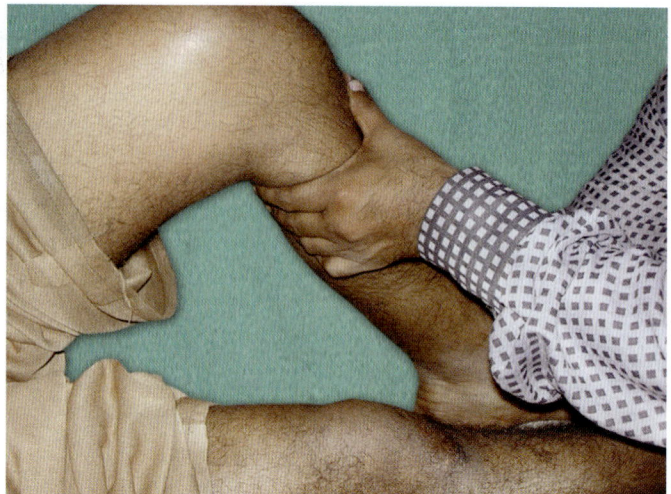

Fig. 19.10: Clinical photo showing anterior drawer test

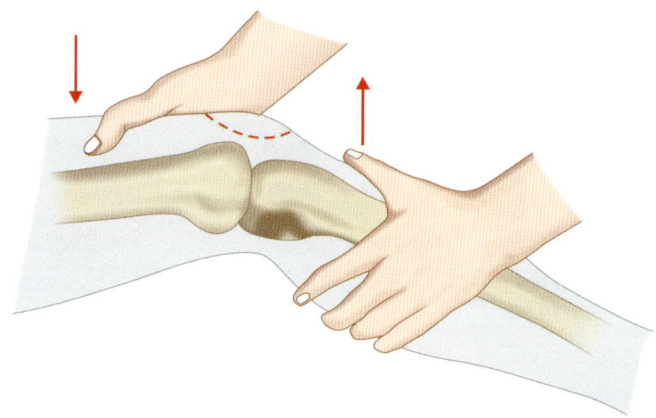

Fig. 19.11: Lachman's test

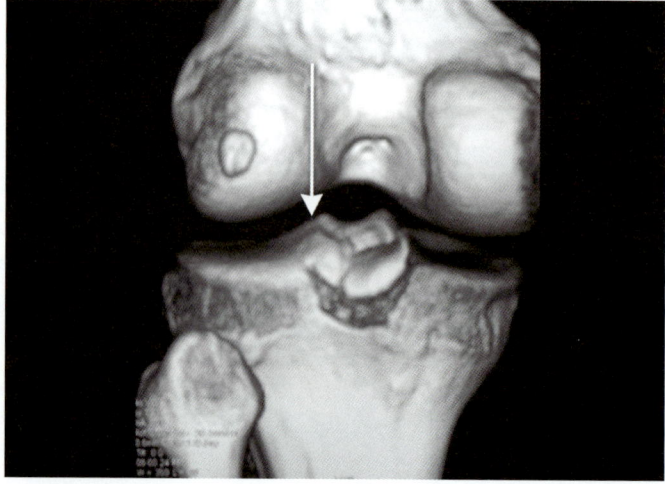

Fig. 19.12: CT Scan showing tibial spine avulsion fracture

is the gold standard investigation for ACL tears and has virtually replaced all others (Fig. 19.13).

KT-1000: This measuring system documents anteroposterior tibial displacement by tracking the tibial tubercle in rotation to the patella. More than 3 mm anterior displacement at 20 lbs predicts an ACL tear with 94% accuracy.

Treatment of ACL Tear

Conservative Measures

This is reserved for Grade I and II tears and consists of rest, long leg casts for 4-6 weeks, NSAIDs, physiotherapy, etc. However the long-term outcomes are poor when compared to surgical reconstructions even in patients older than 50.[1]

Surgery

Surgery is reserved for more severe tears and the techniques vary from primary repair, reinforcements, or reconstruction of the ACL ligament depending upon the extent and duration of time. Arthroscopically assisted ACL reconstruction has been universally advocated due to its superior results.

Fresh: Primary repair is indicated in young adults and athletes. Repair is successful if ACL is torn at its femoral or tibial attachments. It is not successful in mid-position tears. Failure rate is as high as 50%.

Old Cases

- Reinforcement of ACL tear should be augmented except when avulsion is with a fragment of bone. Reinforcement could be either intra-articular or extra-articular or both by using iliotibial band, semitendinosus tendon, etc.
- Reconstruction in chronic ACL insufficiency could be either intra-articular or extra-articular replacement by using quadriceps, tendon, patellar tendon (central 1/3) bone patella tendon bone graft (BPTB) (Fig. 19.14), semitendinosus tendon, gracilis, etc.

These autografts are preferred over allograft, which are reserved for:
- Revision ACL reconstruction
- Rupture of both ACL and PCL.

Surgical Technique of ACL Reconstruction in a Nutshell
- Graft harness and preparation
- Notchplasty
- Tibial tunnel placement
- Femoral tunnel placement
- Graft passage.

Remember
Autografts widely used in reconstruction of ACL tear
- Central 1/3 of patellar tendon (BPTB Graft)
- Semitendinous and gracilis tendons.

Did You Know?
- Semitendinosus graft has been introduced since 2004
- It has now virtually replaced the BPTB graft due to lesser donor site morbidity, and absence of problems like anterior knee pain, slackness of the extensor mechanism, etc.
- However the choice of the graft whether, it is BTPB OR STG the clinical and functional outcome do not alter significantly
- The chances of secondary OA after ACL reconstruction is just around 30%.[1]

Vital Points: ACL Tear
- Common in young active people usually athletes may interfere with activity or it may make activity impossible
- Usually it does not tear in isolation
- Associated with other ligament injuries
- May predispose to menisci lesions
- May predispose to OA changes.

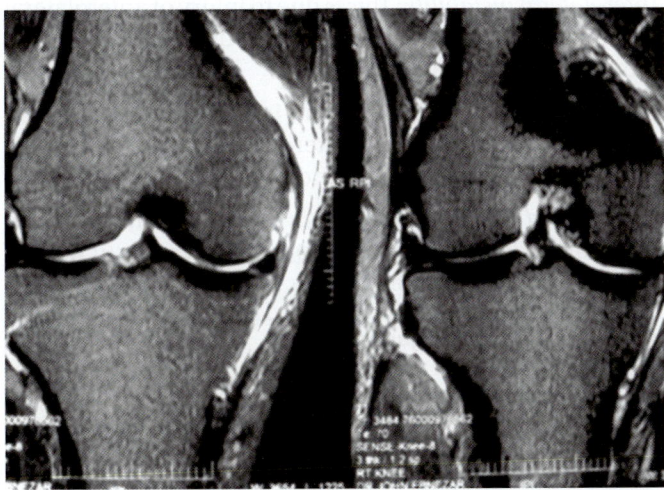

Fig. 19.13: MRI showing ACL tears

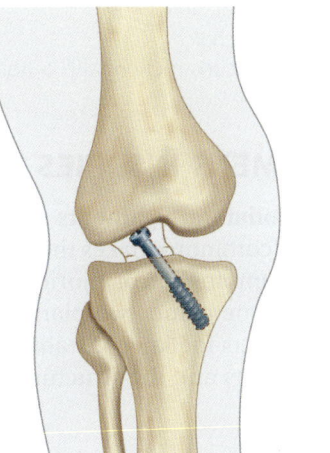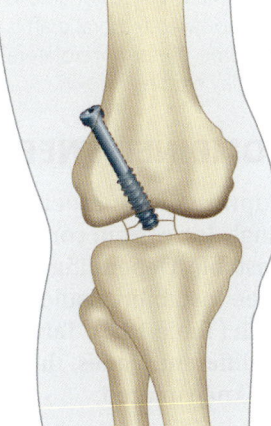

Fig. 19.14: Methods of ACL repair

POSTERIOR CRUCIATE LIGAMENT (PCL) TEAR

It is less common than ACL tear. It is ruptured due to severe rotational injury, dashboard injury, or complete dislocation of the knee. Isolated PCL tear is rare and is accompanied with other ligament injuries.

> **Note:**
> PCL tear accounts for 3–4% of all knee ligament injuries.

Clinical Features

The patient complains of pain, swelling, and tenderness over the popliteal fossa. Clinically, posterior drawer test and sag sign will be positive (Fig. 19.15).

> **Pearl**
> Ninety degrees posterior drawer test is the most important test to diagnose PCL tear.

Investigations: These are similar to ACL tear.

Conservative: Most of the Grade I and II PCL tears can be treated non-operatively.

Surgery: This is indicated in Grade III injuries with posterior translation >10 mm. Reconstruction is done by using medial head of gastrocnemius, etc.

Avulsion of the PCL from the femoral or tibial ends is more common unlike in ACL tears. Here reattachment of the avulsed ligament usually gives good results. Reconstruction is reserved for:
- Midsubstance tears
- Old tears.

> **Graft Options for PCL Reconstruction**
> - Central one-third of patellar tendon
> - Patella tendon allograft
> - Achilles tendon allograft
> - Semitendinosus or gracilis graft
> - Two-tailed femoral graft is the graft of choice
> - Some prefer anterolateral femoral reconstruction with a tibial inlay grafting.

COMBINED KNEE LIGAMENT INJURIES

Rupture of the cruciate and collateral ligaments either singly (rare) or in combination (common) makes the knee unstable. Depending upon the combination of injuries, the knee instability could be either one plane, two planes or both (Table 19.2). Table 19.3 depicts the knee instabilities in different planes, the various tests and the structures of the knee injured.

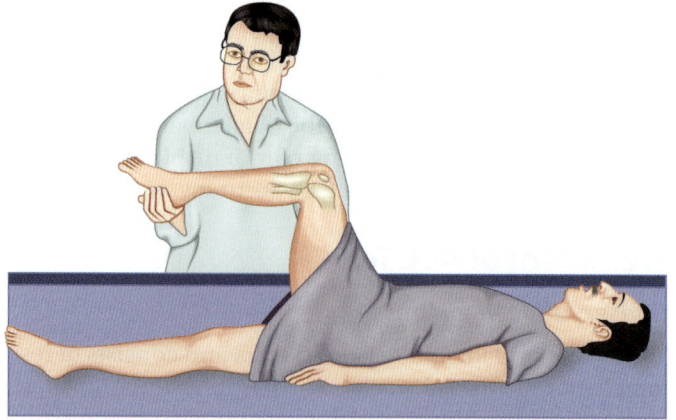

Fig. 19.15: Posterior 'sag sign' for PCL tear

TABLE 19.2: Knee instability in different planes

If only medial structures torn	One plane medial instability
If only lateral structures torn	One plane lateral instability
If ACL and medial structures torn	Two plane anterior and medial instability
If ACL and lateral structures torn	Two plane anterior and lateral instability
If PCL and medial structures torn	Two plane posterior and medial instability
If PCL and lateral structures torn	Two plane posterior and lateral instability

> **Combined Instabilities of Knee**
>
> | | |
> |---|---|
> | If anterior, medial and lateral structures are torn | Anteromedial and anterolateral instabilities |
> | If anterior, posterior cruciates lateral structures are torn | Anterolateral and posterolateral instabilities |
> | If anterior, posterior cruciates and medial structures are torn | Anteromedial and posteromedial instabilities |

Anterolateral instability: This is due to injury of anterolateral structures. Reconstruction is done by using iliotibial band or biceps femoris transfer.

Posterolateral instability: This is due to injury to the posterolateral structures. Posterolateral structures repair or reconstruction is recommended.

Posteromedial instability: This is due to injury to the posteromedial structures. Repair or reconstruction of posteromedial structures is done.

> **At a Glance Cruciate Injuries**
> - ACL commonly tears than PCL (9:1)
> - Commonest mechanism for ACL tear is external rotation with abduction of a flexed knee and for PCL tear dashboard injury

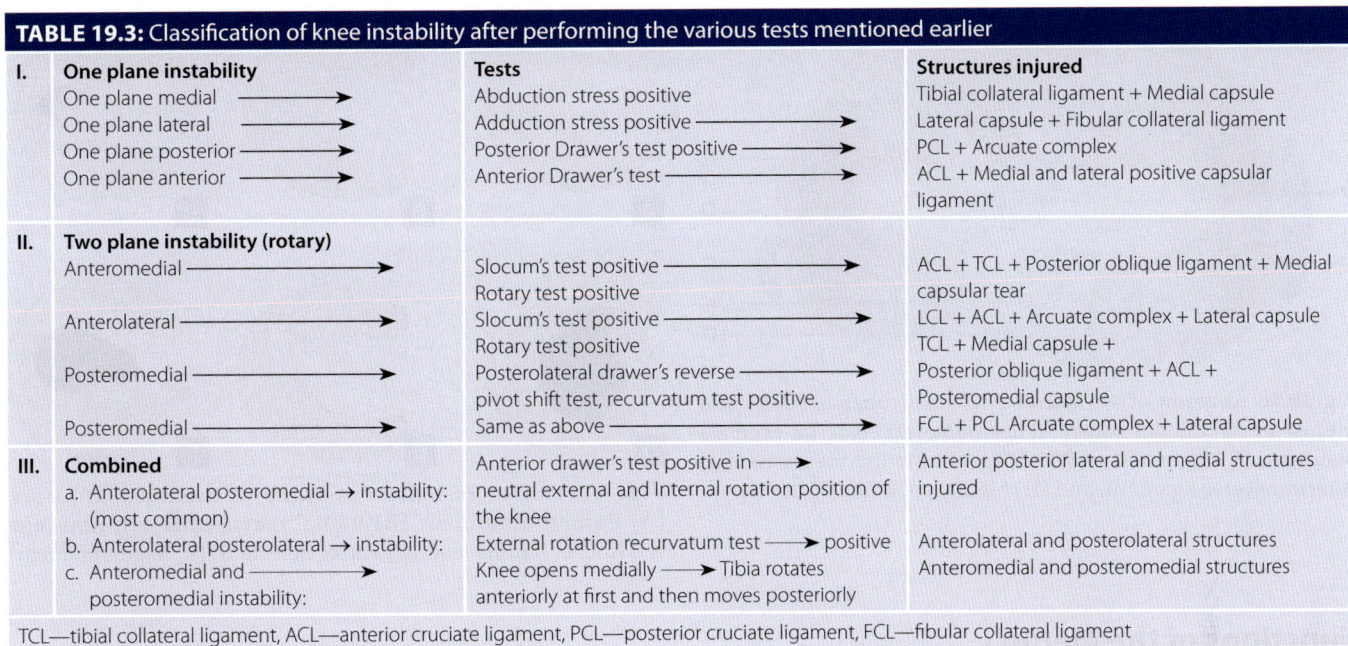

TABLE 19.3: Classification of knee instability after performing the various tests mentioned earlier

	One plane instability	Tests	Structures injured
I.	One plane medial →	Abduction stress positive →	Tibial collateral ligament + Medial capsule
	One plane lateral →	Adduction stress positive →	Lateral capsule + Fibular collateral ligament
	One plane posterior →	Posterior Drawer's test positive →	PCL + Arcuate complex
	One plane anterior →	Anterior Drawer's test →	ACL + Medial and lateral positive capsular ligament
II.	Two plane instability (rotary)		
	Anteromedial →	Slocum's test positive → Rotary test positive	ACL + TCL + Posterior oblique ligament + Medial capsular tear
	Anterolateral →	Slocum's test positive → Rotary test positive	LCL + ACL + Arcuate complex + Lateral capsule
	Posteromedial →	Posterolateral drawer's reverse → pivot shift test, recurvatum test positive.	TCL + Medial capsule + Posterior oblique ligament + ACL + Posteromedial capsule
	Posteromedial →	Same as above →	FCL + PCL Arcuate complex + Lateral capsule
III.	Combined	Anterior drawer's test positive in → neutral external and Internal rotation position of the knee	Anterior posterior lateral and medial structures injured
	a. Anterolateral posteromedial → instability: (most common)		
	b. Anterolateral posterolateral → instability:	External rotation recurvatum test → positive	Anterolateral and posterolateral structures
	c. Anteromedial and posteromedial instability:	Knee opens medially → Tibia rotates anteriorly at first and then moves posteriorly	Anteromedial and posteromedial structures

TCL—tibial collateral ligament, ACL—anterior cruciate ligament, PCL—posterior cruciate ligament, FCL—fibular collateral ligament

- Rarely tears in isolation
- Commonly tears in combinations
- May tear at mid-substance or femoral and tibial attachments
- ACL tear is a common cause of hemarthroses (70%)
- Lachman's test is useful in acute ACL tear
- Drawer's test, rotary test, etc. helps in the diagnosis of combination tears
- Treatment is by three **R's**.
    - **R**epair in fresh cases
    - **R**einforce in old lax ligaments
    - **R**econstruct in old torn ligaments
- Predisposes to instability and osteoarthritis changes.

Collateral injuries
- Medial collateral injury is more common than lateral
- Medial collateral injury is due to valgus force
- Ligament sprain is graded into three degrees
- Stress tests help in the diagnosis
- Usually associated with other ligament injuries
- First and second-degree sprain managed conservatively
- Third degree sprain needs surgical repair
- Old tears need reconstruction or distal transfer.

SEMILUNAR CARTILAGE INJURIES

Anatomy

The semilunar cartilages are two crescent-shaped plates of fibrocartilage that are placed on the condylar surface of the tibia. They are commonly known as medial and lateral menisci and are unique in that not all species have menisci in their knees and not all joints have menisci (Table 19.4). They are vital for the function of the knee joint (Fig. 19.16). The vascular supply to both the menisci is from the lateral, medial, and middle geniculate vessels. The depth of vascular penetration at the periphery is 10–30% width of medial meniscus and 10–25% width of lateral meniscus. In cross-section, they appear triangular, the thicker peripheral portion is vascular and heals well, and the thin central edge is avascular, receiving nutrition by diffusion and hence heals poorly.

TABLE 19.4: Comparative study between medial and lateral meniscus

Features	Medial meniscus	Lateral meniscus
1. Shape	Semicircular	Circular
2. Anterior	Attached to tibial horn intercondylar eminence in front of ACL	To intercondylar eminence of tibia lateral to ACL
3. Posterior horn	Intercondylar area in front of PCL and behind posterior horn of lateral meniscus	To the intercondylar eminence
4. Outer aspect	Attached to posterior fibres of TCL	Separated from FCL by capsule and popliteus
5. Mobility	Less mobile	More mobile

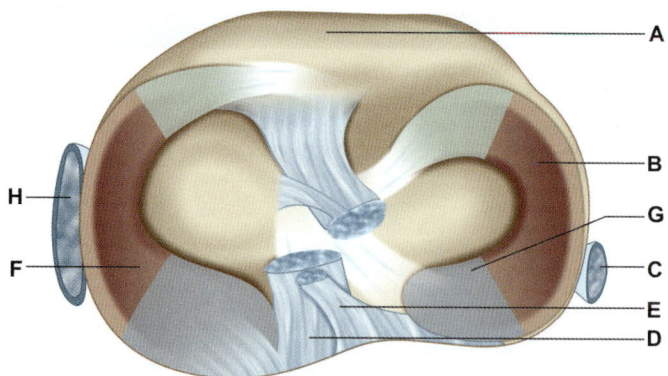

Fig. 19.16: Anatomy of two menisci: (A) Tibial tubercle, (B) Lateral meniscus, (C) Fibular collateral ligament, (D) Posterior cruciate ligament, (E) Ligament of Wrisburg, (F) Medial meniscus, (G) Intertransverse ligament, and (H) Medial collateral ligament

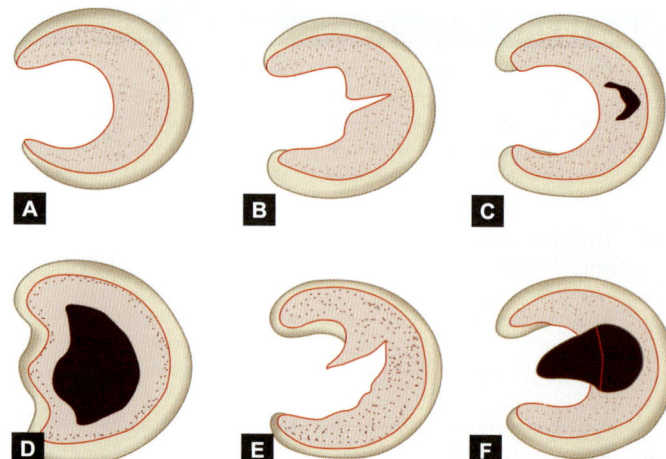

Figs 19.17A to F: Different types of meniscal injuries: (A) Longitudinal tear; (B) Radial tear; (C) Horizontal tear; (D) Bucket handle tear; (E) Parrot beak tear; (F) Segmental tear

Functions of the Menisci

- Contributes towards the stability of the knee joint
- Weight transmission of 40–70% of the load across the knee joint
- Acts as a shock absorber
- Deepens the tibial condyles on which the femoral condyles roll by increasing the contact area by 40%
- Assists in nutrition of the articular cartilage by distribution of the synovial fluid
- Helps the knee in locking mechanism
- Prevents impingement of synovial membrane, capsule, etc.
- Assists and controls gliding and rolling motion of the knee.

MEDIAL MENISCUS INJURY

Medial meniscus is more commonly injured than the lateral and is usually associated with other ligament injuries of the knee.

[1]Smillie's Classification

Medial meniscus injury (Figs 19.17A to F) is seen in over 71% of the cases. In 5% of cases, injury of medial meniscus is bilateral. Lateral meniscus is less commonly injured than the medial meniscus because it is smaller in diameter, thicker in periphery, wide, more mobile, attached to both cruciate ligaments and stabilized posteriorly to the femoral condyle by popliteus.

- *Longitudinal tears* (35%)—in these peripheral attachments tear 10%, complete tear 23% (bucket handle tear), and segmental tear 2% (ant/post)
- *Horizontal tears* (48%)—could be posterior, middle, or anterior
- *Cystic degeneration* (12%)
- *Congenital abnormalities* 5%
- *Regenerative lesions.*

Mechanism of Injury

Mechanism of injury is a rotational force when a flexed knee extends.
- In young, it can occur only when weight is being taken, knee is flexed, and there is a twisting strain. Young active athletes are more prone.
- In middle life, fibrosis has decreased the mobility of meniscus and hence tear occurs with less force.

Predisposing factors: These could be abnormal menisci shape, abnormal stress due to chronic ligament laxity, etc.

Clinical Features

The patient with medial meniscus injury presents with pain on the inner aspect of the knee (Fig. 19.18). History of locking is seen in 40% of the cases and swelling if present is minimal. There is remarkable recovery after the initial acute attack and there could be periodic complaints pertaining to the knee (Flowchart 19.2). One or more clinical

---

[1]**Smillie IS (1974)**, Scotland. His other works: (a) Monograph of knee joint, (b) Osteochondritis diseases.

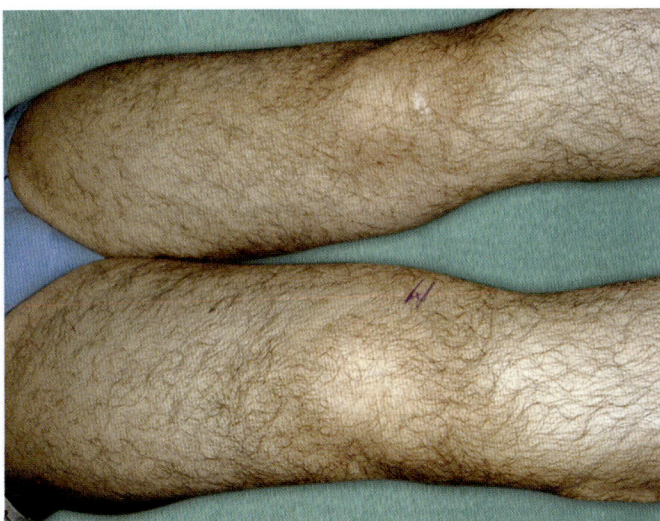

Fig. 19.18: Clinical photo showing medial joint tenderness in medial meniscus injury

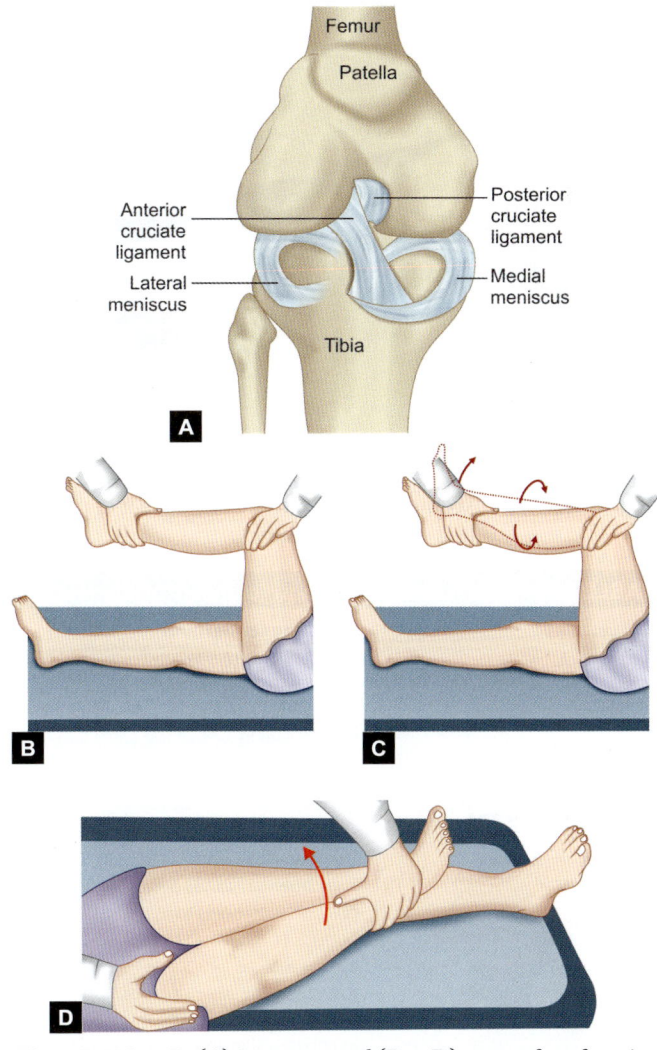

Figs 19.19A to D: (A) Anatomy and (B to D) steps of performing the McMurray's test (see page 240)

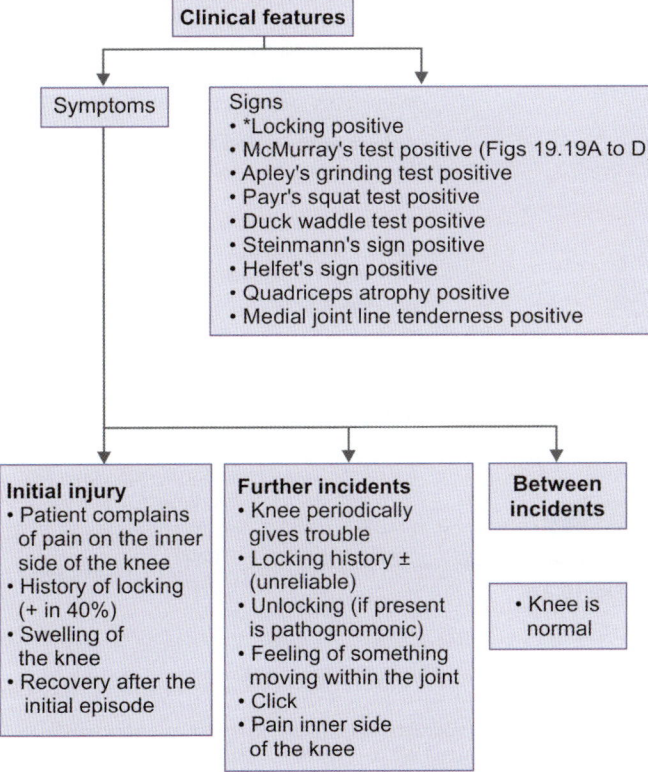

Flowchart 19.2: Clinical features of meniscal injury

signs mentioned in Table 19.5 can be elicited with careful examination of the knee.

Investigations

- Radiograph is usually normal. The views recommended are anteroposterior, lateral, intercondylar notch and sunrise views of the patella.
- Arthroscopy helps to identify the torn meniscus (Fig. 19.20).
- Arthrography may reveal the tear. Double contrast arthrography is 95% accurate.
- MRI is expensive but useful. It is the gold standard in making a diagnosis of meniscal tears (Fig. 19.21).

240   SECTION 2: Regional Traumatology

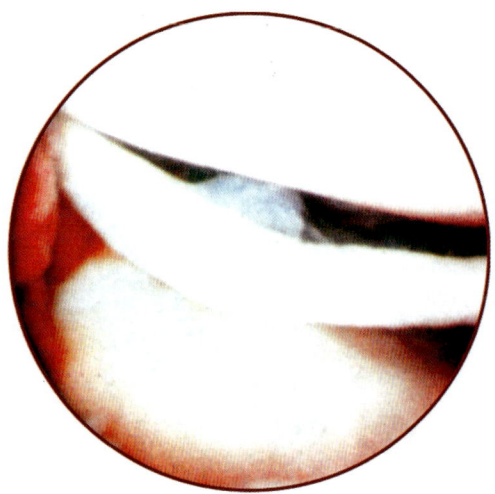

Fig. 19.20: Arthroscopic view of a bucket handle tear of medial meniscus injury

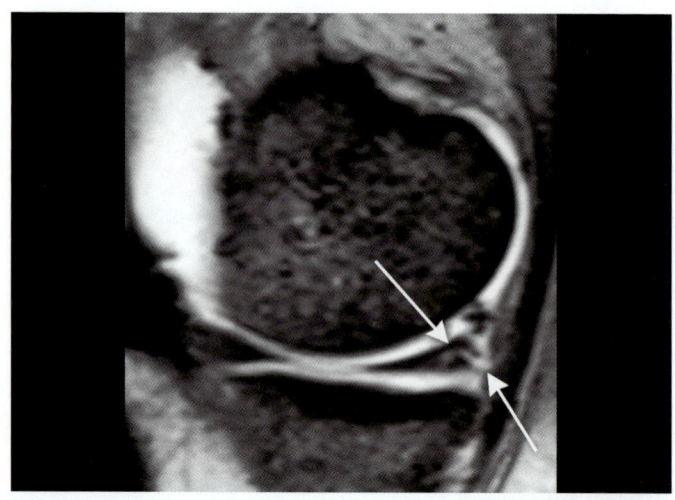

Fig. 19.21: MRI showing tear of the posterior horn of the medial meniscus

TABLE 19.5: Clinical tests for diagnosis of meniscal injuries

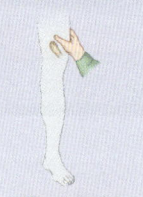 **Fig. 19.22A**	**Joint line tenderness** The medial joint line tenderness is an important clinical sign in detecting medial meniscus injury It is positive in 74% of the cases (Fig. 19.22A)	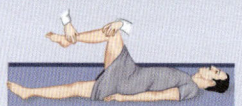 **Fig. 19.22B**	**McMurray's test** Here forced flexion and internal rotation as shown in 1 and external rotation as shown in 2 is done to test the lateral meniscus and the medial meniscus respectively A positive McMurray's test requires both pain and clunk to be felt by the examiner's finger on the medial side (Fig. 19.22B)
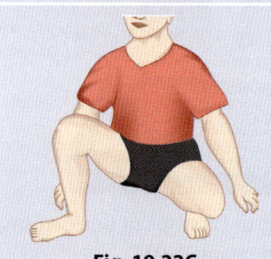 **Fig. 19.22C**	**Duck waddle test** (Fig. 19.22C) The patient assumes a squatting position with heels touching the buttock and is asked to perform a duck walk. The patient will be unable to assume full squatting position in medial meniscus injury. This is called as *childress sign* and is a diagnostic test for posterior horn tear of medial meniscus	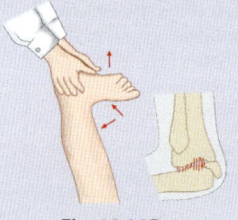 **Fig. 19.22D**	**Apley's compression test** The patient is prone, fixing the thigh against the table the examiner presses the foot and leg downward while rotating the tibia (grinding test) Pain noted during axial compression implies a meniscal lesion
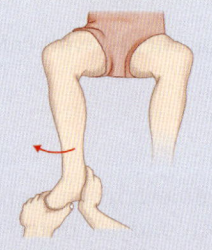 **Fig. 19.22E**	**Steinmann's sign** (Fig. 19.22E) Meniscal pathology may be suspected if medial pain is elicited on lateral rotation (medial meniscus injury) and lateral pain on medial tibial rotation (lateral meniscal injury)	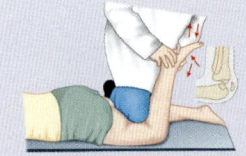 **Fig. 19.22F**	**Apley's distraction test** (Fig. 19.22F) The technique is the same as above but here the examiner pulls the foot and leg upward to distract the joint while again rotating the tibia. Pain noted during axial distraction of joint implies a ligamentous lesion
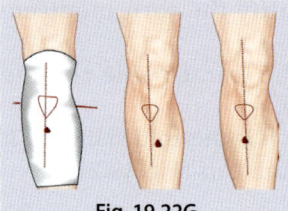 **Fig. 19.22G**	**Helfet's sign** (Fig. 19.22G) In normal knee in sitting position tibial tubercle lies in line with midline of the patella. When extended, lateral tibial rotation puts it in line with lateral border of patella. *Positive sign occurs when the rotation is blocked by a torn meniscus and the tubercle remains centred over the patella in extension*	**Note** 1. The Apley's test is unique among the meniscus tests because of its ability to distinguish between ligamen-tous and meniscal lesions 2. Positive meniscus test confirms the suspicion of out a tear with absolute confidence 3. No one test is diagnostic, hence a combination of tests are carried out. With this, the accuracy rate for diagnosis raises by 60–95% 4. The routine work-up could best include joint line tenderness. McMurray's test and Steinmann's sign	

Differential Diagnosis

Fracture of tibial spine if present may give clue to the possible ACL tear. It also helps to exclude osteochondritis dissecans, osteocartilaginous loose bodies, etc. (Table 19.6).

> **Quick Diagnostic Points**
> **Medial meniscal injuries**
> Medial joint line tenderness — positive 74% of cases
> Apley's grinding test — positive 46% of cases
> Painful hyperextension — positive in 43% of cases
> Steinmann I sign — positive in 42% of cases
> McMurray's — positive in 35% of cases
>
> Hence, no one test is diagnostic. That is why multiple tests are required for diagnosis. See for tests (Table 19.5 and Figs 19.22A to G)

Treatment

Conservative Methods

This is indicated in patients soon after injury with no locking and with infrequent attacks of pain and in tears less than 10 mm, partial thickness tears.

Measures

- Abstinence from weight bearing
- Rest, ice packs, compressive bandage
- Buck's skin traction
- Joint aspiration
- Quadriceps exercises
- If symptom persists, a cylindrical cast may be considered
- *Manipulation under anesthesia:* If joint is locked due to the torn menisci, manipulation under anesthesia is recommended.

Surgery

Indications: Surgery is indicated, if joint cannot be unlocked and if symptoms are recurrent.

Methods

- *Arthroscopic menisci repair:* This is the treatment of choice of late. Repair is indicated if the tear is >10 mm or is unstable on probing. Repair is successful in the outer third (red-red zone) edge of the vascular rim (red-white zone) and even in a few avascular zone (white-white zone) (Fig. 19.23)
- *Closed partial meniscectomy* via an arthroscopy is better than total removal of the menisci by open surgery (Fig. 19.24)
- *Meniscal transplant:* In cases with total menisectomies, cadaver menisci transplant may be considered. However, this is still in the evolving stage.

Complete removal of the menisci incapacitates the knee hence; the emphasis is on conservative surgery than the radical removal.

> **Treatment Facts: Menisci Injuries**
> - Nothing like normal meniscus
> - If minor lesion and asymptomatic better leave it alone
> - Partial meniscectomy better than total
> - Resuturing in appropriate locations
> - Earlier it was said, when in doubt remove, now the concept is when in doubt, observe do not treat.

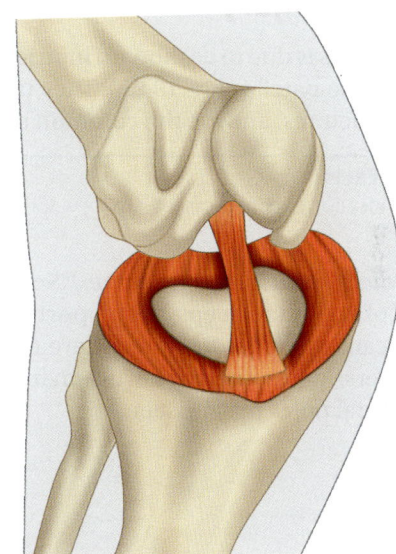

Fig. 19.23: Arthroscopic meniscal repair

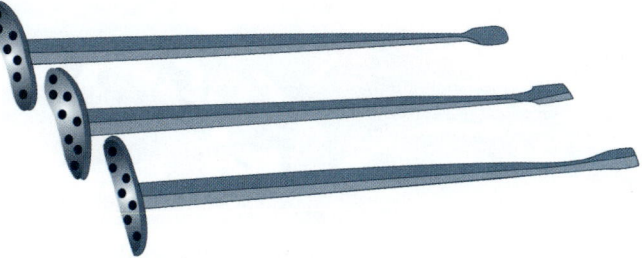

Fig. 19.24: Smillie's meniscus knife used for meniscectomy

TABLE 19.6: Differential diagnosis of locking

1. True locking	Pseudo locking
2. Loose bodies	1. Ligament injuries
3. Recurrent dislocation of patella	2. Chondromalaciae patella
4. Fracture of tibial spine	
5. Meniscal injuries	

> **Note:**
> How important are menisci to the knee?
> Consider the following facts:
> Partial meniscectomy increases stress by 50–60%. Total meniscectomy increases stress by 200–235%.
> Menisci repair may normalize the stress.

FRACTURE OF PATELLA

Patella is the largest sesamoid bone in the body. The clinical picture of a patellar fracture is determined by a combination of definite and equivocal signs.

> **Functions of Patella**
> - Increases the mechanical advantage of quadriceps tendon by increasing the efficiency of extensor mechanism by as much as 50% due to increased lever arm.
> - To aid in the nourishment of articular cartilage
> - To protect the femoral condyles from injury
> - Acts as a hydraulic brake.

Incidence is around 1% of all skeletal fractures.

Mechanism of Injury

Direct trauma: This is due to dashboard injuries and due to direct fall over the patella (Fig. 19.25). They usually cause comminuted fractures, and are the common causes.

> **Incriminating Facts**
> Subcutaneous location of patella makes it more vulnerable for direct injures.

Indirect trauma (Quadriceps contraction): Sudden forceful contraction of the quadriceps as in sports person and athletes can cause patellar fractures. Here the fracture is usually transverse and sometimes avulsion fractures of the proximal or distal poles may be seen.

Age: Common in 20–50 years age group.

Male: Female = 2: 1.

Classification (Figs 19.26A to D)

- Undisplaced:
  - Transverse fracture—these account for nearly 50-80 percent of cases. About 80% occur in the middle-third.
  - Stellate fracture.
  - Vertical fracture.
- Displaced: If displacement is >3 mm and if articular incongruity >2 mm:
  - Transverse—involving upper or lower poles (50–85%).
  - Oblique fracture
  - Vertical fracture (12–27%)
  - Comminuted fracture (30–35%)
  - Polar—could be proximal or distal
  - Osteochondral fractures.

Clinical Features

The patient gives history of trauma following which there is pain and swelling at the knee joint. The patient is unable to

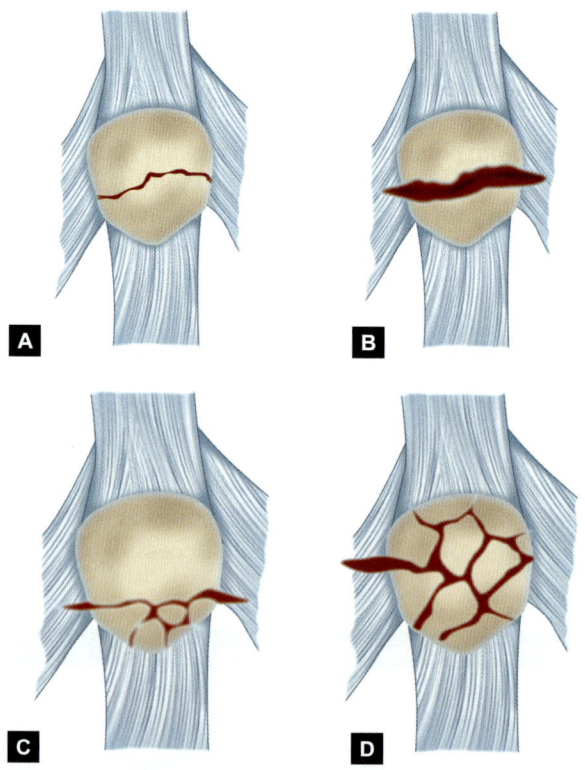

Figs 19.26A to D: Types of patellar fractures: (A) Undisplaced fracture; (B) Transverse fracture; (C) Distal pole fracture; (D) Comminuted fracture

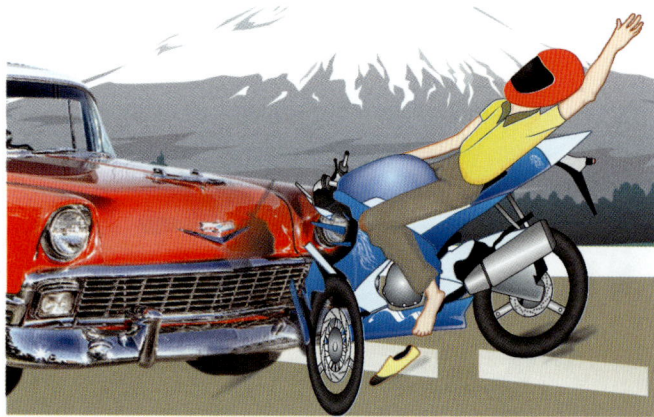

Fig. 19.25: Direct injuries due to road traffic accidents (RTAs) are a common cause of patellar fractures

extend the knee and both the active and passive movements are restricted. On examination, there could be a palpable gap, tenderness, signs of effusion and a positive patellar tap (Figs 19.27A and B).

Investigations

- Radiograph of the knee joint consists of AP view, lateral view (Figs 19.30A and B), intercondylar notch view (Fig. 19.28) and skyline or axial view (Fig. 19.29) to rule out undisplaced vertical fracture.
- CT scan, bone scan, and tomography are other useful investigations.

Note:
Bipartite patella and osteochondral fractures cause confusion in the diagnosis.

Mystifying Facts
- Do you know which patellar fractures are difficult to diagnose clinically? Well, it is the thin vertical fracture of the patella which has a very few clinical signs and symptoms.

Management

Undisplaced Fracture

Nonoperative treatment will produce good results in undisplaced fracture and if displacement is less than 1-2 mm and in intact extensor mechanism and minimal articular step-off (<1-2 mm) and the methods include compression bandage, ice applications, aspiration of hemarthrosis, cylindrical cast in extension (Figs19.31 and 19.32), or long leg cast for 4–6 weeks. Functional cast brace

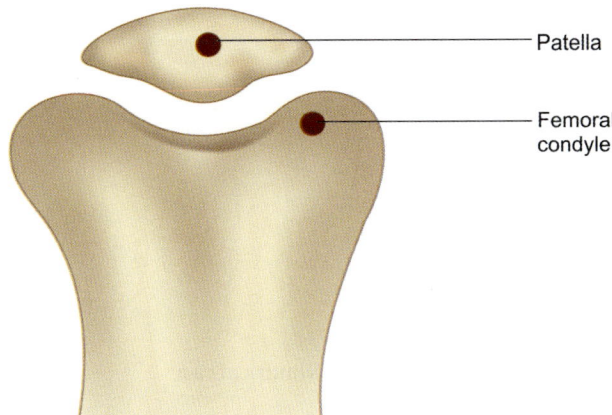

Fig. 19.28: Intercondylar notch view of patella

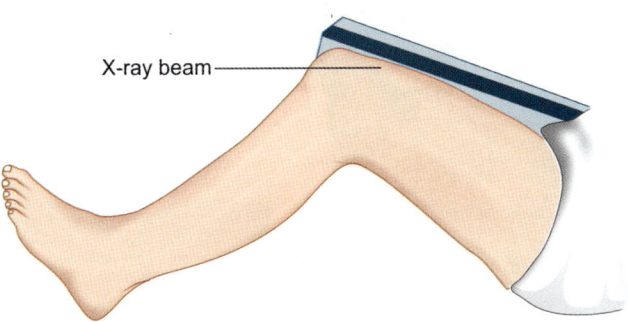

Fig. 19.29: Axial view of the knee

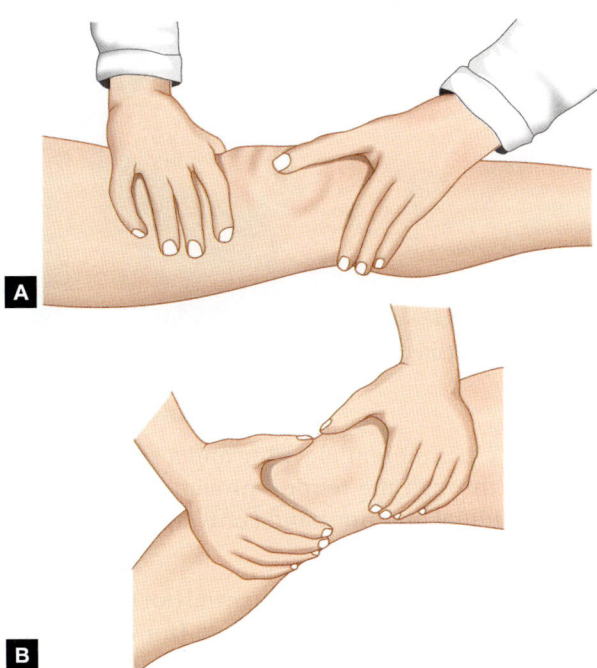

Figs 19.27A and B: Method to elicit: (A) Patellar tap; (B) Fluctuation test

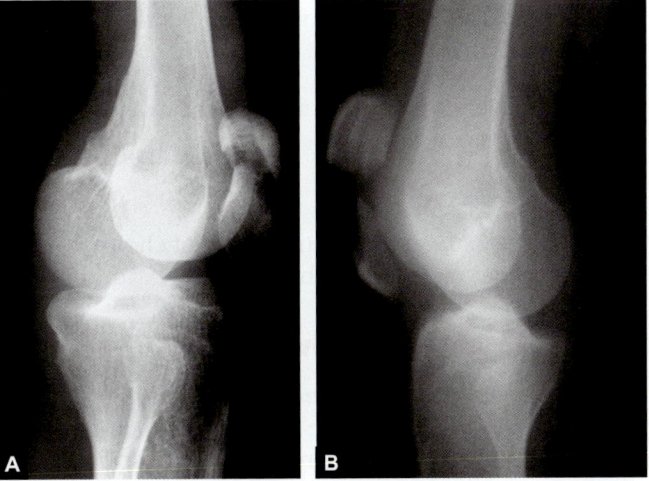

Figs 19.30A and B: Plain X-ray showing fracture patella—proximal pole, middle level and distal pole

244 SECTION 2: Regional Traumatology

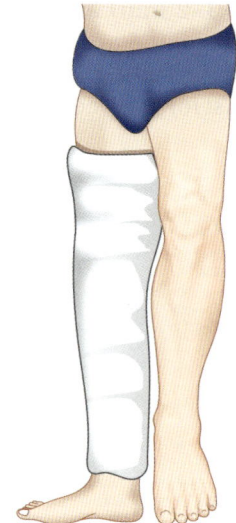

Fig. 19.31: Cylindrical cast

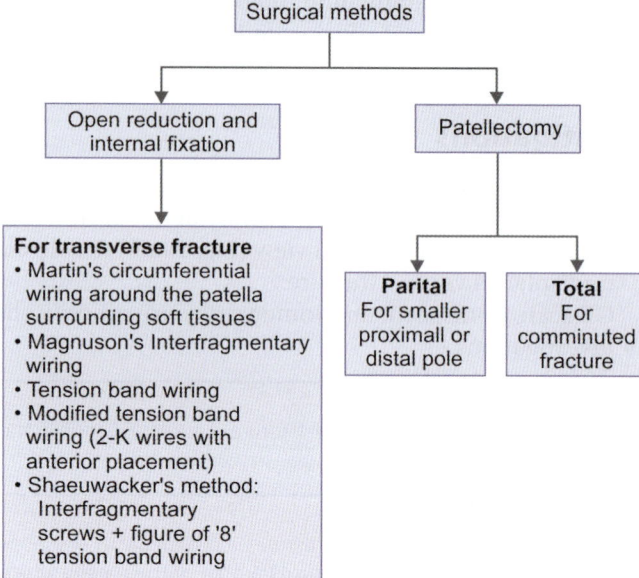

Flowchart 19.3: Surgical methods of fracture patella

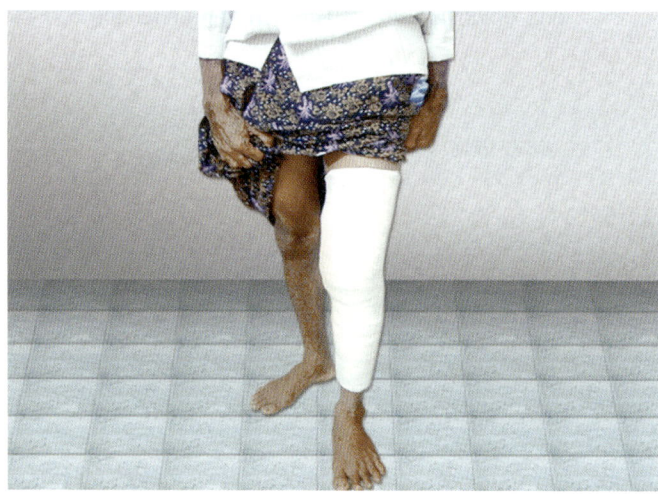

Fig. 19.32: Clinical photo showing cylindrical cast

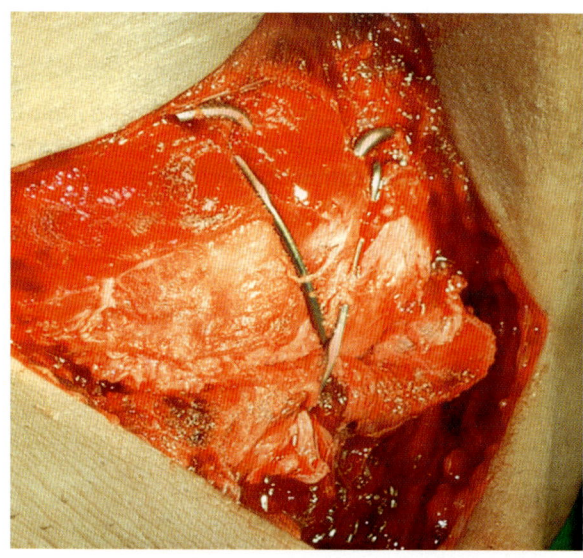

Fig. 19.33: Operative photo showing TBW patella

is also effective. The patient is advised early weight bearing and quadriceps exercises.

Displaced Fracture

In this variety, surgery is the treatment of choice. Surgery is performed as early as possible preferably within 7 days.

Surgical Methods (Flowchart 19.3)

Open reduction and internal fixation: This is indicated in transverse fractures of the patella. Internal fixation is done either by the circumferential wiring or by tension band wiring (Fig. 19.33). The other methods are Pyrford technique of circumferential wiring and a second tension band wiring through the tendon provide better fixation. Lotke longitudinal anterior band (LAB) wiring is another method with good results.

Patellectomy: This could be either partial (for smaller distal or proximal pole fracture) or complete (for comminuted fractures). The emphasis is now on preserving as much patella as possible.

Anterior Tension Band Wiring (ATBW)

ATBW (Figs 19.34 and 19.35) though a popular method of stabilization of mainly transverse patellar fractures, K-wires, offer the following problems:
- Migration of K-wire up and down
- Breakage/protrusion
- Bursa formation.

Cannulated Screws Fixation

These problems are overcome if TBW is done with two cannulated screws instead of 2 K-wires. Other advantages are:
- Early mobilization of the knee
- Less soft tissue reaction
- Rigid stable fixation in osteoporotic bones
- Lag effect of screws provide better compression
- Destructive forces shared equally by screws, and cerclage wire, thereby reducing chances of breakage.

Complications

Postoperative complications: Early fracture dehiscence, postoperative infection, refracture (1–5%), avascular necrosis (25% incidence in proximal pole) are some of the common postoperative complications.

Delayed complications: This is like knee stiffness, osteoarthritis of the patellofemoral and knee joint extensor lag, etc. can occur. Delayed union, nonunion, loss of knee motion, etc. (Fig. 19.36).

Disadvantages of Patellectomy

- Strength of quadriceps returns slowly although knee motion is regained quite fast.
- Obvious atrophy of the quadriceps muscle persists for months and often permanently.
- Protection of the knee by the patella is lost.
- Pathological ossification may develop where the patella is excised.

Extensor lag: This is inability of the patient to perform the last 10° of extension (Figs 19.37 and 19.38). About 80% of quadriceps strength is required to bring about the last 20° of extension. After patellectomy, due to the decreased lever arm, the efficiency of quadriceps is reduced and the patient will be unable to bring about the terminal extension of the knee. Thus, an attempt is made to save as much of patella as

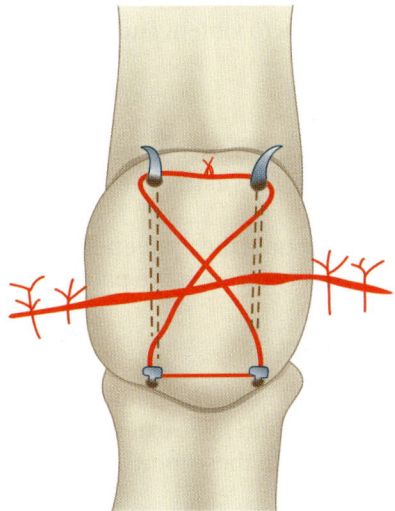

Fig. 19.34: Tension band wiring

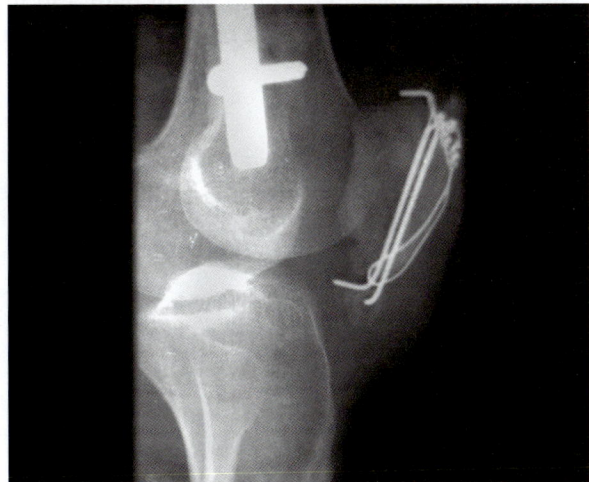

Fig. 19.35: Radiograph showing TBW fracture patella

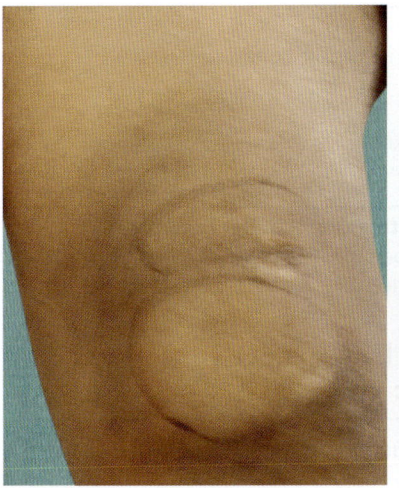 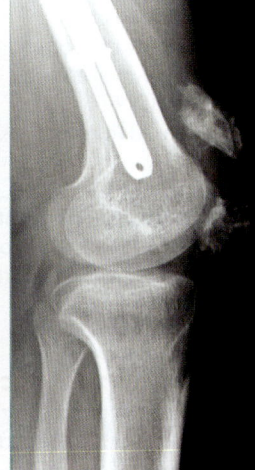

Fig. 19.36: Clinical photo and X-rays showing nonunion patella

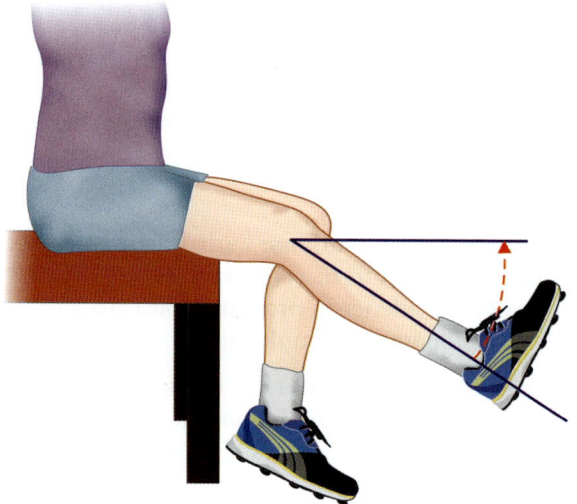

Fig. 19.37: Extensor lag

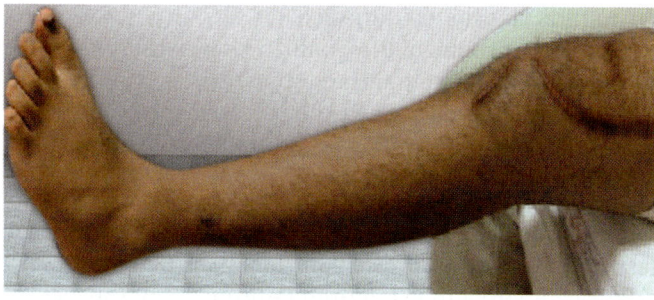

Fig. 19.38: Clinical photo showing extensor lag following patella fracture

possible, all of the patella or at least the proximal or distal half, if practical to preserve the quadriceps efficiency.

Disturbing Facts
Do you know the common sequelae of patellar fractures?
- Patellofemoral arthritis
- Instability of the knee
- Decreased ROM of the knee
- Difficulty with stairs, downhill walking and kneeling.

What is New in The Treatment of Patellar Fractures?
Arthroscopically assisted percutaneous screw fixation for displaced patellar fracture is being tried with varied success.

INJURY TO THE EXTENSOR APPARATUS OF KNEE

The extensor apparatus of the knee is comprised of the following six structures:

- The quadriceps muscle with a group of six extensor muscles and the quadriceps femoris tendon.
- Patella
- Ligamentum patellae (patellofemoral and patellotibial ligaments).
- Patellar bursae and the fat pads
- Capsule and synovial membrane.

Note:
The quadriceps muscle consists of rectus femoris, vastus medialis, lateralis intermedius, articularis genu, and ligamentum patellae.

QUADRICEPS STRAIN

Causes

- Direct blow to the muscle
- Indirect forces due to violent sudden contractions.

Sites

- Rectus femoris is the most commonly injured muscle.
- This is followed by vastus medialis, lateralis, and intermedius.
- Avulsion may occur at the upper pole of patella or tibial tubercle and rarely through the patella.

Clinical Features

- In rectus femoris injury, the patient complains of pain during hip flexion and knee extension as this muscle is known to act on both these joints. Tenderness is present at the site of injury.
- In grade III sprain a gap may be felt at the site of rupture and ambulation is difficult.
- In injuries to the vastus medialis, intermedius and lateralis the patient may complain of pain and limp, terminal stage of flexion and resisted knee flexion is extremely painful.

Treatment

In general, grade I and grade II injuries can be managed conservatively, while grade III injury may require surgical suturing in the event of complete rupture and loss of function (Fig. 19.39).

Treatment Methods

Grade I and II Strain
- Ice therapy and ice packs
- Compression bandaging (Jones)
- Limb elevation

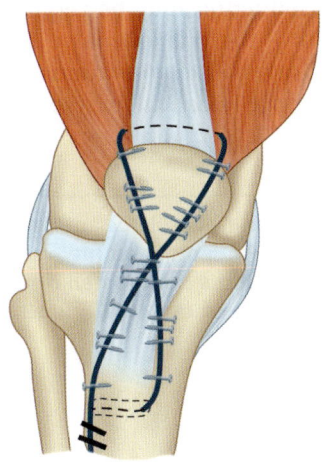

Fig. 19.39: Reconstruction of extensor mechanism

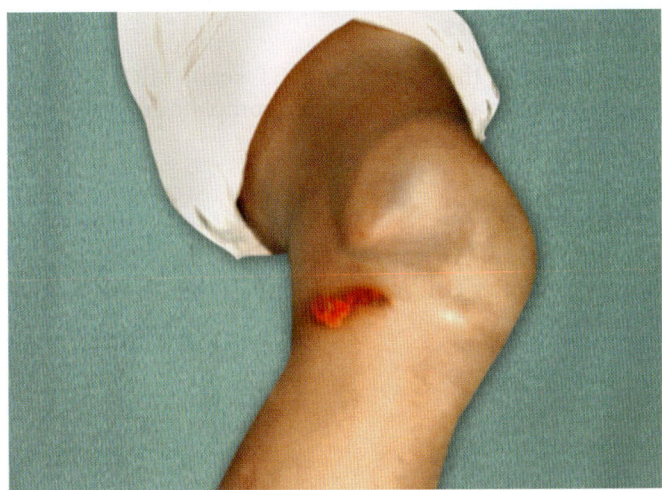

Fig. 19.40: Clinical photo showing acute dislocation on patella

- Mild isometric exercises
- Relaxed passive knee movements
- To improve the strength and mobility of the knee joint, active and active-assisted knee exercises are begun
- Progressive resistive exercises to increase the endurance of the knee muscles
- Gradual weight bearing with assistive devices. The patient should be functionally independent by 6 weeks.

Grade III Strain
- Quadriceps exercises are begun by 5–6 days
- Self-assisted SLR
- By 2nd or 3rd day's nonweight-bearing and partial weight bearing by 3 weeks, full weight-bearing by 6 weeks
- For extensor lag, electrical stimulation helps
- Rest of the measures is the same as mentioned above.

ACUTE DISLOCATION OF PATELLA

Lateral dislocations of patella are very common and are due to lateral force acting on a semi-flexed knee.

Clinical Features

Patient complains of severe pain, swelling, and inability to bend the knee. Patella is seen and felt on the lateral side (Fig. 19.40).

Radiograph of the knee helps to make the diagnosis. MRI helps to assess the short tissue damages.

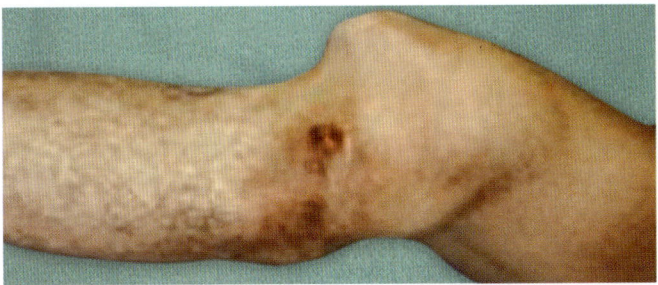

Fig. 19.41: Clinical photo showing acute dislocation of the knee joint

Treatment

Closed reduction and above knee POP casting is done under GA. Immobilization in a long leg cast may be required for a period of 4 weeks.

ACUTE DISLOCATION OF KNEE

This is an uncommon injury and is due to severe violence as in RTA, fall, etc. It is usually associated with injuries to collateral cruciates and meniscus. Patella may also be fractured or dislocated.

Clinical Features

Patient complains of severe pain, swelling, and inability to bend the knee. There could be features of injuries to the neurovascular structures around the knee (Fig. 19.41).

Investigations

Plain X-ray of the knee joint, CT scan, MRI, Doppler studies, etc. are advised to make a complete analysis of the dislocation of the knee.

Treatment

Conservative: An attempt may be made for closed reduction under GA. An above knee POP cast is applied for 12 weeks.

Surgery: Open reduction may be required if the closed reduction fails or if there is extensive ligament injuries, which may require repair, reconstruction or both. Knee is immobilized in above knee POP cast for 12 weeks.

REFERENCE

1. Johannes Struewer, et al. Isolated anterior cruciate ligament reconstruction in patients aged fifty years: comparison of hamstring graft versus bone-patellar tendon-bone graft. International Orthopedics (SICOT). 2013;37:809-17.

20 CHAPTER

Fracture of Tibia and Fibula

This includes fractures of the proximal tibia, shaft and distal tibia (Fig. 20.1).

PROXIMAL TIBIAL FRACTURES

Proximal tibia consists of the medial and lateral condyles along with the upper tibial articular surface and includes the proximal 10–12 cm of the tibia. These fractures are frequently intra-articular and usually unite well considering the cancellous nature of the bone.

Incidence

One percent of all fractures and 8% of fractures in elderly people.

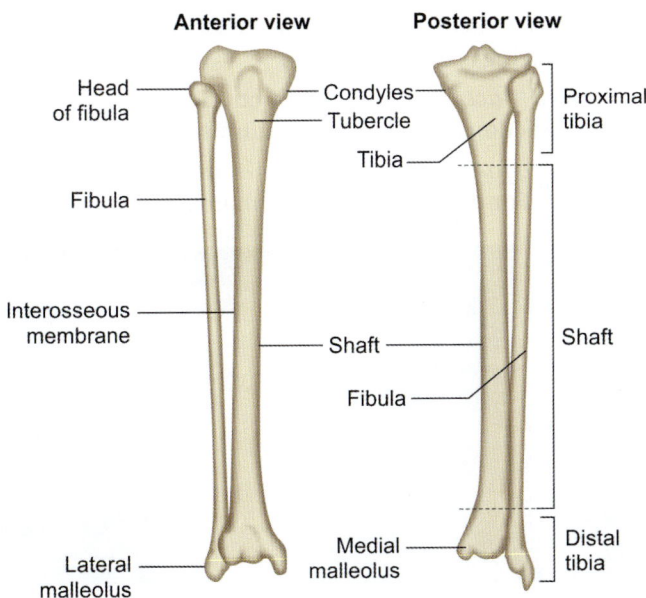

Fig. 20.1: Bony anatomy of tibia and fibula

Mechanism of Injury

It is due to valgus or varus force with axial loading.

Causes

- Fifty-two percent—due to auto-pedestrian injuries (Bumper injuries) (Fig. 20.2).
- Seventeen percent—due to fall from heights.
- Thirty one percent—miscellaneous causes (football or soccer injuries).

> **Interesting Facts: Associated Injuries with Condylar Fractures**
> - Meniscal injury—50 percent
> - Ligament injury—30 percent
> - Peroneal nerve neuropraxia
> - Popliteal artery injury.

Classification

This is shown in Flowchart 20.1.
- Articular variety
- Nonarticular variety.

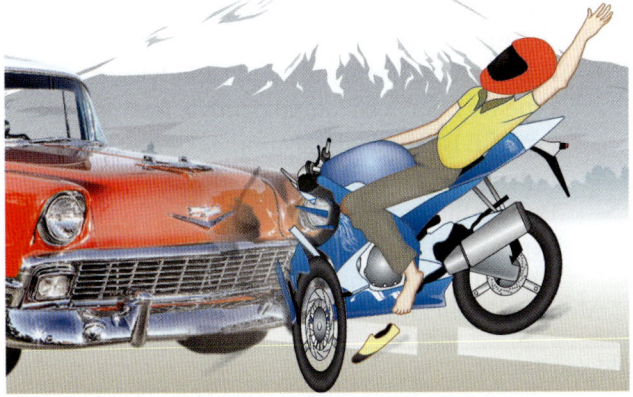

Fig. 20.2: Bumper injuries are a common cause of tibia fractures

Flowchart 20.1: Classification of proximal tibial fracture

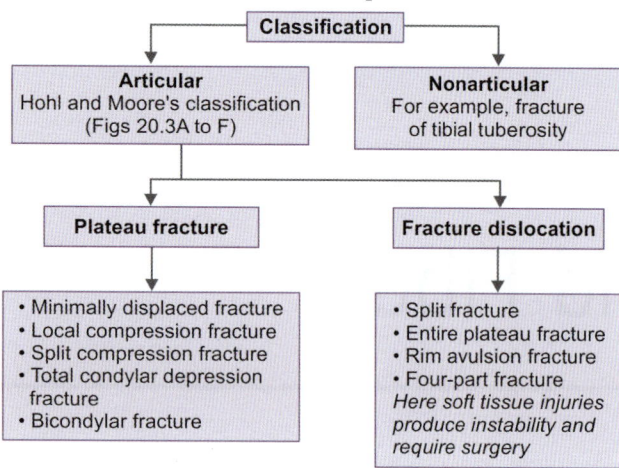

Interesting Facts
- Isolated lateral tibial condylar fracture—55–70%
- Isolated medial tibial condylar fracture—10–23%
- Both plateau fractures—10–30%.

Clinical Features

The patient with proximal tibial fractures presents with pain, swelling, deformity, hemarthrosis, decreased movements of the knee and instability in valgus or varus. There could be features of compartment syndrome of the leg, disturbed peripheral vascular and nerve functions of the leg.

Investigations

The routine AP and lateral radiographs of the knee help to demonstrate majority of tibial condyle fractures. Oblique view may be required to localize the fractures. To study the depth of depression, CT scan is excellent, but 10° caudal plateau view also helps (Figs 20.4A and B). To know the knee ligament injuries, valgus or varus stress films are required. Aspiration may reveal blood or fat. If fat is present, it indicates an intra-articular fracture. Angiography if pulses are feeble or absent.

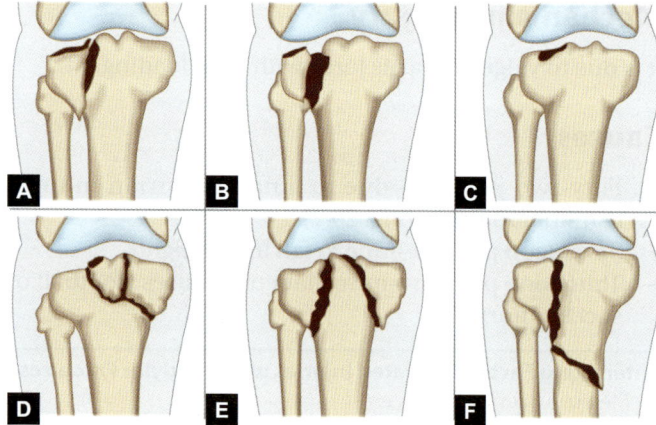

Figs 20.3A to F: Hohl and Moore's classification of proximal tibia fractures: (A) Minimally displaced fracture; (B) Local compression fracture; (C) Split compression fracture; (D) Total condylar depression; (E) Bicondylar fractures; (F) Bicondylar fracture with diaphyseal metaphyseal extension

Other Classifications

- Schatzker's classification: This is widely followed in North America and has six types:
  - Type I : Split fracture of lateral condyle.
  - Type II : Displaced lateral condyle fracture.
  - Type III: Isolated lateral condyle depression.
  - Type IV: Medial condylar fracture.
  - Type V: Bicondylar fractures.
  - Type VI: Bicondylar fracture with diaphyseal metaphyseal extension.
- Modified Hohl and Moore's classification.

Did You Know?
Lateral condyle is fractured 70–80% more often than the medial condyle.

Management

Aim
- To produce a knee that extends fully and flexes to at least 120°.
- Restoration of normal articular surface and ligament repair are both important in preventing late instability.

Conservative treatment is indicated for plateau fractures with <4 mm depression or displacement.

Undisplaced fracture: Above knee, POP cast with 5° flexion or cast bracing is used.

Displaced fracture: Closed reduction, with or without skeletal traction and a long leg cast is used.

In depressed fractures: For less than 8 mm depression, above knee cast. For depression of more than 8 mm with a large

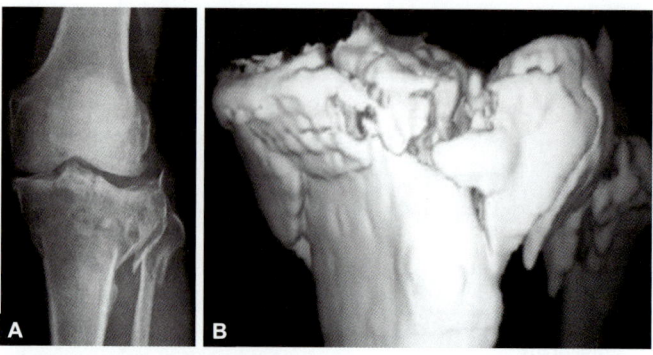

Figs 20.4A and B: (A) Plain X-ray and 3D CT scan of proximal tibial fractures (B)

split fragment, skeletal traction is applied. For more than 8 mm with smaller split fragment, ORIF is done with bone grafting after elevation of the depression.

Surgery

In displaced condylar fractures, bicondylar fractures, split fractures, closed reduction is not useful. Open reduction and internal fixation with cancellous screws, single, or dual buttress plating are the time tested methods (Figs 20.5A and B). External fixation with circular or semi-circular frames is also another useful option. Skeletal traction is useful in grossly comminuted fractures.

Of late lightweight UMEX external fixator frame is being tried with a reasonable success in treating the difficult and comminuted tibial condylar fractures.
Some surgeons advocate dual plating in difficult bicondylar fractures notwithstanding the many complications it opens up because of extensive exposure.

Locking compression plates (LCP) with bicortical screw fixations are being increasingly tried with varied success (Fig. 20.6) especially in osteoporotic fractures.

What is New in the Treatment of Tibial Condylar Fractures?
Arthroscopically assisted evaluation, reduction, and internal fixation are being increasingly tried with varied success recently and hold tremendous promise for the future.

Complications

These include DVT, compartment syndrome, peroneal nerve palsy, popliteal artery laceration, nonunion (rare), malunion and degenerative arthritis (Fig. 20.7).

Do You Know What a Floating Knee is?
Well, it is an ipsilateral fracture of lower end of femur and upper end of tibia.
- It is usually compound
- It is usually associated with vascular injuries
- Surgery is the treatment of choice.

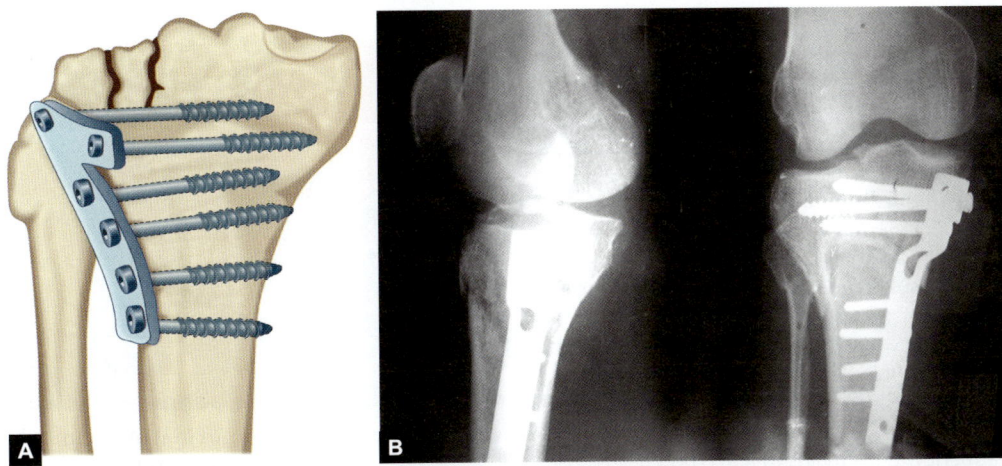

Figs 20.5A and B: (A) Internal fixation of proximal tibia fracture with buttress plate and screws; (B) Radiograph showing buttress plating

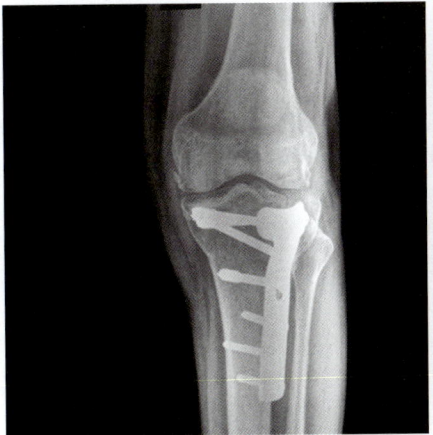 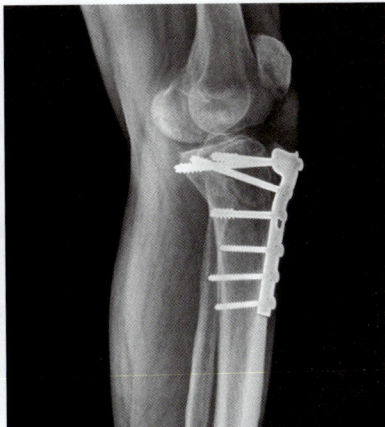 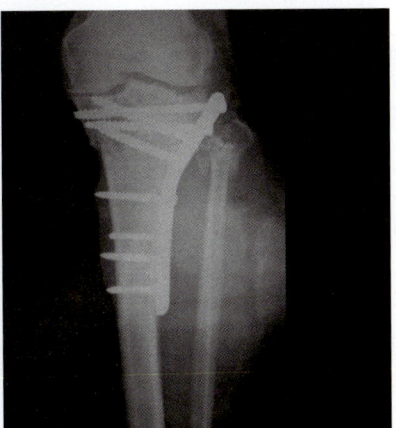

Fig. 20.6: Plain X-ray showing locked compression plating for proximal tibia fracture

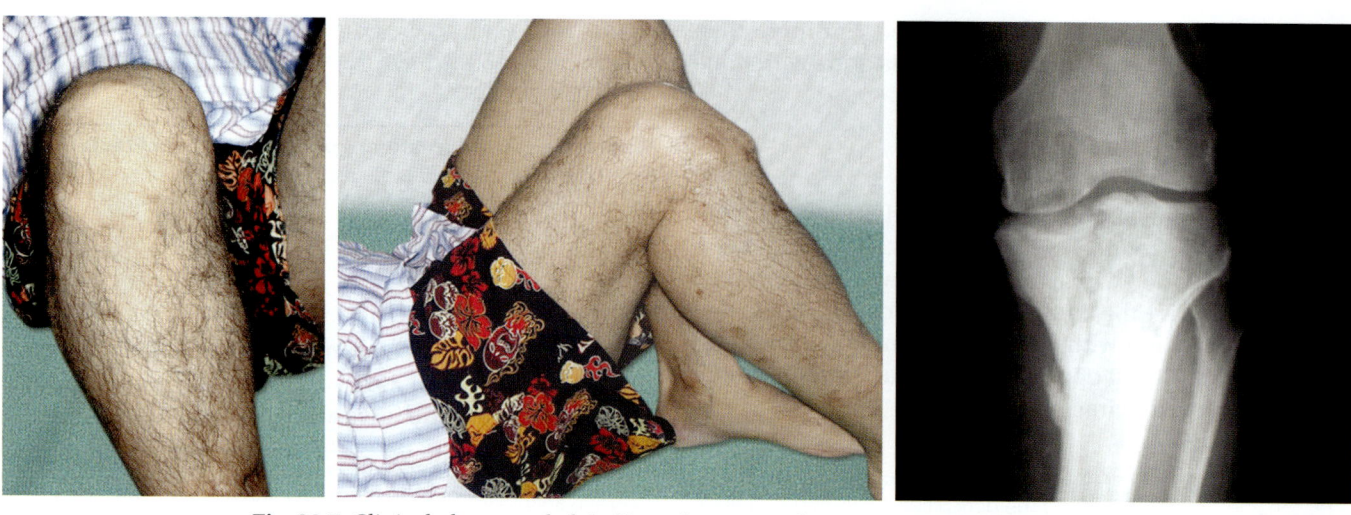

Fig. 20.7: Clinical photos and plain X-ray showing malunion proximal tibia fracture

FRACTURE SHAFT OF TIBIA AND FIBULA

Tibial shaft fractures are the most common long bone fractures and they are famous for high incidence of open fractures.

Features of Tibia Fractures
- Most common of all long bone fractures. Next common to intracapsular fracture neck femur.
- More controversial, exceeded only by fracture neck femur.
- Its one-third surface is subcutaneous and hence incidence of open fracture is high.
- Distal one-third has a deficient blood supply and a fracture in this area is known for delayed union and nonunion.
- Bounded above and below by hinge joints and hence no melanin is acceptable.
- Conservative treatment was the mainstay and is now reserved for low energy stable, simple, undisplaced of less displaced fracture.
- Operative treatment is indicted for most fractures with high energy trauma.

Did You Know?
- Isolated tibia fracture—23%
- Both tibia and fibular fractures—77%
- Seventy seven% of tibia fractures are closed
- Twenty three% are open fractures
- The common site of tibia fractures due to indirect force is the region of the isthmus.

Mechanism of Injury
- RTA—37.5%
- Sports—24.7%
- Assaults—4.5%
- Falls—rest.

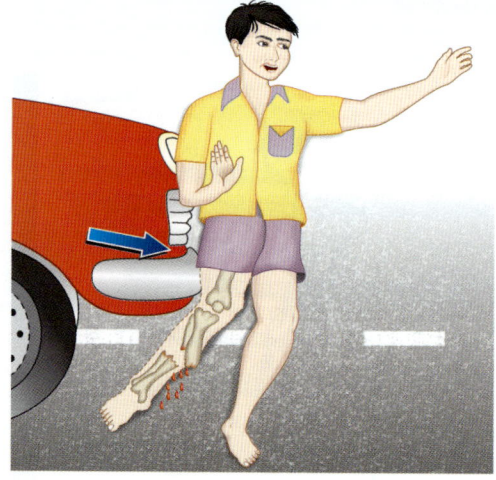

Fig. 20.8: Bumper injuries in RTA commonly cause fracture femur and tibia

Direct violence due to road traffic accidents (most common mode of injury), fall, assault, etc. (Fig. 20.8). Open fractures are common in this mode of injury.

Indirect violence due to falls, twisting force due to sports injuries, usually cause spiral fractures.

Classification
1. Ellis

   Grades of severity   Features

   I   Minor
   - Undisplaced
   - Not angulated
   - Minor comminution
   - Minor open fracture

II Moderate
  - Total displacement
  - Small degree of comminution
  - Minor open wound

  III Major
  - Complete displacement
  - Major comminution
  - Major open fracture

2. Tscherne classification (takes into account soft tissue injuries too)
   C_0 — Simple fracture with no soft tissue injury.
   C_1 — Mild to moderate, fracture with superficial abrasions.
   C_2 — Moderately severe fractures with deep contusions.
   C_3 — Severe fracture with severe destruction of the soft tissues.

> **Interesting Facts: What Holds the Tibia Fractures Together?**
> - Intact fibula
> - Interosseous membrane intact
> - Surrounding calf muscles.

> **Note:**
> Many classifications like the OTA, Tscherne, and Gustilo Anderson classification for open fractures are in vogue.

Clinical Features

In these fractures, the common symptom is pain and the obvious sign is the deformity, apart from other features of fractures (Fig. 20.9). Damage to the blood vessels and nerves is not that common, but fibular neck fracture may injure the lateral popliteal nerve; and if the posterior tibial vessels are injured, compartmental syndrome may develop.

Radiographs

Radiograph for acute cases require AP and lateral views. For delayed cases, AP, lateral and oblique views may be required (Fig. 20.10). Knee joint above and ankle below should always be included.

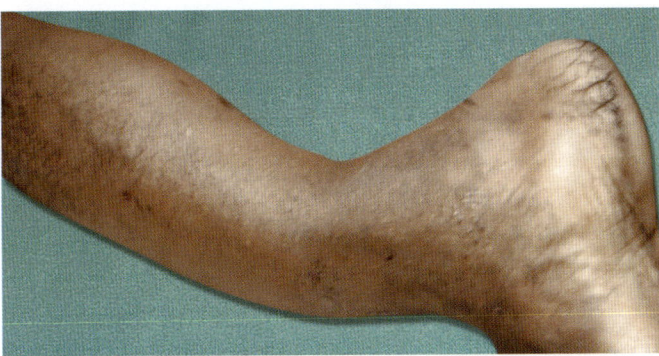

Fig. 20.9: Clinical photo showing deformity in fracture tibia

> **Interesting Facts**
> Do you know fibula bears approximately 12% of the body weight?

Methods of Treatment

Conservative management is done in majority of cases and consists of the following options (Fig. 20.11):

Long Leg Plaster Casts

Indications

- Most closed fractures
- Undisplaced fracture
- Fractures with minor or moderate displacements
- Young adults
- Low energy trauma.

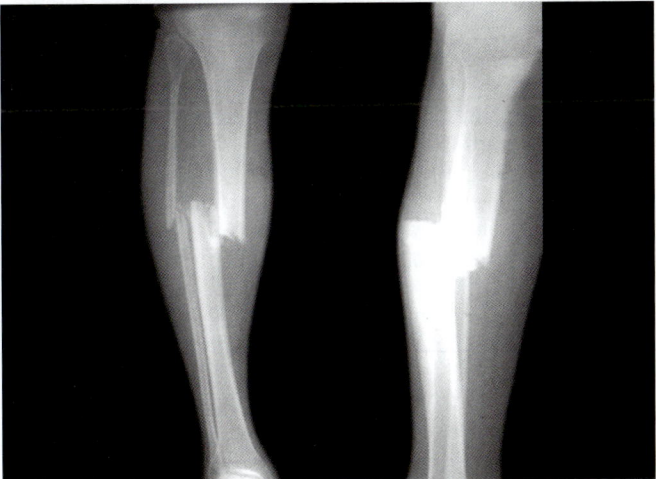

Fig. 20.10: Radiograph showing fracture of tibia and fibula

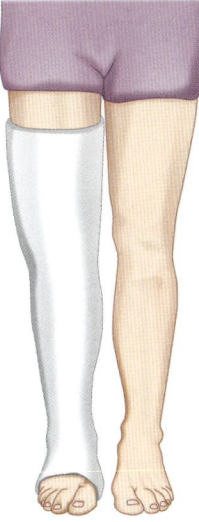

Fig. 20.11: Fracture tibia treated with long leg cast

Methods of reduction in displaced fractures: There are two methods of closed reduction. In the first, the patient is supine and is under general anesthesia. With the limb held parallel to the table, the fracture is reduced by traction and counter traction method (by an assistant) and a long leg cast is applied. The disadvantage with this technique is due to the gravitational forces, posterior angulations develop at the fracture site.

In the second and more commonly followed method (Fig. 20.12), the patient is supine or sitting. The patient is brought to the edge of the table and both the legs are kept dangling. Through a halter, the clinician holds the leg of the patient and manipulates the fracture. A long leg cast is then put with the knee in slight flexion and the ankle at 90°.

Advantages of This Method are:
- Traction and counter traction do not require the services of an assistant.
- The patient's own weight of the leg provides traction through the gravity.
- Easy to compare with the normal leg regarding the accuracy of closed reduction by looking at the control of rotation and angle.

Criteria of Acceptable Reduction
- Rotation should be nearly perfect.
- Ankle and knee joint surfaces should be parallel.
- Acceptable varus or valgus angulations is 5° in AP view.
- Anterior or posterior angulations of 10° in lateral view.
- Even 50% apposition is acceptable provided there is no rotation.
- Shortening of 5–7 mm is acceptable.

Did You Know?
Böhler of Vienna was the first person to use and popularize the long leg casts for tibial fractures.

Concept of Wedge Plasters Correction
For postreduction angulations of the fracture tibia, which is in a plaster cast, the technique of wedge correction of the plaster will enable the surgeon to correct the residual angulations without removing the original plaster cast.

In a postreduction radiograph, the direction of the angulations whether medial or lateral, anterior or posterior is noted. Then an attempt is made to correct the angulations by either opening a wedge or closing a wedge in the cast. In the open wedge plaster correction, the plaster is cut at the opposite end of the angulations and opened thereby correcting the angulations. In the closed wedge technique, a wedge of plaster cast is removed at the apex of the angulations and the plaster cast is closed correcting the angulations (Fig. 20.13).

The open wedge technique is preferred over closed wedge because of the chances of the skin being caught within the plaster edges in the closed technique. After either procedure, the plaster cast is completed and a check radiograph is taken to confirm the correction.

Sarmiento's Total Contact below Knee Cast

After reduction of the fracture and application of a long leg cast for 2–3 weeks, a total below knee cast which is molded around the tibial condyles and patella in the fashion of patellar tendon bearing prosthesis is applied (PTB casts or brace) and movement of the knee joint and weight bearing is permitted (Fig. 20.14). He reported a union rate of 97.5% and the average healing time was 14–15 weeks.

Advantages
- Allows early knee movements
- Sitting can be permitted early
- Ease of ambulation for patients with bilateral fracture.
- Decreases the incidence of delayed union and nonunion.

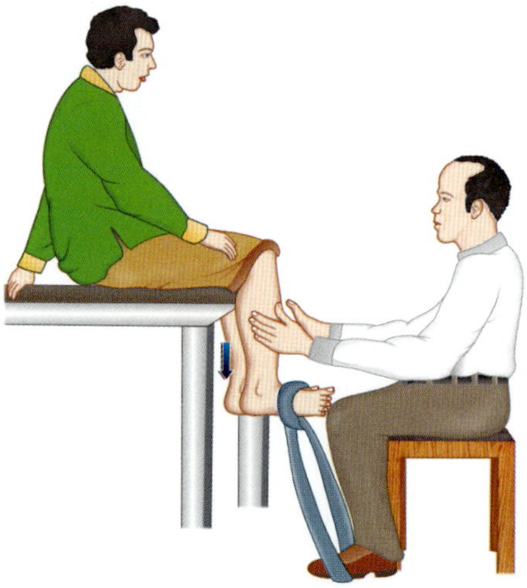

Fig. 20.12: Reduction technique of fracture tibia (No longer practised, except in children)

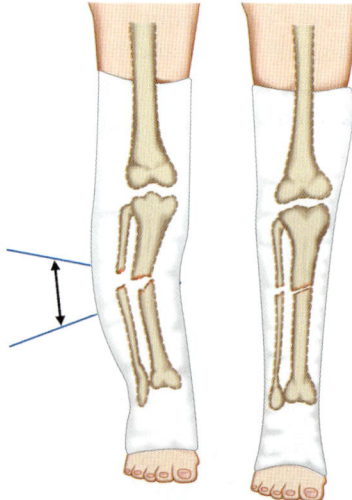

Fig. 20.13: Residual post-reduction angulations corrected by closed wedge plaster technique

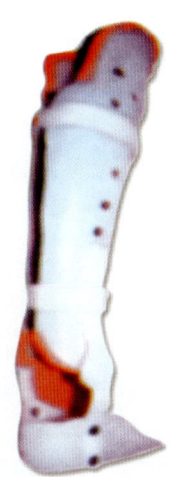

Fig. 20.14: Sarmiento's total contact below knee cast

Functional Braces

This allows movements of both ankle and knee joints, while the PTB cast includes the ankle joint.

Pins above and below the Fracture

Here two Steinmann's pins are passed above and below the fracture site and incorporated within the plaster cast. This method is, however, no longer used except in some remote centers.

Indications

- For moderate and severe fracture
- Unstable fracture
- Open fracture.

Surgical Treatment

As mentioned earlier, only 5% of the cases require operative treatment in tibia fractures.

Absolute Indications

- Tibia fracture with vascular or neural injuries
- Segmental fractures
- Inadequate reduction
- Associated knee problems
- Associated tibia plafond fracture.

Advantages

- Definitive form of treatment
- No loss of position or shortening.
- No post-fracture deformity.
- Joint movements obtained early.

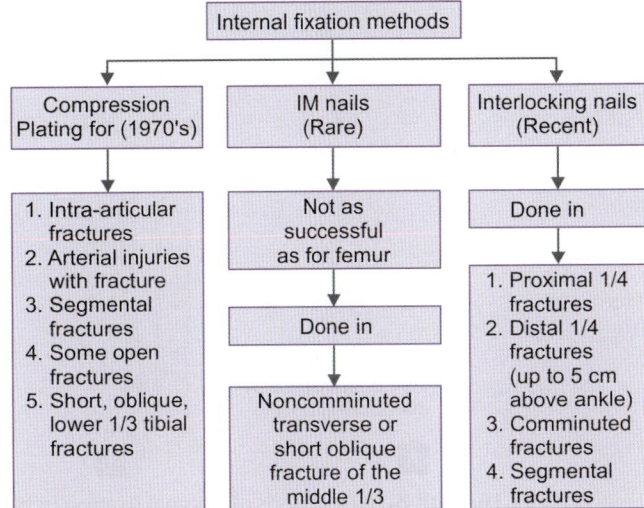

Flowchart 20.2: Internal fixation methods of tibia fractures

Note: ILN could be reamed or unreamed.

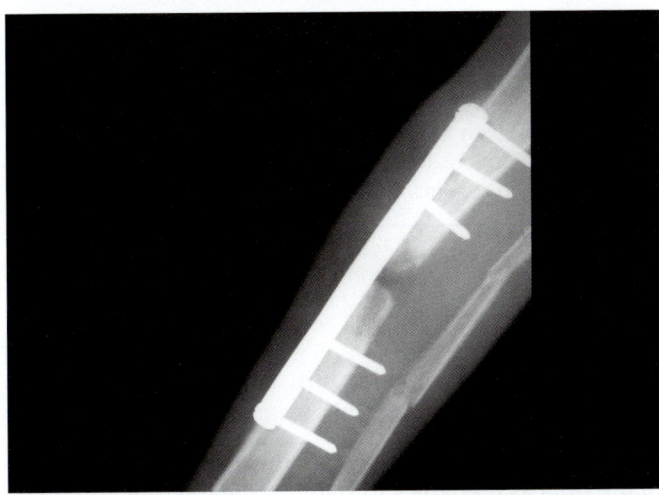

Fig. 20.15: Plating of tibia is no longer the gold standard

Internal Fixation Methods (Flowchart 20.2)

Not so long ago, plating as the internal fixation methods ruled the roost so much, so that tibia fractures were plated right, left and center (Fig. 20.15).

Nevertheless, slowly closed reduction and interlocking nailing emerged as the *Gold Standard* and pushed the technique of plating into oblivion (Fig. 20.16A). It appears that with its obvious advantages interlocking nailing is here to stay (Fig. 20.16B).

The conventional nails are the GK nail and the RT nails with the proximal and distal holes. However, new generation nails are fast emerging as an effective alternative.

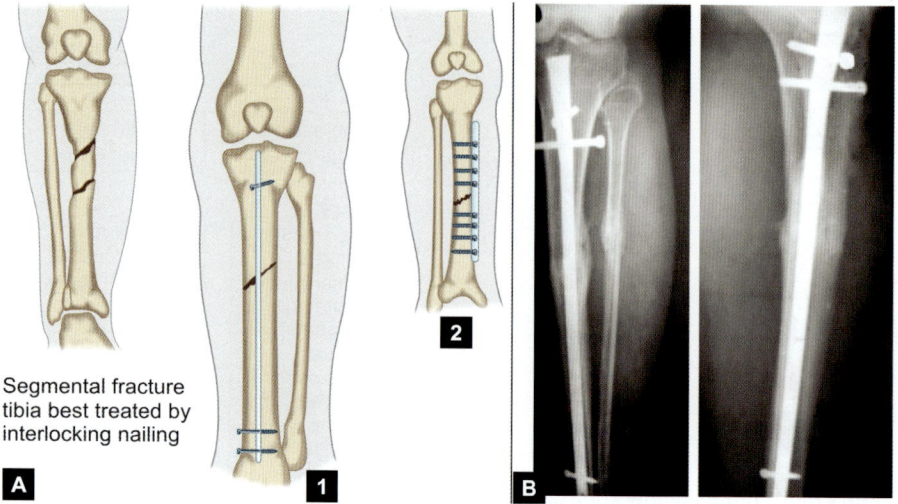

Figs 20.16A and B: (A) Methods of internal fixation in tibia fracture (1) interlocking nailing, (2) DCP plate and screws; (B) Radiograph showing ILN tibia (Gold standard)

Note:
The other most important advantage of ILN nailing is that the fracture need not be opened it can be managed closed.

Know about Newer Generation Nails:
There are nails with multiple holes in different planes, in order to maximize the options for interlocking and to allow nailing of the fractures near to proximal or distal ends.

Vital Points:
Unlocked IM nail is useful only in transverse or short oblique fracture that too only at the isthmus level. These fractures are few and hence it has limited usage.

Caution: Anterior knee pain is the most common complication after ILN of tibia.

Role of external fixators: This is useful in compound fractures of the tibia as it enables to stabilize the fracture and helps to take care of the wound (Figs 20.17A and B).

Types of External Fixators: Four Types
1. *Uniplanar:* Most popular. Easy to apply. Applied on anteromedial surface with 4–6 pins.
2. *Multiplanar:* Quadrilateral or triangular frame. These increase the usage.
3. *Circular frame (Ilizarov).*
4. *Hybrid external fixator:* This combines half rings with tensioned wires.

Complications of Tibia Fractures

Delayed union: This is a common complication and has an incidence of 1–17%. If there is no evidence of union of the fracture even after 20 weeks, delayed union is suspected and is treated with cancellous bone graft.

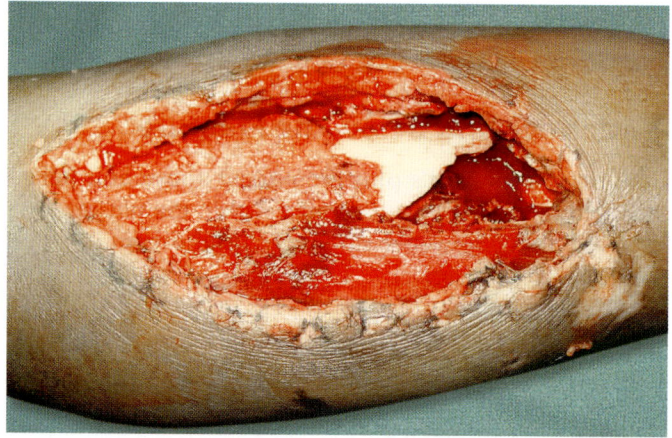

Fig. 20.17A: Clinical photo showing compound fracture tibia

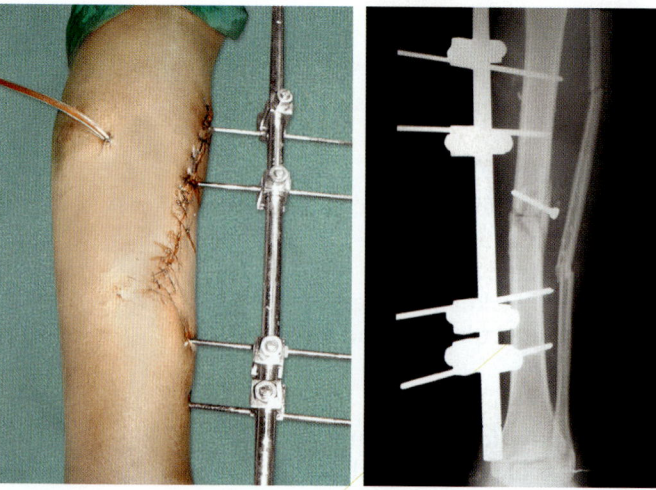

Fig. 20.17B: Clinical photo and X-ray showing debridement and external fixators for compound fracture tibia

Nonunion: This is a notorious problem usually encountered in fractures at the junction of middle one-third and lower one-third. It can be treated by electric stimulation or rigid internal fixation with compression plating and cancellous bone grafting.

Infected nonunion: It poses a tough challenge to the orthopedic surgeons and is best managed by Ilizarov's method of external fixation (Figs 20.18 and 20.19).

Malunion: Because of the parallel hinge knee and ankle joints above and below, malunion of tibia is an unacceptable problem as it may cause early degenerative arthritis (Figs 20.20A and B). Corrective osteotomy is the treatment of choice if the deformity is more.

Shortening: This may be due to malunion or overlap of the fracture fragments, less than 2 cm shortening is acceptable and may be corrected by footwear adjustments, while more than 2 cm shortening may require bone-lengthening procedures (Fig. 20.21).

Infection: Due to the subcutaneous location of the bone, infection is a common complication in these fractures due to a higher frequency of compound fractures following RTAs (Fig. 20.22).

Other complications: Compartmental syndromes, joint stiffness, refractures, fat embolism, and claw toes due to tethering of the long extensors over the callus are the other common complications (Fig. 20.23).

Reflex sympathetic dystrophy (RSD) can be seen but is uncommon.

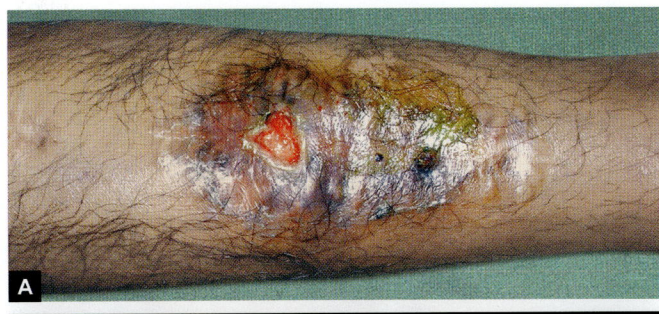
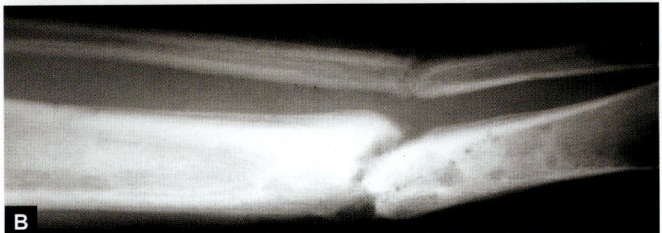

Figs 20.19A and B: Clinical photo of infected nonunion and X-rays

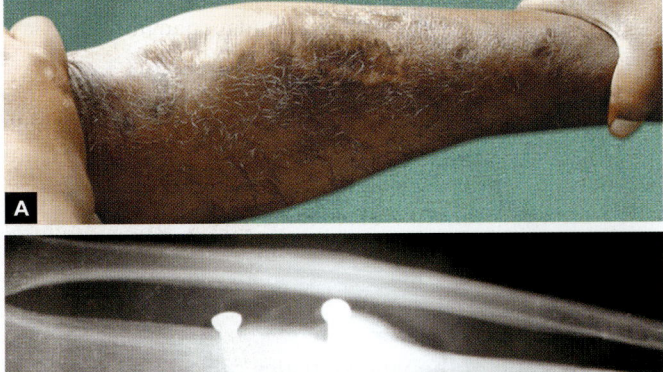

Figs 20.18A and B: Non-union of tibia clinical photo and X-rays

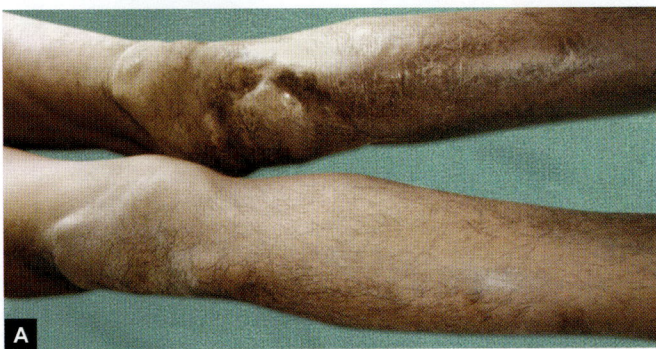
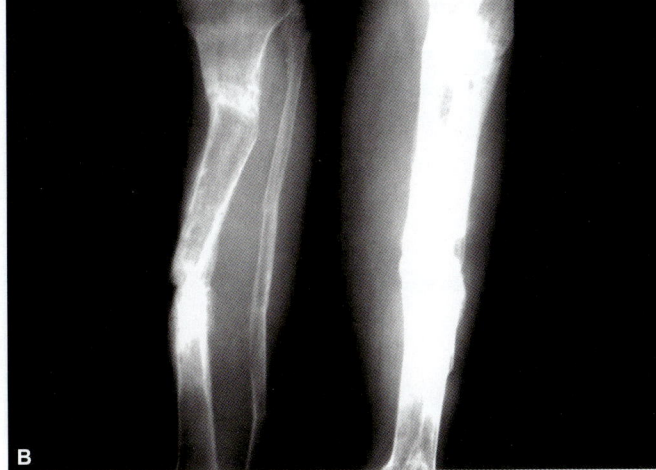

Figs 20.20A and B: (A) Clinical photo showing malunion tibia; (B) Plain X-ray showing malunion

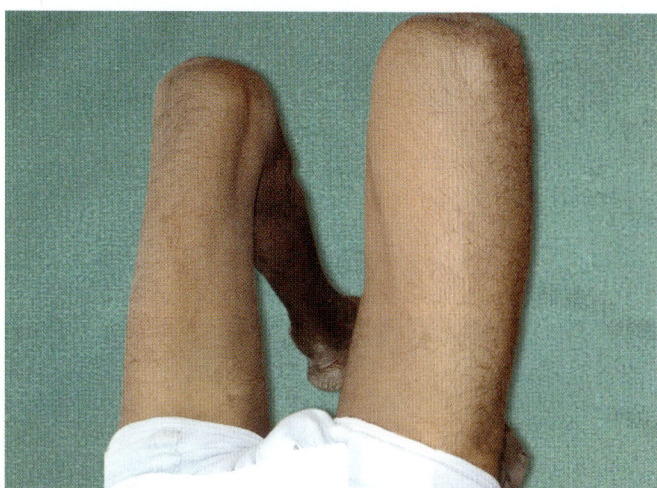

Fig. 20.21: Clinical photo showing shortening of tibia

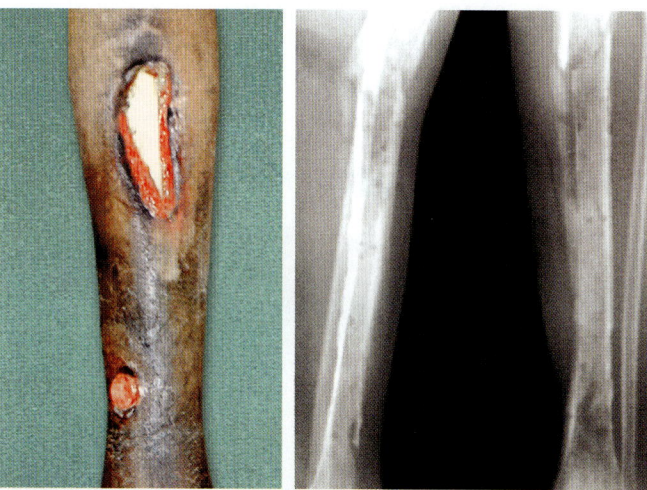

Fig. 20.22: Clinical photo and plain X-rays showing osteomyelitis of tibia (Sequestrum)

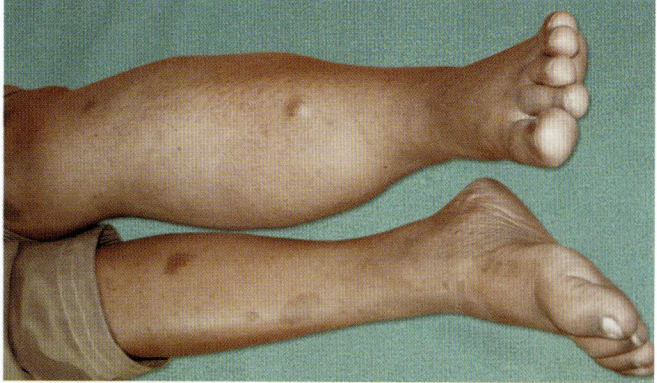

Fig. 20.23: Clinical photo showing compartmental syndrome

Quick Facts
Complications of tibia fracture
- Delayed union
- Nonunion
- Infected nonunion
- Malunion
- Shortening
- Infection
- Compartmental syndromes
- Joint stiffness
- Refracture
- Fat embolism
- Claw toes—due to tethering of long extensors over callus.

A word about Isolated Tibia Fracture
- Occurs in 22% of the cases
- Common in young adults
- Less severe than both bones fracture
- Simple fracture pattern
- Communition is less
- Incidence of open fracture is less
- Only transverse fracture without displacement heals well and can be treated conservatively
- Other fractures tend to be displaced hence fixed internally
- Treatment is more or less similar to both bones fracture.

Now a Word about Isolated Fibular Fractures
- Seen in three situations.
  - Avulsion fracture of proximal fibula
  - Syndesmotic fibular fracture on ankle injuries
  - True isolated fibular fractures
- Nonoperative treatment is enough
- Operative treatment if nonunion develops.

DISTAL TIBIAL FRACTURES

PILON FRACTURES
(Syn: Tibia Plafond Fractures)

These are severe injuries and are predominantly due to high energy axial loading forces following the RTA or fall from height unlike the malleolar fractures, which are mainly due to low energy rotational forces (Figs 20.24A to C). These are also called as distal tibia explosion fractures.

Incidence

Here are some of the vital statistics concerning the pilon fractures:
- It accounts for less than 10% of all lower limb fractures.
- Males are more commonly affected than females.
- Mean age is 35–40 years.

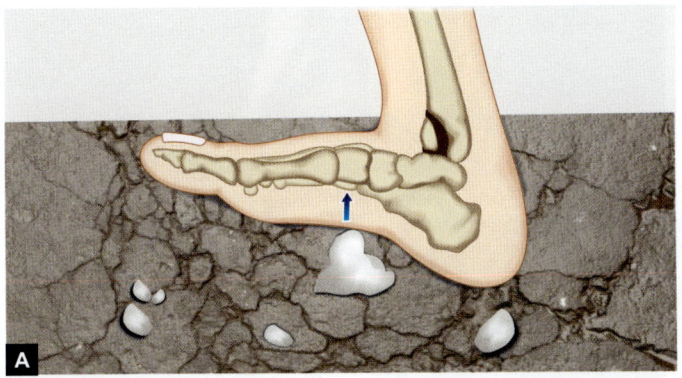
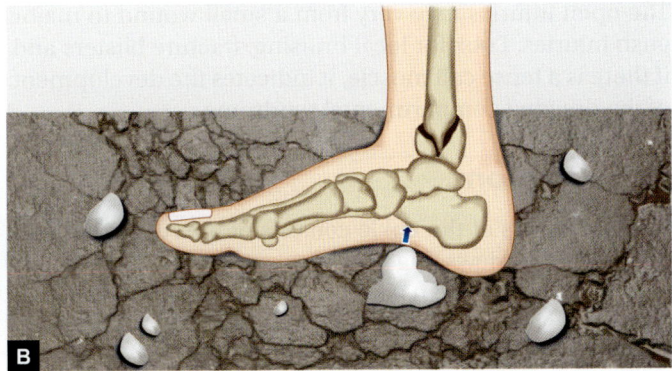
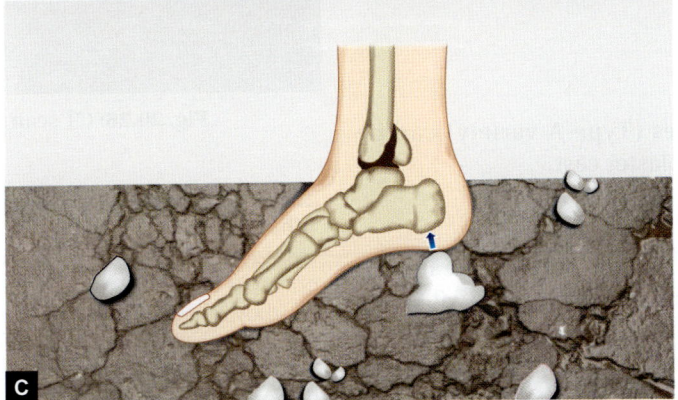

Figs 20.24A to C: Mechanism of injury of pilon fractures

Classifications

The important classifications have been described namely:
- *Ruedi and Allgower classifications* until recently, this were the classification that was widely used. Three varieties are described.
    - Type I: Undisplaced cleavage fracture of the joint.
    - Type II: Displaced but minimally comminuted fractures.
    - Type III: Highly comminuted and displaced fractures.
- *AO/OTA Classification:* This is the most recent classification and it consists of the following varieties (Figs 20.25A to C).
    - Type A: Extra-articular fractures.
    - Type B: Partial intra-articular fractures.
    - Type C: Total intra-articular fractures.

Depending upon the amount of comminution, each variety is divided into three groups. Any of these groups are again divided into three subgroups depending on the fracture characteristics.

The associated soft tissue injuries are classified into four categories from 0–3 from negligible damage to extensive soft tissue damage. Tscherne and Goetzen proposed this classification.

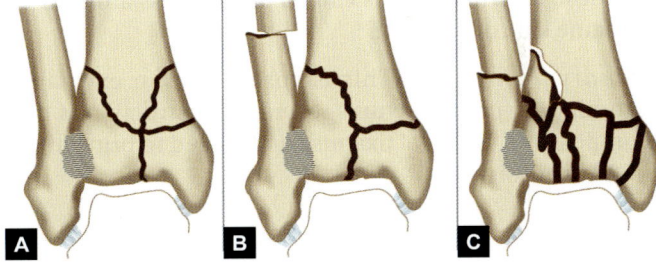

Figs 20.25A to C: Varieties of pilon fractures (OTA varieties)

Note:
In 85% of these injuries fibula is fractured.

Clinical Features

The patient complains of pain, swelling, deformity, and inability to bear weight. Open wounds are a disaster and the patient may complain of cold, clammy feet and loss of sensation.

Findings

Look for the peripheral pulses and the sensations in the foot. There may be gross deformity and swelling of the foot.

The open injuries may vary from a small wound to major gush injuries. Look for local bruising, fracture blisters and if there is a tense calf muscle, it indicates the development of the dreaded compartmental syndrome.

Investigations

Routine X-rays of the ankle consists of the AP, lateral and ankle mortise views (Fig. 20.26).

CT scan is more useful and gives more information about the nature and extent of the injury than mere X-rays (Fig. 20.26).

Treatment

Conservative Methods

Minimally displaced fractures (Type A variety) can be treated conservatively with a plaster cast.

Surgery

Grossly displaced fractures require surgical treatment consisting of open reduction and internal fixation with plate and screws. External fixation is the other useful method of treatment and the methods are:
- Hybrid fixation
- Ilizarov's fixation
- Monolateral fixator.

These external fixators can be used across ankle or on the same side of the joint.

Primary arthrodesis: This is considered in extremely comminuted pilon fractures where reconstruction is next to impossible. External fixators can be used to bring about the arthrodesis.

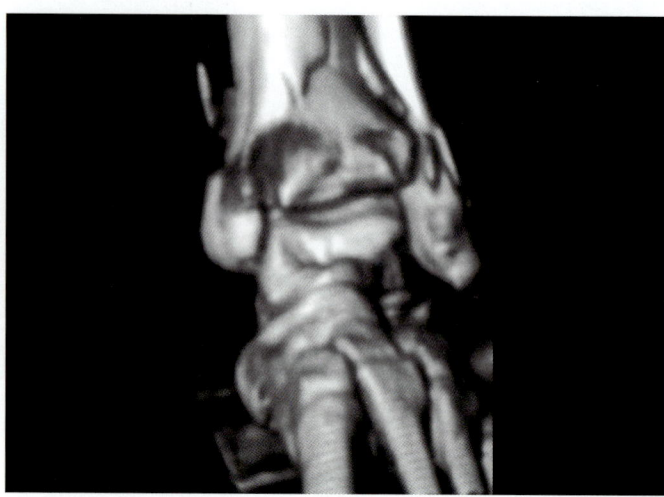

Fig. 20.26: CT scan showing pilon fracture

> **What is New?**
>
> Hybrid external fixator is fast emerging as an effective treatment option for pilon fractures. Here the fractures are reduced and based on CT study, tensioned multiple olive wires are placed in the epiphyseal region of the tibia. These are connected to the half pins located in the diaphysis. From proximal to distal three rings are used, with the distal being at the level of the ankle joint. The distal ring is clam-shelled and placed parallel to the ankle joint. Attach these wires to the rings using posts of various heights.

OPEN TIBIAL FRACTURES

As mentioned previously, open fractures are frequently seen in tibia fractures due to its subcutaneous location.

The principles of treatment, methods of treatment and complications are as discussed in Chapter 3.

21 CHAPTER

Injuries of the Ankle

BRIEF ANATOMY

Ankle Joint Speaks

I am a complex joint made up of distal ends of tibia, fibula, and the talus. The tibiofibular joint functions as a uniplanar hinge joint and in which about 25° of dorsiflexion and 35° of plantar flexion takes place. I am fully congruous in all positions. The stability is provided by the configuration of the ankle mortise and the ligaments, which are arranged in the following three groups:

Medial collateral ligament consists of deltoid ligament with a superficial or deep part (Fig. 21.1A).

Anterior and posterior talofibular ligaments and calcaneofibular ligament (Fig. 21.1B) form lateral collateral ligament.

Anterior tibiofibular ligament, the posterior tibiofibular ligament, the inferior transverse ligament, and the interosseous ligament form syndesmotic ligaments.

It is interesting to note that I am surrounded on all sides by the following structures:
- *Anteriorly:* Tendons of tibialis anterior, extensor hallucis longus, tibial vessels, and nerves, tendons of extensor digitorum longus, and posterior tibialis in that order. These structures are held in position by the superior and inferior retinaculae.
- *Posteromedial:* Tendons of tibialis posterior, flexor digitorum longus, posterior tibial vessels, and nerves and tendon of flexor hallucis longus pass in that order behind and below the medial malleolus. Flexor retinaculae hold them in position.
- *Posterolateral:* Peroneus longus and brevis held in position by superior and inferior peroneal retinaculae.
- *Posteriorly:* It is the tendo-Achilles and plantaris. These tendons are all covered by synovial sheaths. I am the fulcrum at which the leg transmits the body weight to the foot. My peculiarity lies in the fact that I have no muscular covering on any of my sides.

ANKLE INJURIES

Pott described ankle injuries for the first time in 1768.

Interesting 'Incidence Facts' about Ankle Fractures
- More commonly in elderly women
- About 2/3 are isolated malleolar fracture
- About 1/4 are bimalleolar fracture
- Trimalleolar fracture seen only in 7%
- Open fracture 2%.

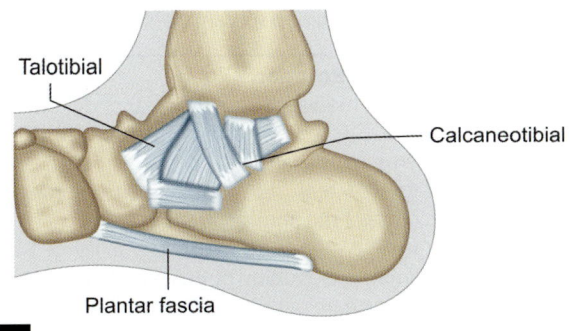 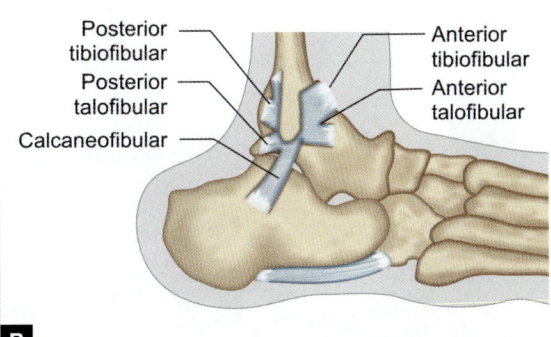

Figs 21.1A and B: Anatomy of ankle ligaments: (A) Medial side; (B) Lateral side

Mechanism of Injury

Ankles are usually injured due to low injury rotational forces due to:
- Twisting injury while walking, running, sports, athletes, etc. are the most common mode of ankle injuries (Figs 21.2 and 21.3).
- Fall from a height: Ankle injuries are indirect injuries here brought about by the displacing talus.

Classification

Ankle injuries are classified after the mechanism causing them. Hence, it is of paramount importance to understand the movement of the ankle to comprehend the classification.

What complicates the issue is the practice of using more than one term to describe the same motion.

There are six movements of the ankle and the hind foot. Plantar flexion and dorsiflexion are the up and down movements of the foot. Movement causing the toes to point inwards is called internal rotation and movement causing the toes to point outwards is called external rotation. Supination is the movement, which raises the medial aspect of the foot and the heel off the ground. In pronation, the motion is to bring the lateral aspect of the foot and the heel from the ground. In adduction, the hind foot is moved towards the midline and in abduction is moved laterally. Pure vertical loading position as in landing, jumping, falling, etc. will cause Pylon fracture by the driving of the talus into the tibia.

Lauge Hansen's Classification

Four major types are described. The mechanism of injury could be adduction force, abduction force or external rotation force. The foot could be in supination or pronation (Figs 21.4A to E). The first word refers to the position of the foot at the time of injury and the second to the direction of injuring force.

Supination Adduction
Stage I : Transverse fracture of lateral malleolus or tear of lateral collateral ligament.
Stage II : Stage I + fracture of medial malleolus.

Supination Eversion
Stage I : Rupture of anteroinferior tibiofibular ligament.
Stage II : Stage I + spiral oblique fracture of the lateral malleolus.
Stage III : Stage II + posterior lip of fracture of tibia (posterior malleolar fracture).
Stage IV : Stage III + fracture medial malleolus or tear of deltoid ligament.

Pronation Abduction
Stage I : Fracture medial malleolus or tear of deltoid ligament.
Stage II : Stage I + rupture of anteroinferior tibiofibular ligament and posteroinferior tibiofibular ligament with fracture posterior lip of tibia.
Stage III : Stage II + oblique supramalleolar fracture of the fibula.

Pronation-External Rotation
Stage I : Fracture medial malleolus or tear of deltoid ligament
Stage II : Stage I + tear of anteroinferior tibiofibular and interosseous ligament.
Stage III : Stage II + tear of interosseous membrane and spiral fracture of the fibula.
Stage IV : Stage III + fracture of posterior lip of tibia due to ligamentous avulsion by posteroinferior and inferior and transverse tibiofibular ligament.

Note:
About 75% of the cases fall into the first two groups.

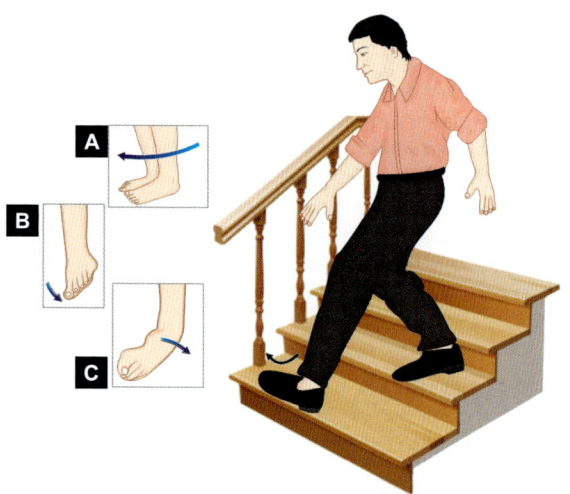

Figs 21.2A to C: Common mechanism of ankle injuries: (A) External rotation force; (B) Abduction force; (C) Adduction force. Inversion injury while getting down the stairs is a common mode of ankle injury

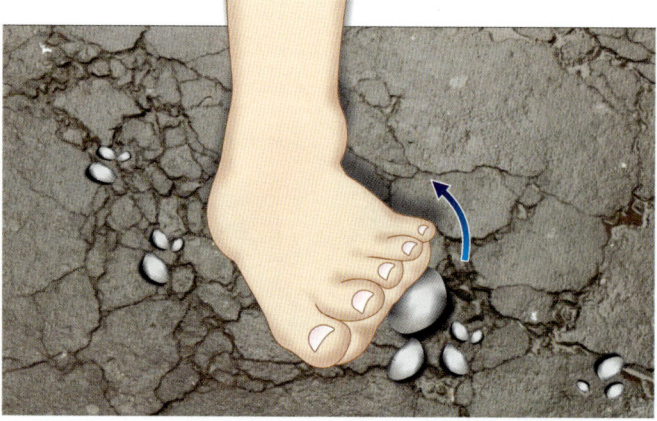

Fig. 21.3: Eversion mechanism of ankle injury

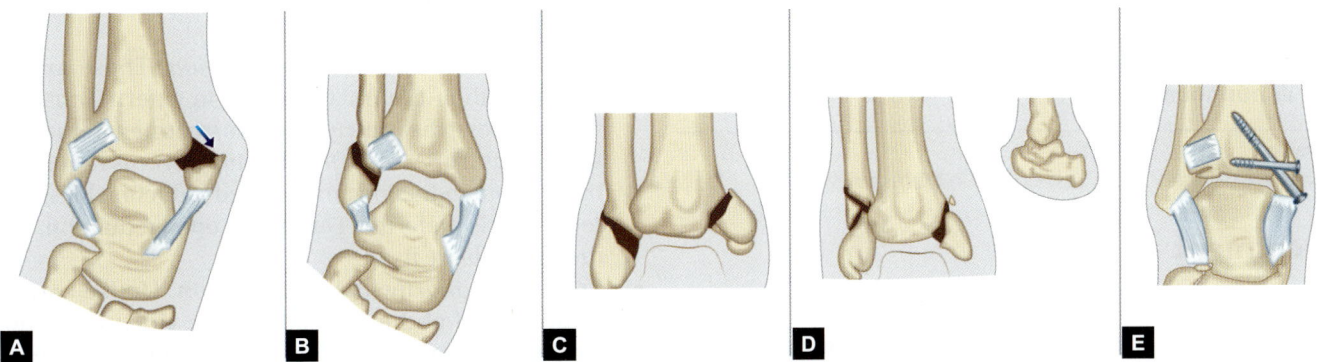

Figs 21.4A to E: Lauge Hansen's classification: (A) Supination adduction; (B) Supination eversion; (C) Pronation abduction; (D) Pronation external rotation; (E) Fracture fixed with malleolar screws

Denis Weber Classification

This is the other classification proposed for ankle injuries and it is based on the level of the fibular fracture, while the Lauge Hansen's system is based on experimentally verified injury mechanism like adduction, abduction, etc.

AO Classification of Malleolar Fractures

Type A : Infrasyndesmotic (Fracture of fibula below the syndesmosis)
Type A : Isolated
Type A2 : With medial mallelol fracture
Type A3 : With posteromedial fracture.
Type B : Transsyndesmotic (Fracture of fibula at syndesmosis level).
Type B : Isolated.
Type B2 : With medial lesion (Malleolar or ligament injury).
Type B3 : With medial lesion and posterolateral tibial fracture.
Type C : Suprasyndesmotic (fracture of fibula above the syndesmosis).
Type C1 : Simple diaphyseal fracture of fibula.
Type C2 : Complex diaphyseal fracture of fibula.
Type C3 : Proximal fracture of fibula.

Clinical Features

The patient usually gives history of inversion injury, following which there is pain, swelling, deformity of the ankle (Fig. 21.5). Movements are decreased, Drawer's test, inversion, and eversion stress tests may be positive. Note the color and condition of the skin. Examine the entire leg.

Investigations

Anteroposterior, lateral and mortise non-weight bearing views of the ankle are recommended in the radiographs

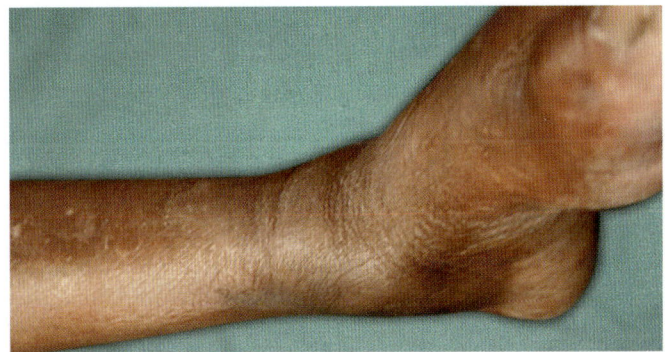

Fig. 21.5: Clinical photo showing ankle fracture

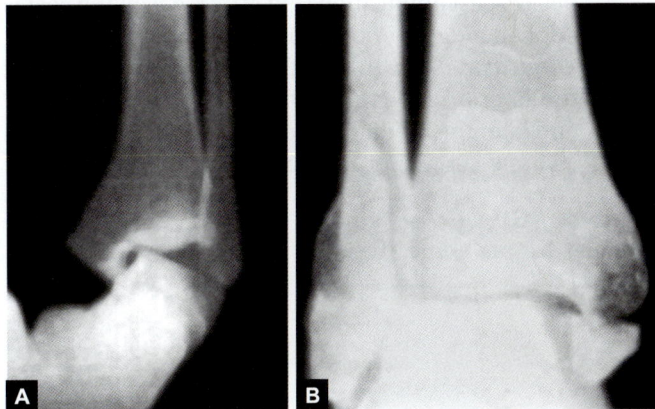

Figs 21.6A and B: (A) Radiograph showing inversion injury of ankle; (B) Bimalleolar ankle fracture

(Figs 21.6A and B). CT scan, MRI, and arthroscopy evaluation is extremely helpful.

Radiographic Parameters of the Normal Ankle

- Talocrural angle—83° ± 4°
- Medial clear space 4 mm

- Tibiofibular clear space < 6 mm
- Subchondral bone line between the distal tibia and medial surface of lateral malleolus should be continuous.

Note:
All these parameters are best studied in Mortise views.

Treatment

Goals

- Anatomical positioning of the talus beneath the tibia.
- To obtain a joint line that is parallel to the ground.
- Smooth articular surface.

If these three things are not achieved, post-traumatic osteoarthritis results.

Stable injuries: No reduction is required, immobilization with only plaster splints till the swelling decreases and then a below knee plaster cast is applied with foot in neutral position.

Unstable injuries: Require reduction and immobilization in plaster casts. The commonly encountered unstable injuries are:

- *Fracture due to external rotation:* This is more common and can be managed both by conservative and operative methods.
    - *Conservative method:* This consists of reversal of the injuring forces by closed reduction and a below knee plaster cast application (Fig. 21.7). A walking cast is applied after a period of one month.
    - *Surgical method:* In this, the malleoli are fixed, first the lateral malleolus is fixed with pin or screws, and later the medial malleolar fracture is fixed with a single screw perpendicular to the fracture line. Below knee splint is given initially and later a cast is applied.
- *Fracture primarily due to abduction:* These are less common than the fractures due to external rotation. Nevertheless, the principles of the treatment remain the same (Figs 21.8A and B). Adduction force is required to bring about reduction and if closed reduction fails, open reduction is preferred. During the open reduction, both the malleoli are fixed.
- *Fracture primarily due to adduction:* Unlike external rotation and abduction, adduction violence is more frequently an isolated event. Wedging of small-comminuted fragments into the fracture line often prevents closed reduction, so that open reduction and internal fixation (ORIF) is required more frequently. Medial malleolus is approached first, since it is more unstable, and the fracture is fixed with two screws, one at right angle to the tibial cortex and another at right angle to the fracture line. Lateral fibular fracture is stabilized with plate and screws.
- *Fracture resulting from primarily vertical compression:* This may be isolated or associated with other forces described above. The anterior and posterior tibial plafond margins are fractured. Two types are described:
    - Posterior marginal fracture for undisplaced fracture, below knee cast is sufficient. For more than 25% of articular surface involvement, ORIF with two screws is preferred.
    - Anterior marginal fracture (tibial plafond injury): It may include a crush of the anterior lip or it may include a major fragment. If crushed, calcaneal traction is given and if there is a large fragment, ORIF is required.

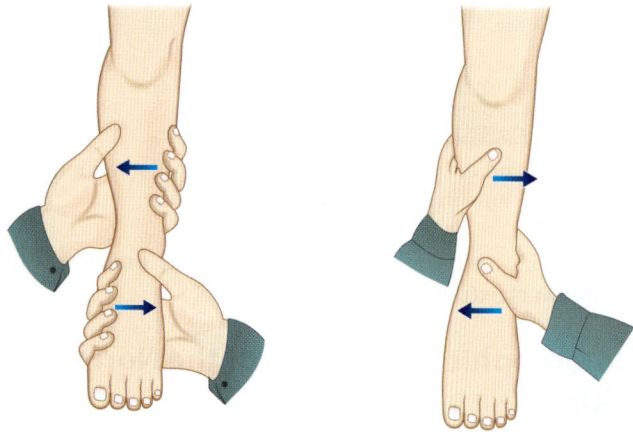

Fig. 21.7: Methods of closed reduction of ankle fractures

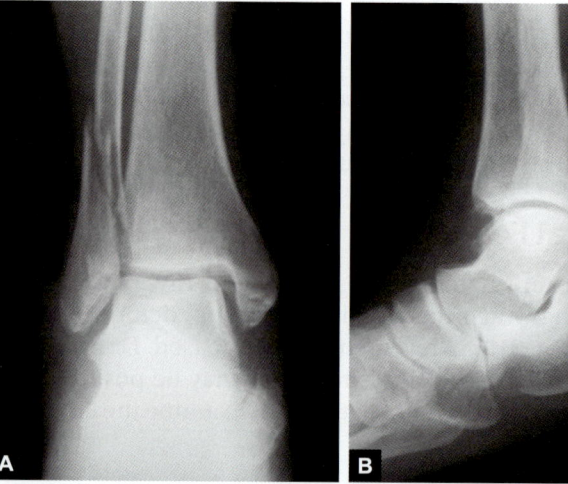

Figs 21.8A and B: Plain X-rays showing pronation abduction ankle fractures

In a Nutshell

The fixation techniques for medial malleolar fractures
- Large fragment fracture—Single lag screw.
- Small fragment fracture—Combination of 4 mm lag screws and a K-wire (Fig. 21.9).
- Low transverse fracture—Tension band wiring or vertical countersunk 4 mm lag screw.

The fixation techniques for lateral malleolar fractures
- For fibular fractures: One-third semi-tubular 3.5 mm plate and screws or multiple 3.5 mm lag screws.
- Long oblique fracture: Two lag screws.
- Low transverse fracture: Single 4.5 mm malleolar screw.
- Both Malleoli: Tension band wiring for lateral malleolar fracture and 4 mm lag screw for associated medial malleolar fracture.

Complications

Complications of ankle fractures include post-traumatic arthritis, reflex sympathetic dystrophy, neurovascular injury (injury to posterior tibial vessels and nerve), nonunion (due to soft tissue interposition), malunion, etc. (Figs 21.10A to C).

ANKLE SPRAINS

These are common injury in sports. If improperly treated, it may result in chronic laxity, pain, or delayed recovery.

Quick Facts: Involvement of Various Structures in Ankle Sprain
- Complete rupture of the anterior tibiofibular ligament (ATFL)—65%
- Both ATFL and calcaneofibular ligament—20%
- Antero inferior tibiofibular ligament (high ankle sprain)—10%
- Deltoid ligament—3%.

TRIMALLEOLAR FRACTURE (Cotton Fracture)

This is a difficult injury complex to treat. The salient features about this fracture are:
- It is due to abduction and external rotation injury.
- There is fracture of the medial, lateral, and posterior malleolus.
- For plain X-ray 50° external rotation view is preferred.
- It more often requires open reduction and internal fixation.
- If the posterior malleolar fragment is less than 25% of the articular surface, then reduction is automatically achieved when the fibular fracture is fixed.
- However, if it is more than 25–30% of the articular surface, then it needs to be reduced and fixed internally.
- The results of fixation are usually inferior to that of bimalleolar fixations.

LATERAL LIGAMENT SPRAIN

This is the most common musculoskeletal injury with an incidence of 1/10,000/day. In 85% of cases, it is due to inversion of supinated plantar flexed foot. The lateral ligament commonly injured is anterior talofibular ligament followed by calcaneofibular ligament. The posterior talofibular ligament is rarely sprained (Fig. 21.11).

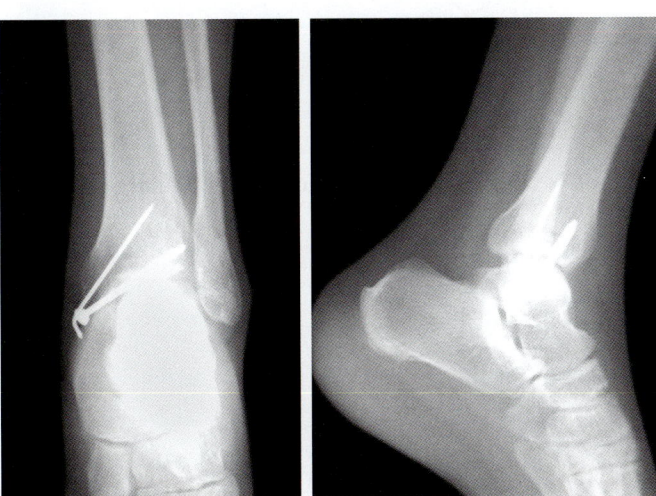

Fig. 21.9: Malleolar fixation with screws and K-wire

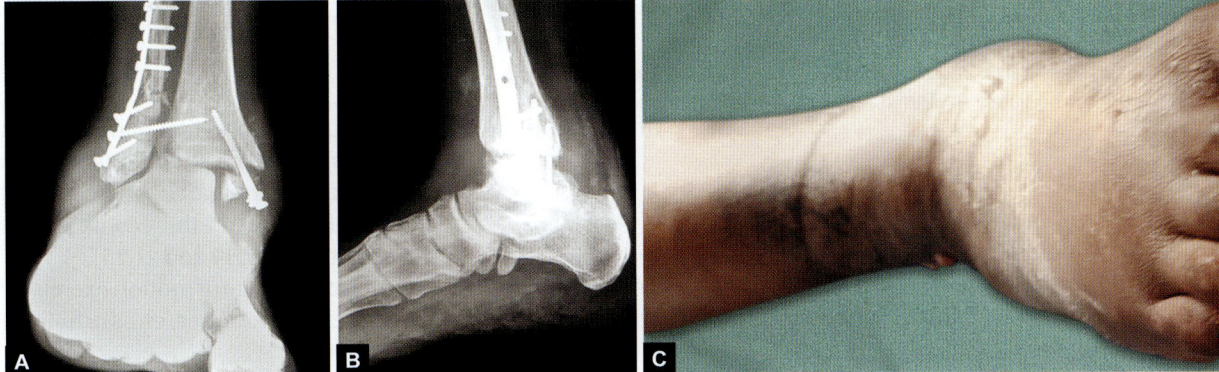

Figs 21.10A to C: Plain X-ray showing malunion and nonunion of ankle fractures. Clinical photo showing the deformity

266 SECTION 2: Regional Traumatology

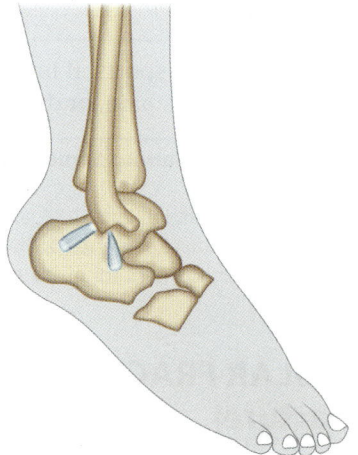

Fig. 21.11: Lateral ligament sprain (Due to adduction injury)

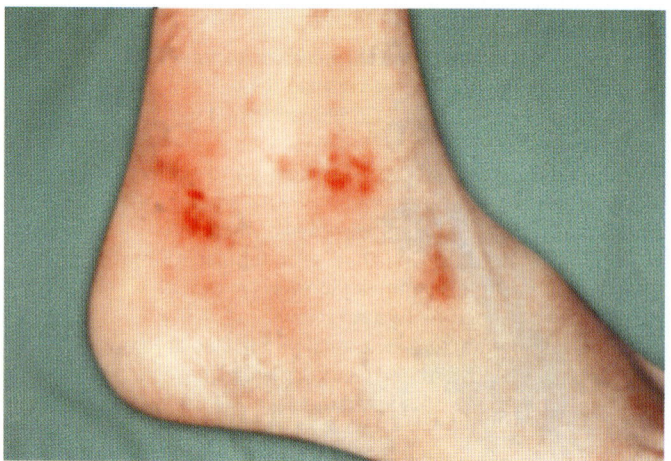

Fig. 21.12: Clinical photograph of ankle sprain

Note:
Lateral ankle sprain is the most common soft tissue limb injury and < 15% actually show a significant fracture.

Clinical Features

The patient complains of pain, swelling, and tenderness over the affected ligament (Fig. 21.12). Anterior drawer test is positive and it is performed by stabilizing distal tibia with one hand, then grasps the posterior heel with the opposite hand, and applies anterior force. If the displacement of talus is more than 8 mm anterior, it suggests laxity of the anterior talofibular ligament. Next, the talar tilt test is performed, if the tilt is more than 5°, it suggests laxity of anterior talofibular and calcaneofibular ligaments.

Radiograph of the Ankle

If the talar tilt of the injured ankle is 10° greater than the uninjured ankle, it is considered as significant.

Vital Facts: Ottawa Rules (Fig. 21.13)
X-rays are required in ankle sprains if:
- There is bony tenderness in the posterior half of lower end of tibia and fibula.
- Tenderness over the fifth metatarsal and navicular bones.
- Inability to bear weight immediately or after 10 days after injury.

Grading of Ankle Sprains

Grade I : No laxity, minimal pain and mild swelling.
Grade II : Mild to moderate laxity, soft tissue swelling, anterior drawer, and talar tilt is slightly positive.
Grade III : Severe swelling and pain, the anterior drawer and talar tilt tests are highly positive.

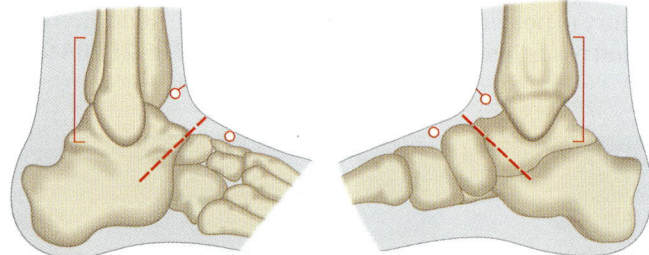

Fig. 21.13: Ankle injuries Ottawa rules

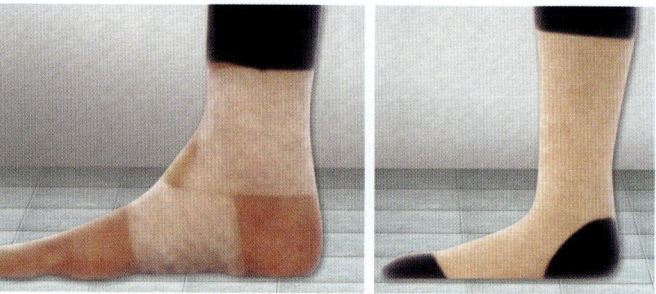

Fig. 21.14: Ankle strap

Treatment

Grade I sprain : Ice therapy, compression bandage, foot and elevation, ankle strap non-steroidal anti-inflammatory drugs (NSAIDs), crutch walking, etc. are the recommended treatment (Figs 21.14 and 21.15).
Grade II sprain : Long leg cast, range of motion exercises, strengthening exercises, etc. are helpful (Fig. 21.16).

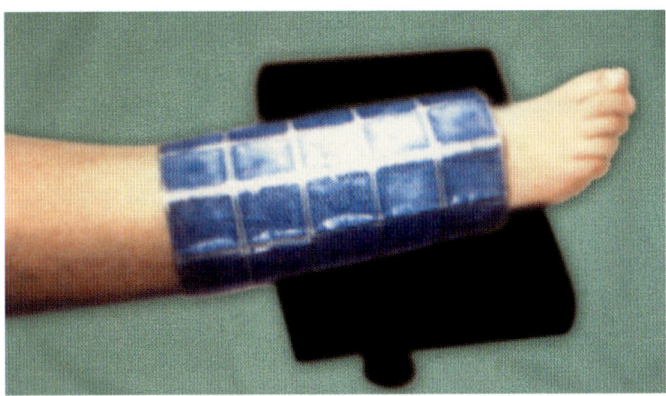

Fig. 21.15: The RICE regimen—rest, ice, compression and elevation

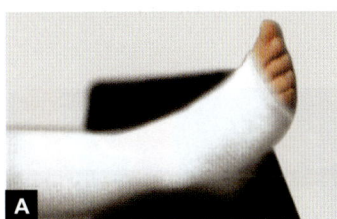 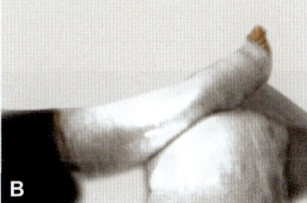

Figs 21.16A and B: (A) Compression bandaging; (B) Elevation for ankle sprain

Grade III sprain : Same lines as mentioned above and sometimes may rarely require surgical repair.

Quick Facts
Treatment of acute ankle sprain in a nutshell (First 48 hours) (PRICE Regime) (see Fig. 21.16)
P – Painkillers
R – Rest
I – Ice therapy
C – Compression bandage (Jones bandage)
E – Elevation at hip level.

MEDIAL LIGAMENT SPRAIN

This is due to pronation eversion injury. In mild sprains, only the superficial part of the deltoid ligament is torn, but in severe forms, the deep part of the deltoid ligament is also torn resulting in a lateral talar tilt. If this exceeds more than 2 mm, significant alteration in the weight bearing mechanism takes place resulting in post-traumatic arthritis. For mild sprains, conservative treatment is sufficient and for severe sprains, surgical reduction and repair are considered.

Do You Know the Sources of Pain after Acute Ankle Sprain?
- Superficial peroneal nerve tension neuropathy.
- Anterior and lateral ankle impingement syndrome.
- Cuboid subluxation.

TENDO-ACHILLES INJURY

There is no other stronger tendon in the body than the tendo-Achilles. Two powerful muscles, the gastrocnemius, and the soleus form it. It is the powerful plantar flexor of the foot. The origin of the name of this tendon is of tremendous historical significance (Box 21.1).

Box 21.1: Do You Know the Interesting Greek Story Behind the Christening of this Tendon as Tendo-Achilles?
Pelus and Thetis were the proud parents of the famous Greek hero, Achilles. His mother desired that his son should be so much fortified with strength that he remains indefatigable in the field of wars. Her coterie of well-wishers suggested to her that if she dips her son completely in the magical river Styx, no force on earth could ever defeat him. Completely obsessed with this thought, she immersed her son in that river by holding him with the tendon above the heel. Apparently, it seemed that she had achieved the impossible but was oblivious of the stark reality that the tendon area in the heel held by her remained undipped in the river and hence was deprived of the magical protection. A seemingly omnipotent Achilles met his Waterloo at the siege of Troy when he was slained by an injury to this tendon during the war. Ironically, though her mother could not make him immortal in war, she gave the idea to the orthopedic surgeons to name this tendon after his son and thus immortalized him.

Note: The moral of this story is whoever tries to play God will be vanquished!

Mechanism of Injury

Acute Rupture

Any direct injury with a sharp object can injure this tendon. Interestingly, in our country, a curious mechanism of injury, thanks to the practice of Indian toilet system, is being described to the utter bewilderment and astonishment of the west. Let us take a closer look at this mechanism.

In the practice of the Indian toilet system, a person is prone to accidental slippage into the water closet of the toilet. Depending on the position of the foot, two types of injury may result:
- *High level injury (68%):* At the moment of slippage, if the foot is dorsiflexed, a high-level open injury is an inevitable outcome (about 3–4 cm above the insertion). However, the positive aspect is that these injuries will heal well after repair (Fig. 21.17A).
- *Low level injury (32%):* Here a panic-stricken patient tries to extricate his foot trapped in the closet in a plantar flexed position. This indiscretion leads to slicing of the tendon at a low level by the overhanging sharp edge of the closet. However, the problems are compounded due to poor healing after repair and due to sloughing of the skin (Fig. 21.17B).

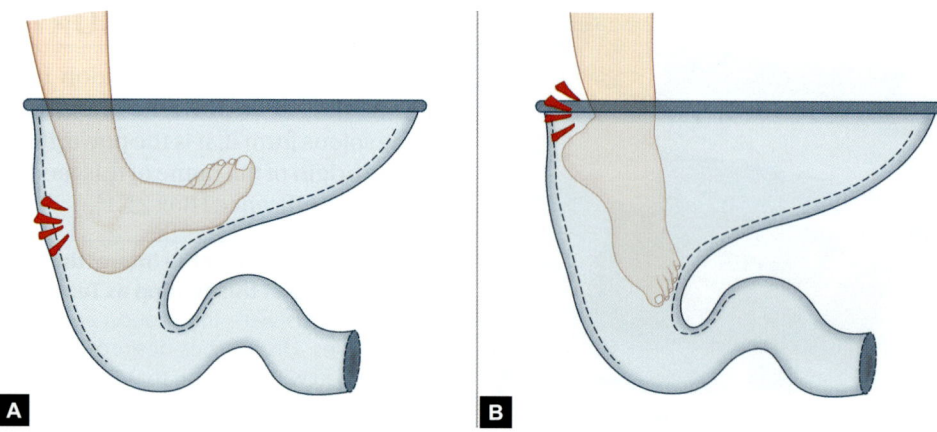

Figs 21.17A and B: Mechanism of injury of tendo-Achilles ruptures: (A) High level injury; (B) Low level injury

Chronic Rupture

This is due to gradual weakening of the tendon over the years. Spontaneous rupture may occur in such situations (Box 21.2).

> **Box 21.2: Vital Facts**
> Predisposing factors leading to chronic TA rupture:
> - Age more than 40 years, people involved in active athletics and sports
> - Weakened athletes
> - Previous history of tendonitis
> - Loss of flexibility of tendo-Achilles.

Clinical Features

In acute tears, the patient complains of pain and swelling in the region of the tendon. The patient is unable to walk.

Signs

Tenderness can be elicited and a gap is felt during a complete tear. Dorsiflexion is exaggerated, but plantar flexion is diminished; but never totally absent due to the residual action of tibialis posterior, toe flexors and the peroneals.

Clinical Tests

- Thompson's test: On squeezing the calf muscles, the foot goes into plantar-flexion. In TA tear, the plantar-flexion is either absent or weak. This test is still the gold standard.
- O'Brien's needle test is also reliable.
- Tip toe test: In incomplete tears, when the patient is instructed to stand over the tiptoes, there will be a definite heel lag.

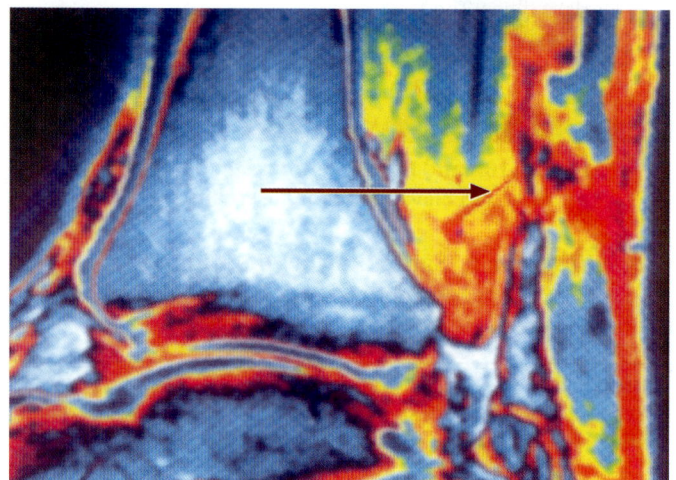

Fig. 21.18: MRI of tendo-Achilles rupture

Investigations

- *X-ray of the Heel:* Lateral view will show soft tissue swelling around the heel.
- *Ultrasound scan* of the tendo-Achilles helps us to detect the tears. It is cheap and useful
- *MRI scan* helps to identify the tears more clearly (Fig. 21.18).

> **Interesting Facts**
> Do you know the common sites of rupture in chronic tears? It is 2–10 cm proximal to the insertion of the tendon in the Os Calcis: This area is weaker than other areas due to relative avascularity.

Treatment

Conservative

Immobilizing the ankle in slight plantar flexion for 6–8 weeks. Though the incidence of infection is less, recurrent ruptures are quite common. Hence, it is second best to surgery.

Surgery

Direct surgical repair (Denholm's repair) and immobilization in a below knee plaster cast with slight plantar flexion is a better alternative (Fig. 21.19). Though recurrent ruptures are less, the chances of infections are high. Hence, extreme caution needs to be exercised to prevent the dreadful infection.

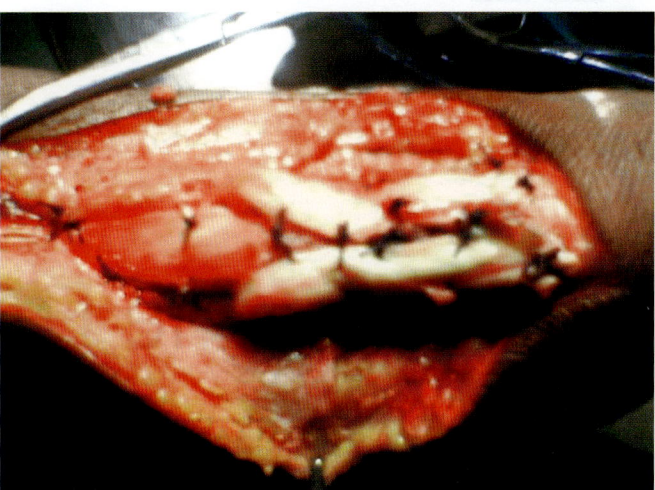

Fig. 21.19: Tendo-Achilles repair by Denholm's method

BIBLIOGRAPHY

1. Harish Gillies. The Management of Fresh Rupture of Tendo-Achilles. JBJS. 1970;52-A:337-43.
2. Hooker CH. Rupture of Tendo-Achilles. JBJS. 1963;45-B(2):360-63.

22
CHAPTER

Injuries of the Foot

FOREFOOT INJURIES

The forefoot complex consists of five metatarsals, sesamoid bones and the bones of the five toes (Fig. 22.1). The joints include metatarsophalangeal and interphalangeal joints. Forefoot plays a very important role both in gait and weight transmission. It is frequently injured in sports persons.

Classification

Fracture of the forefoot is classified as shown in Flowchart 22.1.

Now let us analyze the individual forefoot injuries in detail.

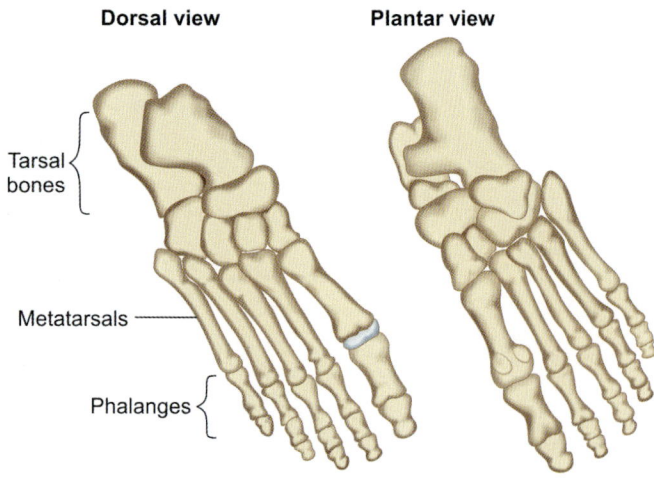

Fig. 22.1: Bony anatomy of the foot

Treatment Goals

Orthopedic Goals

- To restore the normal anatomy of the great toe, phalanx, metatarsal and sesamoid bones.
- In phalanges 2 through 5 toes, perfect alignment is not very crucial.
- Metatarsals two through five needs to be restored as anatomically as possible.

PHALANGEAL FRACTURES

Salient Features

- This is the most common injury of the foot.
- Proximal phalanx is more commonly injured than all other phalanx.
- Proximal phalanx of the fifth toe is most commonly injured.

Mechanism of Injury

- Direct blow due to fall of a heavy object on the toes. This causes transverse or comminuted fractures.
- Indirect forces due to axial loading with secondary varus or valgus forces (stubbing injury). This leads to spiral or oblique fractures.

Clinical Features

The patient presents with pain, swelling, limp, and difficulty to walk and wear the footwear.

CHAPTER 22: Injuries of the Foot

Flowchart 22.1: Fracture of the foot

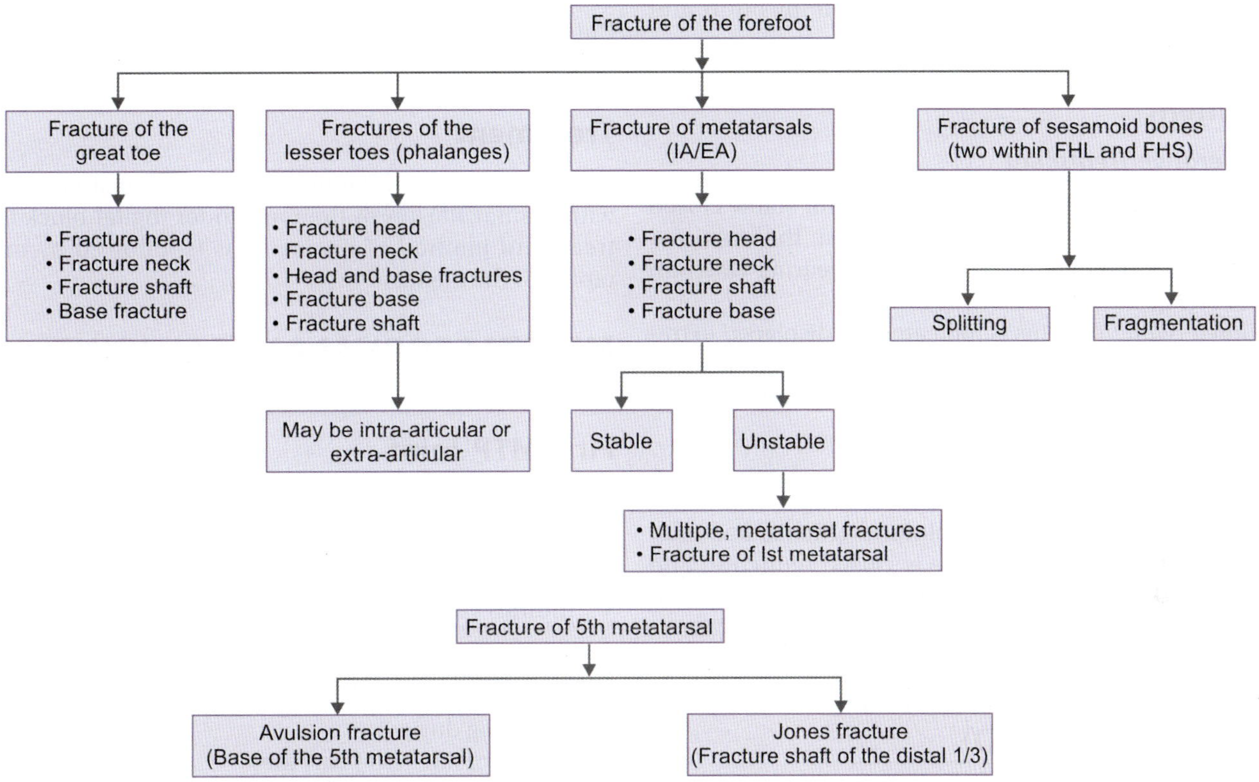

```
Fracture of the forefoot
├── Fracture of the great toe
│     • Fracture head
│     • Fracture neck
│     • Fracture shaft
│     • Base fracture
├── Fractures of the lesser toes (phalanges)
│     • Fracture head
│     • Fracture neck
│     • Head and base fractures
│     • Fracture base
│     • Fracture shaft
│     → May be intra-articular or extra-articular
├── Fracture of metatarsals (IA/EA)
│     • Fracture head
│     • Fracture neck
│     • Fracture shaft
│     • Fracture base
│     ├── Stable
│     └── Unstable
│           • Multiple, metatarsal fractures
│           • Fracture of Ist metatarsal
│           → Fracture of 5th metatarsal
│                 ├── Avulsion fracture (Base of the 5th metatarsal)
│                 └── Jones fracture (Fracture shaft of the distal 1/3)
└── Fracture of sesamoid bones (two within FHL and FHS)
      ├── Splitting
      └── Fragmentation
```

IA—Intra-articular, EA—Extra-articular, FHL—Flexor hallucis longus, FHS—Flexor hallucis superficialis

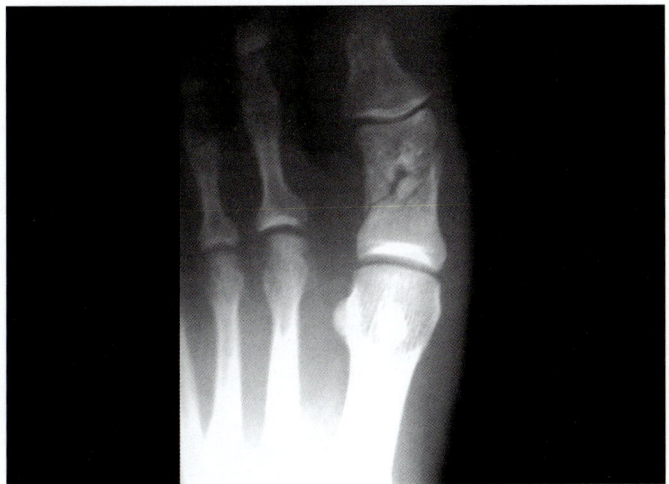

Fig. 22.2: Radiograph showing proximal phalanx fracture

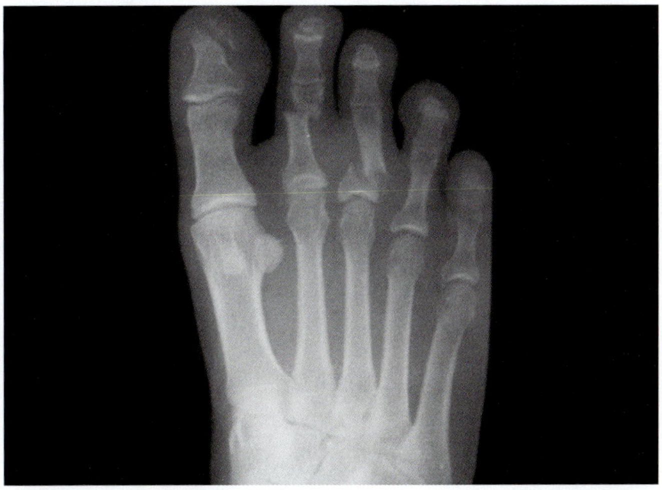

Fig. 22.3: Plain X-ray showing multiple fractures of phalanges

Investigations

Standard AP and lateral films of the forefoot help to make the diagnosis (Figs 22.2 and 22.3).

Classification (OTA)

Group A: Extra-articular and simple diaphyseal fractures.
Group B: Partial articular and diaphyseal wedge fractures.

Group C: Complex articular and diaphyseal shaft fractures. Each group is further subdivided into the position and pattern of fractures.

Treatment

Nonoperative Treatment

- *Immobilization only:* This is indicated for stable closed injuries with no intra-articular extension. The treatment consists of buddy taping and weight bearing with stiff shoes (Fig. 22.4).
- *Closed reduction:* This is indicated for displaced extra-articular or intra-articular fractures. The treatment consists of closed reduction and buddy taping to the medial toe.

Operative Treatment

This is indicated for grossly unstable intra-articular fractures. The treatment method of choice is closed reduction and percutaneous K-wire fixation or open reduction, K-wire or screw fixation (Fig. 22.5).

INTERPHALANGEAL JOINT DISLOCATIONS (IJD)

Salient Features

- It is due to axial loading at the end of the digits
- Majority occur in the proximal joint
- Dorsal dislocation is more common
- May be confused with phalangeal fractures.

Clinical Features

Pain and swelling, stiffness of the toes, dorsoplantar thickening of the toe on palpation are the usual presentation.

Radiograph

Plain X-rays: AP and lateral views help to make the diagnosis.

Treatment

Closed reduction with longitudinal traction along the toes with plantar flexion of the toes under digital block is the treatment method of choice. This is followed by buddy taping to the adjacent toe.

METATARSOPHALANGEAL JOINT INJURIES

First MTP Joint

Salient Features

- Most commonly injured
- Most commonly affected during sports injury
- Injuries vary from minor sprain to frank dislocations.

Mechanism of Injury

Axial loading during:
- Hyperdorsiflexion (Turf toe)
- Hyperplantarflexion (Sand toe)
- Valgus and varus stress.

Clinical Features

Pain over the great toe with weight bearing, tenderness over the MTP joint, ecchymosis, and test for both active and passive stability.

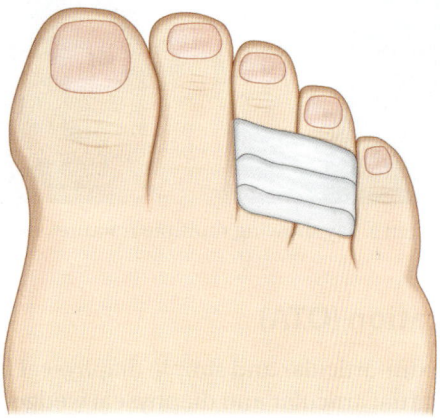

Fig. 22.4: Buddy taping for undisplaced phalangeal fractures of the toes

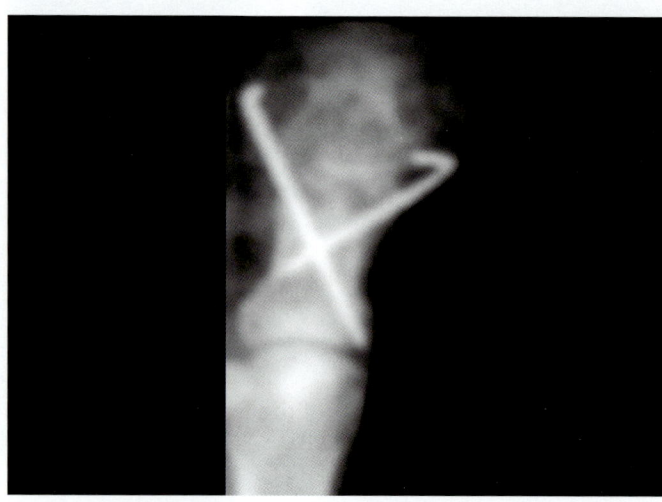

Fig. 22.5: Percutaneous fixation with K-wires

Radiograph

Weight bearing, AP, and lateral views on plain X-rays (Figs 22.6A and B).

Classification

Type I   : Dislocation with intact plantar plate.
Type II : Dislocation with partial disruption of plantar plate.
Type III : Dislocation with complete disruption of plantar plate.

Sprains are classified into Grades I, II and III, depending on the degree of tear.

Treatment

Nonoperative treatment: For stable injuries, RICE regime.

Operative treatment: This is indicated for intra-articular fractures and significant avulsion fractures causing instability. These injuries need open reduction, internal fixation with ligament repair.

INJURIES TO THE OTHER MTP JOINTS

These are hyperdorsiflexion and hyperplantarflexion injuries with axial loading and are rare. The treatment is essentially conservative for minor sprains. Dislocations are treated by closed reduction by finger traps to the affected toe for overcoming the gravitational force. This is successful in 50% of the cases. If this fails, open reduction and pinning may be required.

SESAMOID BONE INJURIES

Two sesamoid bones are present within the flexor hallucis longus and flexor hallucis superficialis tendons of the great toe.

Functions of Sesamoid Bones

- Shock absorber
- Supports weight bearing function of the great toe
- Protects the FHL tendon.

Note:
- Bipartite sesamoid bones are seen in 9–30%.
- Medial sesamoid is more commonly injured.

Mechanism of Injury

- Due to the impact of the foot on a hard surface while the toes are dorsiflexed.
- Stress fracture due to repeated trauma (as in dancers; runners, etc.).

Clinical Features

Pain, tenderness beneath the plantar surface of the sesamoid bone (Fig. 22.7), limp is present.

Investigations

- *Plain X-ray:* AP, lateral and tangential (sesamoid) views
- *CT scan or MRI:* It is more accurate but expensive.

Note:
Did you know that Sachin Tendulkar suffered from sesamoid bone fractures that almost ruined his career?

Treatment

Acute fractures: Soft padding, strapping the MTP joint in neutral or in slightly plantar flexed position.

Sesamoidectomy: This is done if casting fails or if there is persisting pain.

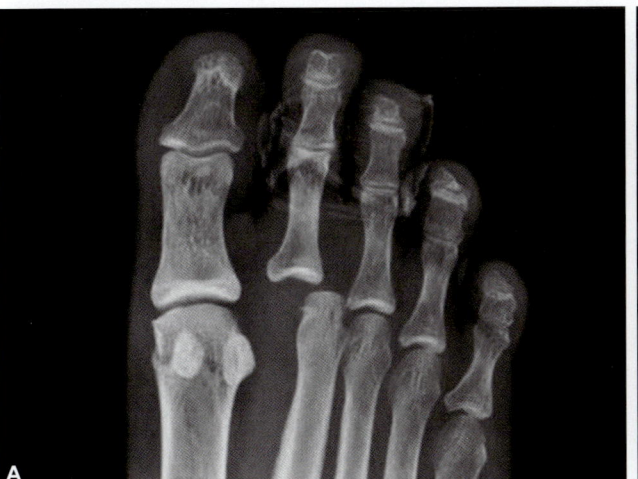
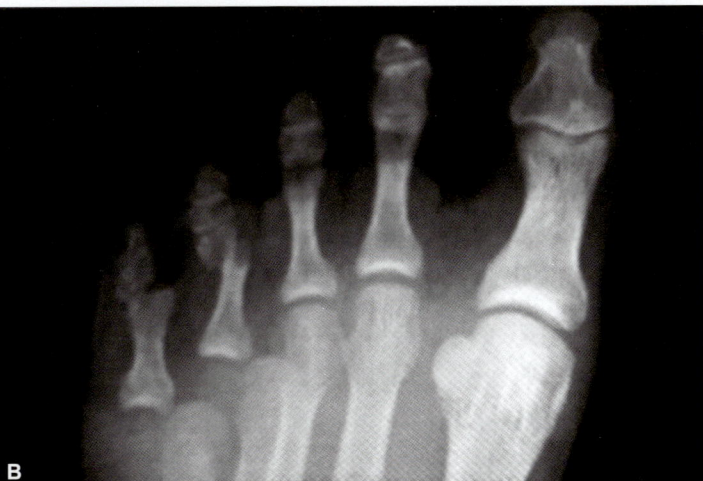

Figs 22.6A and B: Plain X-ray showing dislocation of 2nd, 4th and 5th MTP joints

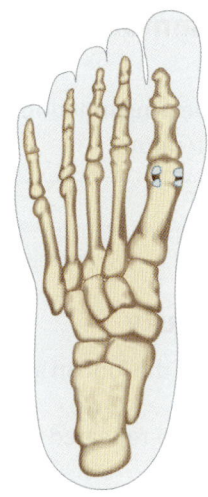

Fig. 22.7: Sesamoid bone fractures

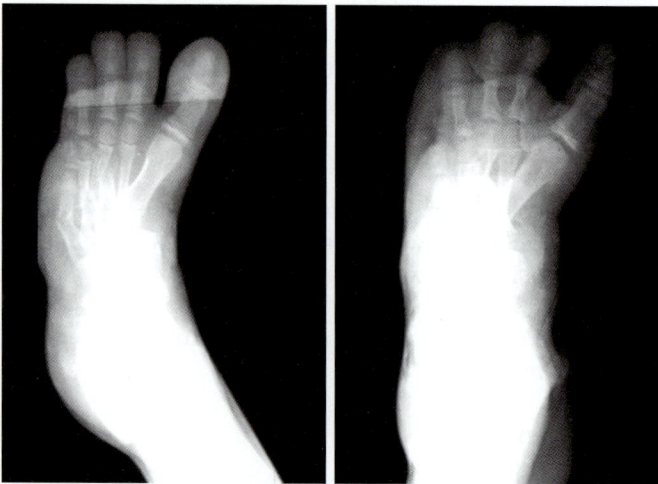

Fig. 22.8: Radiograph showing multiple metatarsal fractures

METATARSAL FRACTURES

Mechanism of Injury

- Direct force—common, due to fall of a heavy object.
- Indirect force—due to twisting forces, avulsion and spiral fractures are caused.
- Avulsion fractures are common at the base of the fifth metatarsal.
- Stress fractures are common at the II and III metatarsals (March fracture).

Clinical Features

The patient complains of pain, swelling, and tenderness over the dorsum of the foot. There could be considerable soft tissue swelling. Limp is present and pain in the foot increases with weight bearing.

Radiograph

Plain X-ray with AP, lateral and oblique views help to make the diagnosis (Figs 22.8 and 22.9).

Classification (OTA)

Group A : Extra-articular and simple diaphyseal fractures.
Group B : Partial articular and diaphyseal wedge fractures.
Group C : Complex articular and diaphyseal shaft fractures.

Treatment

- **First metatarsal:**
  - *Nonoperative methods:* NWB below-knee plaster cast for 6–8 weeks for stable fractures with no loss of bone length.

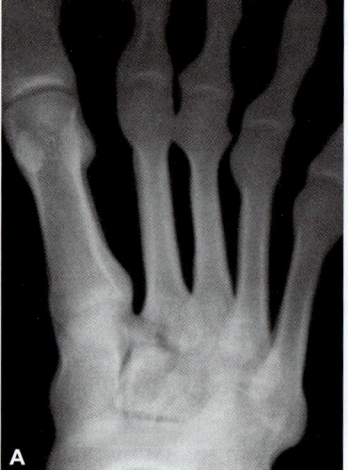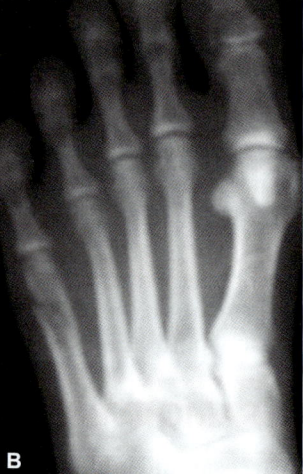

Figs 22.9A and B: Plain X-ray showing: (A) Fracture base of 2nd metatarsal bone; (B) Fracture neck of 5th metatarsal bone

  - *Operative methods:* Displaced and unstable fractures should be treated by closed reduction and percutaneous fixation with K-wires, screws only or with plate and screws (Fig. 22.10).
- **Central metatarsals (2–4):** These injuries are more common than the first metatarsal.
  - *Nonoperative methods:* Fractures with <10 mm long axis angulations and <4 mm transition of shaft with hard or stiff-soled shoes for fractures with >10 degree angulations and >4 mm translation can be treated with closed reduction and gravity, traction or immobilization with hand or stiff-soled shoes.
  - *Operative methods:* Closed reduction and percutaneous K-wire fixation is done for unstable injuries and for multiple fractures.

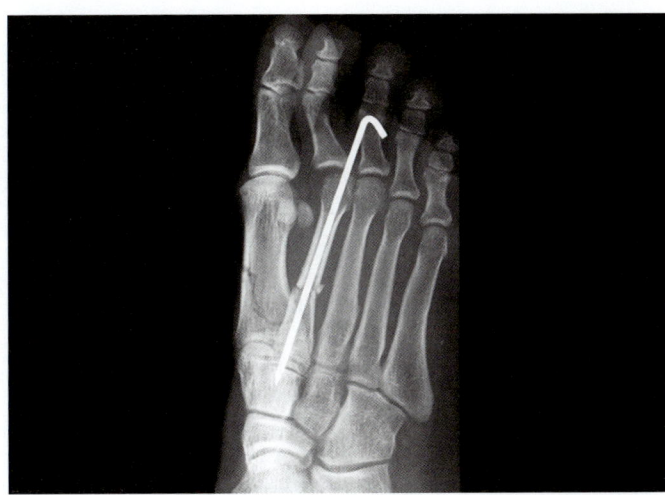

Fig. 22.10: Percutaneous K-wire fixation in metacarpal fractures

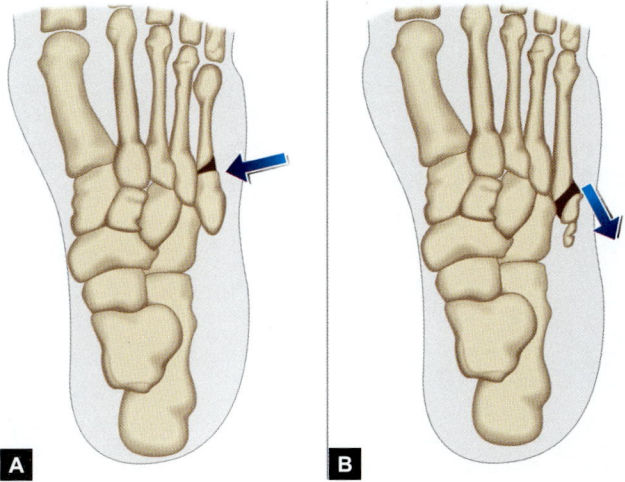

Figs 22.11A and B: (A) Jones fracture; (B) Avulsion fracture of the styloid process of 5th metatarsal bone

FIFTH METATARSAL INJURIES

Mechanism of Injury

- *Direct force:* Rare and is seen in RTAs, sports, etc.
- *Indirect force:* Twisting force injury is more common.

Classification

Fifth metatarsal fractures are divided into:
- Distal spiral or dancer's fracture
- Proximal base fractures. These are further subdivided into:
  - *Pseudo-Jones fracture:* Tip of the styloid process (avulsion fracture).
  - *Jones fracture:* Metaphyseal fracture due to sudden adduction of the forefoot.
- Stress fracture of the proximal fifth metatarsal.

Treatment

Nonoperative treatment is indicated for undisplaced and stable injuries and it consists of:
- Tip of the styloid process or Zone Injury—wearing hard sole or stiff shoes.
- Metaphyseal fractures (Jones)—below knee weight bearing plaster cast for 6–8 weeks.
- Diaphyseal fractures—NWB cast for 3 months.

JONES FRACTURE

It is a fracture of the diaphysis of the fifth metatarsal bone approximately 1.5 cm above the tip of the tuberosity (Fig. 22.11A) at the metaphyseal junction.

Mechanism of Injury

It is an avulsion fracture due to the pull of the peroneus brevis muscle. It is frequently encountered in athletes.

Clinical Features

The patient complains of pain, swelling and limp. On examination, tenderness can be elicited over the base of the fifth metatarsal bone.

> **Disturbing Facts About Jones Fracture**
> - It is often confused with pseudo-Jones fracture.
> - Delayed union and nonunion is a frequent occurrence due to the poor blood supply.
> - Surgery may be required if there is nonunion.

> **Do You Know About Pseudo-Jones Fracture?**
> - This is an avulsion fracture of the styloid process of the fifth metatarsal bone due to the pull of the peroneus brevis muscle (Fig. 22.11B).
> - It heals readily and surgery is rarely required.

Radiology

Radiograph of the foot helps to confirm the diagnosis. It shows a fuzzy periosteal reaction in the metadiaphyseal region after 7–10 days (Fig. 22.12).

Treatment

Conservative: Treatment is essentially conservative and consists of application of a below knee plaster cast for a period of 3–4 weeks.

Surgery: Single K-wire or screw fixation is now being done for displaced fractures (Fig. 22.13).

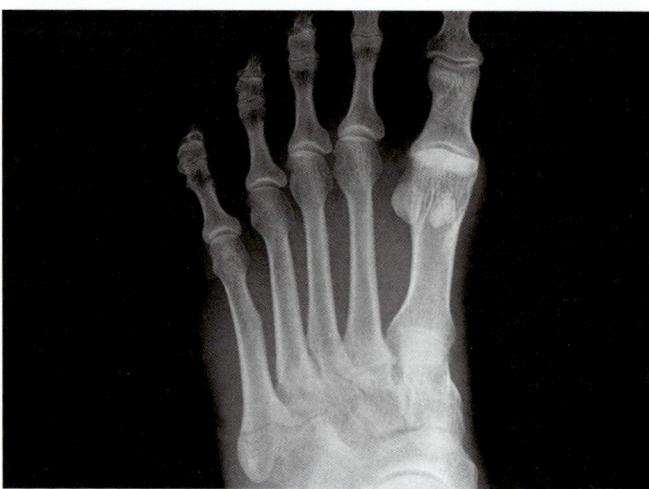

Fig. 22.12: X-ray of metadiaphyseal region

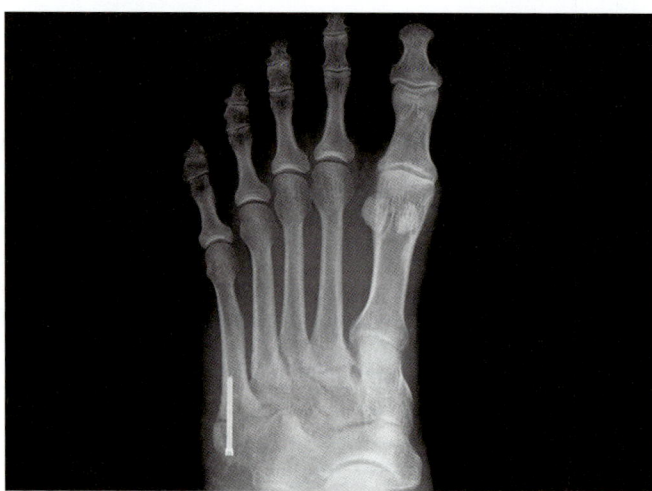

Fig. 22.13: X-ray showing screw fixation of Jones fracture

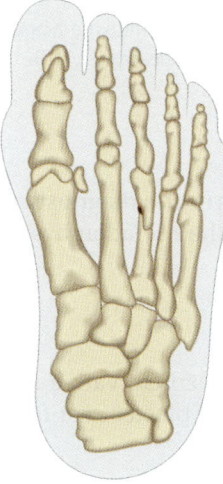
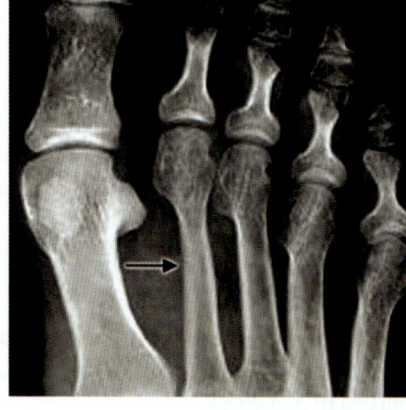

Fig. 22.14: March fracture

MARCH FRACTURE (Insufficiency Fracture)

This is a stress or fatigue fractures of the metatarsals particularly the II metatarsal bone (Fig. 22.14). It is more often encountered in military personnel who indulge in frequent and prolonged marching and hence its name. It is also seen in police officers, dancers, nurses, and surgeons, who require standing or dancing for a long duration. Radiograph helps in the diagnosis and the treatment is rest, NSAIDs, splints, elastic crepe bandage application, etc.

This is an important cause of chronic midfoot pain and it requires prompt identification and treatment.

MIDFOOT INJURIES

Midfoot consists of the navicular, three cuneiform and cuboid bones with their intervening joints. This region of the foot is susceptible to injuries. Midfoot fractures are depicted in Flowchart 22.2.

Mechanism of Injury

There are three common causes of midfoot fractures:
- *Twisting of the forefoot:* This usually occurs in an RTA due to forced foot abduction (twisting injury).
- *Axial loading of a fixed foot:* This can happen in two ways:
  - Fall on an extremely dorsiflexed foot (here an axial compression is applied to the heel).
  - Fall on an extremely ankle equinus (here axial compression is from the body weight).
- *Direct* crushing injuries as in industrial accidents.

Treatment Goals

Orthopedic Goal

- To restore the keystone of the midfoot (i.e. the first and second metatarsal articulation with the medial cuneiform) as it provides stability between the midfoot and forefoot during gait.
- To maintain the medial longitudinal arch of the foot by restoring the length and alignment of the cuneiforms, cuboid and navicular bones. The longitudinal and transverse arches should be maintained as they control the direct distribution of weight of the body or the foot during gait.
- To restore the Lisfranc joint complex.

Note:
Midfoot extends between the Chopart's joint proximally to Lisfranc joint distally.

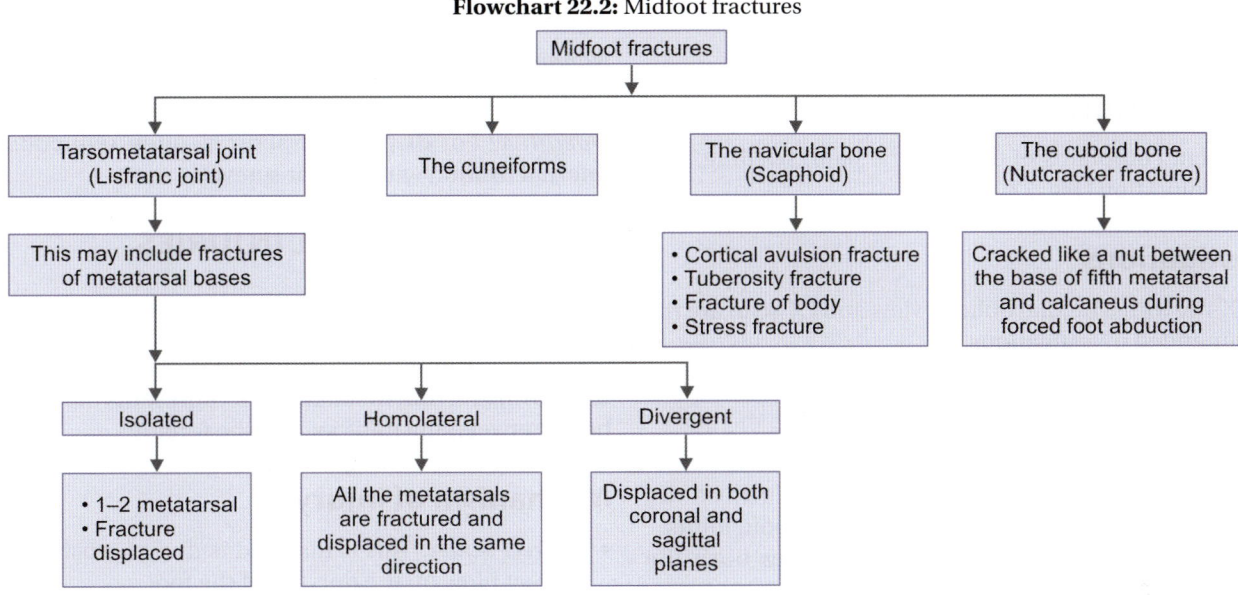

Flowchart 22.2: Midfoot fractures

NAVICULAR BONE FRACTURES

This is the keystone of the medial longitudinal arch of the foot (Fig. 22.15).

Mechanism of Injury

- *Direct blow:* Rare, can cause avulsion or crush injuries.
- *Indirect forces:* Due to fall from height, sports-related injuries or due to RTA.

OTA Classification

Group A: Extra-articular fracture.
Group B: Involvement of the talonavicular joint.
Group C: Involvement of both talonavicular and talocuneiform joints.

Each group is further subclassified depending upon fracture types and position.

Clinical Features

The patient complains of pain, swelling, and limp. Tenderness can be elicited over the navicular bone.

Investigations

AP and lateral X-rays of the joint and CT scan give more reliable information about the fracture pattern.

Treatment

- *Nonoperative treatment:* This is indicated in undisplaced fractures and in fracture with less than 2 mm

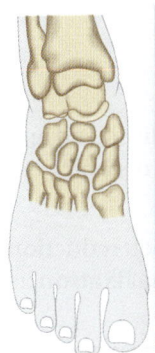
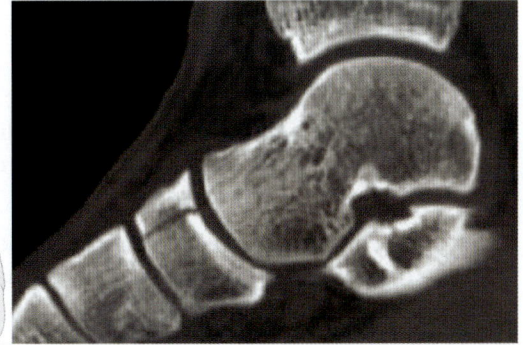

Fig. 22.15: Navicular bone fracture

displacement of the talonavicular joint. The treatment consists of short leg NWB cast for 6–8 weeks.

- *Operative treatment:* This is reserved for displaced fractures with >2 mm separation. Fixation can be achieved most of the times by screw fixation alone. If more than 40% of the articular surface is damaged, talonavicular fusion should be considered.

Complications

- Nonunion
- Avascular necrosis
- Collapse of the arch
- Post-traumatic osteoarthritis.

CUBOID FRACTURES

Mechanism of Injury

- Direct blow

- Indirect force: Forced plantar flexion and abduction (nutcracker effect).

Clinical Features

The patient complains of dorsolateral pain, swelling, and skin discoloration (Fig. 22.16).

Investigations

Plain X-ray with a medial oblique view and CT scan are the recommended investigations.

Classification (OTA)

Group A: Extra-articular.
Group B: Partly intra-articular involving either the calcaneocuboid or the metatarsocuboid joints.
Group C: Completely intra-articular involves both the joints.

Each group is further classified depending upon the fracture pattern and position.

Treatment

Nonoperative method: This is indicated in undisplaced and in fractures < 2 mm separation. The treatment of choice is a below knee cast for 6–8 weeks.

Operative method: For displaced fractures, open reduction and K-wire fixation is indicated. External fixation is recommended for the nutcracker fracture.

> **Note:**
> Cuboid syndrome is a painful subluxation of the calcaneocuboid joint.

CUNEIFORM INJURIES

These are rare injuries and are usually due to indirect forces. More commonly, they are associated with injuries to the tarsometatarsal joints (Fig. 22.17).

Clinical Features

Pain, swelling, tenderness, limp, and pain on weight bearing.

Investigations

Plain X-ray (AP, lateral, oblique views) with CT scan of the foot.

Classification (OTA)

Group A : Extra-articular.
Group B : Partly intra-articular (involves other navicular cuneiform or metatarsal cuneiform joints).
Group C : Involves both articular surfaces.

Treatment

Nonoperative: Short leg cast for 6 to 8 weeks for undisplaced fractures.

Operative: For displaced fractures, open reduction and internal fixation with pins or screws.

TARSOMETATARSAL INJURIES (Lisfranc Injuries)

Lisfranc joint consists of three cuneiform metacarpal articulations and two cuboid metatarsal articulations of the fourth and fifth metatarsals. It represents the transition bone between the midfoot and the forefoot.

Mechanism of Injury

- *Direct injury:* This is rare and is due to crush injury or direct blow on the dorsum of the foot.
- *Indirect injury:* This is more common and three varieties are described (Figs 22.18A and B):
  - Axial loading to the foot in fixed equinus (e.g. football injuries)
  - Axial loading in descending stairs
  - Axial loading following fall from height.

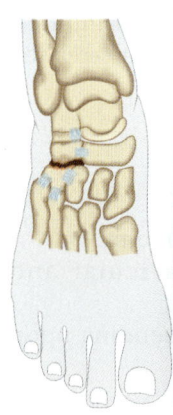
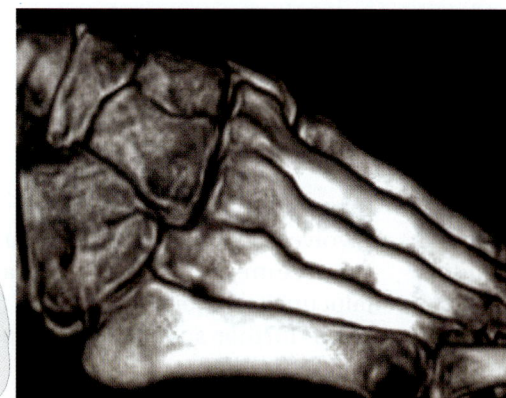

Fig. 22.16: Cuboid bone fracture

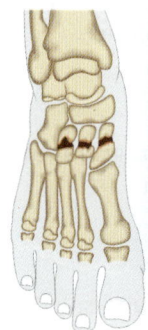
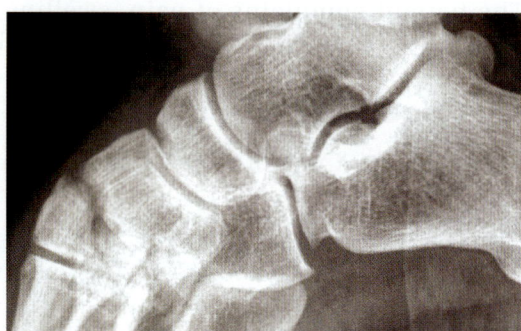

Fig. 22.17: Cuneiform bone fractures

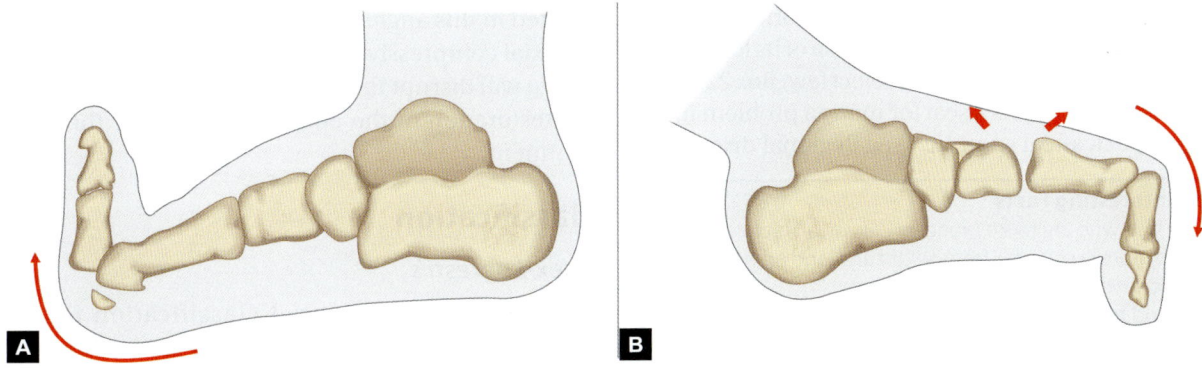

Figs 22.18A and B: Mechanisms of Lisfranc injury

The associated injuries could be fracture of second metatarsal (most common), fractures of cuneiforms, cuboids, metatarsals, and lateral ligament injuries.

Clinical Features

Pain in the tarsometatarsal area. Passive dorsiflexion or plantar flexion produces pain. Single limb heel lift produces pain in the midfoot. Plantar ecchymosis.

Investigations

- Plain X-ray in weight bearing position (AP, lateral and 30° medial oblique position) (Fig. 22.19).
- CT scan provides better visualization and is more accurate in analyzing the injuries.

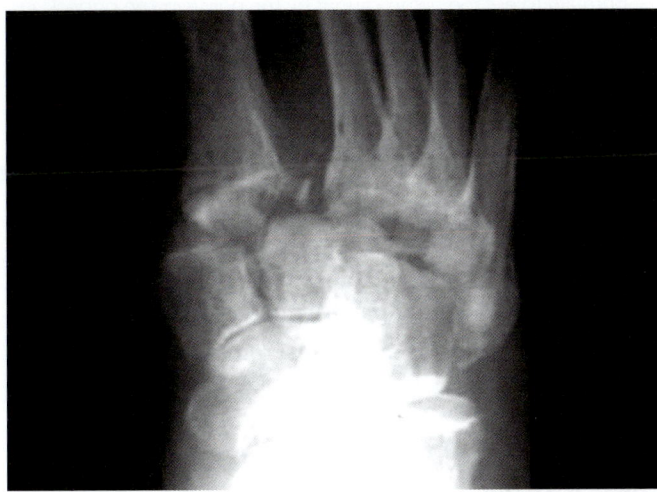

Fig. 22.19: Plain X-ray showing Lisfranc fracture

Classification (OTA)(Figs 22.20A to C)

- *Type I:* Anterior dislocation 1st ray, dorsal and plantar dislocations of the lesser rays.
- *Type II:* Divergent dislocation.
- *Type III:* Homolateral dislocation (medial or lateral).

Treatment

Nonoperative methods: This is indicated for sprains and for <2 mm displacement of tarsometatarsal joint in any plane. The treatment of choice is a below knee POP cast for 6–8 weeks. For sprains—RICE regime.

Operative methods: For displaced injuries, closed reduction, and internal fixation. With K-wires or screws is indicated for displacement <50%. For more than 50 percent displacement, primary fusion is indicated. Open reduction or internal fixation is indicated for widely displaced fractures (Fig. 22.21).

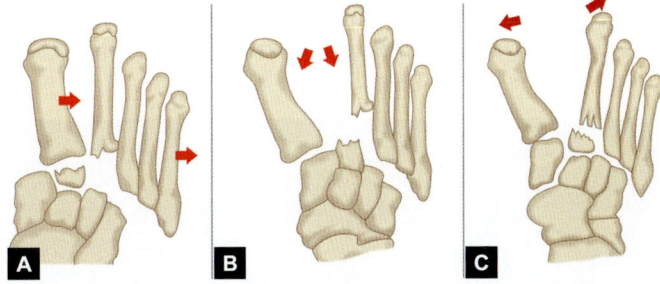

Figs 22.20A to C: Different types of Lisfranc: Injury: (A) Type I; (B) Type II; (C) Type III

HINDFOOT INJURIES

FRACTURE CALCANEUM

Calcaneus is the most often fractured tarsal bone. No ideal method of treatment has been described yet. It is a 'soft' bone residing inside your heel doing the 'hard' jobs like weight transmission and locomotion. It is a 'small' bone cut out for 'big' challenging and difficult roles. Because of its location, it is infrequently fractured (except in a select few, Box 22.1) but because of its function, it is a seat for many a problem in life like heel pain, calcaneal spur, etc. (see Regional disorders).

> **Box 22.1: Interesting Facts**
> The unlucky few, who are more prone for calcaneal fractures are the ones who are more likely to fall from height and land on the feet like:
> - Construction workers of high rise buildings
> - Electrical and telephone linemen working atop the poles
> - Casual laborers engaged in plucking the tender coconuts from the lanky coconut trees
> - Athletes involved in high jump and long jump, etc.
>   Last but not the least, thieves who jump down the houses, after burglary to escape being caught by the police or the public!

Functions

- Supports weight of the body.
- Acts as a springboard for locomotion.

Structure

It has a thin cortical shell except at the posterior tuberosity. Two types of trabecular pattern are described.

Traction trabeculae: This radiates from the inferior cortex.

Compression trabeculae: Converge to support anterior and posterior facets.

Vital Angles

In the lateral view of the radiograph, two angles are important:

Böhler's angle: This is the angle between lines drawn from anterior articular process to the posterior tuberosity. The tuber angle is 25–40° (Fig. 22.22).

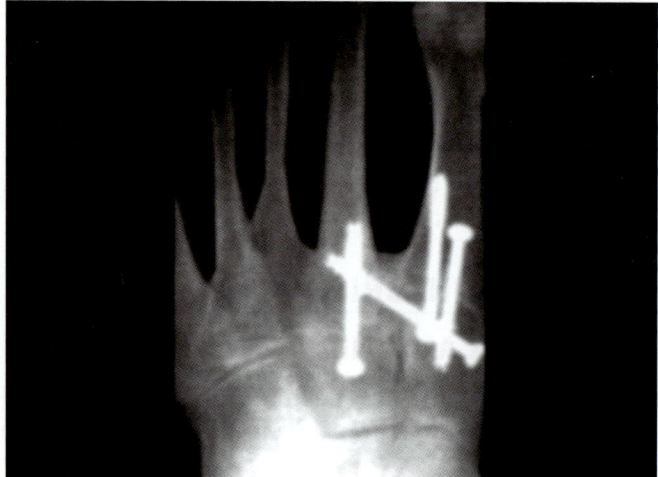

Fig. 22.21: Radiograph showing Lisfranc injury fixed with screws

Crucial angle of "Gissane": The lateral process of talus is wedged in this angle (Fig. 22.23).

Axial compressive forces with talus acting as a bursting wedge will disrupt the subtalar joint.

Restoration of the above two angles is the aim of the treatment.

Classification

Essex-Lopresti's

This is the most accepted classification for fracture calcaneum. It consists of extra-articular fractures (Figs 22.24A to D) (less common accounting for only 25% of the cases) and intra-articular fractures, which is more common (Figs 22.25A to C).

Crosby-Fitzgibbon's: Classification Based on CT Scan Findings (Intra-articular)

Type I   : Undisplaced fracture.
Type II : Displaced intra-articular fractures of the posterior facet (<2 mm).
Type III : Comminuted fractures.

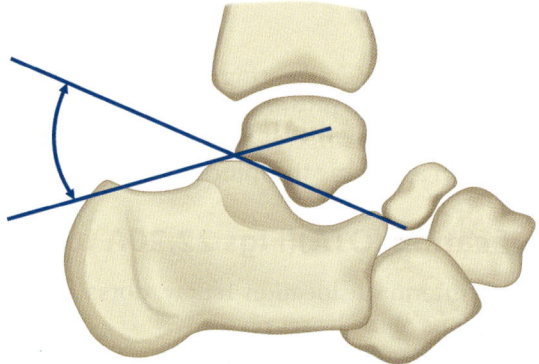

Fig. 22.22: Tuber joint angle (Böhler's angle)

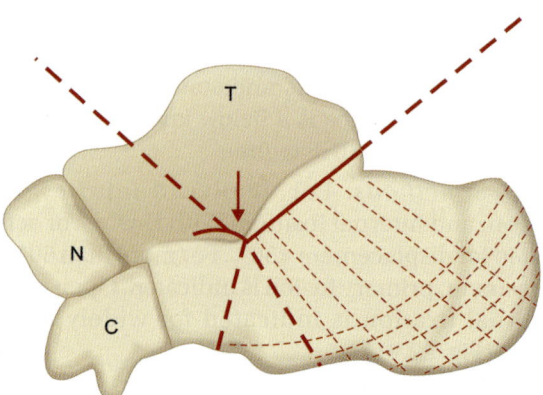

Fig. 22.23: Gissane angle

Note:
Type I : Nonoperative treatment.
Type II : Operative treatment.

EXTRA-ARTICULAR FRACTURES

Mechanism of Injury

Twisting forces cause many of the extra-articular fractures. *Fall from height* with landing on the heels causes vast majority of intra-articular fractures (Fig. 22.26A).

Vital Facts
- Bilateral fractures are seen in 5–9% of cases.
- Ten percent cases have compression fracture of dorsal or lumbar vertebral bodies.
- Twenty-six percent are associated with other injuries of the lower limbs.

Clinical Features

Patient complains of pain swelling, limp, and painful restricted movements of the subtalar and the midfoot joints.

Radiography (Fig. 22.26B)

Plain X-rays of the foot with the following three views are recommended:
- Dorsoplantar or anteroposterior view (Fig. 22.27A).
- Lateral view helps to study the crucial angle of Gissane (Fig. 22.27B).
- Axial calcaneal view (Harris view).
- CT scan is now emerging as the gold standard in evaluation of calceneal fractures.

Classification

- Anterior-fracture of the anterior process.
- Middle:
    - Body fracture
    - Fracture of sustentaculum tali
    - Lateral calcaneal process fracture
    - Peroneal tubercle fracture.
- Posterior:
    - Tuberosity fracture
    - Medial calcaneal tubercle fracture.

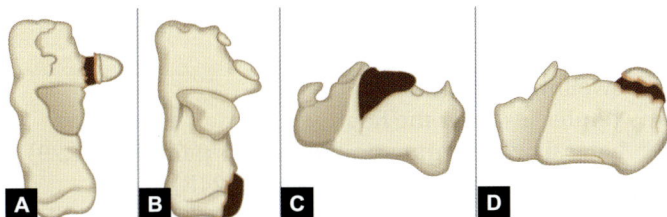

Figs 22.24A to D: Types of extra-articular fractures: (A) S. tali fracture; (B) Medial process fracture; (C) Anterior process fracture; (D) Tuberosity fracture

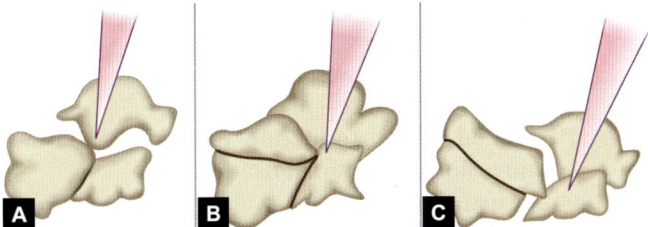

Figs 22.25A to C: Varieties of intra-articular fractures: (A) Undisplaced fracture; (B) Tongue-shaped fracture; (C) Comminuted fracture

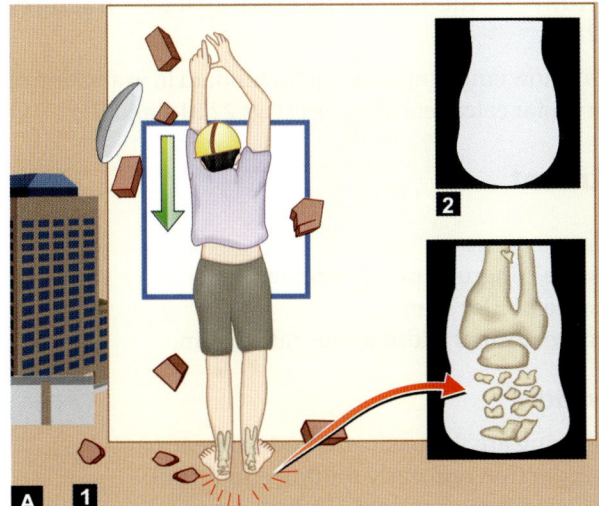
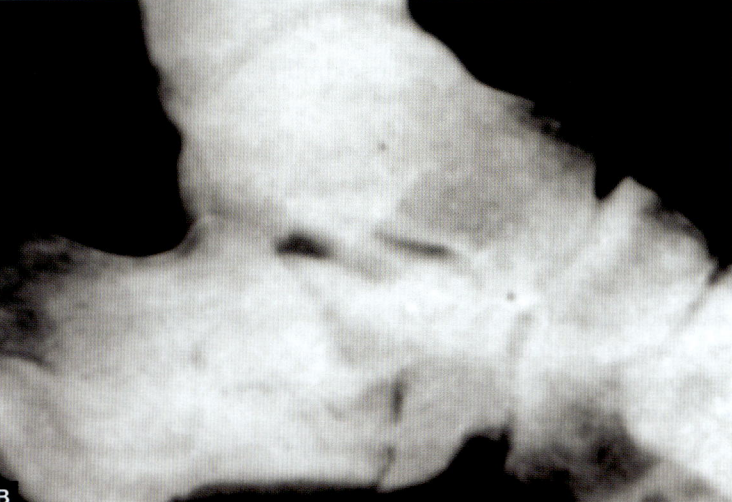

Figs 22.26A and B: (A) 1—Fall from height causes intra-articular fracture of calcaneum, 2—Broadening of the heel; (B) Radiograph showing calcaneum fracture

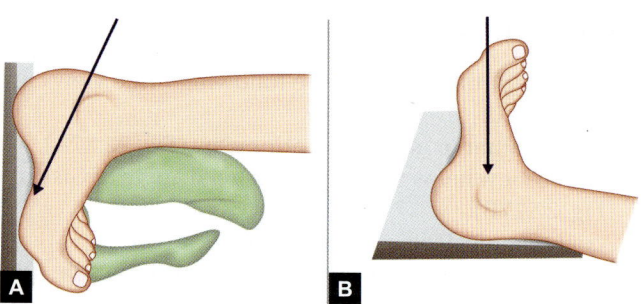

Figs 22.27A and B: Radiographic views: (A) Dorsoplantar view; (B) Lateral view

Treatment

Extra-articular Fractures

- Fracture of anterior process:
  - Avulsion fracture—short leg cast (Fig. 22.28)
  - Compression fracture—should be reduced and fixed with K-wire or screw
- Fracture tuberosity:
  - Undisplaced fracture—short leg cast
  - Displaced fracture—open reduction and internal fixation
- Fracture medial calcaneal process:
  - Undisplaced fracture—plaster cast
  - Displaced—open reduction with medial lateral compression and internal fixation
- Fracture sustentaculum tali:
  - Undisplaced—plaster cast
  - Displaced—open reduction and casting
- Fracture of the body not involving the subtalar joint: Responds well to conservative treatment.

INTRA-ARTICULAR FRACTURES

These account for 60% of all tarsal injuries and 75% of all calcaneal fractures.

Mechanism of Injury

Fall from height: Lateral process of talus acts as a wedge and is forced through the Gissane's angle resulting in four fracture patterns:
- Undisplaced
- Tongue shaped
- Joint depression
- Comminuted.

Clinical Features

- Pain and swelling of the heel, the patient is unable to bear weight, stand or walk, pain and difficulty during inversion and eversion of the heel.

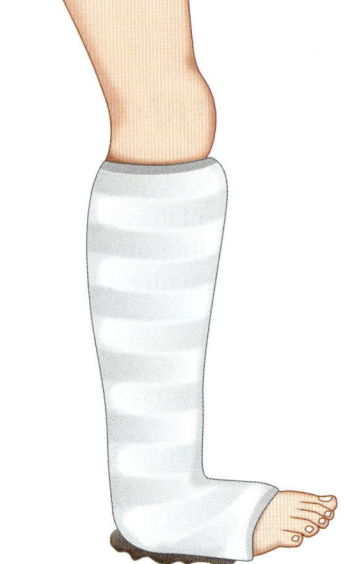

Fig. 22.28: Short leg POP cast with walking heel for calcaneal fracture

Clinical Signs

- Swelling over the heel
- Tenderness over the heel
- Lateral heel compression test elicits pain (Fig. 22.29)
- Broadening of the heel (see Fig. 22.24B)
- Horseshoe swelling on either side the tendo-Achilles
- Distance between the heel and malleoli is reduced.

Investigations

Plain X-rays of the foot as in extra-articular fractures (Fig. 22.30).

CT scan is now emerging as the gold standard in evaluation of intra-articular calcaneal fractures (Figs 22.31A and B).

Treatment

Goals

- Restore congruity of the subtalar joint
- Restore Böhler's angle
- Restore normal width of the calcaneum.

Conservative

The following are the basic methods of treatment:
- No reduction and early motion consists of:
  - Elastocrepe bandage application
  - Foot elevation
  - Weight bearing at the end of 12 weeks.
- Closed reduction and fixation.

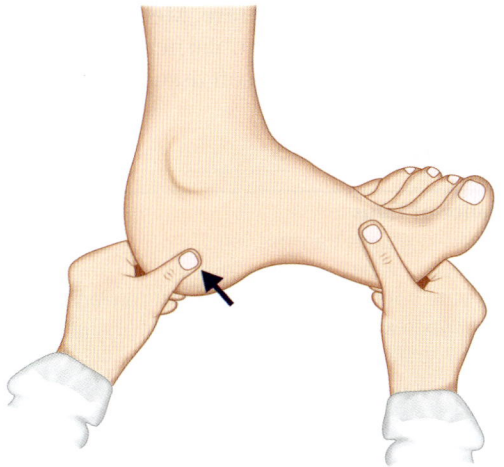

Fig. 22.29: Heel compression test for diagnosing undisplaced or stress fracture of calcaneum

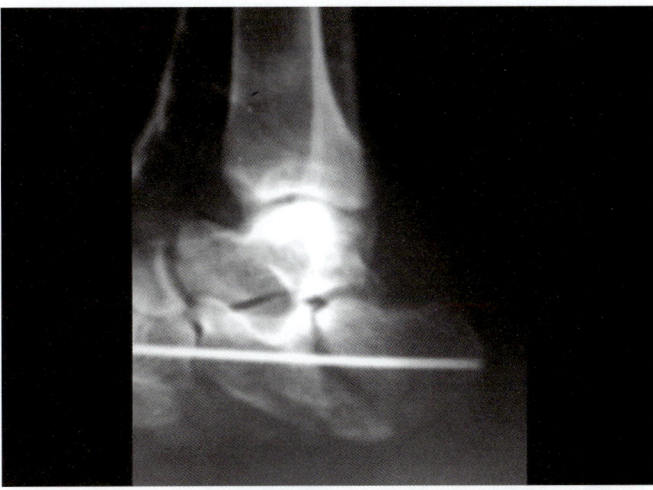

Fig. 22.30: Radiograph showing intra-articular calcaneum fracture

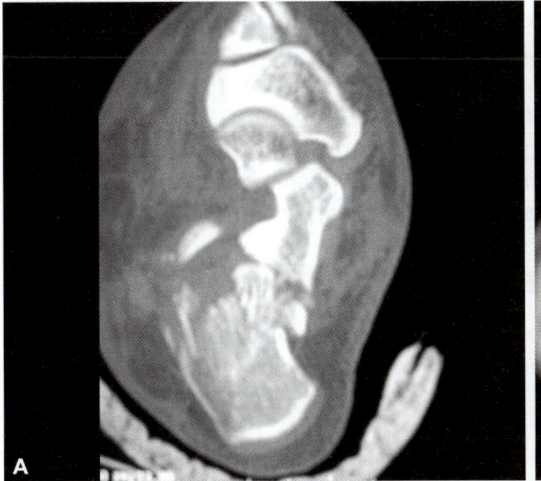
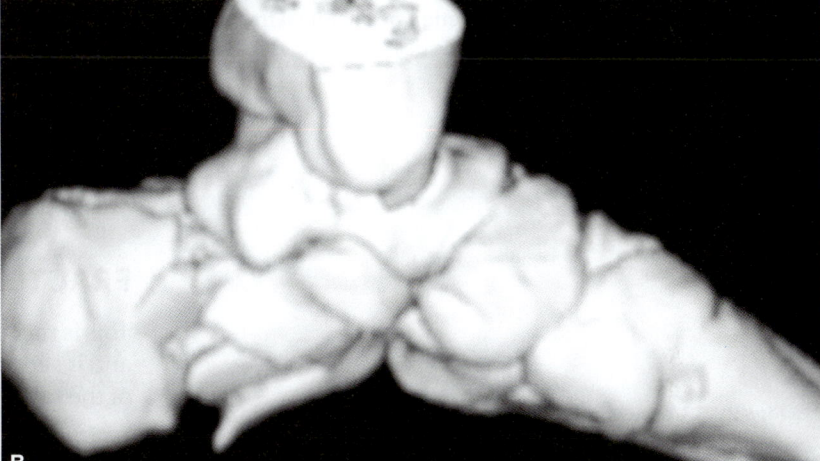

Figs 22.31A and B: CT Scan (3D) showing displaced calcaneal fracture

Omoto Technique of Calcaneal Fracture Reduction (Fig. 22.32)

Common Steps of Reduction

- Under anesthesia (general or spinal), the patient is prone and knee is flexed to 90°.
- With the assistant supporting the thigh, the surgeon compresses the medial and lateral sides of the heel.
- Strong longitudinal traction is now applied along the direction of the leg.
- Varus or valgus force is now applied depending on the displacement.
- Lastly, the calcaneal tuberosity is manipulated in position.
- Compression bandage is finally applied.

Essex-Lopresti method of lifting the fragment with an axial percutaneous pin and retention with K-wires is done (Figs 22.33A and B).

Surgery

Severely comminuted and depressed fracture with subchondral defects requires open reduction and internal fixation with cancellous bone graft to fill the gap (Figs 22.34 and 22.35). Recently, for this purpose, alternatively, biocompatible and less reabsorbable nanocrystalline calcium phosphate cement called Bioban is being tried with successful results in some centers.

Open reduction and internal fixation with plate and screws are difficult and are rarely adopted.

Complications

- Nonunion is rare due to the cancellous nature of the bone
- Malunion is more common
- *Heel pain:* The source of heel pain could be from:

- Subtalar joint due to post-traumatic osteoarthritis
- Peroneal tendonitis due to stenosing tenovaginitis of the peroneal tendons
- Bone spurs due to malunion of fracture and disruption of fat pad of the heel
- Arthritis of calcaneocuboid joint is a major source of pain.
- Nerve entrapment is rare. Medial or lateral plantar branches of posterior tibial nerve or sural nerve may be entrapped due to soft tissue scarring.

FRACTURE TALUS

Importance of Talus
- Takes part in weight transmission
- Has a precarious blood supply
- 3/5th of the bone is covered by articular cartilage
- Sudden hyperextension of the forefoot causes fracture neck called "Aviators Astralagus."

Blood Supply of Talus

- Sixty percent is covered by articular surface, only limited surface is available for vascular perforation
- No muscle originates or inserts into talus
- All the three major arteries of the foot posterior tibial artery, anterior tibial artery, and peroneal artery supply talus
- There is important contribution from capsular and ligamentous vessels
- The branches of these arteries form an anterosuperior and inferior groups. The posteroinferior surface of the body has no blood supply (Fig. 22.36).

FRACTURE NECK TALUS

This is the second most common of all tarsal bone fractures and is second in frequency to the chip and avulsion fracture of the talus.

Incidence is 30% of all talus fractures.

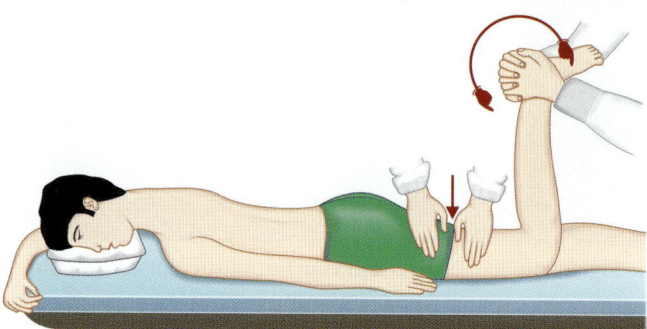

Fig. 22.32: Method of closed reduction of calcaneal fractures (Omoto technique)

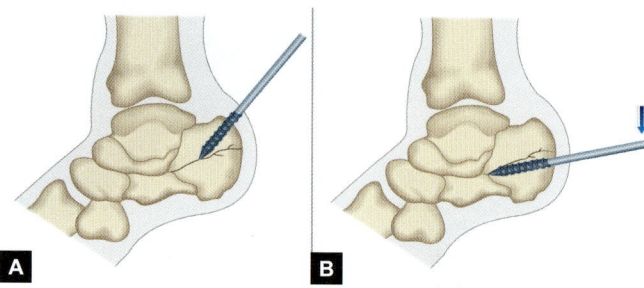

Figs 22.33A and B: Essex-Lopresti method of reduction of calcaneal fractures: (A) Disimpaction; (B) Elevation

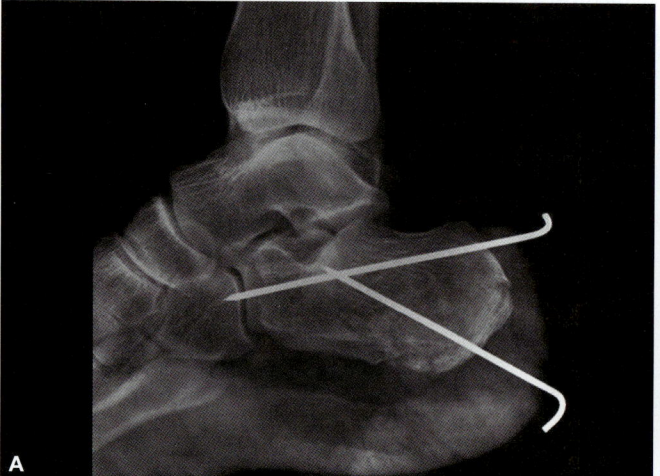
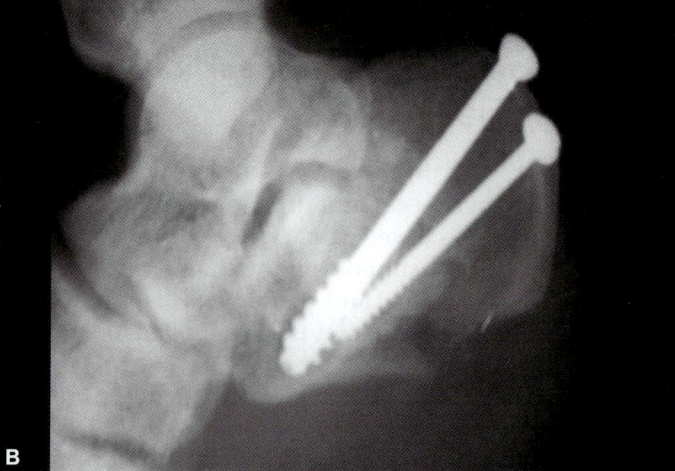

Figs 22.34A and B: Plain X-ray showing fixation of calcaneal fracture with screws

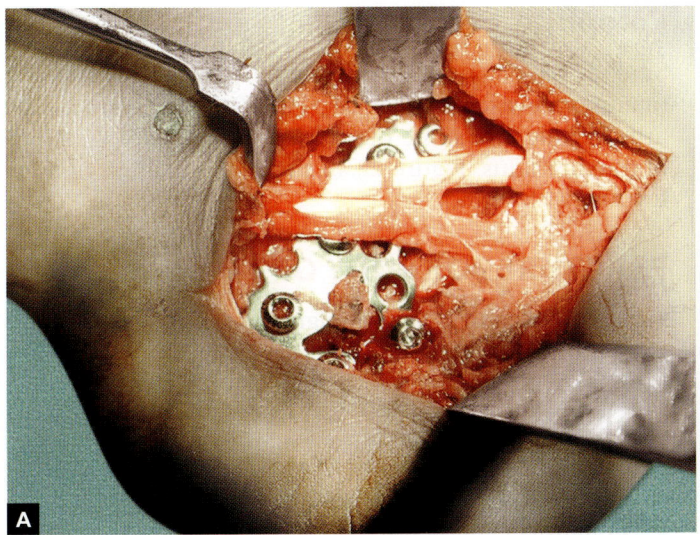
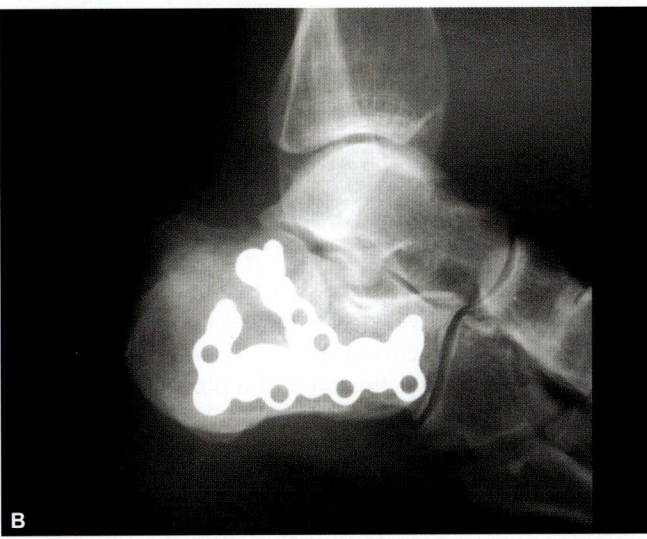

Figs 22.35A and B: Operative photo and plain X-ray showing plating of calcaneal fracture

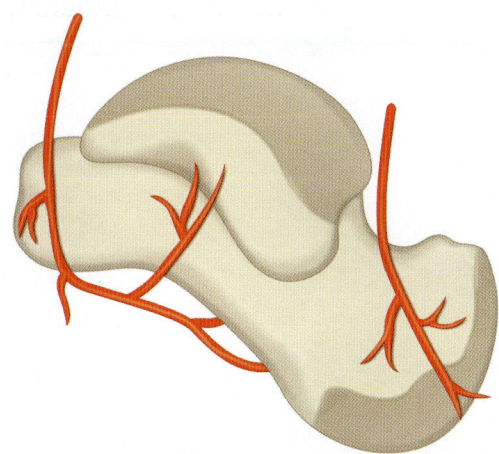

Fig. 22.36: Blood supply of talus

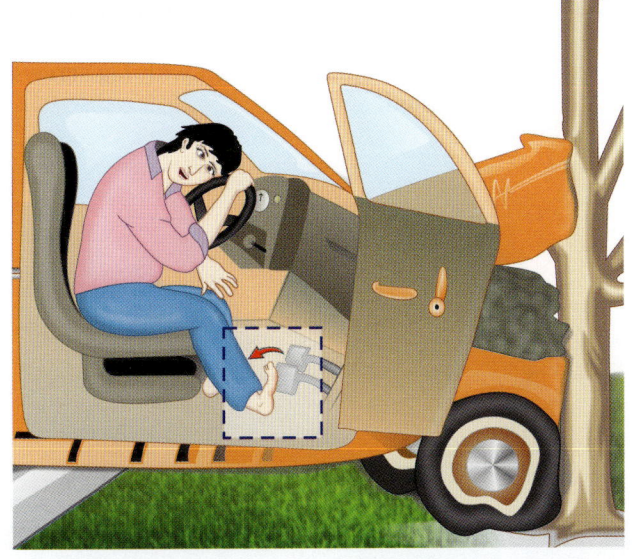

Fig. 22.37: Mechanism of injury of talus neck fractures

Mechanism of Injury

The common mode of injury is hyperdorsiflexion of the foot on one leg (Fig. 22.37). It may be associated with fracture of tarsal bones and fracture of the metatarsal bones.

Earlier, it was more commonly seen in flying accidents, but now it is more commonly seen in RTA due to head-on collision.

Note:
Anderson coined the term Aviator Astragalgus.

Classification (Hawkin's) (Fig. 22.38)

Type I : Undisplaced vertical fracture neck of talus.
Type II : Displaced fracture with subluxation or dislocation of subtalar joint.
Type III : Displaced fracture neck with dislocation of the body of the talus from both ankle and subtalar joints.
Type IV : Displaced fracture neck with dislocation of the head and body of the talus from subtalar/ankle/talonavicular joints.

Clinical Features

The patient usually gives a history of high velocity rudder bar type of accident. The patient complains of pain, swelling, and deformity in displaced fractures. The skin may be kinked or stretched.

Radiography

In radiograph of the fracture talus, the following views are recommended (Fig. 22.39). Anteroposterior view with foot in maximum equinus and 15° pronation, lateral and oblique views of the ankle (Fig. 22.40).

Treatment

Type I : This is best treated by below-knee plaster cast for 6–8 weeks with 6 weeks NWB.

Type II : In this, closed reduction is done by traction in plantar flexion and a plaster cast is put in equinus. Alternatively, closed reduction is followed by percutaneous cannulated screw, fixation to prevent redisplacement of the fragments, which could be possible with earlier treatment. If this fails, ORIF with lag screws is done.

Type III : In these, approximately 25% are open fractures. Debridement is done first and closed reduction is attempted later. If unsuccessful, ORIF with K-wires or open reduction with lag screws is attempted.

Complications

Skin necrosis, infection, delayed union, nonunion, malunion; avascular necrosis (Fig. 22.41), post-traumatic arthritis, etc. are some of the well-known complications of fracture talus. Figure 22.42 shows the fixation of talus fracture with screws.

FRACTURES OF BODY OF TALUS

- Usually due to fall from height
- It is relatively rare
- It may be associated with malleolar fractures.

Types

- Osteochondral fractures of the doom of talus
- Fracture of lateral process

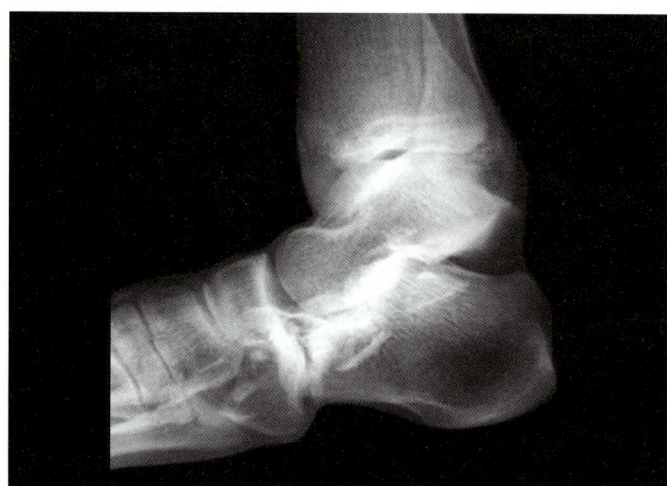

Fig. 22.40: Plain X-ray showing subtalar dislocation

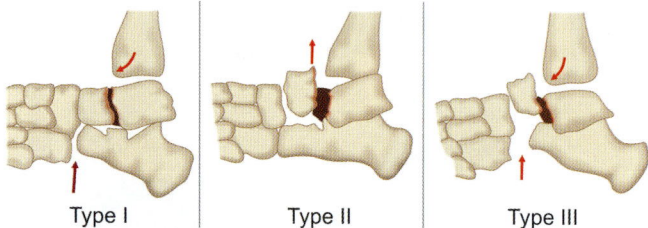

Fig. 22.38: Fracture neck of talus (Hawkin's types)

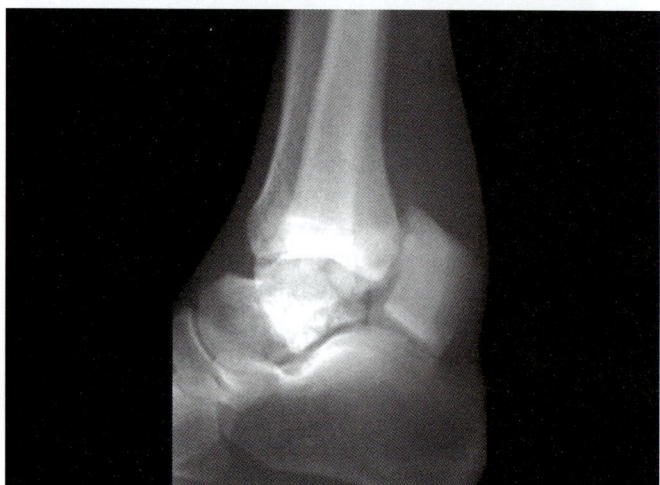

Fig. 22.39: Radiograph of talus fracture

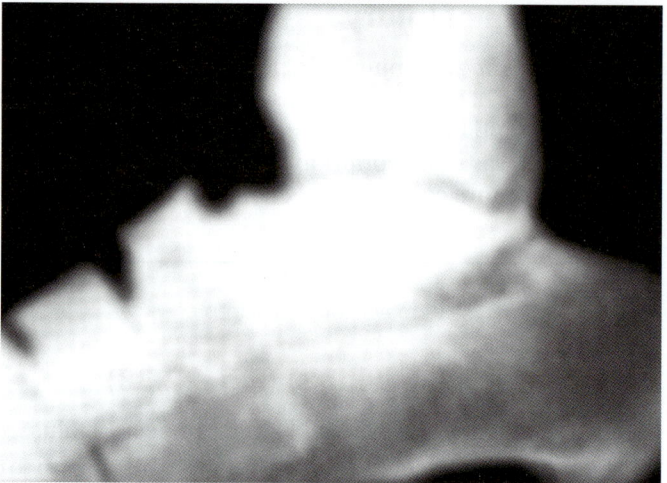

Fig. 22.41: Radiograph showing AVN talus

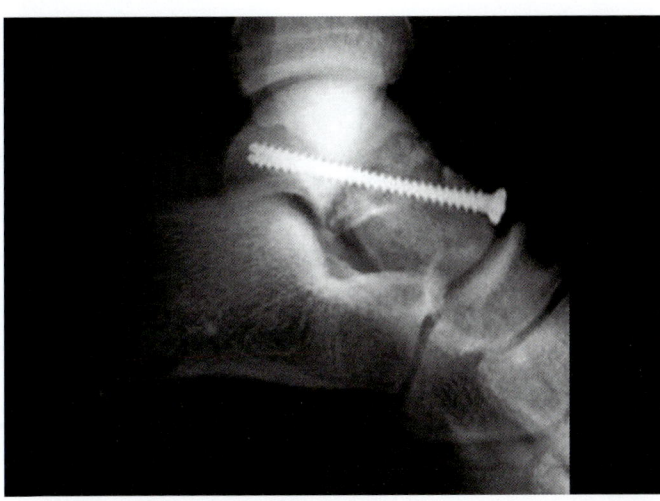

Fig. 22.42: Fixation of talus fracture with screws

- Fracture of posterior process
- Stress fracture of posterolateral body
- Crush fracture.

BIBLIOGRAPHY

1. Adams JC. Outline of Fractures, Including Joint Injuries (8th edn). Churchill Livingstone, Edinburgh; 1983.
2. Amihood S. Posterior dislocation of hip: Clinical observations and review of literature. S Afr Med J. 1974;48:1029.
3. Apley AG, Solermm L. Apley's System of Orthopedics and Fractures (6th edn), Butterworth's: London; 1982.
4. Arnold CC, Linder Holm H. Fracture of the femoral neck. Clin Orthop. 1972;84:116.
5. Boyd HB, George LL. Classification and treatment of trochanteric fractures. Arch Surg. 1949;58:853.
6. Campbell's operative orthopedics, 5th volume. Edited by AS Crens Law (8th edn).
7. Cooney WP. External fixation of distal radial fractures. Clin Orthop. 1983;180:44.
8. Cotton CL. Fractures of the olecranon in adults: Classification and management. Injury. 1973;5:121.
9. Crenshaw AH, Wilson FD. The surgical treatment of the fractures of the patella. South Med J. 1954;47:716.
10. Gingras MB, Clarke J, Evarts CM. Prosthetic replacement in femoral neck fractures. Clin Orthop. 1980;152:147.
11. Grace TG, Eversmann WW (Jr). Forearm fractures: treatment by rigid fixation and early motion. J Bone and Joint Surg. 1980;62-A:433.
12. Hawkins LG. Fractures of the neck of talus. J Bone and Joint Surg. 1970;52-A:991.
13. Hughes JL, Weber H, Wellenegger H, Kuner EH. Evaluation of ankle fractures, non-operative and operative treatment. Clin Orthop. 1979;138:111.
14. J Orge E Alonso, et al. Hip dislocation and associated acetabular fractures. Clinical Orthopedics and Related Research; August 2000.
15. K Sailer, H Umer, R Hourbesch, C Finta, et al. Gamma nail in portrochanteric and subtrochanteric fractures. Source: Orthonet India; Jan 2001.
16. Karlstrom G, Olereud S. Fractures of the tibial shaft: A critical evaluation of treatment alternatives. Clin Orthop. 1974;105:82.
17. Kaufer H. Mechanical functions of the patella. J Bone and Joint Surg. 1971;53-4:1557.
18. Lisfranc joint injuries-RS Kuo, Tejwani, et al. JBJS. 2000.
19. Mann RJ, Neal EG. Fractures of the shaft of the humerus in adults. South Med J. 1965;58:264.
20. Michael RS, et al, Bioban in the treatment of talus fracture. University of Uhn, Germany, European Journal of Trauma. 2002.
21. Neer CS II. Displaced proximal humeral fracture. J Bone Joint Surg. 1970;52-A:1077.
22. Newer Generation Nails for Tibial fractures. Source. Orthnet. 2003;56:5.
23. Reamed Nailing of Gustilo Grade IIIB. Tibial fractures. In: JF Keating, et al. JBJS. 2000.
24. Reckling FW, Cordell LD. Unstable fracture dislocations of the forearm, the Monteggia, and Galeazzi lesions. Arch Surg. 1968;96-999.
25. Rockwood CA, Green DP, 1975.
26. Sarmiento A. Functional bracing of tibial fractures. Clin Orthop. 1974;105:202.
27. Seinshemer F. Subtrochanteric fractures of the femur. J Bone and Joint Surg. 1978;60-4:300.
28. Smith L. Deformity following supracondylar fractures of the humerus. J Bone Joint Surg. 1960;42-A:235.
29. Stoddard A. Manipulation of the Elbow Joint. Physiotherapy. 1971;57:259.
30. Traumatic hip distortions in adults. Edward C Yong, Roger Cornwell. Clinical Orthopedics and Related Research; August 2000.
31. Watson Jones. Fractures and Joint Injuries (6th edn), 2 volumes. Edinburgh: Churchill Livingstone.

23 CHAPTER

Pelvic Injuries, Rib and Coccyx Injuries

BRIEF ANATOMY

The Pelvis Speaks

I am made up of two innominate bones, a portion of spine and sacrum (Fig. 23.1). The innominate bone is formed by fusion of three separate bones, the ilium, ischium, and pubis. Ilium forms the superior part, the ischium the posteroinferior part, the pubis the anteroinferior part. Three bones of mine meet to form the acetabulum. Anteriorly, I am connected by a strong minimally mobile fibrocartilaginous joint called the pubic symphysis. Posteriorly, I articulate with the sacrum through the almost immobile sacroiliac joint. I derive my stability in the posterior aspect from the sacroiliac (SI) and the sacrospinous ligament complex, anteriorly by the pubic symphysis and inferiorly by the muscles and ligaments forming the pelvic floor and perineum.
My main functions are:
- To transmit the forces from the spine to the lower limbs and vice versa.
- In the standing position, I transmit the weight through the ilium and in the sitting position through the ischium.
- I give attachment to the muscles helping in posture and locomotion.
- I protect the vital genitourinary system and lower abdominal viscera.

FRACTURE PELVIS

Stability of the Pelvis

Stability of the pelvis depends on both bony and ligamentous structures. Anterior portion of the pelvic ring neither participates in normal weight bearing nor is it essential for maintenance of pelvic stability. The posterior arch is formed by the sacrum, SI joints, and ilia and is the weight-bearing portion of the pelvis. The posterosuperior SI ligaments provide most of the ligamentous stability of the SI joints.

Stable Pelvic Fracture

These fractures do not involve the pelvic ring and they are minimally displaced.

Unstable Pelvic Fracture

They involve the pelvic ring and are widely displaced. Pelvic fractures pose a problem different from others. Here the emphasis is on recognition of potential complications associated with these fractures, the notable ones being injuries to the major vessels and nerves of the pelvis and major viscera like intestines, bladder and the urethra, severe intrapelvic hemorrhage from fracture of pelvic ring. Mortality from pelvic fracture varies from 10–50%. Proper fracture management decreases the blood loss and controls the hemorrhage. A to F management as proposed by Mac Murthy in multiple trauma patients is important in management of the pelvic fractures.

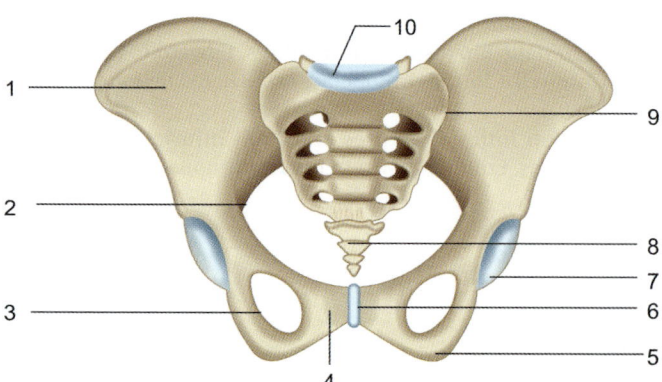

Fig. 23.1: Anatomy of pelvis; (1) Ilium, (2) Arcuate line, (3) Obturator foramen, (4) Pubis, (5) Ischium, (6) Pubic symphysis, (7) Acetabulum, (8) Coccyx, (9) Sacroiliac, (10) Sacrum

> **Vital Practice Points**
> *A to F management of MacMurthy*
> A. **A**irway management
> B. **B**lood and fluid replacement
> C. **C**entral nervous system management
> D. **D**igestive system management
> E. **E**xcretory system management
> F. **F**racture management.

History

Pelvic fractures usually occur due to high-velocity trauma following a road traffic accident (RTA) or due to fall from a height.
The relative incidences are as follows:
- RTA—80.7%
- Fall—16.1%
- Compression fracture—rest.

Mechanism of Injury

There are four mechanisms by which pelvic ring fractures are produced:
- Lateral compression (Fig. 23.2A)
- Anteroposterior compression (Fig. 23.2B)
- Vertical shears forces
- Inferior forces (e.g. fall on buttocks).

The first two mechanisms are common in RTA and may cause stable or unstable fractures. Vertical shear forces are due to fall from a height and will cause grossly unstable fractures.

Fortunately, most pelvic fractures are stable and respond to nonoperative treatment. Unstable fractures need manipulative reduction and stabilization by external fixators and sometimes by internal fixation. A proper evaluation of the fracture by radiograph and CT scan helps to determine the best course of management.

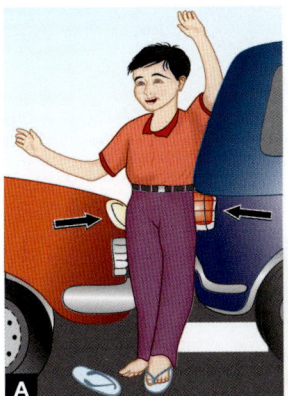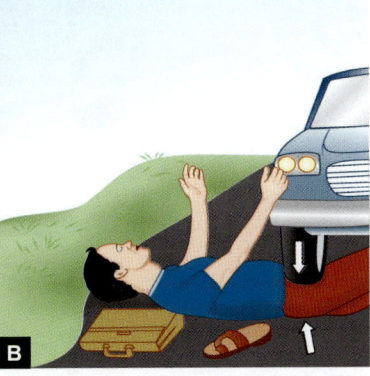

Figs 23.2A and B: Mechanism of pelvic fractures in RTA: (A) Lateral compression; (B) Anteroposterior compression

Classification

Broadly speaking, the pelvic fractures can be placed under two categories.

Fractures not Affecting the Integrity of the Pelvic Ring

Direct blow fractures, which are commonly seen in iliac bone and avulsion fractures frequently encountered in the young, come under this group. Avulsion fractures are commonly seen in anterosuperior and inferior iliac spines and ischial tuberosity (Fig. 23.3).

Fractures Affecting the Integrity of the Pelvic Ring

These are single or double break fractures in the pelvic ring and could be stable or unstable. A stable fracture is one, which resists displacing forces (Fig. 23.4). Obviously, fractures, which cannot resist usual forces, are called unstable fractures and these pose a major therapeutic challenge (Fig. 23.5).

Many classifications have been proposed for pelvic fractures. Key and Conwell's classification is by far the simplest and commonly used classification. It has prognostic importance too.

Key and Conwell's Classification

Fracture of Individual Bones without a Break in the Pelvic Ring

- Avulsion fracture of the:
  - Anterosuperior iliac spine
  - Anteroinferior iliac spine
  - Ischial tuberosity.

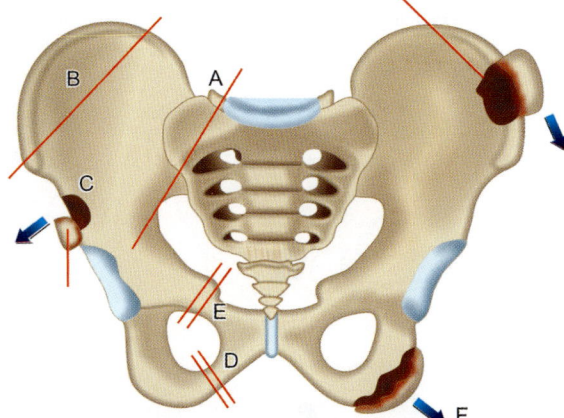

Fig. 23.3: Avulsion fractures and fractures of individual bones not affecting the pelvic ring: (A) Fracture of the sacrum, (B) Fracture of the iliac wing, (C) Avulsion fracture of anteroinferior iliac spine, (D) Inferior rami fracture, (E) Superior ramus fracture, (F) Avulsion fracture of ischial tuberosity, and (G) Avulsion fracture of anterosuperior iliac spine

- Fracture of pubis or ischium
- Fracture wing of ilium (Duverney)
- Fracture sacrum (Fig. 23.6)
- Fracture or dislocation of coccyx.

Single Break in the Pelvic Ring

- Fracture of both ipsilateral rami
- Fracture near or subluxation of symphysis pubis
- Fracture near or subluxation of sacroiliac joints.

Double Breaks in the Pelvic Ring

- Double vertical fracture or dislocation of pubis *(Straddle fracture)*.
- Double vertical fracture or dislocation of pelvis *(Malgaigne's fracture)*.

Acetabulum Fractures

- Undisplaced
- Displaced.

Acetabular fractures are high velocity injuries in young adults and could be undisplaced or displaced. It could involve the anterior or posterior walls or there could be anterior wall or posterior wall fractures (Figs 23.7 and 23.8). The treatment varies from conservative to operative fixation with reconstruction plate and screws.

> **Relative Incidence**
> - Fracture pubic bones are the commonest >69%. Single ramus more common than multiple rami fracture.
> - Malgaigne—11.8% fracture.
> - Multiple crush injuries—10.8% fracture.
> - Wing of ilium—5.4% fracture.

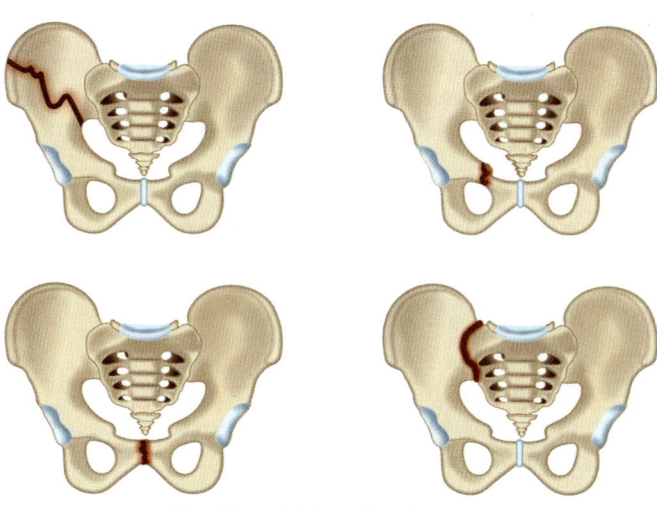

Fig. 23.4: Stable pelvic fractures

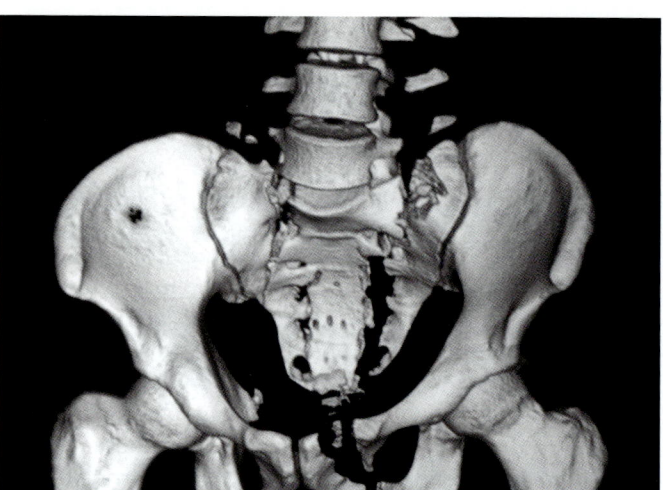

Fig. 23.6: CT scan showing sacral and pelvic fracture

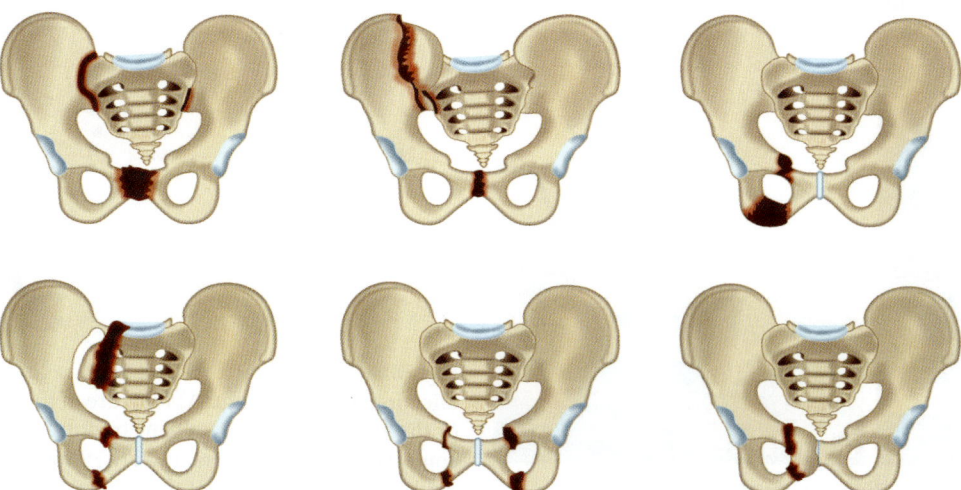

Fig. 23.5: Unstable pelvic fractures

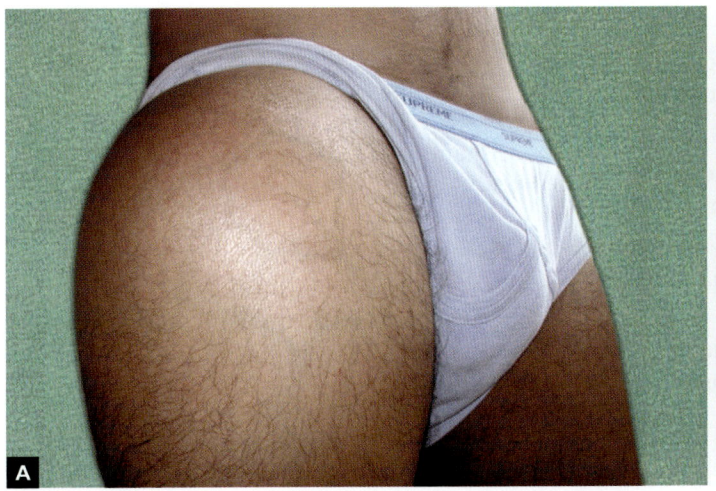 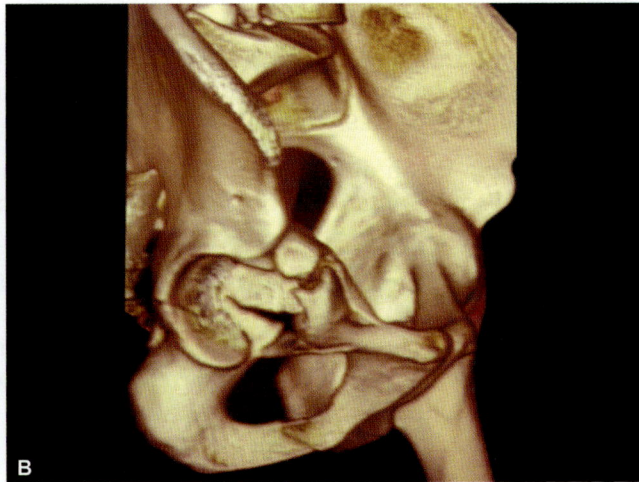

Figs 23.7A and B: Clinical picture and CT sacn of acetabular fracture

Tile's Classification

This is a mechanical classification based on the injury forces.

Type	A	Stable
Type	A1	Fracture pelvis not involving ring
Type	A2	Stable, but minimally displaced
Type	B	Rotationally unstable but vertically stable
Type	B1	Open book injury
Type	B2	Lateral compression—Ipsilateral
Type	B3	Lateral compression—Contralateral (Bucket handle)
Type	C	Rotationally and vertically unstable
Type	C1	Rotationally and vertically unstable
Type	C2	Bilateral
Type	C3	Associated with acetabular fractures

Morel-Lavallee Lesion
This is a closed degloving injury with traumatic shearing of skin from deep fascia. It leaves a large dead space prone for infection.
Treatment consists of debridement and primary closure of soft tissues.

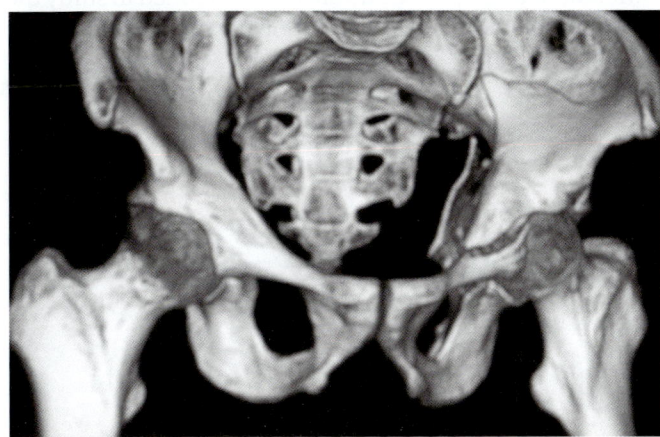

Fig. 23.8: CT scan showing anterior column fracture of the acetabulum

Clinical Features

Symptoms

The patient most often gives a history of high-velocity trauma and usually presents in a state of hypovolemic shock. Features of intra-abdominal injuries and genitourinary injuries are frequently present.

Clinical Signs

The patient may present with all signs of shock. Tenderness over the fracture site and one has to look for three important signs described by Milch.

Quick Facts
Look for the signs of shock in pelvic fracture
- Pale look
- Cold nose
- Sweating
- Tachycardia
- Hypotension
- Cold and clammy skin
- Unconsciousness.

Clinical points: Milch signs
Destot's sign: Large hematoma above inguinal ligament or scrotum.
Roux's sign: Distance from greater trochanter to pubic spine is on affected side.
Earle's sign: On per rectal examination, the bony prominence or a large hematoma can be palpated.

Clinical Tests

Compression test: When a compressive force is applied through the two iliac bones, the patient complains of pain in pelvic fracture (Fig. 23.9A).

Distraction test: When distraction force is applied to the two iliac bones at the anterosuperior iliac spine, the patient complains of pain (Fig. 23.9B).

Direct pressure test: Direct pressure over the symphysis pubis elicits pain (Fig. 23.9C).

Following this, an examination for abdomen and pelvis injuries is carried out and next urethral catheterization or urethrogram is done.

Investigations

Radiography

Different radiographic views are recommended to study the fracture configuration, displacements, etc. in pelvic fractures:
- Plain AP view
- Oblique view—45° oblique projections
- Internal and external rotation view
- Inlet view—40° caudad view
- Outlet view—40° cephalad view.

Figures 23.10 and 23.11 show different types of pelvic fractures.

CT Scan

Further radiographic studies include CT scans and 3-dimensional imaging. This is the gold standard in the evaluation of pelvic fractures (Fig. 23.8).

Management

One should remember that pelvic fractures are usually due to high-velocity trauma and is associated with multiple fractures and multiple system injuries. Resuscitation and correction of hypovolemic shock takes precedence over the management of fracture *per se*. nevertheless, once the general condition is stabilized attention should be given to treat the fracture, which will prevent further blood loss and damage to visceral organs.

Different types of pelvic fractures, their clinical features, and treatment are listed in the Table 23.1.

> **Treatment Points**
> *Three main pitfalls in the treatment of pelvic fracture*
> 1. Treating only fracture overlooking visceral injuries
> 2. Over treating a stable fracture
> 3. Treating an unstable fracture.

Treatment Methods

Initial Treatment

This is carried out as follows:
- Resuscitation and other general measures, to improve the general condition of the patient.
- Blood transfusion and other medical and surgical emergency measures are carried out.

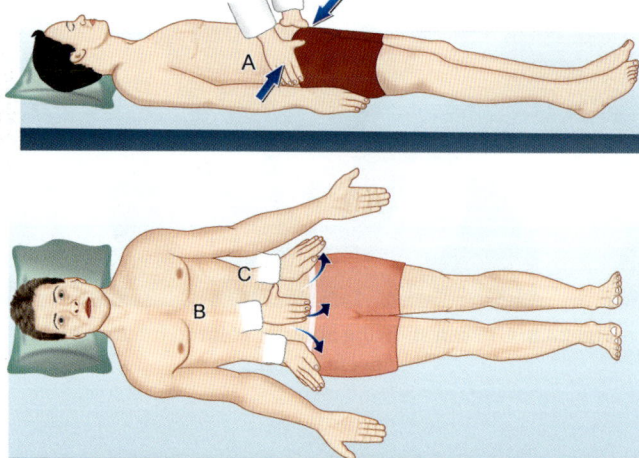

Figs 23.9A to C: (A) Compression test in pelvic fractures; (B) Direct pressure test; (C) Distraction test

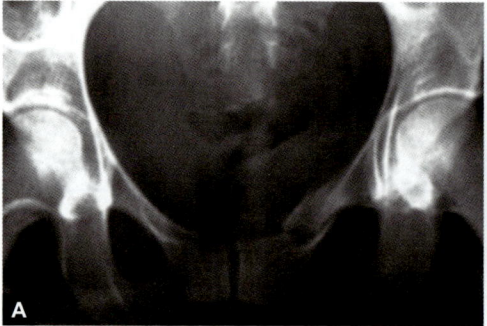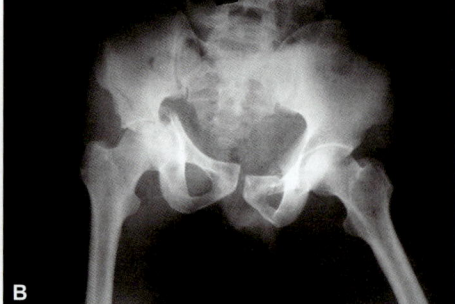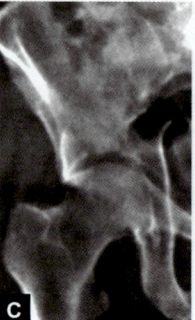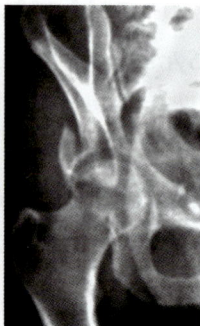

Figs 23.10A to C: Plain X-ray showing various types of pelvic frature: (A) Superior ramus fracture; (B) Fracture acetabulum and separation of symphysis; (C) Pelvic floor fracture

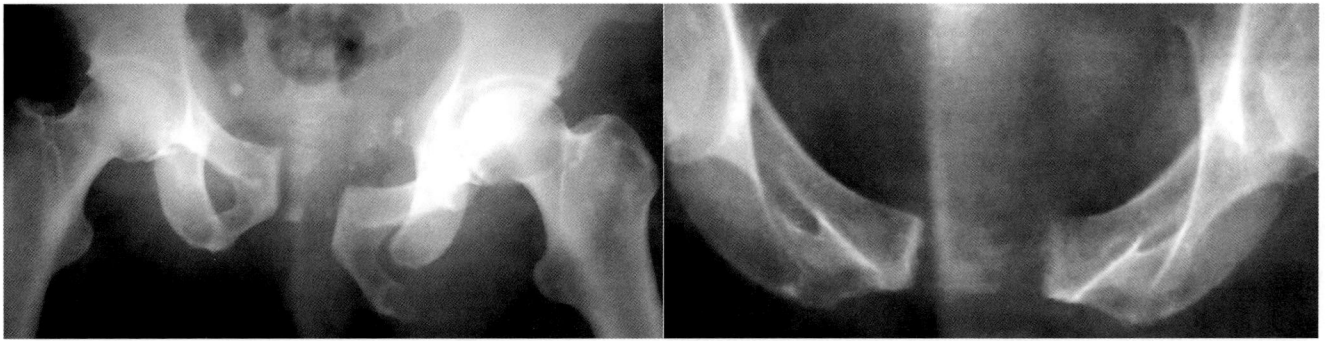

Fig. 23.11: Plain X-rays showing rotation injuries and separation of symphysis pubis

TABLE 23.1: Key and Conwell's types: A comparative study of different types of pelvic fractures, their clinical features, and treatment is presented here

Sl. No.	Type of pelvic fracture	Clinical features	Treatment
Type I	• Avulsion of anterosuperior iliac spine • Avulsion of anteroinferior iliac spine • Avulsion of ischial tuberosity • Single ramus fracture of pubis or ischium • Fracture body of ischium • Stress fracture pubis or Ischium fracture • Fracture iliac wing (6%) • Fracture sacrum • Fracture coccyx	Pain on trying to flex and abduct the thigh Rare Flexion of thigh with knee in flexion ↑ pain Commonest fracture seen in elderly, confused with fracture neck of femur Pain when hamstrings are put in tension Can occur in last trimester of pregnancy Lateral compression force ↑ pain Walking is painful Neurological deficits due to involvement of higher sacral roots Fall in sitting position	Bed rest, hip spica, ORIF rarely done Rest with hip flexed for 2–3 weeks Conservative treatment Bed rest Bed rest Bed rest Strapping of pelvis Undisplaced fracture; bed rest in neurological lesions posterior sacral laminectomy is done Bed rest Cross-strapping of buttocks In severe disability, coccygectomy
Type II	• Fracture of two rami ipsilateral • Fracture or subluxation near symphysis pubis • Fracture or subluxation near SI joint	Flexion, abduction and external rotation (FABER) test is positive. This fracture is common **FABER—Flexion, abduction and external rotation** Tenderness over symphysis pubis + palpable gap + injury to genitourinary tract common. FABER test is positive Straight leg raising test is painful	Bed rest; bucks traction Circumferential strapping Symptomatic treatment and bed rest, pelvic sling, and belt
Type III	• Double vertical fracture (**Straddle fracture**) • **Malgaigne's fracture** (Ipsilateral pubic rami fracture with ipsilateral SI joint dislocation) • Severe multiple fracture of pelvis	Urethral injury—20% Abdominal injury—38% Shortening, external rotation deformity, limb shortening, umbilicus displaced Associated with severe visceral damage	Symptomatic treatment, bed rest, etc. Postural reduction, + traction + pelvic slings • In compound fracture external fixators preferred • Open reduction and internal fixation if associated with multiple system injuries • Rest in bed with sand bags, pelvic slings and traction
Type IV	Fracture acetabulum	Could be displaced or undisplaced, could be a rim fracture or central floor fracture	Skeletal traction through the greater trochanter

Definitive Treatment

Avulsion fractures: Conservative treatment like bed rest, traction, physiotherapy, etc. gives good results. They rarely need surgery.

Undisplaced fractures: Respond to bed rest, traction, pelvic slings (Fig. 23.12), nonsteroidal anti-inflammatory drugs (NSAIDs), etc.

Displaced fractures: Reduction by lateral compression methods as described by Watson Jones is very helpful. Retention is by spica cast, canvas sling, or external fixators (FIg. 23.13).

Role of external and internal fixators: The above methods usually suffice, but the fractures associated with multiple system injuries need to be stabilized either by external fixators or by open reduction and internal fixation (ORIF) (Fig. 23.14). These two methods have the following advantages:
- Gives firm stability
- Helps early mobilization
- Reduces period of bed rest
- Helps early control of osseous bleeding.

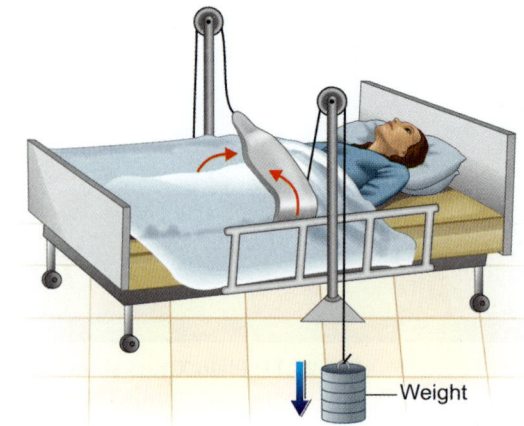

Fig. 23.12: Pelvic sling as a mainstay of conservative treatment in fracture pelvis

Complications

Pelvic fracture is a dreaded injury as it is associated with a plethora of complications. The following are some of them.

Hemorrhage

It is usually intra-abdominal and the incidence is around 20%. The patient usually presents with features of shock. If the pulse is greater than 100/min, it suggests 20% blood volume deficit; if the blood pressure is less than 100 mm systolic, it suggests 30% volume deficit. Diagnostic peritoneal lavage and open paracentesis has an accuracy rate of 98% in intra-abdominal injuries. CT scan is also sensitive and specific.

Treatment is by laparotomy and is indicated if there is continuing blood loss, visceral perforation, expanding palpable suprapubic hematoma.

Injuries of Lower Urinary Tract

Rupture of urethra and rupture of urinary bladder are the common lower urinary tract injuries frequently seen in separation of pubic symphysis and fracture pubic rami. It has an average incidence of 13%. The dictum is *all pelvic fractures must be assumed to have urinary tract injuries until proved otherwise.*

Presence of hematuria is not pathognomonic, but its presence calls for three radiographic studies like retrograde

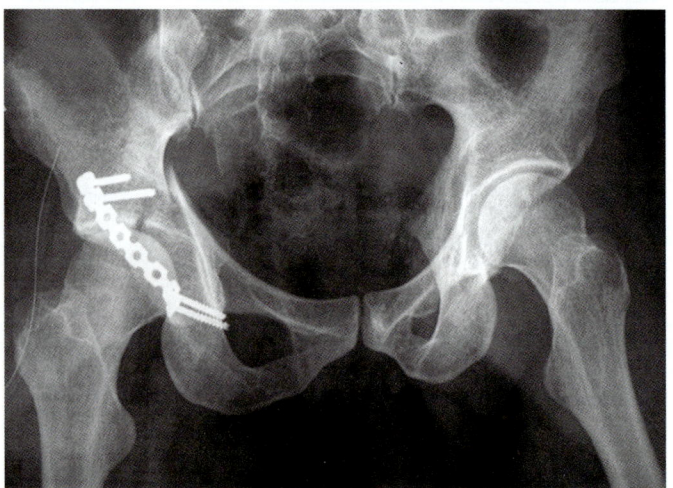

Fig. 23.13: Operative fixation of pelvic fracture with reconstruction plate and screws

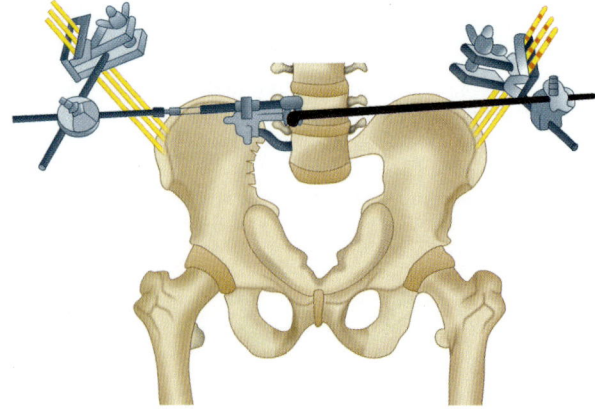

Fig. 23.14: Treatment by external fixation methods in pelvic fractures

urethrogram, cystogram, and IVP. Rupture of anterior urethra is seen in straddle fractures and is not very common. Rupture of posterior urethra is relatively more common and is limited to male. Suprapubic cystostomy, direct repair, railroad repair, urethroplasties are some of the treatment methods.

Bladder injuries are seen in 4% of the cases and are associated with symphysis pubis injuries and rami fracture. Eighty percent injuries are extraperitoneal and calls for direct surgical intervention as quickly as possible.

Other Injuries

Testicular injuries and vaginal lacerations, bowel and rectal injuries and urethral injuries are all common and require immediate surgical intervention.

Other Complications

Loss of reduction, sepsis, thrombophlebitis, delayed union, nonunion, post-traumatic arthritis, fat embolism, major arterial injuries, abdominal wall injury, neurological injuries usually L5, S1 roots due to sacral fracture are the other common complications.

> **Recap: Pelvic Fractures**
> - A fracture feared for its complications
> - RTA accounts for 80% of cases
> - Fracture broadly classified into not affecting and affecting integrity of the pelvic ring
> - Fracture pubic rami, usually single, is the commonest pelvic fracture (69%)
> - Usual presentation is hypovolemic shock
> - Correction of hypovolemia and other general measures takes precedence over fracture management
> - Conservative treatment usually gives good results
> - External and internal fixation is done for specific indications
> - Intra-abdominal and genitourinary injuries are common possibilities and need early recognition and prompt treatment
> - Mortality is 20%.
>
> *Note*: Mortality in closed pelvic fractures is 10-30% and open fractures are 40–50%.

> **Quick Facts: Interesting Pelvic Fractures**
> **Straddle fracture:** Double vertical fractures of pubic-rami.
> **Malgaigne's fracture:** Ipsilateral pubic-rami fracture and SI joint dislocation.
> **Bucket handle fracture:** Pubic-rami fracture with contra-lateral SI joint dislocation.
> **Open back fractures:** Disruption of the pubic symphysis or rami fracture and external rotation of the hemipelvis over an intact posterior SI joints.

INJURY TO THE COCCYX

These are relatively rare injuries, but could be quite troublesome to the patients. This can lead to the development of coccydynia, which is described as a chronic pain in the coccyx.

Mechanism of Injury

It is due to a direct fall on the buttocks (Fig. 23.15). It can also result from seat injuries while driving two wheelers or four wheelers. Of late constant pressure due to prolonged sitting as in the case of computer professionals can give rise to coccydynia.

Clinical Features

The patient usually complains of pain in the buttocks and is unable to sit comfortably. Due to the development of coccydynia the pain may become chronic. The patient also complains of difficulty in traveling and altered sitting postures due to the pain.

Investigations

Plain X-ray of the coccyx especially the lateral view helps to make the diagnosis (Fig. 23.16). However, it is difficult to position the patient for the X-rays. MRI of the sacrococcygeal region is a better option (Figs 23.17A and B).

Treatment

Conservative Measures

The treatment is essentially conservative in nature with periods of bed rest and symptomatic treatment for pain and inflammation.

Physiotherapy Management

Consists of the following steps:
- To relieve pain, thermotherapy likes ultrasound and TENS.

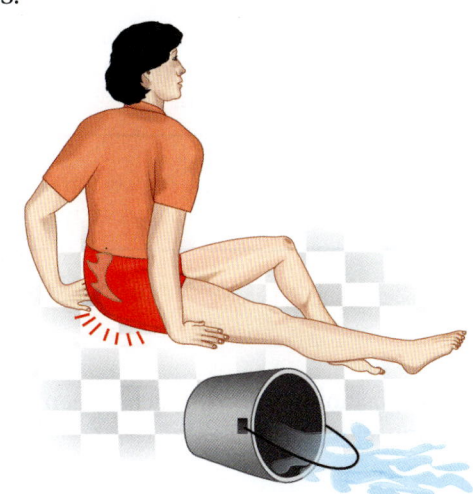

Fig. 23.15: Mechanism of injury in coccyx fractures

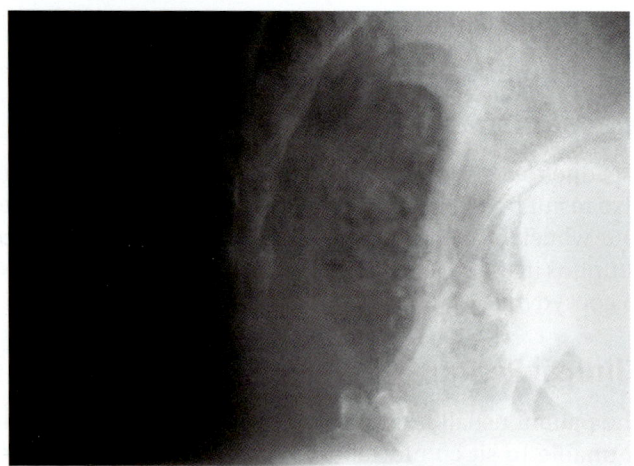

Fig. 23.16: Radiograph of coccyx fracture

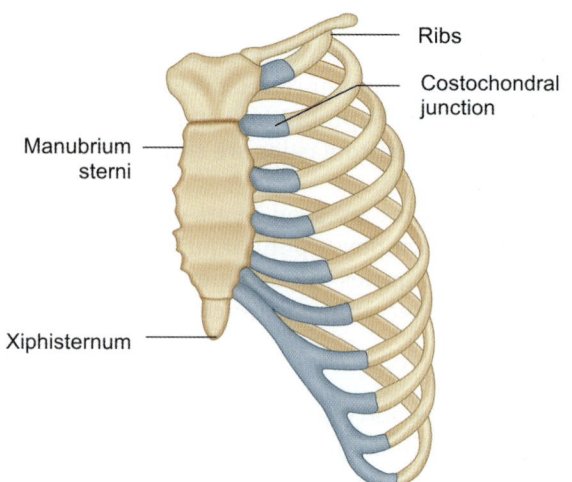

Fig. 23.18: Anatomical features of the ribs

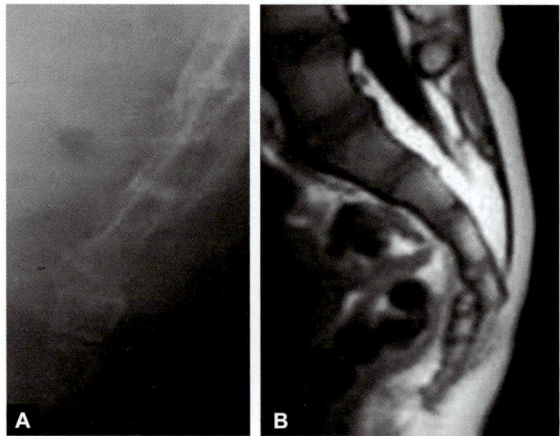

Figs 23.17A and B: Plain X-ray and MRI of sacrococcygeal region showing fracture of coccyx

- To relieve prolonged pressure on the buttocks, sitting on a ring cushion and sitting on alternate buttocks is advised.
- Isometric exercises to the glutei maximus muscle in sitting, lying, and prone positions are advisable.
- *Sitz bath helps to relieve pain.

Note:
*Sitz bath—this consists of sitting in a shallow tub of warm water. Commonly advocated in Piles patients after surgery.

Note:
These injuries are difficult to tackle.

Reasons

- Due to the position of coccyx, which is deep and covered by thick muscles on either side?
- Due to the pressure from sitting. Hence, long sitting posture needs to be controlled.

Injection Therapy

If the pain is unrelieved by the usual conservative and physiotherapy measures, injection therapy consisting of a mixture of local steroids (Depomedorol, Kenacort, etc.) and xylocaine gives excellent relief of pain.

Surgical Excision of the Coccyx

In extreme situations if all the above measures fail then surgical removal of the coccyx may be considered.

RIB FRACTURES

These are relatively rare injuries and are usually due to direct trauma. The rib usually breaks at the angle, which is a point of maximum convexity (Fig. 23.18).

Clinical Features

The patient complains of pain in the affected region and has difficulty in breathing. He also complains of inability to sleep on the affected side or lift weights and has difficulty in traveling or carrying out his day-to-day activities.

Radiology

Plain X-ray of the chest helps to detect the rib fractures with reasonable accuracy (Figs 23.19 and 23.20).

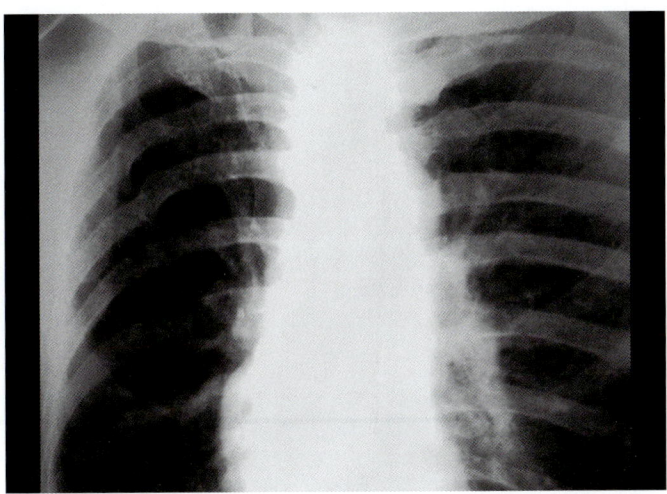

Fig. 23.19: Malunited right 2nd to 4th rib fractures

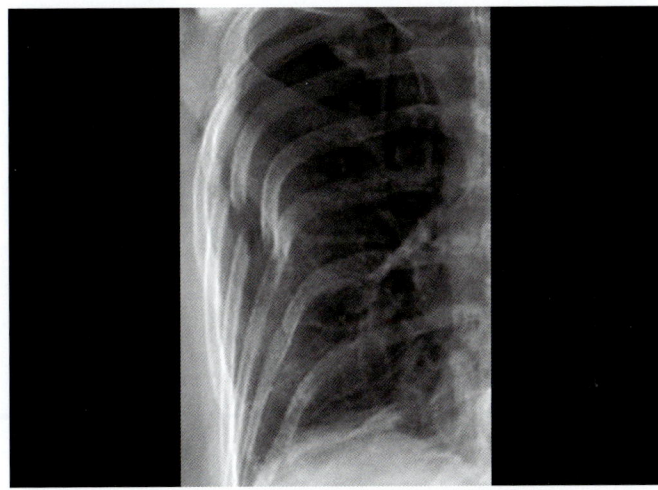

Fig. 23.20: Plain X-ray of rib fracture

Principles of Treatment

It is essentially conservative. Intercostal muscles provide natural immobilization to the fractured ribs and hence no aggressive management is required.

Conservative Measures

Strapping (Fig. 23.21), ultrasound, or TENS, etc. are effective in reducing the pain. Occasionally, a local infiltration of hydrocortisone helps. Very rarely, the fracture fragments may pierce the pleura causing pneumothorax, hemothorax, etc. These are dangerous injuries and needs to be managed aggressively.

Chest Physiotherapy
This essentially consists of deep breathing exercises, which are progressively made more vigorous to improve the mobility of the thorax.

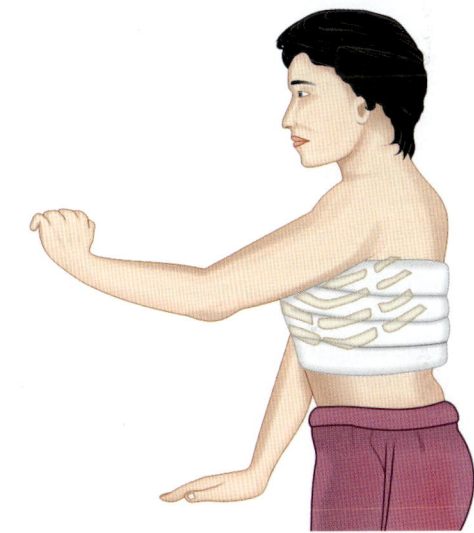

Fig. 23.21: Strapping method for treatment of fracture ribs

CHAPTER 24

Injuries of the Spine

BRIEF ANATOMY

The Spine Speaks

I am a family of 33 bones running from the skull to the pelvis (Fig. 24.1). I have been assigned the twin responsibility of carrying the load of the body and head, thanks to the two-legged posture human beings enjoy and the still more important responsibility of protecting the vital spinal cord.

My neck bones (Fig. 24.2) are called *cervical vertebrae,* bones of upper back and in line with the chest are called *thoracic vertebrae,* and the bones of the lower back are called *lumbar vertebrae*. Each vertebra of mine rest on the vertebra above and below. At these points, they articulate with each other through the *facet* joint, which keeps all my vertebrae in their correct position and in alignment with each other.

I have a spinal shock absorber called the *disc*, which separates each vertebra from the next.

Each vertebra of mine has an *anterior body* and a *posterior neural arch* (Figs 24.3 and 24.4). The body has a tough outer cortex and a cancellous middle portion. It is supported in front and back by anterior longitudinal ligament and posterior longitudinal ligament respectively. The posterior neural arch consists of two pedicles, two transverse processes, a posterior spinous process, and a pair of lamina, which together form the spinal canal along with the posterior surface of the body. In a canal of mine lies the all-important spinal cord.

While ligamentum flavum binds the laminae together, the interspinous ligament binds the spinous processes, and the supraspinous ligament binds the tip of the spinous process. All the structures of mine mentioned so far help me in providing the much-needed stability.

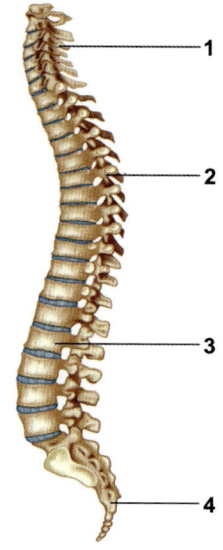

Fig. 24.1: Normal spinal curves: (1) Cervical lordosis, (2) Thoracic kyphosis, (3) Lumbar lordosis, and (4) Sacral kyphosis

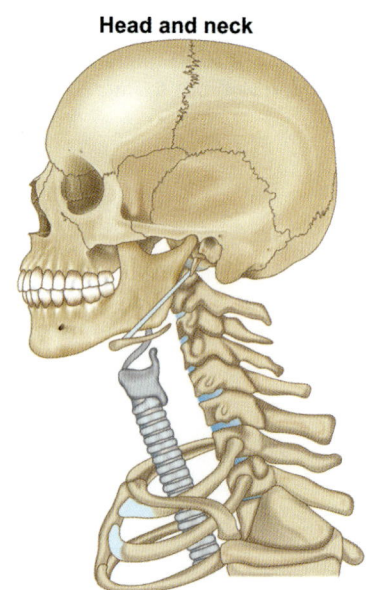

Fig. 24.2: Arrangement of the neck bones

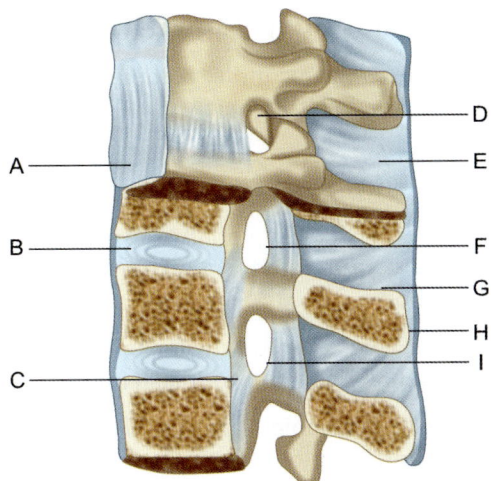

Fig. 24.3: Anatomy of spine: (A) Anterior longitudinal ligament, (B) Intervertebral disk, (C) Posterior longitudinal ligament, (D) Facet joint, (E) Interspinous ligament, (F) Ligamentum flavum, (G) Spinous process, (H) Supraspinous ligament, (I) Intervertebral foramen

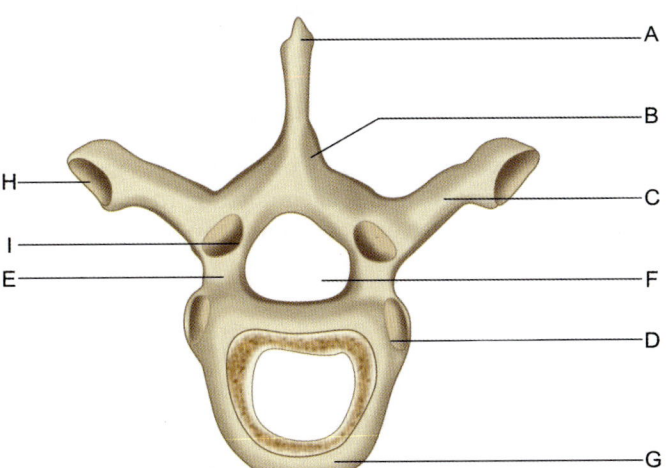

Fig. 24.4: Anatomy of a vertebra: (A) Spinous process, (B) Lamina, (C) Transverse process, (D) Superior articular facet, (E) Pedicle, (F) Spinal canal, (G) Body, (H) Transverse costal facet, (I) Inferior articular facet

When Do We Call Spine as Stable?

A spine, which after the initial injury refuses to be displaced further due to its intact posterior element, is called stable. Conversely, an unstable spine is one, which displaces further due to serious disruptions of the structures jeopardizing the spinal cord.

The *three-column concept* (Fig. 24.5) is the latest description of the spine stability. The *anterior column* consists of anterior half of the vertebral body, anterior part of the disk and anterior longitudinal ligament. The *middle column* consists of posterior half of the body and the disk, the posterior longitudinal ligament. The *posterior column* consists of the posterior vertebral arch consisting of transverse process, spinous process and the accompanying ligaments. One-column injury is stable, two-column injury is unstable, and three columns are invariably unstable. Unstable spine is a dangerous spine for it may injure the spinal cord.

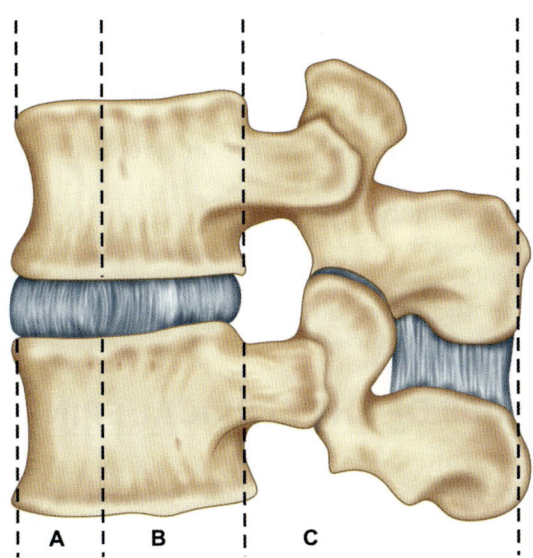

Fig. 24.5: Three-column concept of spine: (A) Anterior column, (B) Middle column, and (C) Posterior column

About Spine
- It is the principal load bearing structure of the head and torso.
- Each portion of the spine has specific functions:
    Cervical spine provides head with limited mobility and protects proximal part of the spinal cord.
    Thoracic spine provides mobility to the upper torso and ribcage and protects the cord.
    Lumbar spine provides the lower torso, its mobility and protects the cord.
- Like the skull, which protects the brain, spinal column protects the cord.
- Spine should be flexible yet strong.
- Spinal cord injury could result in death, quadriplegia, or paraplegia.

Disk Facts: Functions of Disk
- A disk has in the center nucleus pulposus and annulus fibrosus at the periphery
- Binds vertebra together
- Allows motion
- Absorbs shock
- Distributes load between the segments
- Contributes to lordosis
- Comprises approximately 25% of the total length of the spinal column.

Incidence of Spine Injuries

- About 1 million/year in the USA alone.
- Male : Female = 4 : 1
- Injury is common at the cervicothoracic and thoracolumbar regions
- Modes of injury:
  - RTA—45%
  - Falls—20%
  - Sports injuries (diving)—15%
  - Acts of violence—15%.

INJURIES OF THE CERVICAL SPINE

Injuries of the cervical spine are dangerous; and if associated with neurological damage, the results can be devastating. Though diagnostic and treatment methods have vastly improved over years, still injuries of the cervical spine pose the greatest challenge to the skill and acumen of orthopedic and neurosurgeons.

Jefferson pointed out two areas commonly involved in cervical spine injuries, C_{1-2} and C_{5-7}. According to Meyer, C_2 and C_5 are commonly involved. Neurological damage is seen in 40% of cases. In 10% of cases, radiographs are normal.

Causes

Fall from height: It is the most common cause in developing countries.

Diving injuries: Diving into water with insufficient depth or in an inebriated condition.

Road traffic accidents (RTAs): Common cause in developed countries, e.g. whiplash injury (Fig. 24.6).

Gunshot injuries, etc. These injure the cervical spine and the cord directly.

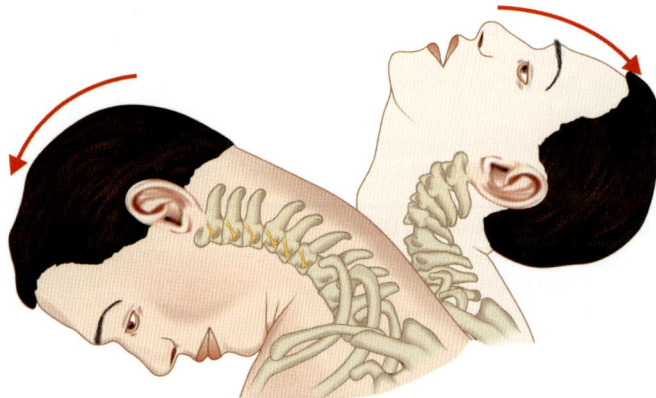

Fig. 24.6: Whiplash injury: Due to sudden deceleration, forceful hyperextension is followed by flexion of the neck

Mechanism of Injury (Figs 24.7A to D)

Pure flexion force: For example, compression fracture of vertebral body, e.g. fall from height.

Flexion rotation force: For example, fall on one side of the shoulder, disruption of facet capsule is seen.

Axial compression: For example, fall of an object on the head results in load compression, e.g. explosive comminuted fracture of C_5 body.

Extension force: For example, avulsion fractures of superior margin of vertebral body, e.g. whiplash injury.

Lateral flexion: For example, fracture pedicle, fracture transverse process and facet joints, etc.

Direct injuries: For example, fracture spinous process and body. Due to assault, gunshot injury, etc.

WHIPLASH INJURY (Syn: Acceleration Injury, Cervical Sprain Syndrome, Soft Tissue Neck Injury)

Definition

It is an unconventional and inconsequential ligamentous injury of the cervical spine allegedly due to an extension injury following a rear-end collision in an RTA (Fig. 24.6).

Incidence

- It is seen in about 25% of rear-end collision of RTAs.
- Seventy% of those affected are women.
- It is common in the 3rd or 4th decades.

Clinical Features

Symptoms

- Upper neck pain that becomes worse with movement.
- Occipital headache.
- Neck stiffness.
- Rarely vertigo, auditory or visual disturbances, etc.

Signs

- Decreased range of neck movements
- Neck muscle spasm is seen.

Note:
Symptoms appear within 48 hours of injury and 57% recover within three months. Final state is reached by one year.

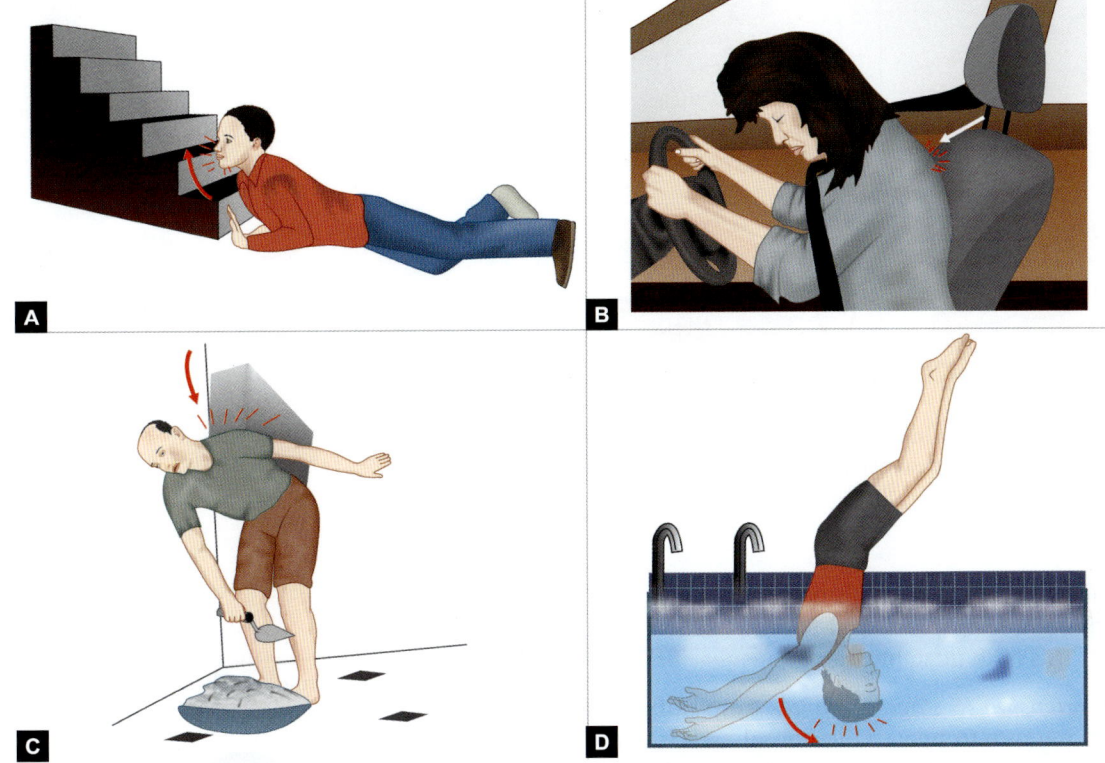

Figs 24.7A to D: Common mechanism of cervical spine injuries: (A) Hyperextension injury; (B) Flexion extension injury; (C) Flexion rotation injury; (D) Hyperflexion injury

Investigations

X-rays are usually normal. MRI helps to make a diagnosis (Fig. 24.8).

Treatment

It is mainly conservative and consists of the following:
- *Drugs:* NSAIDs, muscle relaxants, etc. are given.
- *Collars:* These are recommended for the first three days.
- Short arc active movements are slowly begun.
- Active ROM exercises are slowly commenced.
- After the pain subsides, isometric strengthening exercises are slowly commenced.
- Other modalities take ultrasound, traction, manipulation, massage, etc. also helps.

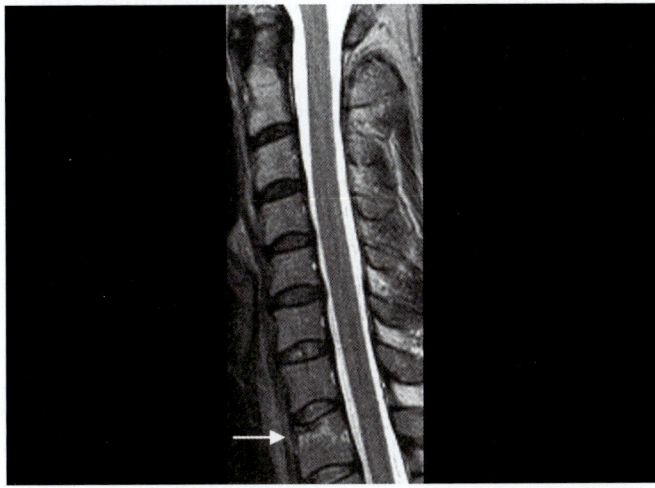

Fig. 24.8: MRI of a Whiplash injury

Allen's Classification of Cervical Spine Fractures (Figs 24.9A to D)

Compressive flexion (5 stages): Ranges from blunting of anterosuperior vertebral margin to posterior displacement into the spinal canal. It is usually a stable fracture but may become unstable if compression is more than 50%.

Vertical compression (3 stages): Ranges from fracture of superior or inferior endplate with centrum fracture of the vertebral body. Stable fracture if compression is less than 50% of the vertebral body.

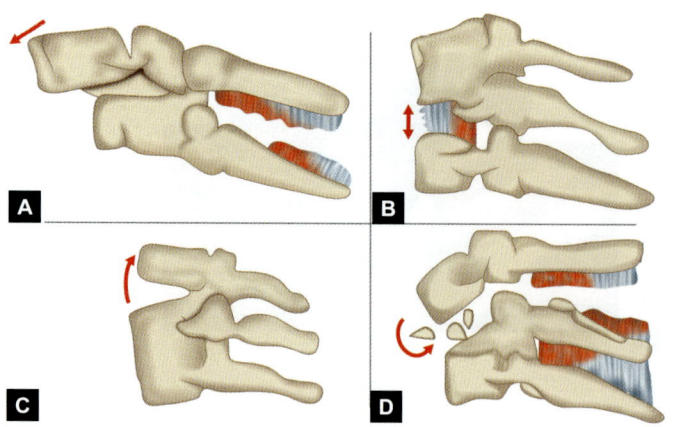

Figs 24.9A to D: Cervical spine injuries: (A) Distraction injury; (B) Compression injury; (C) Hyperextension injury; (D) Compression and distraction injury

Distractive flexion (4 stages): Ranges from failure of posterior ligamentous complex to full-width vertebral body displacement. This is an unstable fracture.

Compression extension (5 stages): Ranges from unilateral vertebral arch fracture to bilateral vertebral arch fracture with full-vertebral body displacement anteriorly. It is unstable.

Distractive extension: Ranges from failure of anterior ligament complex to posterior ligament complex. This is also an unstable fracture.

Lateral flexion: Ranges from asymmetric compression and ipsilateral vertebral arch to fracture without displacement and with displacement. May become unstable.

Note:
All unstable cervical spine fractures have a high incidence of neurological damage.

Clinical Features

The patient usually gives history of trauma following which there will be pain, swelling, and inability to move the neck. There will be tenderness over the involved spinous process and there could be a palpable gap. There may be signs of neurological involvement. Determine the level of cord injury by examining the affected spine (Box 24.1). The injuries to the spinal cord at the cervical region can manifest in the following ways:

Concussion

This is a state of spinal shock and there will be sensory loss, flaccid paralysis, visceral paralysis, reflexes are in abeyance

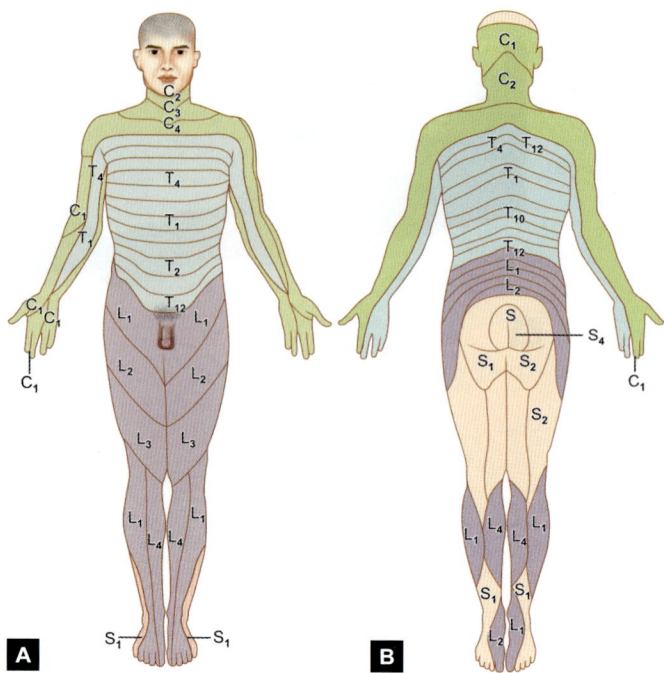

Figs 24.10A and B: Dermatomal levels: (A) Anterior, (B) Posterior

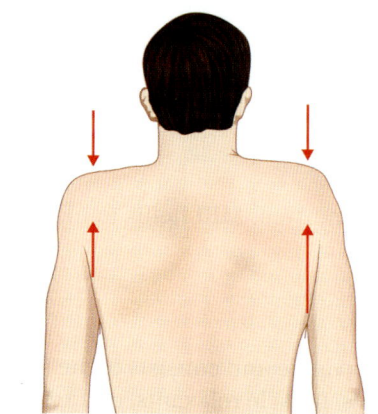

Fig. 24.11: Examination of C_3–C_4 (Trapezius muscle)

and anal reflex is absent. By 8 hours, concussion is known to regress; and by 8-10 days, there is complete recovery.

Nerve Root Involvement

Individual nerve roots could be affected at their respective intervertebral foramen. All the features of peripheral nerve injury with LMN type of lesion are seen. The myotome and the dermatome should be assessed to know the root involvement (Figs 24.10 to 24.17 and Table 24.1).

Cord Involvement

Complete: This leads to quadriplegia or quadriparesis.

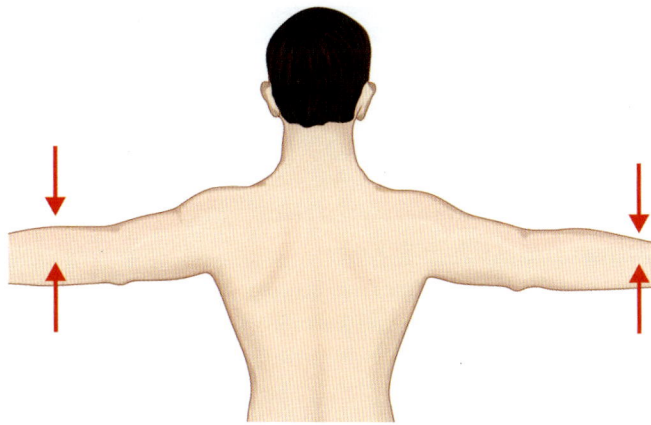

Fig. 24.12: Examination of C_5–C_6 roots (Deltoid muscle)

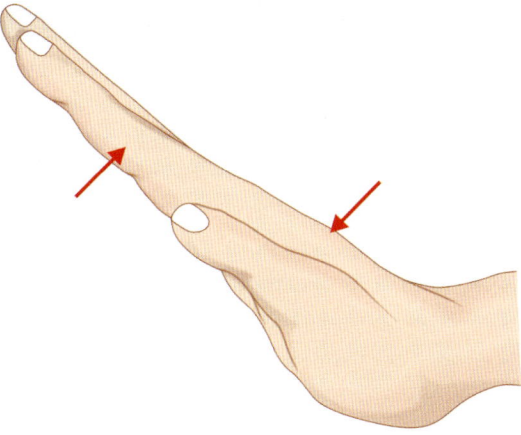

Fig. 24.15: Examination of C_7–C_8 (Wrist extensors)

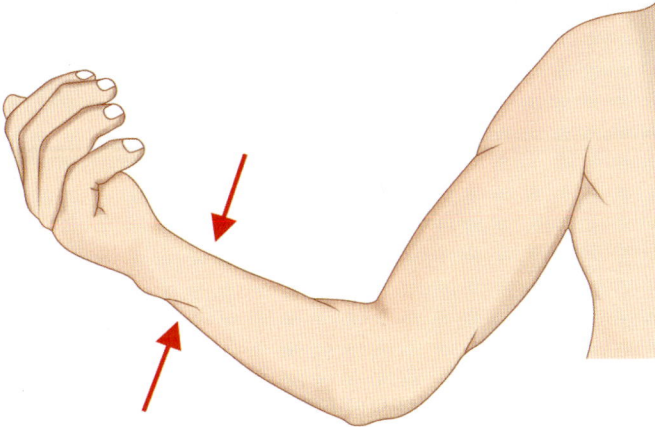

Fig. 24.13: Examination of C_5–C_6 roots (Biceps muscle)

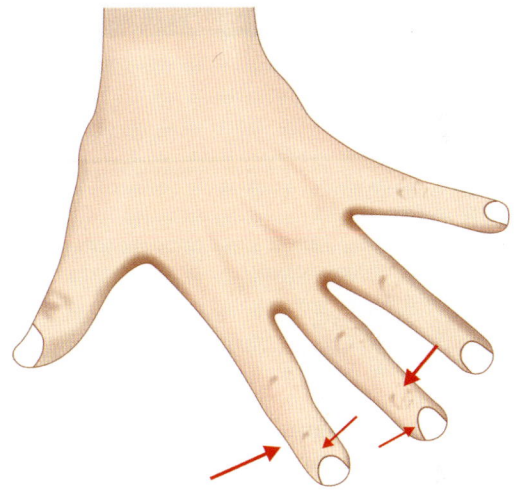

Fig. 24.16: Examination of C_8–T_1 (Dorsal interosseous muscle)

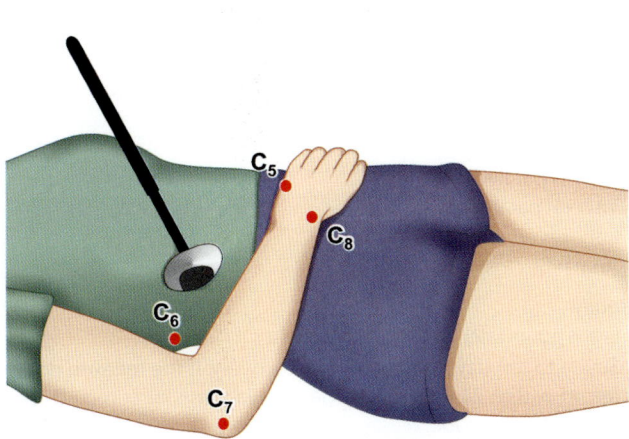

Fig. 24.14: Examination of upper limb reflexes

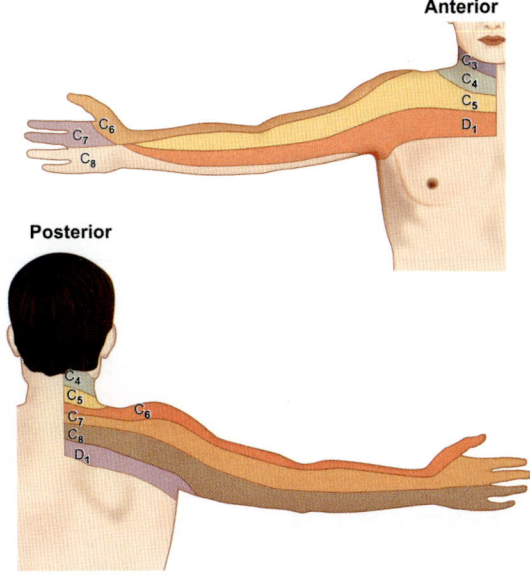

Fig. 24.17: Dermatomal pattern of cervical nerve roots

TABLE 24.1: Root involvement: quick facts

Roots	Sensory system	Motor system
C_2	Sensation decreased over back of the scalp	C_2–C_4 root involvement survival of patient is rare
C_3	↓ sensation over anterior aspect of the neck	-do-
C_4	↓ sensation over lateral aspect of neck and inferiorly over clavicles down to the rib space	-do-
C_5	↓ sensation over the lateral deltoid	↓ voluntary activity of deltoid and biceps
C_6	↓ sensation over the radial aspect of the forearm, thumb, index and middle finger	↓ ECRL, ECRB activity
C_7	↓ sensation over the ulnar border of ring and small fingers	↓ triceps, finger extensors, pronator teres, and FCR activity
C_8	↓ sensation over ulnar border of hand and forearm	↓ FDS or profundus activity
T_1	↓ sensation over the medial aspect of the upper arm	
T_2	↓ over the anterior chest wall above the nipple	Intrinsic function of the hand is intact

Note: FCR—flexor carpi radialis, ECRL—extensor carpi radialis longus, ECRB—extensor carpi radialis brevis, FDS—flexor digitorum superficialis

TABLE 24.2: Cervical spinal cord injury

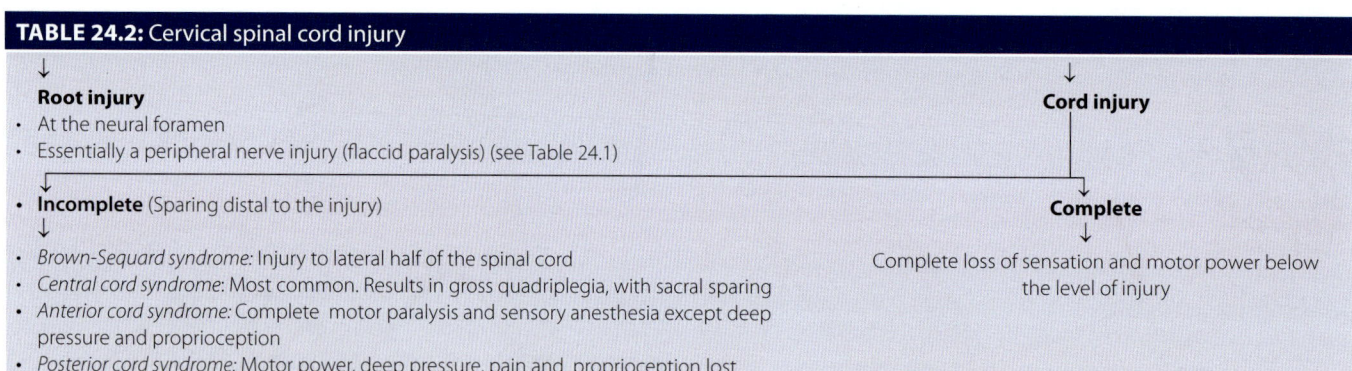

- **Root injury**
  - At the neural foramen
  - Essentially a peripheral nerve injury (flaccid paralysis) (see Table 24.1)
- **Incomplete** (Sparing distal to the injury)
  - *Brown-Sequard syndrome:* Injury to lateral half of the spinal cord
  - *Central cord syndrome:* Most common. Results in gross quadriplegia, with sacral sparing
  - *Anterior cord syndrome:* Complete motor paralysis and sensory anesthesia except deep pressure and proprioception
  - *Posterior cord syndrome:* Motor power, deep pressure, pain and proprioception lost

Cord injury
- **Complete**
  - Complete loss of sensation and motor power below the level of injury

Incomplete: Here the central cord, lateral cord, anterior or posterior cord could be involved (Table 24.2).

Box 24.1: Do You Know How to Find Out the Level of Cord Injury by Looking at the Level of Vertebral Injury?

Bone segment	Cord segment
C_1 to C_7	Add 1 to vertebral level
T_1 to T_4	Add 2 to vertebral level
T_4 to T_{10}	Add 3 to vertebral level
T_{10}	Dorsal segments complete
T_{12}	Lumbar segments complete
L_1	Sacral segments complete
Below L_1	Cauda equina paralysis

Vital Steps
- The lowermost functioning muscle is documented and a functional level is established.
- Next the sacrally innervated skin is examined. Perianal, anal, scrotal, labia, and plantar surface of the toes are examined.
- Perianal sensation may be the only sign to indicate an incomplete lesion.

Other Examinations

Rectal sensation: Loss of sensation around the anus.

Rectal motor: Sphincter contracts, over a gloved finger.

Bulbocavernosus reflex: Involves S_1, S_2 and S_3 nerve roots. Squeeze the glans penis, anal sphincter contracts around the gloved finger.

Initially, following the injury, the above reflexes are absent, indicating spinal shock. Usually, it returns within 24 hours. If not a presumptive diagnosis and determination of a root or cord lesion is made. A diagnosis of a complete or incomplete syndrome is documented.

Cord Concussion
A state of "spinal shock," i.e. temporary electrical dysfunction.
Features
- Sensory loss
- Flaccid paralysis
- Visceral paralysis
- Reflexes are in abeyance
- Anal reflex lost (anal wink lost).

Usually
- Eight hours later concussion regresses
- Seven to ten days later complete recovery. If the reflexes, do not return within 24 hours to 10 days a diagnosis of complete cord transection is made.

Investigations

Radiography: Lateral view is important (Fig. 24.18). If an adequate lateral radiography reveals no fracture or dislocation, then a complete radiographic examination including anteroposterior, open mouth, and oblique projections are performed.

Myelography is of value in incomplete lesion who fails to show progressive improvement.

CT scan makes an accurate diagnosis of hidden fracture. It is not helpful in assessing the soft tissue injury (Fig. 24.19).

MRI evaluates cord injuries better. MRI is found to be very reliable and helpful in assessing the bony, soft tissue damages and injury to the cord very accurately (Fig. 24.20).

General laboratory investigations: Like Hb%, blood group, bleeding time, clotting time, electrolyte status, etc. are done.

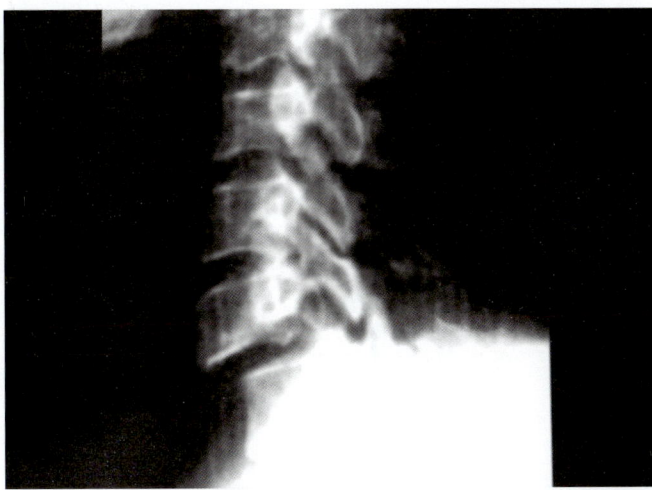

Fig. 24.18: Radiograph showing fracture dislocation of C_6 over C_7

> **Treatment Facts**
> *Goals of treatment of cervical spine injury*
> - Realign the spine
> - Prevent further neurological damage
> - Aid neurological recovery
> - Obtain and maintain spinal stability
> - Aim at early functional recovery.

Treatment Methods

At the Accident Site

Resuscitation and transport is important. In a person lying still without using his neck after an RTA, a cervical spine injury is always suspected until proved otherwise.

The patient is transported with utmost care over a stretcher to the hospital. All unnecessary neck movements should be totally avoided. If the patient needs resuscitation, it has to be carried out with a lot of care.

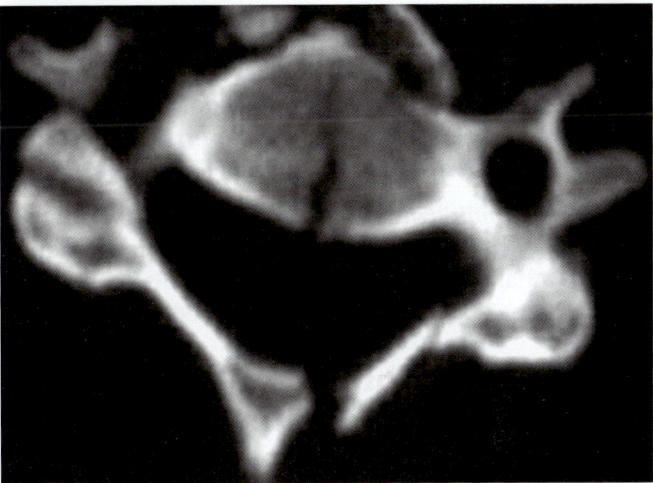

Fig. 24.19: CT showing cervical vertebra fracture

At the Hospital

Nonoperative treatment: Most cases can be treated nonoperatively by halo vest, four postcervical collars, Minerva jacket, cervical collars, etc. (Figs 24.21A to C).

Indications

- Stable cervical spine with no neurological injury. A rigid cervical brace or halo for 8–12 week is usually sufficient.
- Stable compression fracture of vertebral bodies and undisplaced fracture of laminae, lateral masses, or spinous process.
- Unilateral facet dislocations reduced in traction may be immobilized in a halo vest for 8–12 weeks.

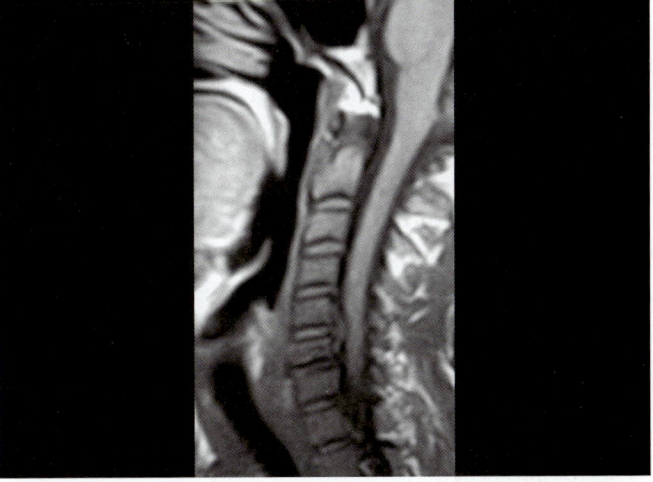

Fig. 24.20: MRI showing compression fracture of 6th cervical vertebra

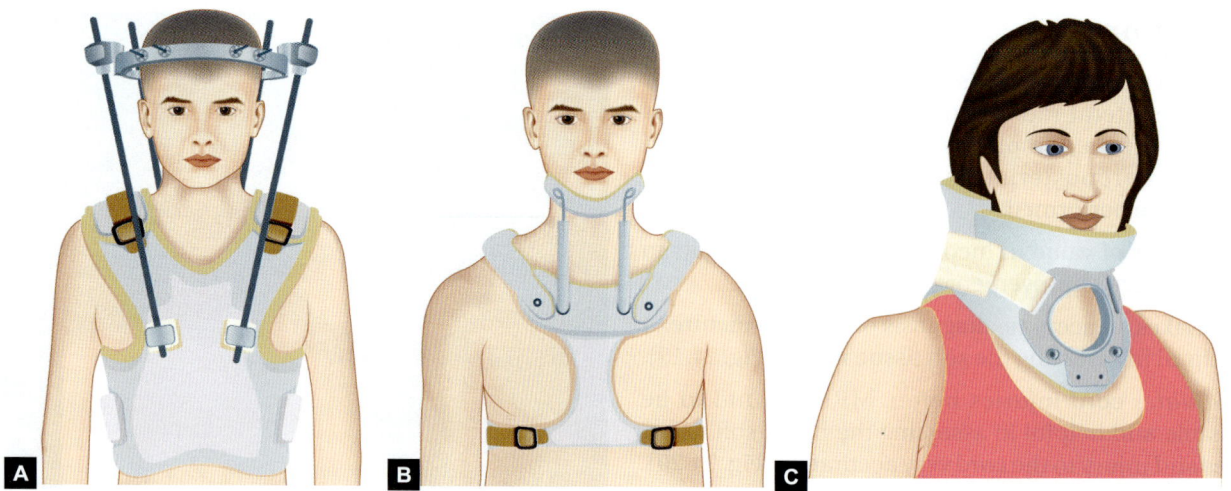

Figs 24.21A to C: Methods of cervical immobilization: (A) Halo vest traction; (B) Four postcervical collar; (C) Cervical collar

Skeletal traction: Reduction with traction is done for unstable fracture (Fig. 24.22). Urgency of reduction is based on neurological loss (Table 24.3). Traction is given for 3–6 weeks and once satisfactory reduction is achieved, the patient is mobilized with a collar, corset, or jacket.

Halo Vest Immobilization: Many unstable cervical spine injuries can initially be managed by cervical traction through a halo ring. After obtaining the alignment of the cervical spine, halo vest may be completed.

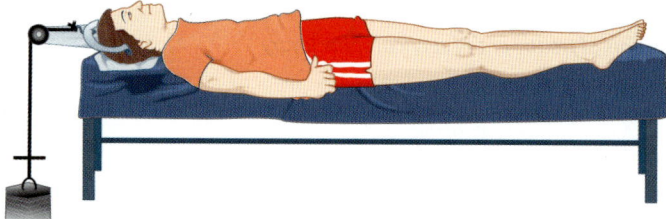

Fig. 24.22: Skeletal traction applied through Crutchfield tongs

Surgical Treatment

Indications: Unstable injuries with or without neurological damage require surgery.

Methods

- In most patients early open reduction and internal fixation (ORIF) is indicated to obtain stability. Cervical spine is stabilized through an anterior or posterior approach. Usually, a posterior approach is used with triple wire stabilization and fusion with iliac bone grafting. This allows rapid mobilization of the patient in a cervical orthosis.
- Anterior decompression consists of removal of the disk and is recommended when disk prolapse is present.
- Anterior cervical plating allows for immediate rigid fixation after decompression and bone grafting. The plates used are H-type or Caspar plates. Recently cervical spine locking plate (CSLP) and reflex anterior cervical plate are providing better fixation and faster rehabilitation.
- Posterior approach preferred for ligamentous instability. Posterior stabilization and rigid internal fixation is provided by systems like Roy-Camillie, Magerl and

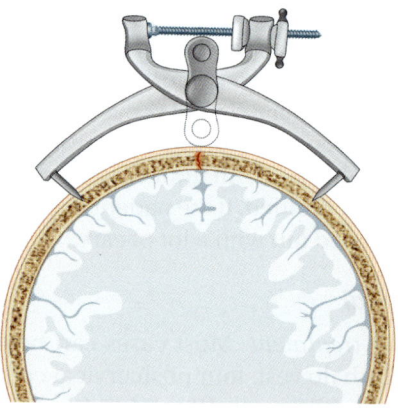

Fig. 24.23: Crutchfield tongs

TABLE 24.3: Skeletal traction

Neurologic loss	No neurologic loss
↓	↓
Urgent skeletal traction through Crutchfield tongs (Fig. 24.23) or Gardner-Wells tongs	No urgency Only maintenance of reduction of skeletal traction
↓	
10 lbs weight for head, 5 lbs weight for each vertebra to a maximum of 40 lbs	
If reduction is obtained, weight is ↓ by 50%. If reduction is not obtained, open reduction is attempted	

Seemann, etc. which has posterior plates and screws, hook plates, etc.
- Anterior approach and corpectomy (removal of the crushed body) for burst fracture with cord compression. After corpectomy, a bone graft or a cage fills up the gap.
- Combined anterior and posterior decompression for posterior instability and anterior compression of the neural elements.

Laminectomy has limited role in the treatment of cervical fracture.

Lateral mass screw fixation provides rigid internal fixation in previous laminectomies or when the spinous processes are damaged, etc.

INDIVIDUAL CERVICAL VERTEBRA FRACTURE OF INTEREST

Burst Fracture of Atlas or C_1

This is popularly known as Jefferson's fracture. It is due to axial loading over the top of the head. Here the patient usually presents with neck pain without neurological deficit. This can be radiologically diagnosed by open mouth odontoid view (Figs 24.24 to 24.26).

Treatment

For stable fracture: Rigid cervicothoracic brace for three months with a Philadelphia cast.

For unstable fractures: Skeletal traction or halo traction for 3–6 weeks followed by application of halo vest.

Rotary Subluxation of C_1 or C_2

Here the patient presents with torticollis and neck pain and is diagnosed radiologically. Treatment is usually by reduction and skull traction.

Odontoid Process Fracture

It is also called Dens fracture.

Anderson and D'olonzo's Classification (Fig. 24.27)

Type I: Oblique fracture of the upper part of the odontoid process. It is uncommon and is treated by cervical cast.

Type II: Junction of odontoid process and body. Common with a nonunion rate of 36%. Requires surgical wiring and fusion.

Type III: Fracture is through the upper part body of the body of vertebra. Cancellous area hence fracture unites well with a halo cast.

Figure 24.28 shows a CT image of the odontoid fracture.

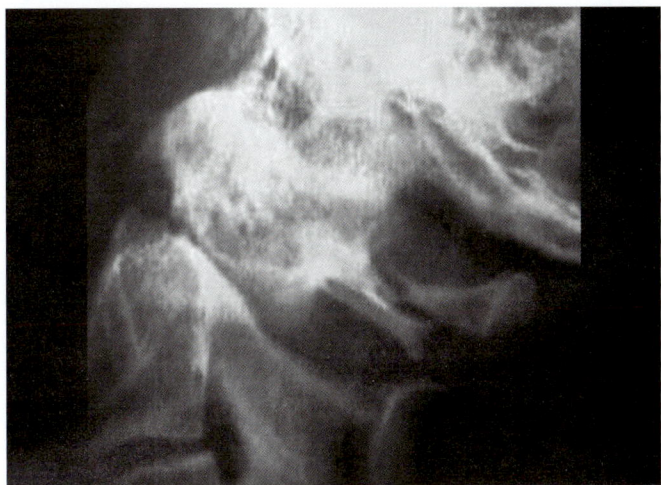

Fig. 24.24: Jefferson's fracture

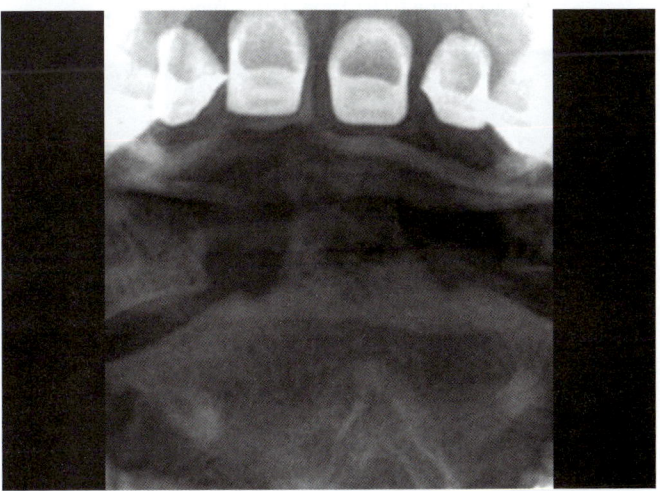

Fig. 24.25: Open mouth view showing Jefferson's fracture

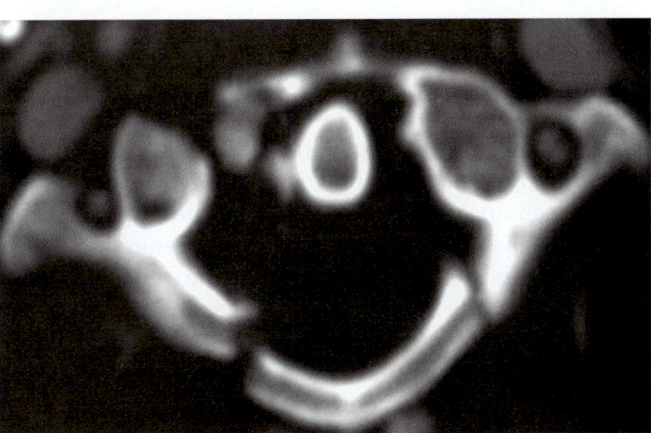

Fig. 24.26: Burst fracture of Atlas or C1

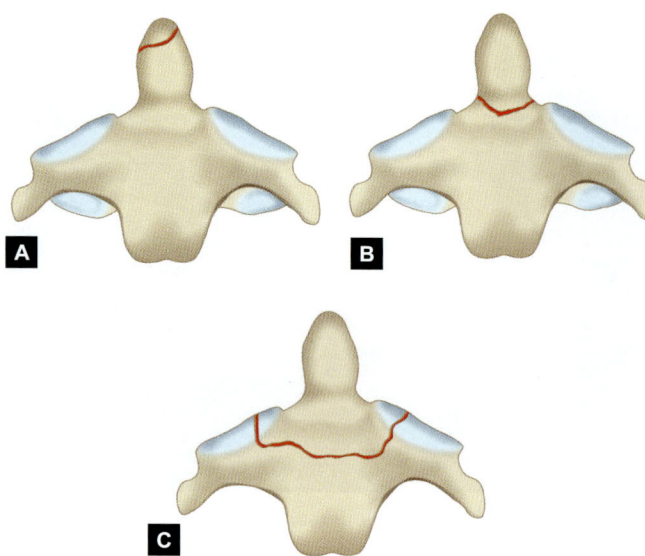

Fig. 24.27: Odontoid process fracture: (A) Type I; (B) Type II; (C) Type III

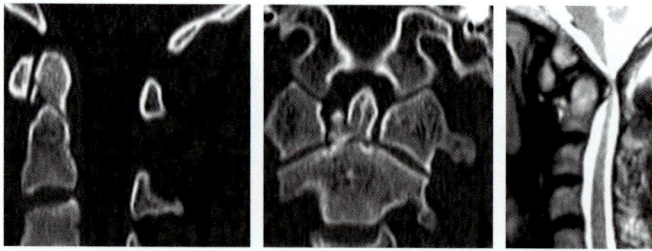

Fig. 24.28: CT Scan and showing odontoid process fracture

Hangman's Fracture

It is a fracture through pedicle at pars interarticularis of C_2 and is due to distraction extension force. There is no neurological deficit and the patient needs rigid cervical support usually through a Philadelphia collar immobilization.

THORACIC AND LUMBOSACRAL SPINE INJURIES

Thoracolumbar spine is generally regarded as extending from 10th thoracic vertebrae to 2nd lumbar vertebrae and is the transitional area between the kyphotic upper thoracic spines to the lordotic lumbar spine. The general anatomy of the vertebral column is more or less the same as in other areas of spine. The three-column concept has already been described. Anterior column is the load bearing structure and the posterior column functions as motion limiters as well as load bearing structures.

Mercifully, the thoracolumbar injuries spare the upper limbs and vital functions. Though a lesser challenge than cervical injury, nevertheless it poses problems, no less risky than the former.

Mechanism of Injury

- Fall from a height
- RTA: Seat belt injury (chance fracture)
- Other causes like gunshot injuries, assault, etc.

McAfee's Classification—3-Column Classification (Figs 24.29A to D)

Wedge Compression

Isolated failure of anterior column due to forward flexion. No neurological deficit.

Stable Burst Fractures

Anterior and middle columns fail. No loss of integrity of posterior elements.

Unstable Burst Fractures

Anterior and middle column fail in compression. Posterior column fail in compression, lateral flexion or rotation. Post-traumatic kyphosis and neural symptoms are present.

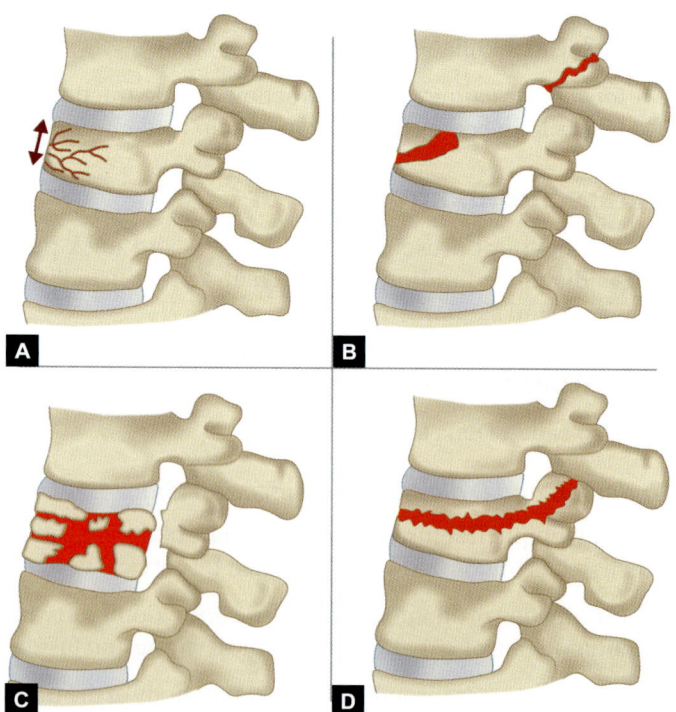

Figs 24.29A to D: Thoracolumbar fractures: (A) Wedge compression; (B) Stable burst fracture; (C) Unstable burst fracture; (D) Chance fracture

Chance Fracture (Seatbelt Injury)

It is seen in people who wear a lap belt without a shoulder harness. Horizontal avulsion fracture of vertebral bodies caused by flexion about an axis anterior to the anterior longitudinal ligament. A strong tensile force (see Fig. 24.7B) pulls entire vertebrae apart.

Flexion Distraction Injury

Flexion axis is posterior to the anterior longitudinal ligament. Anterior column fails in compression. Middle and posterior columns fail in tension. It is unstable because supraspinous, interspinous and ligamentum flavum fail.

Translational Injuries

Malalignment of neural canal, which has been totally disrupted. All three columns fail in shear. At the affected level, one part of sacral canal has been displaced in the transverse plane (Fig. 24.35).

Modified Magerl Classification (AO/ASIF)

Type A: Compression varieties:
- Wedge
- Split
- Burst.

Type B: Distraction:
- Through posterior soft tissues (subluxation)
- Through the posterior arch (chance fracture)
- Through the anterior disk.

Type C: Multidirectional with translation:
- Anteroposterior dislocation
- Lateral (lateral shear fracture)
- Rotational (rotational burst).

Clinical Features

The patient gives history of trauma due to RTA or fall from a height and complains of pain; posterior swelling, tenderness, palpable interspinous gap or a step may be felt (Fig. 24.30). Neurological involvement may vary from paraplegia to individual nerve root involvement (Fig. 24.31). Spinal shock is present for 24 hours during which all the reflexes are lost. Cauda equina paralysis is present if the lesion is below L_1. Exaggerated lumbar lordosis may be seen in old cases.

Investigations

Radiography of the affected spine, this is the preliminary investigation and all three views (AP, lateral and oblique) are taken (Figs 24.32 and 24.33). Fracture of the vertebral body, pedicles, lumbar transverse process, pedicles spinous process, etc. is looked for. Disk space and neural canal narrowing is looked for. With the advent of MRI and CT scan, the role of radiography appears to be diminishing in importance (Figs 24.34A to C).

CT scan and MRI are found to be more useful than radiographs in evaluation of spinal trauma (Figs 24.35 and 24.36). While CT scan helps in studying the bony elements, MRI helps in the study of both bone and soft tissue elements. The damage to the cord is detected accurately and is now being considered as the "gold standard" in the investigation of spine injury.

Mystifying Facts: Radiological Clues about an Unstable Spine
- Loss of vertebral height >50%.
- Kyphosis >30%.
- Spondylolisthesis >3 mm.

Fig. 24.30: Clinical photo showing deformity at the lumbar region and loss of lordosis in a lumbar fracture

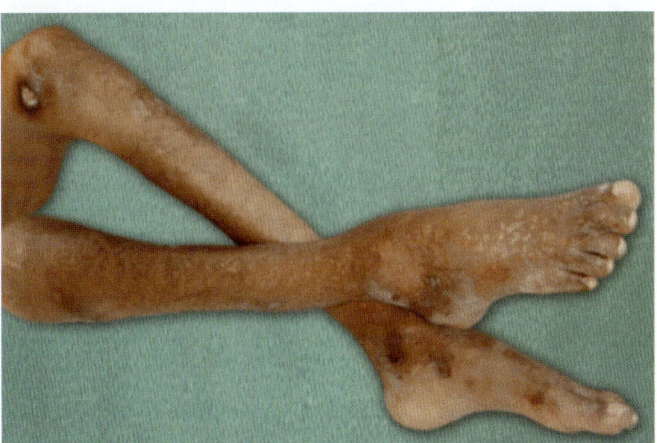

Fig. 24.31: Clinical photo showing neurological damage in thoracolumbar fractures

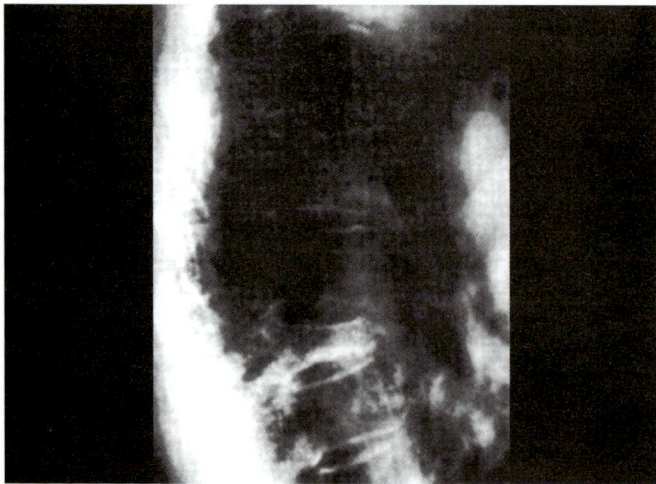

Fig. 24.32: Radiograph showing flexion compression fracture of T_{12} vertebra

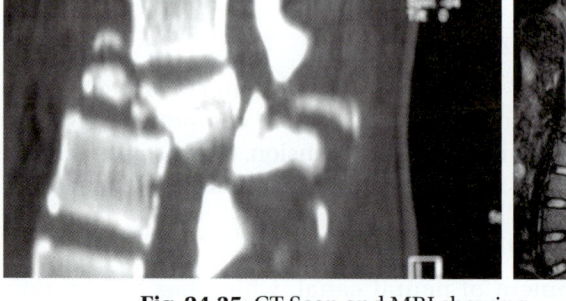

Fig. 24.35: CT Scan and MRI showing translational injury

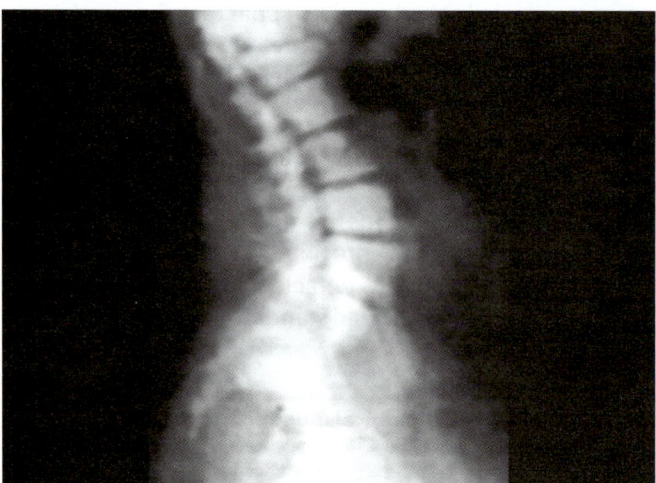

Fig. 24.33: Radiograph showing exaggerated lumbar lordosis due to L_1 fracture

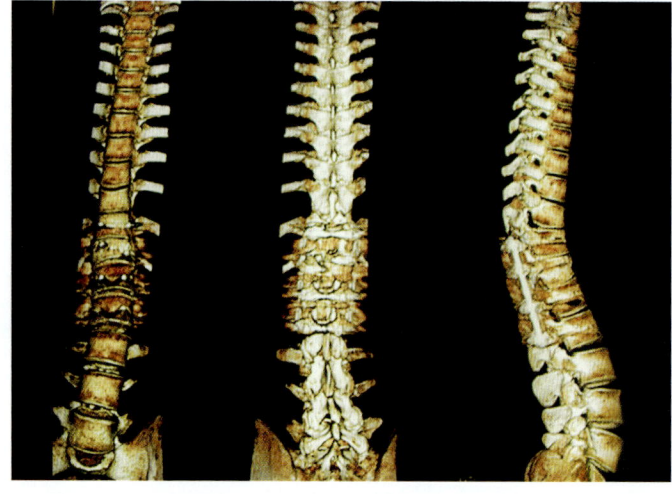

Fig. 24.36: MRI showing posterior fixation of T_{12} vertebral fracture

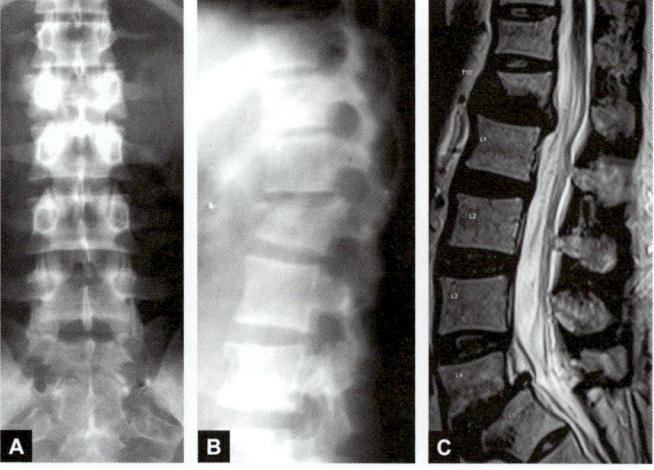

Figs 24.34A to C: Plain X-rays and MRI showing compression fracture L_2 vertebra and T_{12} vertebra (MRI)

Management

This is discussed under two heads.

Management at the site of accident: This consists of careful handling of the patient suspected to have spine injury. Consider all patients with spine injury to have neurological damage, shift them to the hospital with utmost care, and caution avoiding all unnecessary movements.

Definitive treatment at the hospital: The examination and the management measures practiced at the casualty are as follows:

Practice: Caution in handling the neck.

Examination: The general condition and other systems like CNS/CVS/RS/PA/GI tract, etc. Also, examine from head to toe, the presence of other fractures, head, chest injuries, blunt injury abdomen and pelvic fractures.

Evaluate: The spine injury by gentle careful clinical examination. This has to be supplemented by proper investigations like X-ray, CT-scan, MRI, etc.

Assess: Carefully assess the level and extent of neurological damage by examining the dermatome, myotome, and reflexes.

Plan: After evaluating and assessing the damage, plan the line of treatment. The treatment options include non-operative, traction, and operative methods. Now let us carefully took into various treatment modalities.

This varies depending upon the nature of injury and the presence or absence of neurological damage (Flowchart 24.1):

- *For stable fracture without neurological deficit:* Less than 30% anterior wedge, lateral, central compression fracture of the vertebral body is considered as stable fracture. In these injuries, there is no fracture of the posterior cortex of the vertebral body, and there is no disruption of the neural arch.

  Treatment: This is essentially conservative and consists of bed rest, NSAIDs, and external spine supports like brace, corsets, etc. If the vertebral body compression is less than 30%, only corset is used; and if the compression is more than 30% but less than 50%, a plaster jacket along with a corset is preferred (Fig. 24.37).

- *For stable fracture with neural deficit:* It has to be first determined whether the neurological deficit is complete (loss of motor power, sensory loss and absent reflexes) or incomplete (only cord or only spinal nerve roots).

  If neurological damage is incomplete, IV steroids are given for 4 days. Anterior decompression and anterior interbody fusion is done in the first stage, followed by posterior segmental spinal stabilization by either pedicle screws, Hart shill rectangle frame, Luque instrumentation, and etc. can be done one week later (Fig. 24.38). Laminectomy has fewer roles as it makes the spine less stable.

- *Unstable fracture without neurological deficit:* This is best treated by early open reduction, internal fixation and fusion is done preferably within 12–24 hours. It is done with spinal cord monitoring. Internal fixation is either by VSP plates, Hart shill frame, Harrington instrumentation, titanium cages, etc. (Figs 24.39A and B).

- *Unstable fracture with neurological deficit:* Systemic Decadron 4–6 mg/every 6 hours IV for 3 days are given.

Flowchart 24.1: Treatment plan for thoracolumbar injuries

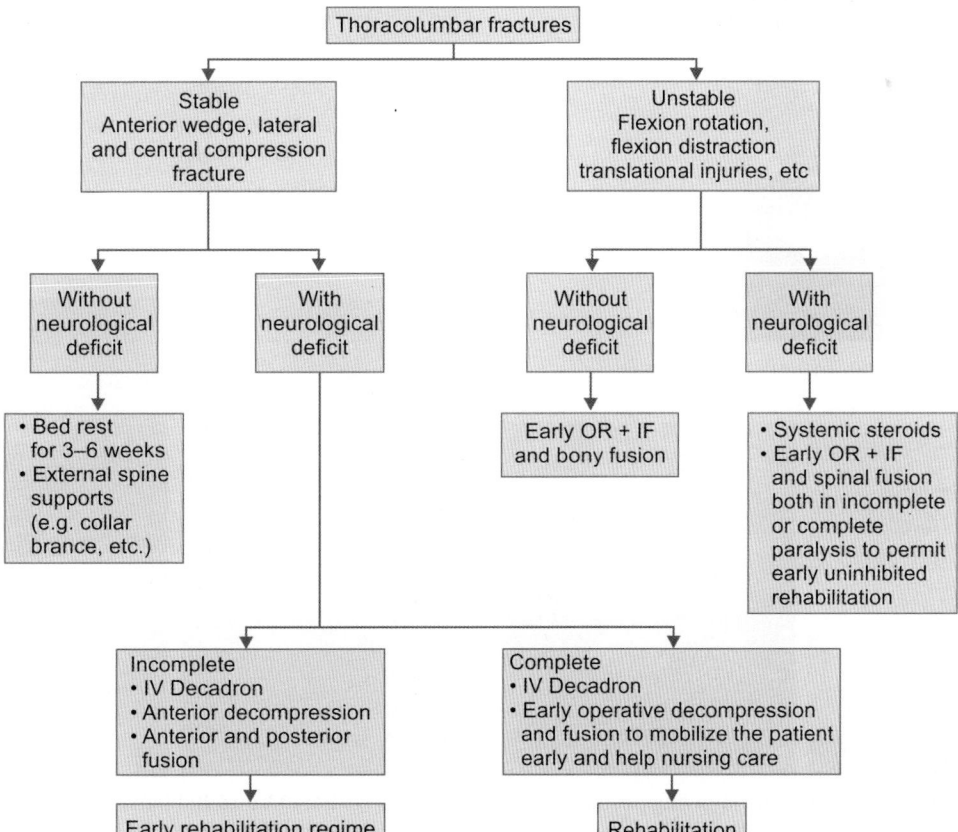

Early open reduction and internal fixation and fusion are done in incomplete neurological deficit cases. This is also desirable in complete neurological deficit to permit early-uninhibited rehabilitation. Segmental spinal stabilization with Luque or Hart shill frame is recommended.

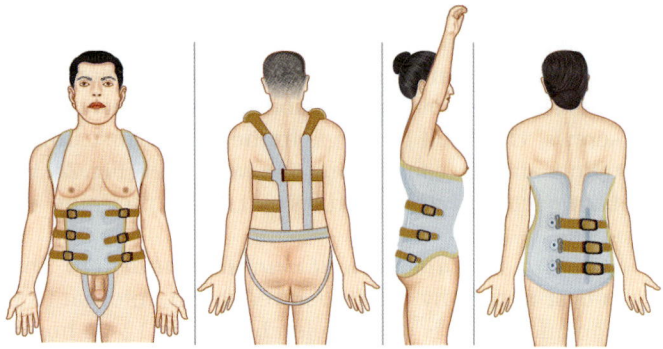

Fig. 24.37: Spinal braces for the treatment of stable thoracolumbar injuries

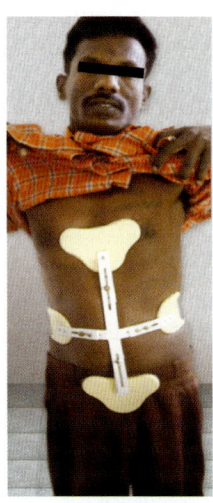

Fig. 24.38: Anterior hyperextension brace

Fixation Choices

Posterior spinal instrumentation for lumbar fractures: Luque screw segmental spinal instrumentation is found to be very effective (Figs 24.40A and B).

Anterior spinal instrumentation for fractures from T_{10} to L_3 and used as a lateral vertebral body device. However, the procedure is more morbid and is associated with dangerous complications like vascular injury, etc. Anterior plate system can be used to manage the thoracolumbar burst fracture and strut grafts can easily be placed with this approach.

Anterior vertebral body excision: This is indicated in vertebral burst fractures of more than two weeks duration and who are not a candidate for posterior instrumentation. This is followed by strut grafting and internal fixation.

> **What is New in the Treatment of Vertebral Compression Fractures?**
>
> *Vertebroplasty:* This procedure consists of injecting liquid bone cement under high pressure through large spinal needles into the acutely painful compressed and collapsed osteoporotic vertebral body (Fig. 24.41). This is done mainly to relieve pain due to collapse of the body, strengthen it further to prevent future collapse and not done to restore the body height. Vertebroplasty is known to reduce pain in 70–90% of patients. This can be used along with the usual fixation methods to improve the stability.
>
> *Balloon kyphoplasty:* This is different from vertebroplasty in restoring the collapsed height of the compressed vertebral body by inflating a balloon inserted through small instruments through the pedicle. After restoring the height, a cavity is created, the balloon is deflated and withdrawn, and the remaining cavity is filled with bone cement or graft under low pressure. This stabilizes the vertebra internally and relieves pain.
>
> Both the above procedures are indicated in painful acute vertebral compression fractures in which the medical management has failed.

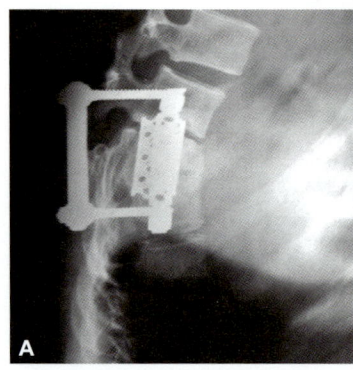
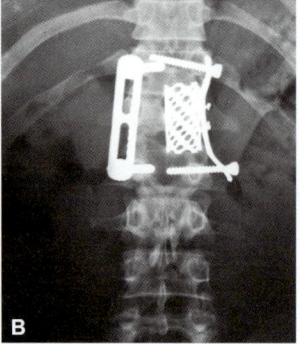

Figs 24.39A and B: (A) Radiograph showing posterior instrumentation (Lateral view); (B) Fixation with cage (AP view)

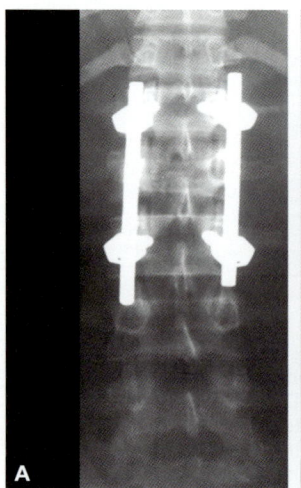
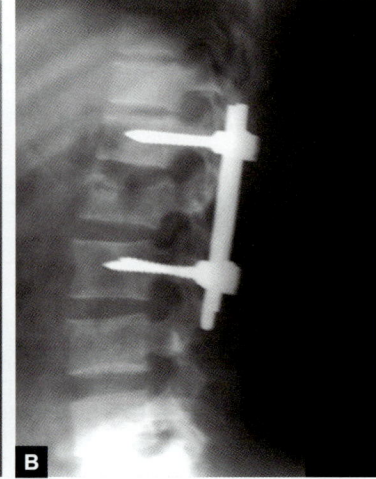

Figs 24.40A and B: Plain X-ray showing posterior instrumentation for L_2 vertebral fractures

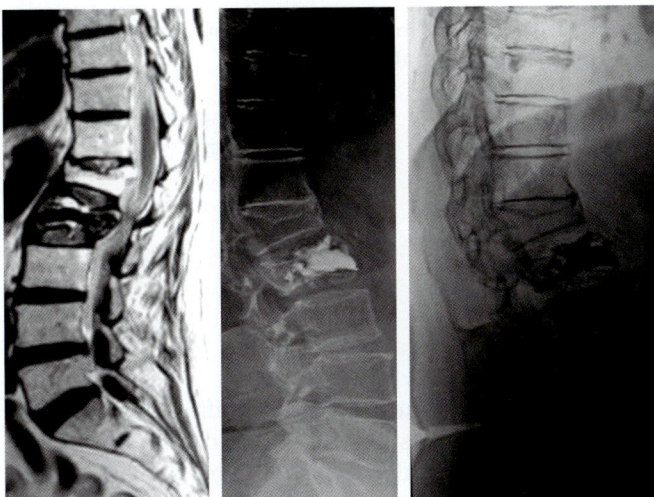

Fig. 24.41: Vertebroplasty for compression fracture L_{1-2} vertebra

SPINAL CORD INJURY

Spinal cord could be damaged due to injuries of spine extending from cervical vertebrae to the thoracolumbar junction. Below this, the cord ends and the cauda equina begin.

Incidence

- Spinal cord injuries are seen in 10–25% of cases of spinal column injuries.
- They are more common at the cervical level (40%) than the lumbar level (20%).

Pathology

The pathology may vary from extradural hemorrhage to cord concussion, laceration to cord crushing. Lesion has longitudinal, sagittal, and coronal dimensions. Amount of neural damage has no relationship to radiographic appearance (Fig. 24.42).

Clinical Classification of Neurological Damage

- Complete paralysis
- Sensory paralysis
- Motor paralysis useless
- Motor paralysis useful
- Recovery.

Injury at the cervical level: This has already been discussed and may vary from concussion, root injuries, incomplete and complete cord transection.

Injuries at the thoracic level: This could result in paraplegia.

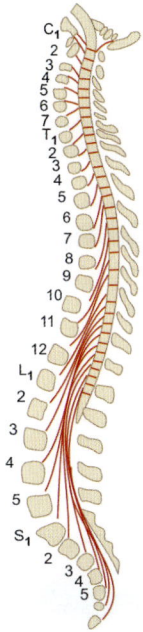

Fig. 24.42: Spinal cord ending at L_1 cauda equina starting at this point

Injuries at the thoracolumbar region: Due to injuries at the thoracolumbar junction, three things can occur:
- Complete cord division and nerves intact
- Complete cord division and partial nerve division
- Complete cord division and complete nerve division.

Injuries below L_1 causes cauda equina paralysis.

Clinical Assessment

General examination: This consists of examination of the head, chest, pelvis, and other systems for incidence of injuries and recording the vital statistics.

Neurological examination: Examine the level of the vertebral injury and find out the level of the corresponding cord injury (see box). Now each muscle group and dermatome has to be checked (Figs 24.43A and B). In cases of cervical cord injury, survival is impossible if the cord is injured above C_4 level due to paralysis of the diaphragm and respiratory muscles. In injuries below C_4 and above C_7, the level of lesion can easily be detected by examining the respective myotome, dermatome, and reflexes. In cases of injury at the thoracolumbar junction, a mixed picture of both cord and root lesion may emerge and there could be an UMN and LMN feature in the lower limbs. Below the L_1, it is the nerve roots, which are damaged, and it is easy to identify the injured nerve root by a careful examination of myotome, dermatome, and reflexes of the lower limb. Slightest voluntary movement and sensation below the level of cord lesion indicate cord continuity with better prognosis.

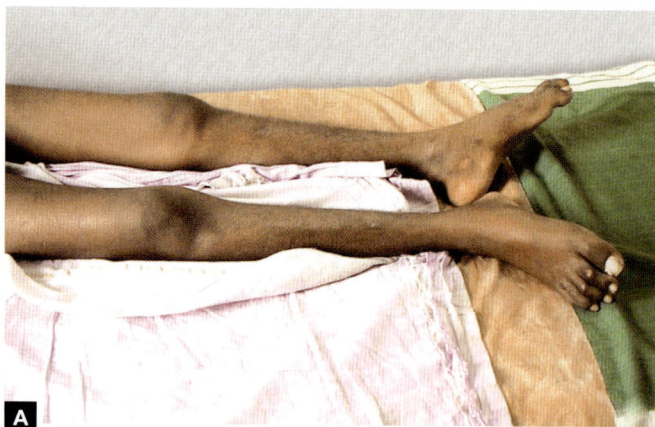
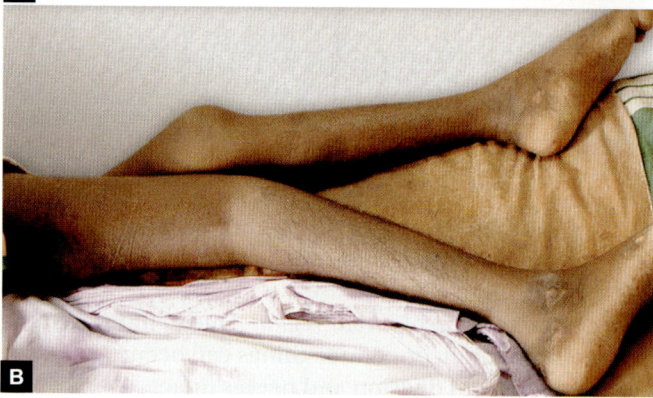

Figs 24.43A and B: Clinical photo showing spastic paraplegia

If paralysis is complete even after 8 hours and if there is symmetrical returning of reflexes and priapism in male, it indicates an unfavorable prognosis.

Return of reflex activity (e.g. anal reflex, bulbocavernosus reflex, and plantar response): Return of reflex activity below the lesion indicates that the spinal shock has passed off and remaining paralysis and anesthesia may be due to injury to the long tracts of cauda equina.

Total sensory and motor paralysis after 8 hours with return of reflex activity indicates that distal part of spinal cord has been separated from cerebral control.

Nerve Wracking Points: Remember the Neurological Facts
- Cervical spine level as mentioned previously
- Between T_1 and T_{10}: Paralysis of trunk and lower limb muscles.
- At T_{10}: Paraplegia and the corresponding cord damage are at L_1.
- Between D_{11} and L_1: Paraplegia and here the lumbar and sacral sections of the spinal cord are damaged along with their nerve roots.
- Below L_1: No cord damage, only root damage leading to cauda equina paralysis.
So to arrive at the proper level of spinal and cord damage, remember this rule:

Do You Know How to Find Out the Level of Cord Injury by Looking at the Vertebral Injury?

Bone segment	Cord segment
C_1 to C_7	Add 1 to vertebral level
T_1 to T_4	Add 2 to vertebral level
T_4 to T_{10}	Add 3 to vertebral level
T_{10}	Dorsal segments complete
T_{12}	Lumbar segments complete
L_1	Sacral segments complete
Below L_1	Cauda equina paralysis

Investigations

This consists of plain radiograph of the affected part and all three views—anteroposterior, lateral, and oblique are done. MRI and CT scan are also done and their role has already been described (Fig. 24.44).

Treatment

- First aid as already discussed
- Management of vertebral fracture and dislocations as discussed in individual injuries.
- Rehabilitation programs in neurological injury following spinal fracture are as follows:

Paralyzed Bladder

Bladder injuries could be either UMN type or LMN type (Table 24.4).

UMN Type (Automatic Bladder)

This is seen in injury above S_2 due to complete transection of the cord. Here the bladder is distended and there is no real sensation of vesical filling and the bladder is controlled by

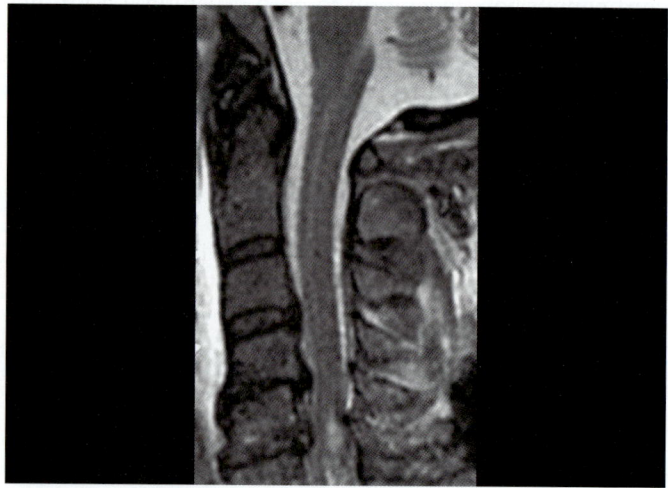

Fig. 24.44: MRI showing damage to the cervical spinal cord

TABLE 24.4: Characteristic features of UMN and LMN bladder injuries

Bladder	Automatic	Autonomous
Type	UMN	LMN
Level	Above S_2	S_2 and below
Reflex center of bladder	Takes over	Lost
Controlled by	Reflex center	Intrinsic plexus of bladder
Emptying by	Involuntary	Voluntary
Residual urine	Minimal	Large >200–300 cc

Goal in either case is to attain an automatic reflex emptying of the bladder.

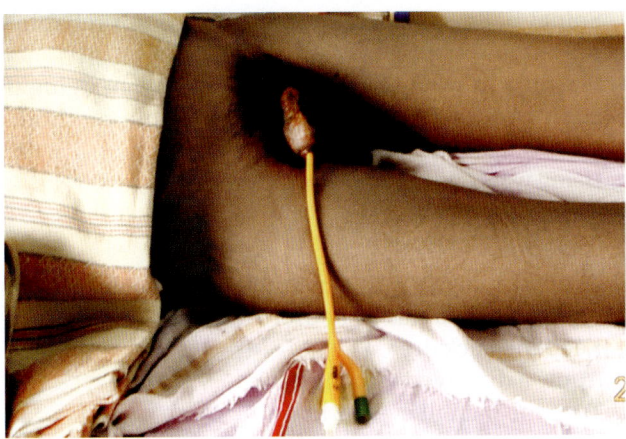

Fig. 24.45: Bladder management in a paraplegia patient

the reflex centers. There is automatic involuntary emptying and no residual urine is left.

LMN Type (Autonomous Bladder)

This occurs in injuries at or below S_2. The bladder reflex center is destroyed. It now depends on the intrinsic plexus in the musculature of the bladder wall (detrusor ganglion). Here, emptying is to be done by manual pressure or by trained contraction of abdominal musculature. There is a large amount of residual urine in this condition.

Treatment: In either condition mentioned above, the treatment method aims at obtaining automatic reflex emptying. This is done as follows:
- Urinary retention catheter is placed in the bladder for 24–48 hours.
- After 48 hours, intermittent catheterization is started, to develop the automatic reflex emptying of the bladder.
- Persons with traumatic quadriplegia have an UMN bladder controlled by reflexes through conus medullaris.
- If intermittent catheterization is not available, bladder range of motion exercises are performed by clamping the catheter tube for 50 minutes and opening for 10 minutes every hour to allow the bladder to develop a reflex pattern of emptying.
- If reflex emptying with residual bladder urine volume of less than 100 cc does not occur within 6–9 months, urological procedures like external sphincterotomy or bladder neck resection is done to achieve a balanced bladder.
- Urinary diversion through ileal loops, etc. is not superior to reflex emptying of the bladder and hence is not recommended (Fig. 24.45).

All possible attempts should be made to remove the catheter and have a catheter-free reflex emptying of the bladder.

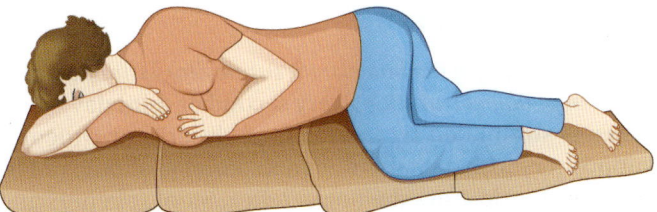

Fig. 24.46: Bed posture (side lying) to prevent formation of bedsores

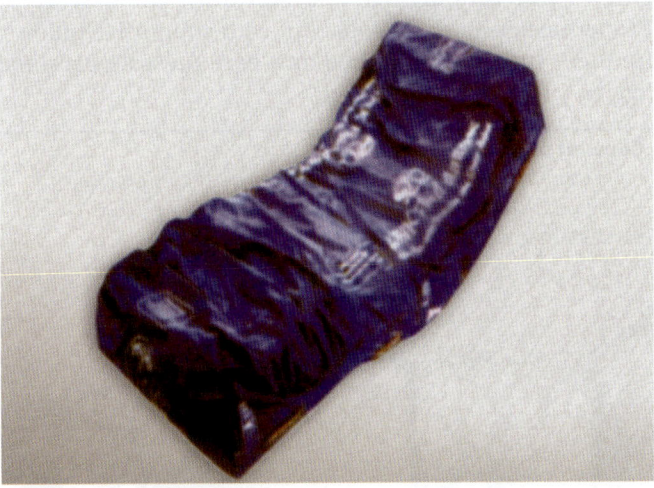

Fig. 24.47: Waterbed, a boon for prevention of bedsores

Bedsore Management

Preventing Bedsores (Figs 24.46 and 24.47)

Nursing goals: Education of the patients and relatives.
- Only sure method of preventing pressure ulcers is strict nursing care and gradual shifting of responsibility of the skin care to the patient's family.

- Spinal beds, mattresses, and pads are not reliable to prevent pressure sores.
- Sleeping in prone position with a pillow bridging the bony prominences is the most reliable method of preventing bedsores.
- Using water bed also helps prevent bedsores.

Managing Bedsores

While prevention is the best mantra, the following measures are recommended once a bedsore develops (Fig. 24.48):
- Keep the back dry
- Apply a dry powder to the back
- Turn the patient every 2 hours
- Use water or air beds
- Do periodic dressings taking all aseptic precautions.

Bowel Program

Reflex emptying of the bowel with suppository stimulation is the goal of bowel training: Every second or third day bowel reflex is stimulated by insertion of glycerin or Dulcolax suppository with digital stimulation. Enemas should not be given as this destroys the bowel reflex. Stool softeners and mild laxatives may be necessary.

Beds: A conventional hospital bed and pillow is preferred. Side-to-side rotating bed is used during the first week. Proper positioning of the patient with supportive pillows, frequent turning in the bed and care towards personal hygiene is very much needed.

Concept of Rotating Beds
- All spine injuries are placed on rotating beds in the causality
- The bed rotates 40° on either side
- Rotation stopped only for 2 hours in 8 hours

- Safety straps and pads are applied firmly
- Extremity exercises are permitted
- Compression stockings to prevent thromboembolism
- Spirometry is done every 2 hours
- All investigations, MRI, X-ray, etc. can be carried out
- The patient can be mobilized once the condition and the spine are stable.

Vital Facts
Who require rotating bed treatment?
- Two to three column injury patients
- Bony injuries without posterior ligamentous disruption
- For individuals who are neurologically normal and improving.

Advantages

- The patient is comfortable
- Nursing care becomes easy
- Investigations, exercises, etc. can safely be done.

Family education: The family members of the victim are trained to take care of the victim's bowel, back, bladder, and bed. They are also encouraged to give all the necessary moral support, which is so essentially required to rehabilitate the patient back to normalcy.

Physical therapy: This consists of putting joints through all the range of movements by passive stretching and exercises. Parallel bar walking, walking with the help of walkers or crutches is encouraged (Fig. 24.49). Wheel chair transfer activities are encouraged for injuries from C_6 level onwards.

Occupational therapy: If possible, the patient is allowed to return to his original work with minor adjustments if necessary. Nevertheless, if the patient, however, is unable

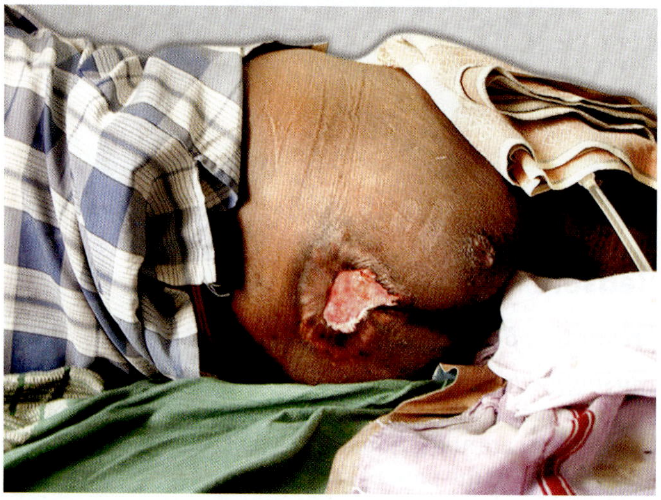

Fig. 24.48: Clinical photo of a bedsore

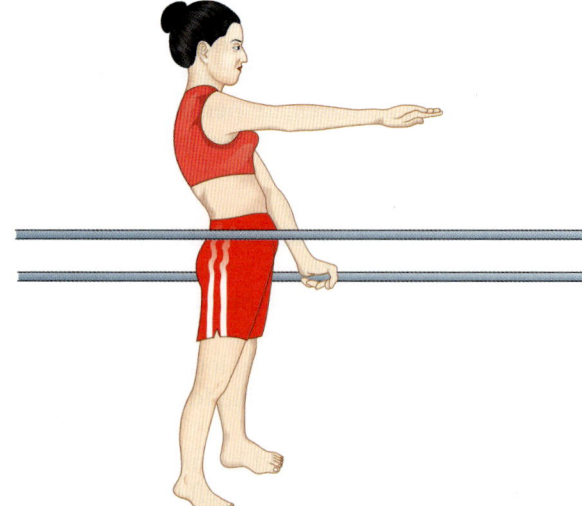

Fig. 24.49: A paraplegic patient learning to balance and walk within a parallel bar

TABLE 24.5: Rehabilitative measures for neurological injury

Level	Disabilities	Measures
$S_{2,4}$	Only bowel and bladder injured	Bladder and bowel program
$L_4–S_1$	Bladder, bowel and prolonged sitting impaired	Short leg braces
$L_{1,2,3}$	Bladder, bowel and walking impaired	Walking with long leg brace
T_{7-12}	UMN bladder	Long leg brace and wheelchair
$T_2–T_6$	Bowel, bladder, walking, sitting impaired	Wheelchair is a must
$C_7–T_1$	Up to the level patient can become independent in all activities of daily living	Wheelchair is a must
C_5	Assistance to all activities of daily living required	Electrical chair is required
Above C_5	Total dependence + impaired breathing	

This table shows the level of spinal injuries, their corresponding disabilities and the measures to be followed.

to return to his original work, an alternative employment depending upon his present status of health is suggested.

Social therapy: The attitude of the people towards these patients should not be of sympathy, but of support and encouragement. The right attitude of the society towards these unfortunate victims will go a long way in rehabilitating them back to normal.

Table 24.5 shows various rehabilitative measures to be taken in patients with paraplegia.

CAUDA EQUINA SYNDROME

Cauda equina syndrome is seen in injuries below the level of first lumbar vertebra. It is essentially injury to the nerve roots below L_1.

Causes

- Tumors of the spine
- Pott's disease
- Protrusion of disk—large midline disk prolapse at 4–5
- Fracture dislocation of the thoracolumbar spine.

Clinical Features

Symptoms

The patient complains of back pain, perineal pain, difficulty in micturition, impotence in male, etc.

Sensory signs: The most salient feature of a cauda equina lesion is an area of *saddle-shaped hyperesthesia and later anesthesia* (involving buttocks, anus, and perineum) (Fig. 24.50).

Motor signs: Flaccid paralysis below the knee.

Reflexes: Ankle jerk is lost and the knee jerk is increased due to the weakness of the opposing hamstrings.

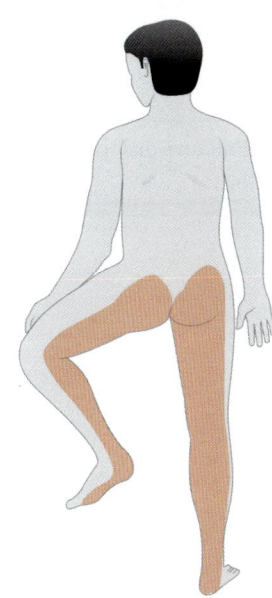

Fig. 24.50: Cauda equina lesion

Bladder symptoms: Common problems are retention of urine with overflow. Even after a severe cauda equina, lesion reflex micturition is established later, reflex being mediated through the vesical plexus.

Anal sphincter relaxation: leading to incontinence of the bowels.

Investigations

Plain X-ray, CT scan, MRI of the affected part is recommended (see Fig. 24.34).

Treatment

Prompt surgical intervention is the treatment of choice. This consists of operative stabilization of the fractures, bowel, back and bladder care and other rehabilitating measures have already been described above.

Prognosis in Spinal Cord Injuries

Ten-year survival rate in spinal cord injury is 86%.

Vital Facts
Do you know the chief causes of death in spinal cord injuries?
Well it is:
- Pneumonia
- Suicides.

Interesting Facts
Do you know what 'SCIWORA' is?
Well it is spinal cord injury without radiological abnormality. It is more common in children <10 years.

BIBLIOGRAPHY

1. Crutchfield WG. Fracture dislocations of cervical spine. Am J Surg. 1937;38:592.
2. Crutchfield WG. Skeletal traction in the treatment of injuries to the cervical spine. JAMA. 1954;155:29.
3. Davis L. Treatment of spinal cord injuries. Arch Surg. 1954;69:488.
4. Dickson JH, Harrington PR, Erwin WD. Harrington instrumentation in the fractured, unstable thoracic and lumbar spine. Texas Med. 1973;69-91.
5. Holds worth FW. Traumatic paraplegia. In: Platt H (Ed). Modern Trends in Orthopedics (2nd series), New York: Paul B, Hoeber Inc; 1956.
6. Holds worth FW. Fractures, dislocations, and fracture-dislocations of the spine. J Bone Joint Surg. 1970;52-A:1534.
7. Jefferson G. Fracture of the atlas vertebra: Report of four cases and a review of those previously recorded. Br J Surg. 1920;7:407.
8. Kelly RP, Whitesides TE (Jr). Treatment of lumbodorsal fracture dislocations. Am Surg. 1968;167:705?
9. Maffee PC, Youn HA, Lasada NA. The unstable burst fracture. Spine. 1982;7:365.
10. Watson-Jones R. Fractures and joint injuries (4th edn), Baltimore: Williams and Wilkins Co. 1952;1,1955,2.

25 CHAPTER

Peripheral Nerve Injuries

BRIEF ANATOMY

About Spinal Nerve

The dorsal and ventral nerve roots arising from the spinal cord join at the intervertebral foramen to form a spinal nerve. In the thoracic segments, these mixed spinal nerves retain their autonomy and supply one intercostals segment both dermatome and myotomal. In virtually all other segments, spinal nerves join with others to form a plexus. There are 31 pairs of spinal nerves consisting of 8 cervical, 12 thoracic, 5 lumbar, 5 sacral and 1 coccygeal.

A spinal nerve has three components: motor, sensory and sympathetic. The sympathetic components of all 31 mixed spinal nerves leave along the 14 motor roots (12 thoracic and 2 lumbar roots). Each spinal nerve now divides into *anterior and posterior* rami. The anterior rami of the upper four cervical nerves form the *cervical plexus* and the lower four cervical together with upper thoracic nerves form the *brachial plexus*. The anterior rami of the first three lumbar nerves and part of the fourth lumbar nerve form the *lumbar plexus*. The sacral anterior rami along with the anterior rami of the fifth lumbar and part of fourth lumbar form the *lumbosacral plexus*.

The posterior rami supply the paraspinal muscles and the skin of the back. They are smaller than anterior rami except for upper three cervical posterior rami. The spinal nerves are then distributed to the limb buds through several peripheral nerves. *Therefore, a peripheral nerve is also a mixed nerve like the spinal nerve* (Fig. 25.1).

Dermatome is an area of skin supplied by a single spinal root.

Myotome represents a muscle unit supplied by a single spinal root.

MICROSCOPIC ANATOMY

Each nerve fiber or axon with a diameter greater than 1 μm has a myelin sheath. The axon is a direct continuation of dorsal root ganglion cell, an anterior horn cell, or postganglionic sympathetic cell. It is encircled by its Schwann cell sheath. In the unmyelinated fibers, the Schwann cell alone acts as a sheath and in myelinated fibers it forms a multilaminated structure that encloses the myelin sheath. A delicate fibrous tissue called the endoneurium surrounds the axon with its Schwann cell and myelin sheath. A denser layer of fibrous tissue called the perineurium encloses a bundle of these fibers (called funiculi). The entire group of funiculi with their surrounding perineurium is encased as a mixed spinal or peripheral nerve in a denser *epineurium* (Fig. 25.2).

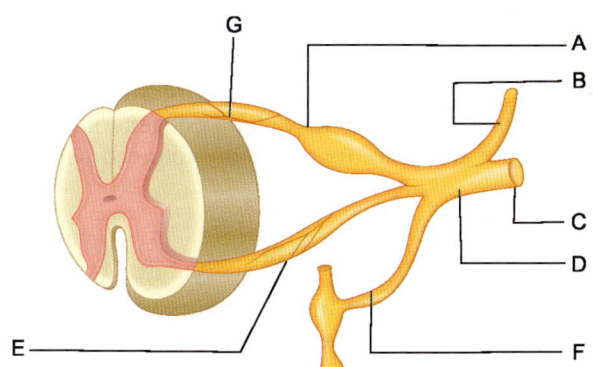

Fig. 25.1: Components of a mixed spinal nerve: (A) Dorsal root ganglion on the sensory root, (B) Posterior rami, (C) Anterior rami, (D) Mixed spinal nerve, (E) Motor root, (F) Gray ramus communicans from the sympathetic ganglion, (G) Sensory root

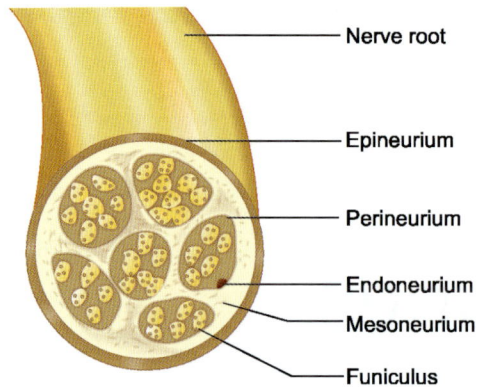

Fig. 25.2: Cross-section of a spinal or peripheral nerve root

Blood supply to the nerve fibers enters through the *mesoneurium*.

GENERAL PRINCIPLES OF NERVE INJURY

NERVE DEGENERATION

Any part of the neuron detached from its nucleus degenerates and is destroyed by phagocytosis. This process of degeneration distal to a point of injury is called *secondary* or *wallerian degeneration*. Reaction in proximal end is called *primary* or *retrograde degeneration*. Time required for degeneration varies between sensory, motor, and is related to the size and myelination. In secondary degeneration, response is obtained to faradic stimulation up to 18–72 hours. After 2–3 days, distal segment is fragmented and the myelin sheath starts degenerating. By seven days, macrophages clear the axon or debris and are completed within 15–30 days. Schwann cells undergo mitosis from seventh day onwards and start filling the areas previously occupied by axon and its myelin sheath. Primary retrograde degeneration proceeds for at least one internodes or more. Histological, it is identical to wallerian degeneration. More proximal the site of injury, more pronounced will be the changes.

NERVE REGENERATION

Axonal sprouting starts from 24 hours after the injury. Unmyelinated initially but later on it gets myelinated. Now if the endoneurium is intact, sprouts will readily pass along their former courses and after regeneration may innervate their previous end organs. If the endoneurium is interrupted, then the sprouting axons may migrate aimlessly throughout the damaged area into the epineurial, perineurial regions forming a *stump neuroma* or *neuroma in continuity* or they may enter into the other empty endoneural tubes or newly formed endoneural tubes only to terminate in myotomal or dermatomal areas of their own. Hence, recovery is difficult if entire axon is transected and filled with scar tissue.

CLASSIFICATION OF NERVE INJURIES

Seddon's Classification (1943) (Table 25.1)

Seddon identified three types of nerve injuries: The first one is a mere contusion; the second is the transection of axons only, and the third complete transection of the nerve. This classification is less accepted clinically.

Sunderland's Classification (Table 25.2)

Accepted clinically and arranged in ascending order of severity from 1–5. Various degrees represent injury to myelin, axon, endoneurium, perineurium, and the entire trunk.

Etiology

General Causes

Metabolic diseases, collagen diseases, malignancies, endogenous or exogenous toxins; thermal, chemical or mechanical trauma, etc. can cause injury to the peripheral nerves.

Local Causes

Forty percent of bone and joint injuries are associated with peripheral nerve lesions.

Types

Primary: This is due to injury of a peripheral nerve resulting from the same trauma that has injured a bone or joint.

Secondary: This is due to involvement of the nerve in infection, scar, callus, etc.

TABLE 25.1: Seddon's classification		
Neuropraxia	Axonotmesis	Neurotmesis
• Minor contusion of the peripheral nerve	• Axon breakdown anatomic section • Endoneurium is intact	• Complete • No recovery
• Axis cylinder is preserved	• Spontaneous recovery is expected	
• Temporary		
• Recovery is complete		

TABLE 25.2: Sunderland's classification of nerve injuries

Degrees	I°	II°	III°	IV°	V°
Axon	Contusion	Disrupted	Disrupted	Disrupted	Disrupted
Endoneurium	Intact	Intact	Disrupted	Disrupted	Disrupted
Perineurium	Intact	Intact	Intact	Few fibers preserved	Disrupted
Entire nerve	Intact	Intact	Intact	Intact	Disrupted
Myelin	Intact	Intact	Intact	Intact	Disrupted
Motor march: Recovery of the motor innervation in a progressive manner from proximal to distal	• No motor march • No Tinel's sign • Complete restoration of function	• Motor march present • Tinel's sign present • Good recovery	• Motor march • Tinel's sign present • Incomplete recovery	• No Tinel's sign or motor march • No recovery	• No recovery • Grade VI° is a mixture of above injuries from I° to V°

Incidence of Peripheral Nerve Injuries
- Radial nerve is commonly injured
- Ulnar nerve 30%
- Median nerve 15%
- Peroneal nerve.
- Lumbosacral plexus 3%
- Tibial nerve.

Clinical Diagnosis

It is difficult to evaluate a nerve injury immediately after a severe trauma. The diagnostic approach towards a peripheral nerve injury should essentially consist of the following steps:

Listen: Carefully listen to what the patient has got to tell you about the history of the injury. Many a times mere listening can help clinch you the diagnosis. Here are some samples:

History	Nerves affected
I'm suffering from leprosy	Ulnar, median and sciatic nerves
I took an injection in the arm or buttocks	Arm—Deltoid nerve. Buttocks—Sciatic nerve
I traveled in a bus overnight	Sciatic nerve compression
I cut my wrist by a glass piece	Neuropathy
I suffered from arm bone fracture	Medial nerve injury
I broke my elbow in a fall	Radial nerve injury
I have suffered a hip dislocation due to dashboard injury	Radial nerve injury median/ulnar injury and sciatic nerve injury

Look: This is the second step in the diagnosis of PNI. After listening to the story, look for the typical tell-tale evidences. Each nerve injury is associated with a particular attitude. Look for those (see box).

Feel and touch: This helps you to detect damage to the sensory component of a nerve. The affected skin could be cold or clammy. Patient may not be able to feel the temperature touch, vibrations, and pressure in the affected areas. Loss of sweating is an ominous sign.

Move: Instruct the patient to move the limb and joints distal to the site of injury. Inability to do so totally reveal complete nerve damage, slight movements possible suggests less than complete damage to the nerve.

Beware of the trick movements a patient may resort to overcome the loss of a particular muscle function. This is a diagnostic "pitfall" one should carefully avoid.

Knock: Using a knee hammer, 'knock' over the knee, ankle, elbow, etc. to elicit the appropriate reflexes. They are normally absent in peripheral nerve injuries.

Measure: With a measuring tape, measure the muscle girth of the limbs for wasting.

Investigate: After following this various clinical steps, certain investigations need to be done to confirm the diagnosis and plan the appropriate line of treatment.

Quick Facts:
It is difficult to evaluate a nerve injury immediately after a severe trauma. However, typical attitudes and simple screening test help clinch the diagnosis with reasonable accuracy.

Typical deformities
- Wrist drop → Radial nerve injury
- Claw hand → Ulnar nerve injury
- Foot drop → Lateral popliteal nerve injury
- Ape thumb → Median nerve injury
- Winging of scapula → Thoracodorsal nerve injury
- Pointing index → Median nerve injury
- Policeman tip → Brachial plexus injury

Simple screening tests
- In ulnar nerve injury, loss of pain at tip of the little finger
- In median nerve injury, loss of pain on the tip of index finger
- In radial nerve injury, inability to extend the thumb (Hitchhiker's sign).

Diagnostic Tests

Electromyography

Electromyography (EMG) helps to record the electrical activity of a muscle at rest and during activity (Figs 25.3A to C).

Intact muscle: There is no electrical activity in an intact muscle at rest. During a weak contraction, the electrodes record a single action potential. In powerful muscle contractions, these motor action potentials superimpose to give an interference pattern.

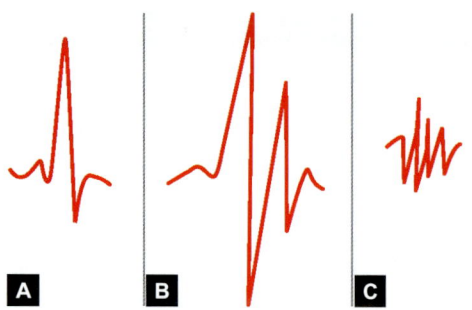

Figs 25.3A to C: Pattern of electromyography curves: (A) Normal insertional activity; (B) Positive waves (5–14 days); (C) Denervation fibrillation after (15–30 days)

Injured or denervated muscle: These muscles show denervation potentials, which are spontaneous electrical activity at rest. These are primitive responses, which is normally suppressed by the stronger nerve action potentials. These denervation potentials normally appear by 1–2 weeks after injury. If they have not appeared by 15–20 days after muscle denervation, it indicates a good prognostic sign.

> **Quick Facts: EMG**
> - Normal insertional activity immediately after section
> - Positive waves seen after 5–14 days
> - Denervation fibrillation after 14 days
> - Spontaneous fibrillation after 15–30 days of interruption.

Uses and limitations of EMG: Electromyography helps to detect the presence or absence of nerve injury if present whether it is complete or incomplete and whether any regeneration is taking place or not. EMG does not give the level of injury or the degree of injury accurately.

Strength duration curve: A muscle usually responds to an electric stimulus. However, greater strength of current is required to excite a denervated muscle than normal muscle. Minimum current required to elicit a muscle contraction is called the "rheobase" and is expressed in mill amperes. The "chronaxie" is the duration of current required to excite a muscle with a current strength of double the rheobase. This is expressed in milliseconds.

To know the excitability of a muscle in relation to the current strength and its duration, the muscle is stimulated by decreasing the duration of the current from 300 milliseconds to 1 millisecond and a consequent increase in the strength of the current required is detected and plotted on a graph as the strength duration curve.

Utility of Strength Duration Curve (SDC)

Normal muscle: A normal muscle responds to stimuli from duration of 300 millisecond to 1 second without any increase in the strength of the current. However, if it is less than 1 millisecond, increase in the strength of the current is required. This curve is called the *nerve curve*.

Completely denervated muscle: Records a muscle curve and here either more strength or longer duration stimulation is required to produce a contraction.

Partially denervated muscle: The curve here lies in between the two curves mentioned above. However, there is an upward kink, which denotes the superimposition of the two basic types of curves.

Limitations of EMG: EMG merely indicates whether the muscle is innervated or not. It gives no specific indications as to the level of injury or degree of injury.

Nerve Conduction Studies

Stimulation of a peripheral nerve by an electrode placed on the skin overlying the nerve will readily evoke a response from the muscle innervated by that nerve. Immediately after section, stimulation distal to the point of injury will elicit an essentially normal response for 18–72 hours after injury until wallerian degeneration sets in. This failure of response after about 3 days excludes "neuropraxia." Slowed conduction at a specific point indicates "compression neuropathy."

Tinel's Sign

This is an important sign, which helps in recording the rate of regeneration of the nerve clinically.

Procedure: Gentle percussion is done along the course of injured nerve. Tingling sensation is experienced by the patient in the distribution of injured nerve rather than the area per cussed, and the sensation should *persist* for several seconds following the stimulation. Positive Tinel's sign indicates regenerating axonal sprouts have not obtained complete myelinization. Response fades as myelinization takes place. Distal progression of the response and the rate of the progression have been used by some to establish prognosis (rate of recovery should be 3 cm per month). Presence of this sign is encouraging. Even a few regenerating sensory fibers can result in positive Tinel's sign. Thus, its presence cannot be taken as an absolute evidence of recovery.

Sweat Test (Starch Test)

Presence of sweating within *autonomous zone suggests that complete interruption of the nerve has not occurred.

---

*Small area of complete anesthesia after section of a peripheral nerve or root

Skin Resistance Test

It is another method of evaluating autonomic interruption by using Richter's thermometer.

Electrical Stimulation

Faradic stimulation is of little value (because even normally innervated muscles may fail to respond).

Galvanic stimulation: Recording of chronaxie and strength duration curve by galvanic stimulation is more helpful in evaluating nerve injuries.

Management

General Principles

Resuscitation is carried out first, if the patient is in shock. General condition is improved by the emergency management measures. A thorough debridement of the wound is carried out; and if the wound is clean, direct suturing of the perineurium or epineurium or epiperineurium of both the cut ends carries out primary repair of the nerve. If the wound is contaminated, nerve is repaired after 3–6 weeks. In closed fractures with peripheral nerve injuries, conservative management is the treatment of choice. Careful assessment of the recovery is made and early surgical exploration is done if the recovery is not satisfactory.

Conservative Management

This consists of the following essential steps:

Splinting of the limbs: Different splints are required to immobilize the limbs in various nerve injuries.
- Upper limb:
  - Brachial plexus injury—aeroplane splint.
  - Axillary nerve injury—shoulder abduction splint.
  - Radial nerve injury—cock-up splint (Fig. 25.4).
- Lower limb: Common peroneal nerve injury—foot drop splint (see Fig. 25.26).

Passive movements of all joints are done to prevent contractures.

Physiotherapy: Massage, exercises, stimulation, etc.

Care of the skin, etc.

Operative Management

This consists of various types of nerve repair (Figs 25.5A to D), tendon transfers, arthrodesis, etc.

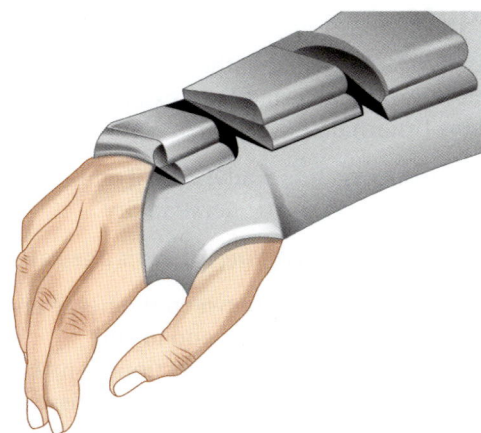

Fig. 25.4: Wrist cock-up splint (Static type)

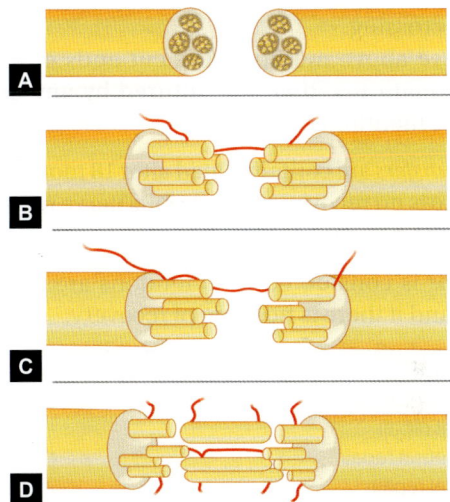

Figs 25.5A to D: Types of nerve repair: (A) Epineural neurorrhaphy; (B) Perineural neurorrhaphy; (C) Epiperineural neurorrhaphy; (D) Interfascicular nerve grafting

Types of Nerve Repair

Primary repair is done within 6–8 hours after injury and if the wound is clean cut.

Delayed primary repair is done between 7 and 18 days after injury and if the wound is contaminated.

Secondary repair is carried out 18 days after injury, if the injury is seen late, failure of conservative treatment, incomplete injury, etc.

Techniques

Endoneurolysis: It is freeing of the nerve entrapped within the scar tissue either external scar (external neurolysis) or within nerve (internal neurolysis).

Partial neurorrhaphy: This is advisable if one-half of a large nerve is disrupted, e.g. sciatic nerve injury.

Neurorrhaphy and nerve grafting if there is a gap after injury.

Methods of closing the gaps between the nerve ends if the nerves cannot be approximated end to end
- Mobilization of the nerves by sectioning its cutaneous branches and freeing it from the fibrous tissue around.
- Positioning of the extremities in functional position.
- Transposition of the nerves, e.g. ulnar nerve transposition.
- Bone resection
- Nerve grafting by using sural nerve
- Nerve crossing.

By these above methods, the cut ends of the nerves can be brought together and sutured by any one of the techniques mentioned above.

Tendon transfers are contemplated after 18 months of injury when there is no recovery after various nerve repair techniques or if the patient presents late.

Arthrodesis is considered if no tendons are available for transfers and if there is no hope of recovery.

> **Quick Recap:**
> Methods of nerve suture
> - Epineural repair
> - Epiperineural repair
> - Perineural repair
> - Fascicular repair.

> **Quick Summary:**
> - Peripheral nerve is a mixed nerve
> - Sunderland's classification is clinically accepted
> - Forty percent of bone and joint injuries are associated with peripheral nerve lesions
> - Radial nerve is the most common peripheral nerve to be injured
> - Screening test helps in quick diagnosis
> - In closed injuries conservative management is the treatment of choice
> - In open injuries, primary nerve repair if the wound is clean and if the wound is contaminated delayed primary nerve repair or secondary repair is done.

ULNAR NERVE INJURY

The Ulnar Nerve Speaks
I am the largest branch of the medial cord of the brachial plexus with a root value of C_8–T_1. I arise at the level of pectoralis minor muscle, run through the axilla, and lie in the medial compartment of the arm. I pierce the medial intermuscular septum at the level of coracobrachialis and lie in the posterior compartment of the arm. I pass over the posterior aspect of the medial epicondyle and enter the forearm through the two heads of flexor carpi ulnaris via the elbow. I lie beneath the flexor carpi ulnaris muscle within the forearm. At the junction of middle and lower one-third of forearm, I give a dorsal sensory branch, which winds round the forearm and passes dorsally to supply the dorsum of the ulnar border of the hand, the little finger, and medial half of ring finger. Later, I pass through the Guyon's canal at the wrist formed by the pisohamate ligament and the hook of the hamate. On the exit from the canal, I split into a superficial and deep branch. I supply the following muscles during my course:
- In the arm—Nil.
- In the forearm—Flexor carpi ulnaris and medial half of flexor digitorum profundus (Fig. 25.6). I supply both these muscles at the proximal third. As already mentioned, I give off a dorsal sensory branch at the distal third.
- In the hand—superficial branch supply palmaris brevis and digital branches to volar aspect of little finger and medial half of ring finger. Through the deep branch, I supply the hypothenar, the dorsal and the palmar interossei, two medial lumbricals and the adductor pollicis muscles.

In short, I supply ulnar flexors of the wrist, deep finger flexors of the little and ring fingers and mainly I supply the intrinsic muscles of the hand comprising hypothenar, lumbricals, and interossei muscles.

Role of lumbricals: Mainly flexes the metacarpophalangeal joints and extends the proximal interphalangeal joint.

Role of interossei: Palmar interossei adducts the fingers and dorsal abducts the fingers. Through the dorsal digital expansion, they aid the action of lumbricals.

Role of hypothenar: Abducts and helps in the movement of apposition of little finger.

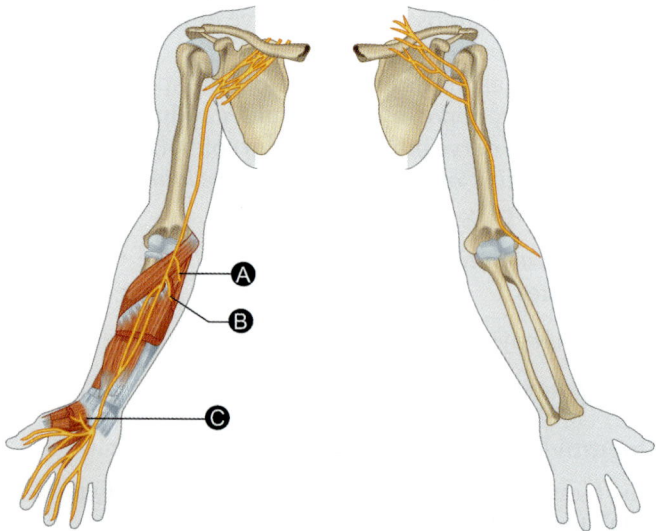

Fig. 25.6: Course of the median and ulnar nerves and their supply, (A) Flexor carpi ulnaris, (B) Flexor digitorum profundus, (C) Intrinsic muscles of the hand

Causes of Ulnar Nerve Injury

General Causes

These are as described in the general principles of peripheral nerve injury.

Local Causes

These are more important and could be in the following areas:

Causes in the axilla
- Crutch pressure
- Aneurysm of the axillary vessels.

Causes in the arm
- Fracture shaft of humerus
- Gunshot and penetrating injuries.

Causes at the elbow
- Compression by the accessory muscle (anserina epitrochlearis)
- Fracture lateral epicondyle of humerus
- Repeated occupational strains
- Recurrent subluxation of the nerve
- Compression by the osteophytes as in rheumatoid and osteoarthritis
- Cubitus valgus deformity due to various causes results in repeated friction of the nerve giving rise to tardy (late) ulnar nerve palsy.

Causes in the forearm
- Fracture both bones forearm
- Incised wounds, gunshot wounds, and penetrating injuries of the forearm.

Causes at the wrist
- Compression by osteophytes
- Fracture hook of the hamate
- Compression by ganglion
- Wrist injuries.

Causes in the hand
- Blunt trauma
- Penetrating injuries
- Occupational—people operating high-speed drills in rock mining, etc
- Associated ulnar artery aneurysm
- Ulnar nerve injuries give rise to *claw hand* deformity either true type or ulnar claw hand.

CLAW HAND

It is a deformity with hyperextension of the metacarpophalangeal joints and flexion of the interphalangeal joints of the fingers.

Types and Causes

Two varieties are described: One is a true claw hand involving both median and ulnar nerves and the second an ulnar claw hand or claw-like hand due to ulnar nerve injury (Flowchart 25.1 and Fig. 25.7).

Pathomechanics

Loss of intrinsic muscle function due to ulnar nerve injury results in loss of flexion at MP joints and extension of IP joints of the fingers.

In a bid to bring about the flexion of the MP joints, the long finger flexors overact pulling the IP joints and wrist into more flexion. This causes a tenodesing (pulling) effect on the long finger extensors. The extensors cannot extend the IP joints without the stabilization of the MP joint in neutral or slightly flexed position, which is normally brought about by

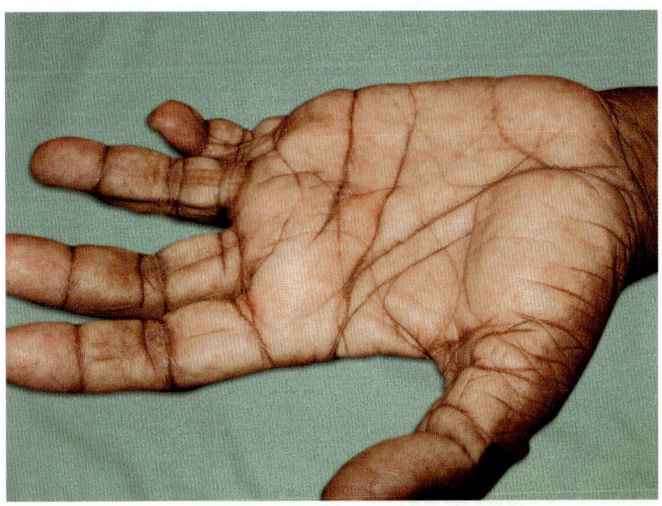

Fig. 25.7: Ulnar claw hand (Clinical photo)

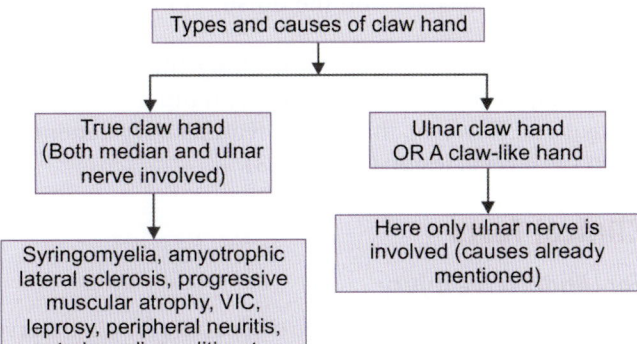

Flowchart 25.1: Types and causes of true claw hand and ulnar claw hand

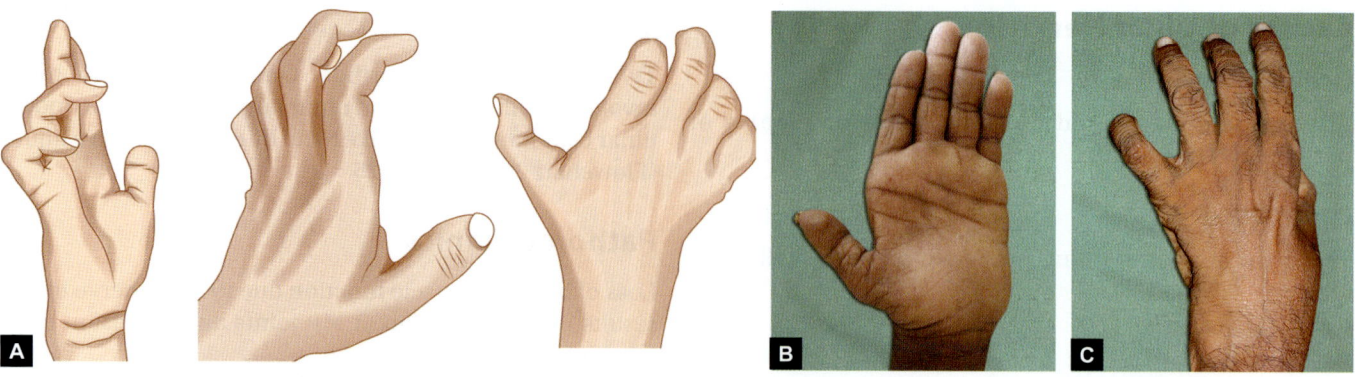

Figs 25.8A to C: (A) (1) Ulnar clawing, (2) Total clawing, and (3) Wasting of intermetacarpal spaces; (B) Hypothenar muscle wasting (Clinical photo); (C) Intermetacarpal spaces (Clinical photo)

the intrinsic. This along with the compensatory over action of the long finger extensors to bring about the lost extension of the MP joints results in hyperextension of the MP joints and the classical deformity.

This is called the intrinsic minus hand: The thumb is also adducted by its long extensors because the intrinsic and the abductors are paralyzed.

Problems of Claw Hand
- Hyperextension of MP joints (not the only primary or most disabling deformity).
- Grasp decreased by 50% due to loss of power of flexion at MP joints.
- Pinch decreased due to loss of stabilizing effect from the intrinsics
- Roll up maneuver lost
- Many surgical procedures are devised to block hyperextension of MP joints as it is still considered as the primary deformity.

Note:
MP—Metacarpophalangeal, IP—Interphalangeal.

Clinical Features

These include the classical deformity, loss of sensation along the ulnar nerve distribution and wasting of the hypothenar muscles, intrinsic muscles of the hand leading to hollow intermetacarpal spaces on the dorsum of the hand (Figs 25.8A to C).

A test for loss of sensation along the distribution (Fig. 25.9) of the ulnar nerve in the hand and fingers is carried out. However, the clinical features vary depending upon the level of lesion (Table 25.3).

Clinical Tests

For Ulnar Nerve Injury

[1]*Froment's sign:* This is a reliable clinical test for ulnar nerve injury (Figs 25.10A and B). Three muscles (first palmar

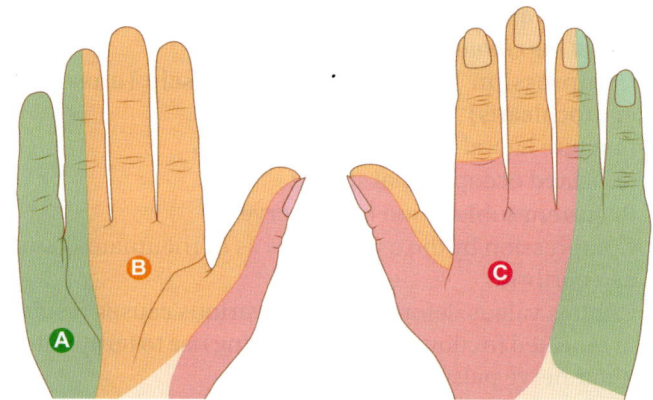

Fig. 25.9: Sensory distribution of the hand: (A) Ulnar nerve distribution, (B) Median nerve distribution, (C) Radial nerve distribution

TABLE 25.3: Levels of lesion	
High above the level of elbow, entire nerve function is lost	
Low	
1. *Below the elbow* at the junction of middle and lower third of forearm	*Spared*: Function of FDP and FCU PB. *Lost*: Motor-HTM, Its, Lum, • Sensory—dorsal aspect of hand (medial border) and one and half fingers
2. *Proximal to Guyon's canal*	*Spared*: FDP, FCU and dorsal sensation. *Lost*: Same as above + loss of volar sensation
3. *Distal to Guyon's canal*	*Spared* FDP, FCU, HTM, PB, dorsal and volar sensations *Lost*: Interossei and lumbricals
FCU—flexor carpi ulnaris, FDP—flexor digitorum profundus, HTM—hypothenar muscles, PB—palmaris brevis, Lum—lumbricals, Its—interossei	

---
[1]**Jules Froment** (1878-1946), France. He was a Professor of Clinical Medicine.

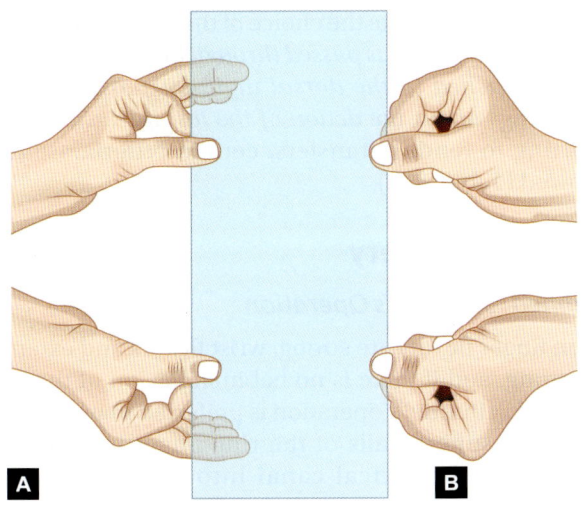

Figs 25.10A and B: Froment's sign: (A) Normal; (B) Ulnar nerve injury

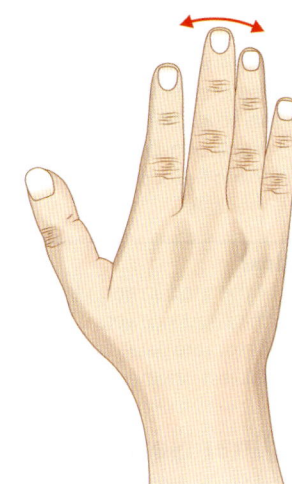

Fig. 25.12: Egawa test

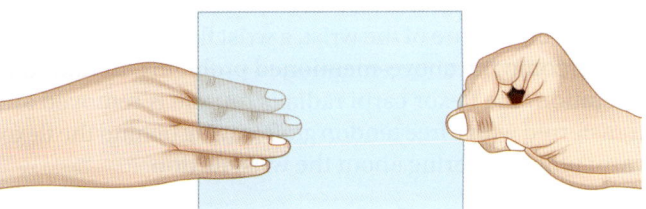

Fig. 25.11: Card test

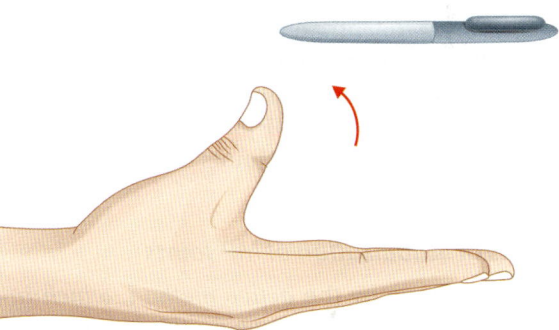

Fig. 25.13: Pen test

interossei, adductor pollicis, and flexor pollicis longus) are required to hold a book between the thumb and other fingers. In ulnar nerve injury, the first two muscles are paralyzed and now to hold the book, the patient has to depend only on flexor pollicis longus, which flexes the thumb prominently. This is the positive Froment's sign.

Card test: Inability to hold a card or paper in between fingers due to loss of adduction by the palmar interossei (Fig. 25.11).

Egawa test: With palm flat on the table the patient is asked to move the middle finger sideways (Fig. 25.12). This is a test for the dorsal interossei of middle finger.

In total clawing median nerve is also injured. Following tests will help to detect the median nerve injury.

Pen test: The patient is unable to touch the pen due to the loss of action of abductor pollicis brevis (Fig. 25.13).

Pointing index or Oschner's clasp test: When both the hands are clasped together, index and middle fingers, fail to flex due to the loss of action of long finger flexors of the index and middle fingers, which are supplied by the median nerve (Fig. 25.14).

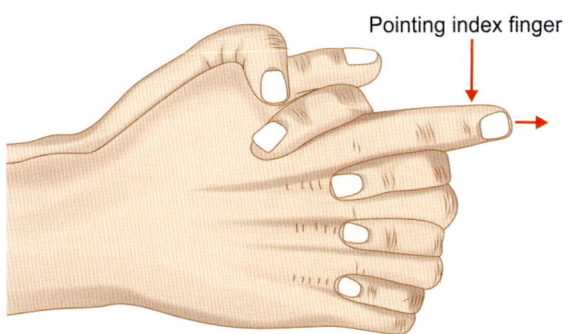

Fig. 25.14: Oschner's clasp test

Benediction test: For the same reason mentioned above, the patient is unable to flex the index and middle finger on lifting the hand (this is the position a clergyman uses to bless the couple during marriage (Fig. 25.15). Hence, called the benediction test).

Note:
Median nerve supplies the following muscles:
- *In the forearm:* Pronator teres, flexor carpi radialis, palmaris longus, flexor digitorum superficialis, flexor digitorum profundus, flexor pollicis longus, and pronator quadratus.
- *In the hand:* Abductor and flexor pollicis brevis, opponens pollicis middle and index lumbricals.

What is Ulnar Paradox?
The higher the lesion of the median and ulnar nerve injury, the less prominent is the deformity and vice versa. This is because in higher lesions the long finger flexors are paralyzed. The loss of finger flexion makes the deformity look less obvious.

Treatment of Ulnar Nerve Injury

In acute injuries, the treatment is as discussed in the general principles.

For Claw Hand Deformity

Principles of treatment: All the treatment measures aim at blocking the hyperextension at the metacarpophalangeal joint. Once this joint is stabilized, the long extensors will bring about the extension of IP joints. The long finger flexors will help in flexion of the MP joints along with their action of finger and wrist flexion.

Methods of Stabilization of MP Joints

This can be done by the *active method, which involves tendon transfer,* or by *passive method, which* involves arthrodesis, capsulodesis, or tenodesis.

Active method: This is by tendon transfers. A neighboring healthy tendon is brought to replace the action of the lost intrinsic. The available normal tendons and the existing local situations dictate the choice of the tendon. *Whichever the tendon chosen, it is passed through the lumbrical canal and is attached to the dorsal digital expansion, which then brings about the action of the lost intrinsics.* Before resorting to tendon transfers, certain criteria are to be followed (Table 25.4).

Choice of Surgery

Modified [2] S Bunnel's Operation

When finger flexors are strong, wrist flexors and extensors are strong, and if there is no habitual flexion of the wrist, modified S. Bunnel's operation is preferred in which flexor digitorum superficialis of the ring finger is transferred through the lumbrical canal into the dorsal digital expansion.

Riordan's Operation

When flexion of the wrist has become habitual or if there is a flexion contracture of the wrist, a wrist flexor can be spared to overcome the above-mentioned problems. In Riordan's operation, the flexor carpi radialis muscle is removed and transferred with a free tendon graft leaving behind the flexor carpi ulnaris to bring about the wrist flexion.

Brand's Operation

When the finger flexors are weak, the wrist flexors are also weak and when the wrist extensors are strong extensor carpi radialis longus or brevis is transferred by a free tendon graft.

Fowler's Operation

When finger flexors, wrist extensors and wrist flexors are not available for transfer, extensor digitorum longus tendon of

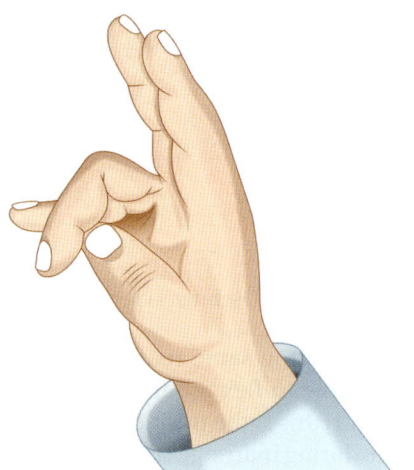

Fig. 25.15: Benediction test

TABLE 25.4: Criteria for tendon transfer
The donor tendon should fulfill the following criteria before it is selected for transfer: <ul><li>The tendon should have a muscle power grade 5 preferably. If not at least grade 4 because after the transfer it loses its muscle power by one grade</li><li>It should have its own nerve and blood supply</li><li>Transfer should be done from the synergistic group because rehabilitation will be easier. The tendon should be routed in a straight line and should be ensured to have sufficient padding to prevent wear and tear</li><li>Tendon should be sutured in moderate tension</li><li>Prior to tendon transfer, joint stiffness, contractures and malunion of bones should be corrected</li><li>Age of the patient should be minimum of 5 years</li><li>The disease should not progress</li><li>Any infection of bone and joints should be controlled</li><li>There should be good range of passive movements available at the joints</li></ul>

---
[2]Sterling Bunnel (1949) UK.

the index and little fingers are transferred by the Fowler's technique.

When no muscle is available for transfer and if the joints are supple, capsulodesis of MP joint or tenodesis is done. If the joints are not supple, arthrodesis in functional position is done.

Tardy Ulnar Nerve Palsy

It is late onset ulnar nerve palsy and could be due to the following causes:
- Malunion or nonunion of lateral condyle fracture of humerus (Figs 25.16A to D)
- Fracture medial epicondyle of humerus
- Dislocation of elbow
- Nerve contusions
- Cubitus valgus
- Shallow ulnar groove
- Hypoplasia of humeral trochlea
- Recurrent subluxation due to inadequate fibrous arch.

Treatment is by anterior transposition of the ulnar nerve.

Entrapment Neuropathy

Entrapment sites: The ulnar nerve could be entrapped in any one of the following sites during its anatomical course:
- Supracondylar process medially
- Arcade of Struthers (near medial intermuscular septum)
- Between two heads of flexor carpi ulnaris
- Guyon's canal.

> **At a Glance: Ulnar Nerve Injury**
> - Ulnar nerve root value is C_8T_1
> - Injury causes ulnar clawing
> - Total clawing when median nerve is also affected.
> - Froment's sign is a reliable test
> - For quick clinical evaluation after injury, the tip of the little finger is tested for sensation
> - Ulnar paradox—higher the lesion less is the deformity and vice versa
> - Correction is by tendon transfers if all criteria are met
> - If no tendons are available for transfer, MP joint is stabilized by capsulodesis, tenodesis, or arthrodesis
> - All surgeries aim at correcting the hyperextension at MP joint.

RADIAL NERVE INJURY

The Radial Nerve Speaks

I am the continuation of the posterior cord of the brachial plexus and I am its largest branch. My root value is $C_{5-8}T_1$. In the axilla, I lie behind the axillary artery, pass posterior to the humerus beneath the teres major, and enter in the interval between the long and medial head of triceps. I wind round the spiral groove, pierce the lateral intermuscular septum at the junction of the distal third and the middle third, and come to lie in the anterior compartment of the arm. Here I lay between the brachioradialis and extensor carpi radialis longus and at the level of the lateral epicondyle, I split into superficial branch and posterior interosseous nerve. Superficial branch is my direct continuation, which runs distally in the forearm under cover of brachioradialis and about two inches above the wrist it pierces the deep fascia, turns dorsally and laterally, and reaches the dorsum of the hand supplying three and half fingers until the level of middle phalanges. My posterior interosseous branch penetrates the supinator muscle through the arcade of Frohse, runs distally in the forearm, and lies on the interosseous membrane. It ends as a pseudoganglion over the wrist joint. I supply the following muscles in my course (Fig. 25.17):
- *Above the spiral groove:* All the three heads of triceps and anconeus.
- *In the spiral groove:* I give off three cutaneous branches, posterior cutaneous nerve of the arm, posterior cutaneous nerve of the forearm and lower lateral cutaneous nerve of the arm.
- *Between the spiral groove and lateral epicondyle:* I supply brachialis, brachioradialis, and extensor carpi radialis longus.
- *Before piercing the supinator:* I supply extensor carpi radialis brevis and part of supinator.
- In the supinator I supply the rest of it. After emerging out of the supinator, I supply all the remaining extensor muscles of the forearm and abductor pollicis longus.

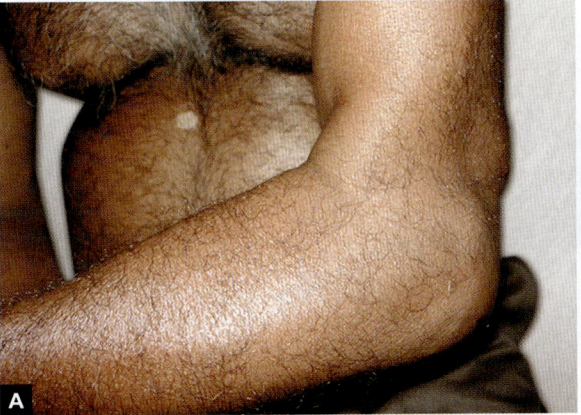
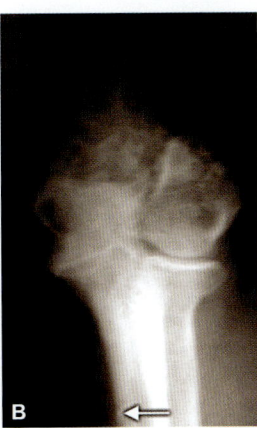
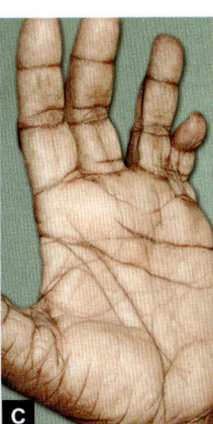
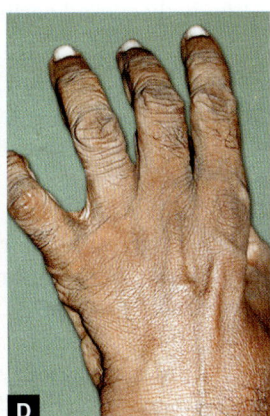

Figs 25.16A to D: X-ray showing malunited lateral condyle fracture of the humerus leading to tardy ulnar palsy

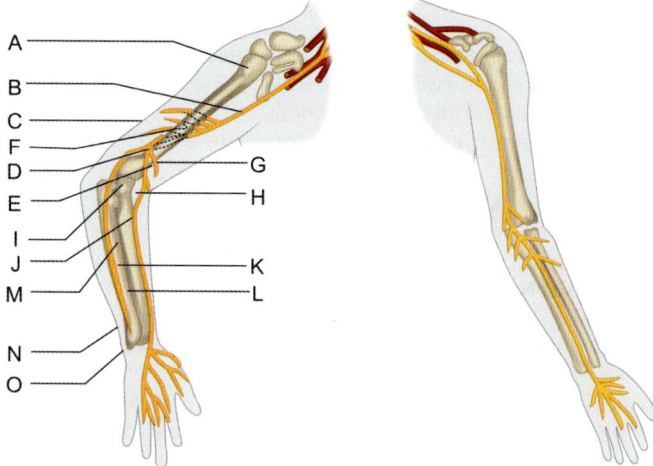

Fig. 25.17: Course and supply of radial nerve: (A) Medial head of triceps, (B) Long head of triceps, (C) Lateral head of triceps, (D) Brachioradialis, (E) Extensor carpi radialis longus, (F) Extensor carpi radialis brevis, (G) Anconeus, (H) Supinator, (I) Extensor digitorum longus, (J) Extensor digitorum minimi, (K) Extensor carpi ulnaris, (L) Abductor pollicis longus, (M) Extensor pollicis longus, (N) Extensor pollicis brevis, and (O) Extensor indices

Thus, you can say that I supply all the muscles on the lateral and dorsal aspects of the forearm, except the brachioradialis and extensor caropiradialis longus, through the posterior interosseous branch of mine.

Radial Nerve can be Entrapped at the Following Sites:
- In the arm—fibrous arch of lateral head of triceps.
- In the forearm—arcade of Frohse.
- At the elbow—radial tunnel syndrome at origin of extensor carpir adialis brevis.
- At the wrist—scar tissue compressing the superficial radial nerve.

Causes for Radial Nerve Injury

General
Already discussed earlier.

Local
In the axilla
- Aneurysm of the axillary vessels
- Crutch palsy.

In the shoulder
- Proximal humeral fractures
- Shoulder dislocation.

In the spiral groove 5'S
- Shaft fracture
- Saturday night palsy (Fig. 25.18)
- Syringe palsy (Fig. 25.19)
- Surgical positions (Trendelenburg)
- 'S'march's (Esmarch) tourniquet palsy.

Saturday night palsy (Also called weekend palsy)
In this condition, there is compression of the radial nerve between the radio-spiral groove and the lateral intermuscular septum.

It is known after an event which typically happens on a Saturday night weekend when in an inebriated condition, a person slumps with his mid-arm compressed between the arm of the chair and his body (see Fig. 25.17).

Did You Know About Honeymoon Palsy?
- You have heard about Saturday night palsy, but have you heard about honeymoon palsy?
- Well, it is sleep palsy and is seen in young couples where a bed partner's head compresses the radial nerve, while resting in the crook of the partner's arms!

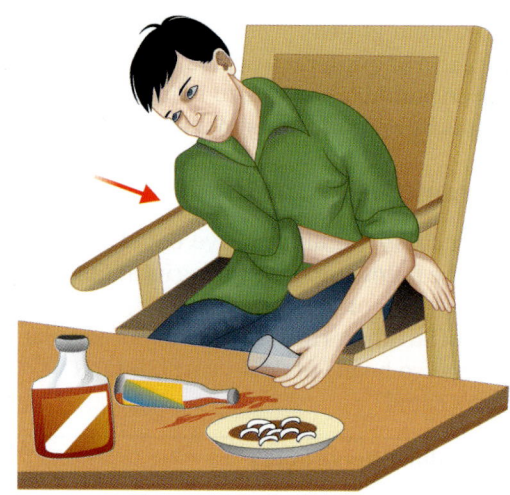

Fig. 25.18: Saturday night palsy (Patient's mistake)

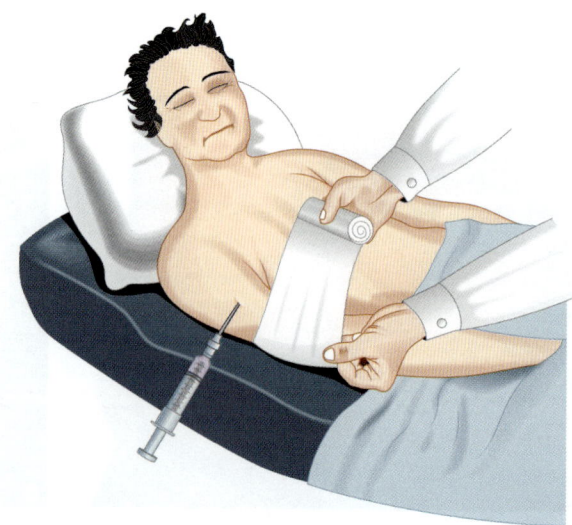

Fig. 25.19: Injection and tourniquet palsy (Doctor's mistake)

Between Spiral Groove and Lateral Epicondyle

- Fracture shaft humerus (Fig. 25.20)
- Supracondylar fracture humerus
- Lateral epicondyle fracture of the humerus
- Penetrating and gunshot injuries
- Cubitus valgus deformity.

At the elbow
- Posterior dislocation of the elbow
- Fracture head of radius
- Monteggia fractures.

Causes in the forearm
- Fracture both bones forearm
- Penetrating and gunshot injuries.

Levels of Lesion

Levels of Lesion	Features
High: Above spiral groove *Low:* Type I	Total palsy
Between: The spiral groove and the lateral epicondyle	*Spared:* Elbow extensor *Lost:* Motor • Wrist extensor • Thumb extensor • Finger extensors *Sensory:* Dorsum of first Web space
Low: Type II Below the elbow	*Spared* • Elbow extensor • Wrist extensor *Lost:* Motor • Thumb extensor • Finger extensor *Sensation* first web space

Clinical Features

If the lesion is high, the patient will present with wrist drop (Fig. 25.21), thumb drop and finger drop. He will be unable to extend the elbow. If the lesion is low the elbow extension is spared; but the wrist, thumb, and the finger extensions are lost, but *the patient can extend the IP joints of the fingers because of the action of the intrinsic muscles of the hand*. Sensation along the posterior surface of the arm and forearm is lost in high lesions and in low lesions the above sensations are spared, but there is loss of sensation over the first dorsal web space.

In acute injuries, it is difficult to evaluate the injury to the radial nerve. In such situations, the Hitchhiker's sign (inability to extend the thumb) is used as the screening test.

Investigations

Radiograph of the injured part and all other investigations mentioned in the general principles are carried out.

Treatment (Flowchart 25.2)

Early cases: As mentioned in the general principles for closed fractures, conservative treatment is adopted. The patient is put on a cock-up splint or dynamic splints (see Figs 25.4, 25.22 and 25.23). This is followed by active and passive physiotherapy. In failed conservative treatment, operative treatment is considered after a period of 12–18 months.

In open fractures, surgery is the treatment of choice. If the wound is clean, primary nerve repair is done, and if the wound is contaminated, delayed primary or secondary nerve repair is resorted to.

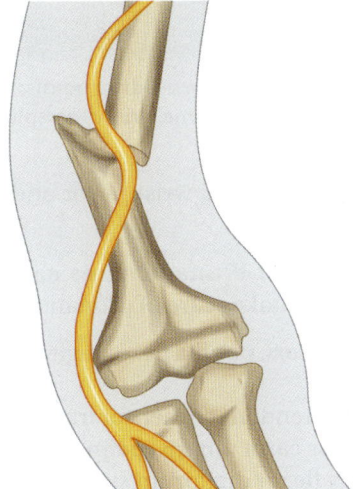

Fig. 25.20: Entrapment of radial nerve in between the fracture fragments of the humerus (nobody's mistake)

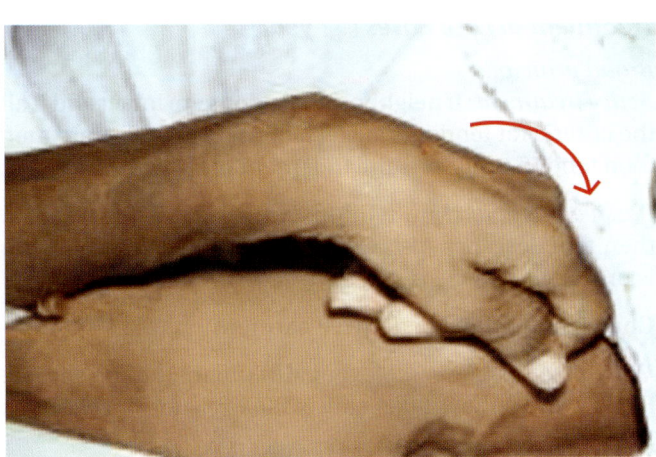

Fig. 25.21: Wrist drop (Clinical photo)

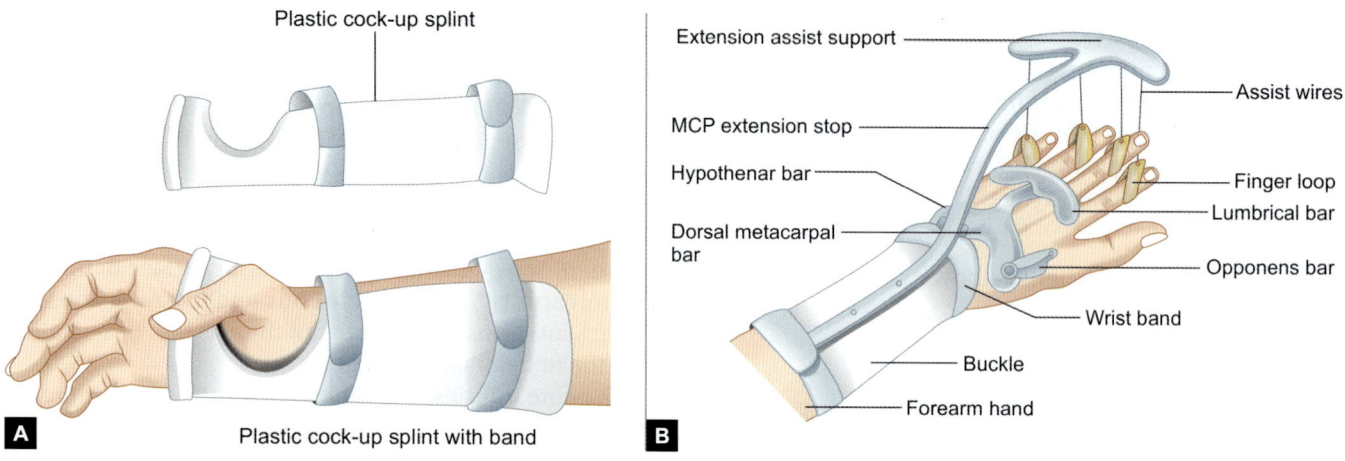

Figs 25.22A and B: Wrist drop splints: (A) Static or cock-up splint; (B) Dynamic splint

Flowchart 25.2: Treatment algorithm of radial nerve injury

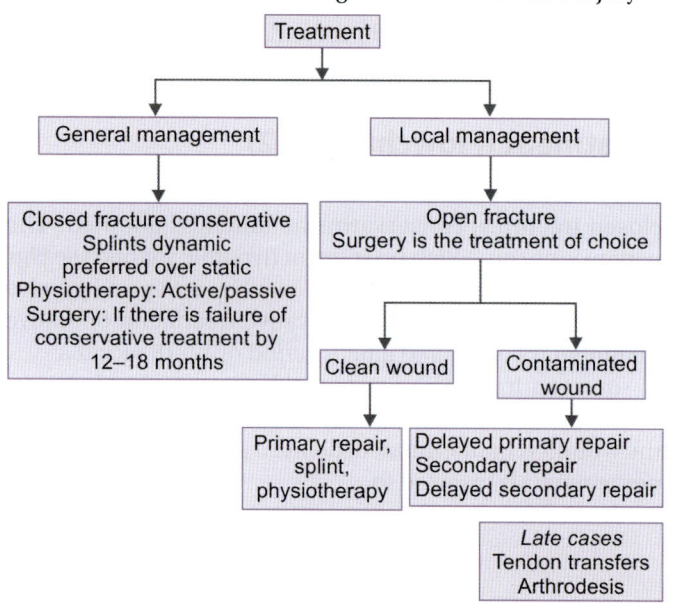

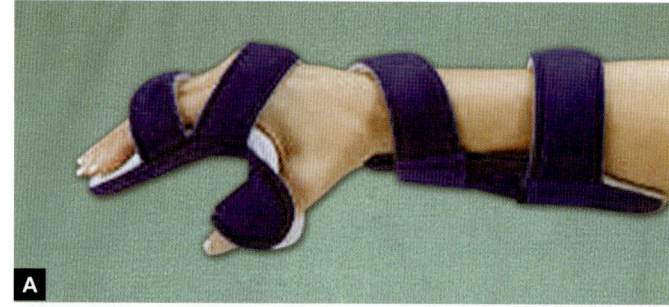

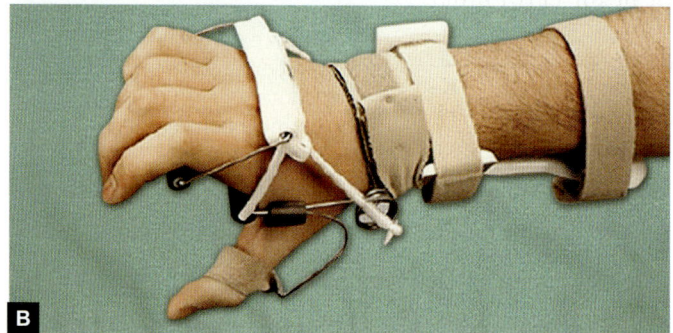

Figs 25.23A and B: Types of wrist drop points: (A) Static wrist splint; (B) Dynamic wrist drop splint

Treatment of Late Cases (>1 year)

Broad principles
Active treatment: If neighboring tendons are intact and if all the criteria for tendon transfers mentioned earlier are met, then tendon transfer is the treatment of choice.

Passive method: If no tendons are available for transfer, then tenodesis or wrist arthrodesis in functional position is preferred.

Choice of tendons in active treatment

From the wrist flexors: Flexor carpi ulnaris can be spared. Flexor carpi radialis takes care of the wrist flexion. Palmaris longus is not a very strong wrist flexor and hence can be spared.

From the pronators: Pronator teres can be spared as pronator quadratus takes care of pronation.

From the finger flexors, rarely a flexor digitorum superficialis can be chosen.

Therefore, the tendons chosen for transfer in radial nerve injuries are flexor carpi ulnaris, palmaris longus, pronator teres, and rarely flexor digitorum superficialis.

Tendon Transfer Techniques

High lesion: For elbow extension transfer of latissimus dorsi or pectoralis major to the triceps muscle can be done, if the patient needs active extension to use the crutches. Otherwise, gravity alone helps in passive extension of the elbow and is sufficient if the patient does not prefer to use the crutches.

Low lesions

Type I
- For wrist extension ° pronator teres transfer.
- For finger extension ° flexor carpi ulnaris split into four slips and transferred dorsally into four fingers.
- For thumb extension and abduction ° palmaris longus transfer.

Type II: Here wrist extension is spared and hence the plan is:
- For finger extension ° flexor carpi ulnaris transfer (split into 4 slips).
- For thumb extension ° palmaris longus transfer.
- For thumb abduction ° pronator teres transfer.

Omer's technique: Consists of splitting flexor carpi ulnaris into five slips and transferring into all the five fingers instead of four.

Boye's technique: Uses flexor digitorum superficialis instead of flexor carpi ulnaris to bring about extension of four fingers.

> **Problems in Radial Nerve Injury**
> - Wrist drop
> - Thumb drop
> - Finger drop only at MCP joint but extension at IP joint is possible due to action of interossei
> - Sensation over dorsal first web space is lost
> - In high lesions inability to extend the elbow and loss of sensations over posterior surface of arm and forearm are additional problems.

> **Radial Nerve Injury at a Glance**
> - Continuation of posterior cord of the brachial plexus.
> - Most common peripheral nerve to be injured.
> - Most common site of injury is the distal end of humerus.
> - Thumb extension test (Hitchhiker's sign) is the screening test.
> - In radial nerve injury extension at finger IP joint is still possible.
> - For early cases in closed fractures conservative treatment.
> - For open fractures operative treatment and repair.
> - For late cases, tendon transfers if neighboring tendons are available and if all the criteria are met.
> - If no tendons are available, wrist arthrodesis is done in functional position.

> **Interesting Nerve Palsies Concerning Radial Nerve**
> Did you know about handcuff palsy, dog handler's palsy, or Cheiralgia paresthetica?
> Well, all these are due to compression of the sensory branch of the superficial radial nerve at the level of the distal one-third of the forearm where it pierces the deep fascia and becomes dorsal.

INJURY TO SCIATIC NERVE

> **The Sciatic Nerve Speaks**
> I am the **thickest** nerve in the body with a root value of $L_{4,5}$ $S_{1,2,3}$. I enter the glutei region through the greater sciatic notch and pass between the greater trochanter of femur and ischial tuberosity. From here, I enter the thigh and in the middle, I divide into *common peroneal* and *the tibial part*. Before doing so, I supply biceps, semitendinosus, semimembranosus, and adductor magnus. The *common peroneal part is the smaller of* my two terminal divisions. This runs along the medial border of biceps, leaves the popliteal fossa at the lateral angle, passes behind the head of the fibula, winds round the neck and divides into *superficial (musculocutaneous nerve)* and *deep peroneal nerve*. The superficial nerve descends in the substance of peroneus longus and supplies the peroneal muscles, skin over the lower part of front of the leg, whole of the dorsum of the foot except the first web space and most of the toes. The deep peroneal nerve supplies all the four muscles of the anterior compartment and divides into *medial terminal branch* and *lateral terminal branch*. The former supplies the first web space (Fig. 25.24) and the latter *ends as a ganglion* after supplying extensor digitorum brevis and second dorsal interosseous. The medial terminal branch also supplies the first dorsal interossei.
>
> The tibial component of mine supplies muscles of the posterior compartment of the leg and provides cutaneous distribution to the entire sole of the foot (Fig. 25.25).

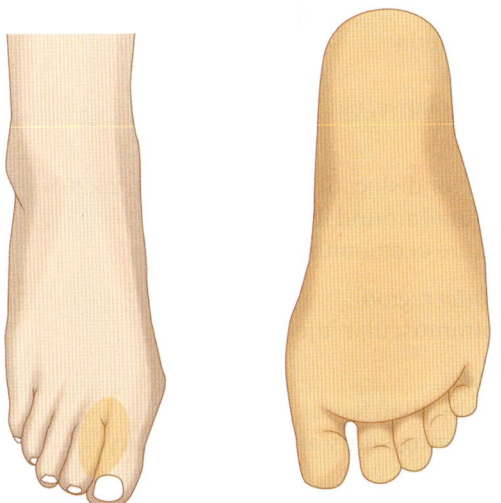

Fig. 25.24: Dorsal web space is supplied by anterior tibial nerve. Sole of the foot is by posterior tibial nerve

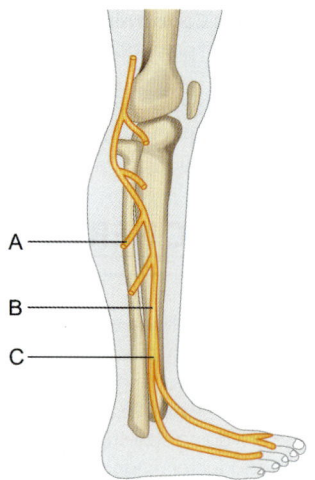

Fig. 25.25: Course and supply of common peroneal (lateral popliteal) nerve; (A) Tibialis anterior, (B) Extensor hallucis longus, (C) Extensor digitorum longus

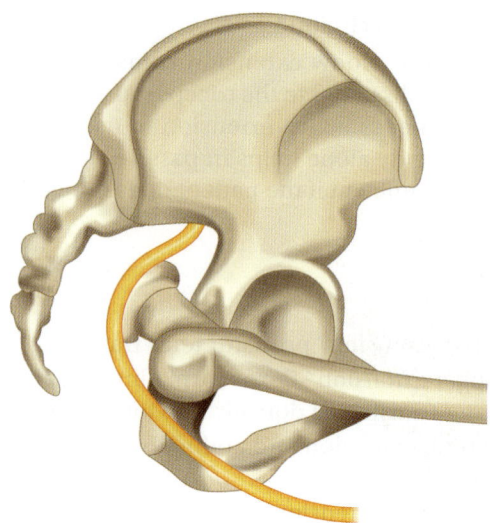

Fig. 25.26: Injury to sciatic nerve due to posterior dislocation of hip joint

FOOT-DROP

Causes of Foot-drop

General

Causes have been already mentioned, the important one being leprosy as a cause of foot-drop.

Local

Causes are seen along the course of the nerve.

At the spine
- Spina bifida
- Tumors
- Disk prolapse, etc.

At the hip
- Posterior dislocation of the hip (Fig. 25.26)
- Fractures around the hip
- Fracture acetabulum.

At the glutei region
Deep intramuscular injections.

At the thigh
- Fracture shaft femur
- Penetrating injury and gunshot injury.

At the knee (Common causes)
- Forcible inversion of the knee
- Dislocation of knee.
- Fracture lateral condyle of tibia
- Lateral meniscal cysts and tumors
- Dislocation of superior tibiofibular joint
- Tight plaster casts around the knee
- Poor padding during traction
- Surgical damage during application of skeletal traction.
- *Direct injuries*—gunshot injuries, incised and penetrating injuries, etc.

Levels of Lesion	
High lesion (Above knee)	Both tibial nerve and common peroneal nerve is paralyzed
Low lesion (Below knee)	*Spared:* Peroneus longus and brevis
Type I Anterior tibial nerve injury	*Lost:* Tibialis anterior, extensor hallucis longus, extensor digitorum longus and peroneus tertius *Sensation:* Over first web space is lost
Type II Musculocutaneous nerve injury	*Spared:* All the above muscles innervated by anterior tibial nerve *Lost:* Peroneus longus and brevis *Sensation:* Over outer leg and foot.

Clinical Features

The resulting deformity following injury to the above nerves is foot-drop. This could either be complete (in sciatic nerve or lateral popliteal nerve injury) or incomplete (injury to either superficial or deep peroneal nerve).

In high lesions, it is a total foot-drop and in low lesions, the foot-drop is usually incomplete. In low type I, the patient cannot dorsiflex and invert the foot but eversion is possible, front of the leg is wasted (Fig. 25.27). In low type II, the patient cannot evert but can dorsiflex and invert the foot. There is wasting of the outer half of the leg (Fig. 25.28).

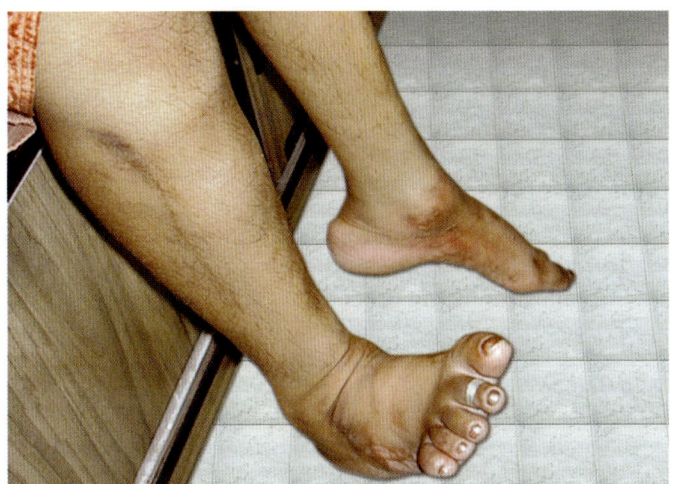

Fig. 25.27: Clinical photo showing right foot-drop

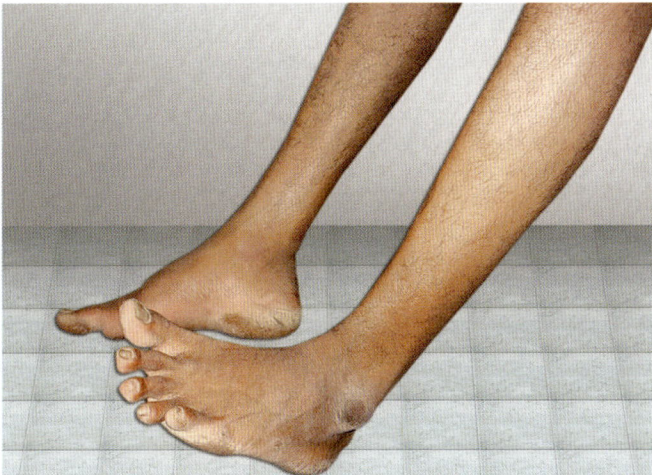

Fig. 25.28: Foot-drop (Clinical photo) showing wasting of muscles

Flowchart 25.3: Treatment algorithm of foot-drop

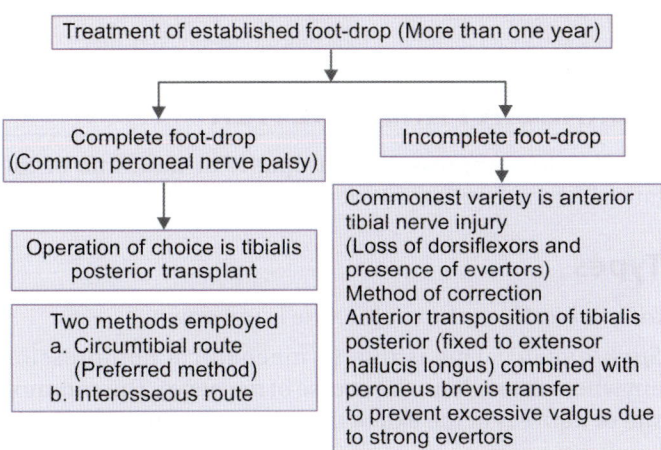

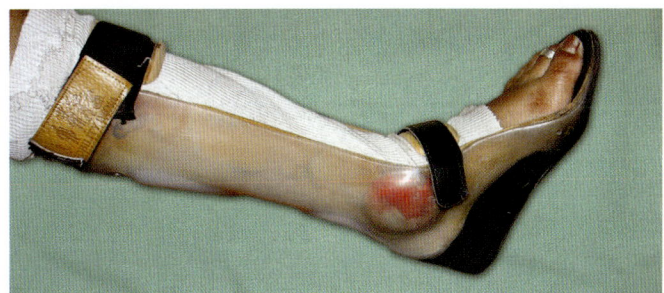

Fig. 25.29: Showing static foot-drop splint

In type I, injury sensation over the dorsal web space is lost and in type II, injury it is lost over outer leg and foot. The gait typical of foot-drop is a *high stepping gait*.

Treatment (Flowchart 25.3)

Early

The lesions show a high incidence of recovery. Hence, conservative treatment with a view to encourage recovery (at least for 1 year) should be carried out.

Splintage of knee in 20° of flexion and ankle in 90° for night-time. In the daytime, walking is allowed by using a "Foot-drop appliance."

Foot-drop appliances are of two varieties (Figs 25.29 and 25.30):
- Dynamic—spring shoe (Fig. 25.31)
- Static—backstop shoe (Fig. 25.32).

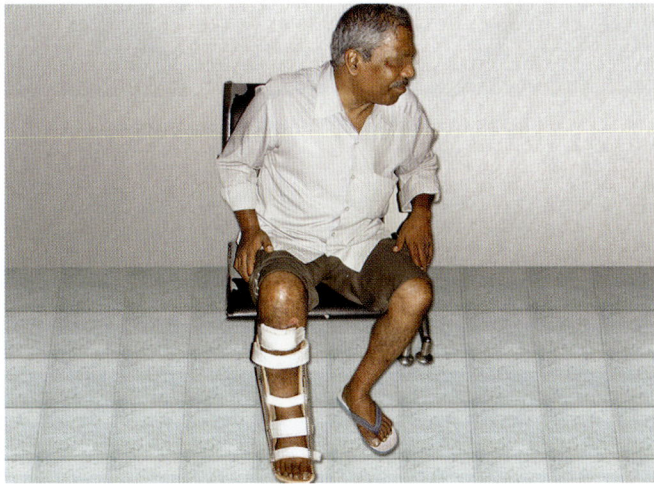

Fig. 25.30: Dynamic foot-drop splint

Along with the splintage, general treatment to correct the underlying etiology is undertaken. Steroids are also known to help.

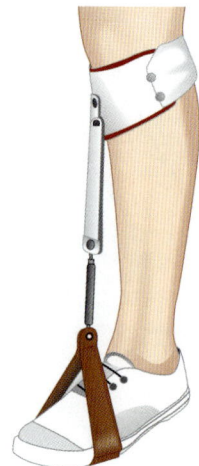

Fig. 25.31: Dynamic foot-drop splint

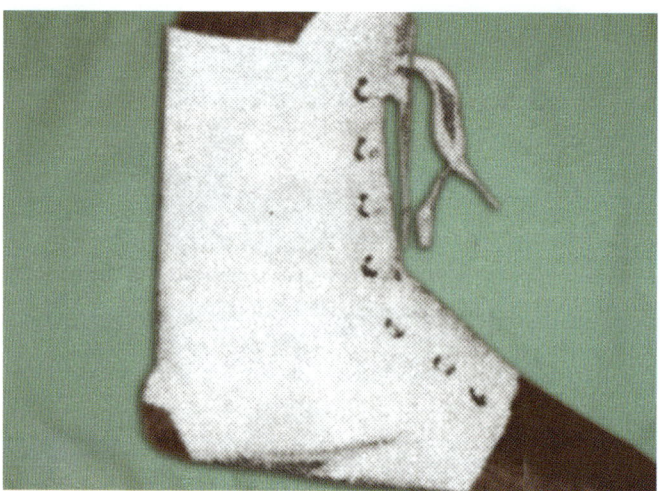

Fig. 25.32: Foot-drop splint (Static variety)

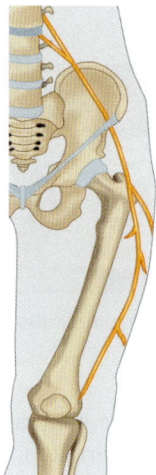

Fig. 25.33: Course of the lateral femoral cutaneous nerve

Late

Common peroneal nerve stripping is done in leprosy. It is done in a thickened, tender nerve in a tuberculoid case with history of recent paralysis.

Choice of Surgery

- Tendon transfers—for mobile foot-drop.
- Tendo-Achilles lengthening—in fixed equinus.
- Subtalar stabilizing procedure—for fixed varus.
- Triple arthrodesis—for fixed varus at the subtalar joint.

> **At a Glance**
> - Sciatic nerve is the thickest nerve in the body.
> - Common peroneal nerve also called as lateral popliteal nerve is commonly injured at the fibular neck.
> - Leprosy is the commonest general cause
> - Foot-drop could be complete or incomplete
> - High stepping gait is characteristic
> - Dynamic foot-drop splint is the mainstay of conservative treatment
> - Conservative treatment is indicated up to one year
> - Tendon transfer for mobile foot-drop contemplated after 1 year.

MERALGIA PARESTHETICA

It is due to compression neuropathy or neuroma of the lateral femoral cutaneous nerve (Fig. 25.33).

Types

Idiopathic: Here, the exact cause is unknown.

Spontaneous: This is due to mechanical compression anywhere throughout the course of the nerve. The common site of injury is at the exit of the nerve at the pelvis.

Iatrogenic: This is commonly seen after orthopedic surgeries like anterior iliac crest bone grafting and anterior pelvic procedures and prone positioning for surgeries.

Clinical Features

This is characterized by pain, numbness, and paresthesia along the anterolateral aspect of the thigh.

Diagnostic Test

If there is relief of pain and paresthesia after injecting local anesthetic, the diagnosis is clinched.

Treatment

Conservative

Idiopathic type: Improves by removal of the compressive agents, non-steroidal anti-inflammatory drugs, and local steroid injection.

Iatrogenic type: Care should be exercised during pelvic surgery.

Operative

If pain persists in spite of the above treatment, surgery is indicated. The procedures include neurolysis or transection of the nerves.

BRACHIAL PLEXUS INJURIES

Everything about brachial plexus is complex, its anatomy (Fig. 25.34), mode of injury, the diagnosis, management, and prognosis. It is a narrowing experience for both the patient and the surgeon. Among the more famous causes of brachial plexus, injury is the birth injury in children and bike injury in adults.

> **Note:**
> 2B's: **B**irth injury in children
> **B**irth injury in adults

Causes

Brachial Plexus Injuries (Figs 25.35A and B) could be:

Closed: Here the injury could be due to birth trauma or bike trauma as mentioned above.

Open: It is a rare injury and could be due to penetrating or gunshot injuries.

> **Note:**
> Other less important causes of brachial plexus injuries:
> - Traction injuries
> - Tumor removal
> - Abnormal pressures due to faculty postures
> - Postirradiation scenario
> - Surgical excision of cervical ribs
> - Shoulder dislocations.

TYPES OF LESIONS

Supraclavicular Lesion

Preganglionic Lesion

This is an unfortunate situation wherein the nerve roots are avulsed from the spinal cord. The cause could be either birth or bike trauma as mentioned earlier. The characteristic feature of this lesion is the presence of Horner's syndrome (Fig. 25.36).

> **Interesting Facts: About Horner's Syndrome**
> What constitutes a Horner's syndrome? (All P's)
> - Ptosis of the eyelid
> - Pupils, which are small and constricted

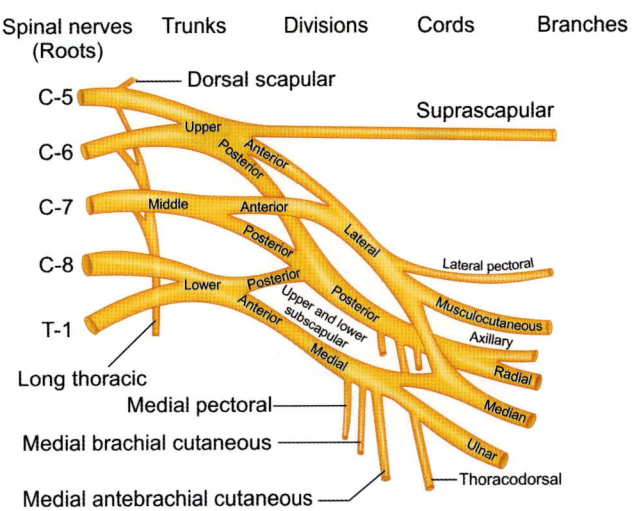

Fig. 25.34: The normal anatomy of brachial plexus

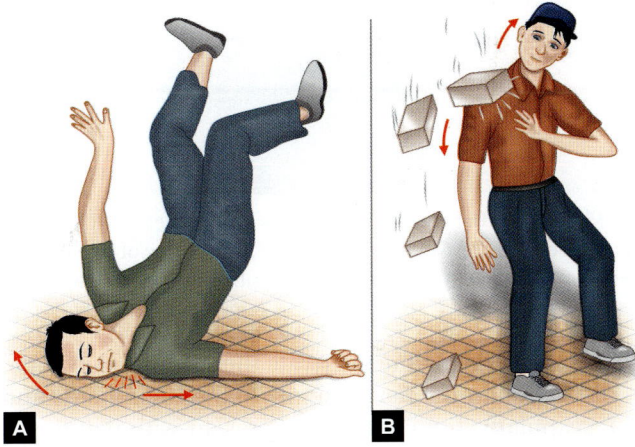

Figs 25.35A and B: Mechanism of brachial plexus injury

> - Protrusion of the eyeball, which is slight
> - Pain even at rest
> - Positive sensory action potentials
> - Poor prognosis.

Postganglionic Lesions

Here there is no Horner's syndrome. The prognosis is slightly better than the preganglionic lesion. A positive Tinel's sign may be elicited in this lesion.

Clinical Assessment of Brachial Plexus Injury

It is important to assess whether the brachial plexus injury is pre-ganglionic or postganglionic.

In preganglionic lesions
- Horner's syndrome is present (Fig. 25.36A).

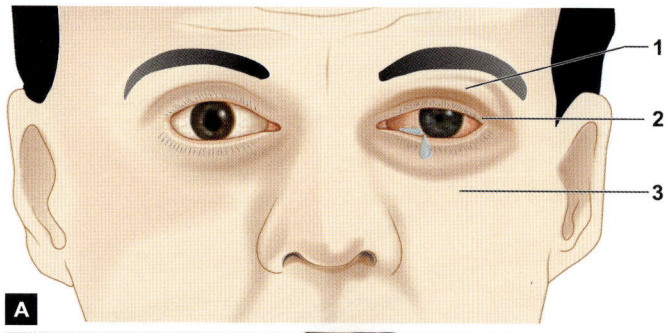

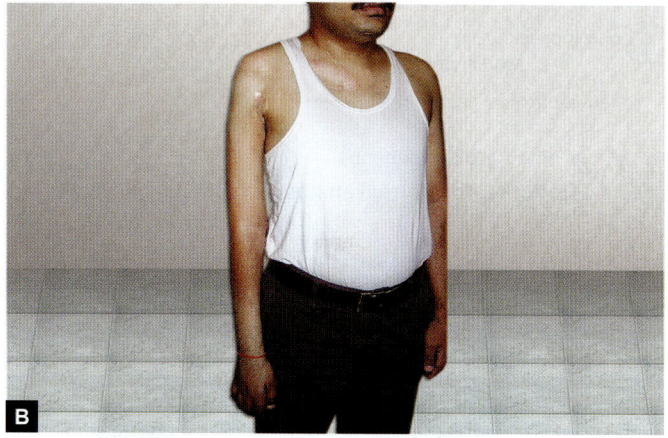

Figs 25.36A and B: Features of Horner's syndrome: (A) (1) Drooping of the eyelid, (2) Constricted pupil, (3) Absence of sweating in the surrounding skin; (B) Flail upper limb (Clinical photo)

- The patient is unable to elevate the scapula (due to the disruption in the nerve supply to the Rhomboids and L scapulae). The patient may present with flail upper limb (Fig. 25.36B).

In postganglionic lesions
- No Horner's syndrome.
- The patient is able to elevate the scapula.
- Tinel's sign is present in the later stages.
  (Tapping above the clavicle, produces tingling sensation in the anesthetic limb).

Investigations

These are less reliable than the clinical tests. However, X-ray to rule out neck fractures, CT scan to study the cross-section anatomy, MRI to study the soft tissue damages, myelogram (shows meningocele in avulsion, but hazardous) and electrical studies are some of the investigations which give useful information during a brachial plexus injury.

The electrodiagnostic tests include EMG, nerve conduction study, SEP (somatosensory-evoked potential), percutaneous electrical stimulation, etc. EMG is by far the most reliable and effective test, which successfully identifies the roots, involved.

Treatment

During the Initial Stages

- *Splinting*
  - *For complete paralysis:* A flail arm splint (FAS) designed by Framton is advised (Fig. 25.37).
  - *For incomplete lesions:* Here splints with necessary modifications as per the situations can be used.

- For pain control, TENS is best suited
- To prevent contractures and deformities, a careful passive ROM exercises under suitable guidance is recommended.

> **Quick Facts: About FAS**
> - It immobilizes the shoulder in abduction
> - It prevents glenohumeral joint subluxation
> - It permits five different positions of the elbow
> - It provides a platform for the forearm on which split hook, etc. can be applied
> - It can be operated through a cable to the shoulder strap attached to the opposite normal limb
> - It is cosmetically acceptable.

During the Later Stages

Measures to strengthen the muscles: If there are movements, efforts are made to strengthen the muscles by repeated self-resistive exercises, PNF techniques, etc.

Re-education of the muscles: This is done by encouraging movements of the shoulder, percutaneous electrical stimulation, stimulating techniques like icing, brushing, etc.

Modifying: The splints and dynamizing it helps.

TENS to control pain.

After 2 years, reconstructive surgeries are planned for the residual paralysis and deformities.

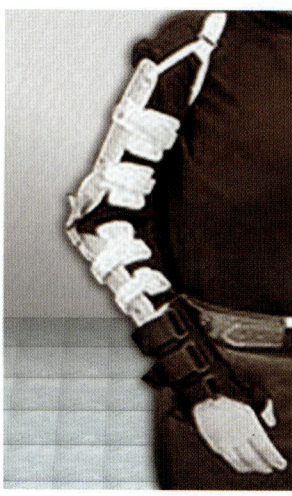

Fig. 25.37: Flail arm splint

Surgical Measures

Acute phases: In preganglionic lesions wherein the roots have avulsed from the cord, surgical exploration serves no purpose. However, suture or nerve grafting can be considered in postganglionic lesions.

Late stages (> 2 years): Reconstructive surgeries are planned after 2 years when the recovery can no longer take place. Surgeries are planned according to the residual paralysis.
- *For shoulder function:* Trapezius transfer to the neck of the humerus to improve abduction is advised.
   Arthrodesis of the shoulder is done in functional position.
- *For elbow function:* Steindler's flexorplasty (transfer of latissimus dorsi or pectoralis major to biceps).
- *For wrist and finger extension:* After the surgery, the patient is put on a detailed regime for re-educating the transplanted muscle.

ERB'S PALSY

This is due to injury to the C_5 nerve root and rarely the C_6 nerve root is injured. It occurs either very early in life due to birth trauma (obstetric palsy, due to faulty application of forceps) or in young adults due to bike trauma.

Effects of the Injury

At the shoulder here, there is paralysis of the deltoid, rhomboids, supra- and infraspinatus and teres minor muscles. This results in the loss of shoulder abduction and external rotation.

At the elbow, biceps and brachialis muscles are paralyzed. This results in loss of flexion of the elbow joint.

At the forearm: Supinator, muscles are paralyzed resulting in loss of supination of the forearm.

Clinical Features

The combined effect of the injury is an arm hanging loosely by the side of the trunk. The shoulder is internally rotated, the elbow is in extension, the forearm is pronated, and the wrist is in flexion. This characteristic posture is popularly known as *Policeman or Waiter's tip* (Fig. 25.38). Apart from this, there may be sensory loss on the outer aspects of the arm and forearm both in the front and back.

Management

Splinting

This is done by using an abduction or aeroplane splint. (Fig. 25.39) The shoulder is maintained in abduction

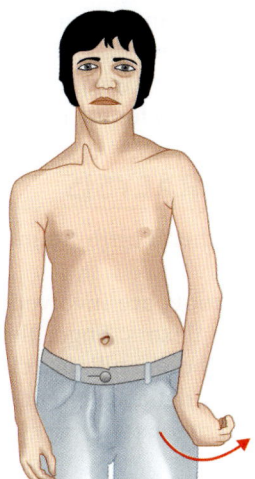

Fig. 25.38: Waiter's or Porter's tip position in Erb's palsy

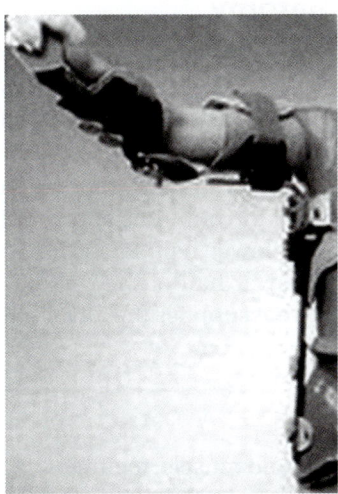

Fig. 25.39: Aeroplane splint

and external rotation, elbow in 90° of flexion, forearm in supination and wrist in extension.

Measures to Prevent Contractures

A full range of passive movements to the affected joints helps prevent the contractures. This is a home treatment program and should be taught to the mother.

Electrical

Stimulation of the affected muscles by using bilaterally symmetrical PNF stimulus helps to activate them.

Surgery

This is rarely indicated as most of the cases recover spontaneously with the above treatment. Some of the recommended surgical measures are:
- Exploration and repair of the nerve roots

- Tendon transfers to improve abduction and external rotation of the shoulder
- Release of soft tissue contractures
- De-rotation osteotomy for the rotational deformity.

KLUMPKE'S PARALYSIS

This is also due to either a birth trauma or a bike trauma (Fig. 25.40).

The $C_8 T_1$ nerve roots are involved and there will be paralysis of the wrist flexors, finger flexors, and intrinsic muscles of the hand. These results in a claw hand deformity. The clinical features and management are discussed in the section on ulnar and median nerve injuries.

AXILLARY NERVE INJURY

Relevant Anatomy

It takes origin from the posterior cord of the brachial plexus and winds round the lower border of the subscapularis. It goes through the quadrangular space and lies medial to the surgical neck of the humerus and divides into anterior and posterior branches. The anterior branch winds around the surgical neck of the humerus and supplies the deltoid muscle except the lower half. Posterior branch supplies the teres minor, lower half of the deltoid and ends as a cutaneous nerve that supplies the lower half of the deltoid region.

Clinical Features

Wasting of the deltoid muscle, regiment badge anesthesia, inability of the patient to abduct the shoulder are some of the classical features.

Investigations

Electrodiagnostic tests help in the accurate detection of the site and extent of the lesion.

Treatment

Treatment is essentially conservative management followed by physiotherapy and exercises.

INJURY TO THE LONG THORACIC NERVE (Winging of the Scapula)

Highlights
- It is also called as scapula alata
- Here the medial border of the scapula is positioned laterally and posteriorly.
- It is called as winged scapula because the inferior angle of the scapula protrudes backwards instead of lying flat.

Causes

- Weakness of the serratus anterior muscles
- Impingement of the long thoracic nerve
- Damaged trapezius muscle or denervation of its nerve supply
- This may be due to injury to the above structures due to repetitive lifting, fall on the shoulders, sports injuries, brachial plexus neuropathies, iatrogenic division of the long thoracic nerve, severe traumatic depression of the shoulder, facioscapulohumeral dystrophy, fall from the bike, etc.

Relevant Clinical Findings

- Classical winged deformity (Fig. 25.41).
- On pushing against the wall the scapula stands out prominently.
- There may be difficulty in lifting the arm above the head.

Treatment

Conservative treatment consists of physiotherapy, exercises, and shoulder rehabilitation.

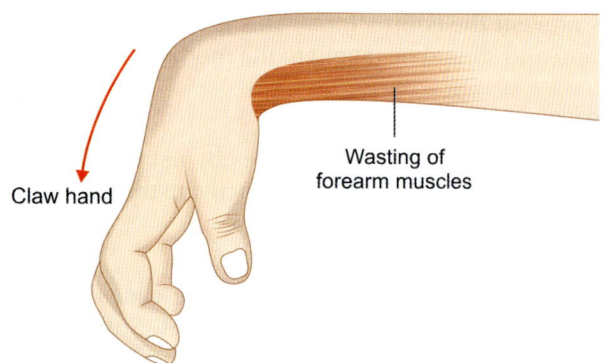

Fig. 25.40: Klumpke's paralysis

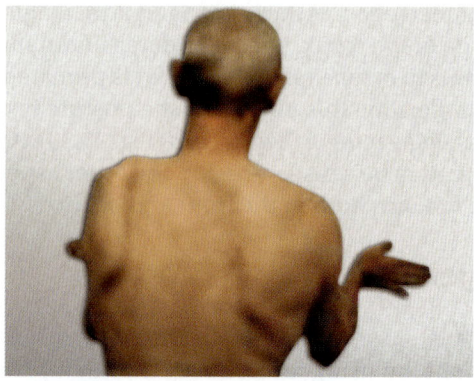

Fig. 25.41: Winging of the scapula (Clinical photo)

Surgical treatment is recommended in resistant cases. The recommended procedures are pectoralis major muscle transfer in isolated serratus anterior palsy or scapulodesis in failed transfers.

BIBLIOGRAPHY

1. Bunnel S. Surgery of the Hand (3rd edn), Philadelphia: JB Lippincott Co; 1956.
2. Grossman MD, Ducey SA, et al. Meralgia Paraesthetica.
3. Kahn EA. Direct observation of sweating in peripheral nerve injuries. Surg Gynecol Obstet. 1951;92:22.
4. Leffert RD. Brachial plexus traction injuries. Clin Orthop. 1988;237:24.
5. Lewi SD, Miller EM. Peripheral nerve injuries associated with fractures. Ann Surg. 1922;76:528.
6. Moldarcer J. Tind's sign: Its characteristics and significancies: J Bone JA Surg. 1978;60-A:412.
7. Mukherjee SR. Tensile strength of nerves during healing. Br J Surg. 1953;41:192.
8. Ober FR. Tendon transplantation in the lower extremity. N Engl J Med. 1933;209:52.
9. Omer GE, Spinner M. Peripheral nerve testing and suture techniques. In American Academy of Orthopedic Surgeons, Instructional Course Lectures. St Louis: CV Mosby Co; 1975.p.24.
10. Perry WB. Rehabilitation of the hand (4th edn). Butterworths: London; 1981.pp.126-44.
11. Seddon HJ. Three types of nerve injury. Brain. 1943;66:237.
12. Seddon HJ. The practical value of peripheral nerve repair. Proc R Soc Med. 1949;42:427.
13. Seddon HJ. Nerve grafting. J Bone Joint Surg. 1963;45-B:447.
14. Sunderland S. A classification of peripheral nerve injuries producing loss of function. Brain. 1951;74:491.
15. Sunderland S. Nerve and nerve injuries, Baltimore. The Williams and Wilkins Co; 1968.
16. Watson-Jones R. Primary nerve lesion injuries of the elbow and wrist. J Bone Joint Surg. 1930;12:121.

SECTION 3
Nontraumatic Orthopedic Disorders

- Approach to Orthopedic Disorders
- Deformities and their Management
- Treatment of Orthopedic Disorders
- Regional Conditions of the Neck
- Regional Conditions of the Upper Limb
- Regional Conditions of the Spine
- Regional Conditions of the Lower Limb
- Disorders of the Hand

SECTION 3

Nontraumatic Orthopedic Disorders

26 CHAPTER

Approach to Orthopedic Disorders

As in other branches of medicine, the diagnosis of orthopedic disorders revolves around the following fundamentals (Fig. 26.1).

Therefore, we will try to discuss in brief the three steps of diagnosis in orthopedics.

HISTORY

History is "His- Story," as told by the patient. History taking is an art. Caution has to be exercised in the story "told" and the story "untold." Everything told should be taken with a pinch of salt lest the examiner is misled.

Certain Points of Importance in the History

Age Certain diseases have predilection age groups, e.g. Perthes' disease and acute osteomyelitis are common in children. Avascular necrosis and degenerative disorders are common in the elderly. Some diseases may be seen in all the age groups, e.g. tuberculosis of bone and joints.

Quick Facts: Age vs Orthopedic Disease
<1 year	Congenital dislocation of hip and cerebral palsy
1–2 years	Nutritional rickets
	Poliomyelitis
	Ewing's tumor
5–10 years	Tuberculosis of hip
	Perthes' disease
15–20 years	Slipped capital epiphysis
<15 years	Osteomyelitis
10–20 years	Bone malignancies
30–40 years	Rheumatoid arthritis
>40 yeas	Degenerative disorders
	Prolapsed intervertebral disk (PIVD)
	Multiple myeloma, etc.

Sex congenital dislocation of hip (CDH) is common in females. Congenital talipes equinovarus (CTEV) is more common in males.

Quick Facts: Sex vs Orthopedic Disease
- *Males:* Perthes' slipped epiphysis, traumatic disorders, multiple myeloma, etc.
- *Females:* Rheumatoid arthritis, CDH, osteoporosis, etc.

Onset: It may be sudden or gradual.

Trauma: It could be a predisposing factor or the causative factor.

Traumatic Points
Role of trauma vs orthopedic disorders
Trauma as a causative factor
- Fracture
- Dislocation
- Sprain
- Strain
- Subluxation

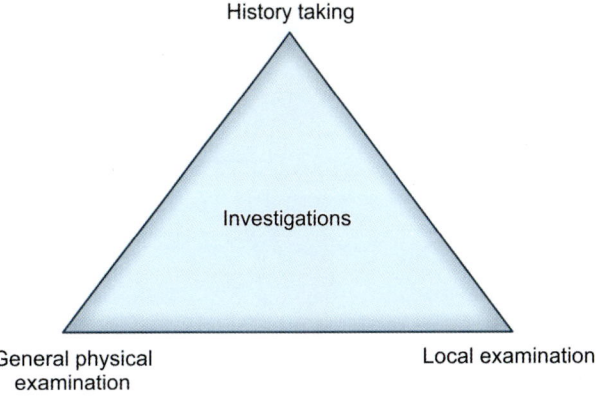

Fig. 26.1: Fundamentals of diagnosing orthopedic disorders

Trauma as a predisposing factor
- TB hip
- Perthes' disease
- Slipped capital epiphysis
- Osteogenic sarcoma
- Acute osteomyelitis, etc.

Fever: It may be high as in acute osteomyelitis or low grade as in tuberculosis.

Pain: This could be continuous or intermittent, low or high grade. One should be on guard about the radiating pains as these often mislead the examiner (Fig. 26.2).

Facts: About Radiating Pains

Region	Radiation sites
Cervical spine	Shoulder, arm, forearm, and fingertips
Upper limbs	
a. Shoulder	Arm and elbow
b. Elbow	Forearm
Thoracic spine	Girdle pains
Lumbar spine	Groin, buttocks, posterior thigh, legs and foot
Hip	Knee

Any constitutional problems: Like weight loss, anorexia, etc. if present are a pointer towards neoplasm, tuberculosis, etc.

Seasonal variation: If present, it is suggestive of rheumatoid disorders. Apart from these points, relevant past history, socioeconomic status and personal history should be taken into account.

An attempt should be now made to place the problem into one of the following categories at the end of history taking.

Is the problem congenital?
If so, it will be present since birth or seen within a few years from birth. A strong family history is elicitable.

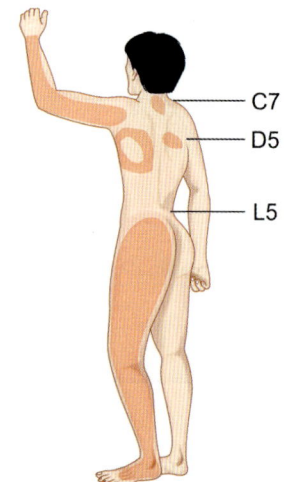

Fig. 26.2: Radiating pain at the upper limbs, chest and lower limbs

Is it developmental?
Here the disease is manifested during the process of development.

Is it an infective disorder?
History of fever, chills, rigors, sweating, etc. are present.

Is it inflammatory disorder?
Seasonal variation, remissions and exacerbation, multiple joint involvement, etc. are present.

Is it a metabolic disorder?
Nutrition, socioeconomic status, generalized skeletal disorder, etc. assume importance in this group.

Is it an endocrine disorder?
Look for other evidences of hormonal imbalance, e.g. Hypothyroidism → cretinism
Hypopituitarism → dwarf, etc.

Is it traumatic?
History of fall, road traffic accident (RTA), assault, etc. is elicited.

Is it degenerative?
Advancing age, slow progress is the hallmark.

Is it neoplastic?
Look for the features of either benign or malignant bone tumors.

If it cannot be categorized into any of the above, then it could be *idiopathic.*

Having made a tentative diagnosis at the end of history, next important step is resorted to.

Diagnostic Facts

• Present since birth	Congenital
• During the development process	Developmental
• History of fever, chills, rigors	Infective
• Nutrition, socioeconomic status	Metabolic
• Other evidences of hormonal imbalance	Endocrinal
• Seasonal variation, multiple joint involvement, etc.	Inflammatory
• History of RTA, fall, assault	Traumatic
• Features of either benign or malignant	Neoplastic
• Advancing age, etc.	Degenerative
• If no obvious complaints	Idiopathic

EXAMINATION

A good systematic clinical examination will help to clinch the diagnosis with certainty. *No sophisticated technology can replace the value of a good clinical examination.* A good clinician will make the diagnosis clinically and will make use of the investigation armamentarium judiciously. *A clinician should command the investigation and not vice versa.*

Examination of the locomotor system involves four steps.

STEP I

Examination of Gait

An examination of the gait is extremely important as it gives vital clues regarding the diagnosis.

Definition: It is a term used to describe the style of walking. This is dependent on not only normal muscles and joints but upon an intact central nervous system (CNS), peripheral nervous system and normal labyrinthine function.

Walking is divided into two phases.

The stance phase: This forms 60% of the gait and here the foot is on the ground (Figs 26.3A to C). It is further subdivided into:
- *Heel strike*—i.e. heel striking the ground.
- *Mid-stance*—here the foot is flat on the ground.
- *Push off*—here the foot is off the ground.

The swing phase: This forms 40% of the gait cycle and here the foot is not in contact with the ground (Figs 26.4A to C). It is further subdivided into:
- *Acceleration*—here leg is in front of the body.
- *Swing through*—here leg continues to swing forward.
- *Deceleration*—swing slows down and the heel is ready for the strike.

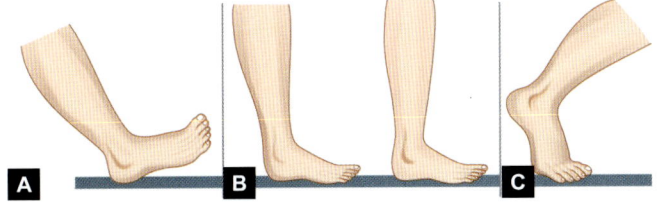

Figs 26.3A to C: Stance phase of gait: (A) Heel strike; (B) Mid-stance; (C) Push-off

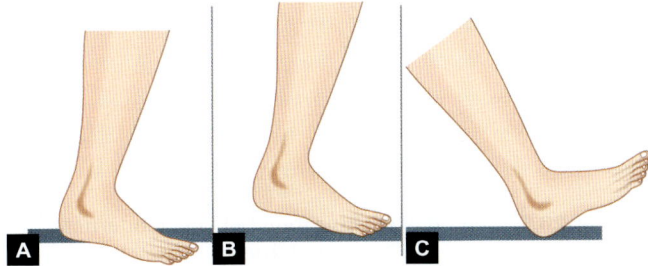

Figs 26.4A to C: Swing phase of gait: (A) Acceleration; (B) Swing through; (C) Deceleration

In normal gait, each leg alternatively goes through a stance phase and a swing phase. Thus, the body is carried forward in normal walking by these rhythmic cycles.

Running gait: Here the sequences are the same as in walking but are faster.

Types of Gait and Probable Diagnosis

Types	What happens	Probable diagnosis
Antalgic gait	Duration of stance phase decreased	Any painful lesion of foot, knee, hip, etc.
Gluteus medius gait	Lurch of body towards the affected side during every stance phase.	Paralysis of gluteus medius
Gluteus maximus gait	Backward lurch	Anterior polio
High stepping gait	To clear the dropped foot from the ground	Foot drop
Scissors gait	Legs cross while walking	Cerebral palsy
Short leg gait	When shortening >2"	Limb shortening (congenital or acquired)
Stiff hip gait	No flexion at hip	Septic arthritis at hip
Quadriceps gait	Limping gait with the hand on the knee	Polio
Trendelenburg gait	Pelvis drops on opposite side of the hip	e.g. congenital or old traumatic dislocation of hip joint, nonunion fracture neck of femur
Calcaneus gait	No push off	Calf weakness
Stiff knee gait	Pelvis raised during swing phase	Stiff knee
Ataxic gait	Child walks with legs apart	Spinal cerebellar ataxia
Hysterical gait	Seen in conversion hysteria	

STEP II

General Physical Examination

A good general physical examination (GPE) from head to toe gives vital clues in the diagnosis of most of the orthopedic disorders, particularly generalized disorders of the skeleton, e.g.
- Metabolic disorders, e.g. rickets, etc.
- Developmental disorders, e.g. osteogenesis imperfecta, etc.

STEP III

Clinical Examination

Symptoms

The following are the usual presenting symptoms in a patient with orthopedic disorder.

Pain: This is the first and the most common complaint. It is a highly subjective complaint and can be classified as mild, moderate, or severe.

The must-ask questions regarding the pain are how did it start? Is it related to trauma? Site of pain? Does it radiate? What are the aggravating and relieving factors? Does it interfere with sleep? etc.

Swelling: It may precede or follow pain. Relevant questions to be asked are site of the swelling, painful or painless. Is it rapidly growing (e.g. malignancy) or slow growing (benign growth)? Is it associated with fever, chills, etc. (e.g. infective origin), single or multiple (e.g. neurofibromas, etc.)?

Deformity: Sudden onset of deformity is usually seen in fresh fractures and dislocations. Long-standing deformities are usually seen in old fractures and other non-traumatic disorders like congenital, developmental, and metabolic conditions. The patient may complain of cosmetic and functional impairment due to the deformity.

Limitations of joint movements: In the initial stages, it may be due to muscle spasm; and in the later stages, it may be due to intra-articular adhesions (e.g. TB, septic arthritis, rheumatoid arthritis, etc.) or extra-articular contractures (like post-burn contractures, Volkmann's ischemic contracture, etc.).

Limp: This could be painful (e.g. arthritis of hip, trauma, etc.) or painless (e.g. CDH, Coxa Vara, etc.). The patient may complain of difficulty or alteration in various day-to-day activities like walking, squatting, running, working, etc.

Limb weakness: This may be due to disuse atrophy, motor problems like polio, motor neuron disease, etc., muscle problems like muscular dystrophies, etc., or due to peripheral or diabetic neuropathies.

Signs

General

Look for the signs of anemia, fever, weight loss, etc.

Local

Deformity: Deformity may be due to an abnormality of bone or joint. If a joint is out of its anatomical position, a deformity is said to exist. In addition, in case of bone, deviation from its normal anatomy is deformity. In cases of old fractures and dislocations, the deformity may be fixed.

> **Remember**
> A fixed deformity is the angle between the neutral position of the normal joint and the position the deformed joint will reach.

Temperature: This is always compared with the normal side. Check with dorsum of the hand, as this is the most sensitive part.

Tenderness: This is elicited by examining from the normal to the affected area and is graded I to IV (Fig. 26.5).

Swelling: The following things are noted in the examination of a swelling.

- Decide the anatomical plane. The plane of the swelling could be either bone (swelling decreases in size when muscle is put into contraction) or could be in the muscle (swelling slightly decreases in size and gets fixed on muscle contraction) or could be between the muscle and the skin (no change in the size at the swelling when muscle is put into contraction). Also, examine the level of the swelling and identify whether it is epiphyseal, metaphyseal, or diaphyseal (Figs 26.6A to D).
- Describe the shape as globular, oval or round, etc.
- Grade the consistency (*see* below).
- Decide whether it is congenital, neoplastic, etc.
- Look for slipping sign, sign of emptying, indentation sign, and expansile impulse.

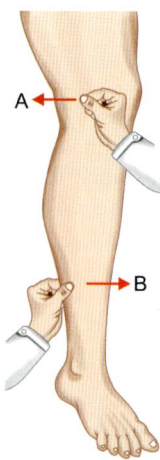

Fig. 26.5: Method of eliciting joint (A) Line tenderness; (B) Bony tenderness

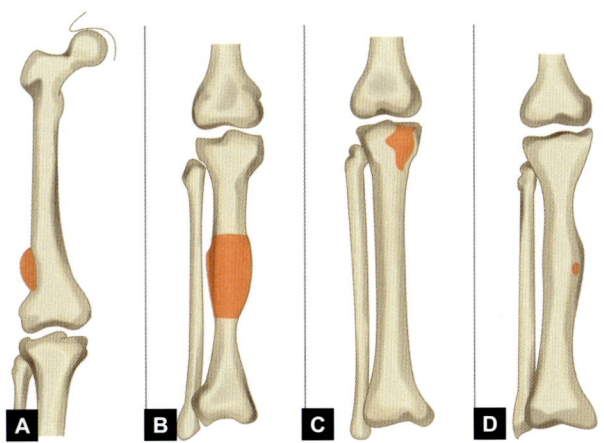

Figs 26.6A to D: Different levels of bony swelling (A) Metaphyseal; (B and D) Diaphyseal; (C) Epiphyseal

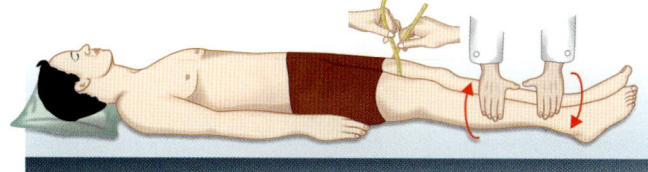

Fig. 26.7: Method of measuring the girth of a limb and checking the movements

> **Remember**
> Grading of consistency
> - Grade I — Very soft (like jelly)
> - Grade II — Soft (as relaxed muscle)
> - Grade III — Firm (like a contracted muscle)
> - Grade IV — Hard (as a contracted biceps)
> - Grade V — Stony and bone hard

Movements of joints:
- Active movement the patient himself moves the joint in one direction and later in the other. The extent of active movement is noted. Both the joints should be tested.
- Passive movement of the joint is tested by the examiner without causing pain. The extent of passive movement is noted (Fig. 26.7).

> **Remember**
> - Limitation of all movements of a joint indicates arthritis.
> - Limitation of certain movements of a joint indicates an extra-articular lesion or mechanical block.
> - If passive movements exceed active movements, paralysis of muscle is likely.

Measurements: Accurate limb length measurements give vital clues regarding the diagnosis. Measurement should be taken for two purposes.

To know the limb length: For this, measurement is taken between two fixed bony points and is always compared with the normal.

Upper limbs
- *Arm length:* From the angle of acromion to the lateral epicondyle of humerus (Fig. 26.8).
- *Forearm length:* From the lateral epicondyle of humerus to the radial styloid process.

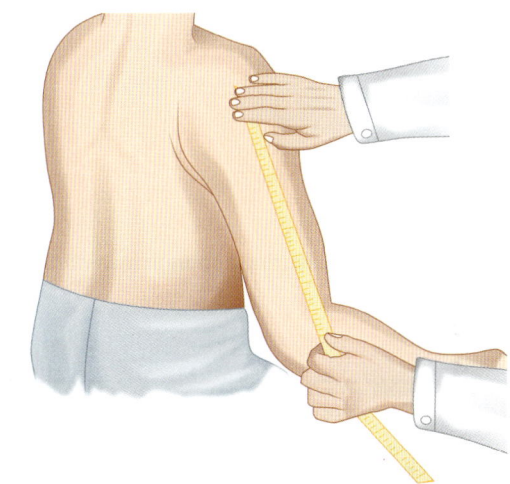

Fig. 26.8: Method of upper arm length measurement

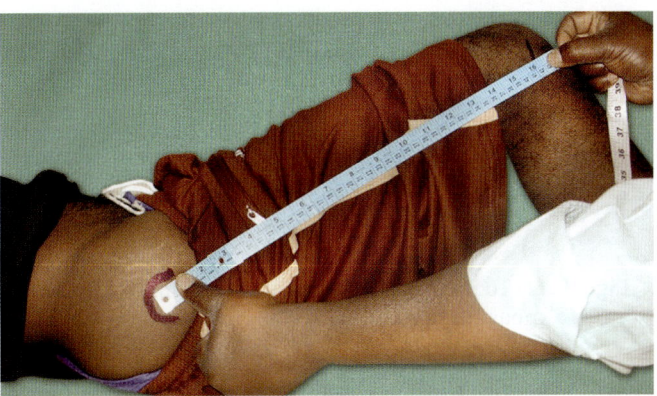

Fig. 26.9: Method of measuring the thigh

Lower limbs
- *Thigh length:* From anterosuperior iliac spine to the medial knee joint line (Fig. 26.9).
- *Leg length:* From the medial knee joint line to the medial malleolus.

To know the apparent length of the lower limbs measurement is taken from the xiphisternum to the medial malleolus (Fig. 26.10).

To know the girth of the limb: To detect wasting of muscles, the circumference of the limb is measured at fixed points

350 SECTION 3: Nontraumatic Orthopedic Disorders

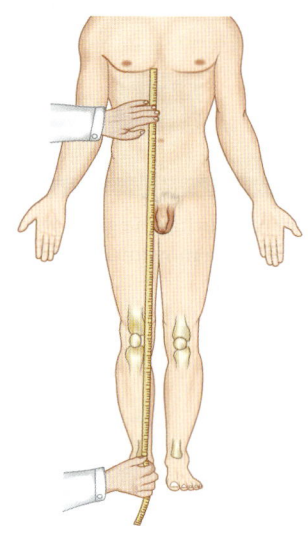

Fig. 26.10: Method of measuring apparent lower limb length

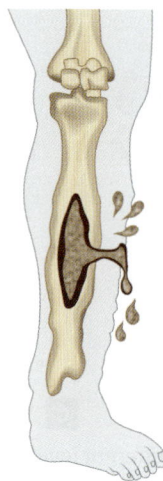

Fig. 26.12: Irregular thickening of bone and discharging sinus due to chronic osteomyelitis

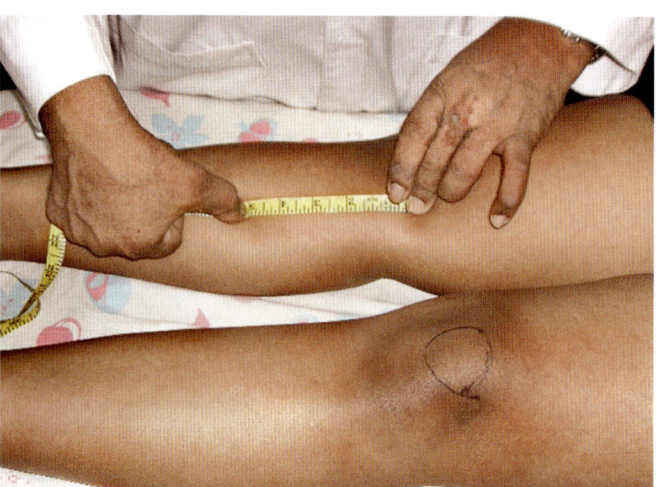

Fig. 26.11: To measure the girth of a limb, mark a point of measurement on both sides and measure

on both sides, e.g. 18 cm above joint line in the thigh (Fig. 26.11).

Irregular thickening of bone and persistent discharging sinus: If this is present along with scars fixed to bone, it indicates chronic osteomyelitis (see box for causes of persistent sinus) (Fig. 26.12).

Peripheral, vascular, and nervous system examination should be done next. This is discussed in appropriate sections.

Quick Facts: Sinus Tracts
Causes of persistent discharging sinus: • Un-obliterated cavities   • Unabsorbed sequestra

- Epithelialization of sinus tract
- Presence of foreign body
- Secondary infection
- Diabetes, steroid therapy, etc.
- Malignant change in the sinus.

INVESTIGATIONS

These help to confirm the diagnosis and in some cases help to make the diagnosis (e.g. crack fracture, etc. can be diagnosed only by X-ray). One has to choose carefully from the following vast armamentarium:

Laboratory investigations: This consists of blood investigations like routine hemogram, urine examination, ECG, chest X-ray, etc.

Special investigations:
- *Radiography:* At least two views of the affected part should be taken; oblique views and some special views are required in some cases.
- *CT scan:* Study the cross-section of the limb anatomy and bones.
- *MRI:* This is the recent gold standard in the investigative armamentarium of bone disorders. It helps to study the bone, soft tissues, medullary spread, etc. with greater accuracy. The only problem is its prohibitive cost.
- *Angiography and biopsy* help in tumor diagnosis.

Thus, a reasonably accurate diagnosis can be made by following the guidelines discussed above.

Steps in the Process of Diagnosis	
At the end of investigation	Final
At the end of examination	Provisional
At the end of history	Guess

27 CHAPTER

Deformities and their Management

DEFINITION

Any deviation from the normal anatomy of a bone and joint is called a deformity.

CLASSIFICATION

The deformities can be classified as shown in the Flowchart 27.1.

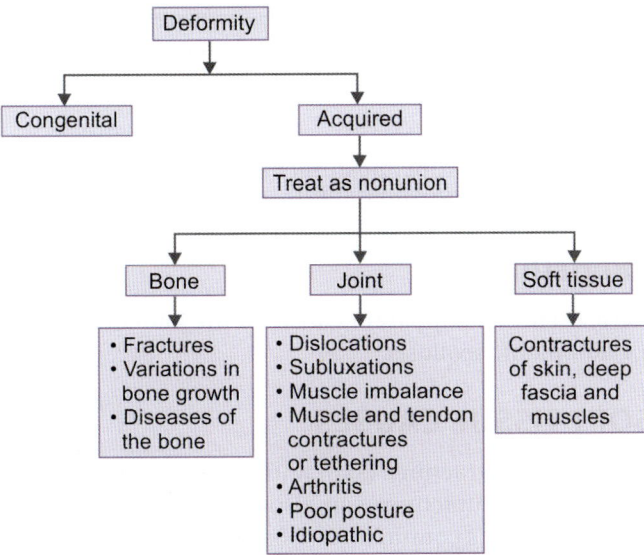

Flowchart 27.1: Classification of deformities

Acquired deformities are more commonly encountered than the congenital variety.

DEFORMITIES SINCE BIRTH (CONGENITAL)

These are due to some genetic abnormalities or environmental variations or both. They may be obvious at birth or may be seen a few years later. Incidence is around 2–3%. They may be so severe that the child is still born or may be so minor that it is not noticeable *(See section on Congenital Deformities)*.

ACQUIRED DEFORMITIES

These could be due to problems in the bone, joint or soft tissues (Figs 27.1A to G).

Clinical Facts: Famous Orthopedic Deformities due to Fractures	
• S-shaped deformity	Supracondylar fracture humerus
• Gunstock deformity	Malunited supracondylar fracture humerus
• Cubitus valgus	Malunited lateral condyle fracture of humerus
• Dinner fork deformity	Malunited Colles
• Mallet finger	Avulsion tip of base of distal phalanx
• Genu varum/valgus	Tibial condylar fractures
• Varus-valgus at ankle	Ankle injuries
• External rotation lower limb	Fracture neck femur, trochanteric fracture, fracture shaft femur, fracture tibia.

BONE CAUSES

The following causes are responsible for deformities in the bone:

Growth Disturbances

Tumor, infections, or trauma near the growth epiphysis can cause unequal stimulus, suppression, or stimulation of growth. This results in bending, shortening, or lengthening of a bone respectively, e.g. osteomyelitis, epiphyseal injuries, tumor, etc.

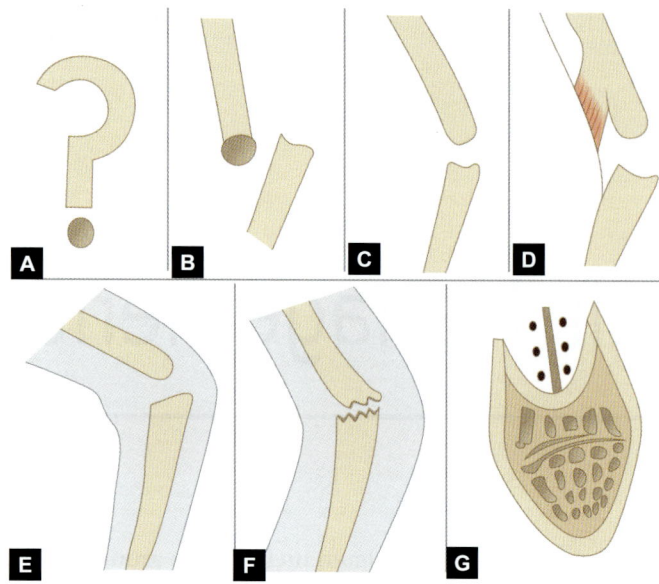

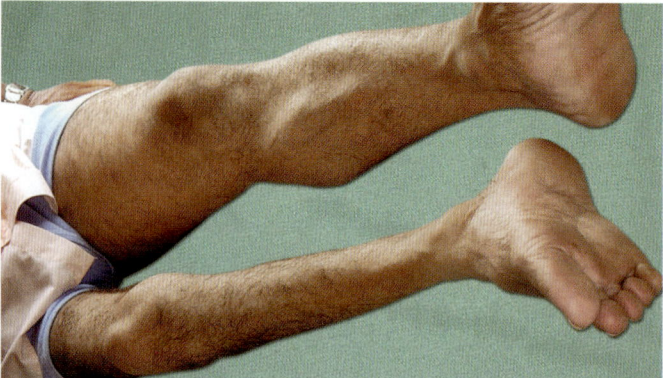

Fig. 27.2: Clinical photo of deformities in polio

Figs 27.1A to G: Causes for deformity: (A) Idiopathic; (B) Dislocation; (C) Muscle imbalance; (D) Muscle tethering; (E) Soft tissue contractures; (E) Fractures; (G) Postural

Bone Disorders

Endocrine disorders, metabolic disorders, developmental disorders are some of the examples with bone deformities.

Fractures

This is by far the most important cause for a bone deformity. All displaced and fresh fractures cause temporary deformity while malunion or nonunion of fractures lead to deformities later.

JOINT CAUSES

The causes for the deformities due to joint are varied.

Dislocation or Subluxation

This is usually due to trauma. It may also be seen due to pathological conditions of the hip, e.g. TB hip.

Muscle Imbalance

Muscles balancing the joint on either side, if they are either overactive (e.g. cerebral palsy) or under active, e.g. polio, deformity of the joint results (Fig. 27.2).

Tethering of Muscles and Tendons

This can take place due to the growth of fibrous tissue following infections or due to callus following fractures. Tethering restricts the joint movements and if held for some time deformity results, e.g. VIC, tenosynovitis of finger flexors, etc.

Arthritis

Any joint may give rise to muscle spasm in the initial stages and fibrous or bony ankylosis in later stages giving rise to deformities, e.g. TB knee, rheumatoid hand, TB hip, etc.

Postural

This is due to improper postural habits like hallux valgus in women due to tight and rigid shoes.

Idiopathic

Here, there is no apparent cause for the joint deformities, e.g. idiopathic scoliosis.

SOFT TISSUE CAUSES

Soft tissue contractures (skin and deep fascia) other than the muscle contractures can also cause joint deformities, e.g. Dupuytren's contractures, post-burn contracture, etc.

Treatment Options

Conservative Measures

These include manipulative correction under anesthesia and retention by splints or casts, gradual correction by traction or splints, etc. (e.g. turn buckle splints). Correction by plaster wedging is hazardous.

Surgical Measures

There are various surgical options available:
- *Ilizarov:* This is the gold standard for deformity correction in recent times
- Soft tissue release by surgical methods
- Tenolysis, tendon lengthening or tendon transfers are successfully employed in polio, cerebral palsy, etc.
- *Arthroplasty* can be crude as a salvage procedure (e.g. girdle stone excision in TB hip) or sophisticated as in total hip replacement or total knee replacement in osteoarthritis, rheumatoid and other disorders
- *Corrective osteotomy* this is a simple but effective procedure to correct joint deformities, e.g. French osteotomy in cubitus varus deformity, etc.
- *Arthrodesis* fusion of the joints in functional positions in badly damaged joints, e.g. TB knee, rheumatoid arthritis, etc.
- *Epiphyseal growth arrests:* When potential for growth is still left, stapling of the epiphysis can be attempted on one side to correct the bending deformity, e.g. in genu varum or valgum.

28 CHAPTER

Treatment of Orthopedic Disorders

There are three time-tested and time-honored treatment methods: (i) masterly inactivity, (ii) conservative methods, and (iii) operative treatment methods of treating an orthopedic disorder.

Masterly Inactivity

It is interesting to observe that nearly 50% of the orthopedic disorders can be managed best by *not doing anything*. To allay the doubts, fears, myths, and misconceptions, a patient has regarding his ailment and assuring him that nothing is seriously wrong with him is all that is required.

This is more of a 'mind' management than 'orthopedic' management and is more a 'human' care than 'health care'!

Conservative Methods

This is the next commonly advocated and recommended method of treatment.

Rest

This implies not total rest but selective rest with avoidance of unnecessary activities and strain. HO Thomas first advocated this and of late due to improved methods of treatment and technology; emphasis is now on early restoration of activities and not passive rest.

Support

This enables the diseased part to heal, provides rest, prevents deformities, relieves pain and also supports the patients psychologically, e.g. plaster splints for fractured limbs, lumbosacral belts and corsets for low backache, calipers in polio, cervical collars for neck pains, knee cap, ankle binders, etc. (Figs 28.1 and 28.2).

Traction

This is a popular method of treating certain chronic orthopedic conditions like low backache, cervical spondylosis, etc. In these conditions, it is known to reduce pain, muscle stiffness, spasm, etc. (Figs 28.3 and 28.4).

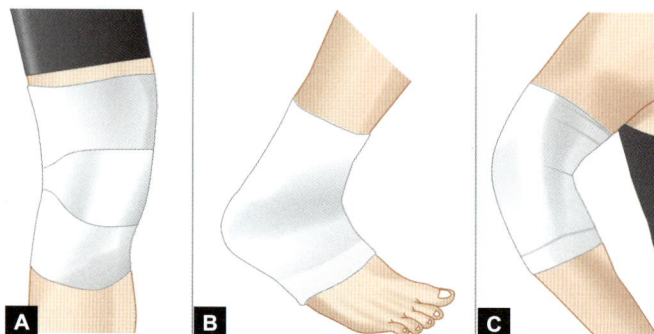

Figs 28.1A to C: Supportive braces: (A) Knee support cap; (B) Ankle support; (C) Elbow support

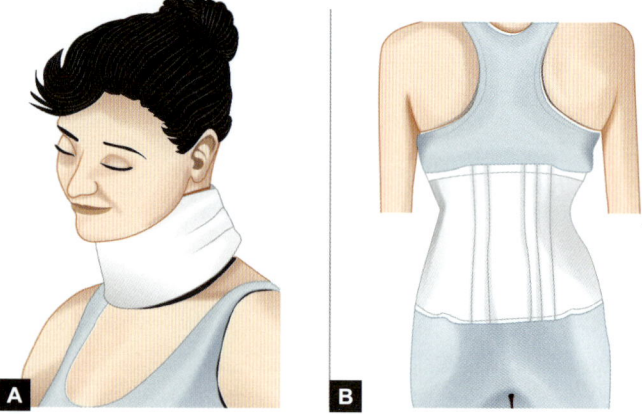

Figs 28.2A and B: Neck and back supports: (A) Cervical collar; (B) Sacrolumbar support

Physiotherapy

Physiotherapy, if properly understood and skillfully executed by trained persons, gives excellent results in treating orthopedic disorders and in postoperative rehabilitation. For optimum results, physiotherapy should be pursued systematically until its final logical conclusion and should not be abandoned in between. Physiotherapy has a great role to play and sometimes is the only treatment option in diseases like polio, cerebral palsy, hemiplegia, paraplegia, etc.

The following are the various physiotherapy options:
- *Active exercises:* Here the patient is made to actively contract his or her muscles and joints against resistance and weight. This helps to mobilize the joints, strengthen the muscles and to improve coordination or balance (Fig. 28.5).
- *Passive exercises:* This can be given by the physiotherapist normally or by machines which can provide continuous passive movements of the joints. This is of immense help to maintain the mobility of all the joints when active movements are not possible due to paralysis or injury to the muscles. Thus, the joints are kept supple and deformities are prevented (Fig. 28.6).

Note: Active muscle strengthening exercise could be either isometric (here muscle does not move and hence no change in length, e.g. pushing against a static object) or isotonic (here muscle actually moves, e.g. quadriceps exercises).

- *Electrical muscle stimulation:* Depending upon whether the nerve supply of a muscle is intact or not, two types of electrical stimulation is chosen:

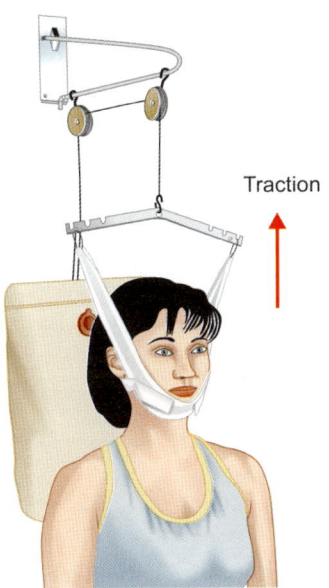

Fig. 28.3: Cervical traction

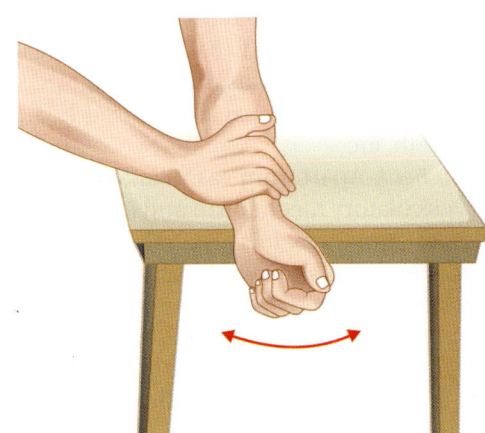

Fig. 28.5: Method of active wrist dorsal and palmar flexion of the wrist joint

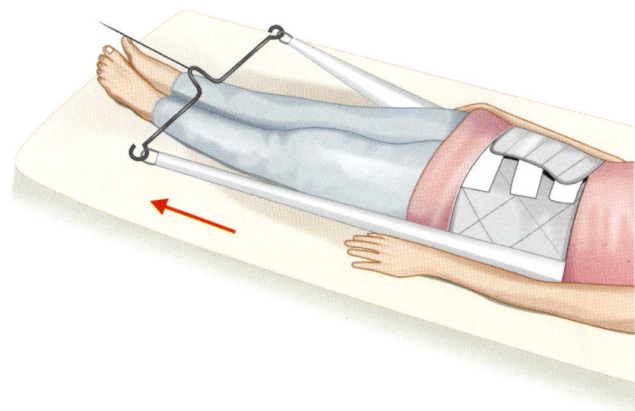

Fig. 28.4: Lumbar traction

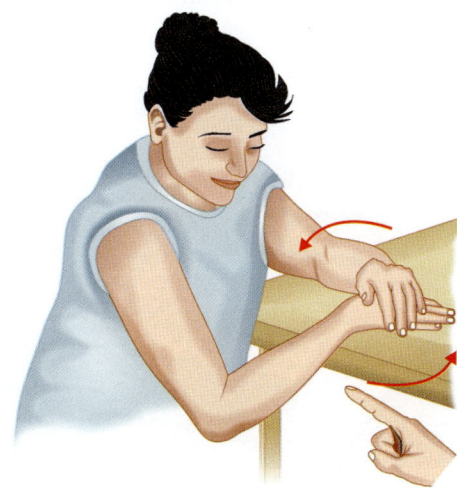

Fig. 28.6: Self-assisted passive wrist flexion and extension with the hand at the edge of a table

- *Faradism:* In this, the nerve supply of the muscle should be intact. In faradism, an electronic stimulator delivers shocks at shorter duration at a frequency of 1 mm at 50 Hg to the muscle through its intact motor nerve root, e.g. for regaining the strength of intrinsic muscles of the hand and foot, quadriceps muscle and to retain the tendons after tendon transfers.
- *Galvanism:* Here the muscle is stimulated directly with shocks of longer durations (100–1000 mm at frequency of 5–15 Hg). When the muscle is denervated after a peripheral nerve injury, etc. this treatment modality helps.

- **Hydrotherapy:** This is particularly useful in patients suffering from rheumatoid arthritis. The warmth and buoyancy of water helps to relieve pain and muscle spasm.
- **Heat therapy** by direct application of heat the local temperature underneath the tissues rises up to 10° inducing vasodilatation, reduced muscle spasm and decreased pain. There are two varieties of heat therapies:
  - *Surface heat:* This heats only the superficial tissues and consists of hot packs, infrared heat, paraffin wax bath, etc.
  - *Deep heat:* Apart from vasodilatation, it stimulates the circulatory mechanism and helps in heating the deeper structures. It is also helpful in treating joint disorders, e.g. shortwave diathermy, ultrasound, interferential heat therapy, etc. (Fig. 28.7).
- **Manipulation:** This term denotes a deliberate attempt by the surgeon to passively move the joints bone or soft tissues. It is useful in three specific purposes:
  - *Manipulation for correction of deformity:* Closed reduction of fractures and dislocations and manipulation of a clubfoot falls under this category. This is done under general anesthesia and after the correction; the part is immobilized in splints, etc. to retain the correction.
  - *Manipulation for joint stiffness:* This is useful in the knee joints, it may be successful in shoulder and foot but responds poorly in cases of elbow and hand. The manipulation should be done gradually under general anesthesia and forcible or abrupt movements should be avoided (Fig. 28.8).
  - *For relief of chronic pain:* Manipulation may help in chronic pain of shoulder tarsal, spine or sacroiliac joints.

Note:
Manipulation should not be done in acute painful conditions for fear of aggravating the problem.

Massage: Delicate, continuous and systematic massage if done regularly has a lot of beneficial effects like relief of pain, soothening effect, etc. (Fig. 28.9).

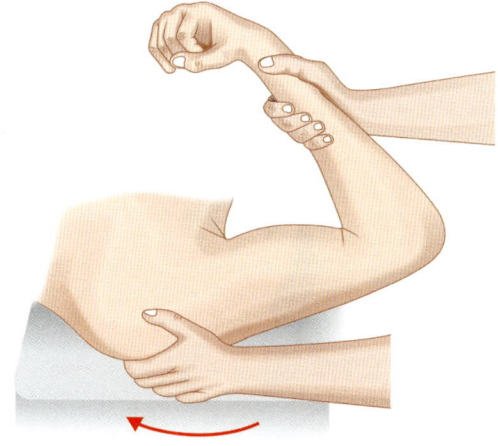

Fig. 28.8: Active assisted shoulder abduction with gravity eliminated

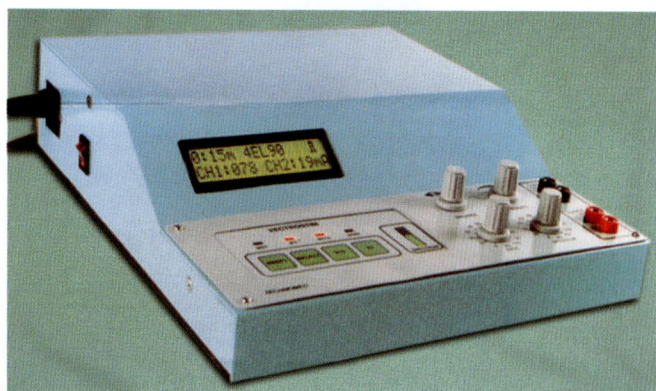

Fig. 28.7: Equipment for interferential therapy (IFT)

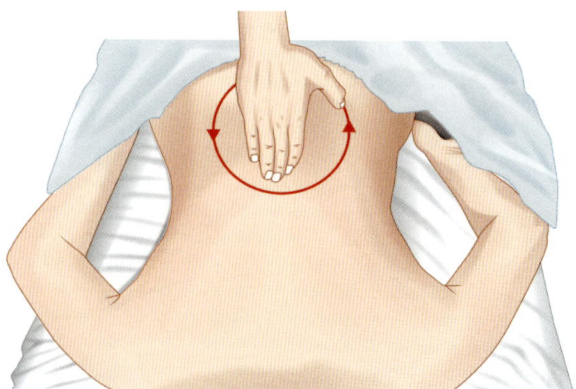

Fig. 28.9: Technique of back massage

Radiotherapy

It has a role in:
- *Inflammatory conditions* like recalcitrant ankylosing spondylitis.
- *Neoplastic conditions,* e.g. Ewing's sarcoma and giant cell tumor recurrence.

Drugs

Drugs though limited have an important role to play in orthopedic practice. The commonly used ones are:
- *Analgesics and anti-inflammatory agents:* These help relieve pain and inflammation. Long-acting drugs are preferred in chronic disorders like rheumatoid arthritis, etc. while short-acting drugs are preferred in acute infections, trauma, etc.
- *Muscle relaxants:* These are useful to relieve painful muscle spasms.
- *Sedatives and anxiolytics:* These are used to induce sleep, alleviate anxiety and to relieve muscle spasm.
- *Antibiotics* these are extremely useful in acute and chronic infections of bones and joints. Broad-spectrum, bactericidal agents are usually preferred.
- *Hormones:* Growth hormones, stilbestrol for metastatic carcinomas, anabolic steroids and estrogens for osteoporosis are some of the examples.
- *Specific drugs:* Vitamin C for scurvy, vitamin D for rickets are some of the examples.
- *Cytotoxic drugs:* These are used as chemotherapeutic agents for malignant tumors.

OPERATIVE TREATMENT METHODS

Operative treatment should be resorted after great deliberations and when all other treatment options have been tried or thought of. Once undertaken, it should not worsen the condition of the patient.

A brief account of various orthopedic surgical techniques is presented here.

Osteotomy (Figs 28.10A and B)

This is a procedure of creating a surgical fracture to achieve the following objectives:
- To correct excessive angulations, bowing or rotation of a long bone.
- To compensate and correct the malalignment of a joint.
- To correct leg length inequality either by shortening or by lengthening.
- To alter the line of weight bearing and increase the stability at the hip joint, e.g. abduction osteotomy.
- To relieve the pain in an arthritic hip, e.g. displacement osteotomy, high tibial osteotomy, etc. (Fig. 28.11).

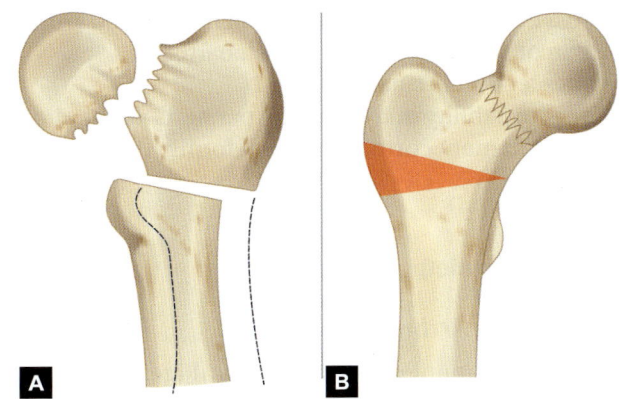

Figs 28.10A and B: Different types of osteotomies: (A) McMurray's displacement osteotomy; (B) Angulation osteotomy

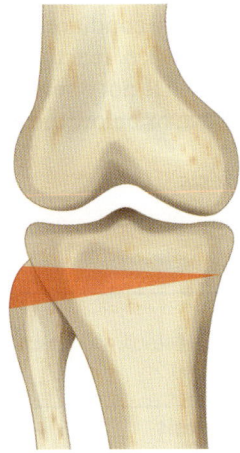

Fig. 28.11: High tibial osteotomy done in OA knee

A Quick Glance at Famous Osteotomies

Upper limbs	*Done for*
• French osteotomy	Malunited supracondylar fracture humerus
• Fernandez and Campbell osteotomy	Malunited Colles' fracture
Lower limbs	
• Salter, Chiari, Pemberton	CDH
• McMurray's, Shanz	Fracture neck femur
• Pauwels	OA hip
• High tibial osteotomy	OA knee
• Dwyer's osteotomy	Clubfoot
Spinal osteotomy	Ankylosing spondylitis

Arthrodesis

Arthrodesis is fusion of the joints by surgical methods. Because it limits the function of the joint, arthroplasty it is more commonly used nowadays. However, it can be used in the following situations:

- Gross destruction of the joints as in rheumatoid arthritis, Charcot's joints or advanced osteoarthritis.
- Quiescent tubercular arthritis
- Gross instability due to muscle paralysis as in polio.
- For permanent correction of a deformity.

Methods

There are three methods:

Intra-articular Arthrodesis

Here joint is opened, articular cartilage is denuded, cancellous bone grafts are packed, joint is kept in a functional position and either fixed internally or externally by plaster, etc. (Fig. 28.12).

Extra-articular Arthrodesis

This is indicated in infective condition of the hip, shoulder or spine. In this, there is no risk of reactivating or spreading the infection as the joint itself is not opened, but bone-to-bone fusion is obtained above or below the joint.

Combined Arthrodesis

This is a combination of the above two procedures (Figs 28.13A and B)

> **Note:**
> Arthrodesis of a joint gives it stability but takes away its mobility. It is like robbing Peter to pay Paul.

> **Practical Facts: Arthrodesis**
> Each joint should be fixed in its functional position as mentioned below to enable the patient to continue using it:
>
> | Joints | Functional positions |
> |---|---|
> | Upper limbs | |
> | Shoulder | 30° Abd/30° flexion/40° internal rotation |
> | Elbow | |
> | • Eating hand (right) | 90° of flexion |
> | • Toilet hand (left) | 70° of flexion |
> | Wrist | 20° dorsiflexion |
> | Forearm | 10° pronation |
> | MP joint | 35° flexion |
> | IP joints | 45° flexion |
> | Lower limbs | |
> | Hip | 15° flexion, no adduction or abduction or rotation |
> | Knee | 20° flexion |
> | • Ankle (men) | 90° or neutral position |
> | • Ankle (women) | 15–20° of plantar flexion |
> | Metatarsophalangeal joints of big toe | Slight extension |

Arthroplasty

Arthroplasty is an operation to construct a new mobile joint. The following are the indications:
- Advanced osteoarthritis or rheumatoid arthritis of hip, knee, shoulder, elbow, hand and foot.
- Quiescent destructive tuberculous arthritis of hip and elbow.
- Fracture neck nonunion in patients of more than 60 years.
- Rarely to correct deformity, e.g. hallux valgus.

Types

There are three varieties of arthroplasties (Figs 28.14 to 28.17) namely:
- *Excision arthroplasty:* Here one or both the articular surfaces are excised; fibrous tissue fills up in the gap thus created and provides mobility (Fig. 28.14A).

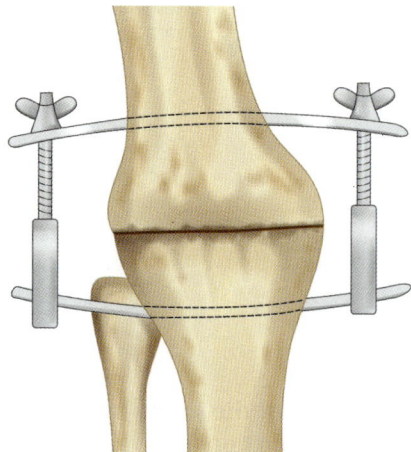

Fig. 28.12: Charnley's compression arthrodesis

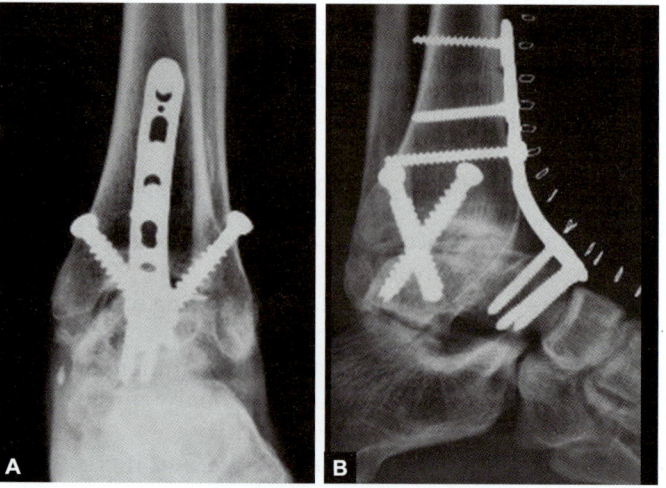

Figs 28.13A and B: Plain X-ray showing combined intra-articular and extra-articular arthrodesis

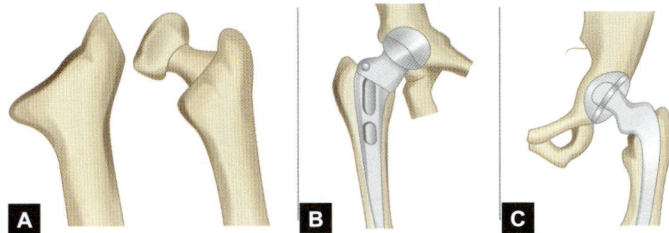

Figs 28.14A to C: Different types of arthroplasties: (A) Excision arthroplasty; (B) Hemireplacement arthroplasty; (C) Total hip replacement

It is usually done in hip, elbow and metatarsophalangeal joint of the great toe.
- *Hemireplacement arthroplasty:* Either of the articulating surface is removed or replaced by prosthesis of similar shape and size, e.g. (Fig. 28.14B) Austin Moore's prosthesis in fracture neck nonunion.
- *Total replacement arthroplasty:* Here both the articular surfaces are excised and replaced by prosthetic components, the larger joint is replaced by a metallic prosthesis, and the smaller joint by high-density polyethylene (Fig. 28.14C). Both the components are fixed by acrylic cement, e.g. total hip replacement for osteoarthritis or rheumatoid hip and partial or total knee replacement for advanced intractable osteoarthritis or rheumatoid arthritis (Figs 28.15 to 28.19).

Bone Grafting Operations

Bone grafting is used in the following situations in orthopedic practice:
- To promote union in cases of nonunion or ununited fractures.
- In arthrodesis of joints for intra-articular or extra-articular fusion.
- To fill a defect or cavity in a bone.

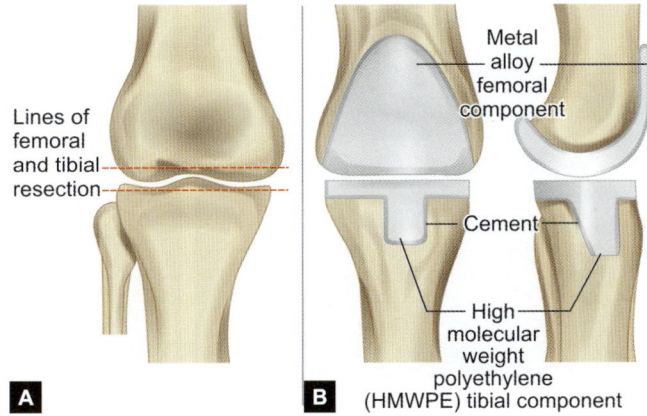

Figs 28.16A and B: Cemented total knee replacement

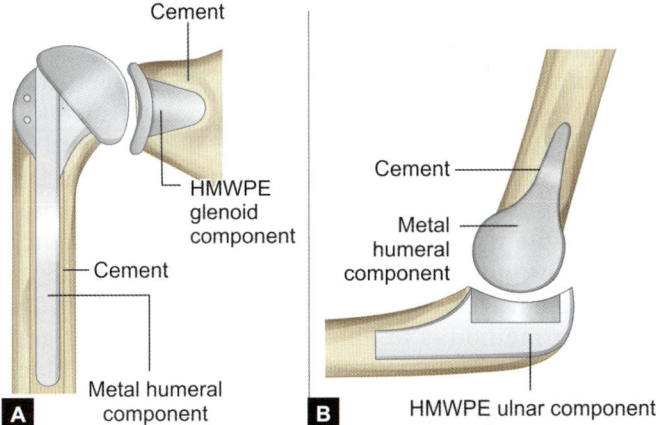

Figs 28.17A and B: (A) Unconstrained total shoulder replacement; (B) Unconstrained total elbow replacement

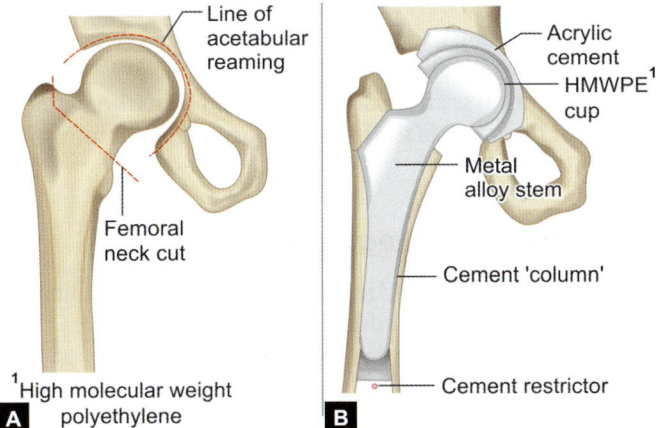

Figs 28.15A and B: Cemented total hip replacement

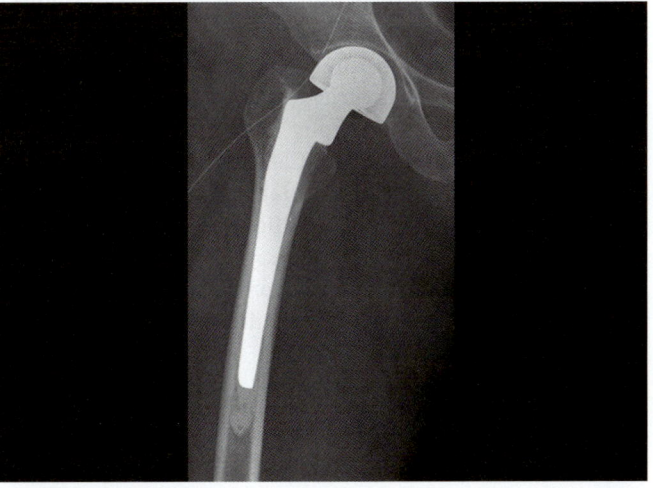

Fig. 28.18: Plain X-ray showing hemireplacement arthroplasty (Bipolar)

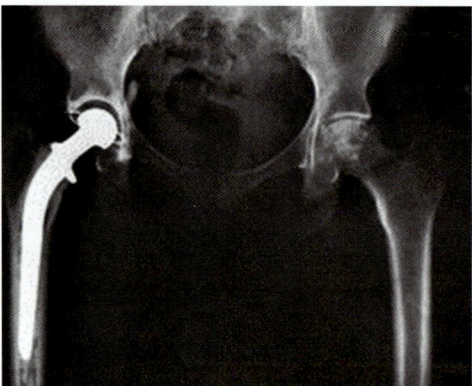 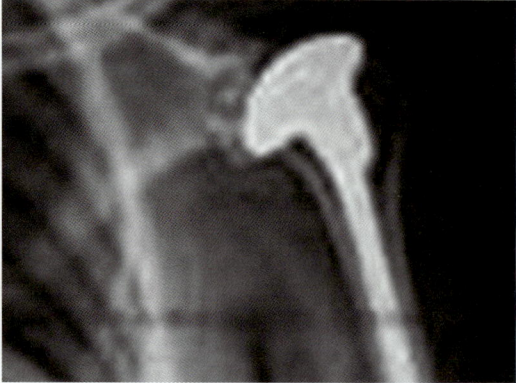 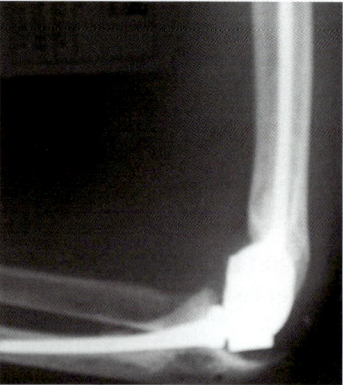

Fig. 28.19: Plain X-ray showing different arthroplasties—hip, shoulder and elbow

Types

There are three types of bone grafts.
- *Autogenous grafts or autografts:* These are bone grafts either cancellous or cortical obtained from different parts of the patient's own body. Cancellous bone grafts are obtained from the iliac crest and the cortical bone graft is obtained from the fibula. Due to improvement in microvascular surgery, it is now possible to obtain a graft with the muscle pedicle with its blood vessel intact and anastomosed to the recipient area, e.g. Meyer's muscle pedicle graft. The other method is to obtain a free vascularized graft where the bone graft is taken along with its blood supply, and the blood vessels are anastomosed to the vessels in the recipient area, e.g. fibula with its blood supply intact.
- *Allograft or homograft or homogeneous grafts:* Here the bone graft is obtained from another person's body usually if the requirement is large as in filling up the gap after a tumor resection (e.g. osteoclastoma) and if graft is insufficient from his or her own body. Allograft is obtained from another person living or dead. The latter is called "cadaveric graft". These bone grafts are usually used fresh or may be stored under aseptic conditions until required. Cadaveric bone is sterilized either by boiling or by irradiation and stored at –70°C in a bone bank after decalcification and preservation with formalin.
- *Xenografting (heterogeneous or heterograft):* Here the bone graft is obtained from animals mainly bovine. It is sparingly used.

Artificial bone: This is made up of hydroxyapatite and is now being used in some centers.

Role of a Bone Graft

It provides a scaffold or a temporary bridge upon which a new bone is laid down. Thus, the bone cells of the graft die and are eventually replaced by a new living bone. Vascularized grafts are incorporated very rapidly.

Tendon Surgeries

This includes:

Tendon transfers: In this operation, the insertion of a healthy functioning muscle is moved to a new site, so that it has a different action. Other intact tendons will take care of the original function of the transferred tendon.

Indications

- Muscle paralysis as in polio or peripheral nerve injury.
- Muscle imbalance as in cerebral palsy
- In rupture or cut tendon where direct suture is not possible.

Tendon grafting: In this, a length of free tendon is used to bridge a gap between the severed ends of the recipient tendon, e.g. reconstruction of flexor tendons severed in the fibrous digital sheaths of the hand.

Free tendon graft is usually obtained from the palmaris longus or from one of the toe extensors at the dorsum of the foot (Fig. 28.20).

Equalization of Leg Length

In patients with unequal leg length as in polio, equalization of leg length can be obtained by:
- Leg lengthening by Ilizarov's technique

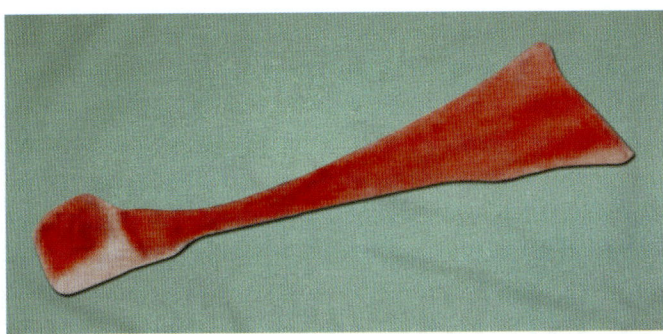

Fig. 28.20: Tendon graft

- Leg shortening, especially in femur or tibia. Not advocated as a routine procedure
- Arrest of epiphyseal growth by stapling in children.

Excision of tumors: This has been discussed in chapter on Bone Neoplasias.

Amputations: See discussions on amputations.

A Quick Recap

Treatment method in orthopedics
Masterly inactivity
Conservative methods:
- Rest
- Support
- Traction
- Physiotherapy
- Radiotherapy
- Massage
- Drugs

Operative methods:
- Osteotomy
- Arthrodesis
- Arthroplasty
- Bone graft procedures
- Tendon surgeries
- Equalization of leg length
- Excision of tumors
- Amputations

29 CHAPTER

Regional Conditions of the Neck

Regional orthopedics deals with a vast array of interesting orthopedic problems. Each region has its own peculiar problems depending on various factors like anatomical, physiological, occupational and others operating in that region. An effort is made in this section to highlight the various regional orthopedic problems. However, a detailed description of the regional disorders is avoided as it is outside the scope of this book. The student is requested to refer bigger books in orthopedics in case he or she desires a detailed study of the regional problems.

TORTICOLLIS (WRYNECK)

Torticollis is defined as the rotational deformity of cervical spine that causes turning and tilting deformity of the head and neck (Fig. 29.1).

Causes

- *Congenital:* (refer Chapter 35, Congenital Disorders for description).

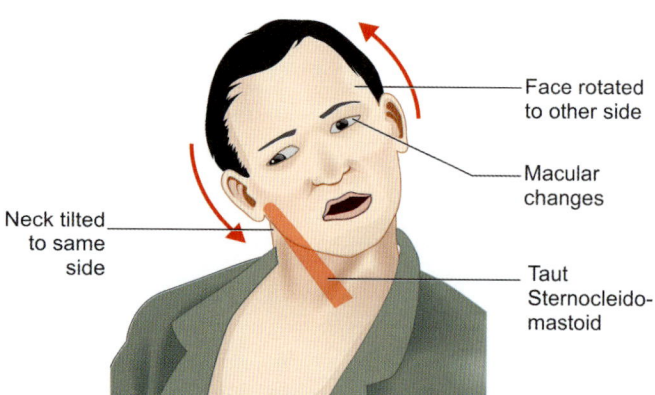

Fig. 29.1: Features of wryneck

- *Infective:* Tuberculosis of cervical spine, acute respiratory tract infection, etc.
- *Traumatic* Sprain, dislocation, and fracture of the cervical spine.
- *Myositis or fibromyositis* of sternocleidomastoid, exposure to cold causes myositis.
- *Spasmodic:* Painful, persistent, or intermittent sternomastoid muscle contraction.
- *Unilateral muscle paralysis,* e.g. polio
- *Neuritis* of spinal accessory nerve
- *Ocular disturbances:* Child turns head to one side to compensate for defective vision.

Clinical Features

Head of the patient is tilted towards the affected side while the chin points to the other side. Sternocleidomastoid muscle is prominently seen. In the later stages, the patient may develop facial asymmetry and macular disturbances in the eye.

Among the acquired causes of torticollis, spasmodic muscle contraction of the sternocleidomastoid is the most common cause.

Management

Conservative

Initially conservative line of treatment is observed. This consists of non-steroidal anti-inflammatory drugs (NSAIDs), muscle relaxants drugs, etc. Physiotherapy like ultrasound, heat, massage is advocated. In acute pain, the patient is encouraged to wear a collar. Gradual neck stretching exercises are advised once the acute symptoms subside.

Surgical

Management is advised after the failure of conservative treatment. It consists of release of sternomastoid muscle from its clavicular attachment as in congenital torticollis and intradural section of both spinal accessory and three cervical roots in cases of torticollis due to spasmodic or neural causes.

THORACIC OUTLET SYNDROME

The space at the thoracic outlet or inlet when it is less than adequate, subjects the neurovascular structures seeking to gain entry into the upper limbs via this space, to undue pressure (Fig. 29.2). The blame for the neurovascular complaints should be placed at the doorstep of the decreased space and not at the structures producing the problems.

This syndrome results from the compression of neurovascular bundle comprising of subclavian artery and vein, axillary artery and vein and brachial plexus at the thoracic outlet. Thoracic outlet is a space between the first rib, clavicle, and the scalene muscles. The above structures are liable to be compressed (Fig. 29.3) when this space gets narrowed either due to hypertrophy of the existing muscles or due to any other cause like congenital, trauma, etc.

Sites of Compression

The sites of compression could be either supraclavicular, subclavicular or infraclavicular.

Supraclavicular: Interscalene triangle between the anterior scalene muscles.

Subclavicular: Interval between the second thoracic rib, clavicle, and subclavius.

Infraclavicular: Beneath an enclosure formed by the coracoid process, pectoralis minor, and costocoracoid membrane.

Rare Causes

Scissor-like encirclement of axillary artery by the median nerve.

Contributing Factors

Dynamic Factors

Arm when in full abduction pulls up the artery by 180° causing compression in the short retroclavicular space.

Static Factors

Vigorous occupation: Increases the muscle bulk and thereby decreases the space.

Inactive occupation: Decreases the muscle bulk and thereby increases the space.

Congenital: Cervical rib decreases the interscalene space and thereby decreases the retroclavicular space.

Traumatic: Malunion or nonunion of fracture clavicle.

Arteriosclerosis.

Anomalies of the first thoracic rib.

Miscellaneous
- Tumor arising from the upper lobe of the lung
- Cervicothoracic scoliosis
- Abnormal variations of the scalene muscles.

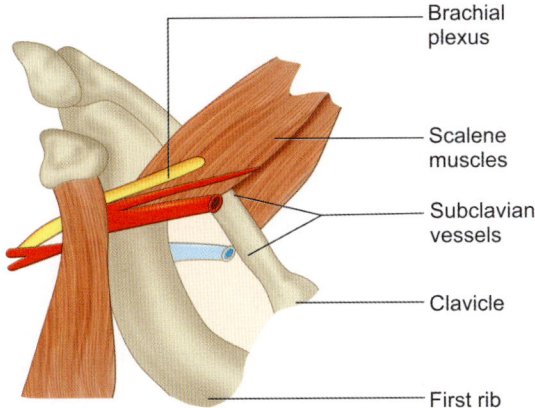

Fig. 29.2: Anatomy of the thoracic outlet

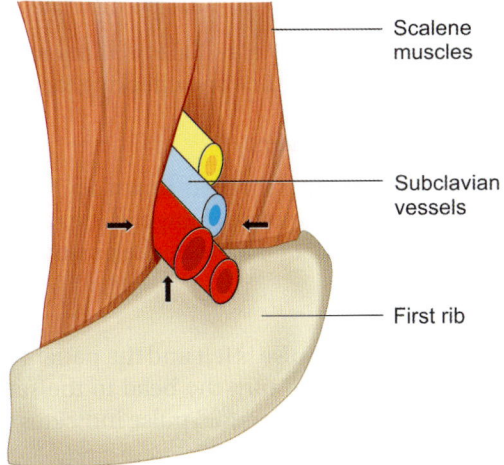

Fig. 29.3: Abnormal scalene muscle insertion causing compression of neurovascular structures

Clinical Features

Obviously, this syndrome poses two major problems. The first one relates to the compression of the major vessels and secondly to the compression of the nerves. The first problem has a *definite clinical entity,* while the second one presents a *vague picture* and makes an accurate diagnosis difficult.

Vascular Problems

Here the compression could be arterial or venous. During the arterial compression, which is mild in the early stages the patient complains of *numbness* of the whole arm with rapid fatigue during overhead exercises. If the compression is significant, the patient will complain of *cold, cyanosis, pallor,* and *Raynaud's phenomenon.* Venous compression leaves the limb *swollen* and *discolored* after exercises, which disappears slowly with rest.

Neurogenic Problems

This involves $C_8 T_1$ segment (Klumpke's paralysis). Patients complain of *paraesthesia* along the medial aspect of the arm, hand, little and ring fingers. There is *weakness* of the hand also.

Tests

Intermittent Claudication Test

The arm is abducted and elevated and fingers are exercised. The inference:
- If pain develops after 1 minute; it is negative (normal).
- If pain develops before 1 minute; the test is positive.
  Compression of subclavian artery in the neck: Radial pulse decreases.

Allen's Test

To determine the adequacy of radial and ulnar arteries, by compressing each one at a time and checking for adequacy.

Costoclavicular Maneuvers

The patient's shoulder is braced down and back. The reproduction of the symptoms, change in the radial pulse, bruit heard in infraclavicular area are the positive findings.

Provocative Tests

Adson's test: The radial pulse is felt and the patient is asked to take a deep breath and turn the head to the same side (Fig. 29.4B). Decrease in the radial pulse indicates positive test.

Wright's test: The same maneuver as above but the head is tilted towards the opposite side (Fig. 29.4A). It should be noted that thoracic outlet syndrome is a diagnosis of

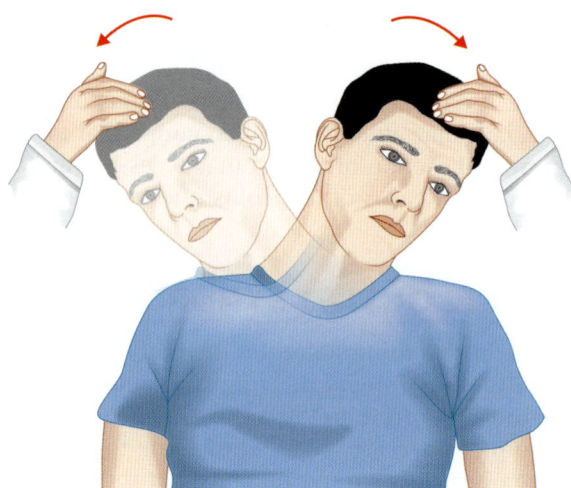

Figs 29.4A and B: Methods of performing: (A) Wright's test; (B) Adson's test

exclusion. First, the cervical pathology should be excluded and later the above tests should be performed as the initial screening procedures.

Complications

Subclavian artery compression → results in post-stenotic dilatation → stasis favors thrombosis → the thrombi break and migrate distally causing embolization → these results in the distal artery blockade causing ischemia and gangrene of the upper limbs.

Investigations

X-ray neck: To rule out intrinsic causes like cervical spondylosis, cervical rib, etc.

Nerve conduction studies: Difficult to determine the nerve conduction velocity through the thoracic outlet, but its biggest value is to rule-out problems like entrapment, e.g. ulnar nerve at elbow, wrist, etc.

Treatment

Conservative Treatment

Consists of rest, physiotherapy, exercises like shoulder shrugging, etc.

Surgical Treatment

Indications: Gangrene and poststenotic dilatation.

Methods

- *Removal of the first thoracic rib:* This is the most effective treatment as it deals with both supraclavicular and infraclavicular etiological factors in this syndrome.

- *Removal of cervical rib:* If this is the cause of compression.
- *Scalenotomy* is indicated in scalenus anticus syndrome.

> **Quick Facts**
> - Sites of compression could be supra, sub, or infraclavicular.
> - Clinical manifestation could be neural, vascular or both.
> - Diagnosis is usually by exclusion and the screening test helps.
> - Excision of the first thoracic rib is the most effective surgical procedure.

CERVICAL RIB

Cervical rib problem is akin to the story of the "Return of the Prodigal Son." However, unlike the chastened prodigal son, cervical rib returns to torment the unfortunate victim!

It is a rib arising from the 7th cervical vertebra, rarely 6th and 5th cervical vertebra.

Incidence: It is 0.46%. Nearly 50% of those are unilateral.

Side: It is more frequent on the right side.

Developmental Factors

In the embryo nerves larger than the ribs interfere with the development of the costal process. When brachial plexus is prefixed, well-developed 4th cervical root and small 2nd thoracic root offer little resistance to the costal process at the 7th cervical root.

In post-fixed brachial plexus, well-developed 1st thoracic root offers resistance to costal process of 7th cervical root. Obviously, cervical rib is more common in prefixed variety.

Types

Four varieties are described:

Complete: The cervical rib reaches up to the first thoracic rib.
Bulbous end: In this, the cervical rib has a bulbous end.
Tapering end: In this, the cervical rib tapers.
Fibrous band: In this, the rib is represented by a thick fibrous band.

Pathological Anatomy

The neurovascular structures, the brachial plexus, and subclavian vessels are hung up by the cervical rib that is inserted into the scalene tubercle of the 1st rib space.

Pronounced drooping of the shoulder in women after middle age, trauma, unusual lifting operations, acute illness make the muscles weak, pulling the plexus and artery distally giving rise to symptoms.

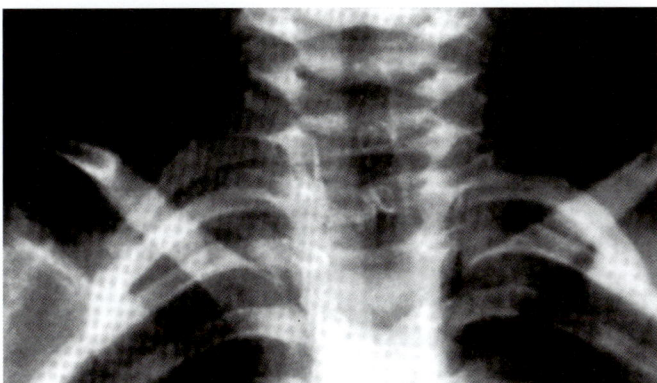

Fig. 29.5: Radiograph showing unilateral cervical rib

Clinical Features

Cervical rib with local symptoms: Show presence of a lump and tenderness in the supraclavicular fossa.

Cervical rib with vascular symptoms: This gives rise to pain in the upper limbs, temperature and color changes, radial pulse are feeble or absent and a feeling of numbness is present.

Cervical rib with nerve pressure symptoms: The nerve pressure symptoms are due to the angulations of the first thoracic nerve root. The patient complains of paresthesia along the medial aspect of the arm, hand and little fingers. There is weakness of the hand muscles also.

Radiograph

X-ray of the neck (AP and lateral views) helps to detect the presence of cervical rib (Fig. 29.5). However, the absence of the rib on the X-ray does not rule out the possibility of the presence of cervical rib. CT scan and MRI helps in better assessment.

Treatment

In mild cases, sling exercises often help. In more severe cases, scalenotomy (resection of scalenus anterior muscle) may be required and is successful in 70% of the cases. In troublesome cases, removal of the cervical rib or the first rib surgically with its periosteum to prevent its regeneration is advocated.

CERVICAL DISK SYNDROMES

This has been dealt in section on Geriatric Orthopedics.

30
CHAPTER

Regional Conditions of the Upper Limb

REGIONAL CONDITIONS OF THE SHOULDER

FROZEN SHOULDER
(Syn: Periarthritis, Adhesive Capsulitis)

Paradoxically shoulder joint privileged as the most mobile joint in the body has its nemesis because of this very advantage. Its mobility makes it very vulnerable to problems, which ultimately "freezes" its movements. Unable to come to terms with the paucity of liberal movements hitherto enjoyed, the hapless patient resigns himself or herself to suffer the agony in silence!

It is defined as a clinical syndrome characterized by *painful restriction* (Figs 30.1A and B) *of both active and passive shoulder movements* due to causes within the shoulder joint or remote (other parts of the body).

History

Dupley first described it in 1872 and called it as *humeroscapular periarthritis.* In 1934, **Codman** coined the term *Frozen shoulder*, and in 1945, **Neviaser** gave the name *adhesive capsulitis*.

> **Epidemiology**
> - Incidence in general population is 2 percent.
> - Incidence in diabetics is 10–35 percent.
> - More common in females than males.
> - Mean age is 40–60 years.
> - Bilateral 12 percent.

Causes

The causes for frozen shoulder could be:
- Primary: Here the exact cause is not known and it could be idiopathic.
- Secondary: According to **Lumberg,** the secondary causes could be:
  - *Shoulder causes:* Problems directly related to shoulder joint which can give rise to frozen shoulder are tendonitis of rotator cuff, bicipital tendinitis, fractures, and dislocations around the shoulder, etc.
  - *Non-shoulder causes:* Problems not related to shoulder joint like diabetes, cardiovascular diseases with referred pain to the shoulder, which keeps the joint immobile, reflex sympathetic dystrophy, frozen hand shoulder syndrome, a complication of Colles' fracture, can all lead to frozen shoulder. The reason could be prolonged immobilization of the shoulder joint due to referred pain, etc.

Pathology

- During abduction, and repeated overhead activities of the shoulder, long head of biceps and rotator cuff undergo repeated strain. This results in inflammation, fibrosis, and consequent thickening of the shoulder capsule, which results in loss of movements (Figs 30.2A and B). *If the movements are continued, then the fibrosis*

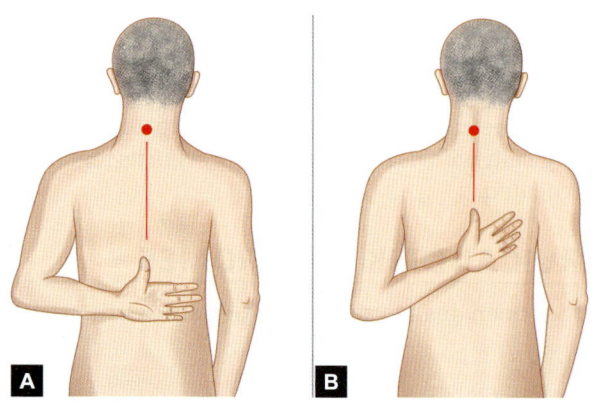

Figs 30.1A and B: Test to detect frozen shoulder (note the distance between the thumbs): (A) Frozen shoulder; (B) Normal

gradually breaks, movements return but never come back to normal.
- Prolonged activity causes small scapular and biceps muscles to waste faster, load on joint increases and degenerative changes sets in. Capsule is fibrosed and shoulder movements are decreased.

Clinical Features

A patient with frozen shoulder clinically presents as follows:
- Decreased range of both active and passive shoulder movements.
- The patient demonstrates a capsular pattern of movement restrictions (i.e. external rotation > abduction > internal rotation).
- Pain is noted at the end stage of stretch.
- Accessory joint play is reduced.
- Resistive tests are generally pain free in the available range of motion.
- Patient is unable to do routine daily activities like combing the hair, in case of women wearing the buttons of their blouse (Fig. 30.3), doing overhead activities (Fig. 30.4), etc.

Facts You Must Know
Diagnosis of frozen shoulder is primarily by clinical examination which records capsular type of restriction of both the active and passive range of motion of the shoulder.

Clinical Stages

There are three classical stages in frozen shoulder, according to **Reeves:**

Stage I (stage of pain): Patient complains of acute pain, decreased movements, external rotation greatest followed by loss of abduction and then forward flexion. *Internal rotation is least affected.* This stage lasts for 10–36 weeks.

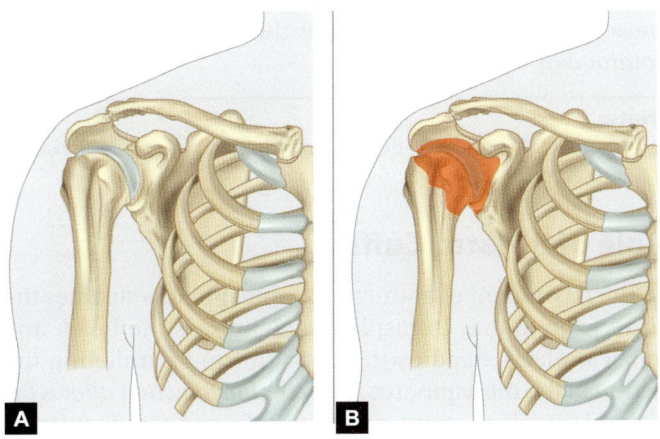

Figs 30.2A and B: (A) Normal capsular pattern; (B) shrinkage of the capsule in frozen shoulder

Note:
Pain in frozen shoulder does not radiate below the elbow (Fig. 30.5).

Stage II (stage of stiffness): In this stage, pain gradually decreases and the patient complains of stiff shoulder. Slight movements are present. This lasts for 4–12 months.

Stage III (stage of recovery): Patient will have no pain and movements would have recovered but will never be regained to normal. It lasts for 6 months to 2 years.

Investigations

Radiograph: X-ray of the shoulder is usually normal; but in a few cases, 'sclerosis' may be seen on the outer edge of greater tuberosity (Golding's sign) (Fig. 30.6).

Arthrogram: It helps in the diagnosis (Fig. 30.7).

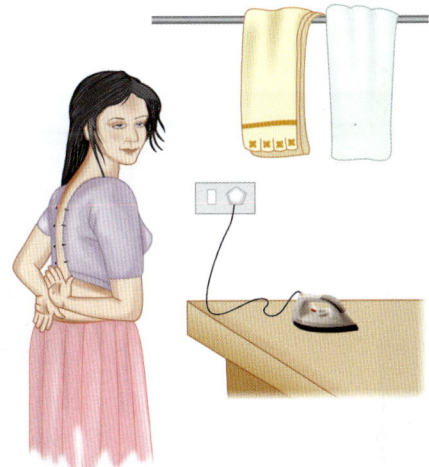

Fig. 30.3: A patient of frozen shoulder is unable to do the daily routine activities like these

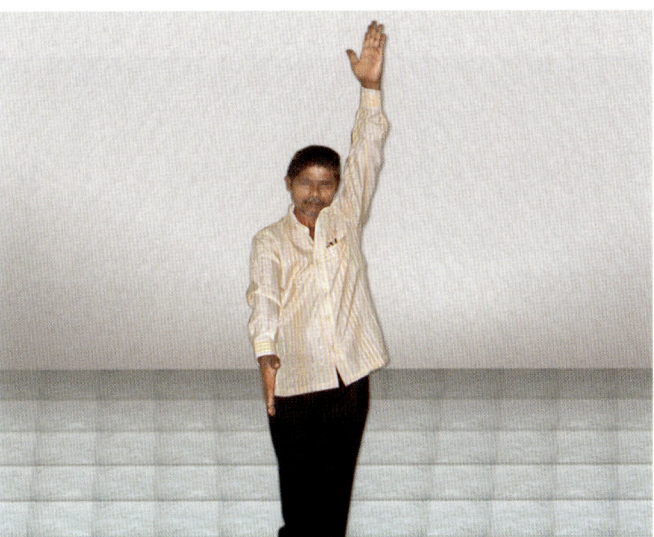

Fig. 30.4: Clinical photo of frozen shoulder, decreased range of movements both active and passive

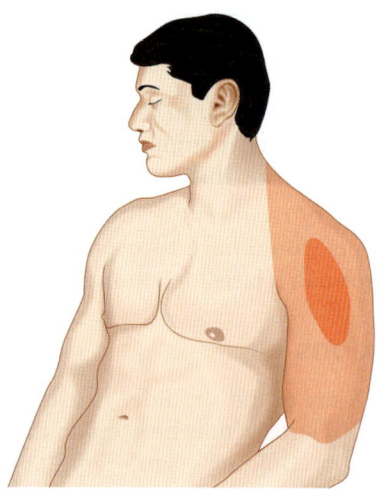

Fig. 30.5: Region of distribution of pain in frozen shoulder (Does not radiate below the elbow)

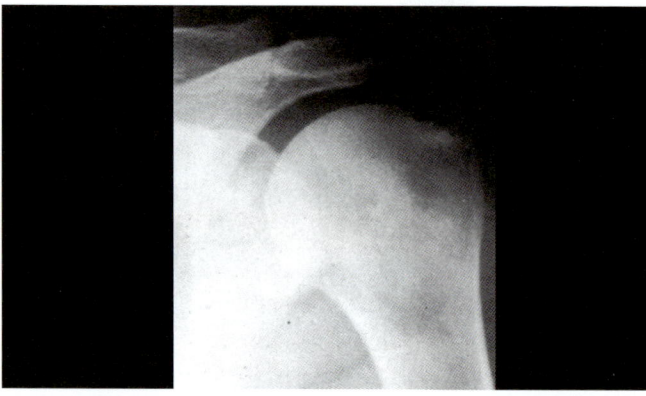

Fig. 30.6: Radiograph showing features of frozen shoulder (Usually normal)

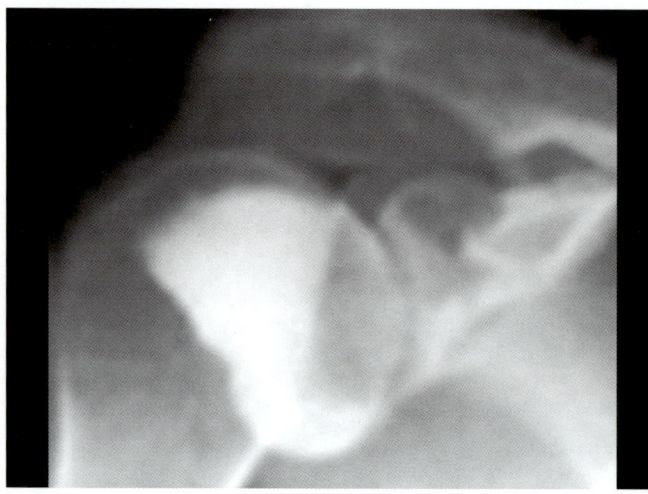

Fig. 30.7: Arthrogram of frozen shoulder

Treatment

Conservative

Stage I: In this stage, long acting once a day non-steroidal anti-inflammatory drugs (NSAIDs) are usually preferred as this condition usually runs a long course (10–36 weeks). Intra-articular steroids may help to provide transient relief of pain only.

Stage II: In this stage, since the pain will have reduced considerably, exercises both active and passive are gradually begun followed by physiotherapy, ultrasound, and heat and shoulder wheel exercises. The role of manipulation of the shoulder is controversial but can be attempted under general anesthesia in this stage.

Stage III: In this stage, active and passive exercises, physiotherapy consisting of short wave diathermy, ultrasound, etc. are continued.

Surgery

- *Arthroscopic distension (Bruisement technique):* This helps to increase ROM after several weeks or months.
- *Arthroscopic releases:* This is indicated in recalcitrant cases where the above measures have all failed.

> **Treatment Pearls**
> - Exercises are most effective than modalities, drugs and steroid injection.
> - Mobilization techniques are the other effective method.
> - Traditional manipulation under GA is a previous successful method.
> - Traditional manipulation under GA is more successful than traction manipulation.

ROTATOR CUFF LESIONS

This includes both impingement syndrome and rotator cuff tears.

Fine adjustments of the humeral head within the glenoid is achieved by coordinated activity of four interrelated muscles (Fig. 30.8) arising from the scapula and is called *rotator cuff.*

> **Note:**
> - Rotator cuff comprises supraspinatus, infraspinatus, subscapularis and teres minor (Mnemonic SITS).

Role of Rotator Cuffs

In the movement of abduction, supraspinatus steadies the head from above, infraspinatus depresses the head, and subscapularis steadies the head in front paralleling the action of the infraspinatus. *This combined action allows the deltoid muscle to swing up the arm from a steady fulcrum irrespective of the position of the scapula* (Figs 30.9A and B).

Impingement Syndrome

It is a problem, which is commonly associated with supraspinatus tendon. Other causes like bicipital tendonitis, and intraspinatus tendonitis, subacromial bursitis, etc. may give rise to rotator cuff problems, but they are not that common (Box 30.1).

Box 30.1: Causes of Impingement Syndrome
- Complete or partial rupture of rotator cuff
- Supraspinatus tendonitis
- Calcific deposits
- Subacromial bursitis
- Subdeltoid bursitis
- Periarthritis
- Bicipital tenosynovitis
- Fracture greater trochanter.

SUPRASPINATUS TENDINITIS

Among the various causes mentioned above, supraspinatus tendinitis is the one that is commonly encountered and this gives rise to the *impingement syndrome*. Impingement occurs beneath the coracoacromial arch. The most vulnerable structures for impingement between the undersurface of the acromion and the head of the humerus are the greater tuberosity, the overlying supraspinatus tendon (Fig. 30.10) and the long head of biceps. The major site of compression is anterior to the angle of the acromion. Hence, the proper term is *anterior impingement syndrome* or painful arc syndrome (Fig. 30.11).

Neer's Stages of Impingement Syndrome
- Edema stage.
- Tendinitis and fibrositis.
- Rotator cuff tears and rupture of biceps tendon.
- Bone changes.

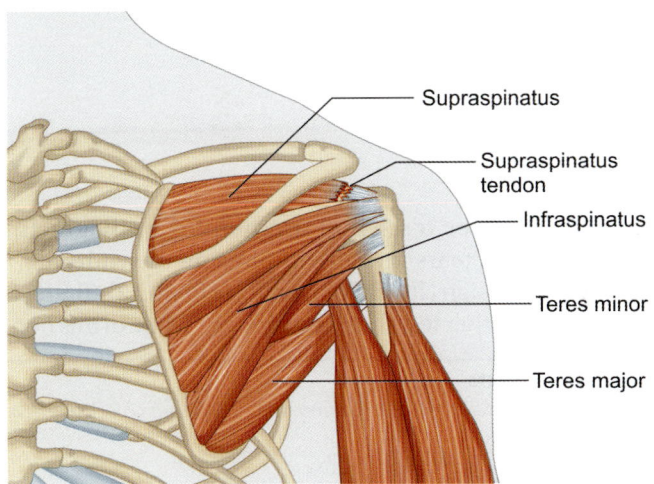

Fig. 30.8: Muscles of the rotator cuff

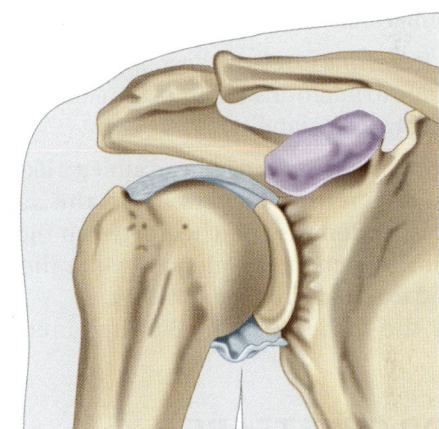

Fig. 30.10: Supraspinatus tear

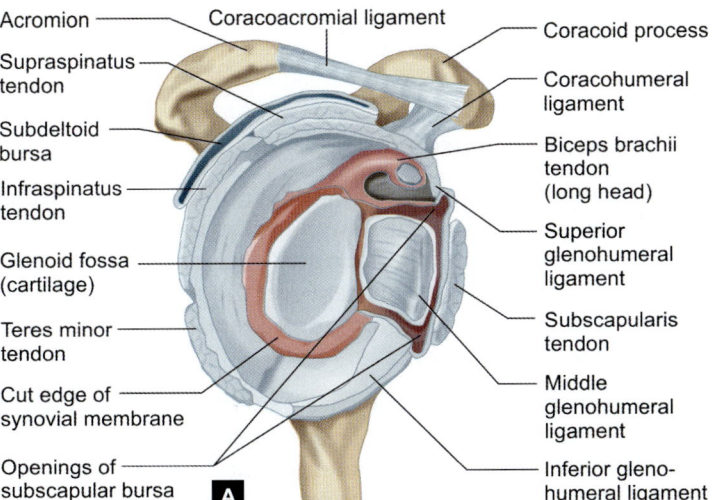

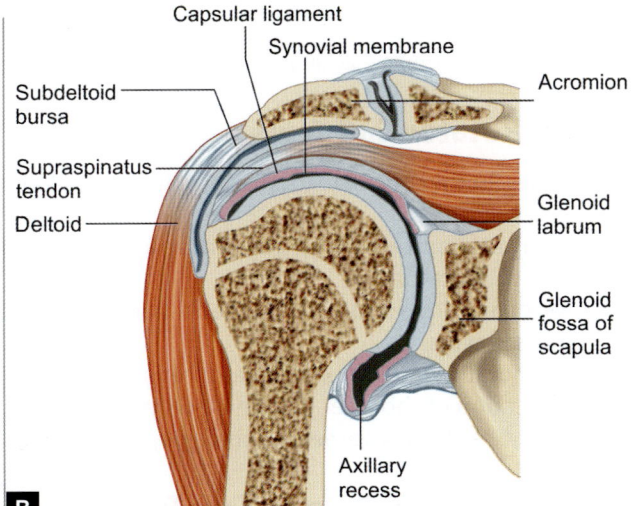

Figs 30.9A and B: Anatomy of the shoulder joint (internal structures): (A) Shoulder joint opened (lateral view); (B) Coronal section through shoulder joint

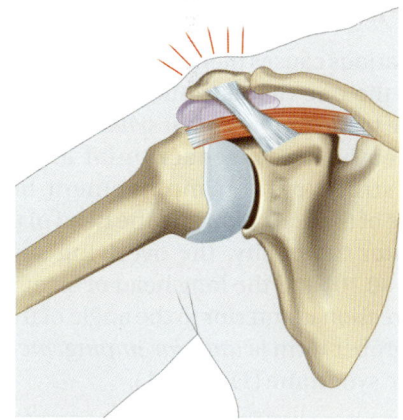

Fig. 30.11: Anterior impingement syndrome

Types of Impingement Syndrome

Primary: Here impingement occurs beneath the coracoacromial arch and is due to subacromial overloading.

Secondary: This is due to relative decrease in the subacromial arch and is due to micro-instability of the glen humeral joint or scapulothoracic instability.

Posterior (Internal): Seen in overhead athletes like throwers, swimmers, and tennis players. Here the supra- and infraspinatus tendons are pinched between the posterior and superior aspects of the glenoid when the arm is in elevated and externally rotated position.

Among the three, primary impingement is more common.

ROTATOR CUFF TEARS

Note:
Incidence of rotator cuff tear, less than 70 years—30 percent; 71–80 years—60 percent; more than 89 years—70 percent.

About Rotator Cuff Tears

The causes for rotator cuff tears, partial or full, are as follows:
- Age >40 years.
- Occupations requiring repetitive and excessive overhead movements.
- Overhead sports and athletes like throwers, swimmers, tennis players, etc.
- Degenerative etiology is the major cause.
- Dislocation of shoulder joint in 40–60 years of age.
- About 2/3rd cases are seen in male population.

Classification of Rotator Cuff Tears

(According to American Arthroscopic Orthopedics)
- Small tear (<1 cm).

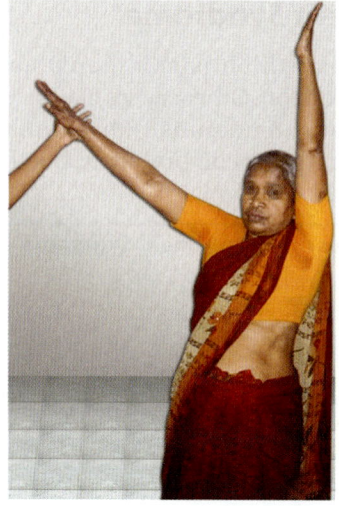

Fig. 30.12: Clinical photo showing painful arc

- Medium tear (1–3 cm).
- Large tears (3–5 cm).

Clinical Tests

Special shoulder tests that are helpful in diagnosing rotational, cuff tears and the impingement syndrome, is the painful arc sign (It is 81% specific) (Fig. 30.12). There are innumerable other tests but is outside the scope of this book.

Interesting Facts
Do you know the clinical facts leading to the diagnosis of RCL tear?
- Age >40 years.
- Previous history of minor trauma.
- Degenerative changes on the X-rays.
- Various clinical tests.
  How accurate are these tests?
  There are 91 percent sensitive and 75 percent specific.
  Pearl: Clinical tests are more accurate and cost effective than a battery of investigations in diagnosing an RCL.

Clinical Features

All patients with impingement syndrome have similar clinical features like pain, swelling, limitation of shoulder movements, muscle atrophy (supraspinatus and infraspinatus), and tenderness over the greater tuberosity, etc. The following grades are described in anterior impingement syndrome.

Grade I: This is common in young adults and athletes in the age group of 18–30 years. Due to overstress and repeated overhead activity, impingement occurs and supraspinatus is inflamed. The painful arc appears here (Fig. 30.13).

Grade II: This is seen in age group of 40–45 years and may be due to supraspinatus tendinitis or subacromial bursitis.

The cause could be either overuse or degeneration and osteophyte formation.

Grade III: It is seen in patients over 45 years of age and may be due to occupational overuse, fall, and sudden increase in activity, atrophic degenerative changes in the cuff and rarely due to acute tear of the rotator cuff.

Investigations

X-rays of the shoulder: This helps to detect bony avulsions, spurs, calcific deposits, sclerotic areas, etc. (Box 30.2) (Figs 30.14A and B).

Arthrogram: Single contrast arthrogram is considered as the gold standard in diagnosing rotator cuff tears.

Ultrasonography: This is highly reliable in diagnosing rotator cuff pathology with a sensitivity of 98 percent.

MRI: This is also very accurate (81%) but expensive (Fig. 30.15).

> **Mystifying Facts About X-Ray Changes in Rotator Cuff Lesions**
> - ↓ Subarachnoid space ⁻ 6 mm
> - Anterior spurring of ACM joint
> - Humeral head degeneration
> - Sclerotic inferior acromion (eyebrow sign)
> - Hooking of the acromion.

Management

Conservative Treatment

It consists of heat, massage, NSAIDs, local infiltration of hydrocortisone, subacromial steroid injections, exercises both active and passive, temporary immobilization, etc. *Ninety percent will recover with these measures.*

Surgical Treatment

Indications: Failure of conservative treatment for three months, if the patients are young and active, and if there is increasing loss of shoulder function, surgery is indicated.

Methods

- Arthroscopic repair in small and partial tears.
- Open methods in major tears.

Depending upon the etiological factors, the following surgical techniques are described: Excision of adhesions and manipulation of shoulder, excision of calcium deposits, repair of incomplete tear, acromioplasty (Fig. 30.16), acromionectomy for more disabling pain with normal range of movements, direct suture for complete rupture of rotator cuff, rotation, and transposition of flap, free graft, etc. Results are good in 85–90 percent.

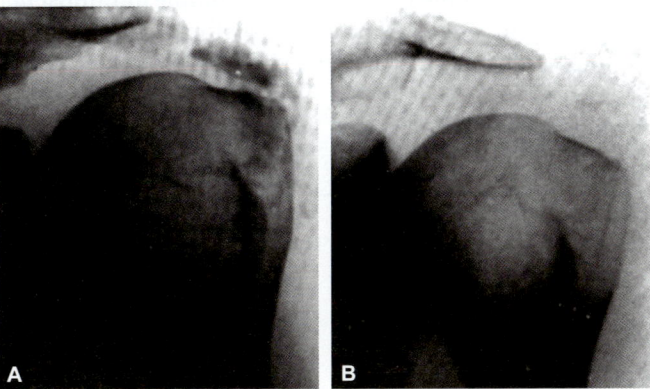

Figs 30.14A and B: Radiographs showing changes in the rotator cuff tears: (A) Calcific depositis; (B) Degenerative changes

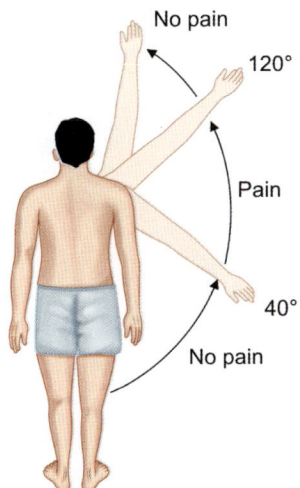

Fig. 30.13: Pain occurs in the impingement syndrome between 40–120° of shoulder abduction as it is in a position that the supraspinatus tendon is impinged against the undersurface of the acromion and head of the humerus. Rest of the movements are painless (painful are syndrome)

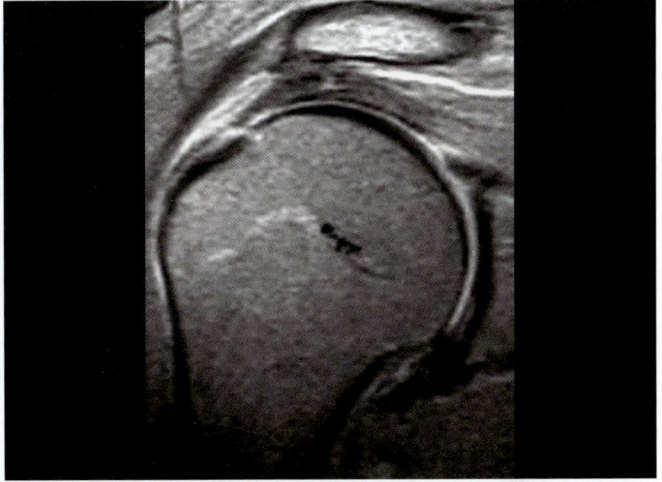

Fig. 30.15: MRI showing rotator cuff tear

Differential Diagnosis of Impingement Syndrome

- Frozen shoulder.
- Cervical spondylosis.
- ACM and shoulder joint arthritis.
- Bursitis.
- Snapping scapula.
- Suprascapular neuropathy.

DELTOID CONTRACTURE

Deltoid, the powerful shoulder abductor, if fibrosed, results in a grotesque looking shoulder with severe functional impairments (Fig. 30.17).

Causes

Deltoid contracture could be congenital or acquired and the latter is more common. Among the acquired variety, the possible causes are:
- Due to anatomical aberration of multiple intramuscular septae in the intermediate portions of the deltoid, repeated intramuscular injection into the deltoid results in fibrosis.
- Chronic infection due to the injected drugs.
- Pressure ischemia.

> **Disturbing Injection Facts**
> The muscles commonly used for IM injections:
> - Deltoid muscle
> - Triceps muscle
> - Anterior abdominal muscles
> - Gluteal muscles
> - Quadriceps muscle
>
> Among these, deltoid, glutei, and quadriceps are the commonly injected muscles. However, post-injection contractures are more common in quadriceps followed by deltoid.

> **Do You Know?**
> The most common cause of muscle contracture in our country is PPRP (Post-polio residual paralysis).

> **Interesting Facts about Post-injection Muscular Contractures (Indian Contribution)**
> - Post-injection muscle contractures are not very common.
> - Though reported all over the world, India is perhaps the leader.
> - The credit of 'first reporting' in India belongs to Bhattacharya.
> - Largest number reported is by TK Shanmugasundaram.
> - No specific injectable has been incriminated but tetracycline was found to be the culprit in most number of cases by Shanmugasundaram.

Clinical Presentations

A patient with deltoid contracture typically presents as follows:
- Inability to keep the arm in contact with the chest in the anatomical plane of the scapula.
- When the arm is forcibly brought into contact with the chest, winging of the scapula happens.
- Dimple or puckering of the skin over the deltoid may or may not be seen.
- On palpation, a thick intermediate fibrotic deltoid muscle can be felt.
- Shoulder function is not severely affected.

If the above clinical findings are supported by a strong history of repeated IM injections into the deltoid muscle, the diagnosis is more or less certain.

> **Mystifying Facts**
> *Beware of the diagnostic pitfalls:*
> - Neglected ADS (Anterior dislocation of shoulder).
> - Serratus anterior palsy.
> - Old injury to the proximal humeral epiphysis.
> - Poliomyelitis.

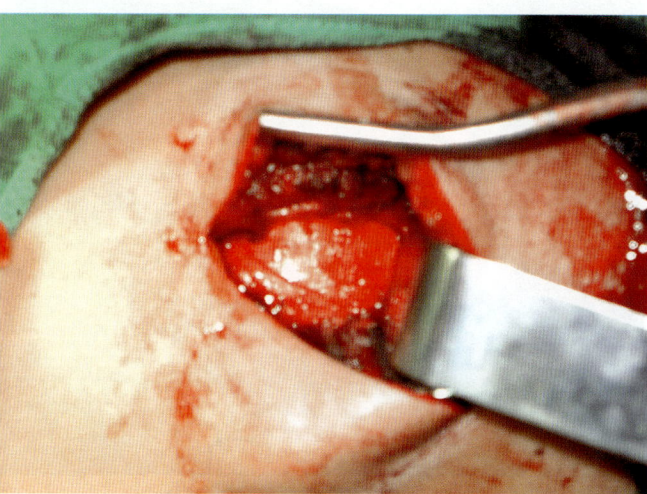

Fig. 30.16: Operative photo showing acromioplasty

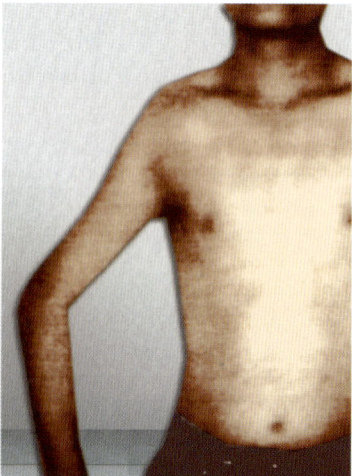

Fig. 30.17: Features suggestive of deltoid contracture (Clinical photo)

Investigations

Plain X-ray, MRI, etc. helps in the diagnosis.

Treatment

Prevention

This is better than the best of curative measures and consists of avoiding unnecessary and indiscriminate deltoid IM injections.

Curative

Surgical release of the fibrotic bands by closed fasciotomy technique of Shanmugasundaram gives excellent results. Open surgical release either the transverse or oblique division of the contracted muscle is indicated in more severe cases.

Rehabilitation

To facilitate faster recovery of shoulder function and to correct winging of the scapula, repeated stretching and straightening exercises are recommended.

REGIONAL CONDITIONS OF THE ELBOW

TENNIS ELBOW

I am sure everyone is fascinated by tennis. We may not get a place under the sun with Roger Federer, Nadaf, Pete Sampras, Leander Paes, Sania Mirza and others, but certainly, we may get an appointment with an orthopedic surgeon for a problem common in them, that too without playing tennis! Yes, the obvious reference is towards *tennis elbow* (Fig. 30.18).

> **Note**
> Sachin Tendulkar should be credited for popularizing and creating lots of awareness and controversies about tennis elbow at least in our country!

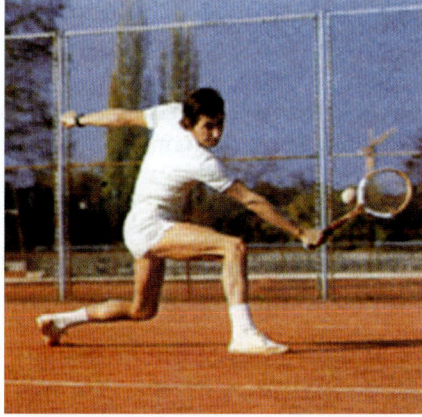

Fig. 30.18: Tennis elbow (A professional hazard)

History

It was first described from the *Writer's cramps* by Range in 1873. It was Madris who called it as "tennis elbow" shortly thereafter.

Definition

Tennis elbow syndrome encompasses lateral, medial, and posterior elbow symptoms (Flowchart 30.1). The one commonly encountered is the lateral tennis elbow which is known as the classical tennis elbow and is the *pain and tenderness on the lateral side of the elbow*, some well-defined and some vague, that results from repetitive stress.

Flowchart 30.1: Types of tennis elbow

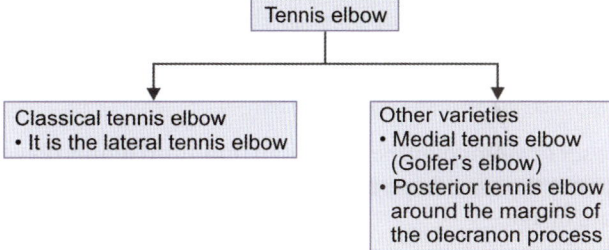

> **Vital Points**
> *Location of pain in tennis elbow*
> - Lateral epicondyle (75%)
> - Lateral muscle mass (17%)
> - Medial epicondyle (10%)
> - Posterior (8%).

Lateral Tennis Elbow

It is a lesion affecting the tendinous origin of common wrist extensors (Fig. 30.19). It is more common in men than women are and is believed to be a degenerative disorder.

Causes

Epicondylitis: This is due to single or multiple tears in the common extensor origin, periostitis, angiofibroblastic proliferation of extensor carpi radialis brevis (ECRB), etc.

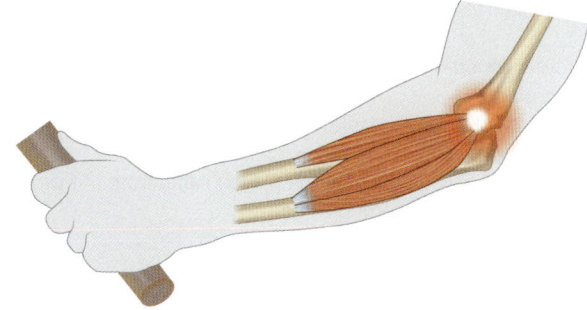

Fig. 30.19: Repetitive stress at common extensor origin in tennis players

Inflammation of adventitious bursa: Between the common extensor origin and radiohumeral joint.

Calcified deposits: Within the common extensor tendon.

Painful annular ligament: It is due to hypertrophy of synovial fringe between the radial head and the capitulum's.

Pain of neurological origin, e.g. cervical spine affection, radial nerve entrapment, etc.

> **Mystifying Fact**
> Extensor carpi radialis brevis (ECRB) is the most commonly involved structure in lateral epicondylitis.

> **Seen in**
> - All levels of tennis players.
> - In world class players "SERVE" appears to be the cause.
> - In less than world class players "backhand stroke."
> - Seen in other sports also.
> - May be occupational, etc.
> - More common in the dominated arm.

Causes in tennis players: More than one-third tennis players all over the world are affected with this problem over 35 years of age.

> - Novice.
> - Playing several games per week.
> - More than 35 years of age.
> - Equal sex incidence.
> - Backhand stroke (38%).
> - Serve (25%).
> - Forehand stroke (23%).
> - Backhand volley (7%).
> - Overhead smash (4%).
> - Forehand volley (3%).

> **Contributing Factors**
> - Little playing experience.
> - Consistent missing of "*sweet spot*" while hitting.
> - Poor stroke techniques: Use of arm instead of body.
> - Poor power or flexibility.
> - Heavy stiff racket, large handle size, too tight racket stringing.
> - Heavy duty wet balls.
> - Playing surface—balls bounce quicker off the cement court.

> **Did You Know?**
> Though called tennis elbow, it is more common in non-tennis players (95%). Causes can be:
> - Throwing sports.
> - Swimming.
> - Carpentry, plumbing, textile workers.
> - Housewives.
>
> However, up to 50 percent of tennis players suffer from this problem at some time in their sporting career.

Pathophysiology and Related Symptoms

Stage I: There is acute inflammation but no angioblastic invasion. *The patient complains of pain during activity.*

Stage II: This is the stage of chronic inflammation. There is some angioblastic invasion. *The patient complains of pain both during activity and at rest.*

Stage III: Chronic inflammation with extensive angioblastic invasion. *The patient complains pain at rest, night pains, and pain during daily activities.*

Etiology

Problems in tennis players: More than one-third tennis players all over the world are affected with this problem over 35 years of age are obviously due to faculty playing techniques.

Non-tennis players: Ironically tennis elbow is more common in non-tennis players. This unfortunate group is comprised of housewives, carpenters, miners, drill workers, etc. India's Cricketing Legend Sachin Tendulkar and Sreesanth have made tennis elbow very popular across the country and the world.

Indian housewives: This is the third largest group suffering from this condition. The household chores like washing, brooming, cooking, etc. require repeated extension of the elbow leading to the development of this condition (Fig. 30.20).

Computer related injuries: This is emerging as the recent epidemic among computer professionals across the globe due to repetitive stress while using laptops, mouse, etc.

Clinical Features

Patient complains of pain on the outer aspect of the elbow and has difficulty in gripping objects and lifting them. Sportspersons will have difficulty in extending the elbow. The following are some of the useful clinical tests:

Clinical Tests

Local tenderness on the outside of the elbow at the common extensor origin with aching pain in the back of the forearm (Fig. 30.21).

Cozen's test: Painful resisted extension of the wrist with elbow in full extension elicits pain at the lateral elbow (Fig. 30.22).

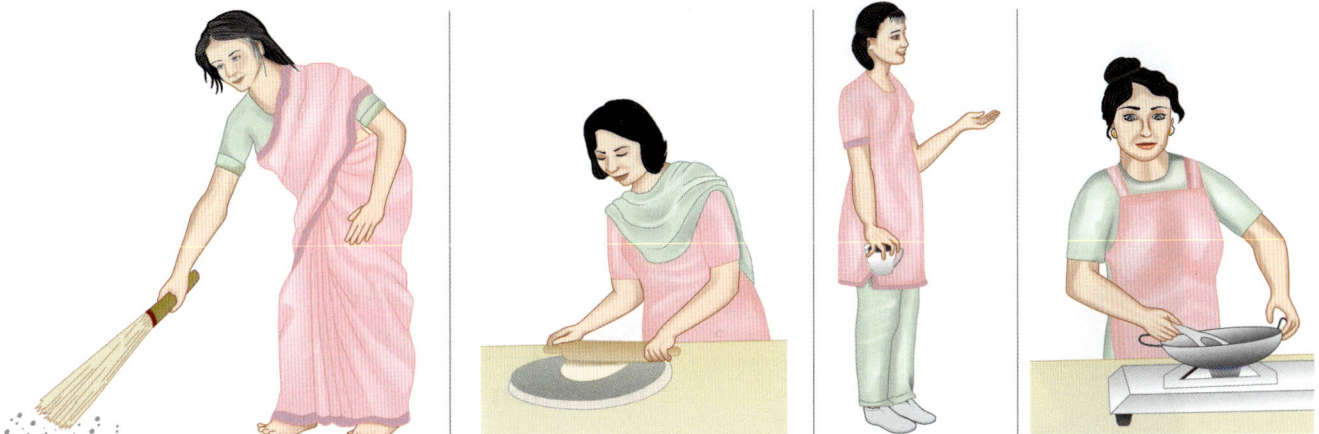

Fig. 30.20: All these activities carried out by our traditional Indian housewives can lead to tennis elbow

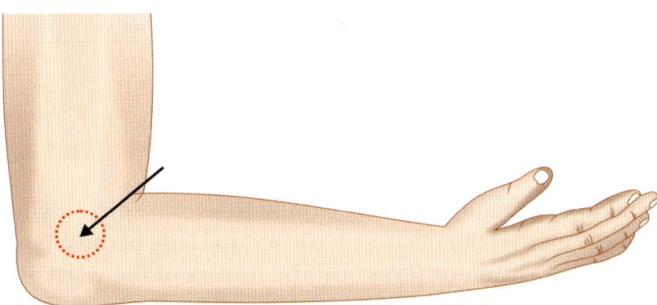

Fig. 30.21: Arrow showing site of tenderness in tennis elbow

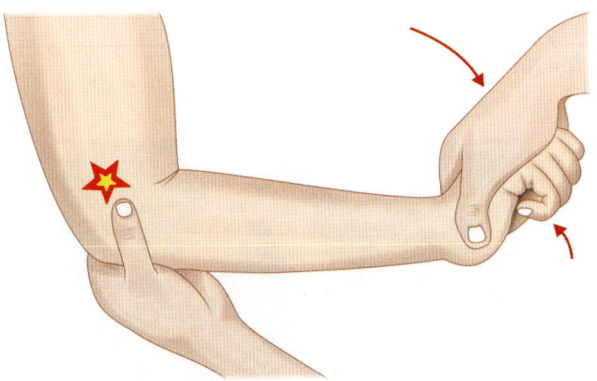

Fig. 30.22: Method of performing the Cozen's test

Elbow held in extension, passive wrist flexion, and pronation produces pain.

Maudsley's test: Resisted extension of the middle finger (Remember the letter 'M') elicits pain at the lateral epicondyle due to disease in the extensor digitorum communis.

Investigations

Radiograph

The AP, lateral and radiocapitellar views are the recommended views. In most cases, it is normal. However, in 16 percent of the cases, a faint calcification along the lateral epicondyle can be detected.

Ultrasonography

This is increasingly being done with good success of late.

Treatment

Conservative Management

It consists of rest and physiotherapy. In tennis players exercises, light racket, smaller grip, elbow strap, etc. are helpful (Fig. 30.23). Injection of local anesthetic and steroid are useful in 40 percent of cases.

Mill's Maneuver

This is the final option before surgery. About 10 percent of the cases do not respond to conservative treatment. In them, a forceful extension of a fully flexed and pronated forearm after injection may be attempted.

Surgical Management

Indications

- Severe pain for 6 weeks at least.
- Marked and localized tenderness over lateral epicondyle.
- Failure to respond to restricted activity or immobilization for at least 2 weeks.

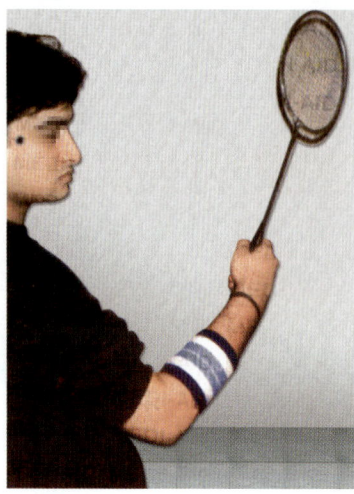

Fig. 30.23: Elbow supports to be used in tennis elbow

Surgical Methods
- Percutaneous release of epicondylar muscles.
- Bosworth technique of excision of the proximal portion of the annular ligament, release of the origin of the extensor muscles, excision of the bursa, and excision of synovial fringes.

> **What is New in the Treatment of Tennis and Golfer's Elbow?**
> - The use of extracorporeal shock wave therapy (ESWT): About 2,000 shock waves of 0.04-0.12 nj/mm^2, three times at monthly intervals for 6 months are found to be effective in cases with failed conservative treatment for at least 6 months.
> - Arthroscopic release: Of ECRB with failed conservative treatment for nearly 6 months. It is minimally invasive and helps in early rehabilitation.
> - Autologous blood injections: In refractory cases, injections of 2 ml of autologous blood and 0.5 percent bupivacaine has been tried with good success in some centers.
> - Counterforce bracing (called the tennis elbow or forearm band): These forces release the forces in the ECRB region.
> - Rehabilitative exercises: These are wrist flexion, extension, forearm supination and pronation, wrist radial and ulnar deviations at three sets of ten repetitions everyday for 2–6 months is known to give good results.
> - Ultrasound-guided percutaneous needle therapy: This consists of ultrasound-guided corticosteroid injection and needle debridement of the structures around lateral epicondyle.
>
> *Indications:* In small tears, not responding to conservative therapy and if too small for surgery.
>
> *Advantages*
> - Minimally invasive procedure.
> - Restoration of function is rapid.
> - The option of surgery is still open.
>
> In expert's hands, it has a success rate of 65 percent.

> **Quick Facts**
> *Significant relief of symptoms in tennis elbow:*
> - Changing tennis strokes — 92 percent
> - Stretching exercises — 84 percent
> - Use of splints — 83 percent
> - NSAIDs/steroid — 85 percent
> - Physiotherapy — 50–75 percent
> - Rest more than 1 month — 72 percent

GOLFER'S ELBOW (Syn: Epitrochleitis, Medial Tennis Elbow)

Definition
It is a tendinopathy of the insertion of the epitrochlear muscles [flexors of the fingers of the hand flexor carpi radialis (FCR) and pronators]. It is more commonly seen in golf players (Fig. 30.24).

> **Did You Know?**
> Golfer's elbow is also called Swimmer's elbow.

Clinical Features
Medial epitrochleitis is very similar to lateral epicondylitis (tennis elbow) but occurs on the medial side of the elbow, where the pronator teres and the flexors of the wrist and fingers originate. Tensing of these muscles by resisted wrist and finger flexion in pronation will provoke the pain and tenderness (Fig. 30.25).

Tenderness is often less well localized than in tennis elbow.

> **Do You Know?**
> Tennis elbow is nine times more common than Golfer's elbow.

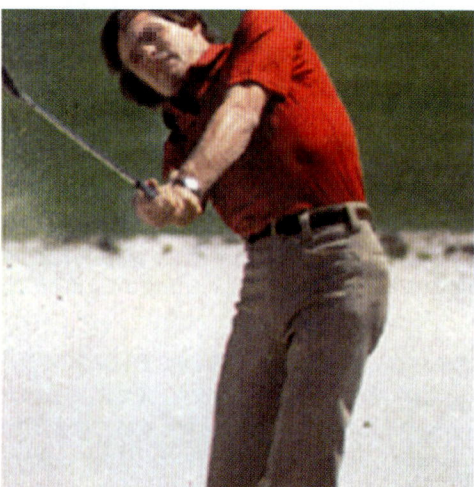

Fig. 30.24: Golfer's elbow

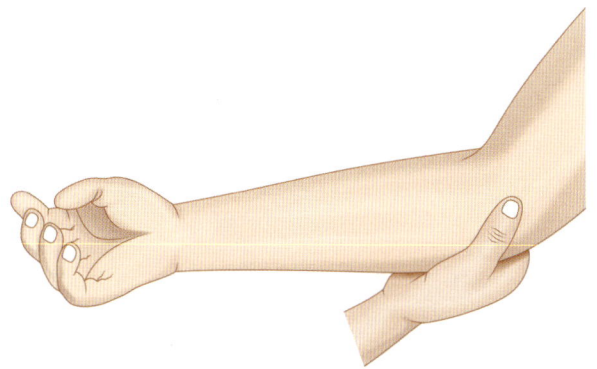

Fig. 30.25: Method of eliciting tenderness in Golfer's elbow

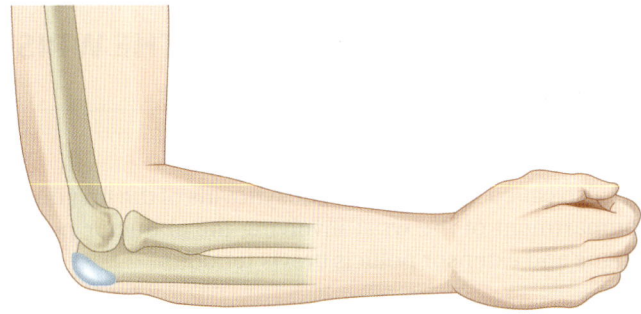

Fig. 30.26: Olecranon bursa

Treatment

It is the same as for tennis elbow, but the treatment is even less satisfactory.

> **Lesser-known but Interesting Elbow Conditions**
> You know about tennis and Golfer's elbow, but do you know about:
> *Boxer's elbow:* This is also called as hyperextension overload syndrome or olecranon impingement syndrome and is due to the repetitive valgus hyperextension by a boxer during jabbing.
> *Little leagues elbow:* This is a medial epicondyle avulsion fracture. It is seen commonly in children and adolescents involved in throwing sports.

OLECRANON BURSITIS
(Syn: Student's Elbow, Miner's Elbow or Draughtsman Elbow)

This is a chronic inflammation of the olecranon bursa (Fig. 30.26). It may be the result of repetitive minor injuries or irritation, microcrystalline deposition. Infection occurs due to chronic friction as in students who tend to keep their elbows repeatedly over the table, bench, etc. over long periods during writing, reading, etc. (Fig. 30.27).

Clinical Features

It usually manifests as a swelling over the tip of the olecranon (Fig. 30.28). There may be pain, if there is inflammation. Inspection or palpation usually easily detects it.

Investigations

- *X-ray* shows soft tissue shadow
- *Aspiration and culture* of the bursal fluid is necessary in order to exclude the possibility of an infectious etiology.
- *USG* of the elbow is a useful diagnostic tool.

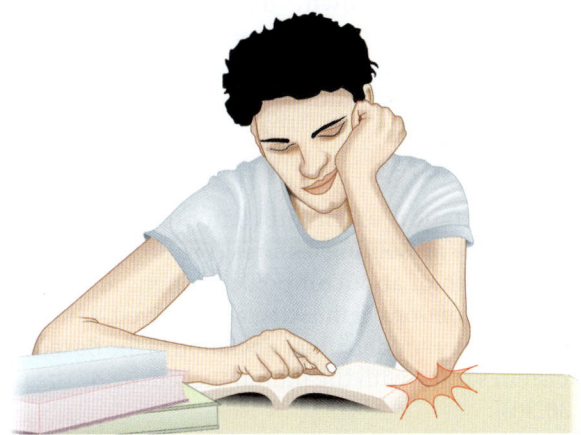

Fig. 30.27: Are you guilty of reading like this? Well you could develop student's elbow!

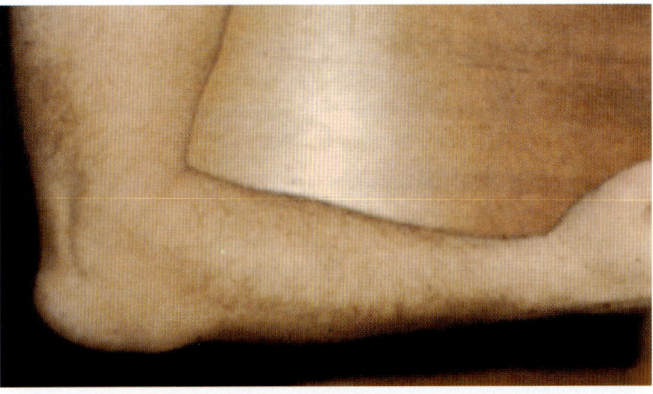

Fig. 30.28: Clinical picture of olecranon bursitis

Treatment

Treatment is essentially conservative and consists of NSAIDs, local steroids, etc. Surgical excision is done in chronic cases. Microcrystalline-induced bursitis has a good prognosis and the symptoms usually resolve after a few days, whether treated or not. However, bursitis due to repeated minor irritation is more difficult to treat.

REGIONAL CONDITIONS OF THE WRIST AND HAND

DE QUERVAIN'S DISEASE

It is also called as stenosing tenosynovitis of the first dorsal compartment of the wrist involving the abductor pollicis longus and extensor pollicis brevis tendons.

Etiology

Exact cause is not known. [1]de Quervain's disease is commonly seen in women between 30 and 50 years of age, and may be due to repeated overuse of the wrist. Trigger finger is common in conditions like rheumatoid arthritis.

Clinical Features

Pain and limitation of the movements of the involved tendons are the presenting features (Fig. 30.29). In this, the common sheath of abductor pollicis longus and extensor pollicis brevis tendons at the wrist are involved. Tenderness can be elicited by sudden ulnar deviation of the flexed hand [Finkelstein's test—with the thumb tucked inside the palm (Fig. 30.30)].

> **Pitfalls**
> *Do you know that Finkelstein's test is not pathognomonic of de Quervain's disease? It is also positive in:*
> - First carpometacarpal arthritis.
> - Wartenberg's syndrome.
> - Arthritis of radiocarpal and intercarpal joints.

> **Interesting Facts**
> *Do you know about intersection syndrome? Well, it is tenosynovitis of the II dorsal compartment.*

Investigations: Plain X-ray may show a soft tissue shadow and USG is a more reliable diagnostic tool.

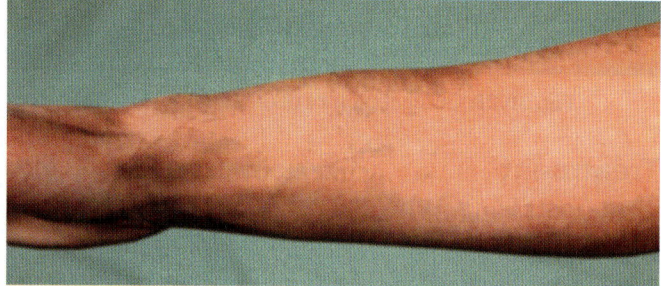

Fig. 30.29: Clinical photograph of de Quervain's disease

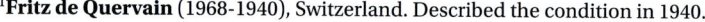

[1]**Fritz de Quervain** (1968-1940), Switzerland. Described the condition in 1940.

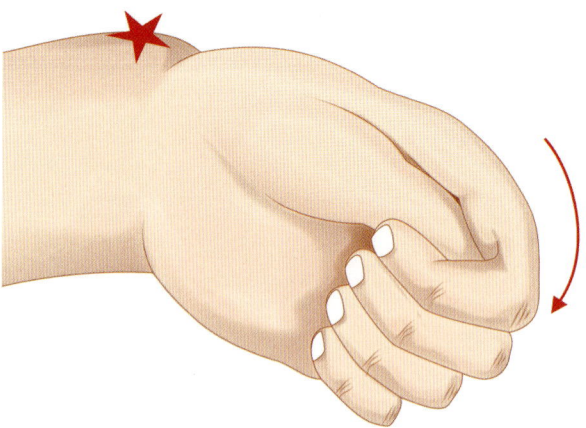

Fig. 30.30: Finkelstein's test

Treatment

Conservative Methods

This treatment consists of rest, NSAIDs, physiotherapy, local infiltration of hydrocortisone, wrist immobilization, etc.

Surgery

Division of the appropriate retinaculum if the above measures fail.

> **Mystifying Facts**
> *Do you know the reasons for failure of conservative treatment in de Quervain's disease?*
> - Anomalous tendons.
> - Multiple slips of abductor pollicis longus tendon.
> - Multiple sub-compartments within the first wrist compartment. This is seen in 75 percent of the cases.

TRIGGER FINGERS AND THUMB

It is a stenosing tenovaginitis, in which the sheath of a flexor tendon thickens, apparently spontaneously, to entrap the tendon.

It is locking of the finger in a position of flexion, (Fig. 30.31) that occurs at the retinaculae of the flexor tendons of the fingers and the thumb (Fig. 30.32) in the palm. The A_1 pulley is also thickened and fibrosed (Fig. 30.33). In the palm, the flexor muscles are sufficiently strong to continue forcing the tendon through the diminished gap in the flexor retinaculum. The flexor tendon consequently gradually develops a constriction under the retinaculum and a bulge distal to it. Finally, the flexor muscles may force the bulge through the retinaculum, but the extensor muscles may be insufficiently powerful to extend the finger hereafter. The finger now snaps as it passes through the constriction and finally locks in a position of flexion from which attempts

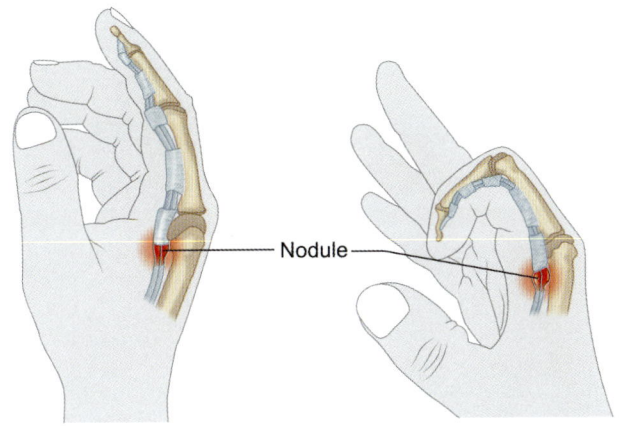

Fig. 30.31: Trigger finger

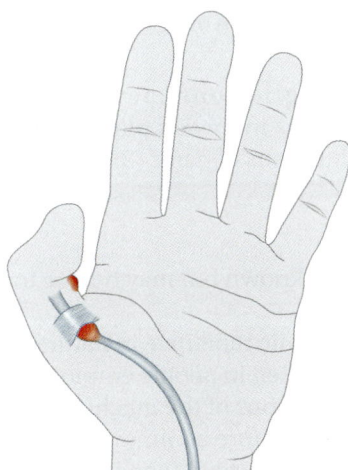

Fig. 30.32: Trigger thumb

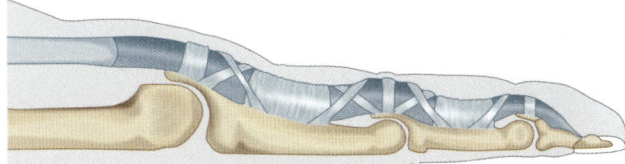

Fig. 30.33: Flexor retinaculae (pulleys) of the finger which may be responsible for trigger fingers

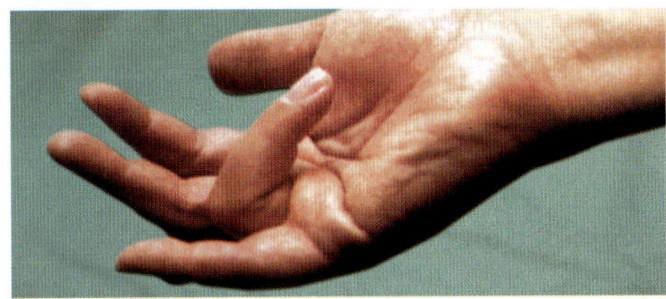

Fig. 30.34: Clinical photograph of a trigger finger

to passively extend the fingers are painful (Fig. 30.34). These are common in women. Congenital trigger fingers are seen in 25 percent of cases and may present as late as 2 years of age.

Treatment

- Splinting of the fingers.
- Use of NSAIDs, physiotherapy, etc.
- Administration of locally acting steroid injection.
- Finally, if all the above measures fail, surgical excision of A_1 pulley is indicated.

What is New in the Treatment of Trigger Finger?
Percutaneous release of trigger fingers using a specially designed knife in difficult cases.

GANGLIA (GANGLION CYST)

The term *Ganglia* is derived from a Greek term meaning *Cystic tumor*.

Definition

It is defined as a localized, tense, painless, cystic, swelling, containing clear gelatinous fluid (Fig. 30.35A).

Origin: The clear gelatinous fluid may be due to leakage or subsequent fibrous encapsulation of synovial fluid through the capsule of a joint or a tendon sheath (Fig. 30.35B).

Sites: It is commonly seen over dorsum of the wrist, flexor aspects of the fingers and dorsum of the foot.

Did You Know?
It accounts for 50–70 percent of all soft tissue tumors of the hand and wrist.

Quick Facts: Ganglion
- Dorsal wrist ganglia accounts for 60–70 percent of all hand ganglia. It arises from scapholunate ligament.
- Volar ganglion—18–20 percent.
- Ganglion at the flexor tendon.
- Sheath at A_1 pulley—10–12 percent.

Predisposing factors: Chronic repetitive stress and sometimes injury. It is more prevalent in women (M: F = 1:3).

Clinical Features

Swelling over the dorsum of the wrist is the only complaint. However, patient may complain of pain and enlarged swelling affecting the movements of the wrist in the event of complications.

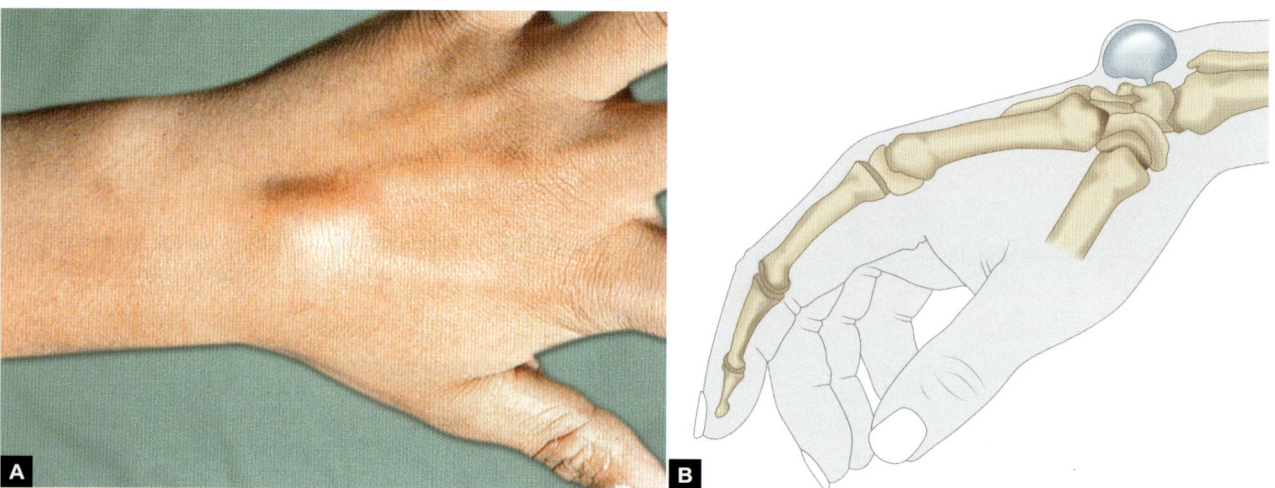

Figs 30.35A and B: Clinical photograph showing: (A) Ganglion; (B) Origin of a ganglion

Investigations

Plain X-ray of the part and laboratory examination of the aspirated fluid can be done. USG helps.

Treatment

It may resolve spontaneously over a period. Excision is indicated if it is causing symptoms.

Biblical Facts
What role the Holy Bible has in orthopedics? Well in ancient days, it was used to bang the ganglion into submission!

What is New?
Treatment of Ganglia: Arthroscopic release of the dorsal wrist ganglia is a sensible option than open excision for the following advantages:
- Minimal scarring
- Safe
- Faster rehabilitation
- Early mobility.

Did You Know?
In some dorsal wrist ganglia is usually due to capsular abnormality in the region of interosseous scapholunate ligament.

DUPUYTREN'S CONTRACTURE

Dupuytren's[2] contracture is defined as proliferative fibroplasias of the subcutaneous palmar tissue, forming nodules of cords along its ulnar border. *This fibroplasias results in finger contractures, thinning of subcutaneous fat, adhesions of skin to the lesion, pitting of skin, and knuckle pads on the dorsum of proximal interphalangeal (PIP) joints.*

The following lesions may be associated with Dupuytren's, lesions in medial plantar fascia in 5 percent and plastic indurations of penis (3%).

Causes

Exact cause is not known but may be due to:
- Heredity.
- Trauma of chronic repetitive in nature.
- Occupational, seen in people employed in rock drilling due to the vibrations of the machine.
- Males—10 times more common in males.
- Whites are affected more than blacks.
- Frequent and severe in epileptics and alcoholics (42%).
- Onset is usually less than 40 years of age.

Pathogenesis

Nodules and cords develop due to fibroplasias and hypertrophy of already existing fibers of palmar fascia on its ulnar border.

Clinical Features

Usually begins with ring finger at the distal palmar crease and later involves little finger. Flexion of metacarpophalangeal (MCP) and PIP joints occur (Fig. 30.36) Discomfort is rare, itching or occasional pain over the nodules may be present.

Prognosis: Poor Prognostic Facts
- *Hereditary:* In patients with family history, the lesion progresses fast. Hence, heredity is a poor prognostic factor.
- *Sex:* In women, it begins late and progresses slowly.

---

[2]**Baron Guillaume Dupuytren** of France (1817). His other contributions: (1) Described neurological manifestation of spina bifida occulta. (2) Subungual exostosis. (3) Callus and its formation. (4) Upward and outward dislocation of foot.

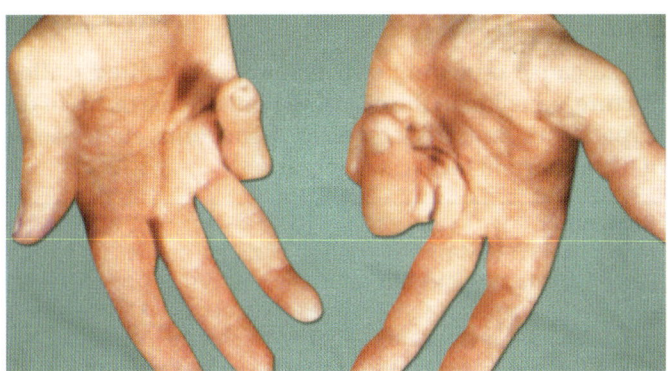

Fig. 30.36: Contractures of MCP and PIP joints of ring and little fingers in Dupuytren's disease (Clinical photo)

- *Alcoholics or epileptics:* Severe, rapid and recurs.
- *Bilateral.*
- *Behavior of the disease in the past.*

Do You Know the Actual Structures Involved in Dupuytren's Contracture?
- Palmar fascial (few fibers).
- The pretendinous bands.
- The superficial transverse ligament.
- The spiral band.
- The natatory ligament.
- The lateral digital sheet.
- The Grasham's ligament.
- The Cleland's ligament.

Investigations

Laboratory and X-rays are not helpful. USG and MRI helps but are seldom done.

Treatment

Observation: Consists of no treatment with observation being done at every three months interval.

Radiotherapy: It is given only during early fibroblastic phase.

Surgery: It is the best-known treatment and is delayed until actual contractures develop.

A procedure chosen depends upon the degree of contractures, age, occupation, status of the palmar skin, presence, or absence of arthritis of the finger joints, etc. More severe the involvement, more extensive is the surgery.

Surgical Methods

Subcutaneous fasciotomy: This is preferred in elderly, arthritis patients and if the general condition is poor. Results are good when lesion is mature than diffuse. It may be used as a preliminary step to fasciectomy. This procedure has a 72 percent recurrence rate.

Partial selective fasciectomy: This is indicated only when the ulnar two fingers are involved. This is a commonly done procedure, morbidity is less and is associated with less complications. Recurrence rate is 50 percent, needs another surgery in 15 percent of the cases.

Complete fasciectomy: This is rarely done and is associated with hematoma, joint stiffness, delayed healing, and recurrence.

Fasciectomy with skin grafting: This is done in young people with epilepsy, alcoholism, and in cases of recurrence after excision.

Amputation may be considered if flexion contractures of PIP joint are very severe.

Resection and arthrodesis is indicated for severe contractures of the PIP joint. This is better than amputation as it prevents amputation neuroma.

CARPAL TUNNEL SYNDROME

Carpal tunnel syndrome was first described by Sir James Paget[3] in 1854, but the term was coined by Moerisch.

Anatomy

Bones bound the carpal tunnel on three sides and a ligament on one side (Fig. 30.37). The floor is an osseous arch formed by the carpal bones and the transverse carpal ligament forms the roof.

Contents

Tendons of flexor digitorum superficialis and profundus in a common sheath, tendon of flexor pollicis longus in an independent sheath and the median nerve (Fig. 30.38).

Synovitis of the above tendons can generate pressure on the nerve.

Note:
Know that 9 tendons and 1 nerve pass through the carpal tunnel.

Causes

General

Inflammatory—For Example rheumatoid arthritis.
Endocrine—hypothyroidism, diabetes mellitus, menopause, pregnancy, etc. are some of the important endocrine causes.
Metabolic cause—gout.

---
[3]**Sir James Paget**, London (1814-1899). His other contributions: (1) Paget's disease. (2) Apophysitis of tibial tubercle.

382 SECTION 3: Nontraumatic Orthopedic Disorders

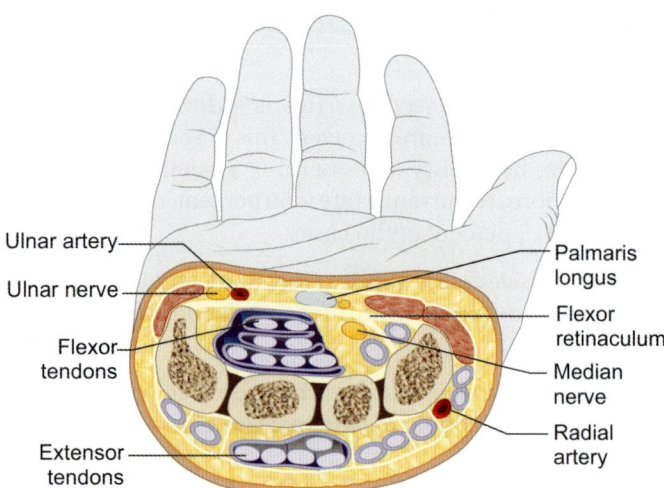

Fig. 30.37: Anatomy of the carpal tunnel

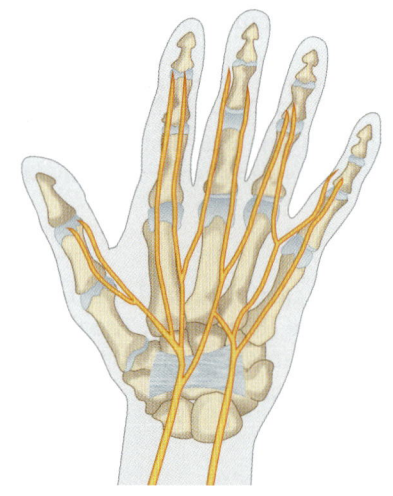

Fig. 30.38: Median nerve coursing through the carpal tunnel

Local

These cause crowding of the space. Malunited Colles' fracture, ganglion in the carpal region, osteoarthritis of the carpal bones, and wrist contusion, hematoma, etc. are some of the important local causes.

> **Remember**
> Mnemonic PRAGMATIC for causes of carpal tunnel syndrome [(*P*—Pregnancy, *R*—Rheumatoid arthritis, *A*—Arthritis degenerative, *G*—Growth hormone abnormalities (acromegaly), *M*—Metabolic (gout, diabetes myxoedema, etc.), *A*—Alcoholism, *T*—Tumors, *I*—Idiopathic, *C*—Connective tissue disorders (e.g. amyloidosis)].

Clinical Stages or Features (Figs 30.39A and B)

Stage I: In this stage, pain is usually the presenting complaint and the patient complains of characteristic discomfort in the hand, but there is no precise localization to the median nerve. There may be history of morning stiffness in the hand.

Stage II: In this stage, symptoms of tingling and numbness, pain, paresthesia, etc. are localized to areas supplied by the median nerve.

Stage III: Here, the patient complains of clumsiness in the hand and impairment of digital functions, etc.

Stage IV: In this stage, sensory loss in the median nerve distribution area can be elicited and there is obvious wasting of the thenar eminence.

Clinical Tests

These are provocative tests and act as important screening methods and as an adjunct to the electrophysiological testing.

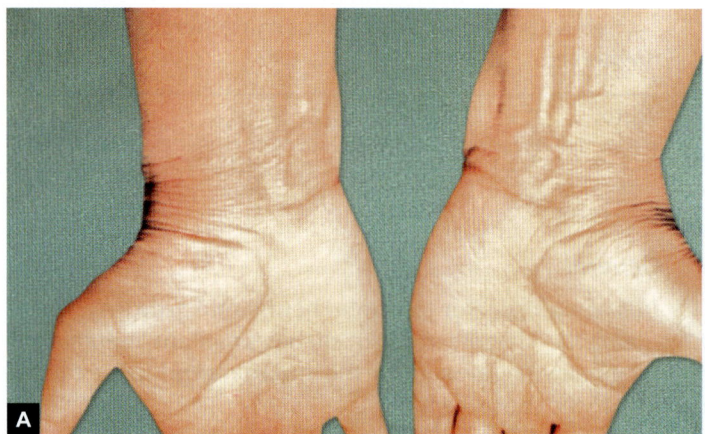
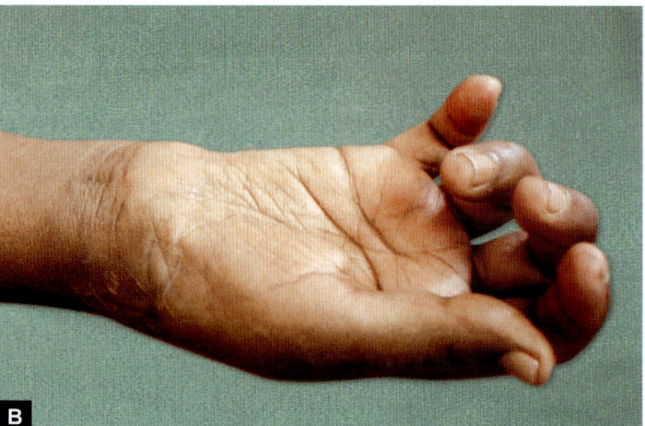

Figs 30.39A and B: Clinical photograph of: (A) Bilateral carpal tunnel syndrome; (B) Deformity

Wrist flexion (Phalen's test): The patient is asked to actively place the wrist in complete but unforced flexion. If tingling and numbness are produced in the median nerve distribution of the hand within 60 seconds, the test is positive. It is the most sensitive provocative test (Fig. 30.40). It has a specificity of 80 percent.

Tourniquet test: A pneumatic blood pressure cuff is applied proximal to the elbow and inflated higher than the patient's systolic blood pressure. The test is positive if there is paresthesia or numbness in the region of median nerve distribution of the hand. It is less reliable and is specific in 65 percent of cases only.

Median nerve percussion test: The examiner gently taps the median nerve at the wrist (Fig. 30.41). The test is positive if there is tingling sensation, seen only in 45 percent of cases.

Median nerve compression test: Direct pressure is exerted equally over both wrists by the examiner (Fig. 30.42). The first phase of the test is the time taken for symptoms to appear (15 sec to 2 min). The second phase is the time taken for the symptoms to disappear after release of pressure.

Investigations

Plain X-ray helps identify malunited wrist fractures. USG and MRI gives additional information. Nerve Conduction studies is a more reliable indicator of nerve compression.

Other Tests

Two-point discrimination test: This test is positive in about one-third cases.

Electrodiagnostic tests are not very infallible with 10 percent individuals having normal values.

Treatment

Non-operative methods

In the initial stages, non-steroidal anti-inflammatory drugs are given. If it is unsuccessful, steroids like prednisolone for 8 days starting with 40 mg for 2 days and tapering by 10 mg every 2 days are tried. Use of carpal tunnel splint is also advocated (Fig. 30.43). Physiotherapy also helps.

Injection Treatment

This is indicated in patients with intermittent symptoms, duration of complaints less than one year and if there is no sensory deficits, no marked thenar wasting, etc. In the injection therapy, a single infusion of cortisone with splinting for 3 weeks is tried.

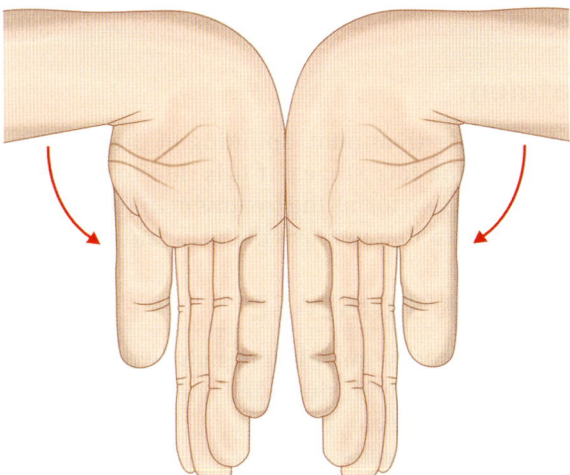

Fig. 30.40: Phalen's test

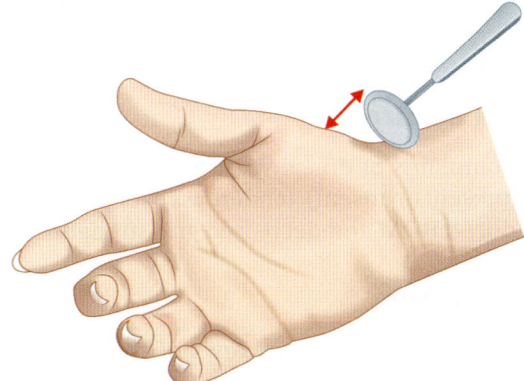

Fig. 30.41: Median nerve percussion test

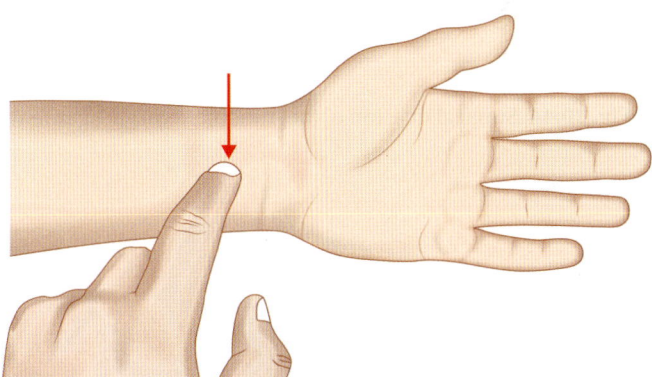

Fig. 30.42: Median nerve compression test

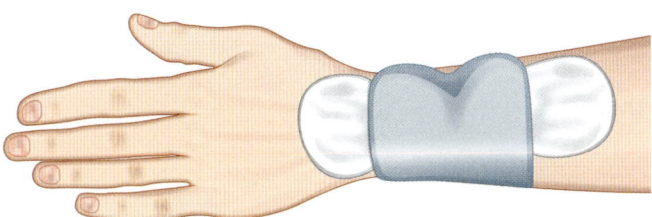

Fig. 30.43: Carpal tunnel splint

Surgery

This consists of division of flexor retinaculum and transverse carpal ligament and is indicated in failed nonoperative treatment, thenar atrophy, sensory loss, etc. (Fig. 30.44).

> **What is New in the Treatment of Carpal Tunnel?**
> **Chow's technique**
> This is an endoscopic release of the carpal ligament. It is a reliable alternative for the open procedure and has a success rate of 93.3 percent.

COMPOUND PALMAR GANGLION

This is a condition, which affects the flexor tendons of the fingers mainly the ulnar bursa. It is usually due to tuberculosis though rheumatoid arthritis may also be a cause. The term *compound* is derived from a swelling one above and below the flexor retinaculum (Fig. 30.45).

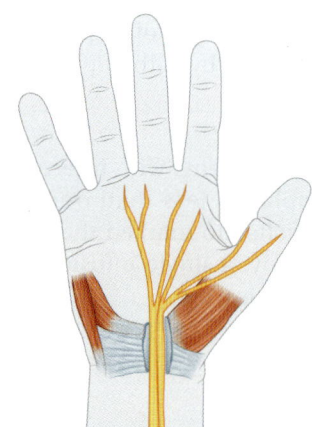

Fig. 30.44: Surgical division of the transverse carpal ligament

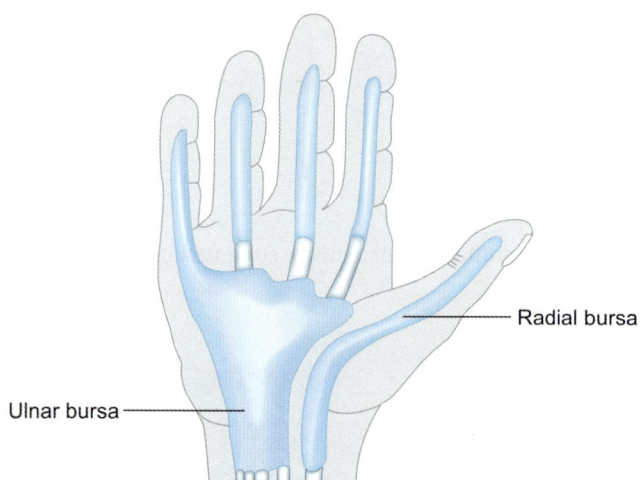

Fig. 30.45: Ulnar bursa site of compound palmar ganglion

Here, the endothelial lining of the sheath is substituted by granulation tissue containing miliary tubercles. The presence of *melon seed* bodies is a hallmark of this condition. Effusion may be seen and in the late stages, the tendons may rupture.

> **Quick Facts: About Melon Seed Bodies**
> - Hallmark of compound palmar ganglion.
> - Resemble grains of boiled sago.
> - Gives rise to a soft, coarse crepitations.
> - Made up of fibrin, cellular debris, and occasional TB bacilli.

Clinical Features

Those affected with this condition are usually less than 40 years and pain is not a feature. An hourglass swelling with cross-fluctuation may be noticed. There may be features of median nerve compression, but there is definite evidence of wasting of the hand and forearm muscles.

Investigations

Routine laboratory tests, plain X-ray of the wrist and hand, biopsy, etc. are some of the recommended investigations.

Treatment

Anti-tubercular treatment, splinting of the forearm and exercises in the late stages, if it is due to tuberculosis. Complete excision forms the treatment in rheumatoid. Synonyms: avascular necrosis of the lunate.

KEINBOCK'S DISEASE

It is related to overuse and ulnar negative wrist variance and may be associated with sickle cell anemia, steriod abuse, gout, cerebral palsy etc
- Age: 2nd-5th decade.
- Male preponderance.

> **Why and How?**
> It is because of the vulnerable lunate blood supply: single nutrient vessel, or poorly organized intraosseous anastamoses (Fig. 30.46).

Clinical Features

Patient complains of dorsal wrist pain, swelling, warmth (may be present or absent), tenderness over the radiolunate joint, reduced ROM and decreased grip strength.

Investigations

X-ray—PA, lateral, oblique views of the wrist, usually demonstrates sclerotic lunate (Fig. 30.47).

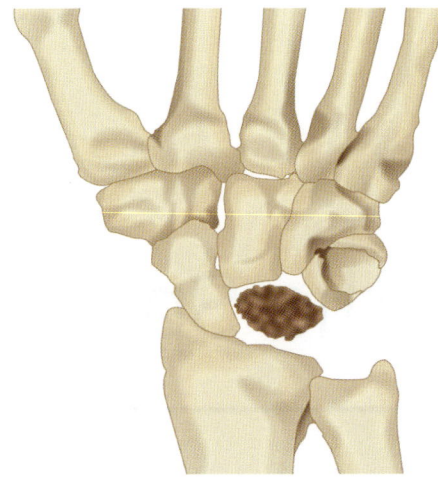

Fig. 30.46: Keinbock's disease

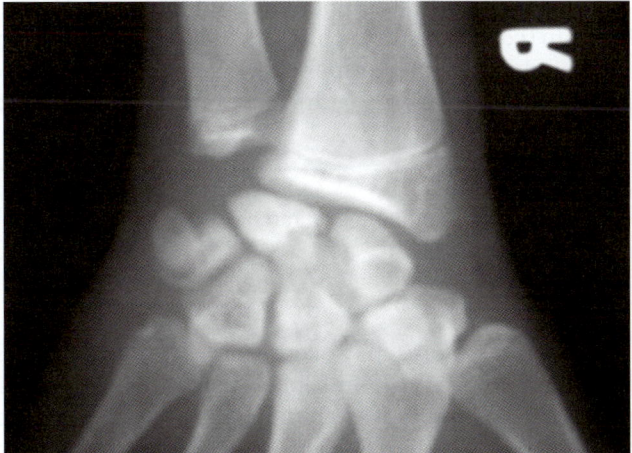

Fig. 30.47: Plain X-ray showing Keinbock's disease

Early stages may be normal or minimal sclerosis. One need to evaluate for ulnocarpal impaction.

MRI: demonstrates avascular changes in the lunate.

CT Scan: Demonstrates degree of fragmentation and collapse.

Bone scan diagnostic at 48 hours (100% sensitive, 98% specific).

Lichtman Classification
- Stage 1: The lunate appears normal on X-ray or there may be a nondisplaced fracture; MRI demonstrates loss of signal consistent with osteonecrosis.
- Stage 2: Increased lunate radiodensity without loss of contour; lunate not collapsed.
- Stage 3A: Increased lunate radiodensity and fragmentation without loss of carpal height.
- Stage 3B: Lunate fragmentation with proximal migration of the capitate and rotation of the scaphoid.
- Stage 4: lunate severely collapsed and fragmented, secondary arthritic changes in the wrist.
(Lichtman DM, JBJS 59A;899:1977).

Treatment
This is largely based on the stages of the disease

Stage 1: The treatment of choice is splinting, activity modifications, NSAIDs. However, ulnar lengthening or radial shortening for patients with negative ulnar variane can be considered.

Stage 2: The treatment of choice is 4 + 5 extensor compartmental vascularized bone graft. However, Proximal row carpectomy can be considered

Stage 3 A: The treatment of choice is treatment: 4 + 5 extensor compartmental vascularized bone graft. Scaphocapitate arthrodesis, or scaphotrapeziotrapezoid arthrodesis can be considered.

Stage 3B: The treatment of choice is treatment: scaphocapitate arthrodesis, or scaphotrapeziotrapezoid arthrodesis proximal row carpectomy can be considered.

Stage 4: The treatment of choice is proximal row carpectomy. Consider: scaphocapitate arthrodesis, and scaphotrapeziotrapezoid arthrodesis can be considered.

Differential Diagnosis
- Ulnocarpal impaction syndrome.
- Preiser's disease.

Complications
- Stiffness.
- Loss of motion.
- Weakness.
- Carpal tunnel syndrome.
- Persistent pain.
- Instability.
- Degeneration in adjacent joints.

BIBLIOGRAPHY

1. Bhattacharya S. Abduction of contracture of shoulder from contracture of intermediate part of deltoid. Report of 3 cases. J Bone Joint Surg (BE). 1966;48B:127-31.
2. Shanmugasundaram TK. Post-injection, fibrosis of skeletal muscle: A clinical problem. A personal series of 169 cases. Int Orthop. 1980;4:31-7.

Keinbock's Disease Review References
- Weiss AP, Weiland AJ, Moore JR, Wilgis EF. Radial shortening for Kienbock's disease. J Bone Joint Surg Am. 1991;73:384-91.
- Morgan WJ. JAAOS. 2001;9:389.

31 CHAPTER

Regional Conditions of the Spine

SCOLIOSIS

By definition, scoliosis is the lateral curvature of the spine in the upright position in the coronal plane. The lateral curvature is usually accompanied by some rotational deformity. Only man boasts of an erect posture. Nature has designed four physiological curves in the so-called erect spine, cervical and lumbar lordosis, dorsal curve in the thoracic spine and the sacral region. Thus, when the spine develops a lateral curve, it is abnormal. It throws the well-adjusted spinal mechanism out of gear and poses the following problems:
- A cosmetically unacceptable deformity.
- Deranges the load and force transmission mechanism through the spine.
- Jeopardizes the functions of vital organs like lungs, heart by overcrowding the ribs.
- Managing—it is cumbersome and unrewarding experience most of the times.

Thus, a scoliotic curve makes the spine 'crooked' and a 'crooked spine is a wicked spine,' if one considers the above problems it poses.

> **Mystifying Facts**
> Do you know the difference between scoliosis and spinal asymmetry?
> - Lateral curve <10° — is spinal asymmetry.
> - Lateral curve >10° — is scoliosis.

Varieties

Structural scoliosis: *In structural scoliosis, the curves are fixed and nonflexible and fail to correct with side bending.* Lateral bending of spine is asymmetric or involved vertebrae are fixed in a rotated position or both.

Nonstructural scoliosis: In nonstructural scoliosis, the curves are flexible and readily correctible with side bending. It is frequently seen as a compensatory mechanism to a leg length discrepancy, fixed flexion deformity of the hip (compensatory scoliosis), local inflammation or irritation due to acute lumbar disk disease and prolapsed disk (sciatic scoliosis) or due to poor postural habits (postural scoliosis).

> **Note:**
> - Postural scoliosis is the most common variety of nonstructural scoliosis.
> - Idiopathic scoliosis is the most common variety of structural scoliosis.

Structural scoliosis may occur from a variety of causes. Idiopathic scoliosis accounts for 90 percent of all scoliosis and appears to represent a hereditary disorder, but the exact mechanism of its production is unknown. Broadly speaking, there are two types of scoliosis:
- Idiopathic (unknown cause).
- Known cause. The important among these are:
  - *Congenital scoliosis:* This is due to defect in segmentation, which is usually due to a lateral bar or due to a defect in the formation, including hemivertebrae or double hemivertebrae. These curves usually progress very fast and require surgical fusion on both the convex and concave sides of the curve.
  - *Paralytic scoliosis:* This is due to muscle imbalance on either side of the trunk, the most common cause being anterior poliomyelitis. Cerebral palsies, muscular dystrophies, etc. are the other common causes.

Some of the other causes are mentioned at the end of the chapter.

Idiopathic Scoliosis (Unknown Cause)

This is the most common (75–90%) and three varieties are recognized—infantile, juvenile, and adolescent (Table 31.1). Though the exact cause is not known, role of genetics is hotly debated. Overall incidence is 1–4 people/thousand.

TABLE 31.1: Types of idiopathic scoliosis

Infantile	Juvenile	Adolescent
• >70–90 percent	• 15 percent	• 2–3 percent
• <3 years	• 4–10 years	• 10–16 years
• Curve is progressive or resolving	• Thoracic curve usually to the right	• F: M = 3.6:1
Treatment	**Treatment**	**Treatment**
• Curves <20° observation	• <20° observation	• Surgical correction
• >20° bracing	• >20 percent Milwaukee brace	
• If severe surgical fusion	• If> 60° surgical correction and fusion	

Clinical Features

Though idiopathic scoliosis can occur at any age, it usually appears clinically between 10 and 13 years. It is more common in females (10%). The disease is usually asymptomatic and is usually accidentally discovered. The diagnosis is usually made on routine physical examination (Figs 31.1A and B).

Method of examination: For the examination, the patient should be undressed to the waist or wear a bathing suit and a routine should be followed. The shoulders and iliac crest are inspected to determine whether they are at the same level. The scapulae, ribcage, and flanks are then observed for symmetry. The spinous processes are palpated to determine their alignment. Rib hump or abnormal paraspinal muscular prominence indicates spinal rotation. Rib hump leads to asymmetry of the trunk and is called angle trunk rotation (ATR). It is measured by using a scoliometer.

The patient is then made to bend forward to see for the disappearance of the curve (Adam's test).

Scoliotic Facts

Structural curve: This is a laterally curved spine that lacks normal flexibility.

Primary care: This is the earliest curve to appear.

Compensatory curve or secondary curve: This is the curve, which develops above or below the primary curve in an effort to balance the spine.

Major curve: This is the largest structural curve.

Minor curve: This is the smallest curve.

Apical vertebra: This is the most deviated vertebra from the vertical axis of the patient.

End vertebrae
- The uppermost vertebra whose superior surface tilts maximally towards the concavity of the curve.
- The lowermost vertebra whose inferior surface tilts maximally towards the concavity of the curve.

Quick Facts

Curve patterns in idiopathic scoliosis (Figs 31.2A to D)

Curve	Apical vertebra
Cervical	C_1–C_6
Cervicodorsal	C_7–T_1
Thoracic	T_2–T_{11}
Thoracolumbar	T_{12}–L_1
Lumbar	L_2–L_4
Lumbosacral	L_5–S_1

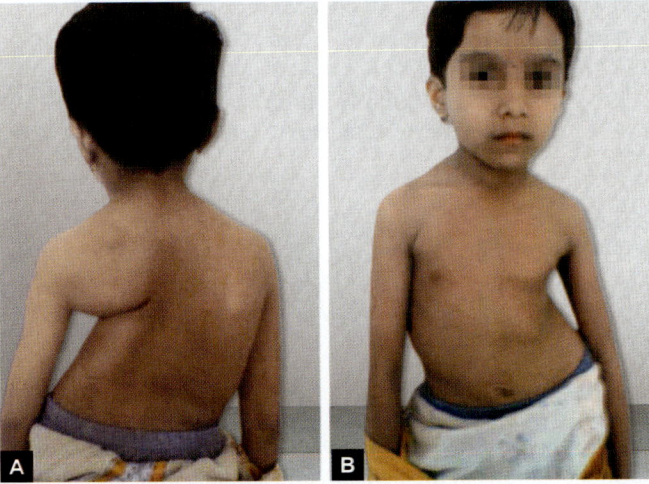

Figs 31.1A and B: Scoliosis: (A) Viewed from back; (B) Viewed from front (Clinical photos)

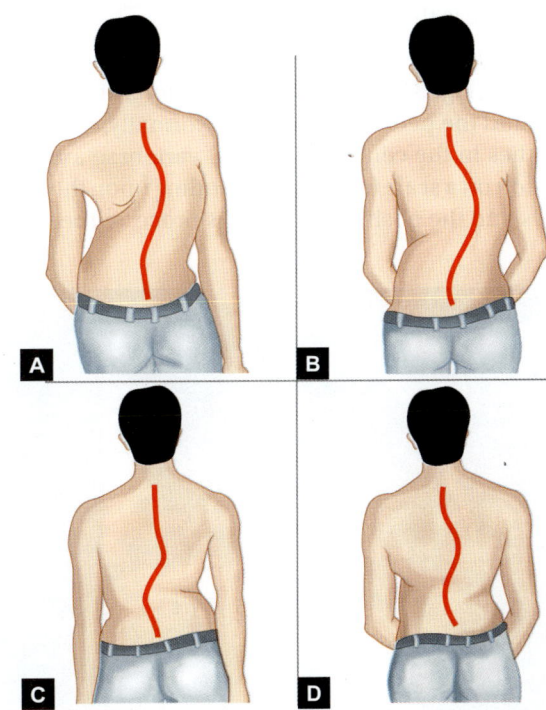

Figs 31.2A to D: Various types of scoliosis: (A) Thoracic; (B) Thoracolumbar; (C) Double curve thoracic and lumbar; (D) Lumbosacral

> **How to Describe a Scoliotic Curve?**
> Remember the mnemonic PLEAD
> P—Pattern (primary, secondary, etc.)
> L—Location (thoracic, thoracolumbar lumbar)
> E—Etiology (idiopathic, congenital, paralytic, etc.)
> A—Apex (thoracic lumbar)
> D—Direction (right, left).

Radiology

Radiographic evaluation of the spine is the only available method to determine the severity of the curve. It is repeated at intervals to determine the progression of the curve. In radiography of the spine, the following views are taken.

PA view of the spine (Fig. 31.3), standard lateral radiography of the spine, right and left bending films of spine and the Stagnara derotation view, which is an oblique view of the spine. The radiological parameters of importance are:

Cobb's method to measure severity of the curve: The upper and lower vertebrae are identified (Fig. 31.4). The upper end vertebra is the highest one whose superior border converges towards the concavity of the curve and the lower end vertebra is the one whose inferior border converges towards the concavity. Intersecting perpendicular line from the superior surface of the superior end vertebrae and from the inferior surface of the inferior end vertebrae is drawn. The angle of deviation of these perpendiculars from a straight line is the 'angle of the curve'.

Nash and Moe's method to measure vertebral rotation: In the PA view (Figs 31.5A and B), the positions of the spinous process and the pedicles are noted. Normally, the spinous process lies in the center. The apical vertebrae are graded for rotation on a scale from 0–4, depending upon the pedicle shadows and the position of spinous process. The spinous processes are identified and classified according to the amount of rotation.

Reisser's sign: This is a classification of the ossification of the iliac epiphysis, which usually starts from the anterior superior iliac spine and progresses posteriorly towards the posterior iliac spine. Reisser's stage 4 corresponds with cessation of spine growth and stage 5 correlates with cessation of height increase. *The importance of this sign is the completion of growth can be radiologically assessed which indicates no possibility of the curve progression.*

> **Reisser's Classification**
> It uses ossification of iliac apophysis to grade the remaining skeletal growth. The ossification progresses from lateral to medial:
> Type I   —   Ossification of lateral 25 percent
> Type II —   Ossification of lateral 50 percent
> Type III —   Ossification of lateral 75 percent
> Type IV —   Ossification of lateral 100 percent
> Type V   —   Fusion of ilium

Rib angle of Mehta: The rib vertebral angle is constructed by the intersection of a line perpendicular to the apical vertebral end plate with a line drawn from the mid-neck

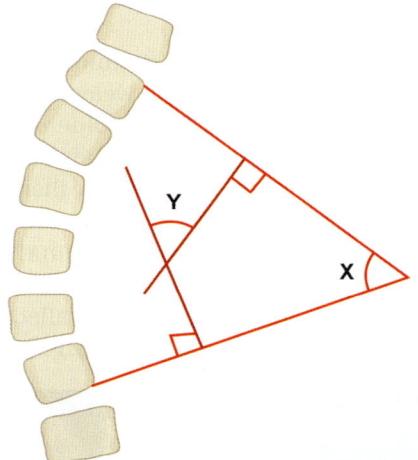

Fig. 31.4: Cobb's method of measuring severity of a curve (Y = angle)

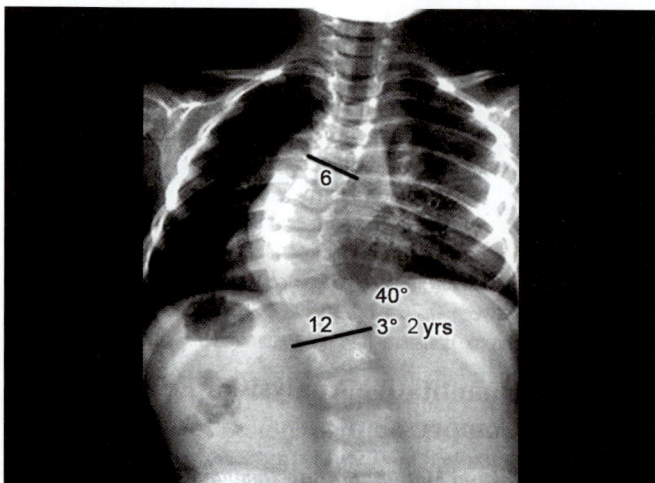

Fig. 31.3: Radiograph showing a paralytic scoliosis

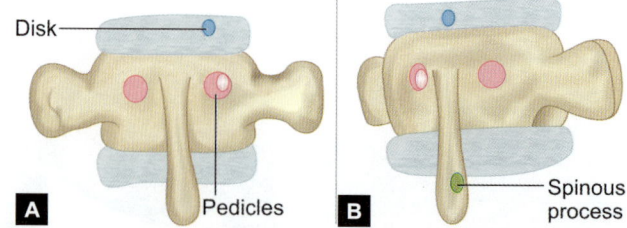

Figs 31.5A and B: (A) Normal PA view of the spine showing the normal positions of the pedicles and spinous processes; (B) The pedicles and spinous processes shadows are altered and indicate vertebral rotation in scoliosis

to the mid-head of the corresponding rib. The rib vertebral angle (RVAD) is the difference between rib vertebral angle of the convex and concave side of the apical vertebra. If the initial RVAD is less than 20°, progression is unlikely; and if initial RVAD is more than 20°, the curves tend to progress (Fig. 31.6).

CT scan and MRI helps in more accurate diagnosis (Figs 31.7A and B).

Original Structural Curves are Distinguished from Secondary Curves by the Following Criteria:
- Vertebrae in structural scoliosis are displaced to the convexity of the curve; but in secondary curve, they are displaced to the concavity of the secondary curve.
- When there are three curves, middle one is structural.
- When there are four curves, two middle ones are structural.
- The greater curve or the one towards which the trunk is shifted is the structural curve.
- The curve that is flexible and corrective is the non-structural curve.

Compensation

If head is to be balanced above the pelvis when the patient is erect, it is done so by any curve or curves that develops in the opposite direction. *The formation of curves in the opposite direction is called compensation.* The angle of the secondary curves should be equal to that of the primary curve. If it exceeds, it is called overcompensation.

Treatment

The most important aspect in the treatment of scoliosis is early detection of the curve. A curve that is obvious in standing position has already approached 30–40°. *Detecting a curve before it reaches 20° is of utmost importance because curves over 20° tend to progress.* Frequent re-examinations are essential. The treatment depends on the age of the patient and the severity of the curve.

Nonsurgical treatment: Observation is the primary treatment of all curves and more so for curves less than 20 degrees. *At present, radiography is the only definite documentation of curve size and progression.*

Generally Accepted Guidelines for Observation
- Curves of less than 20° in skeletally immature persons are examined every 6 months.
- Curves less than 20° in skeletally mature persons require no further evaluation.
- Curves more than 20° in skeletally immature patients should be examined every 3–4 months. Orthotic treatment for curves more than 25°.
- Curves more than 30–40° in skeletally mature persons do not require treatment. However, they are examined radiographically for progression every 2–3 years.

Orthotic treatment: This is effective in skeletally immature persons (Fig. 31.8A). For mild or moderate curves, [1]Milwaukee brace, Boston brace, Reisser's turn buckle cast, localizer cast, etc. are used, and the 20° level is considered still for bracing.

Remember
The 'Orthotic' leaders: Mnemonic BMC
    B—**B**oston braces (TLSO)
    M—**M**ilwaukee brace
    C—**C**harleston brace
Most effective among these is the Boston brace.

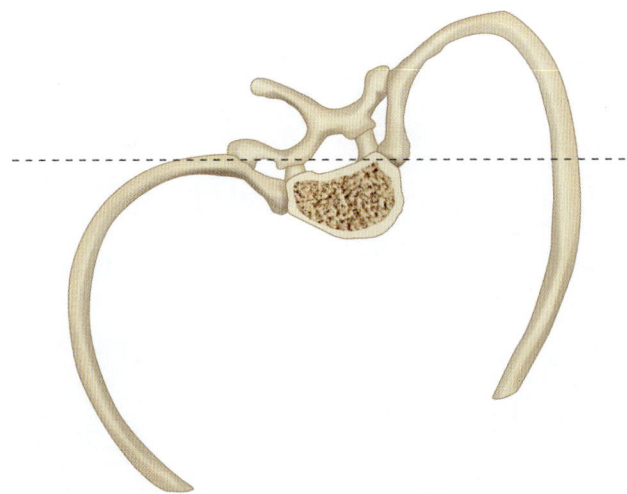

Fig. 31.6: Rib distortion due to vertebral rotation

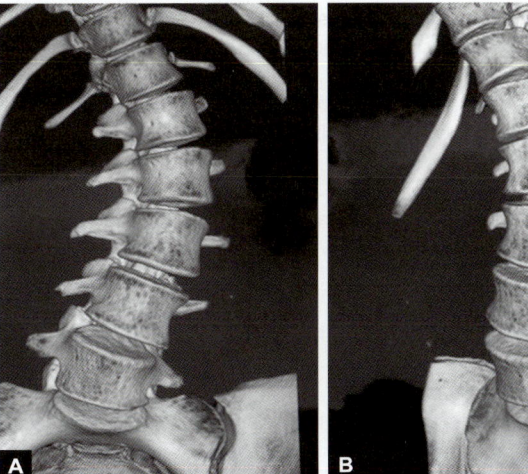

Figs 31.7A and B: CT scan showing lumbar scoliosis

---

[1]Milwaukee brace was developed in 1945 for more efficient and comfortable passive correction of the scoliosis.

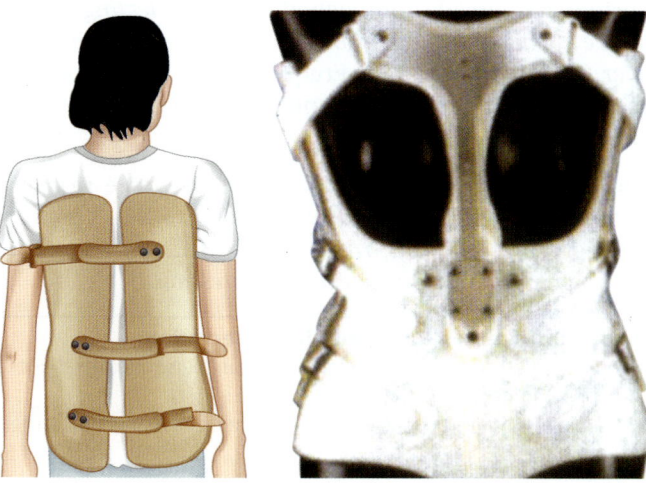

Fig. 31.8A: Orthotic treatment of structural scoliosis—Boston brace

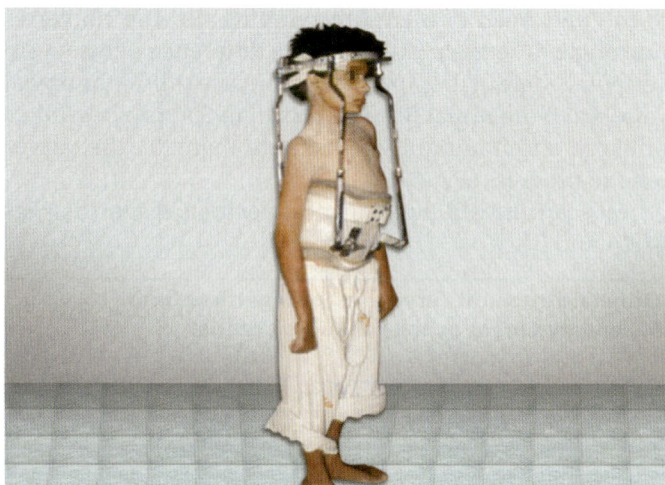

Fig. 31.8B: Halopelvic distraction apparatus used for skeletal traction in correction of structural scoliotic curves

Do You Know?
Complications of bracing?
- Most common: Discomfort and rejection due to poor appearance.
- Skin breakdown
- Excessive sweating
- Allergic skin reaction
- Increased gastric pressure and gastroesophageal reflex
- Spontaneous sternum fracture.

Other non-operative measures: Exercises, traction and electrical stimulation have been unsuccessfully tried in adolescent variety.

Traction
Traction helps to stretch the contracted structures prior to surgery. Methods of traction could be either non-skeletal or skeletal. Skeletal traction is provided by halopelvic or halofemoral traction (Fig. 31.8B).

Mystifying Facts: About Braces
- Do you know what curves respond best to bracing?
  - Curves <40°
  - Less severe lumbar hyperlordosis
  - Curves with thoracic lordosis
  - Hyperkyphosis
  - Risser's curve is 0
- How much is the efficacy of bracing?
  It is about 74 to 81 percent when worn for 23 hours/day until skeletal maturity.
- How do braces act?
  By derotating the spine using the rib or transverse process as the lever
- What are the corrective forces?
  The primary corrective forces are the 'lateral forces' in the braces.

Surgical treatment: This is indicated for high degree thoracic curve, which is inflexible and is associated with secondary changes in the ribs. Casts are not effective in thoracic spine. Spinal surgery is also indicated when the curve is over 60° and aims at obtaining fusion at the spine (see box) (Fig. 31.9). Surgical methods are showing in Flow chart 31.1.

Do You Know in Scoliosis?
- *The proper indications for surgery?*
  - Curves >50° in the mature patients
  - Curves >10° with marked rotations
  - Double major curves >30°
- *The most common form of surgical intervention in idiopathic scoliosis.*
  Well, it is the segmental instrumentation with multiback system (CD).

Quick Facts
- Scoliosis is lateral curvature of the spine.
- Idiopathic variety accounts for 90 percent of the cases.
- Female preponderance.
- X-ray is the only definite documentation of curve size and progression.

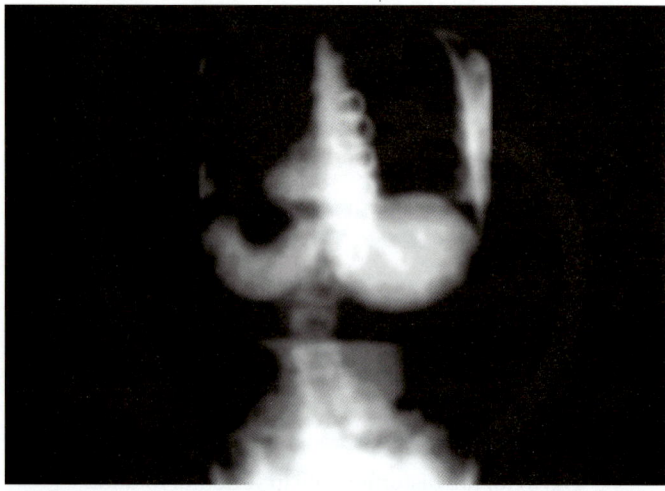

Fig. 31.9: Radiograph showing scoliosis surgical correction by segmental instrumentation

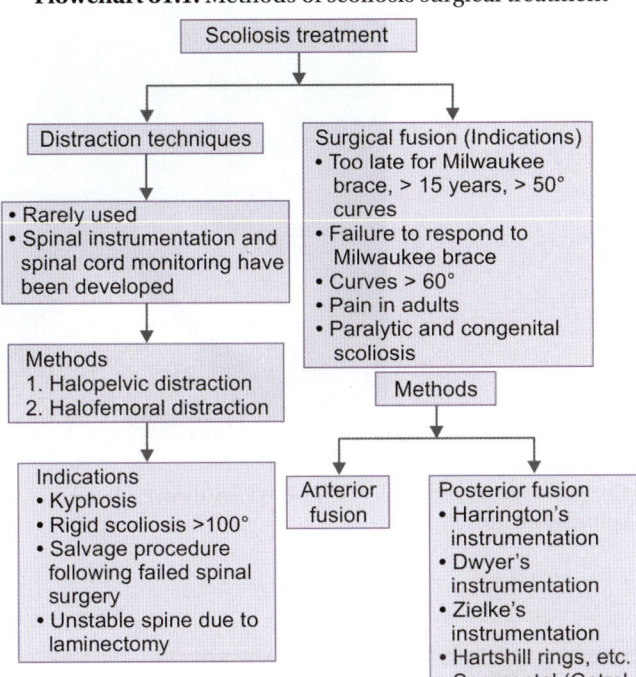

Flowchart 31.1: Methods of scoliosis surgical treatment

Interesting Facts

Remember 3 'O's in the treatment of idiopathic scoliosis:
- Observation for curves <20°
- Orthosis for curves for >20°–50°
- Operations for curves >50°.

In a Nutshell

Treatment options in scoliosis

Congenital	—	Surgery/bracing
Paralytic	—	Wheelchair seating systems
	—	Bracing, surgery
Idiopathic	—	3 'O's mentioned earlier
Marked rotation	—	Bracing
Degenerative		
<60 years	—	Postural correction, exercises, Corset, etc.
>60 years	—	Surgery

Alternative therapies: Exercises, electric stimulation, biofeedback, tractions, manipulations, etc.

Unfavorable Prognostic Facts in Scoliosis
- Congenital/juvenile/paralytic
- >20–40° curve
- Thoracic curve
- 2–4 degree of rotation
- Risser's sign 0/immature
- Female
- Premenarchial
- Presence of osteoporosis
- Rapid increase in curve size
- Single short curve
- Previous discectomy, laminectomy, etc.

- The most important aspect of treatment is early detection.
- Curves <20° need observation.
- Curves >20° require treatment.
- Curves between 20 and 40° can be treated by Milwaukee brace, which has to be worn 23 hours per day for a period of at least two years.
- Curves >40° need surgical correction and fusion.

Facts About Curve Progression
- Curves <20° will improve spontaneously in over 50 percent of cases.
- No accurate method to predict the outcome of curve.
- Twenty percent curves <30° will progress.
- Progression is more common in young children.
- Bigger the curve at detection, higher is the chance of curve progression.
- Curve in females and double curves are more likely to progress.

Scoliosis of known cause: Congenital/paralytic.

Neuromuscular scoliosis
- *Neuropathic causes:* Spinal cord injury, poliomyelitis, progressive neurological disorders, syringomyelia, myelomeningocele, and cerebral palsy are some of the neuropathic causes.
- *Muscular* AMC and muscular dystrophy are some of the important muscular causes.
- *Neurofibromatosis.*
- *Miscellaneous:* Multiple epiphyseal dysplasia, osteogenesis imperfecta, etc.

SPONDYLOLISTHESIS
(Spondylos—Spine; Olisthein—To Slip)

It is the story of a "slipping" spine causing "gripping" problems to both the patient and the clinician. That animals never suffer spondylolisthesis is proof enough to declare that this condition is a curse of erect posture, which only man prides to possess!

Definition

It is defined as slow anterior displacement of a vertebra at the lower lumbar spine, generally accepted as the lowermost vertebra L_5 slipping forward on the first sacral segment S_1 (Figs 31.10A and B).

Essential lesion is the interruption in the concavity of the pars interarticularis.

Spondylolysis: In this, the defect in the pars exists but without the forward slipping. This could be due to a fracture, stress fracture or nonunion.

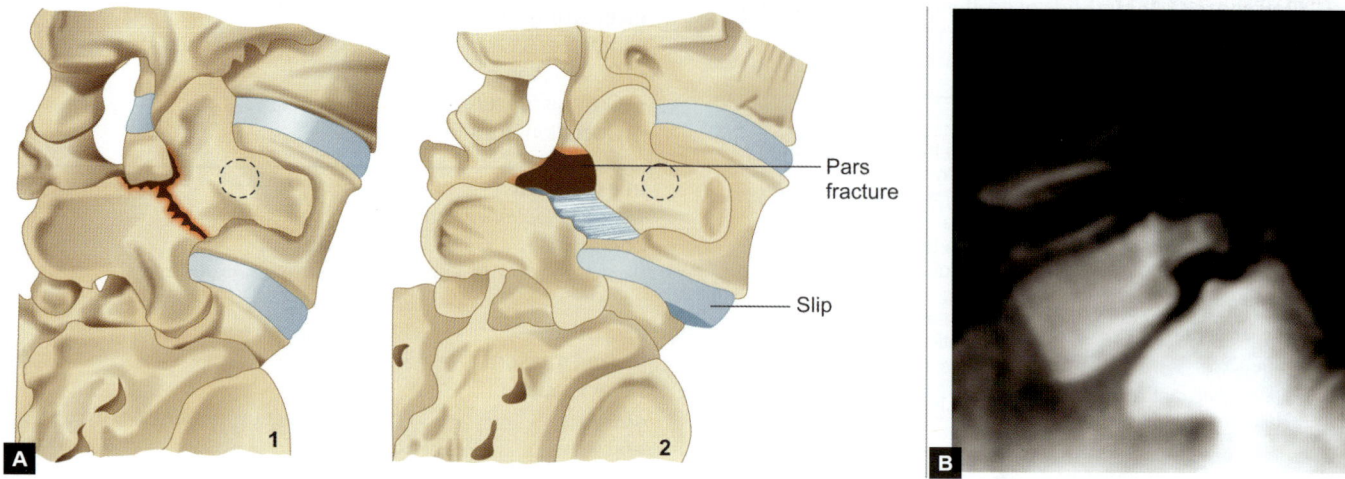

Figs 31.10A and B: (A) (1) Fracture or discontinuity in the pars (spondylolysis), (2) Spondylolisthesis; (B) Radiograph showing spondylolisthesis

> **Interesting Facts About Spondylolysis**
> - About 50 percent of the patients who present with isthmic spondylolysis do not progress to spondylolisthesis.
> - Spondylolisthesis is the most common cause of low backache in childhood.

Classification (Wiltse, Macnab, and Newman)

Different varieties are described (Figs 31.11A to F).

Dysplastic: Congenital abnormalities of the upper sacrum or the arch of L_5. These permit the olisthesis to occur.

Isthmic (true): The lesion is in the pars and is the most common variety. Common in children. Rarely seen before 8 years. At adolescent growth spurt, sudden increase in activity, gymnastics, carrying heavy bags, etc. may lead to a fatigue or stress fracture of the pars, which may give rise to the slip.

Types

- Lytic fatigue fracture of the pars in children.
- Elongated but intact pars.
- Acute fracture of the pars due to trauma.

Degenerative: This is due to long-standing intersegmental instability. Here pars are intact but the facet joints degenerate and allow the forward slip.

Traumatic: This is due to fracture in other areas of the bony hook rather than the pars.

Pathological: There is a generalized or localized bony disease in this variety.

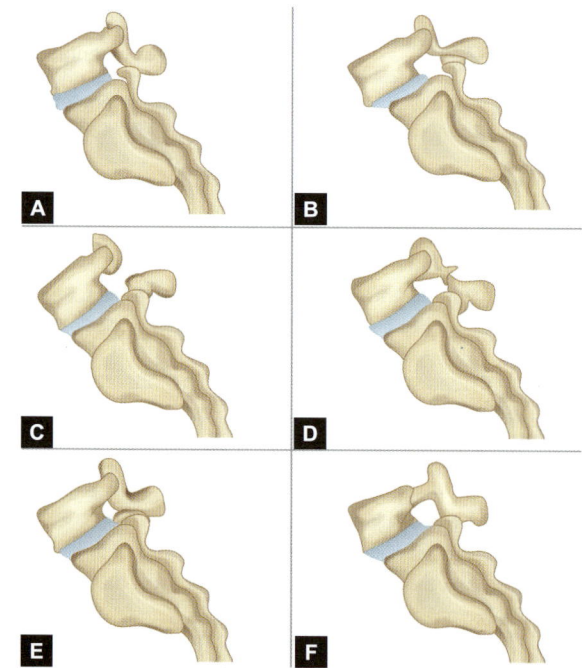

Figs 31.11A to F: Varieties of spondylolisthesis: (A) Normal; (B) Congenital; (C) Isthmic; (D) Traumatic; (E) Degenerative; (F) Pathological

Clinical Features

The clinical features of different varieties of spondylolisthesis are shown in Table 31.2. However, increased lumbar lordosis and transverse furrow over the lower back are unmistakable features of spondylolisthesis (Figs 31.12A and B). A step is palpable at the site of lesion (step sign) (Fig. 31.13).

CHAPTER 31: Regional Conditions of the Spine

TABLE 31.2: Clinical features of different spondylolisthesis

	True spondylolisthesis (Isthmic)	Congenital	Degenerative
Clinical features	• Asymptomatic or low back pain. History of trauma present in 50 percent • Common history of injury in adults and children	• Pain—low backache, buttocks, feet, toes, thighs and legs	• Known as pseudospondylolisthesis • Intermittent symptoms and is common in the elderly patients five times more common in women and affects 4 to 10 percent of the population
Deformity	• ↑ lumbar lordosis • Palpable step at L_5–S_1 • Torso is short • Abdomen protruded forwards • Transverse furrow at L_5 • Sacrum is vertical • Buttocks flat and Hamstring tightness • L_5 spinous process prominently felt. Scoliosis in 13%	• Scoliosis, pelvic waddle present • Buttocks are flat • Stiffness of spine present • Cannot bend beyond the lower thigh	• Pain in the back, buttock or thigh
Neurology	• L_5 nerve root is involved, but rare	• L_5 or S_1 nerve root is involved	• L_5 rare • Neurological claudication may be present • L_{3-4} common
Obstetrics	• Narrowing occurs at the outlet		
X-ray	• Lateral view is characteristic • Oblique view—shows Scottish Terrier's sign	• Development of sacral neural arch, superior sacral articular process is defective • Sacral root is not well developed	• Hyperactivity at L_{4-5} • No motion at L_5–S_1 • Displacement is <30 percent
Myelography	• Partial or complete block at L_5		• Hour glass configuration

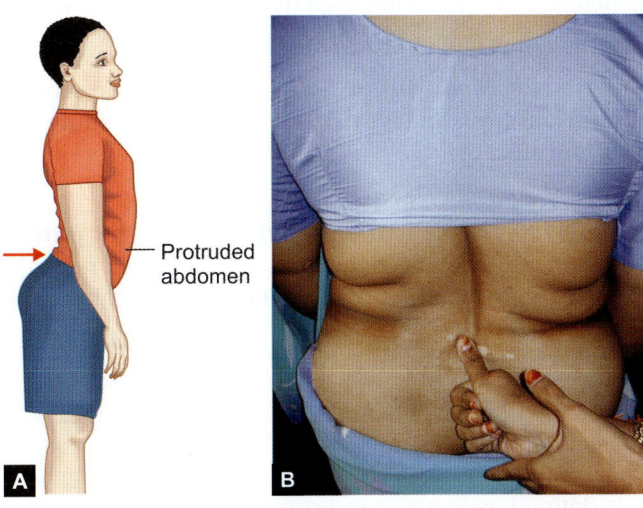

Figs 31.12A and B: Clinical signs in spondylolisthesis: (A) Increased lumbar lordosis; (B) Step sign (Clinical photo)

Investigations

Radiograph of the spine is the investigation of choice (see Fig. 31.10B). Anteroposterior and lateral films are helpful. However, oblique view of the lumbar spine demonstrates the defect in the pars very accurately as a "Scottie dog" sign. The Scottie dog's neck, which represents the pars defect, is broken in the isthmic variety (Fig. 31.14).

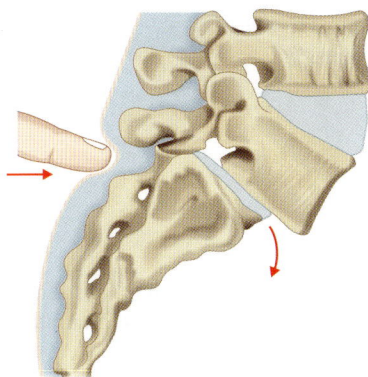

Fig. 31.13: Method of eliciting step sign

The edges of the defect are smooth and rounded and suggest a pseudoarthrosis rather than acute fracture.

Radiological Grading
Meyer ding's grading* (Fig. 31.15)
G1   25 percent forward displacement
G2   25–50 percent
G3   50–70 percent
G4   >75 percent
*Percentage of slip calculated by the upper vertebral displacement over the lower vertebral body, on a lateral view plain X-ray of the LS spine.

CT scan and MRI are more reliable investigation.

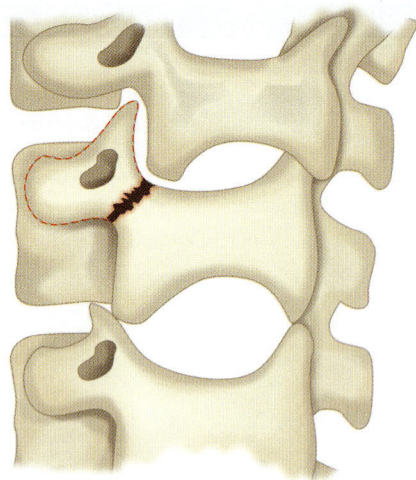

Fig. 31.14: Scottish Terrier sign (fracture of pars in oblique view)

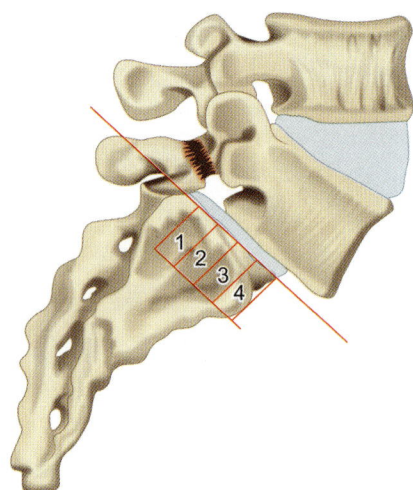

Fig. 31.15: Meyer ding's grading (1932) of spondylolisthesis. The amount of slippage is graded 1–4 on a plain lateral X-ray of the spine

Treatment

Conservative Treatment

Clinically, spondylolisthesis is divided into three groups, asymptomatic, mild-to-moderate and severe varieties, based on the severity of symptoms. Table 31.3 shows the different methods of conservative treatment to be employed in the above three clinical varieties of spondylolisthesis.

Surgical Management

Indications
- Failure of conservative therapy.
- Signs of root compression.

TABLE 31.3: Different methods of conservative treatment

Asymptomatic	Mild-to-moderate	Severe
• Correction of poor posture • Elimination of stressful occupation • To avoid certain special sports activities	• Alleviation of anxiety • Analgesics and muscle relaxants • Deep heat • Exercises	• Rest • NSAIDs • Gradual exercises to strengthen the trunk and hamstring muscles

- Progressive slipping.
- Slip of more than 30 percent even when painless.
- Persistent pain in the back, thigh, or persistent sciatica.

Methods of Surgery

Posterolateral fusion: This is the best method of fusing the slipped vertebra because it preserves the supporting soft tissues and has a high rate of fusion.

Posterior fusion: In this method, postoperative and additional slip is frequent until the fusion is solid. This also has a high rate of pseudoarthrosis and has to be done with intertransverse fusion.

Laminectomy: This mainly helps to relieve the neurological deficits and has to be followed by posterolateral fusion.

Laminectomy and intertransverse fusion.

Anterior interbody fusion: This is indicated for subtotal spondylolisthesis and is a risky and difficult procedure with doubtful efficacy.

Methods of Fusion and Stabilization:
Fusion is achieved in spondylolisthesis by putting autologous cancellous bone graft and Hart shill rectangle frame or Steffee plate and screws help obtain stabilization (Fig. 31.16).

KYPHOSIS

Definition

It is defined as increase in normal posterior convexity of the thoracic spine and is referred to as 'hyper-kyphosis' (Fig. 31.17A).

Causes

Localized injury or disease: Like fracture, Potts' disease, secondary in the spine, etc.

Generalized bone diseases: Ankylosing spondylitis, osteomalacia, Paget's disease, acromegaly, etc. are some of the examples.

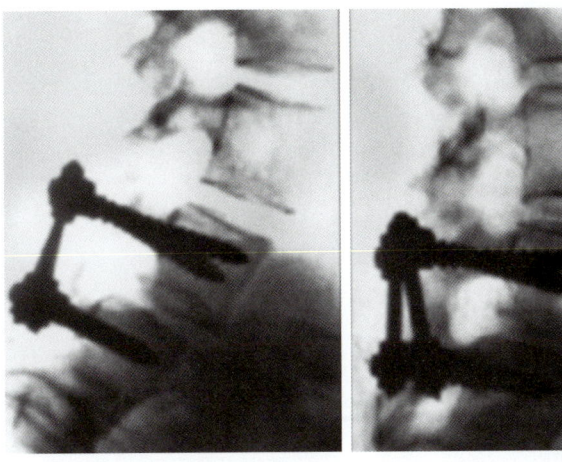

Fig. 31.16: Radiographs showing posterior spinal stabilization by Steffee plate and screws

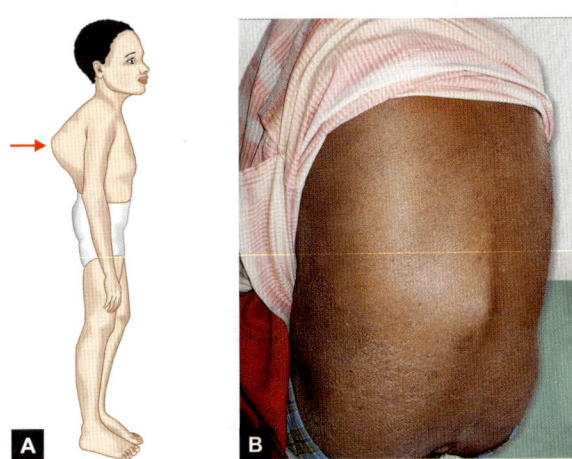

Figs 31.17A and B: Thoracic kyphosis: (A) Arrow showing gibbus; (B) Clinical photo of gibbus

Defective Growth or Poor Postural Habits

Children: Stooping posture while reading.

Adolescents: Vertebral epiphysitis (Scheuermann's) seen in boys 14–17 years of age.

Adults: Bending occupation, e.g. porter, cobbler, etc.

Old men and women: Senile osteoporosis.

> **Vital Facts: About Scheuermann's Disease**
> - Adolescent kyphosis.
> - Cobb's angle >45°, wedging of 5° and at least three adjacent apical vertebrae involved.
> - Slightly more common in females.
> - Cause unknown, familial.
> - Deformity is the main complaint than pain.
> - Typical X-ray finding—Schmorl's node.
> - ***Treatment:*** Milwaukee brace in immature spine. In severe deformity and in adults, surgical decompression and stabilization is advised.

Types

Knuckle

Prominence of single spinous process indicating collapse of single vertebra, e.g. TB spine/Kummel's disease, etc.

Angular

Two to three vertebral body is collapsed, e.g. late stage of TB, secondary carcinoma, etc. (Fig. 31.17B).

Round

Several vertebrae are involved and hence gives a round appearance, e.g. in children—Scheuermann's disease, in old age—senile kyphosis.

Clinical feature: Deformity is the usual complaint. Pain may rarely be seen. Loss of heights in advanced cases.

Methods of Examination

Inspection: Look from the side and note if the thoracic curvature is regular, now determine if the kyphosis is mobile, or fixed.

> **Tests for Mobility**
> When do you say postural kyphosis is mobile?
> - When the patient bends forward, deformity increases.
> - When the patient braces the shoulder back, deformity decreases. If the above two tests are negative, kyphosis is fixed.
>
> **What is Gibbus?**
> Acute kyphosis is called gibbus and is due to single or two level vertebral involvements.

Investigations

Plain X-ray of the thoracic spine, CT scan, MRI, laboratory tests are some of the important investigation methods to evaluate the severity of kyphosis.

Treatment

In mild deformities, anterior hyperextension bracing is indicated. In severe deformities, surgical decompression and stabilization is advised.

LUMBAR CANAL STENOSIS

This is dealt in the section on Geriatric Orthopedics.

Regional Conditions of the Lower Limb

REGIONAL CONDITIONS OF THE HIP

COXA VARA

Definition

It is an abnormality of the proximal end of femur, which is characterized by decreased neck shaft angle (Fig. 32.1A).

Normal coxa vara is due to differential growth pattern of capital femoral and greater trochanteric epiphysis. In coxa, valga the neck shaft angle is increased (Fig. 32.1B).

Note:
Normal neck shaft angle is 135°.

Classification

Congenital

- Congenital coxa vara.
- Congenital short femur with coxa vara.
- Congenital bowed femur with coxa vara.

Acquired

According to the site of disturbance.

- *Capital coxa vara:* This is seen in Perthes' disease, chondro-osteodystrophy, cretinism, septic arthritis of hip, etc.
- *Epiphyseal coxa vara:* Slipped capital femoral epiphysis (Fig. 32.2).
- *Cervical coxa vara:* This is seen in malunited trochanteric fracture, pathological hip conditions like:
   - *Children:* Rickets, bony dystrophies, etc.
   - *Adults:* Osteomyelitis, osteoporosis, Paget's disease, fibrous dysplasia, etc.

Part of generalized skeletal dysplasias: This is seen in mucopolysaccharidosis, multiple epiphyseal dysplasias, achondroplasia, cleidocranial dysostosis, etc.

Disadvantages of Coxa Vara

- Normal apposition between joint surfaces is lost.
- Trochanter is displaced upwards, impinges on the side of pelvis.

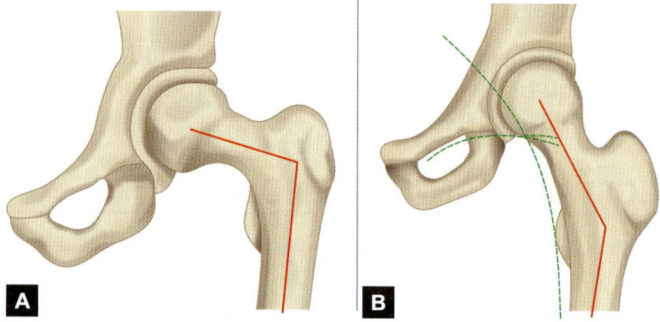

Figs 32.1A and B: (A) Coxa vara; (B) Coxa valga

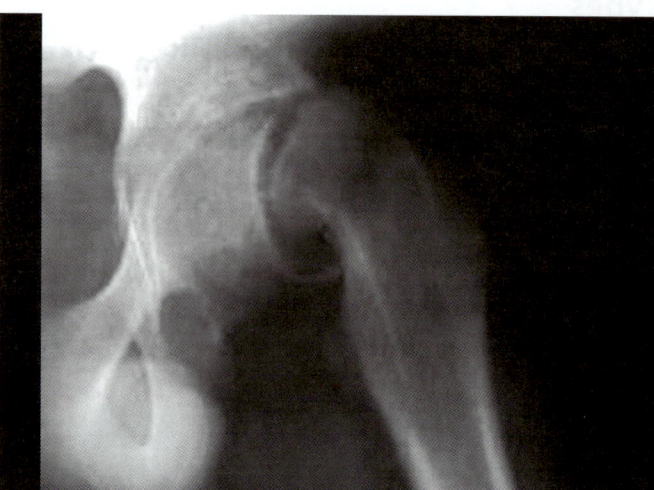

Fig. 32.2: Coxa vara due to slipped femoral epiphysis

- Marked shortening of the limb.
- Waddling gait.

Clinical Features

Small stature, limp, waddling gait, upward shift of greater trochanter, decreased rotation and abduction of hip, pain, stiffness and flexion contractures are some of the important clinical features of coxa vara.

Radiography

Radiographic features are: neck shaft angle is less than 90°, length of the neck is decreased, head is unusually translucent, and triangular fragment of bone is seen occupying lower part of the head close to the neck (Figs 32.3 and 32.4).

Treatment

It consists of corrective osteotomy at the intertrochanteric level. Usually, a lateral valgus wedge osteotomy is preferred. Macewen and Shands' corrective osteotomy corrects both coxa vara and retroversion of the femoral neck.

LEGG-CALVÉ-PERTHES DISEASE (Syn: Osteochondritis Deformans Juvenilis and Coxa Plana)

Legg-Calvé-Perthes[1] disease is a complex pediatric hip disorder and has some controversial aspects. Although its precise etiology remains unknown, the pathogenesis and pathology are fairly well understood. The prognosis for a child with this disease has improved considerably than in the past.

Definition

It is *a disorder affecting the capital femoral epiphysis*. It is the most common form of osteochondroses, characterized by avascular necrosis (AVN) and disordered enchondral ossification of the primary and secondary centers of ossification. It is associated with potential long-term morbidity.

Predisposing Factors

Genetic aspects increased incidence of 2–20 percent in families of Perthes'.

Abnormal growth and development: Perthes' disease may be a manifestation of an unknown systemic disorder rather than an isolated abnormality of the hip joint. The bone age of children with Perthes' disease is typically lower than their chronological age by 1–3 years; as a result, the affected children are shorter than normal.

Environmental factors: Majority of children belong to the poorer class.

Sex: Eighty percent affected are males (4:1).

Trauma to the hip joints.

Etiology

The etiology remains unknown, but it is *currently accepted that the disorder is caused by an interruption of the blood supply to the capital femoral epiphysis, causing avascular necrosis.*

Pathogenesis

Capital femoral epiphysis: The following are the changes seen in the capital femoral epiphysis:

Initial ischemia is followed by revascularization and pathological subchondral fracture occurs due to trauma

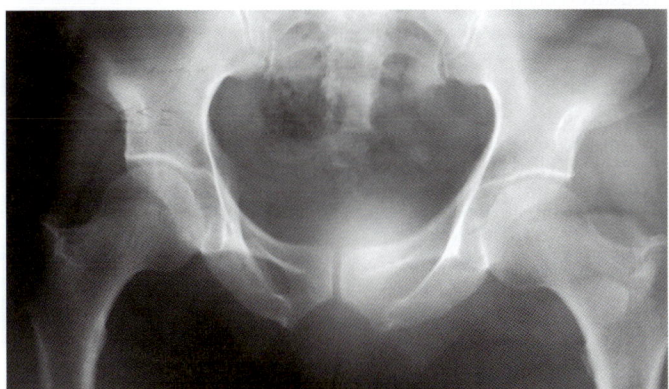

Fig. 32.3: Plain X-ray showing coxa vara

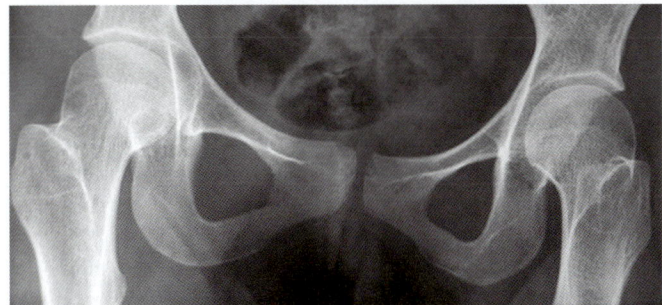

Fig. 32.4: Plain X-ray showing coxa valga

---

[1]**George Clemens Perthes** (1869-1927), a German Orthopedic Surgeon described it independently. **Legg, Arthur Thornton, Massachusetts** (1910) and **Jacques Calve** (1910) of France also described it and called it as coxa plana.

or vigorous active movements. This results in a second mechanical ischemic episode, which heralds the onset of true form of Perthes. Again, slow revascularization called *creeping substitution* takes place and the head is molded due to the forces acting on it (biologic plasticity).

Epiphyseal growth plate changes: The two ischemic episodes mentioned above also take place here.

Metaphyseal changes: Four characteristic changes are seen in the metaphyseal area: presence of adipose tissue, osteolytic lesions, disorganized ossification, and extrusion of growth plate.

Ultimate result: Following the epiphyseal growth plate and metaphyseal changes, the following results are seen:
- Altered longitudinal growth of the proximal femur.
- Coxa vara and coxa magna.
- High greater trochanter and short femoral neck results in functional coxa vara.
- Shortening by 1–2 cm.
- Trendelenburg gait is due to disturbed hip abductor mechanism (Flowchart 32.1).

Clinical Features

It is usually common in boys between 4 and 8 years (mean age 7 years) but can also occur less than 2 years and more than 12 years. *If the child is older than 12 years, it is not true Perthes' disease but rather adolescent avascular necrosis.*

Flowchart 32.1: Pathogenesis of Legg-Calvé-Perthes disease

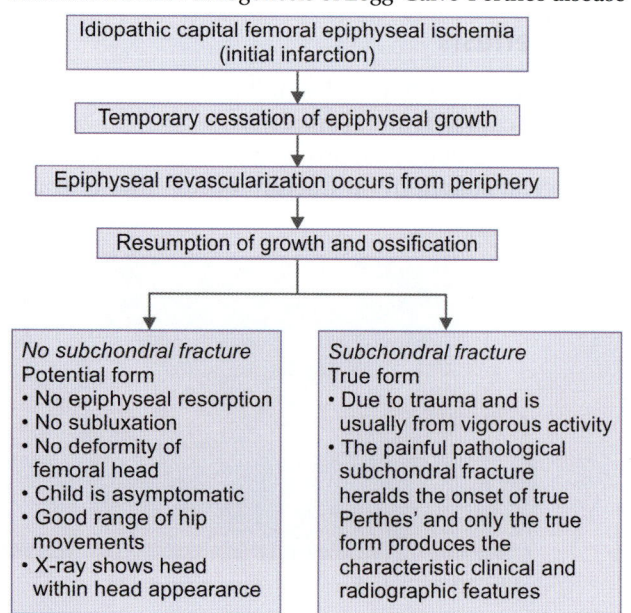

Symptoms
- Painless limp (classical presentation).
- Mild pain in the hip or anterior thigh or knee.
- History of trauma may be present or absent.
- Onset of pain may be acute or insidious.

Signs
- Antalgic gait.
- Muscle spasm (detected by roll test).
- Proximal thigh atrophy (by 2–3 cm).
- Limitation of abduction and internal rotation.
- Short stature.

Clinical Tests

Internal rotation test (Figs 32.5 and 32.6) for hip shows decreased internal rotation.

Trendelenburg test is positive.

Abduction test: Abduction is limited on the affected side (Figs 32.7 and 32.8).

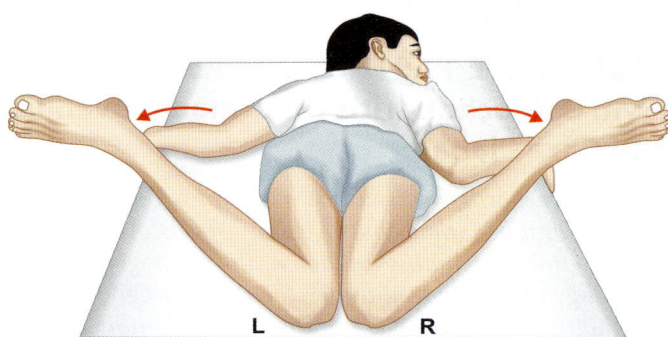

Fig. 32.5: Limitation of internal rotation of right hip. Hip rotation is best assessed in prone position because any restriction can be measured easily

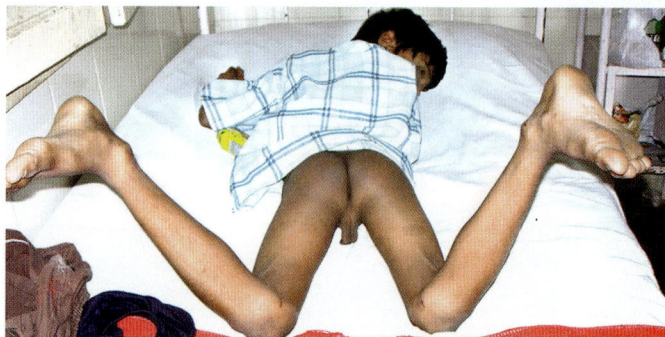

Fig. 32.6: Clinical photo showing loss of internal rotation in Perthes

CHAPTER 32: Regional Conditions of the Lower Limb

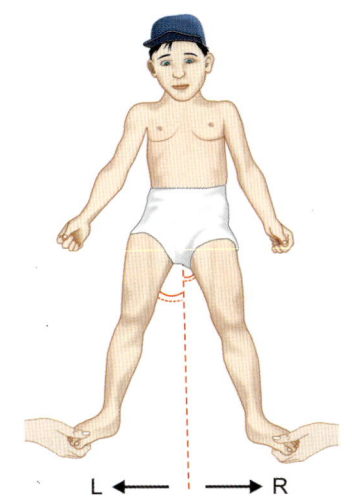

Fig. 32.7: Limitation of abduction of the right hip in Perthes' disease

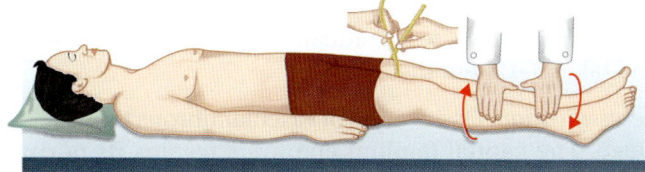

Fig. 32.9: Roll test to detect muscle spasm in Perthes' disease (right) and recording of muscle wasting (left)

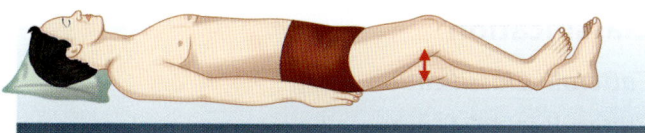

Fig. 32.10: Fifteen degrees of fixed flexion deformity of the hip which is characteristic in Perthes' disease

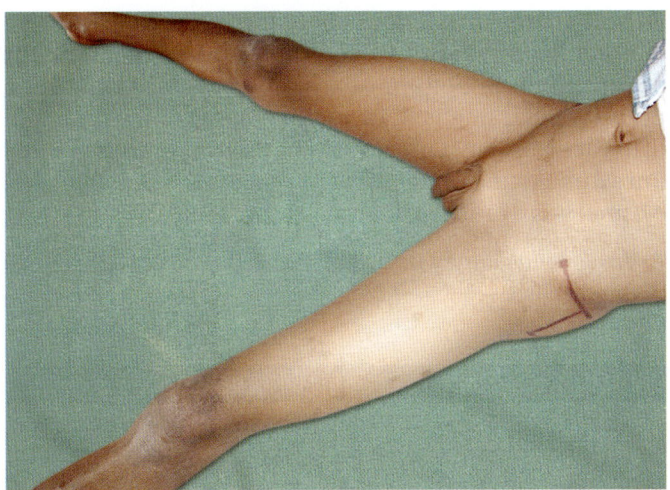

Fig. 32.8: Clinical photo showing loss of abduction in Perthes

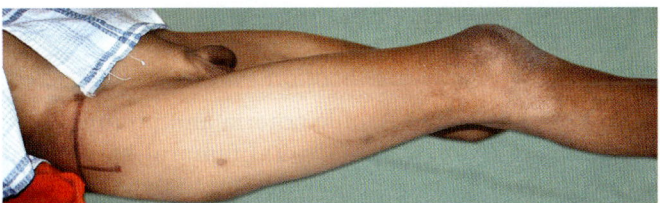

Fig. 32.11: Clinical photo showing FFD hip in Perthes

TABLE 32.1: Major radiographic characteristics in Perthes'	
Group I	Involvement is limited only to the anterior portion of epiphysis
Group II	Whole epiphysis is involved with the exception of intact lateral margin of epiphysis
Group III	Involvement of even the lateral margin of epiphysis
Group IV	Whole head involvement

Roll test: Passive rotation of the lower limb is done to detect the muscle spasm (Fig. 32.9). This is positive.

Thomas test: Reveals typically 15° fixed flexion deformity (FFD) of hip (Figs 32.10 and 32.11).

Radiographic Characteristics (Waldenstrom)

Perthes' disease is divided into five distinct radiographic stages (Table 32.1).

Cessation of growth of the capital femoral epiphysis: Occurs after the initial ischemic episode and lasts for 6–12 months.

Subchondral fractures: Causes collapse of the head and causes ischemia (Fig. 32.12). Visible on the radiograph for an average of three months.

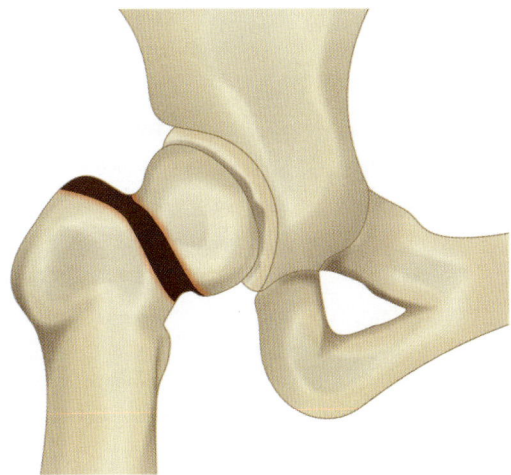

Fig. 32.12: Subchondral fracture in Perthes' disease

Resorption: The necrotic epiphyseal bone beneath the subchondral fracture is gradually and irregularly resorbed and takes 6–12 months.

Re-ossification: Ossification of vascular fibrous tissue takes place. The capital femoral epiphysis regains its normal strength, takes 6–24 months.

Healed or residual stage: The femoral head is healed with or without residual deformity.

Classification

Catterall[2] Classification

Catterall in 1971, proposed a four-group classification system for Perthes' disease based on the radiographic appearance and extent of the involvement of the femoral head. *This classification has been extremely useful in retrospective analysis of the results of treatment and has a very limited prognostic value (Table 32.2).*

Salter-Thompson's Classification

It simplifies the radiographic criteria and permits early diagnosis of the extent of capital femoral epiphyseal involvement. It is an accurate method to determine the prognosis and decide the form of treatment.

This classification is based on the presence of subchondral fracture and radiographic crescent sign:

Group A (Catterall Gr I and II): In this, less than half of the capital femoral epiphysis is involved.

Group B (Catterall Gr III and IV): In this, more than half of the capital femoral epiphysis is involved.

The presence of an intact and viable lateral margin of capital femoral epiphysis indicates good prognosis and its absence suggests poor prognosis.

Herring classification: This is shown in Table 32.3.

Stulberg Classification

- Gold standard for rating residual femoral head deformity and joint congruence.
- Recent studies show poor interobserver and intraobserver reliability.

Radiographic Assessment

This is necessary to determine the progress of the disease, sphericity of the femoral head, epiphyseal extrusion or collapse, and response to the treatment (Fig. 32.13). Plain radiographs are usually adequate but rarely arthrography, MRI may be required.

Salter's extrusion angle: This angle helps to assess the femoral head extrusion (Fig. 32.14). A horizontal line is drawn from the bottom of acetabular "tear drop" and a perpendicular line is drawn at the lateral ossified margin of the acetabulum. Lines drawn from intersections of these lines through the midpoint of physis give extrusion angles. Normal is 50° or more.

Arthrography: It may be useful in the early resorption stage of the disease.

TABLE 32.2: Catterall's radiological classification of Perthes'

Group	I	II	III	IV
Epiphysis				
Anterior	Negative	Part	Positive	Positive
Posterior	Negative	Negative	Positive	Positive
Medial	Negative	Negative	Positive	Positive
Lateral	Negative	Negative	Positive	Positive
Subchondral fracture				
AP view	Negative	seen	# seen	# seen
Lateral	Positive	# seen	# seen	# seen
Prognosis	Good	Good	Less favorable	Poor

Abbreviations: Positive—Affected; Negative—Not affected; #—Fracture.

TABLE 32.3: Lateral pillar (Herring) classification

Group A	Lateral pillar maintains full height with no density changes identified	Uniformly good outcome
Group B	Maintains >50% height	Poor outcome in patients with bone age >6 years
B/C Border	Lateral pillar is narrowed (2–3 mm) or poorly ossified with approximately 50% height	Recently added to increase consistency and prognosis of classification
Group C	Less than 50% of lateral pillar height is maintained	Poor outcomes in all patient

- Determined at the beginning of fragmentation stage, usually occurs 6 months after the onset of symptoms
- Based on the height of the lateral pillar of the capital femoral epiphysis on AP imaging of the pelvis
- Has best interobserver agreement
- Designed to provide prognostic information
- Limitation is that final classification is not possible at initial presentation due to the fact that the patient needs to have entered into the fragmentation stage radiographically

---

[2]**Anthony Catterall** (1971), described the natural history and monograph of this disease.

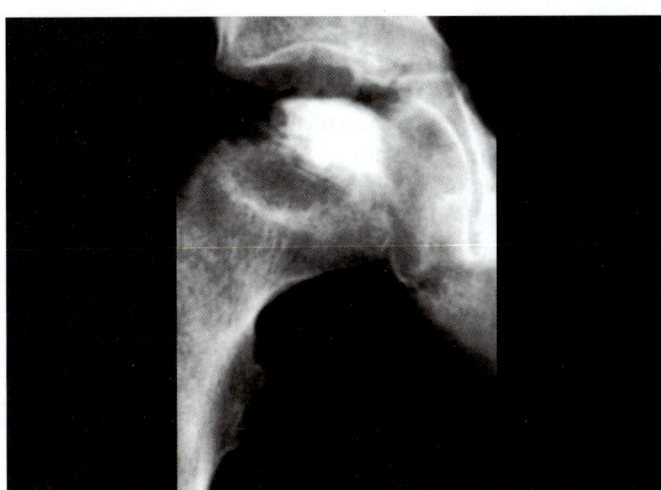

Fig. 32.13: Radiograph showing Perthes' disease

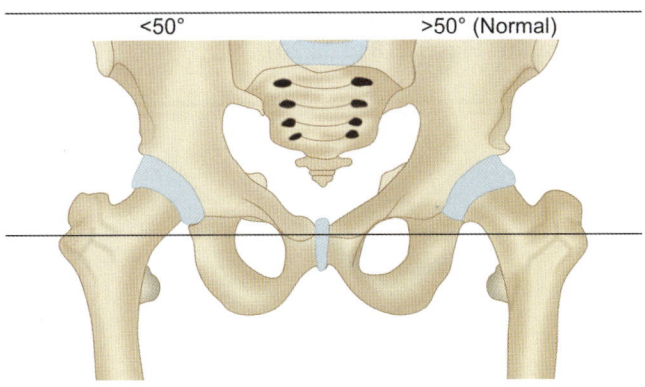

Fig. 32.14: Salter's extrusion angle

Radionuclide bone scan: It is used to detect potential form of Perthes' disease.

MRI: It may be helpful in defining area of epiphyseal infarction and femoral head contour.

Management

Perthes' disease is a local, self-healing disorder of the femoral head. Prevention of the femoral-head deformity and secondary degenerative osteoarthritis is the only justification for treatment.

Treatment Methods (Flowchart 32.2)

Elimination of hip irritability can be done by 1 to 2 weeks period of bed rest, sling, suspension, traction, etc.

Restoration and maintenance of hip motion can be done by physical therapy active and passive. Abduction exercises may be helpful.

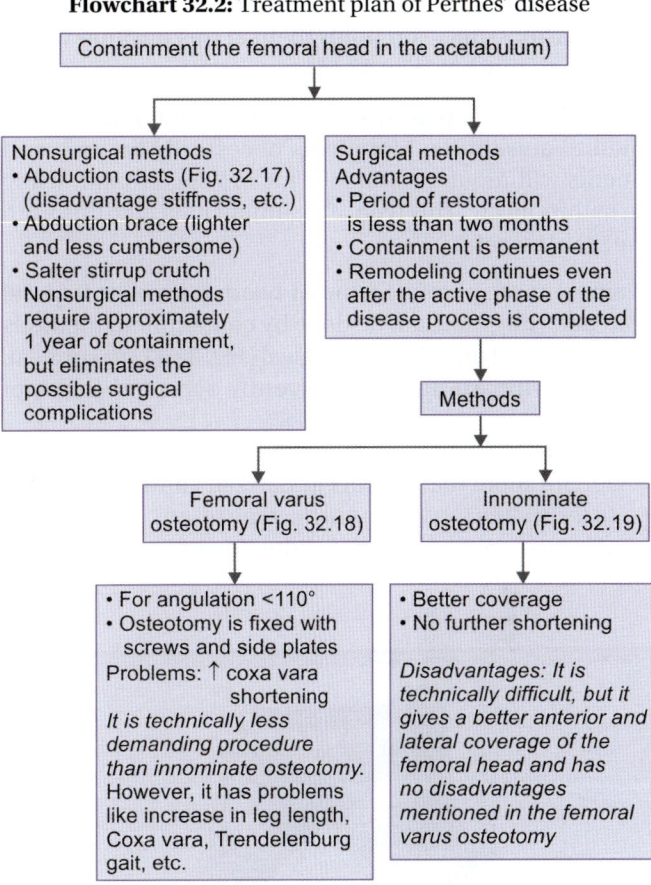

Flowchart 32.2: Treatment plan of Perthes' disease

Prevention of the extrusion and collapse by bed rest, abduction splints, etc.

Splints Used in Perthes

The Scottish Rite Brace

This is one of the most commonly used braces for treating Perthes disease. It as a pair of thigh cuffs separated by a telescoping spreader bar and a hinged suspension belt, and it is designed to be worn over the clothing. It is lightweight and easily removable for rest or bathing (Fig. 32.15).

Disadvantages: It lacks built-in hip flexion, causing patient movements that prevents the coverage of the femur anterior head. Also it does not rotate the hips internally, and most patients tend to naturally rotate the hips externally when walking in the brace, compromising femur anterior head coverage.

The Petrie Cast

This is another most commonly used brace design for Perthes disease. The cast places both legs in a fixed position at maximum abduction, meaning that they are spread apart as wide as possible, and holds them at this position with a rigid separating bar (Fig. 32.16).

Disadvantages: It requires regular physical therapy under epidural anesthesia. Mobility is necessarily limited, and patients will require assistance for moving around, using the bathroom etc. This type of treatment typically lasts from three to six weeks.

Attainment of spherical femoral head to prevent femoral head deformity and can be done by containment methods (see box) which may be nonsurgical (Fig. 32.17) or surgical. The following are the four currently accepted forms of management:
- *Observation* is indicated for children less than 6 years, and for more than 6 years in Caterall I and II.
- *Intermittent symptomatic treatment* consists of observation, bed rest and abduction exercises.

Definitive early treatment: Nonsurgical or surgical containment of the femoral head early in the course of the disease is indicated when the:
- Age at onset is more than 6 years or older.
- Catterall III and IV grades.
- Lateral extrusion of the capital femoral epiphysis.

Prerequisites are good to full range of hip motion, no residual irritability, and the femoral head must also appear round or almost round.

Late Surgical Management for Deformity

For a significant femoral head deformity, which prevents reduction into the acetabulum or remodeling after treatment with standard containment methods, an alternative must be considered and may consist of one of the following techniques: Muscle release and abduction casts, partial excision of the femoral head or cheilectomy, proximal femoral valgus osteotomy and greater trochanter advancement (Figs 32.18 to 32.20).

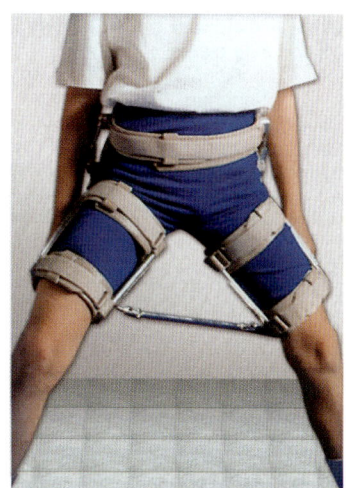

Fig. 32.15: Showing Scottish Rite brace

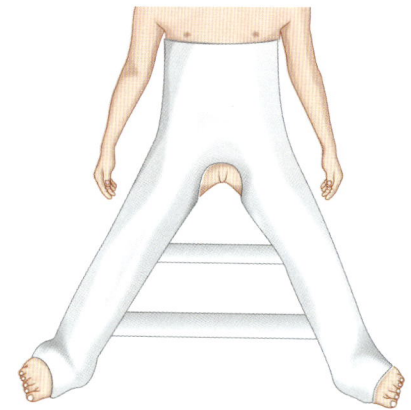

Fig. 32.17: Abduction cast is a nonsurgical method of containment in Perthes' disease

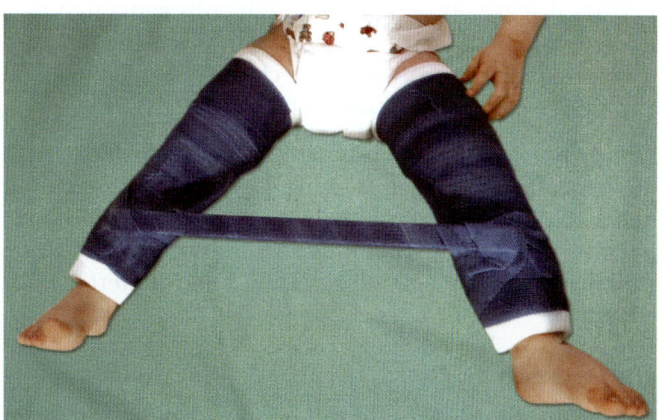

Fig. 32.16: The Petrie cast

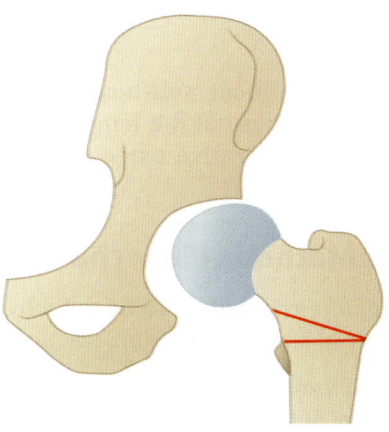

Fig. 32.18: Femoral varus osteotomy

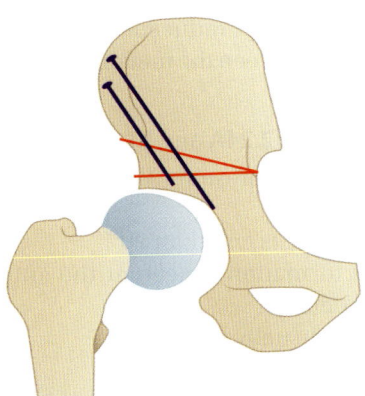

Fig. 32.19: Innominate osteotomy

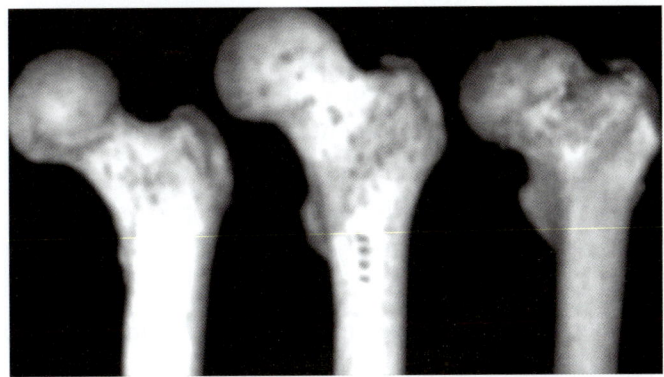

Fig. 32.21: Cadaveric specimen of a slipped capital femoral epiphysis

SLIPPED CAPITAL FEMORAL EPIPHYSIS (Syn: Epiphyseal Coxa Vara; Adolescent Coxa Vara)

Slipped capital femoral epiphysis (SCFE) occurs during adolescent rapid growth period when epiphysis plate is weak and the capital epiphysis is displaced down and back (Fig. 32.21). Müller first described it in 1889.

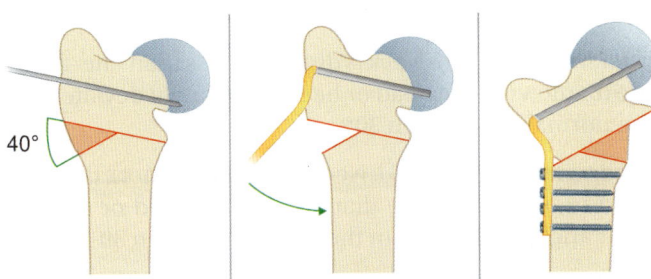

Fig. 32.20: AO technique of varus femoral osteotomy

Prognosis
Poor prognostic factors are:
- Sex—female.
- Age of the clinical onset if more than 6 years.
- Catterall group III and IV.
- Loss of femoral head containment.
- Persistent loss of motion.
- Premature epiphyseal growth plate closure.

Quick Facts: Perthes' Disease
- Commonest osteochondroses.
- Eighty percent affected are males between the age group 4–8 years.
- Two episodes of infarction.
- First episode cause is not known.
- Second episode is due to subchondral fracture.
- Subchondral fracture heralds onset of true Perthes'.
- Painless limp is the characteristic symptom.
- Decreased abduction, internal rotation is present.
- Catterall's grading helps plan the treatment.
- Salter and Thompson's grading has prognostic value.
- It is a local self-healing disorder.
- The main goal of treatment is to attain a spherical femoral head either by non-surgical or surgical methods.

Etiology

Predisposing Factors

Age: It is common in 10–17 years of age.

Sex: Male : Female are 5:2 ratios.

Body type: Female—slender long built, and male—obesity type.

Location: Left hip is involved in 58 percent of the cases.

Trauma: Trivial or none at all.

Theories of Causations
- *Harris hormonal theory:* Due to hormonal imbalance between the increased growth hormone and decreased sex and thyroid hormone.
- *Traumatic theory:* Epiphyseal line is the weakest part of the normal adolescent bone.
- *Theory of periosteal thinning:* Periosteum, which is thick in children, thins out during adolescence.

Clinical Types

Acute (11%): Sudden onset and the symptoms are less than two weeks duration.

Chronic (60%): Symptoms are present for more than two weeks. X-ray shows callus and remodeling.

Acute on chronic (23%): Symptoms are present for one month and there is a recent sudden increase in pain following trivial injury.

Preslip (6%): X-ray shows irregular wide epiphysis.

Clinical Features

This depends on the stages of the slip as shown in Table 32.4.

Investigations

Radiographic Changes

Early Changes

- Marginal blurring of the proximal metaphysis.
- Lower margin of metaphysis is included within the acetabulum normally but excluded in the early epiphyseal slip.
- *Trethowan line:* Line drawn along the superior margin of the neck, transects the epiphysis normally (Figs 32.22A and B), but will be above it in slip.
- Depth of epiphysis is reduced.
- There is a step between the metaphysis and the epiphysis (Fig. 32.23).

Late Changes (Figs 32.24A and B)

- Trethowan sign is present.
- Head is atrophic.
- Neck shaft angle is less than 90°.
- New bone formation is seen at the anterior superior part of the neck.
- Joint space is usually clear.
- Shenton's line is broken.

CT scan and MRI: This is very useful in assessing the degree of slips, etc.

Classification of Slipping

Mild slipping (51%): Neck is displaced less than one-third of the diameter of the head or head-shaft angle deviates from the normal by less than 30°.

Moderate slipping (22%): Neck is displaced more than one-third to one-half of the diameter of the head or the head shaft angle deviates from the normal between 30 and 60°.

TABLE 32.4: Showing stages in SCFE and clinical features		
Preslipping Stage	Chronic-slipping stage	Stage of fixed deformity
• Discomfort in the groin • Stiffness/limp • No objective finding • Medial rotation of the hip is decreased	• Pain ↑ • Antalgic gait • All movements ↓ particularly. Abduction and internal rotation • Varus + Adduction + External rotation deformity is present • Shortening is present • Extension and external rotation↑ • Waddling gait is present • Trendelenburg's gait is positive	• No pain • No spasm • Limb shortening + • External rotation + • Adduction deformity

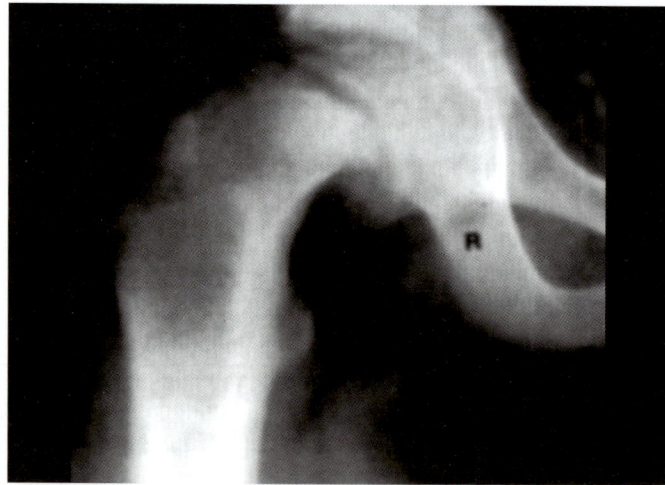

Fig. 32.23: Radiograph showing SCFE (Early changes)

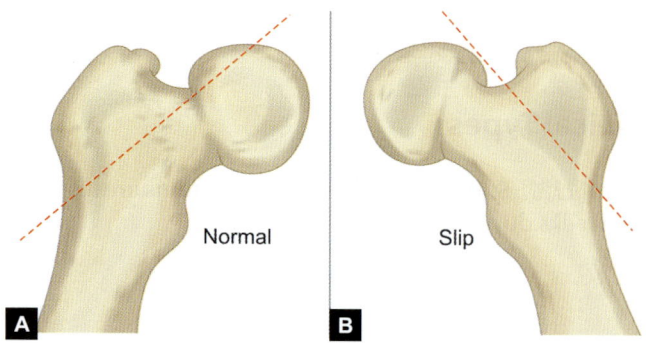

Figs 32.22A and B: Trethowan sign

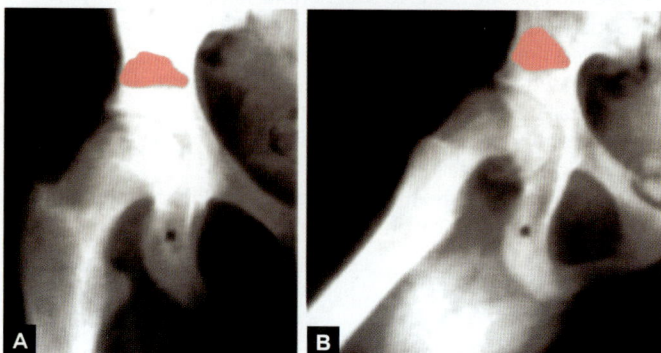

Figs 32.24A and B: Radiographs showing SCFE (Late changes)

Severe slipping (17%): Neck is displaced more than one-half diameter of the head or head shaft angle is more than 60° from normal.

Treatment

- If epiphysis has begun to displace, there is no safety until the epiphyseal line has fused.
- When there is minor displacement, epiphysis is fused at once by pining in displaced position.
- Acute major slip: Emergency reduction is done under (GA) or reduction is obtained by traction and fixed with pins.
- Irreducible displacement: This is treated by open reduction and cervical osteotomy.
- Old fixed displacement: This is treated by a corrective osteotomy at the intertrochanteric or subtrochanteric level.

Complications

Avascular necrosis (13%) of the femoral head and chondrolysis are the usual complications. Secondary osteoarthritis may be seen at later stages.

Hip pointer: This is a contusion over the iliac crest due to a fall directly on it in sports like football, gymnastics, basketball, etc.

REGIONAL DISORDERS OF THE KNEE

Deformities around the knee joint could be in two planes. In the coronal plane, we may encounter genu valgum and genu varum deformities; and in the sagittal plane, antevertum and recurvatum deformities (Figs 32.25A to E).

Strange it may seem but a normal knee is a crooked knee. Nature identifies a 6° physiological outward deviation of the knee (valgum) as normal and not a straight knee! Only when the crookedness of the knee increases (genu valgum) or decreases (genu varum) or when it bends backwards (recurvatum) that it is considered abnormal and is a cause of worry. A person affected by any one of these conditions is brought on his "knees" and is forced to seek remedial measures to be up on his "knees" normally again!

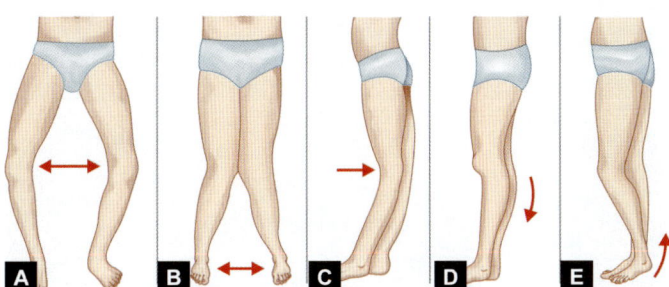

Figs 32.25A to E: Various knee deformities: (A) Genu varum; (B) Genu valgum; (C) Genu recurvatum; (D) Triple deformity; (E) Fixed flexion deformity

GENU VALGUM (KNOCK-KNEE)

Definition

It is an outward deviation of the longitudinal axes of both tibia and femur. Apex of the curve or angulations of the knee are medial (Fig. 32.26).

Incidence

Seventy-five percent children have genu valgum up to 4 years of age. This is called physiological genu valgum, which usually disappears by 7 years.

Types

It is broadly classified into physiological and pathological, the latter could be unilateral or bilateral (Table 32.5).

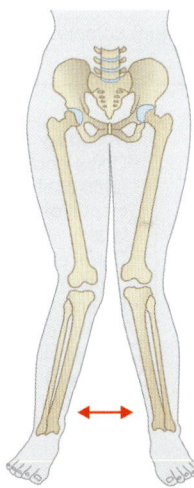

Fig. 32.26: Genu valgum or knock-knee deformity

TABLE 32.5: Causes of genu valgum	
Unilateral	Bilateral
• Trauma	• Physiological (disappears by 4 years)
• Osteomyelitis	• Pathological
• Tumors	• Congenital disorders
	• Idiopathic (most common)
	• Developmental disorders (e.g. epiphyseal dysplasia)
	• Endocrine disorders (e.g. thyroid disorders)
	• Metabolic disorders (e.g. rickets)
	• Paralytic disorders
	• Traumatic disorders
	• Infective disorders
	• Degenerative disorders
	• Inflammatory disorders (e.g. rheumatoid arthritis)

Clinical Features

Genu valgum complex: The primary deformity in a genu valgum is *a medial angulation of the knee* (Fig. 32.27). In response to this, secondary deformities develop in the femur, tibia, and foot. Primary and secondary deformities together form the genu valgum complex (Flowchart 32.3).

> **Quick Facts: Idiopathic Genu Valgum**
> The following are its features:
> - Commonest variety.
> - Invariably bilateral.
> - Deformity is the only complaint.
> - Occurs at the age of 2–3 years.
> - Recovers by the age of 6 years.

Assessment of Genu Valgum Deformity

Clinical Assessment

Intermalleolar gap: The severity of the deformity is measured by noting the intermalleolar distance.

Flowchart 32.3: Genu valgum complex

```
                    Genu valgum complex
                    /                 \
        Primary deformity         Secondary deformities
        Medial angulation         • Distal ends of femur and proximal
        of the knee                 ends of tibia are rotated externally
                                    by pull of biceps and tensor fascia
                                    lata
                                  • Distal end of tibia develops a
                                    compensatory internal torsion
                                  • Lateral dislocation of patella
                                  • Lateral structures shortened,
                                    medial structures elongated
                                    (of knee)
                                  • Pronated flat foot
```

Method: In the spine position, the patella is brought to vertical by rotating both the legs and made to touch lightly at the knee. Then holding both the knees in position, the distance between the two malleoli is measured. The acceptable normal limit is 8–10 cm. In genu valgum deformity, it will be more than 10 cm.

Plumb line test: Normally, a line drawn from anterosuperior iliac spine (ASIS) to middle of the patella, if extended down strikes the medial malleolus. In genu valgum, the medial malleolus will be outside this line.

Knee flexion test: This is to detect the cause of genu valgum whether it lies in the femur or tibia. If the deformity disappears with flexion of the knee, the cause lies in the lower end of femur and if it persists on flexion, the cause lies in the upper end of the tibia.

Radiographs

Clinical assessment of genu valgum is less accurate in adults and an assessment by radiology is preferred. X-ray of the entire lower limb is taken with the patient weight bearing (Fig. 32.28). The angle formed between the femoral and tibial shafts is measured on the radiographs and allowing for a normal angle of 6°, genu valgum is calculated.

Treatment of Genu Valgum (Table 32.6)

Mild cases: Child is seen at intervals of 3 months and the progress is recorded. These cases usually require no treatment, and raising the inner side of the heels by 4–5 mm may possibly relieve strain on ankles. The knock-knee braces may be useful. If by the age of 4 years, intermalleolar distance is 10 cm or more, operation may become necessary and unless deformity is increasing rapidly, operation is best postponed until the child is 10 years old.

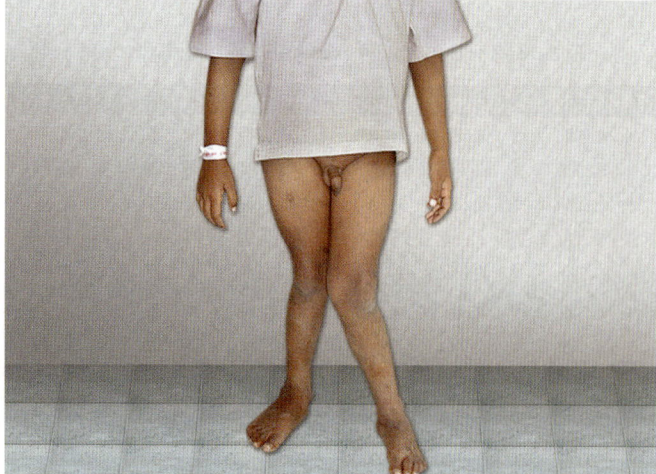

Fig. 32.27: Clinical photo showing genu valgum deformity

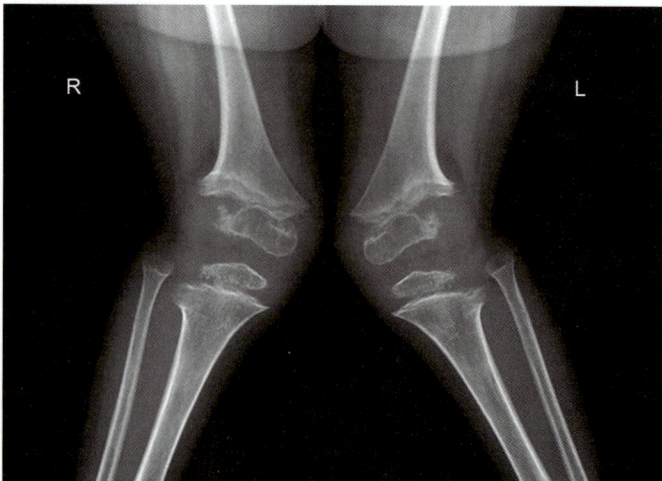

Fig. 32.28: Plain X-ray showing genu valgum

TABLE 32.6: Treatment of genu valgum	
Mild (< 8 cm IM distance at 4 years)	*Severe (> 10 cm IM at 10 years)*
• No treatment	Surgery
• Raise medial heel by 4–5 mm	• Unilateral genu valgum
• Knock knee brace (outer Iron bar, inner strap) ↓	• Intermalleolar distance >10 cm at 10 years ↓
Epiphysis arrest	**Osteotomy**
• Done before Skeletal maturity	• Done after skeletal maturity
• Lateral epiphysis should be intact as seen in X-ray	• Medial closed wedge osteotomy if limb is longer or normal
• Staple the medial epiphysis to arrest the growth	• Lateral open wedge osteotomy if limb is short
Abbreviation: IM, Intermalleolar	

Severe Cases

- If lateral portion of epiphyseal plate is intact as seen in the radiographs, it contributes to the longitudinal growth at a reduced rate. This situation is suitable for stapling of the medial epiphysis, which arrests the growth on the medial side, allows the growth on the lateral side, and thus helps to correct the deformity.
- After skeletal maturity, an osteotomy must be performed at the site of maximum deformity of tibia or femur. If limb is long, *medial close wedge osteotomy* is done. If limb is short, *lateral open wedge osteotomy* is done. Knock-knee deformity more than 10 cm at the age of 10 years is an indication for surgery.

Treatment Facts of Genu Valgum
- <4 years—No treatment.
- 4–10 years—Heel raise, knock-knee brace.
- 10–14 years—Epiphyseal stapling.
- 14–16 years—wait until skeletal maturity, as it is too late for stapling and too early for osteotomy, as it may recur.
- >16 years—Osteotomy.

Quick Facts: Genu Valgum
- Medial angulations of the knee.
- Seventy-five percent is physiological up to 4 years of age.
- Idiopathic is the most common type.
- Deformity is the only complaint.

GENU VARUM (BOW LEGS)

Definition

It is defined as *lateral angulation of the knee. The longitudinal axis of femur and tibia deviates medially*. The deformity involves tibia alone or the femur or tibia and fibula both (Fig. 32.29).

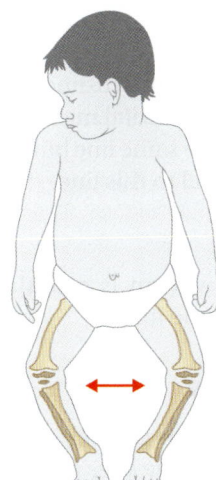

Fig. 32.29: Genu varum with increased intercondylar distance. Genu varum is said to exist if there is approximately 3 cm gap between the medial femoral condyles when the malleoli are together

Types and Causes

Unilateral
- Due to growth abnormalities of upper tibial epiphysis.
- Infections like osteomyelitis, etc.
- Trauma near the growth epiphysis of femur.
- Tumors affecting the lower end of femur and upper end of tibia.

Bilateral

Physiological (is corrected by four years).

Pathological:
- Congenital causes.
- Postural abnormalities.
- Developmental disorders.
- Metabolic disorders (rickets rare).
- Endocrine disorders.
- Degenerative disorders (e.g. osteoarthritis of knee). This is a common cause.
- Occupational disorders (e.g. in jockeys).
- Idiopathic.
- Paget's disease.
- 'Blounts' disease (tibia vara).

Clinical Measurements of the Deformity

Child
- The patient is examined supine with knee extended, patella facing the ceiling and the medial malleoli touching each other. If the separation of knee exceeds

more than 3 cm or if it is unilateral, it should be investigated.
- A line is drawn from anterosuperior iliac spine through center of patella to medial malleolus. Normally, all the structures are in the same line but in genu varum medial malleolus is medial to this line.

Adults

The angle of genu varum is calculated on a standing radiograph of the whole limb.

Clinical Features

Genu varum complex: The primary deformity in genu varum is *lateral angulation of the knee (Fig.32.30)*. In response to this, secondary deformities develop in the tibia and the foot. This together is known as genu varum complex (Table 32.7).

> **Note:**
> *What is apparent genu varum?*
> Due to anteversion of femoral neck, there is medial rotation of the femur and the child looks bow-legged. Nevertheless, with the patella facing forwards, the "varus deformity" disappears.

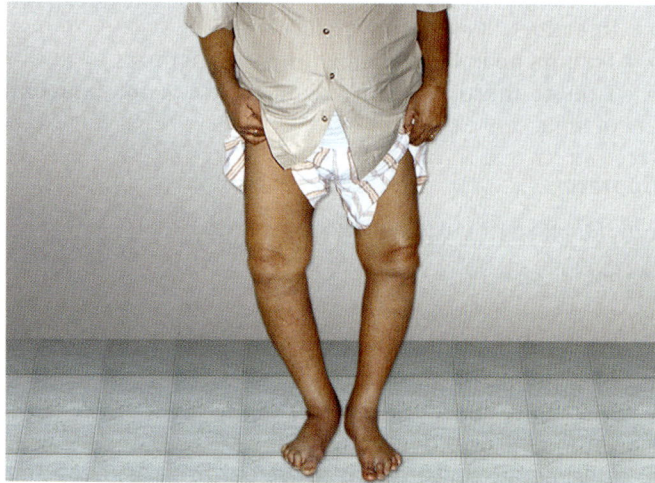

Fig. 32.30: Clinical photo showing genu varum deformity (Bilateral of knees)

TABLE 32.7: The primary and secondary deformities in genu varum

Primary deformity	Secondary deformities
Lateral angulations of the knee	**Associated abnormalities** • An internal torsion of distal tibia • In toeing of both the feet • Patella face outward while walking • Tight medial and lax lateral • Structures of the knee

Radiograph

Radiograph of the whole limb should be done to assess the severity of genu varum (Fig. 32.31).

Treatment

- Treatment should be conservative until four years of age. Knee-ankle-foot outhouses with the medial bar and the lateral strap are used.
- Correction of early deformity is done by dynamic bracing or splints. After four years, significant deformity should be corrected by surgery. Lateral epiphyseal stapling (Fig. 32.32) when the child is within the growth period and supracondylar medial open or lateral closed wedge osteotomy is done after skeletal maturity.

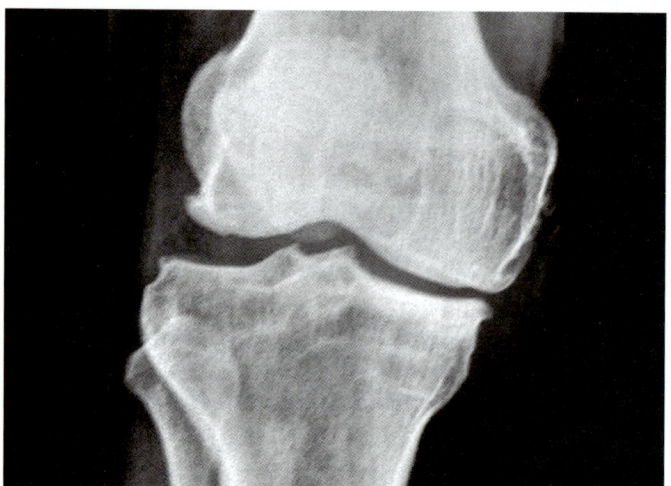

Fig. 32.31: Plan X-ray showing genu varum due to OA knees

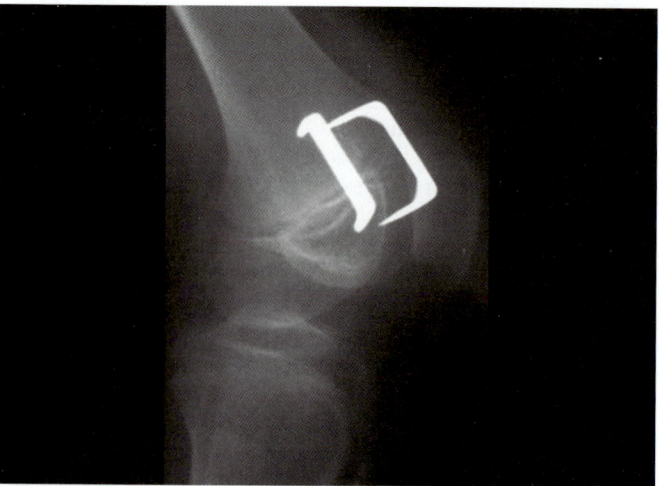

Fig. 32.32: Plain X-ray showing epiphyseal stapling

GENU RECURVATUM

Definition

Genu recurvatum is defined as *backward bending of the knee*. Up to 5° of genu, recurvatum is sometimes seen in women with lax ligaments and is usually generalized. Here, the popliteal fossa is convex instead of concave.

Causes

Congenital: Discussed in congenital disorders.
Quadriceps contracture is the most common cause in acquired genu recurvatum and is discussed below.

There are two varieties:
- Congenital variety.
- Post-injection contractures of infancy and childhood.

Quadriceps contracture in early childhood has an age of onset between one and seven years.

Neurological disorders: Polio, cerebral palsy, etc.

Malunited fractures around the knee.

Clinical Features

- Limitation of knee flexion from mild to severe.
- Effusion and other evidence of knee abnormality are absent.
- Sometimes, a dense band that becomes tense during flexion of the knee could be palpated in the proximal part of the patella.
- Patella is always located more proximally and sometimes laterally.
- Other features include; it is usually bilateral, common in identical twins, more common in females, and extremely resistant to conservative treatment.

Post-injection Contractures in Infancy

This was first described in 1962 by Miki.

Features

- Repeated injections and infusions to the thigh soon after birth.
- Dimples present in the skin at the sites of injections.
- Common in twins and prematurity (because they often make injections necessary and in infants anterior thigh is commonly the preferred site).
  The muscles usually involved are:
  - Vastus lateralis
  - Rectus femoris
  - Vastus intermedius: Vastus medialis is not involved because injections are not given to this muscle.

Clinical Tests to Measure Genu Recurvatum

- It is to be measured in the weight bearing position from the lateral side.
- The long axis of the thigh (from the tip of the trochanter to the midpoint of the lateral femoral condyle) is drawn.
- The long axis of the leg is drawn next (from the middle of the lateral tibial condyle and the lateral malleolus).
- The angle between these two lines is the angle of recurvatum.

Radiograph

Radiograph of the affected knee is recommended.

Treatment

Surgery is the treatment of choice and is usually indicated in established contractures, as conservative treatment is not beneficial. Early recognition and prevention through passive exercises while the child is receiving injections is the best preventive measure. Surgery is indicated early in habitual dislocation of the patella and in established contractures to prevent late changes in the femoral condyles and patella.

Methods

Thompson's quadriceps plasty (V-Y plasty) is the commonly done procedure.

Kullman and Leonart's surgery: Proximal release of rectus femoris in an isolated contracture of rectus femoris.

BURSAE AROUND THE KNEE

Knee is a complex joint in the body subserving complex functions. To do so, it requires a host of ligaments, muscles, menisci, etc. To serve the knee efficiently and longer, these structures need to be cushioned properly from the bony surfaces. As long as the knee is being used normally, no problems are encountered. Violation of the physiological actions by way of over and abnormal use frustrates and irritates these cushions, which are nothing but bursae around the knee-giving rise to various interesting clinical problems (Fig. 32.33).

Bursae are sacs lined with membrane similar to synovium. They are located over the joints and bony prominences and may or may not communicate with the joint. They reduce the friction and protect the delicate structures from pressures. When subjected to repeated pressure, they give rise to bursitis. There are two types of bursae, one that is normally present and second, an

adventitious bursa, which develops due to trauma, friction, pressure, etc. Adventitious bursa differs from true bursa by the lack of true endothelial or synovial lining.
Bursa around the knee is as follows:

Anterior

Suprapatellar: Always communicates with the knee joint.

Prepatellar bursitis (Housemaid's knee) (Figs 32.34A and B) is seen in the lower half of patella and upper half of ligamentum patella.

Infrapatellar seen in the lower half of ligamentum patella (Clergyman's, Parson's, or Carpet layer's knee or Vicar's knee) (Fig. 32.35).

Lateral

Cyst of lateral meniscus.

Medial

- Cyst of medial meniscus.
- Bursa anserine—between the tibial collateral ligament and tendons of the semimembranosus, gracilis, semitendinosus.

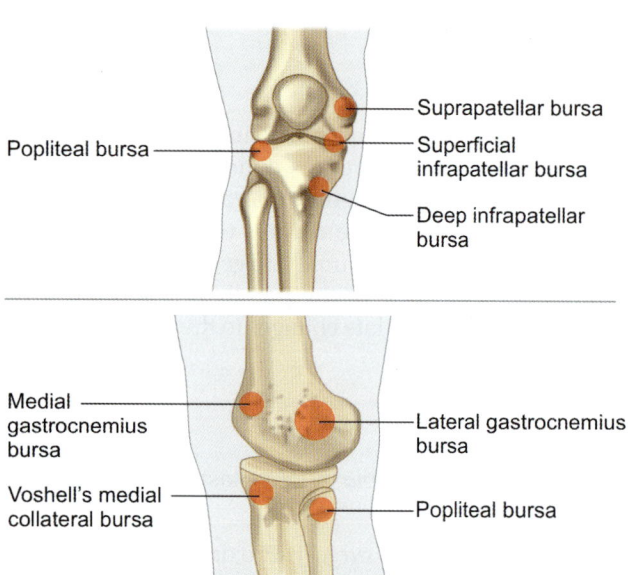

Fig. 32.33: Bursae around the knee

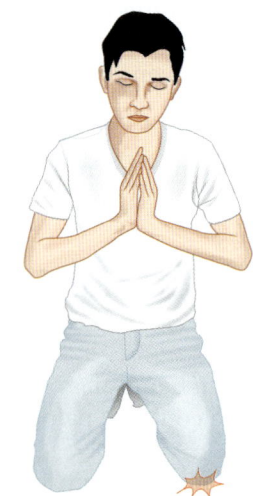

Fig. 32.35: When a clergyman prays for others, his knee weeps in silence (Clergyman's knee)

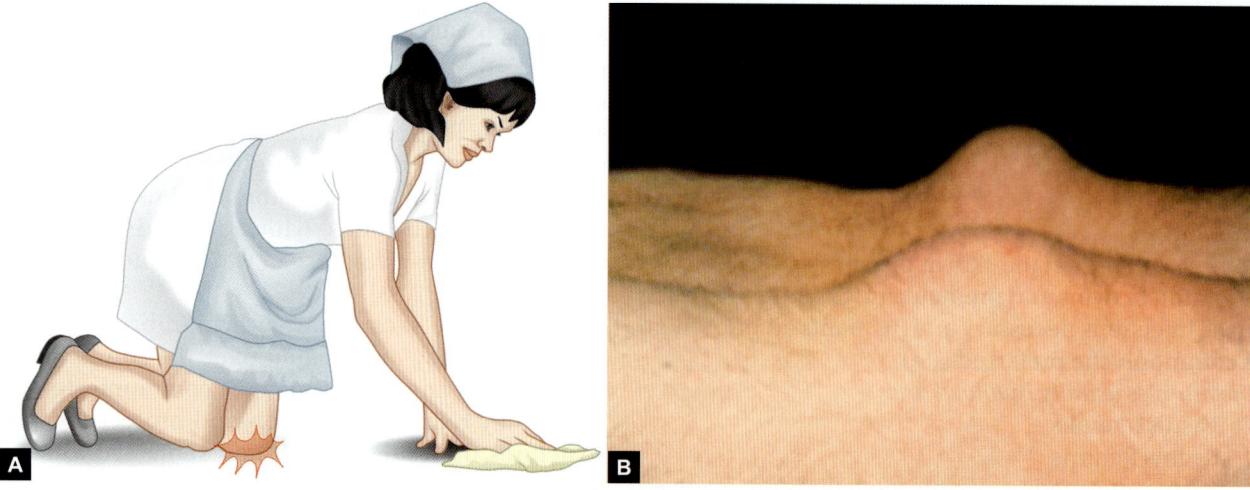

Figs 32.34A and B: (A) This is how a housemaid insults her knee; (B) Clinical photograph of a prepatellar bursitis

Posterior

- Semi-membranosus bursitis.
- Baker's cyst.
- Lymphangiectasia.
- Aneurysm of popliteal artery.
- Neuromyxofibroma.

POPLITEAL CYST (BAKER'S CYST)

Adam first described this in the year 1840 and later by [3]Baker in 1877.

> **What is Baker's Cyst?**
> The exact origin is not known, but it is a distended bursa arising from any one of the structures below:
> - Between hamstrings and collateral ligaments.
> - Between hamstrings and tibial condyles.
> - Each head of gastrocnemius.

Commonly symptoms are seen in bursa of the medial head of gastrocnemius and semi-membranosus bursa.

How is it Produced?

- In 30 percent of cases, herniation of synovial membrane through posterior part of capsule takes place (Fig. 32.36A).
- Escape of fluid through the normal communication of bursa with knee (either semi-membranosus or medial gastrocnemius) is the other mode (Table 32.8).
- Indeterminate site in about 10 percent of cases.

> **What is a Giant Cyst?**
> It is a huge popliteal cyst commonly seen in rheumatoid arthritis.
> *Treatment*
> - One to two days of nonsurgical treatment.
> - Later, arthrography and cyst is excised.
> - Synovectomy is done later to prevent recurrence.

In adults, intra-articular pathology is seen in 50 percent, of these 50 percent are caused by a lesion in the posterior one-third of medial meniscus and the remaining from some other pathology of the knee.

Clinical Features

These are similar to internal derangement of the knee, like pain, stiffness, swelling, giving way, etc. There is a swelling seen in the popliteal fossa and the clinching point in the diagnosis is that the swelling disappears on flexion and appears on extension of the knee (Fig. 32.37).

Duck waddle test is useful to detect pathology in the posterior part of the medial meniscus.

TABLE 32.8: Difference between Baker's cyst in children and adults

Children	Adults
No communication with the joint	Communication is present
Intra-articular pathology are rare	Commonly seen in 50 percent of cases?
No recurrence even with complete removal of the cyst	Recurrence is common
Postoperative immobilization is not required	Postoperative immobilization is required

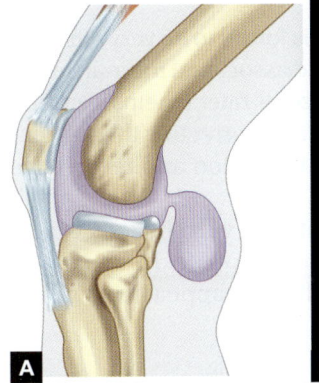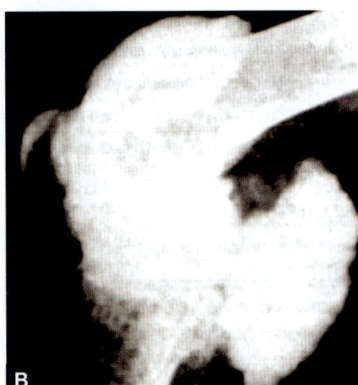

Figs 32.36A and B: (A) Baker's cyst arises from the herniation of the synovial membrane through the capsule; (B) Arthrography showing ruptured popliteal cyst

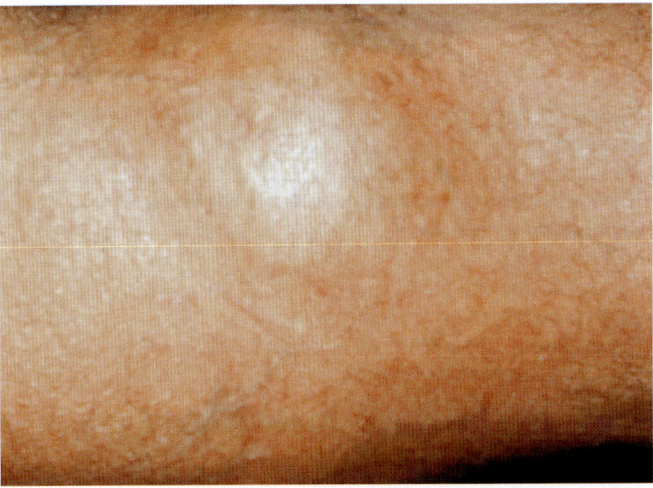

Fig. 32.37: Popliteal cyst (Clinical photo)

Investigations

- *X-ray of the knee joint:* Prominent soft tissue swelling over the popliteal fossa.

---

[3]**William Morrant Baker** (1838-1896) of England. Described Baker's cyst in 1877.

- *Ultrasound:* This is a very effective diagnostic tool with 100 percent sensitivity.
- *MRI:* This is the next best.
- *Arthrography:* This is invasive but very effective (Fig. 32.36B).

Treatment

The treatment of choice is excision of the bursa and closure of the capsular orifice by:
- Scarification of the edges and suture.
- To close the gap by a graft from tendinous part of the gastrocnemius, etc.
- *Arthroscopic treatment:* This is found to be very effective treatment of popliteal cyst and associated intra-articular pathology with 95 percent success rate. It helps in curing the intra-articular pathology and correcting the valvular mechanism responsible for formation and recurrence of the popliteal cyst.

One-third to one-half of patients with Baker's cyst is children. It is rare after seventh year of life. Hence, delay in excision is followed by gradual disappearance of the cyst.

RECURRENT DISLOCATION OF PATELLA

It is a condition caused by recurrent dislocation of patella usually to the lateral side. This is usually preceded by an episode of acute traumatic dislocation of the patella and probably has not healed properly after the initial trauma.

It has to be differentiated from another entity called habitual dislocation of patella in which the patella dislocates with each flexion and extension movements of the knee.

> **The Predisposing Factors Responsible for Recurrent Dislocation of Patella:**
> - Patella Alta
> - Genu valgum
> - Hypoplastic lateral condyle of femur
> - Tight lateral structures of the knee joint
> - Lax medial patellar retinaculum
> - Femoral anteversion
> - External femoral torsion
> - Genu recurvatum
> - Abnormal insertion of vastus medialis
> - Patellar tendon laterally inserted
> - External tibial rotation
> - Hypoplastic patella
> - Atrophy of vastus medialis
> - Hypertrophy of vastus lateralis
> - Generalized joint relaxation

Clinical Features

The patient gives history of diffuse pain in the knee joint, which is worsened by going up and down the stairs or hills. He or she complains of a feeling of insecurity in the knee and may feel the joint is about to give way or the patella is about to go out! On examination in addition to the predisposing factors mentioned above, there may be a mild swelling and crepitus in the joint. The apprehension test is positive. In this test, the patient's knee is held flexed at 30° and an attempt is made to push the patella laterally. In a positive test, the patient complains of pain and resists the attempt. Next, the Q-angle (Fig. 32.38) is determined. If the Q-angle is more than 10°, medial transplantation of the patellar tendon is recommended.

> **Interesting Facts: About Q-Angle**
> Do you know what Malicious Malalignment syndrome is? Well, when all of the following are present together, it constitutes the MMS:
> - Excessive femoral anteversion
> - External tibial torsion
> - Genu valgum
> - Increase in Q-angle.

Radiographs

The following radiographic views are necessary: AP view, lateral view, infrapatellar view and the intercondylar notch view or the tunnel view. In the lateral view, the Blumensaat's line (Fig. 32.39) is drawn which represents the bony roof of the intercondylar notch. Normally, the lower pole of the patella just touches that line. If the patella is above this line, a diagnosis of high riding patella is made.

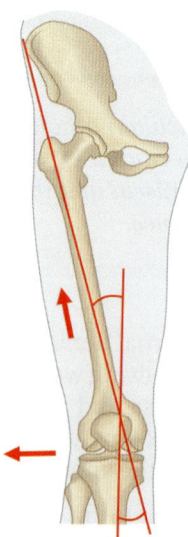

Fig. 32.38: Showing Q-angle

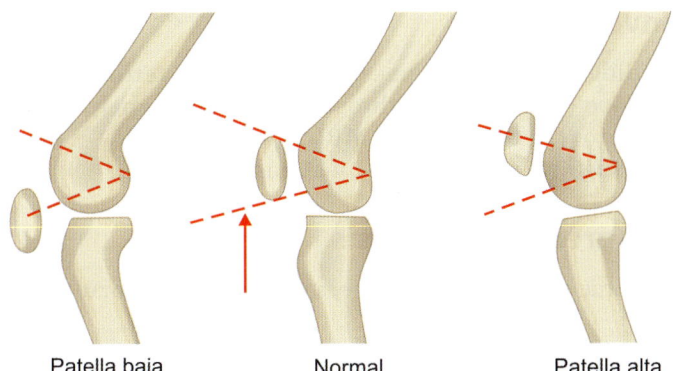

Fig. 32.39: Showing the Blumensaat's line

Again, in the lateral view, the ratio between the length of the patella and the length of the patellar tendon is determined. If it is more than one, it suggests patella Alta. This is also known as Insaal's line.

Treatment

A Nonsurgical or Conservative Measure

This consists of quadriceps exercises, supportive elastocrepe bandages, nonsteroidal anti-inflammatory drugs (NSAIDs), etc. and is found to be successful in only 50 percent of the cases.

Surgical Methods (Fig. 32.40)

These are successful in the remaining cases and can be conveniently grouped under four methods (Table 32.9):
- Proximal realignment of structures like the capsule of the knee, quadriceps, etc. (e.g. Campbell's operation).
- Distal realignment of structures like patellar tendon, tibial tuberosity, etc. (e.g. Roux-Goldthwait's operation).
- Both proximal and distal realignment of structures around the knee.
- Patellectomy and realignment of extensor mechanism, e.g. West and Soto-Hall.

Treatment of Habitual Dislocation

This is essentially surgical and consists of the release of tight lateral structures and repairs of lax medial structures.

CHONDROMALACIA PATELLA

It is defined as a blistering, cystic change of the patellar cartilage and it usually affects the medial facet of the patella. This condition is commonly associated with vastus medialis tendinitis.

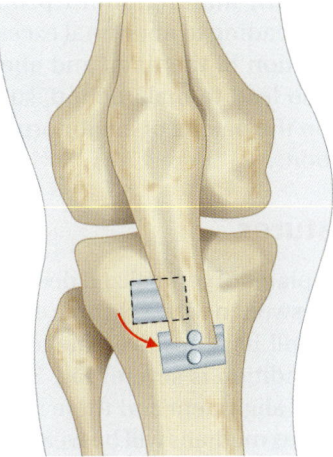

Fig. 32.40: Surgical method of treating recurrent dislocation of patella (Houser's method)

TABLE 32.9: A brief account of the surgical procedures	
Surgery	what is done?
Campbell's	Proximal to the knee, the capsule is stripped and carried from medial to the lateral side
Roux-Goldthwait's procedure	Here lateral structures of the knee are released and the patellar tendon is split and the lateral half is transferred medially
Galeazzi's procedure	Here the semitendinosus tendon is tenodesed to patella
Houser's procedure (Fig. 32.27)	Here the tibial tuberosity is shifted down and medial
Elmslie-Trillat Procedure	Here release of lateral knee structures, plication of medial structures and medial transfer of tibial tuberosity is done
Hughston's procedure	It is a combination of the above procedures
West and Soto-Hall procedure	This includes patellectomy and is done as a last resort

It is caused by the combination of several factors, which ultimately push the patella out of its groove on the femur. It is attributed to a decrease in sulfated mucopolysaccharide in the ground substance.

> **Did You Know?**
> Aleman coined the term 'chondromalacia patella' in 1928.

Factors

The following features may give rise to chondromalacia patellae.

Weakness of the vastus medialis muscle, high Q-angle that causes vastus imbalance and over action of the lateral vasti, malalignment produced by foot pathomechanics leading to abnormal excessive pronation and internal rotation of the tibia, and aberrations of the anatomy can also lead to malfunction, such as irregular-shaped facets on the patella or an abnormally high vastus medialis insertion.

Clinical Features

The patient complains of generalized deep pain in the knee. The knee may be swollen with a chronic effusion of synovial fluid and there will be a positive patellofemoral grinding test when the condition is severe (Fig. 32.41). The patella will appear out of alignment and there may well be a high Q-angle. The vastus medialis will be weak, radiographs will occasionally show spurring and the patient will be unable to do squats. In this condition, the typical complaint is that of pain in the knees after prolonged sitting as in watching a movie or while traveling.

> **Interesting Facts: About Movie Sign**
> If your knees play a spoilsport while you are engrossed watching a movie, watch out, you may be suffering from the irksome chondromalacia patellae! (Fig. 32.42)

Investigations

Radiographs of the knee shows irregular retro-patellar surface (Fig. 32.43). Arthroscopy is an extremely useful diagnostic technique. MRI is another very useful investigative option (Figs 32.44A and B).

Differential Diagnosis

Chronic synovitis of the knee, sprain of the retinacula, etc.

Treatment

Treatment consists of ice and ultrasound massage of the painful area, realignment of the mal-tracking of the patella by orthotic therapy and arthroscopic shaving of the retropatellar surface gives excellent results.

LOOSE BODIES IN THE KNEE (Joint Mice)

Important causes of loose bodies in the knee are:

Non-traumatic
- TB arthritis.
- Rheumatoid arthritis.

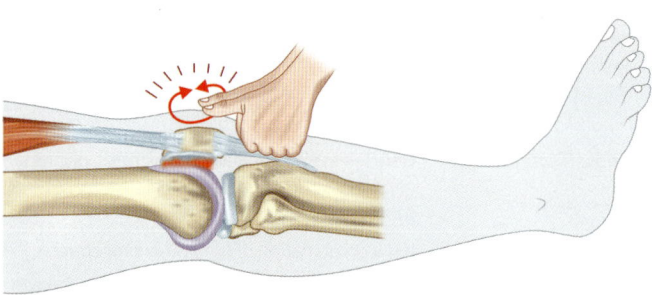

Fig. 32.41: Method of performing grinding test in chondromalacia patella

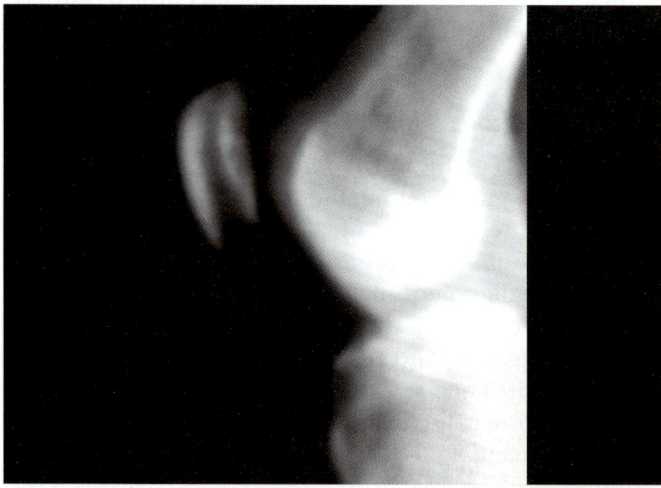

Fig. 32.43: Radiograph showing chondromalacia

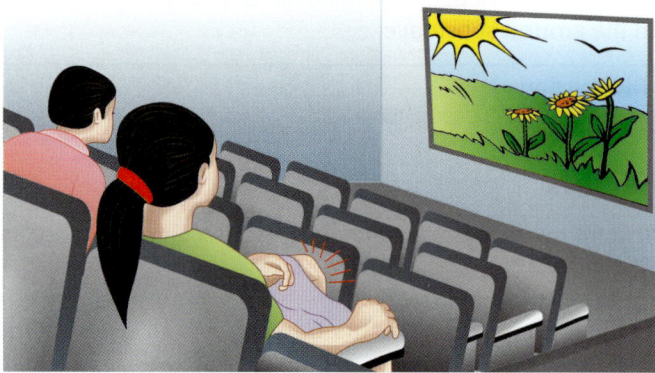

Fig. 32.42: Movie sign, a hallmark of chondromalacia

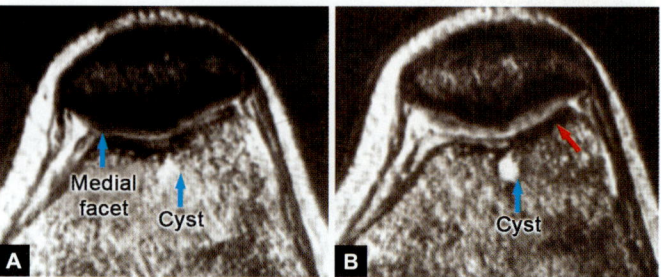

Figs 32.44A and B: MRI showing chondromalacia

- Osteoarthritis.
- Osteochondritis dissecans.
- Synovial chondromatosis.
- Hemarthrosis.
- Hemophilia.

Traumatic
- Intra-articular fracture.
- Meniscal injuries.
- Organized hemarthrosis.
- Detached articular cartilages.
- Foreign bodies.

Clinical Features

- A sense of giving way.
- A feeling of something is moving within the joint.
- Pain and effusion within the knee.
- Locking episodes.

Investigations

This consists of X-ray, diagnostic arthroscopy, MRI, etc. X-ray and MRI showing loose bodies in the knee (Figs 32.48 and 32.49).

Treatment

Arthroscopic removal of the loose bodies is the treatment method of choice and is considered the Gold Standard (Fig. 32.45).

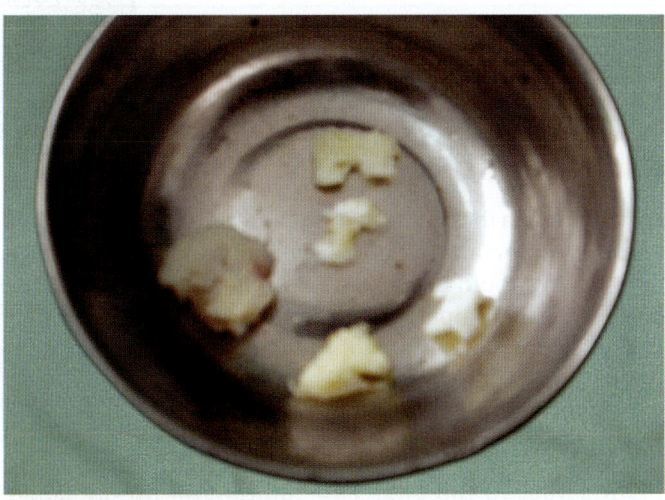

Fig. 32.45: Loose bodies removed through arthroscopy

LESSER-KNOWN BUT IMPORTANT REGIONAL CONDITIONS OF THE KNEE

JUMPER'S KNEE

This is a patellar tendonitis involving the lower pole of the patella due to overuse of the patellofemoral extensor mechanism. Superior pole of the patella and the site of the insertion at the tibia tubercle can also be rarely involved.

Clinical Features

The presentation is very typical and consists of pain at the onset of activity; this reduces during activity and recurs at the completion of the activity.

Treatment

Some of the recommended measures are:
- Rest to the knee.
- RICE regimen, NSAIDs and physiotherapy helps.
- *Exercises*: Isometric quadriceps exercises, inferior patellar glides, isotonic quadriceps exercises, hamstring stretching, and eccentric quadriceps stretching are some of the recommended exercise measures.
- Proper orthotic shoes and orthotics to correct hyperpronation.

OSGOOD-SCHLATTER DISEASE

This is an apophysitis of the insertion of the tibial tubercle leading to tendinitis initially and avulsion later.

Clinical Features

There is a localized tenderness over the tibial tubercle, quadriceps is weak and hence the knee extension is poor and the patella rides higher.

Radiograph

Plain X-ray of the knee especially the lateral view helps in making the diagnosis (Fig. 32.46).

Treatment

It is the same as for jumper's knee. In recalcitrant cases, local steroid injections may help.

SINDING-LARSEN-JOHANSSON SYNDROME

This is an apophysitis of the patellar tendon at the insertion of the patellar tendon into the distal pole of the patella.

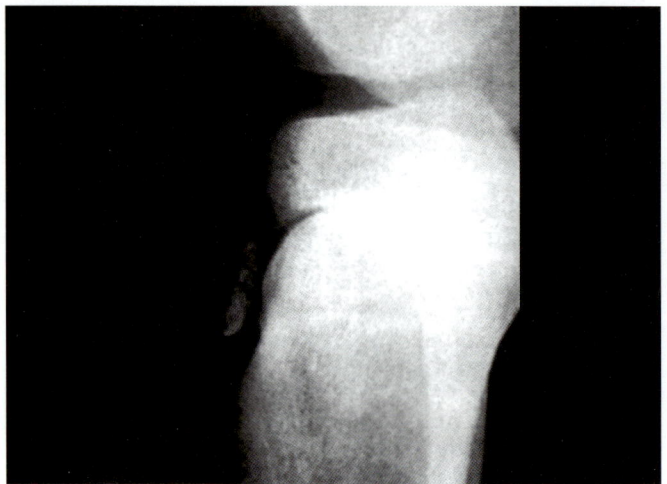

Fig. 32.46: Radiograph showing Osgood's disease

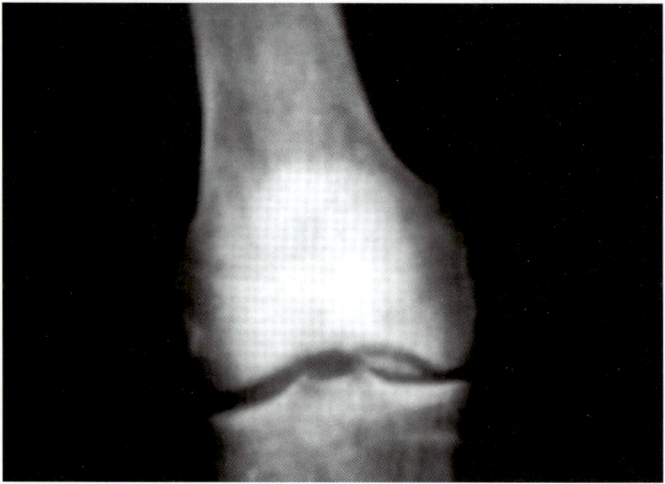

Fig. 32.47: Radiograph showing osteochondritis dissecans

ILIOTIBIAL BAND (ITB) SYNDROME

You already know that ITB is a tendinous and fascial continuation of the tensor fascia latae. It is often inflamed in over-the-hill runner due to repeated friction. Later, knee pain, tenderness over the ITB band and positive Ober's test all help to clinch the diagnosis.

PLICA SYNDROME

This is a fold of synovium present in the suprapatellar, infrapatellar, and mediopatellar aspects of the knee. It could be injured during knee trauma, ACL tear, and hemarthrosis leading to knee pain. However, it is unclear whether it is the cause or sequel of other knee pathologies mentioned above.

OSTEOCHONDRITIS DISSECANS

In this condition, avascular necrosis occurs in an area of subchondral bone followed usually by degenerative changes in the overlying cartilage. Though it can occur in any joint, it is most commonly seen in the knee joint. This avascular bone undergoes necrosis, gets detached, and forms a loose body. In fact, this is the most common cause for loose bodies within the knee (see box) (Fig. 32.47).

> **'Loose' Facts: Do You Know the Sources of Loose Bodies within the Knee?**
> - Osteochondritis dissecans—50 percent.
> - Fractured articular surfaces—11 percent.
> - Synovial chondromatosis—2 percent.
> - Source unknown in 33 percent.
> - Osteophytes, damaged menisci, etc. in a few cases.

Causes

Many causes are cited and are controversial:
- Exogenous trauma.
- Endogenous trauma.
- Ischemia.
- Abnormal ossification within the epiphysis.
- Genetics.
- Combination of these.

Common site: Lateral aspect of the medial femoral condyle near the attachment of posterior cruciate ligament.

Age groups
- In young patients before epiphyseal closure. Treatment outcome is good.
- In adults, here treatment outcome is poor.

> **Note:**
> It is rare in patients <10 years and older >50 years of age.

Sex: Male to female ratio is 2 : 1.

Clinical Features

It is different in the two age groups and consists of vague pain and discomfort in the knee, swelling, catching, popping, and locking could occur. After complete separation, loose bodies can be palpated. Tenderness can be elicited over the anteromedial surface of the femoral condyle by deep palpation after flexing the knee.

Investigations

Plain X-rays of the knee (AP, lateral and tunnel view), arthrogram, arthroscopy, bone scan, MRI, etc. are some of the important investigation tools (Fig. 32.48). Plain X-ray also helps to detect the loose bodies of the knee joints (Fig. 32.49).

Treatment Methods

Conservative

This depends on the age of the patient and degree of involvement. Treatment method varies from conservative in children to operative in adults.

Surgery

The operative methods are arthroscopic excision, curettage, pinning, debridement, grafting, etc. The outcome of the treatment is good in children and is not so good in adults.

HOFFA'S SYNDROME (Syn: Fat Pad Syndrome)

It is affection of the infra-patellar fat pad due to direct trauma to the anterior knee. It could also be due to sudden entrapment following forced knee extension.

Clinical Features

The patient complains of pain and swelling of the infra-patellar fat pad. Tenderness can be elicited on either side of the patellar tendon and at the anteromedial and anterolateral joint lines.

Investigations

Plain X-ray and ultrasonogram helps to make the diagnosis.

Treatment

This is essentially conservative and consists of the following measures:
- Protection of the anterior knee.
- Physiotherapy measures: TENS, ultrasound, SWD, etc. Heat therapy helps.
- Quadriceps strengthening exercises is helpful.

INFANTILE QUADRICEPS CONTRACTURE

Introduction

Knee joints have always been a marvel of engineering. Come to think of it everyday from the moment we get up till we retire to bed we are on our knees. For we Indians high flexion activities like squatting is a way of life. If for some reasons muscles that bring about flexion and extension of the knees develop contractures severe disability develops. A straight and stiff knee due to quadriceps contracture is a disabled knee. Mercifully extension contractures are less than flexion contracture. Contracture in a muscle could be due to fibrosis or scarring that could cause shortness of the muscle with respect to bone and joints. This leads to limitation of joint movements and fixed deformities.

Causes

Quadriceps contracture could develop due to congenital or acquired causes. It is the latter that is more common. Now let us explore the causes:

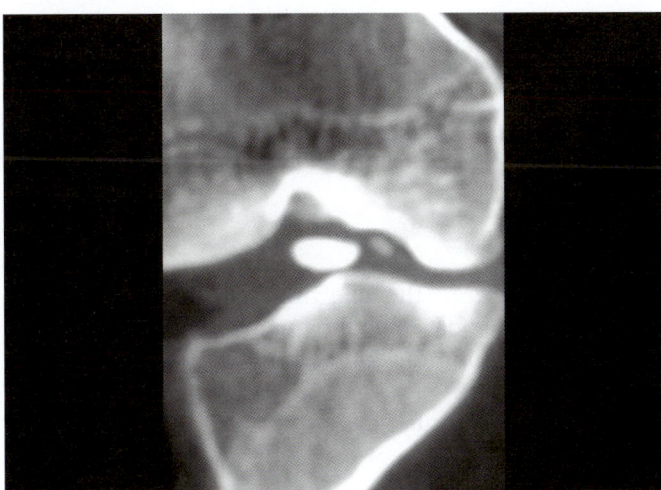

Fig. 32.48: MRI of the knee showing osteochondritis dissecans with loose bodies

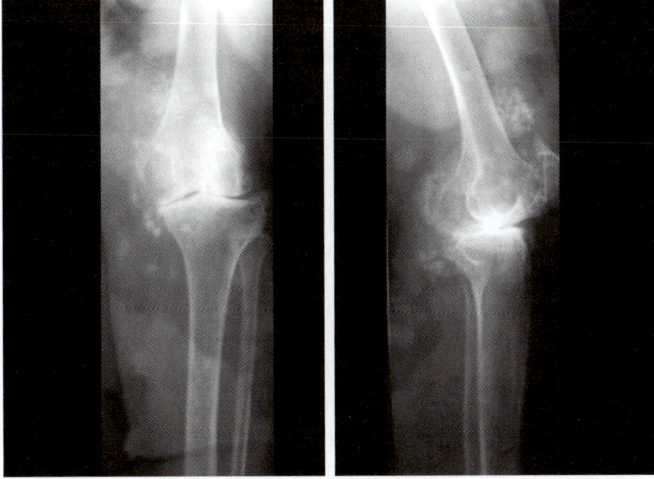

Fig. 32.49: Radiograph showing loose bodies in the knee

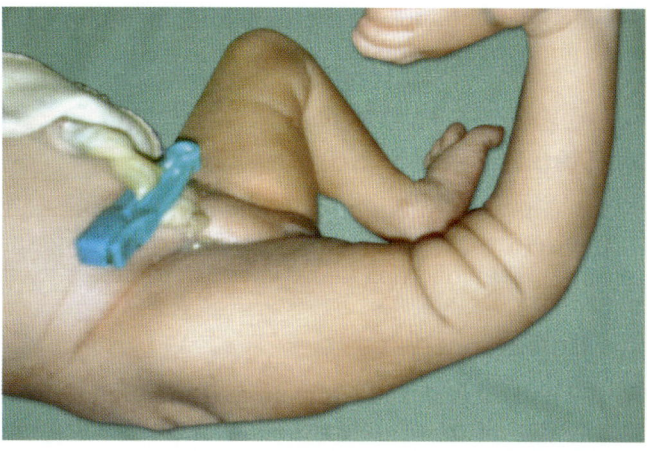 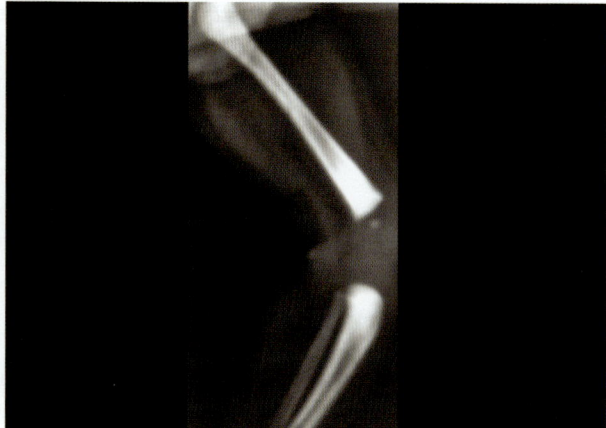

Fig. 32.50: Clinical photo and X-ray of congenital genu recurvatum

Congenital

- Arthrogryposis multiplex congenita.
- Congenital genu recurvatum (Fig. 32.50).
- Spina bifida.

Acquired

- Infants: Repeated injections into the quadriceps.
- Fracture of the femur with quadriceps adherent to the callus.
- Prolonged immobilization of the knee in a plaster cast following an injury to the lower limb.
- Injections and chronic osteomyelitis of the femur.
- Injury to the quadriceps muscles.

Post-injection Quadriceps Contractures

This is the most common variety of acquired quadriceps contracture.

Historical Facts of Interest

- Hinkwosky first reported it in 1961 in 12 children.
- Fairbank and Brett first said it could be congenital.
- Gunn in 1964 first established a link between repeated intramuscular injection into the thigh and quadriceps contracture.

Important Past Clinical History

- This is usually always a history of severe infections in infancy like severe bronchopneumonia, septicemia, acute gastroenteritis, CHD, neonatal jaundice, etc. Thus, a careful evaluation of the past history is of extreme importance.
- For the above infections, there is history of repeated intramuscular injections into the thigh.
- Over the formative years, the child slowly loses its ability to flex the knees.

> **Incriminating Infamous Injections**
> - Tetanus toxoid (Most common in Japan).
> - Antibiotics.
> - Vitamin K.
> - Ascorbic acid.

Predisposing factors: The following factors contribute to the development of post-injection quadriceps contractures:
- Low socioeconomic conditions.
- Poor nutrition.
- Prolonged recumbency.

Sites of Contractures

- Vastus intermedius (due to the poor blood supply among the quadriceps groups).
- Vastus lateralis.
- Tendinous band along the anteromedial border of the vastus lateralis.
- Rectus femoris especially in Japan where injection are given in front of the thigh.

Pathomechanics

Due to the sheer bulk of the medications injected into the less bulky quadriceps muscle of an infant and due to the toxicity of the drugs, the capillaries and muscle bundles are compressed leading to muscle necrosis and subsequent fibrosis. The muscle tends to develop as the child grows older and progressive loss of flexion is seen.

The following structures are involved according of Nicoll:
- Fibrosis of vastus intermedius lies down the rectus femoris to the femur proximally and in the suprapatellar pouch.

- Adhesions between the patella and the femoral condyle.
- Lateral expansions of the vasti fibrosed, shortened and adhered to the femoral condyle.
- There could be actual shortening of the rectus femoris muscle.

Clinical Features

- History of repeated intramuscular injection into the thigh.
- History of previous some diseases in the infancy.
- At birth both the knees appear normal.
- Gradual limitation of the flexion, both active and passive, is then noticed by the parents.
- In Asian countries, parents first become concerned when their child fails to squat.
- A child walks with a straight knee gait.

Clinical Signs

Examination of the child should be carried out from the front, back, and sides.

From the Front

- Wasting of the front of the thigh.
- Absence of skin creases over the knee.
- Small patella.
- High riding patella.
- Forward inclination of the pelvis.
- Injection scars are visible in the mid-thigh. These become prominent on flexion of the knee.
- White patches and dimpling of the skin are due to subcutaneous atrophy.
- Genu recurvatum may be seen with growth and subluxation could result.
- Habitual dislocation is usually seen.
- In a dislocated position of the patella, knee flexion is full.

From the Sides

- Exaggerated lumbar lordosis.
- Prominent abdomen.
- Forward inclination of the pelvis.

Clinical Tests

In the Supine Position

- *Thomson's test:* It is frequently positive (Figs 32.51A and B).
- *Ely's test:* The knee is slowly flexed in a supine position. It does up to a point and later the hip on the same side will automatically flex and is seen to rise up from the bed indicating that the rectus on that side is tight.
- Patella is firmly held in the midline and the knee is flexed. Not more than 30 degrees of flexion is possible. Further flexion is possible on allowing the patella to dislocate laterally.

In the Prone Position

Reverse Ely's test: The trunk and the thigh are in contact with the table and the knees are hanging on the edge (Fig. 32.52). As the knee is flexed, lordosis slowly increases.

In the lateral position: Ober's test. This is usually positive.

Radiographs

The knee is normal in early stages. In the later stages, the following changes may be seen (Fig. 32.53).
- Displacement of patella.
- High riding patella.
- Hypoplastic patella.
- Flattening of the femoral condyles.
- Genu recurvatum.
- Anterior dislocation of the tibia.
- Degenerative changes seen in the joint late.

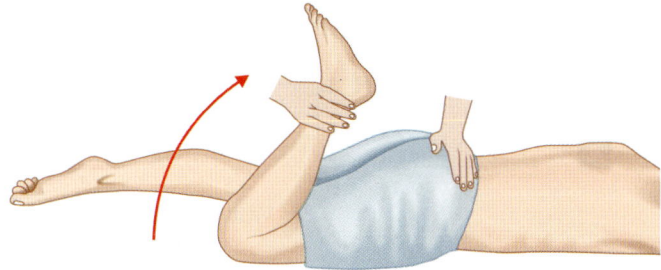

Fig. 32.52: Method of performing the Reverse Ely's test

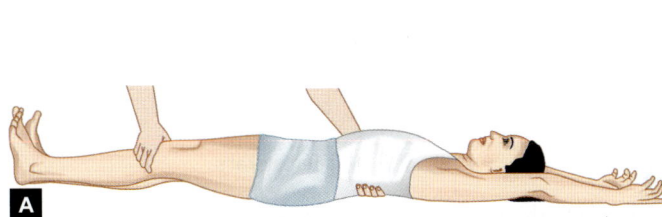

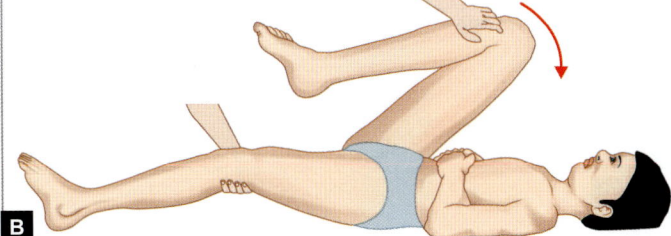

Figs 32.51A and B: Method of performing the Thomas test

Treatment

Conservative Methods

Physiotherapy and stretching has very little in the management of established quadriceps contracture and is mentioned here only for completion.

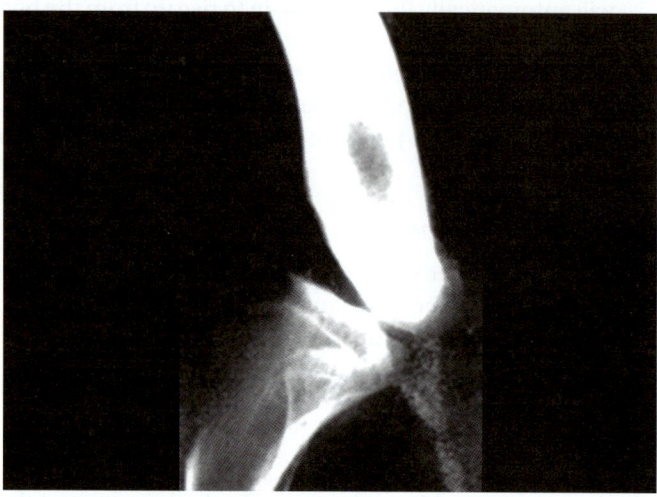

Fig. 32.53: Radiographic changes in infantile quadriceps contracture
Source: Sengupta, Textbook of Orthopedics, GS Kulkarni, 1st edition.

Surgery

This is the treatment of choice. Surgical lengthening of the quadriceps can be done either proximally or distally.

Surgical Methods

Proximal release:

This is indicated during the early stages of contractures when there are no significant changes seen in the joint (Figs 32.54A to D), Sengupta recommends proximal release.
- This helps to eliminate extensor lag and prevent hemarthrosis of the knee.
- Here the affected muscle is in the upper lateral part of the thigh involving mostly the vastus lateralis and intermedius muscles.

Procedure

- A curved incision is taken along the base of the greater trochanter and down the mid-thigh laterally. The length of the incision depends upon the degree of contractures.
- The contracted iliotibial tract and the tendon of fascia lata are transversally cut.
- Now the vastus lateralis is released along the origin from the greater trochanter, trochanteric line, and intermuscular septum.

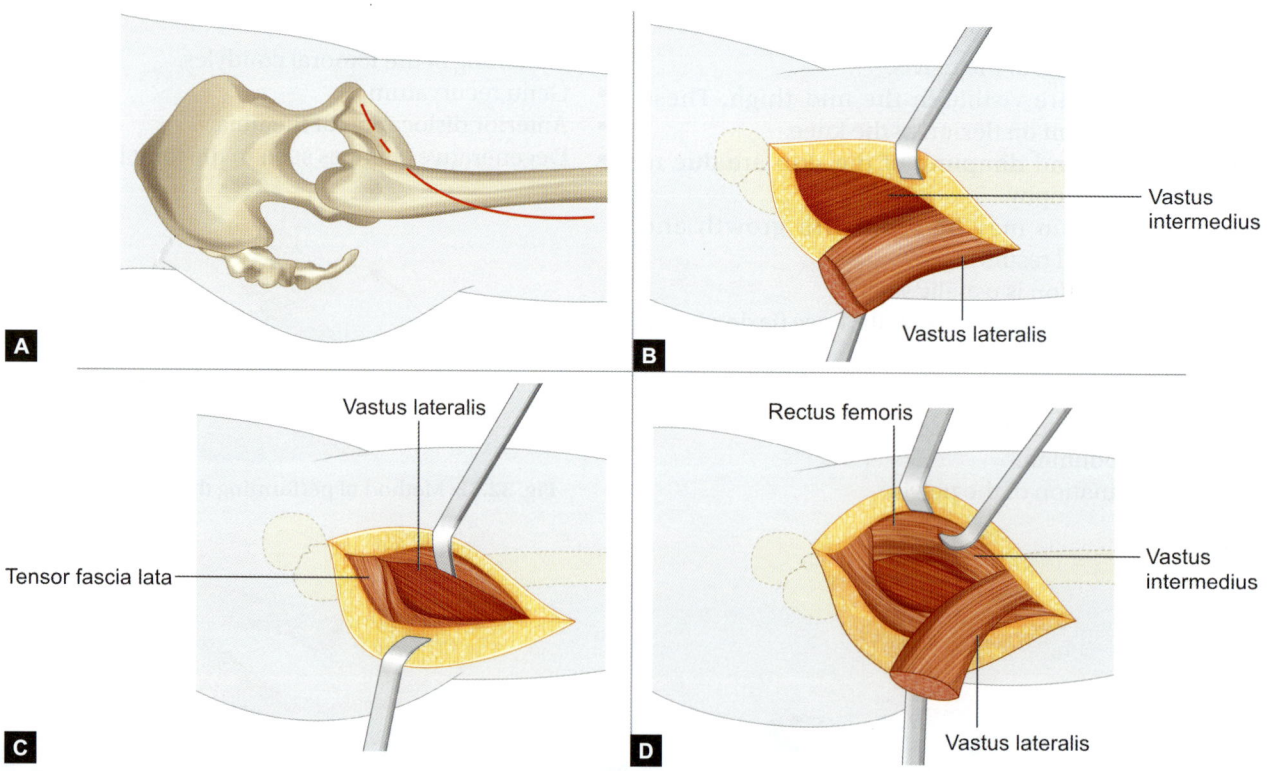

Figs 32.54A to D: Surgical technique of proximal quadriceps contracture release
Source: Sengupta, Textbook of Orthopedics, GS Kulkarni, 1st edition.

- The intermedius is released next.
- The knee is gradually bent and the remaining adhesion is now released.
- And finally if the rectus femoris is contracted, it is released.
- Complete flexion of the knee should now be possible.

Postoperative Protocol

- The knee is maintained in full knee flexion for 4 weeks in a plaster slab.
- Quadriceps exercises are then begun.
- After 3–4 weeks, child is allowed to walk.
- After 12–14 weeks, it can be allowed to get up from the squatting position.
- Knee stretching exercises should be continued throughout the growth period.

Distal Release: Thompson's Quadriceps Plasty

This is the most commonly done procedure in India. The steps of the procedure are as follows:

- Antero-lateral incision in the distal third of the thigh and the knee.
- Vasti is exposed and separated from the recti and also on the either side of the patella and partially excised.
- Remaining adhesions are slowly released by gradually bending the knee.
- If the rectus muscle is contracted-Y plasty is done.

Disadvantages

- Knee hemarthrosis.
- Extensor lag (Fig. 32.55).

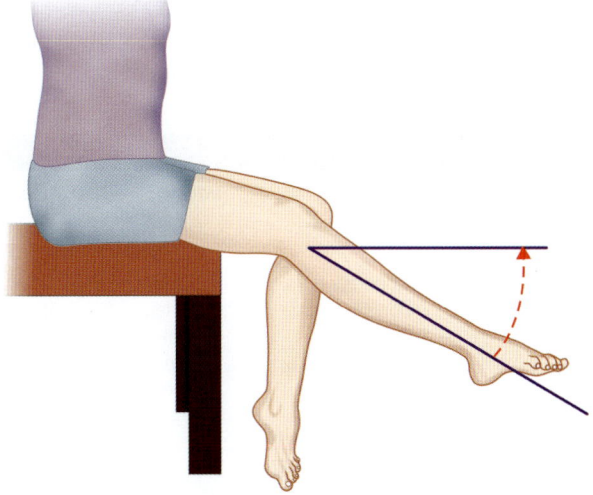

Fig. 32.55: Extensor lag

Postoperative Rehabilitation

- The leg is kept in plaster cast in a flexion of 70–90 degrees for 2–4 weeks.
- Later active and passive range of movements' exercises is begun.
- Knee stretching exercises are carried out for a prolonged period.

Other Procedures

- If genu recurvatum has developed, supracondylar femoral osteotomy can be done.
- In severe cases, knee arthrodesis is indicated.
- If only rectus femoris in involved (knee movement is full with the hip flexed but restricted when hip is extended). Through a longitudinal skin incision, the fibrotic rectus femoris are cut transversely (Sasaki et al.).
- In recurrent dislocation of patella, reefing of the medial capsule of the knee may need to be done in addition to the above procedure. This surgery is performed after the child is 6 years of age. If recurrence still continues, gracilis tendon may be transferred to the superomedial aspect of the patella.

Prognostic Factors

Poor prognosis is indicated by:
- Genu recurvatum.
- Elderly patient.
- Post-polio quadriceps.

Results

Criteria: Active and passive extension of the knees.

Grading

- *Good:* 90–135 degrees.
- *Fair:* 45–90 degrees plus extension lag present.
- *Poor:* More extension lag + decrease power in the quadriceps.

REGIONAL DISORDERS OF THE FOOT

ARCHES OF THE FOOT

The tarsal and metatarsal bones of the foot are bound by ligaments and arranged in the form of two arches, longitudinal and transverse. Integrity of these arches is maintained by:
- Shape of the bones.
- Tension of the ligaments and plantar aponeurosis.

- Muscular action of both short and long muscles through bracing action of their tendons.

Longitudinal Arch

Longitudinal arch is of greater height and has a wider span along the medial side of the foot than the lateral. It has two pillars, anterior and posterior. The posterior pillar is short and solid and is formed by calcaneus alone. Rest of the tarsal bones and metatarsal form the anterior pillar. The anterior pillar has two columns, medial and lateral. Head of the talus forms the keystone of the summit and is situated between the deep socket formed by anterior end of calcaneum and navicular and is supported by the plantar calcaneonavicular ligament called the spring ligament.

All other ligaments on the plantar surface of the bones of foot play a part in maintaining the arches of the foot and they are assisted by extensive insertion of tibialis posterior and peroneus longus and especially by the plantar aponeurosis, which joins the two ends of the arch and acts as a "tie beam" (Fig. 32.56A).

Transverse Arch

Transverse arches of the foot lie along the line of tarso-metatarsal articulations. Inferior surfaces of the cuneiforms and metatarsal are narrow transversely and are held tightly together by plantar and interosseous ligaments and by tendons of peroneus longus. This arrangement gives the plantar surface in this region a much smaller transverse radius of curvature than the dorsal surface, thus, forming a well-defined transverse arch (Fig. 32.56B).

Two conditions of clinical importance discussed in this chapter relates one to exaggerated longitudinal arch called the pes cavus and the other to loss of medial longitudinal arch called the pes planus (Fig. 32.60).

PES CAVUS

Pes cavus is a deformity characterized by an excessively high longitudinal arch that results from an equinus position of the forefoot in relation to the hind foot (Fig. 32.57B).

In this condition, finger can be slipped under the navicular bone and it penetrates a distance of greater than 2 cm from the vertical edge of the foot.

Pathogenesis

- Weakness of intrinsic muscles of the foot.
- Over activity of the intrinsic.
- Muscle imbalance:
  – Weak anterior tibial muscle and normal peroneus muscle.
  – Weakness of the calf muscles.

Pathologic Anatomy

This consists of dropping of the foot, contractures of the plantar fascia, varus of the heel and clawing of the toes.

Classification

This is depicted detail in Table 32.10.

Clinical Features

This consists of high medial longitudinal arch (Fig. 32.58), first metatarsal drop, and pronation, tight plantar fascia, cock-up deformities of all the toes at the MTP joints, varus heel, and clawing (Fig. 32.59) of the toes (late feature).

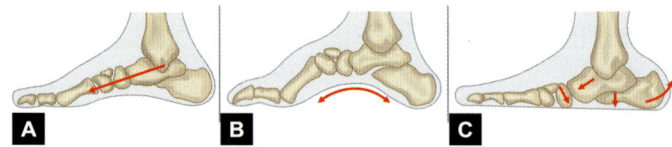

Figs 32.57A to C: Foot arch deformities: (A) Normal foot; (B) High-arched foot; (C) Flatfoot

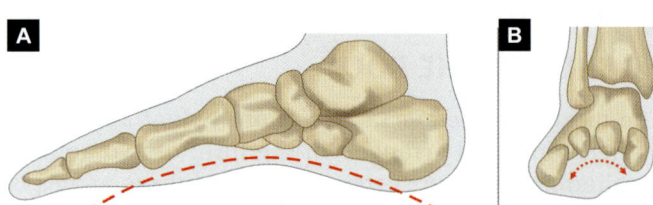

Figs 32.56A and B: Arches of the foot: (A) Longitudinal; (B) Transverse

TABLE 32.10: Classification of pes cavus

Idiopathic	Secondary	Trauma	Others
• Commonest type (80%) • Develops after 3 years of age • Male: Female 1 :1 • May be seen in spina bifida	• Spinocerebellar hereditary degeneration • Freidreich's ataxia • Poliomyelitis • Diseases of conus medullaris • Spina bifida • Cerebral palsy • Progressive peroneal palsy	• Direct trauma to the foot or the leg • Compartmental syndromes	• Myopathies • CTEV • Plantar fibromatosis

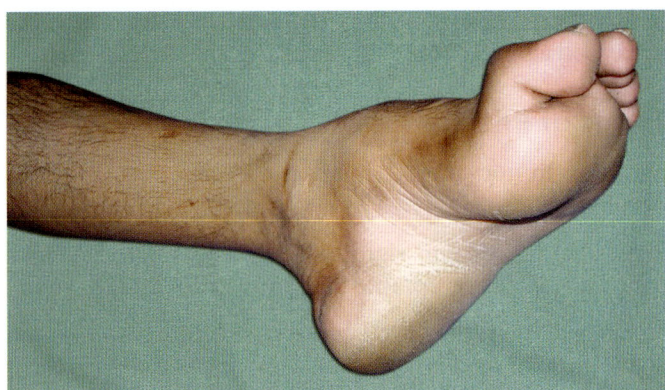

Fig. 32.58: Pes cavus (Clinical photo)

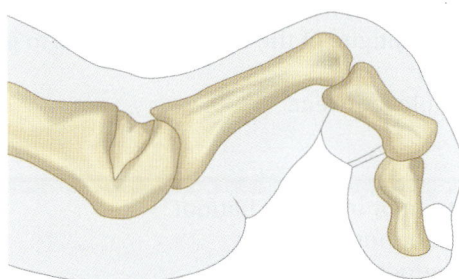

Fig. 32.59: Claw toes (Extension of the first phalanx and plantar flexion of second and third)

Radiographs

AP view

Talocalcaneal angle is decreased.

Lateral View

Angle between two lines, one through the first metatarsal and another through the talus or calcaneus is decreased.

Treatment

Correction of the primary deformity, which is equines, and probation of the foot is done first. Secondary deformities like contracted plantar fascia, clawed toes and virus of the heels are corrected next.

Early Stages

Require conservative treatment. Consisting of painkiller, physiotherapy exercise, footwear modifications, etc.

Late Stages

Surgery is required, soft tissue release in children, bony surgeries in adults. Table 32.11 for degree of claw toes corresponding deformities and for their respective treatment.

TABLE 32.11: Degrees of pes cavus, their corresponding deformities, and treatment

Degree	Deformities	Treatment
First	• Foot is normal • Deformity appears when foot is relaxed • Flexible and corrected by pushing I MT bone manually up	• Daily manipulations • Exercises • Anterior arch bar • Night splint
Second	• Equinus and pronation of I MT is fixed • Clawing of large toe • Early contractures of the plantar fascia	• Steindler's operation • Jones transfer • EHL is transferred to the neck of I MT • Arthrodesis in adults
Third	• All five metatarsals are in equinus • Calcaneus begins to invert • No bony deformities	• Extensor shift operation • Dwyer's osteotomy in children
Fourth	• All the components of deformities become pronounced and resist passive correction • Some midtarsal movements are preserved	• Japa's V-shaped osteotomy • Anterior tarsal wedge osteotomy
Fifth	• Extreme degree of cavus foot • All components are fixed • Toes are dislocated dorsally • Plantar fascia is markedly contracted	• Bone wedge corrections of hind foot and midfoot and triple arthrodesis

Abbreviations: MT, Metatarsal; EHL, extensor hallucis longus.

PES PLANUS

Definition

Pes planus (flatfoot); (Fig. 32.60B) refers to loss of medial-longitudinal arch of the foot (see Fig. 32.57C).

Associated Abnormalities

- Heel valgus.
- Mild subluxation of the subtalar joint.
- Eversion of the calcaneus at the subtalar joint.
- Lateral angulations at the metatarsal joint.
- Supination of the forefoot.
- Shortened tendo calcaneus.

Types

Flatfoot is essentially congenital and acquired and has been depicted in Table 32.12.

Clinical Features

Medial arch is obliterated, navicular bone is prominent, and fingers cannot be inserted under the arch and sole of the foot and area of weight-bearing increases and may show increased callosity (Fig. 32.61).

Types of Pes Planus

Flexible: On non-weight bearing, normal appearing arch develops.

Rigid: Could be semi rigid or fixed. During non-weight bearing, normal acceptable medial arch does not develop.

Static type: This is the most common type; the reasons could be faulty postural activity of muscles, equinus deformity of the foot, and varus deformity of the foot.

Predisposing factors
- General muscle hypotonia.
- Excessive fatigue of the foot muscles due to prolonged standing.
- Unsuitable footwear.

Types
- Foot strain or incipient flatfoot.
- Mobile flatfoot.
- Rigid flatfoot.

Peroneal or spasmodic flatfoot: It is common in young adolescents. Patient complains of acute onset of pain, the tightness, spasm of peroneal muscles, and eversion of foot. It is commonly associated with calcaneonavicular bar. It can also be associated with conditions like tuberculosis, rheumatoid arthritis, which causes spasm due to reflex muscle reaction.

Radiograph

Consisting of the routine AP, lateral and oblique views helps to assess the extent of the disease and helps plan the treatment (Fig. 32.62).

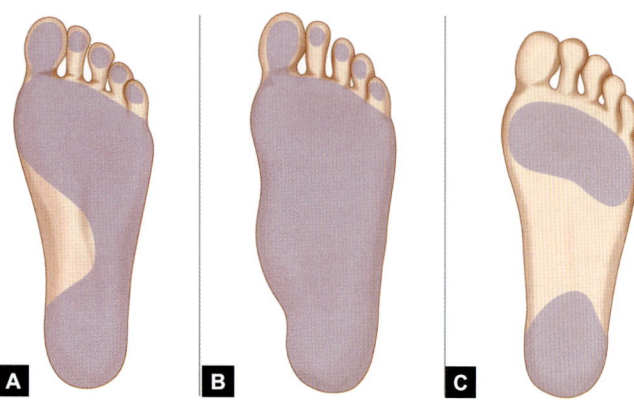

Figs 32.60A to C: Podoscopic appearance of: (A) Normal foot; (B) Flatfoot; (C) Pes cavus

TABLE 32.12: Varieties of pes planus	
Congenital causes	*Acquired causes and varieties*
• Calcaneovalgus foot	• Traumatic flat foot (fracture calcaneus; traumatic Potts' fracture)
• Vertical talus deformity	• Relaxed or static flatfoot (commonest)
• Talocalcaneal bar	• Rigid flatfoot, fibrous or bony ankylosis from any cause
• Congenital ligament laxity	• Spasmodic flatfoot due to spasmodic contraction of the peroneal muscles

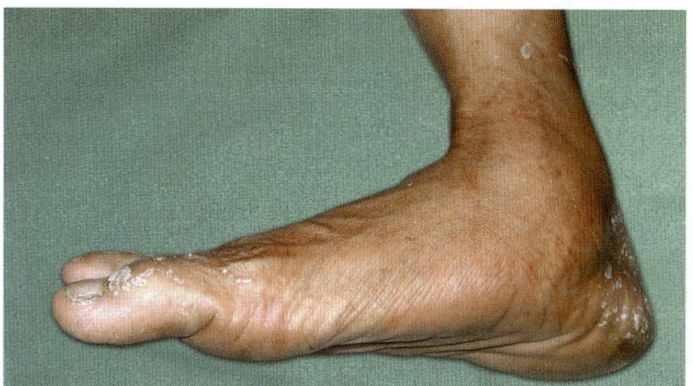
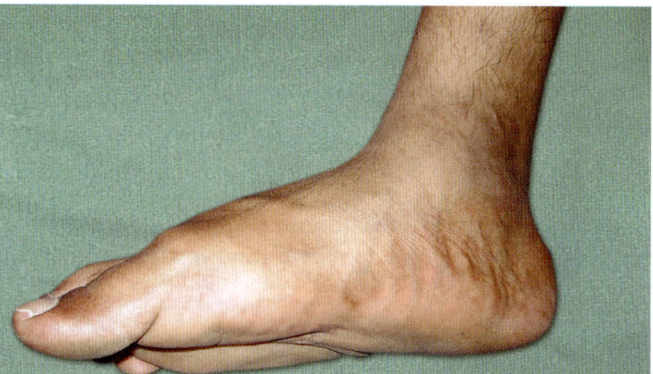

Fig. 32.61: Clinical photo showing flat foot

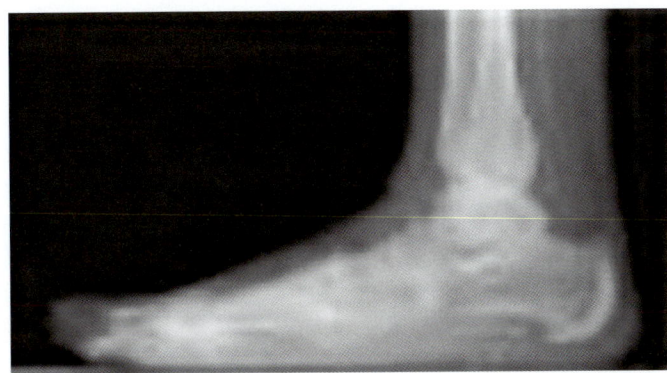

Fig. 32.62: Radiograph showing pes planus

Treatment Plan

Fifteen to twenty percent adults have flexible pes planus, which are asymptomatic.

Up to 3 years, orthopedic shoes with Thomas heels, medial heel wedges and navicular pads.

Between 3 and 9 years of age
- *Asymptomatic* cases need parent education
- Symptomatic cases require:
  – Orthopedic shoes for mild cases
  – Custom prosthesis for severe cases.

10–14 years age group
- *Asymptomatic* cases require no treatment.
- *Symptomatic* cases require molded orthoses worn in a sturdy shoe.

Surgical Correction

Principles
- This is done to relieve the disabling pain after exhausting every means of conservative management and not for cosmetics alone.
- The patient should accept loss of inversion and eversion.
- Subtalar joint should be included for arthrodesis of the painful flatfoot.

Techniques
- Miller's flatfoot procedure.
- Modified Hoke-Miller's flatfoot procedure.
- Durban's flatfoot plasty.
- Triple arthrodesis.
- In congenital variety displacement osteotomy of calcaneum.
  Except for the calcaneal osteotomy, all these procedures require arthrodesis of at least one metatarsal joint.

FOOT PAIN

Foot pain is a common public health problem and can be seen in fore, mid or hind foot as shown in Flowchart 32.4.

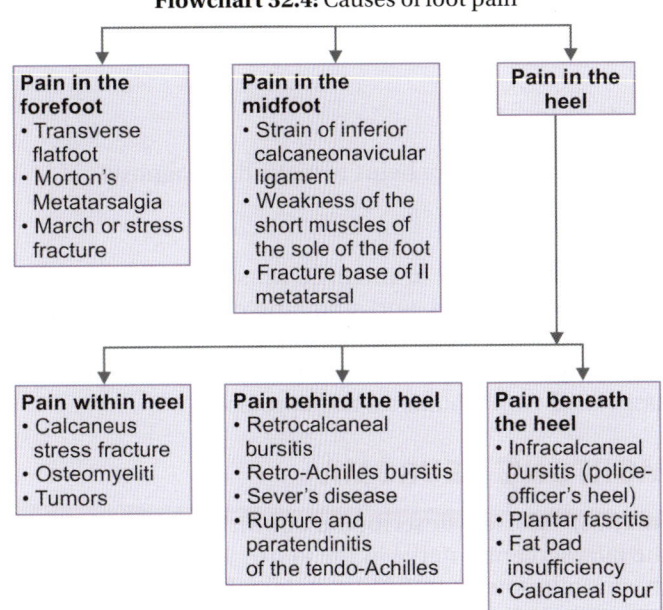

Flowchart 32.4: Causes of foot pain

METATARSALGIA

Definition

It is defined as pain beneath the metatarsal heads or shafts. It may be due to trauma, inflammation, and static causes.

Types

Static metatarsalgia: Found with developmental anomalies like metatarsus primus varus, hallux valgus, metatarsus hypermobilis, and obesity and debilitating illness.

Relaxation metatarsalgia: Interosseous muscle flex the MTP joints ° extend the toes ° draw the metatarsals together. Failure of these muscles causes splaying of the foot. The extra-weight borne by the metatarsal heads throws a strain on the transverse ligament of the metatarsal heads and pain results.

Compression metatarsalgia: Due to crowded footwear and this causes neuritis.

Fracture of II metatarsal bone: An old fracture of the base of the second metatarsal bone (transverse and undisplaced) is a common cause of chronic mid foot pain. It usually remains undetected. Treatment ranges from immobilization, electrical stimulation to surgical bone grafting.

Clinical Features

In relaxation metatarsalgia (commonest variety), the patient complains of pain beneath the metatarsal heads, compression of the foot increases the pain (Fig. 32.63). Splayfoot, atrophy of the interosseous muscles, and clawing of the toes are the other features.

Radiograph

Plain X-ray of the foot helps to make the diagnosis.

Treatment

Treatment consists of intrinsic muscle exercises, well-designed shoes, pad, and strapping changed at intervals of one week, support of inner sole with pad, and oblique osteotomy of the metatarsal necks for metatarsalgia associated with metatarsal head prolapse.

MORTON'S NEUROMA

In 1876, [4]Morton described a condition of pinching of the lateral plantar nerve in the fourth web space between the mobile fourth to fifth metatarsal heads of the foot (Fig. 32.64). However, it is more common in the III web space and rare in the first.

Cause: Neuroma is secondarily due to the irritation of the intermetatarsal plantar digital nerve as it travels beneath the metatarsal ligament and is due to the entrapment by the distal extent of the transverse inter-metatarsal ligament which produces perineural fibrosis.

Prevalence: More common in women than men.

Onset of symptoms: It is usually in the fifth decade of life.

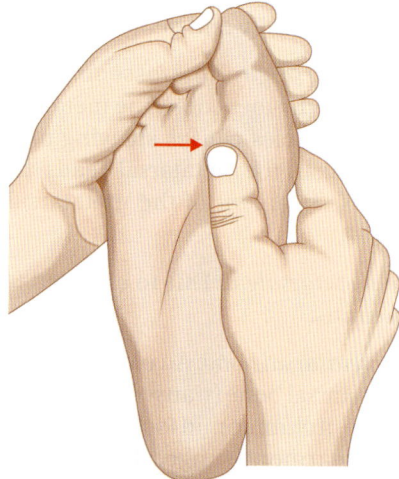

Fig. 32.63: Method of eliciting tenderness in metatarsalgia

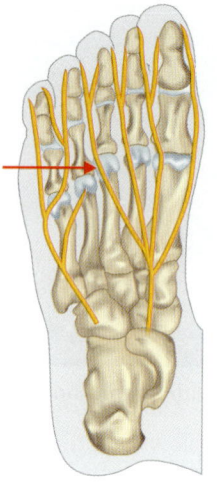

Fig. 32.64: Morton's neuroma

Clinical Features

The patient complains of pain in the region of the third and fourth metatarsal heads, by walking pain increases and decreases by rest. There could be deep burning pain and extension of paresthesia into the toes.

Tests

Mulder's click: When neuroma is squeezed between the metatarsal heads, a click is felt. This is common in women and is usually unilateral.

Extension test: Passively extend the MTP joints. This tightens the ligament and compresses the nerve eliciting pain.

Provocation tests: Deep palpations in the intermetatarsal space provoke pain.

Investigations

- It is mainly a clinical diagnosis and there is rarely a necessity of any investigations to arrive at a diagnosis.
- However, investigations are required in the following situations:
  - To confirm the diagnosis
  - In cases of double lesions
  - To assess the location
  - To find out the size of the lesion
  - Medicolegal considerations before surgery.
- Investigation Options:
  - MRI—It has a high sensitivity rate of 82.9%.
  - Ultrasound—It is less useful than MRI and has a sensitivity rate of 56.5%.
  - CT scan
  - Injection of local anesthetics

---

[4]**George Thomas Morton** (1835-1903) of Philadelphia, USA.

– Electrophysiology
– Histopathological examination: Helps in definitive diagnosis.

(Ref: Torres-Claramunt et al, Indian Journal of Orthopedics, May 2012, Vol. 46, Issue 3, 321-324)

Treatment

Nonoperative Treatment

This consists of shoes with metatarsal bars (Fig. 32.65), local infiltration of hydrocortisone, wide toe box (use is unpredictable), etc. are some of the common nonoperative methods of treatment. Neurodynamics helps in some cases.

Surgical Treatment

This is mainly excision of the neuroma in the third web space and this has an 83 percent success rate (Fig. 32.66).

Did You Know?
HO Thomas discovered metatarsal bar.

PAINFUL HEEL

The following are some of the causes of pain in the heel (Fig. 32.67):
- Traumatic disturbances.
- Developmental and pathological disturbances.
- Epiphysitis of the calcaneum (Fig. 32.68).

Differential Diagnosis of Heel Pain
Posterior Heel Pain
- Retrocalcaneal bursitis
- Hageland's deformity (pump-bump)
- Tendo-Achilles or tendonitis
- Calcification within the Achilles tendon
- Referred pain from a soleus muscle triggers point
- Radiculopathy of S_1.

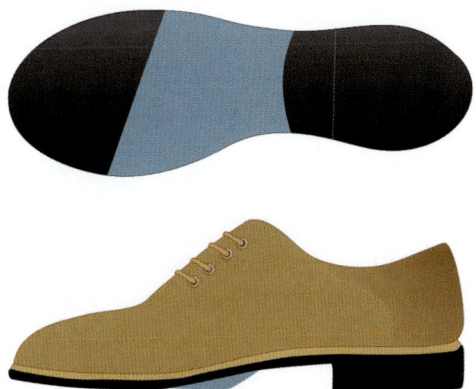

Fig. 32.65: Incorporation of metatarsal bars, under the sole of the footwear

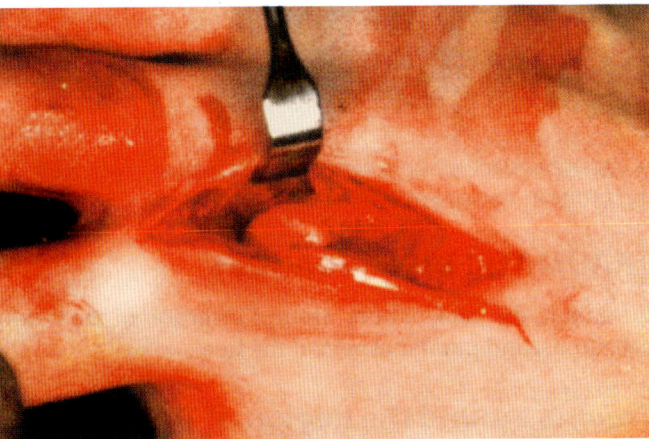

Fig. 32.66: Operative exposure Morton's neuroma

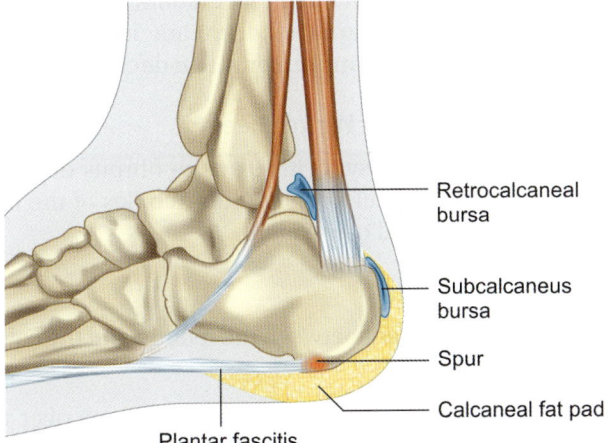

Fig. 32.67: Causes of heel pain

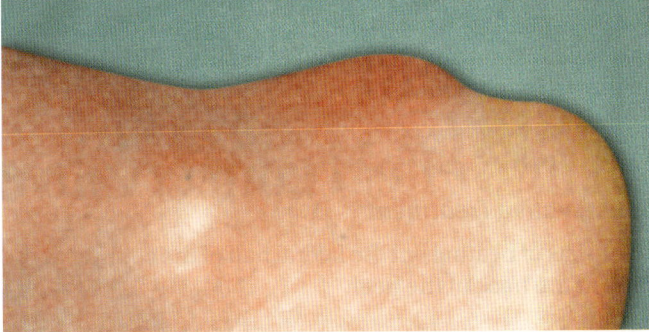

Fig. 32.68: Pump-bump due to friction from the back of the pump shoes (Clinical photo)

Plantar Heel Pain
- Inflammation or microtrauma of the plantar fascia.
- Entrapping neuropathy of tibial nerve or its branches and sciatic nerve.
- Fat pad atrophy.
- Heel spur.
- Stress fracture of calcaneum.
- Tarsal tunnel syndrome.

- Systemic problems like rheumatoid, etc.
- Radiculopathy of S_1.
- Irritates of the first branch of lateral plantar nerve or nerve to abductor digiti minimi (Baxter's nerve).
- Plantar heel bursitis.
- Thrombosis of the plantar medial venous plexus.
- Post-traumatic fat pad insufficiency (after due to calcaneal fracture).

TRAUMATIC DISTURBANCES

Trauma to the back of heel, around insertion of the tendo calcaneus, and plantar aspect of the heel.

Trauma around the Region of Tendo-Achilles

Tenosynovitis of tendo-Achilles, formation, and initiation of enlarged bursa, and partial tendon tears. In all the above cases, pain increases on movements and decreases by rest.

Hageland's Disease or Winter Heel

In this condition, tenosynovitis leads to fibrous deposits, which press on the back of the tendo-Achilles of the heel on wearing a boot and cause pain.

Bursa Enlargements

Normal bursa is present between the tendon and the calcaneus.

Adventitious bursa is subcutaneous and forms over the most prominent part of the posterior surface of the bone. It accounts for early 39 percent of the cases of pain in the heel. A tender hard lump usually forms over this and is called the *knobby heels*. It is seen in children and adolescents in whom it is liable to develop due to friction by the ill-fitting boot.

Treatment

Conservative Treatment

It consists of beating out the lateral half of the counter of the shoe at the back of the heel.

Surgery

It is the treatment of choice and consists of removal of the prominent posterosuperior angle of the calcaneum and any exostoses. In younger children, excision of a large wedge shape of bone is found to be useful.

Partial Tears of Tendo-Achilles

Here pain is due to fibrous tissue or periostitis.

Treatment

This consists of rest, and below-knee cast in full equinus for 3 weeks, later for 2 weeks in neutral position.

DEVELOPMENTAL AND PATHOLOGICAL DISTURBANCES OF THE HEEL

PLANTAR FASCIITIS (Subcalcaneal Pain)

This is defined as pain on the plantar surface of the heel and is the most common cause of posterior heel pain (Fig. 32.69).

> **Do You Know the Source of Pain in Plantar Fasciitis?**
> - Plantar fascia
> - Subcalcaneal bursa
> - Fat pad
> - Tendinous insertion of the intrinsic muscles
> - Long plantar ligament
> - Medial calcaneal branch of tibial nerve
> - Nerve to abductor digiti minimi

Clinical Features

The patient complains of pain in the heel, which is more in the morning. It gradually subsides as the patient takes a few steps. The pain increases on prolonged standing, walking, etc.

Types: See Flowchart 32.5.

Clinical Tests

Tenderness can be elicited on the medial aspect of the posterior heel. Passive stretching of the toes increases pain in the heel (Figs 32.70A and B).

> **Mystifying Facts: Why is Plantar Heel Pain More in the Morning?**
> During sleep, foot is in plantar flexed position causing shortening of the plantar structures. Sudden dorsiflexion in waking up from the night's sleep stretches the structured abruptly causing pain.

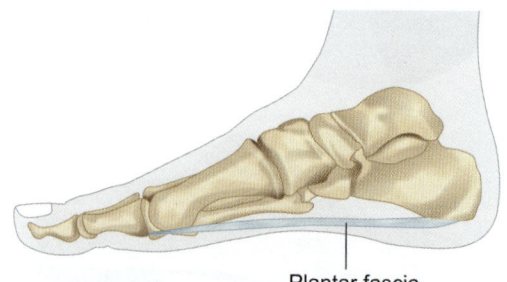

Fig. 32.69: The plantar fascia

Flowchart 32.5: Types of plantar fasciitis

```
Types of plantar fasciitis
    │
    ├──────────────────────┐
Insertional plantar fasciitis    Diffuse plantar fasciitis
    │                            │
Called the heel pain        Pain felt diffusely over
    syndrome                the heel and the sole
    │                           of the foot
Pain is felt at the
medial calcaneal tubercle
(Point tenderness)
```

Radiographs

Consisting of the routine AP, lateral and oblique views are advised. However, the X-ray does not show any changes in plantar fasciitis. It helps to detect calcaneal spur and other heel pathologies.

Treatment

- *Measures to reduce pain and inflammation* taping, temporary, or permanent shoe orthotic, heel cushion, weight management, etc. Physiotherapy also helps.
- Night splints to reduce pain (Fig. 32.72).
- *Measures to improve the neurodynamics of the tibial nerve*—active calf muscle stretching and calf soft tissue mobilization.
- Joint mobilization with talocalcaneal glides.
- Strengthening the muscles that support the arch namely—the posterior tibial, peroneal, and intrinsic muscles.
- No response to conservative treatment for three months—LIHC (local infiltration of hydrocortisone) is indicated.
- No response to conservative treatment for 6 months—surgery (partial plantar release) is advised.

Rehabilitation Methods

- Massage the heel by hand.
- Rolling of the foot over a tennis ball.
- Stretching exercises of the tendo-Achilles and hamstrings and intrinsic muscle exercises of the foot.
- Wearing silicon heel cups and MCR footwears helps to reduce shock and thus pain (Fig. 32.71).

What is New?
- Endoscopic plantar fasciotomies have a success rate of 85 percent.
- For recalcitrant heel pain instead of surgery 1000 impulses of low energy extracorporeal shock wave treatment (3 applications) is found to be effective.

Quick Facts: Treatment of Plantar Fasciitis in a Nutshell
I line
- NSAIDs.
- Heel pad/cushion.
- Stretching exercises of the ankle and foot.

II line
- Local infiltration of hydrocortisone.
- Custom molded foot orthotic.
- Soft supportive shoes.
- Foot strapping.
- Stretching exercises.
- Night brace or AFO or short leg walking cast.

III line
Surgery if the entire regime mentioned above fail after one year.

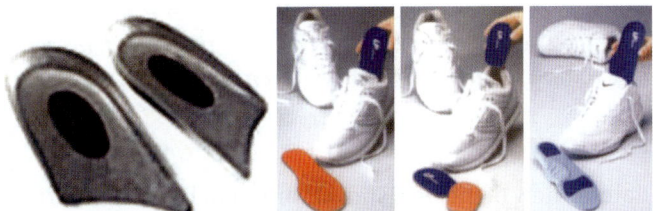

Fig. 32.71: Heel cups for cushioning in heel pain

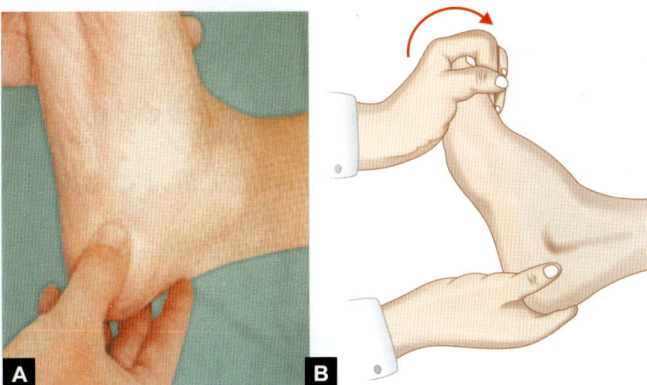

Figs 32.70A and B: (A) Method of eliciting tenderness in plantar fasciitis; (B) Passive stretching of toes increases pain

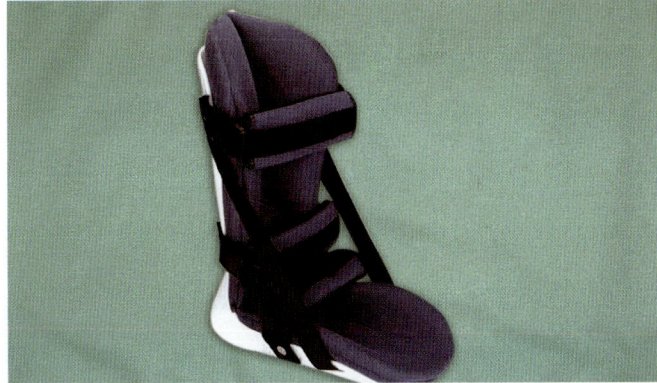

Fig. 32.72: Clinical photo showing night splints used in plantar fasciitis and spurs

CALCANEAL SPURS

It is a spike of bone at the anterior edge of the calcaneal tuberosity (usually medial).

It may be seen on the posterior aspect of the calcaneum also and is called the retrocalcaneal spur (Fig. 32.73).

Causes

- Due to repeated attacks of plantar fasciitis.
- Due to repeated trauma.
- Constant pulls of the shortened plantar fascia.
- Ill-fitting footwear (Figs 32.74A and B).
- Fibromatosis of the plantar fascia.

> **Important Spur Facts**
> - Nearly 80 percent of patients with plantar fasciitis have plantar heel spurs.
> - About 10 percent of the general population has asymptomatic heel spurs.
> - Though believed, it is actually not the source of pain.
> - Many patients with "suspected painful heel spur syndrome" have actually plantar fasciitis.
> - Spur has no therapeutic or prognostic significance.

Clinical Features

The patient complains of pain over ball of the heel, tenderness on plantar aspect of the heel (Fig. 32.75), slight swelling at the attachment of plantar fascia. *It is due to fibrositis or traumatic detachment of plantar fascia and does not give rise to symptoms per se and the pain when present is due to the causative condition and not the spur.*

Radiographs

Lateral view of the heel show prominent bone spike arising from the calcaneum (Figs 32.76 and 32.77).

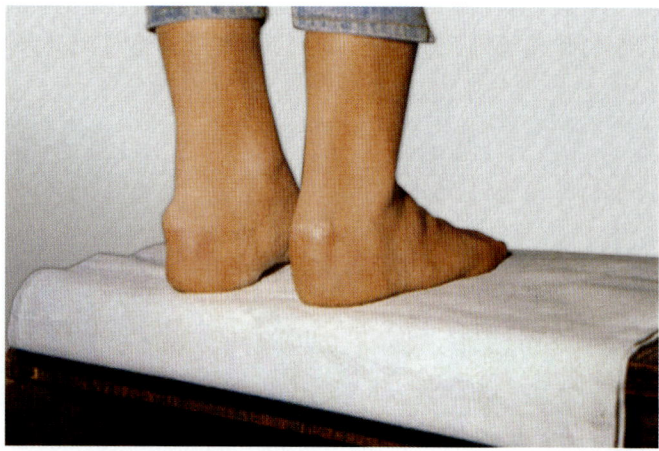

Fig. 32.73: Retrocalcaneal spur (Clinical photo)

Pitfall: *Only 50 percent of the patient with heel pain show calcaneal spurs on X-ray.*

Treatment

Conservative methods include treating the causative factor, rest, NSAIDs, local infiltration of hydrocortisone

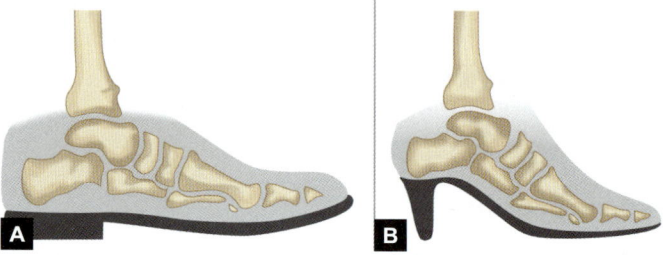

Figs 32.74A and B: (A) Correct footwear; (B) Improper footwear which distorts the normal arches of the foot

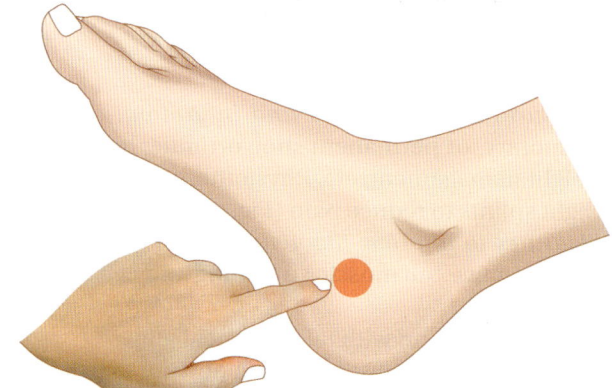

Fig. 32.75: Point of tenderness in plantar fasciitis and calcaneal spur

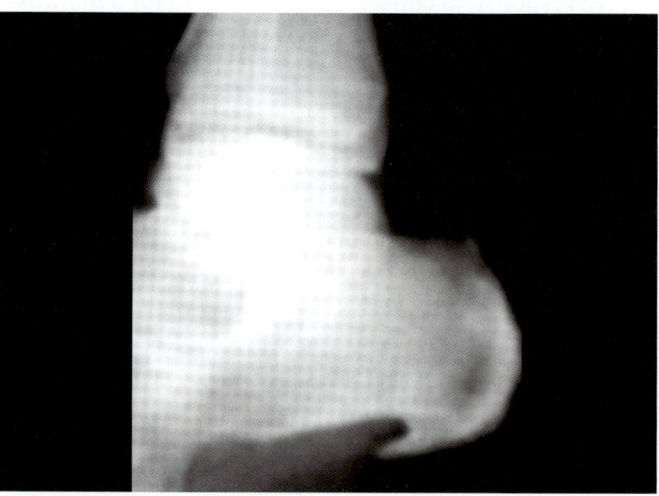

Fig. 32.76: Radiograph showing calcaneal spur (best seen in the lateral view)

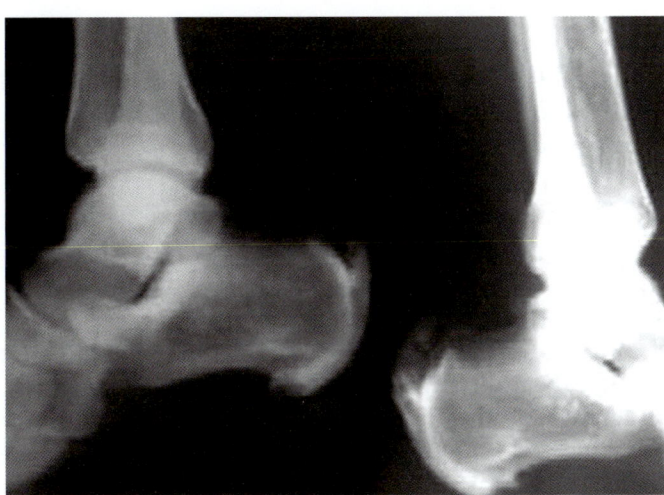

Fig. 32.77: Plain X-rays lateral view showing bilateral calcaneal and retrocalcaneal spurs

and microcellular rubber (MCR) used for the sole of the footwear (Fig. 32.78).

Surgery is indicated when no relief is seen with the conservative treatment.

Methods

- Osteotomy of the calcaneus.
- Decompressing operation with multiple drill holes in the calcaneus.
- Excision of the medial inferior tuberosity.

> **What is New in the Treatment of Calcaneal Spur?**
> - Endoscopic treatment of calcaneal spur syndrome.
>   **Indications:** Recalcitrant heel pain.
>   **Procedure:** Medial endoscopy and lateral instrumentation.
>   - Debridement of posterior roof of the calcaneal arch.
>   - Removal of calcaneal spurs.
>   - Lateral to medial release of plantar fascia.
>   - Debridement of the periosteum of calcaneal tuberosity.
>   - Release of nerve to abductor digiti minimi.
> - Low-dose acoustic shock waves delivered by a machine called an Ossatron. The acoustic waves may work by stimulating increased blood flow to the area, decrease inflammation, and help the tissue to heel.

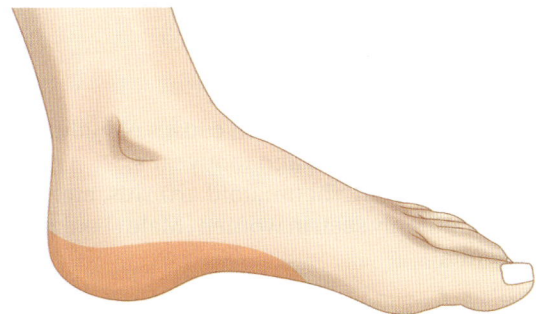

Fig. 32.78: UC-BL shoe inserts to relieve heel stress in plantar fasciitis and calcaneal spur

FAT PAD INSUFFICIENCY (Atrophy of Fat Pad)

Salient Features

- Seen in older athletes.
- Also seen in younger athletes with multiple cortisone injections.
- Pain and tenderness is diffuse over the heel.
- Flattening of the fat pad on standing.

Clinical Features

Patient complains of pain in the heel, limp, difficulty in standing for a long-time, etc. On examination, there is flattening of the heel, broadening and the calcaneum can be easily felt.

Radiograph

X-ray of the heel in the lateral view shows loss of soft tissue shadow.

Treatment

- NSAIDs.
- Ice therapy.
- Polyethylene or polypropylene heel cup for increased cushion and support.

CALCANEAL STRESS FRACTURE

This is common in athletes who jump and run repeatedly and faulty training techniques. Patient complains of diffuse heel pain and the heel compression test is positive. Treatment is essentially conservative in nature.

Joint arthritis develops due to calcaneal fracture or due to TB, syphilis, gonococcal arthritis, etc.

EPIPHYSITIS OF THE CALCANEUM ([5]SEVER'S DISEASE)

This is commonly seen in 9–13 years It is common in boys and is due to inflammation of bursa beneath the tendo-Achilles tendon.

---
[5]**James Warren Sever**, Boston, USA (1878-1964). Described this condition in 1912.

Clinical Features

It is usually asymptomatic, but there could be pain behind the heel due to the development of infection or fracture of the epiphysis following trauma to the heel.

Plain X-ray of the Hind foot especially the lateral view is recommended and it helps to detect the epiphysitis (Fig. 32.79).

Treatment

Consists of rest and footwear correction and this usually helps.

Fibromatosis of the Plantar Fascia

In this condition, nodule formation is seen which becomes painful with pressure and weight bearing. It is similar to Dupuytren's contracture, and is seen commonly in patients with antiepileptic drugs.

LESSER-KNOWN BUT IMPORTANT FOOT CONDITIONS

PLANTAR FIBROMATOSIS (LEDERHAM SYNDROME)

Definition

It is proliferative fibroplasias of the plantar aponeurosis similar to Dupuytren's contracture.

Presentation

Nodules can be felt on the medial non-weight bearing side of the aponeurosis.

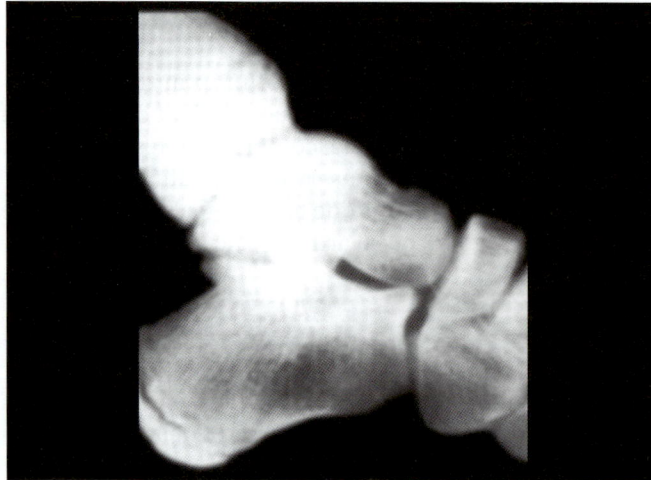

Fig. 32.79: Radiograph showing Sever's disease

Treatment

For small lesions, conservative treatment including shoe modifications is recommended. For large painful lesions, wide surgical excision is recommended.

PUMP-BUMP
Salient Features

- It is not a true tendonitis.
- It is an inflammation of the superficial bursa situated over the insertion of the tendo-Achilles (see Fig. 32.69).
- It is usually due to rubbing of the back part of the pump shoes and is more common in women.

DANCER TENDINITIS

It is tendonitis of the flexor hallucis longus and is seen in ballet dancers.

HALLUX VALGUS

It is a deviation of the great toe at the metatarsophalangeal joint away from the midline (Figs 32.80A and B).

Secondary Problems

Due to primary problem, some secondary changes develop namely:
- Varus of first metatarsal bone.
- Adduction of the phalanges.
- A protective adventitious bursa may develop over the medial aspect of the joint (called the bunion).
- Hypertrophy of the medial end of the first metatarsal head.
- OA changes in the first MTP joint.
- New bone formation at the end of the I MTP joint.
- Extensor hallucis tendon may be displaced laterally.
- The bunion may be ulcerated and infected due to friction from tight footwear.

Causes

These are some of the important causes of hallux valgus:
- Wearing of tight socks and footwear's.
- Diseases like gout, rheumatoid arthritis, etc.
- More commonly seen in women (Male : Female = 1 : 10).
- Congenital.

Clinical Features

Often, deformity is the only complaint (Fig. 32.81). However, in some longstanding cases, there could be pain in the great

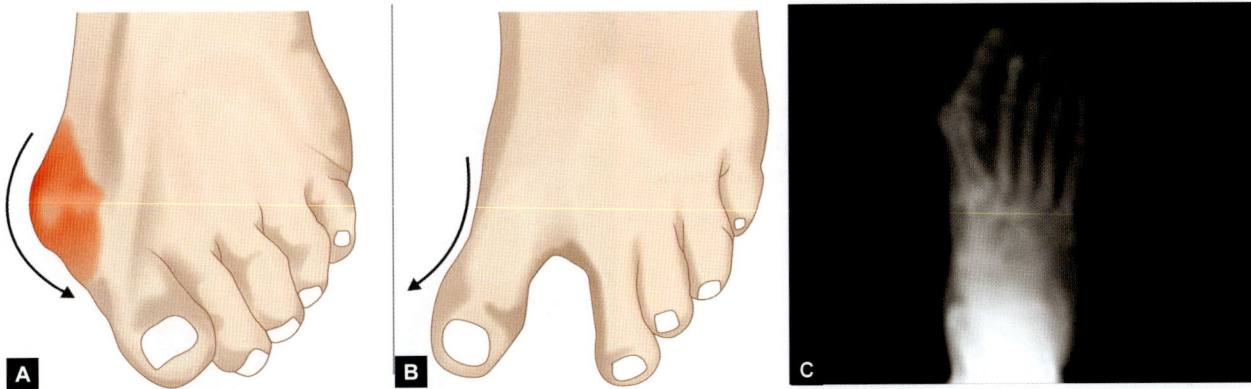

Figs 32.80A to C: (A) Hallux valgus; (B) Hallux varus; (C) Radiograph of hallux valgus

toe and there could be a significant swelling on the medial side due to bunion. Friction of the bunion due to the ill-fitting footwear could lead to skin ulceration.

Radiographs

Consisting of the routine AP, lateral and oblique views helps to assess the extent of the disease and helps plan the treatment (Fig. 32.80C).

Treatment

Mild Cases

Physiotherapy measures and footwear correction suffices in mild cases.
- Relaxed passive stretching of the abductors of great toe.
- Active exercises to the foot intrinsic muscles.
- Proper weight-bearing methods.
- Footwear's with straight inner border with a wedge between the I and II toe helps.
- Faradic footbath is recommended.

Severe Cases

Surgery is the treatment of choice and includes:
- *Keller's operation:* Excision of the head of the first metatarsal and proximal portion of the proximal phalanx.
- *Mayo's operation:* Here only head of the I metatarsal bone is excised.
- *Arthroplasty:* Excision of the I MTP joint with bunion.
- *Arthrodesis* of the I MTP joint is also done.

HALLUX RIGIDUS

In this condition, there is pain and stiffness in the MTP joint of the great toe.

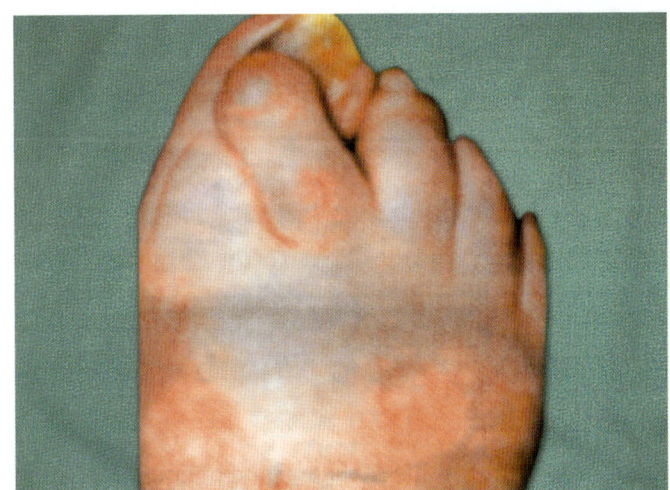

Fig. 32.81: Clinical photograph of hallux valgus

Causes

- Repeated injuries to the great toe.
- Improper footwear.
- Familial and common in females.

There may be erosion of the articular cartilage and formation of exostosis.

Clinical Features

Patient may complain pain and stiffness of the great toe and of difficulty in gait, wearing footwear, etc.

Radiographs

Consisting of the routine AP, lateral and oblique views help to assess the extent of the disease.

Treatment

Mild Cases

- Conservative measures like painkillers, etc.
- Thermotherapy helps to reduce pain and spasm.
- Footwear modifications like metatarsal bars, soft soles, etc.
- POP cast may be required in some cases.

Severe Cases

This may be treated by:
- Arthroplasty of the I MTP joint.
- Arthrodesis of the I MTP joint.

HAMMER TOES

Definition

It is a toe deformity with PIP joint flexion. It could be flexible or fixed (Fig. 32.82).

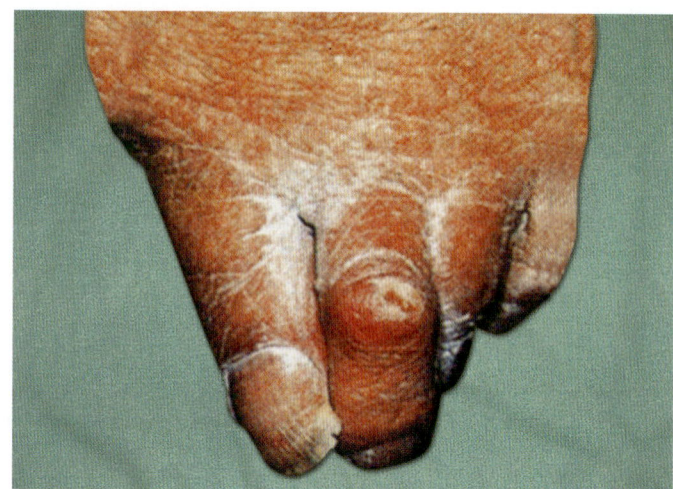

Fig. 32.82: Clinical photograph of hammer toe

Clinical Features

Most often, deformity is the only complaint. Pain sometimes results from a callus on the dorsum of the PIP joint or under the head of the metatarsal. Hammering of the second toe often is accompanied with hallux valgus deformity (Fig. 32.83A).

Radiographs

Consisting of the routine AP, lateral and oblique views help to assess the deformity.

Treatment

This includes:
- Stretching of the dorsal extrinsic in a position of plantar flexion and MTP extension.
- Intrinsic muscle strengthening exercises.
- Extra depth shoes.

CLAW TOES

Definition

It is an extension deformity of the MTP joint with simultaneous flexing or clawing of the toes at both the proximal and distal inter-phalangeal joints (Fig. 32.83B).

Causes

It is due to muscle imbalance in which the active extrinsic are stronger than the deeper intrinsic (lumbricals and interosseous). This happens usually in a neurological disorder. It is usually seen in pes cavus.

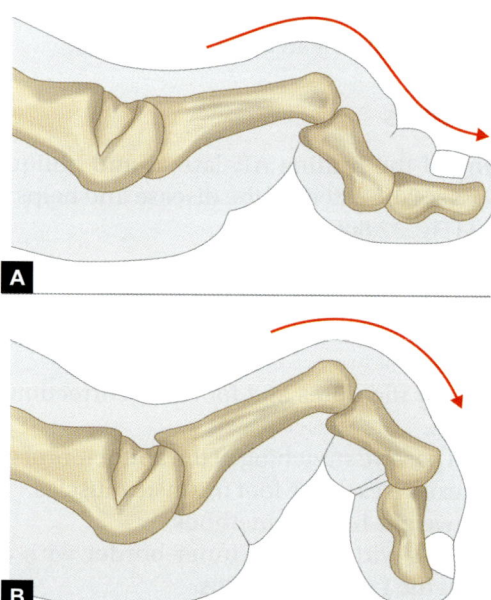

Figs 32.83A and B: (A) Hammer toe; (B) Claw toe

Clinical Features

Deformity is the main complaint. Patient may also complain of difficulty in gait, wearing foot wears, development of callosities, foot pain, etc. (Fig. 32.84).

Radiographs

Consisting of the routine AP, lateral and oblique views helps to assess the extent of the disease and helps plan the treatment.

- NSAID's are recommended in severe pain.
- Local infiltration of corticosteroids is indicated in unrelenting pain.
- Below knee cast—If there is fracture of the scaphoid bone.
- Sesamoidectomy if the above treatment methods fail.

> **Effective Conservative Treatment for all Forefoot Conditions**
> - Metatarsal pad or cut-out under orthosis to change the pressure under the tender area.
> - Changing the ill-fitting shoes.
> - Maintaining the correct arch position by support and exercises.
> - Intrinsic muscle strengthening exercises to improve flexion and extension of the MTP and IP joints.

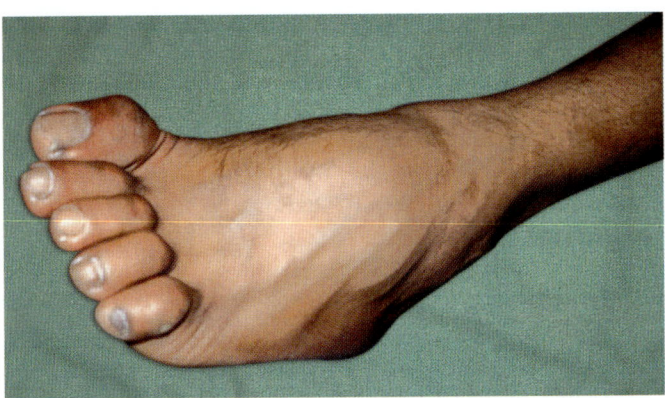

Fig. 32.84: Clinical photograph of claw toes

Treatment

In flexible claw toes, the treatment is similar to hammer toes.

SESAMOIDITIS

Definition

This is an inflammation in the two small sesamoid bones that are situated in the tendon of the flexor hallucis brevis muscle under the first MTP joint.

Causes: it may be because of overuse in sports, athletes and may rarely be due to direct trauma.

Associated Problems

Since the medial digital plantar nerve runs close to the medial sesamoid bone, it is often irritated.

Clinical Features

- Ambulating is extremely painful.
- First MTP joint is tender to palpate.
- Pain increases on extension of the great toe.
- There could be swelling at the head of the first metatarsal.

> **Did You Know?**
> Sachin Tendulkar suffered from Sesamoid bone problems not once but twice in his illustrious career which almost threatened his playing the game of cricket!

Investigations

This consists of X-ray of the foot, MRI, bone scan, etc.

Treatment

This consists of the following measures:
- Footwear modifications.
- Non-weight bearing for few weeks.

BIBLIOGRAPHY

Arthroplasty

Hip

1. Bakenbaugh RD, Ilstruip DM. Total hip arthroplasty: a review of 333 cases with long-term follow-up. J Bone Joint Surg. 1978; 60-A: 306.
2. Berrin T, Dorr LD, Perry J, Grontley J, Hull DB. Functional evaluation of total hip arthroplasty with a 5 to 10-years follow-up evaluation. Clin Orthop. 1985;195:252.
3. Charley J. The long-term results of low friction arthroplasty. J Bone Joint Surg. 1972;54-B:61.
4. Charley J. Total prosthetic replacement of the hip in attention to physiotherapy. Physiotherapy. 1968;54:406.
5. Gitelis S, et al. The influence of early weight bearing on experimental total hip arthroplasties in dogs. Clin Orthop. 1982;169:29.
6. Jensin JS, Mathiesen B, Jvede N. Occupational capacity after hip replacement. Acta Orthop Scarda. 1985;56:135.
7. Johnston RC, Smidt GL. Hip motion measurements for selected activities of daily living. Clin Orthop, 1970; 72:205.
8. Mcbeath AA, Bahrke MS, Batra Batze B. Walking efficiency before and after total hip replacement as determined by oxygen consumption. Bone Joint Surg. 1980;62A:807.
9. Yoslow W, Simone HD. Hip replacement rehabilitation. Arch Phys Med and Rehab. 1976;57:175.

Total Knee Arthroplasty

1. Ewald FC, et al. Kinematics total knee replacement. J Bone Joint Surg. 1984;66-A:1032.
2. Good Fellow J, O'Connor J. The mechanism of the knee and prosthetic design. J Bone and Joint Surg. 1978;60-B: 358.
3. Insall JN, Binnazzi R, Soudry M, Mestriner WA. Total knee arthroplasty. Clin Orthop. 1985;192:13.
4. Kapanji LA. The physiology of the joints. New York, Churchill Livingstone. 1971;2.
5. Laughman RK, Stauffer RN, Istrup DM, Chao EYS. Functional evaluation of total knee replacement. J Orthop Res. 1984;2-307.

6. Morrison JB. Function of the knee joint in various activities. Biomed Eng. 1969;4:573.
7. Scott WN, Tria AJ. Principles of surgical technique in knee arthroplasty. Orthop Clin North Am. 1982;13:131.

Total Ankle Arthrosplasty

1. Alexakis P, Smith RC, Wellisch M. Irradiations for ankle fusion vs. total ankle replacement versus plantar fusion. Orthop Trans. 1977;1:87.
2. Morris JM. Biomechanics of the foot and the ankle. Clin Orthop. 1977;122:10.
3. Newton SE III. Total ankle arthroplasty: A 4 years study. Orthop Trans.1977;1:86.
4. Sammaroo GJ, Burstein AH, Frankel VH. Biomechanics of the ankle: A kinematics study. Orthop Clin North Am. 1975;4:1.
5. Stauffer RN. Total joint arthroplasty of the ankle. Mayo Clin Proc. 1979;54:570.

Total Shoulder Arthroplasty and Elbow

1. Cofield RH. Total shoulder arthroplasty. The Neer prosthesis. Orthop Trans. 1979;3:262.
2. Neer CS. Reconstructive surgery and rehabilitations of the shoulder. In: Kelly (Ed), et al. Textbook of Rheumatology. Philadelphia; 1981.
3. Saunders WB, Bryan RS. Total replacement of the elbow joint. Arch Surg. 1977;112:1092.

Painful Heel Syndrome

1. Campher JW, Inman VT. Treatment of plantar fasciitis and calcaneal spurs with 4C-BL shoe insert. Clin Orthop. 1974;103:57.
2. DuVris HL. Heel spur (Calcaneal spur). Arch Surg. 1957; 74:536.
3. Furey JG. Plantar fasciitis, the painful heel syndrome. J Boneard Joint Surg. 1975;57-A:672.
4. Graham CE. Painful heel syndrome: Rationale and treatment Foot Ankle. 1983;3:261.
5. Hicks JH. The mechanics of the foot. Part II. The plantar aponeurosis and the arch. J Anat. 1954;88:25.

Arthrodesis

1. Ahank I. Arthrodesis and arthroplasty of hip joint. Acta Orthop Gland. 1963;33:253.
2. Barr JS, Record EE. Arthrodesis of the ankle joint. Indications, operative technic, and clinical experience. N Engl J Med. 1953;248:53.
3. Carnesale PG. Arthrodesis of the hip; A long-term study. Orthop Digest. 1976;4:12.
4. Charnley J. Compression arthrodesis. Edinburgh, E and S, Livingstone Ltd; 1953.
5. Charnley J, Lowe HB. A study of the end results of compression arthrosis of the knee. J Bone Joint Surg. 1958;40-B:633.
6. Clawson RS, McKay DW. Arthrodesis in the presence of infection. Clin Orthop. 1976;114:209.
7. Moure FH, Smith JS. Arthrodesis of the knee joint. Clin Orthop. 1959;13:215.
8. Nelson CL, Evarts CM. In Arthroplasty and Arthrodesis of the Knee Joint. Orthop Clin North Am. 1971;2:245.
9. Putt V. Arthrodesis for tuberculosis of the knee and of the shoulder. Chir Organ Mov. 1933;18:217.

Regional Disorders

Frozen Shoulder

1. Bosworth DM. Supraspinatus syndrome. Symptomatology, pathology, and repair. JAMA. 1941;117:422.
2. Delta Prota RJ, Evarts M. Rotator cuff tears. Contemp Orthop. 1982;4:327.
3. Duncan BF. The frozen shoulder syndrome rehabilitations approach to treatment. Contemp Orthop. 1983;6:69.
4. Grey RG. The natural history of idiopathic frozen shoulder. Journal Bone Joint Surg. 1978;60-A:564.
5. Haggart GE, Dignam RJ, Sullivan TS. Management of the frozen shoulder. JAMA. 1956;161:1219.
6. Lee MH, Wright V, Longron EB. Periarthritis of shoulder controlled trial of physiotherapy. Physiotherapy. 1973;59:312.
7. Maitland GD. Treatment of glenohumeral joint by passive movement. Physiotherapy. 69:3.
8. Mosley HF. Ruptures of the rotator. GH Br J Surg. 1951; 38-340.
9. Neer CS II. Impingement lesions. Clin Orthop. 1983; 173:70.
10. Neviaser RJ. Painful conditions affecting the shoulder. Clin Orthop. 1983;173:63.
11. Depalima AF. The painful shoulder. Postgrad Med. 1957; 21:368.

Tennis Elbow

1. Coonrad RW, Hooper WK. Tennis elbow: its coarse natural history conservative and surgical management. J Bone Joint Surg. 1973;55-A:1177.
2. Cyriax JH. The pathology and treatment of tennis elbow. J Bone Joint Surg. 1936;18:921.
3. Dungar BF. Rehabilitation of the tennis elbow syndrome. Contemp Orthop. 1983;7:61.
4. Field FW, Field SM. Treatment of tennis elbow. Use of a spinal trace. JAMA. 1966;195:67.
5. Gardner RC. Surgery for tennis elbow: A five-year follow-up. Orthop Rev 1974; 3:45.
6. James EY, Chow AMD. Carpal tunnel. Chow technique. Source: Orthonet, May-June 1999.
7. Norklood LA, Shock JA, Andrews JK. Acute medial elbow ruptures. Am J Sports Med 1981; 9:16.

Olecranon Bursitis

1. Canoso JJ. Idiopathic or traumatic olecranon bursitis; clinical features and bursal fluid analysis. Arth Rheum. 1977;20:1213.
2. Jaffe L, Fetto JF. Olecranon bursitis. Contemp Orthop B. (5)51:1984.

Cervical Disk

1. Bloom MH, Ranaji FL. Anterior anterovertebral fusion of the cervical spine: A technical note. J Bone and Joint Surg. 1981;63-A: 842.
2. Bucy PC, Hein burger RF, Oberhill HK. Compression of the cervical spinal cord by herniated intervertebral discs. J Neurosurg. 1948;5:471.
3. Bun JWD. Rupture of the intervertebral disc in the cervical region. Proc R Soc Med. 1948;41:513.
4. Coventry MB, Ghormley RK, Kernohan JW. The intervertebral disc, its microscopic anatomy, and pathology part II: Changes in the intervertebral disc concomitant with age. J Bone and Joint Surg. 1945; 27:233.
5. Garna A. Cervical traction, an ancient modality. Orthop Rev. 1984;13:429.
6. Scoville WB. Types of cervical disc lesions and their surgical approaches. JAMA. 1966;196:105.
7. Shertz HH, Watters WC III, Zeiger L. Evaluation, and treatment of Natz pain. Orthop Clin North Am. 1982; 13:439.

Scoliosis

1. Blount WP, Schmidt AC, and Bidwell R. Making the Milwaukee brace. J Bone Joint Surg. 1958;40-A:526.
2. Cobb JK. Outline for the study of scoliosis. In: JW Edwards (Ed). American Academy of Orthopedic Surgeons. Instrumental Course Lectures, Vol 5, Ann Arbor; 1948.
3. Drummond D, et al. Interspinous process segmental spinal instrumentation. J Paediatr Orthop. 1984;4:397.
4. Goldstein LA. The surgical management of idiopathic scoliosis. Clin Orthop. 1973;93:131.
5. Harrington PR. Treatment of scoliosis. Correction and internal fixation by spine instrumentation. J Bone and Joint Surg. 1962;44A:591.
6. Kisser JC. The iliac apophysis; as invaluable sign in the management of scoliosis. Clin Orthop. 1958;11:111.
7. Kleinberg S. Scoliosis: Pathology, etiology and treatment, Baltimore: Williams and Wilkins Co; 1951.
8. Mehta MH. Radiographic estimation of vertebral rotation in scoliosis. J Bone Joint Surg. 1973;55-B:513.
9. Moe JH. Methods of correction and surgical techniques in scoliosis. Orthop Clin North Am. 1972;3:17.
10. Stagnara P. Scoliosis in adults: Surgical treatment of severe forms. Excerpts Med Found International Congress Series No. 1969;192.
11. Thulbourne T, Gillespie R. The rib-hump in idiopathic scoliosis measurement, analysis, and response to treatment. J Bone and Joint Surg. 1976;58-B:64.
12. Wyer AF. Experience of anterior correction of scoliosis. Clin Orthop. 1973;93:191.

Kyphosis

1. Blackborne JS, Velikas EP. Spondylolisthesis in children and adolescents. J Bone Joint Surg. 1977;59-B:490.
2. Bosworth DM, Fielding JW, Demarest L, Bonaquist M. Spondylolisthesis: A critical review of a consecutive series of cases treated by arthrodesis. J Bone Joint Surg. 1955;37-A:767.
3. Bradtord DS, et al. Anterior strut-grafting for the treatment of kyphosis. Review of experience with 48 cases. J Bone Joint Surg. 1982;64-A:680.
4. Kiriluwto O, Sartavirta S, Salenius P, Morri P, Pytkkanen P. Posterolateral spine fusion, a 1-4 years follows-up of 80 consecutive patients. Acta Orthop Siard. 1985;56:152.
5. Mezerding HW. Low back ache and sciatic pain associated with spondylolisthesis and protruded intervertebral disc; incidence, significance and treatment (symposium). J Bone and Joint Surg. 1941; 23:461.
6. Moe JH. Treatment of adolescent kyphosis by non-operative and operative methods. Mantoba Med Rev. 1965;75:481.
7. Wiltse LL, Newman PH, Macnab I. Classification of spondylolysis and spondylolisthesis. Clin Orthop. 1976; 117:23.
8. Witlse LL, Jackson DW. Treatment of spondylolisthesis and spondylolysis in children. Clin. Orthop. 1976; 117:92.
9. Wittse LL, Winter KB. Terminology and measurement of spondylolisthesis. J Bone Joint Surg. 1983;65-A:768.

Hallux Valgus

1. Albrechkht E. Pathology and treatment of hallux valgus. Russki Vrach. 1911;10:14.
2. Bragman J, Corless J, Gross A, Langer F. A review of surgical procedures for hallux valgus, Foot Ankle. 1980; 1:39.
3. Clutton HH. The treatment of hallux valgus St Thomas Rep. 1994;21:1.
4. Writhton J. A ten-year review of Keller's operation at the Princes Elizabeth Orthopedic Hospital-Exeter. Clin. Orthop. 89:207-1972.

Knee

Arthroscopic Treatment of Popliteal Cyst

1. Valerio Samsone, MD Allesantra DC Ponti, Orthonet, Arthroscopy, May-June 1999.

Pes Planus

1. Harris RT, Beath J. Etiology of peroneal spastic flat foot. J Bone Joint Surg. 1948;30-13:624.
2. Jay Kumar S, Cowell HR. Rigid flatfoot. Clin Orthop. 1977;122:77.
3. Jones RL. The human foot: an experimental study of its mechanics and the role of its muscles and ligaments in the support of the arch. Am J Anat. 1941;68-1.
4. Milkstrom J, Williams RA. Shoe correction and orthopedic foot supports. Clin. Orthop. 1983;70:30.
5. Stabeli LT, Griffin L. Corrective shoes for children: A survey of current practice. Pediatrics. 1980;65:13.

Morton's Neuroma

1. Cohen HH. Mortan's metatarsalgia (interdigital neuroma). Bull Hosp Joint Dis. 1952;13:206.
2. Morris MA. Morton's metatarsalgia. Clin orthop. 1977;127:203.
3. Metatarsalgia: Morris G Nix K, Goldman PP, Department of Pediatrics, Philadelphia, 2000.

Sesamoid Bones of the Forefoot

1. Jahss MH. The sesamoids of the hallux. Clin Orthop. 1981;157:88.
2. Morris JM. The biomechanics of the foot and the ankle. Clin Orthop. 1977;122:10.
3. Orr TG. Fracture of great toe sesamoid bones. Ann Surg. 1918;48:609.
4. Parra G. Stress fractures of the sesamoids of the foot. Clin Orthop. 1960;18:218.

Chronic Heel Pain

1. Praveen K, Vohra DPM. Open heel surgery Vs Endoscopic plantar fasciotomies. Journal of American Pediatric Medical Association Feb. 1999.
2. Rosenfeld I. Chronic heel pain - Treatment by Ossatron. Source: Readers' Digest Feb. 2001.

Infantile Quadriceps Contracture

1. Hnevkovsky the progressive of the vastus intermedius muscle in children. J Bone Joint Surg. 1961;43B:318-25.
2. Fairbanks TJ, Barrett AM. Vastus intermedius contracture in early childhood: In marries report identical twins. J Bone Joint Surg. 1961;43B:326-34.
3. Gunn DR. Contracture of the quadriceps muscle: Discussion on the etiology and relationship you recurrent dislocation of the patella. J Bone Joint Surg. 1964;46B:492-70.
4. Hagen R. Contracture of the quadriceps muscle in children: Report of 12 you marry, Minutes Orthop. Scand. 1968;39:565-78.
5. Lloyd-Roberts GC, Thomas TG. The etiology of quadriceps contractures in children JBJS. 1964;46B:498.
6. Makhani JS. Quadriceps fibrosis: Complication of intramuscular injections in the thigh. Indian J Pediatric. 1971;38:54-60.
7. Nicoll EA. Quadricepsplasty. JBJS. 1963;45B:483.
8. Lenart G, Kullmann L. Isolated contracture of the rectus femoris muscle. Clin. Orthop. 1974;99:125-30.
9. Mukherjee PK. Injection fibrosis on the quadriceps femoris muscle in children. J Bone Joint Surg. 1980; 62A:453-56.
10. Sasaki T, Fukuhara H, lisaka H, Monji J, Kanno Y, Yasuda K. Postoperative evaluation of quadriceps contracture children: comparison of three different procedures. J Paediatr Orthop. 1985; 5:702-07.
11. Sengupta S. Pathogenesis of infantile quadriceps fibrosis and its correction by proximal release. Pediatric Orthop. 1985;5:187-91.
12. Thompson TC. Quadricepsplasty to improve knee function. JBJS. 1944;26:366.

33 CHAPTER

Disorders of the Hand

Hand is a very important organ of the body. Disorders affecting the hand could lead to loss of hand function in various forms and degrees. Thumb itself accounts for over 40 percent function of the hand. It is imperative that the problems affecting the hand should be diagnosed and managed correctly. The following are the various disorders affecting the hand.

CONGENITAL ANOMALIES OF THE HAND

Some of the important congenital anomalies of the hand are:

Polydactyly: It is a duplication of one or more digits and may require amputation for cosmetic purposes (Fig. 33.1).

Syndactyly: This is fusion of digits and usually occurs between the middle and ring fingers and is 3 times more common in males. The fusion may be only in the skin or all the structures. In the latter case, surgery is done early at 18 months age and in the less severe former case, surgery is done after 5 years.

Macrodactyly: This is a rare congenital anomaly and is characterized by enlargement of all structures especially of the nerves of a single or more digits. It is often associated with neurofibromatosis, lymphangioma, arteriovenous malformation, etc.

Congenital trigger digits: Thumb is more commonly involved. It is frequently bilateral and is due to flexion contracture of the distal joint of the thumb. More than 30 percent of these cases resolve after first year and the remaining may require surgical release after 2 years of age.

Streeter's dysplasia: This is a syndrome of congenital constrictions, which may affect any part of the body. In the hand, it may range from simple constriction to congenital amputation. To prevent distal circulatory compromise, it frequently requires surgical release by Z-plasty.

Camptodactyly: This is a flexion contracture of the proximal interphalangeal joint especially of the little finger. It may rarely be seen in other fingers too. Severe deformity in older patients requires tendon-lengthening procedures. Clinicodactyly is angulation of the finger in radioulnar direction. Mild clinicodactyly is seen in normal children, while the severe ones are associated with mental retardation.

Cleft hand (also called Lobster claw hand): This is frequently bilateral and is associated with cleft foot, cleft lip, cleft palate, etc. There are two varieties: in the first type, a deep palmar cleft separates the two central metacarpals; and in the second type, the central rays are absent. Both the varieties require surgical excision and Z-plasty.

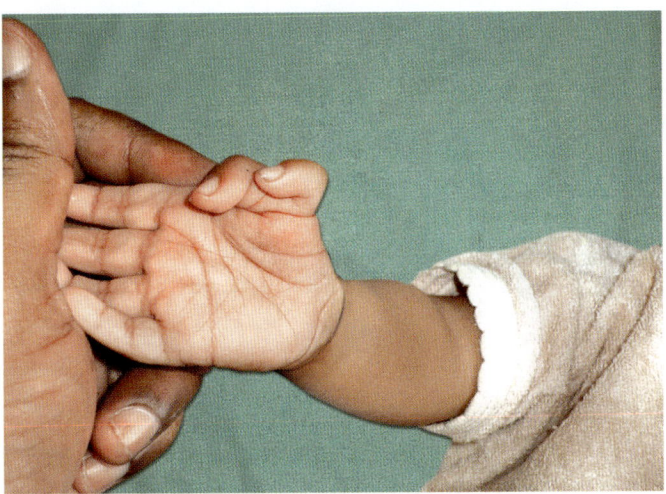

Fig. 33.1: Clinical photograph of polydactyly

Mirror hand (reduplication of ulna): Here the ulna and carpus are reduplicated and there may be seven or eight fingers with no thumb. Pollicization of a finger solves the problem of the absent thumb.

Congenital radioulnar synostosis (refer page 475).

Madelung's deformity (refer page 476).

Congenital absence of radius or ulna: Congenital absence of radius is more common than that of ulna. The radius may be completely absent or in parts. The forearm is short, wrist is highly unstable, and the hand is deviated radially. It requires complex and difficult surgical corrections.

This deformity of radius absence is also called radial club hand and the absence of ulna is called the ulnar club hand (1 : 4).

Kirner's deformity: This is a spontaneous injuring of the terminal phalanx of the fifth digit. It is a rare disorder and is more often seen in females.

INFECTIONS OF THE HAND

The effects of hand infection can be as devastating as major trauma. Trivial injuries like a scratch, a prick, small punctured wounds, etc. cause hand infections. *Staphylococcus aureus* (80%), *Streptococcus pyogenes* and gram-negative bacilli are the famous trio who inflict the infective unmitigated disaster in the hand. The sequel of these infections is edema, abscess, necrosis, fibrosis, and lastly contractions leading to a grotesque, debilitating hand. The presence of an abscess seems to send a message to the surgeons, *"Drain Me, or I'll drain myself!"* Hence, an abscess caused should be drained; the surgeon only has to decide the proper time and incisions. Early use of potent antibiotics has considerably downed the threat of serious hand infections.

As elsewhere before we delve into the discussions on individual hand infections, it helps considerably to know the principles of treatment:
- Hands should be kept elevated to facilitate gravity to drain and thereby prevent edema and swelling of the hand.
- Following the treatment, the hand needs to be placed in functional position (*see* Fig. 33.3) for optimum results.
- Early and appropriate use of IV antibiotics prevents pus formation (within 24–48 hours).
- If pus is formed, let it out through proper incisions at the appropriate time.
- Local anesthetic may help the spread of infection and adds more fluid to the already existing swelling. Hence, general anesthesia or regional block is preferred.
- Tourniquet is indicated, but exsanguinations are not preferred as it helps spread the infection (alternatively, elevation of hand for three minutes is ideal).
- Do not forget the all-important hand aftercare, which has a direct bearing on the outcome of the hand function.

With the principles of treatment as a backdrop, let us now consider the important hand infections in order of importance.

PARONYCHIA

Paronychia (Fig. 33.2) is an infection of the eponychium and could be acute or chronic. Acute paronychia has the distinction of being the most common infection of the hand. *S. aureus* is the culprit and it is usually due to a hangnail, unsterile manicure instruments, and reckless nail pairing. The infection normally begins at one corner, tracks down to the opposite end via the eponychium or nail (40%).

Clinical Features

Agonizing pain, marked tenderness and a conspicuous red looking swelling are the hallmarks of acute paronychia.

Treatment

Conservative measures and early antibiotic therapy is the mainstay of initial treatment. However, if abscess has formed and if the pus is at one end, incise it, if under one nail corner, remove that corner; and if it has shifted to the opposite end, excise proximal one-third of the nail. If encountered with a floating nail, write its obituary by taking it out totally, as it is dead and gone!

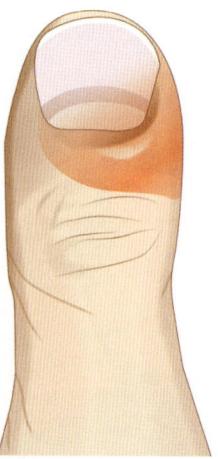

Fig. 33.2: Paronychia

Note: Chronic paronychia which is regarded as a complication of acute paronychia is usually not so! It is usually seen in syringomyelia or in people who do not wear rubber gloves during washing!

APICAL SUBUNGUAL INFECTION

Here the space between the distal phalanx and the nail plate gets infected. An injury or pinprick could lead to this. Pain is excruciating and the tenderness is felt most below the nail free edge and the pus is usually left pointing towards this free edge. Initially, conservative treatment helps but in the stage of pus formation, drainage is done by a small V-shaped incision. Rarely a chronic sinus develops and the phalanx could develop osteomyelitis.

DISTAL PULP SPACE INFECTION (Syn: Felon)

Next to acute paronychia, this is the most common hand infection. It usually follows a pinprick, with the index finger and thumb being the common unfortunate victim.

Surgical anatomy: Multiple fibrous septae travel from skin to bone partitioning the fat-filled distal pulp space into tiny compartments (Fig. 33.3). One such septum also cordons of the space at the distal finger flexor crease. The terminal branches of the digital artery after giving a branch to the basal epiphyseal plate runs through this compartment. The evil effects of this arrangement could lead to the following undesirable consequences:
- Since it is a tight compartment, any swelling increases the pressure causing excruciating pain.
- If superficial, penetrates the skin causing skin necrosis and if deep penetrates the periosteum causing osteomyelitis.
- Thrombosis of the digital arteries leads to osteomyelitis.
- It may in rare events cause flexor tenosynovitis or infective arthritis of the DIP joint.

Clinical Features

The patient initially complains of dull pain more so in the dependent position and swelling. Loss of sleep due to nocturnal pain is a usual feature after about 2 days. Pressure over the involved part increases pain. Abscess may develop in later stages if left unattended.

Treatment

Treatment consists of antibiotics in the initial stages and if the pain lasts for more than 12 hours, incision helps (Fig. 33.4). If the abscess is pointing volar wards, a longitudinal midline incision is taken; and if the abscess is deep, a longitudinal incision at the side cutting through the partitions is preferred. If osteomyelitis develops in the distal phalanx, sequestrectomy is done if the sequestrum is well-formed and separated.

MIDDLE AND PROXIMAL VOLAR SPACE INFECTION

These also follow pinpricks and may be confused with tenosynovitis of the flexor tendons (Fig. 33.5). Spread to the adjacent web space is common. Clinical features and treatment are almost similar.

INFECTION OF THE WEB SPACES

What are these web spaces?
These are three triangular areas filled with loose fat between the ends of the fingers. Infection reaches these areas either through a skin-crack or a blister or through the lumbrical canal courtesy an abscess in the proximal volar space.

Clinical Features

The patient first presents with severe constitutional symptoms and edema of the back of the hand. Once the infection localizes, the following signs become evident:

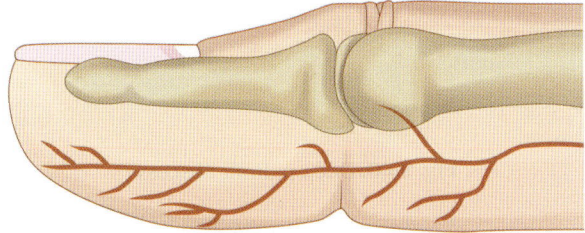

Fig. 33.3: Multiple fibrous septa in distal pulp space

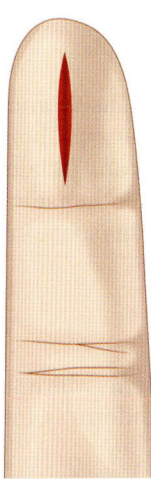

Fig. 33.4: Surgical incision for draining felon

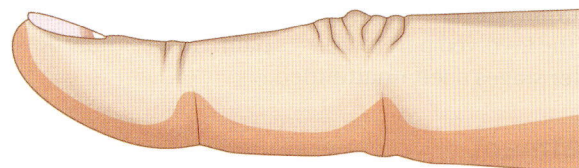

Fig. 33.5: Middle volar space infection

- The base of the affected finger is swollen.
- In severe cases, the adjacent finger is separated.
- Skin over the affected space shows purplish discoloration.
- A fan-shaped blush extends from the web to the dorsum.
- Maximum tenderness is found in the web and base of the finger.

Treatment

Conservative Treatment

Antibiotics and hand immobilization helps in the initial stages.

Surgery

In the later stages, incision and drainage become very essential. Though the swelling is more toward the dorsum, the dangerous part of the abscess remains nearer the palm. If not incised, it may spread into the middle palmar space via the lumbrical canal. Two incisions may be required for drainage, one on the dorsal surface between the metacarpal heads and the other on the palm distal to the distal palmar crease. The web should be left unincised.

DEEP PALMAR ABSCESS

This is rare and accounts for only 1 percent of all hand infections.

Surgical Anatomy

This is a space lined by fascia and in between the flexor tendons above and metacarpal bones below. The fascia of the hypothenar muscles and its lateral border by the fascia of the adductor and other thenar muscles forms its medial border. A fascia divides this space into middle palmar space and a thenar space.

Clinical Features

The patient usually presents with a severe systemic reaction. There is a local pain, tenderness, loss of active movements of the middle and ring fingers and there is generalized gross swelling of the hand and fingers, which resemble an inflated rubber glove (also called frog hand). Similar symptoms are seen in a thenar abscess, but the thumb web is more swollen, index finger is held flexed and active movements of both the index and thumb is lost. With the increasing swelling, the concavity of the palm becomes flat and later convex before it bursts open (Fig. 33.6).

Diagnostic Test

In a deep palmar abscess, passive stretching of the metacarpophalangeal joint is painful while that of interphalangeal joint is painless. In tenosynovitis of the flexor tendons, the passive stretching of both the MP and the IP joints are painful.

Treatment

After the initial conservative treatment, the abscess in the middle palmar space is drained by a central transverse incision at the level of the distal palmar crease in line with the middle finger extending ulna wards towards the hypothenar eminence. Abscess in the thenar space is drained by a curved incision in the thumb web parallel to the border of the first dorsal interosseous muscle.

TENOSYNOVITIS

These are serious infections and are due to infection of the fibrous sheaths and synovial lining of the flexor tendons of the hand.

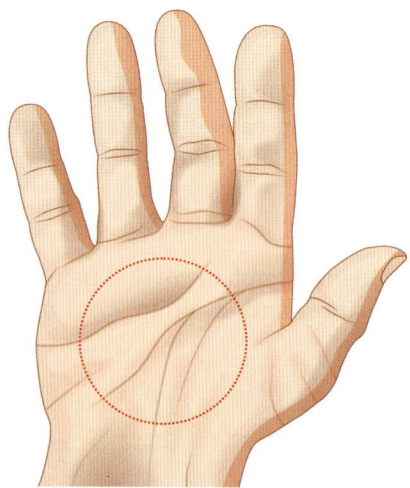

Fig. 33.6: Deep palmar abscess

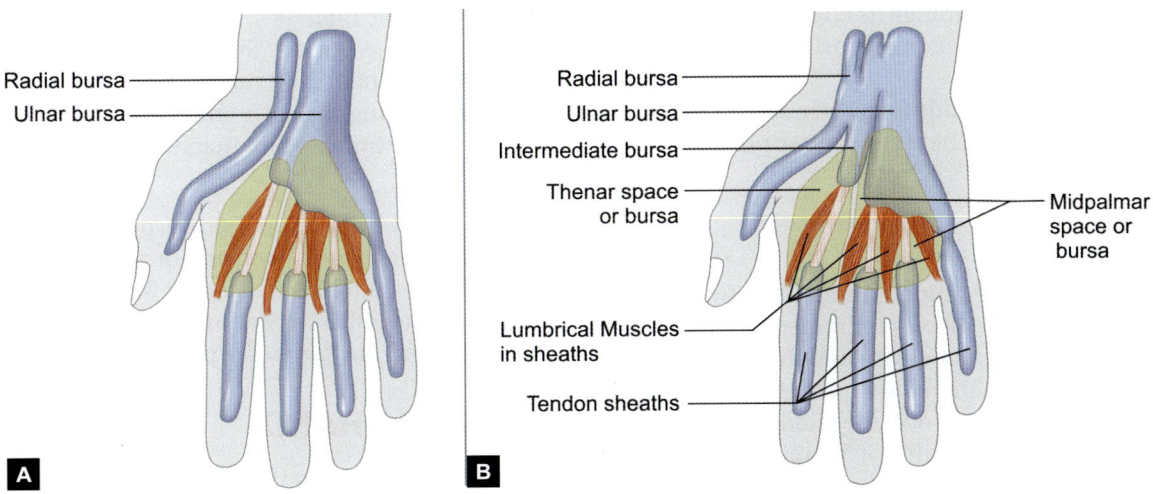

Figs 33.7A and B: (A) Radial; (B) Ulnar bursae of the hand

Surgical Anatomy

The fibrous and synovial sheaths of the flexor tendons of the hand are arranged in two groups: the radial and ulnar bursae (Figs 33.7A and B). The radial bursa is the smaller of the two and it lines the flexor tendon of the thumb and extends 1–2 cm above the wrist up to the distal end of the tendon. The ulnar bursa encloses the synovial sheaths of the index, middle, ring, and little fingers. Distally, those for the index, middle and ring fingers, it extends up to the level of transverse palmar cause; and for the little finger, it extends throughout the length of the tendons. The ulnar bursa encloses tendons of flexor digitorum superficialis and profundus of the above fingers. These two bursae may communicate with each other.

Etiology

The causative organisms are usually due to *S. aureus* or *S. pyogenes*. Penetrating injuries of the tendon sheaths, extension of the infection from its terminal pulp space, etc. are some of the common modes of infection. The consequences of tenosynovitis are disastrous, as it may lead to adhesions, rupture if infection is severe, and loss of gliding movements.

Clinical Features

The patient complains of pain, swelling, and the affected finger is motionless. Active or passive extensions of the fingers are very painful. The classical local signs include

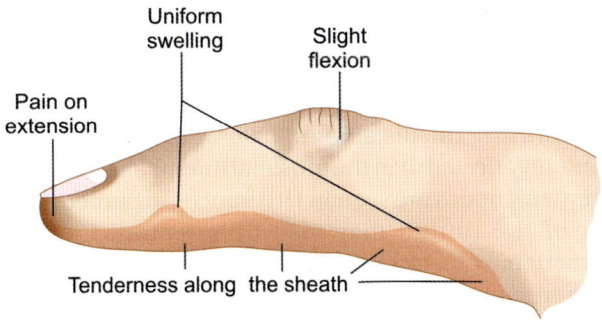

Fig. 33.8: Tenosynovitis of a finger showing its four typical features

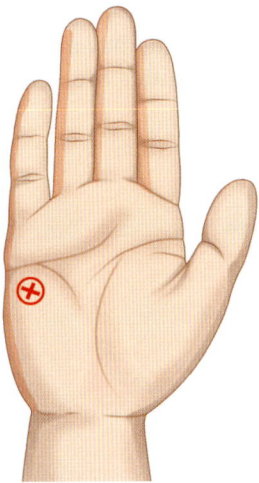

Fig. 33.9: Kanavel's sign

the swelling of the finger through its entire length, flexion of the finger with marked pain on extension, and tenderness over the sheath.

In tenosynovitis of the little finger (Fig. 33.8), tenderness can be elicited at a point in between the two palmar creases. This is called the 'Kanavel's sign' (Fig. 33.9).

Treatment

Early treatment with antibiotics is started. In the early stages of pus formation, abscess is drained by a transverse incision at the distal palmar crease and the proximal edge of the sheath is opened. Then the sheath is opened distally through a midcarpal incision over the middle phalanx. If the infection has progressed far, then a full midlateral incision may be required. Sloughed tendons require excision.

ARTHRITIC HAND

The following arthritic conditions affect the hand.

Rheumatoid arthritis: The rheumatoid hand is discussed on page 568.

Osteoarthritis: The distal interphalangeal joints are more commonly affected than the proximal interphalangeal joints. Heberden's nodes are seen in DIP joints. Carpometacarpal joint of the thumb may also be affected. Cartilage destruction, spur formation, and limited motion are the common sequel (see Fig. 47.24).

Lupus erythematosus: This involves the skin over the nose as well as tendons and joints. Periarticular soft tissue and tendons are affected very severely; joints are grossly deformed at the metacarpophalangeal joints.

Psoriasis: Psoriatic arthritis has an incidence of about 7 percent and the deformities are similar to rheumatoid arthritis.

Reiter's syndrome: This is described as a triad of conjunctivitis, urethritis, and synovitis. Synovitis is asymmetrical and heel pain, back pain, and nail deformities are seen. More common in young males, it attacks the lower limbs more than the upper limbs. More than 90 percent resolve on its own.

Gout: It usually presents as a single, painful, red joint in an adult male. The joint is swollen, hot, tender, and is usually confused to a cellulitis or abscess and drained. This is a disease due to massive deposits of monosodium urate crystals around the joints (see page 582).

PARALYTIC HAND

This is mainly due to peripheral nerve involvement of the upper limbs. Discussed at great length in the chapter on peripheral nerve injuries.

BIBLIOGRAPHY

1. Beasley RW. Principles of tendon transfer. Orthop Clin North Am. 1970;2:433.
2. Beasley RW. Surgery of the hand and finger amputations. Orthop Clin North Am. 1981;12:763.
3. Carter SJ, Mersheimer WL. Infections of the hand. Orthop Clin North Am. 1981;455.
4. Clinkscales GS (Jr). Complications in the management of fractures in hand injuries. South Med J. 1970;63:704.
5. Jones JM, Schenck RR, Chesney RB. Digital replantation and amputation: comparison of function. J Hand Surg. 1982;7:183.
6. Riordan DC. Tendon transfers in hand surgery. J Hand Surg. 1983;8:748.
7. Verdan CE. Practical considerations for primary and secondary repair in flexor tendon injuries. Surg Clin North Am. 1964;44:951.
8. Wakefield AR. The management of flexor tendon injuries. Surg Clin North Am. 1960;40:267.

SECTION

4

Common Back Problems

➲ Low Backache and Repetitive Stress Injury

34 CHAPTER

Low Backache and Repetitive Stress Injury

INTRODUCTION

Low backache is a very common problem and has a ubiquitous distribution. Among the galaxy of causative factors, both spinal and extra spinal, the most common cause of low backache seems to be the lumbar disk disease. Bad posture plays a very significant role in the genesis of this disease. So much is the contribution of bad posture towards this problem that one can categorically conclude that low backache is all about disk degeneration predisposed by poor posture. A thorough expertise of the posture, disk disease, and back care will enable the student to understand and treat this malady in his or her both patients and household. Other causes of low backache are merely mentioned and the students are suggested to refer suitable chapters for details.

Note:
Low backache refers to pain from the low lumbar areas, lumbosacral area, and both the SI joints.

EPIDEMIOLOGY OF BACKACHE

Backache, which was known as an ancient curse, is now known as a modern international epidemic. Eighty percent of the population is affected by this symptom at sometime in life. Impairments of back and spine are ranked as the most frequent cause of limitation of activity in people younger than 45 years. In 2 percent of the population, backache is the presenting complaint in general practitioner's clinic. In 78 percent men and 89 percent women, specific cause was not known. It was believed that bad posture was responsible for most of these cases. The cost to the society and the patient for treatment, compensation, etc. is very high.

POSTURE

Posture is defined as the positional relationship of the different regions of the body to each other. It is divided into:
- Standing
- Sitting
- Recumbent positions.

The features of normal posture are as follows:
- Moderate lordosis of cervical and lumbar spines.
- Kyphosis of the thoracic and sacrococcygeal sections.
- Forward pelvic inclination of 30°.
- Neutral rotation of femur.
- Plumb line dropped from the mastoid process passes through the middle of the shoulder and hip, just anterior to the knee and lateral malleolus of the ankle.

PATHOLOGICAL PHYSIOLOGY

In the course of evolution from quadruped to orthograde animal, the relatively straight spine develops forward (neck and low back) and backward curves (thoracic and sacral) as it yields to the forces of gravity. Paraspinal and glutei muscles maintain the erect posture. There is a continuous minimal muscular contraction called the postural tone.

These physiologic curves give the spine its S shape. It is imperative to maintain this S curve in all our erect activities failing which spine becomes unbalanced (Fig. 34.1).

When the spine becomes displaced and unbalanced, a greater number of muscle fibers are called into play at more frequent intervals to keep the spine straight. Thus, fatigue develops earlier. This fatigue causes muscle insufficiency because of which the spine sags putting the strain on the ligaments and posterior articulating facets. Changes occur at the facet joints and the lumbosacral junction.

Posture of the hip joint is the key to that of the whole body because it determines the pelvic inclination, the pelvis being the foundation for the spine and rotation of the legs. Normal angle is 28–31°.

Functional Anatomy

In the upright position spine has a stabilizing function. The body weight is transmitted through the shoulder girdle to the thorax and abdominal cavity, the hydraulic action of which enables the weight to be carried towards the pelvis. Bad posture with lax abdominal muscles impairs the function of the hydraulic system overloading several segments of the spine (Figs 34.2A and B). In all upright position other than that of the physiological vertical axes, the strain on the structures like disks and ligaments is quite high. Furthermore, stabilization of the muscles is less good during movements, especially if performed abruptly or associated with lifting of a weight. Thus, it can be concluded that postural defects, overloading and abrupt unbalanced movements are frequently responsible for backache (Fig. 34.3).

> **Remember**
> - Posture is an entity seen only in human beings, thanks to the two-legged posture.
> - Backache is a very common malady next only to headache and affects nearly 80 percent of the population.
> - Most common cause of backache is bad posture, which increases the strain on the disks and ligaments causing faster disk degeneration.
> - Any abrupt, unbalanced, and unwarranted movements upset the stabilizing function of the back muscles increasing load on the disks.
> - Hence, bad posture, overloading and abrupt unbalanced movements are the causes of disk rupture or prolapse.

Structures Involved in Backache (Figs 34.4A to C)

- *Vertebral bodies:* Micro-crush fractures, and spondylosis.
- *Intervertebral disks:* Disk degeneration and prolapse.
- *Posterior intervertebral joints:* Degenerative lesions, synovitis, sprain, etc.
- *Ligaments and small intervertebral muscles*: Elongation, excessive use, reflex contractures.
- *Posterior longitudinal ligament*: Elongation and irritation by discal protrusion.
- *Nerves:* Irritation or compression of the spinal nerve roots by disk herniation or irritation of the sensory nerves of the various paravertebral structures.

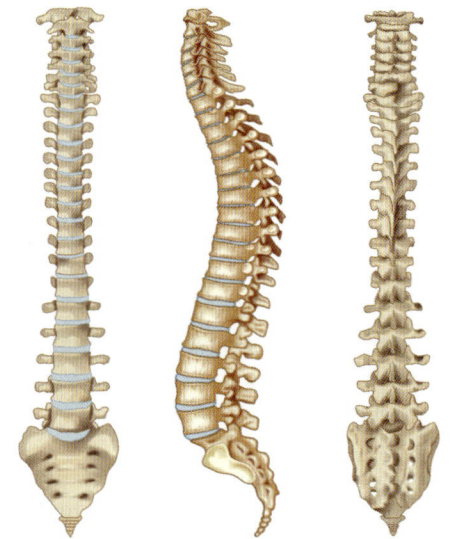

Fig. 34.1: Normal appearance of vertebral column

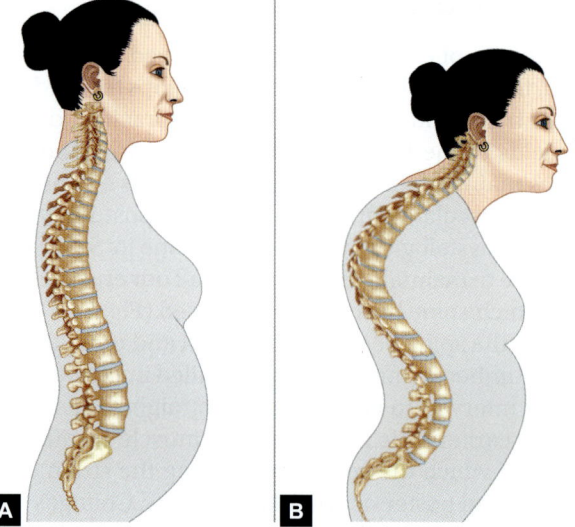

Figs 34.2A and B: Postures: (A) Normal posture; (B) Bad posture

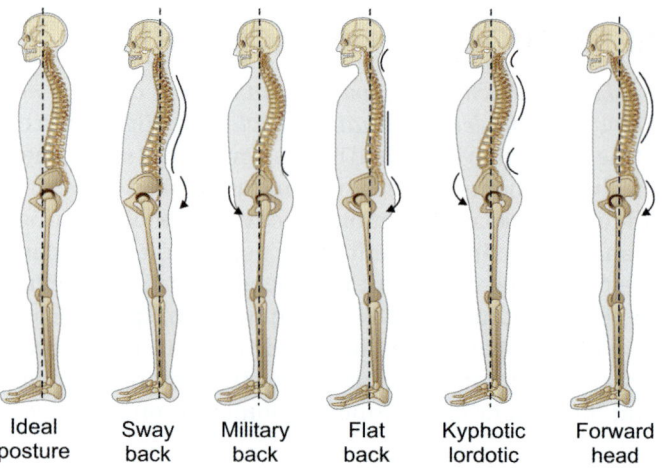

Ideal posture — Sway back — Military back — Flat back — Kyphotic lordotic — Forward head

Fig. 34.3: Common postural problems

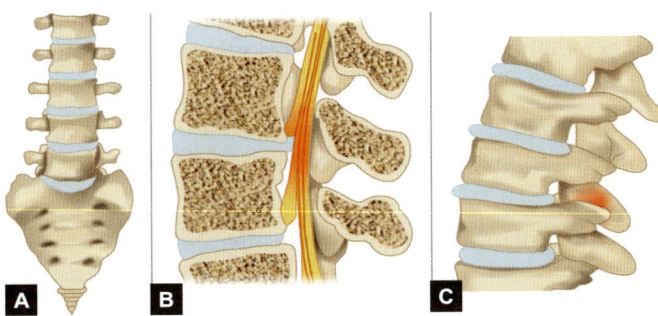

Figs 34.4A to C: Structures involved in low backache: (A) Osteophytes seen in lumbar spondylosis; (B) Compression on PLL and nerves due to disk protrusion; (C) Disk disease and facet joint arthritis

> **Remember**
> *Factors keeping the spine healthy*
> - Genetics.
> - Muscle strength and balance.
> - Flexibility.
> - Posture.
> - Body weight.
> - Adaptation to stresses.

LUMBAR DISK DISEASE AND DISK PROLAPSE

DISK ANATOMY

Development of spine starts from the third week of intrauterine life and continues until third decade of life. There are 23 disks throughout the spine, absent only in atlantoaxial articulation. It is thinnest in the thoracic region and thickest in the lumbar. Each disk is interposed between the bodies of a pair of vertebrae (see Fig. 34.1). Body of each vertebra is covered by a thin end plate of a bone, which is perforated by numerous tiny holes. This in turn is covered by a hyaline cartilage, which may be considered as the outermost portion of the disk.

Anteriorly and laterally, the bodies and the disks are bounded firmly by the anterior longitudinal ligament and posteriorly by the posterior longitudinal ligament, which is weak. The intervertebral disks in adults are avascular; the cells within it are sustained by diffusion of nutrients into the disk through the pores in the bodies. Movements and weight bearing help in diffusion. Degeneration of the disk may be prompted by changes in the permeability of the cartilage end plate.

The disk consists of two parts; centrally, it is *nucleus pulposus*, which is made-up of collagen fibrils, fibrocytes, chondrocytes, gelatinous matrix, and water and salt. Peripherally, it has *annulus fibrosus, which* is a fibro cartilaginous tissue. It is thick anteriorly and thin posteriorly more so in the posterolateral aspect. *Hence, poster lateral disk prolapse is more common.* The fibers of annulus are joined by diagonal fibers also known as Sharpe's fibers.

Neural fibers in the outer rings of the annulus contain branches of the sinovertebral nerve dorsally and ventrally branches from the sympathetic chain.

With age, water content of the disk decreases, fibrous tissue and cartilage cells increase, and the nucleus becomes granular and friable.

> **Mystifying Facts About the Disks**
> - There is no disk between C_1 and C_2
> - It is avascular and gets its nutrition through local diffusion
> - The nutrition of the disk is best in side lying position
> - Eighty percent of the nutrition process takes place in the first one hour of night's rest
> - The outer annulus fibrosus of the disk is innervated by the sinovertebral nerve and gray ramus communicants of the sympathetic chain.

DISK PHYSIOLOGY

Disk apart from giving the spine its mobility functions as a shock absorber. Following loss of disk, the vertebral body reacts to abnormal pressure forces by hypertrophy bone formation at the surface revealed as sclerosis and osteophyte formation. Schmorl's node is the disk material, which has escaped into the body through the pores and is walled off by the fibrous tissue.

> **Remember**
> *About disk*
> - It gives spine the mobility.
> - It acts as a shock absorber.
> - It is fibrocartilaginous.
> - It increases the height of the spine by 25 percent.
> - Centrally, it has a nucleus pulposus and peripherally annulus fibrosus.
> - It is avascular.
> - Annulus fibers are weak posteriorly; hence, posterolateral disk prolapse is more common.
> - With age, water content of the disk falls.

NATURAL HISTORY OF LUMBAR DISK DISEASE

All spines degenerate with advancing age and so does the intervertebral disks. Degenerative process is divided into three stages:

Stage of Dysfunction

- Seen between 15 and 45 years of age.
- Circumferential and radial tears are seen in the disk annulus.
- Localized synovitis of the facet joints is seen.

Stage of Instability

- Seen between 35 and 70 years of age.
- There is an internal disruption of the disk.
- Progressive disk resorption takes place.
- Degeneration of facet joints with lax capsules, subluxation, and joint erosions are seen.

Stage of Stabilization

- Seen over 60 years of age.
- Progressive development of hypertrophic bone about the disk and facet joints leading to segmental stiffening or frank ankylosis is seen.

Disk herniation is considered as a complication of disk degeneration in stages II and I (Fig. 34.5). Spinal stenosis is a complication in late instability and early stabilization stages. Disk can herniate either into the body as Schmorl's node or posteriorly towards the canal compressing the nerve roots.

CLASSIFICATION OF PROLAPSED INTERVERTEBRAL DISK (FIG. 34.6)

Disk bulging or protrusion: This refers to some eccentric accumulation of nucleus with slight deformity of the annulus.

Prolapsed disk is the one in which eccentric nucleus produces a definite deformity as it works through the fibers of the annulus.

Extruded disk: Here, the disk comes out into the canal and impinges on the adjacent nerve root (Fig. 34.7).

Sequestrated disk: Here the nuclear material has separated from the disk itself and potentially migrates.

> **Interesting Facts**
> Do you know at what levels lumbar disk prolapse most commonly occur does?
> $L_{4-5} > L_5S_1 > L_{3-4} > L_{2-3} > L_{1-2}$

ETIOLOGY OF DISK HERNIATION

The etiology consists of risk factors and the definitive causes resulting in disk herniation.

Risk Factors

- Jobs requiring heavy and repetitive weightlifting (Fig. 34.8).
- Use of machine tools.
- Operation of motor vehicles.
- Cigarette smokers and tobacco consumers.
- Anxiety and depression.
- Stressful occupation as in doctors, police, etc.
- Women with greater number of pregnancies.
- Obesity and other cardiovascular risk factors.
- Monotonous work, working overtime, etc.
- Improper postural habits.

> **Do You Know the Relative Load on Your Spine Measured at L_{3-4}?**
> - Lying on the sides (25%)
> - Standing 100 percent

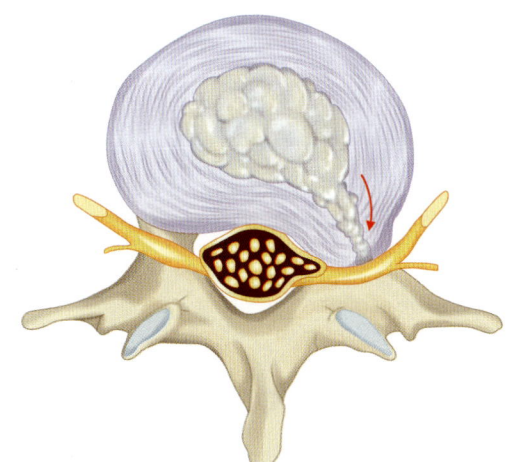

Fig. 34.5: Posterolateral disk herniation

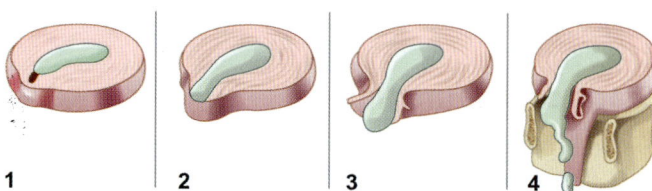

Fig. 34.6: Types of prolapse disk: (1) Bulge disk, (2) Prolapse disk, (3) Extruded disk, and (4) Sequestrated disk

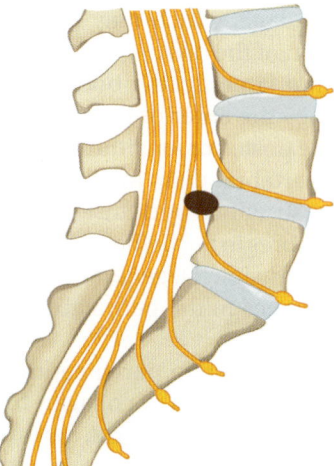

Fig. 34.7: Disk prolapse compressing the nerve root

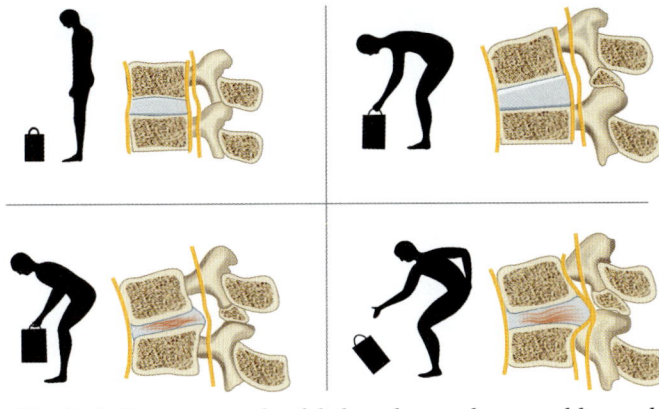

Fig. 34.8: Common mode of disk prolapses due to sudden and improper weightlifting

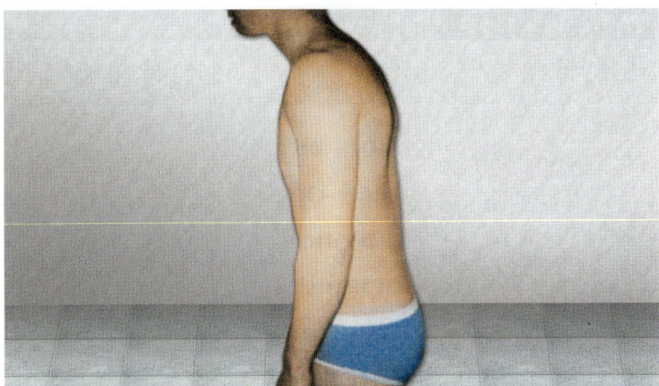

Fig. 34.9: Clinical presentation in a patient with disk slip (Clinical photo)

- Seated 145 percent
- Standing with forward bend — 150 percent
- Sitting with forward bend — 180 percent

Generally,
- Load is better in supported sitting than unsupported sitting
- Lumbar support decreases the load.

Definitive Causes

- Degenerative changes make the disk susceptible to trauma. Any trauma, which suddenly increases the pressure, will result in rupture of the posterior fibers of the annulus, e.g. weightlifting, fall on the buttocks, direct trauma to the back, twisting movements and occupation involving flexion and lifting motions.
- Disk may also rupture during pregnancy, labor and after prolonged bed rest due to disk softening.
- Disk rupture without any cause is due to degenerative process.

Remember
About disk disease
- It is due to aging process.
- It passes through three stages.
- There are four types of disk prolapse.
- Disk prolapse is a complication of stages I and II.
- Herniation can take place into the body or posteriorly into spinal canal.

Clinical Features

Clinical features can be discussed under three headings:

Low backache: Back pain is common in the second decade, disk disease and disk herniation in the third or fourth decade. *The usual history of lumbar disk herniation is of repetitive low back pain, radiating to the buttocks and decreased by rest.* Pain is increased by flexion episode, sitting, straining, sneezing, coughing, etc. Pain is decreased by rest and in semi-Fowler position (Fig. 34.9).

Radiculopathy: This refers to pain in the distribution of the sciatic nerve and is invariably due to disk herniation. This is called as sciatica. *Leg pain equal to or more than the back pain evidence the radicular pain from the nerve root compression due to herniated disk.* Pain usually begins in the lower back radiating to the sacroiliac regions, buttocks, and thigh. The radicular pain usually extends below the knee.

Nerve root compression: About 95 percent of the disk prolapse takes place through the L_{4-5} region compressing the L_5 nerve root (Fig. 34.10). The other nerve roots commonly involved are L_4 and S_1 due to disk prolapse between L_{3-4} and L_5–S_1 respectively. Table 34.1 shows the various clinical manifestations following nerve root compression.

Remember One Question Test: Radicular Pain
Between the knee and the ankle, where is the pain?
- Front → L_4
- Side → L_5
- Back → S_1

EXAMINATION OF THE BACK (TABLE 34.2)

Inspection: Note any postural defects like scoliosis, lordosis, or kyphosis. In intervertebral disk size prolapse (IVDP) there

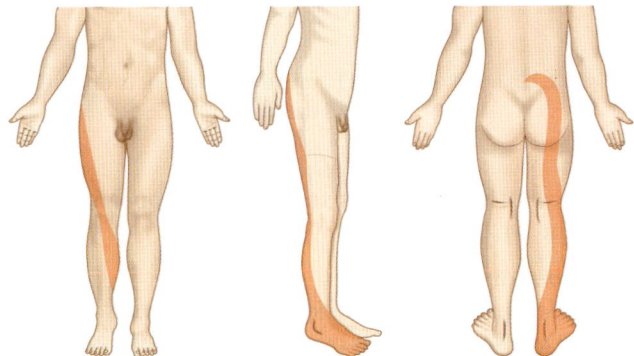

Fig. 34.10: Dermatome pattern from above downwards belong to L_4 L_5 S_1 nerve roots respectively

TABLE 34.1: Level of disk prolapse and nerve root compression

Disc prolapse between	Pain Reflexes loss	Radiation *SLRT	Sensory loss	Motor loss		
L_3 and L_4 L_4 nerve root is involved	Lumbar region	Along the antero-medial aspect of the thigh	Medial shin	Quadriceps	Knee jerk	Normal
L_4 L_5 95% disk prolapse occur here L_5 root involved	Lumbar region, groin, sacroiliac region	Lateral thigh, leg, dorsum of the foot and hallux	Hallux area	Extensor hallucis muscle	Medial hamstrings	Reduced
L_4 and S_1 S_1 root is involved	Same as above	Buttocks, posterior thigh, leg and lateral foot	Lateral foot	Gastrocnemius	Ankle jerk	Reduced

Easy way to remember
L_4 root involvement—remember '4' heads of quadriceps. Hence, knee jerk lost (Fig. 34.11)
L_5 root involvement—remember '5' toes—Great toe and lateral 4 toes lose extension (Fig. 34.12)
S_1 root involvement—remember 'A' of tendo-Achilles. Hence, ankle jerk lost (Fig. 34.13)

*SLRT—straight leg raising test

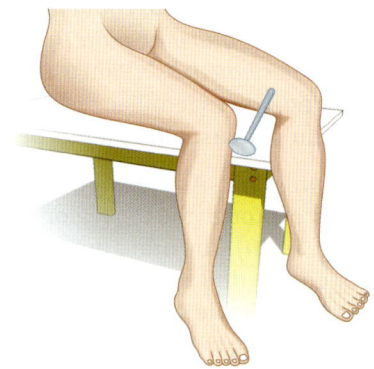

Fig. 34.11: Involvement of L_4 myotome (Patient is unable to extend the knee and loss of knee reflex)

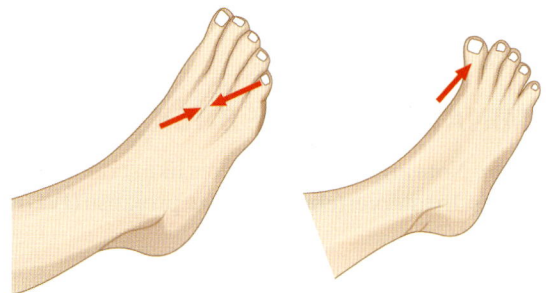

Fig. 34.12: Involvement of L_5 myotome, patient is unable to extend the toes

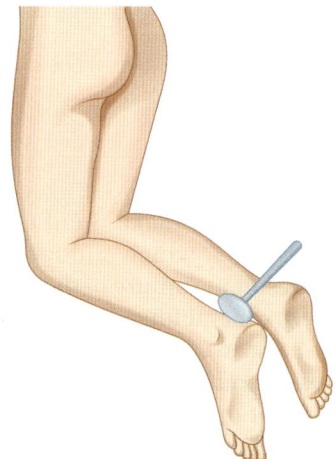

Fig. 34.13: S_1 myotome involvement loss of ankle jerk and plantar flexion

- Palpable tender indurations of small intervertebral muscles.
- Tenderness at the level of posterior articulation of the involved segment and pain on percussion of affected intervertebral space.

b. *Movements:* All the movements of the spine are tested and found to be restricted in all directions.

Evaluation of neurological system: The dermatome and the myotomal distribution are carefully analyzed (see Table 34.1) to detect the level of lesion.

Clinical tests: These tests are based on the stretching of sciatic nerve over the prolapsed disk:
a. Forward bending to touch the toes.
b. Sitting and alternatively extending one leg and then the other.
c. *Slump test* sitting bent forward and extending one leg and then the other.

will be loss of lumbar lordosis and the back appears flat (Figs 34.22 and 34.23).

Palpation consists of:
a. *Tenderness:* Look for the following points:
  - Diffuse tenderness over the lower back
  - Localized tender infiltrates of the skin and subcutaneous tissue.

CHAPTER 34: Low Backache and Repetitive Stress Injury

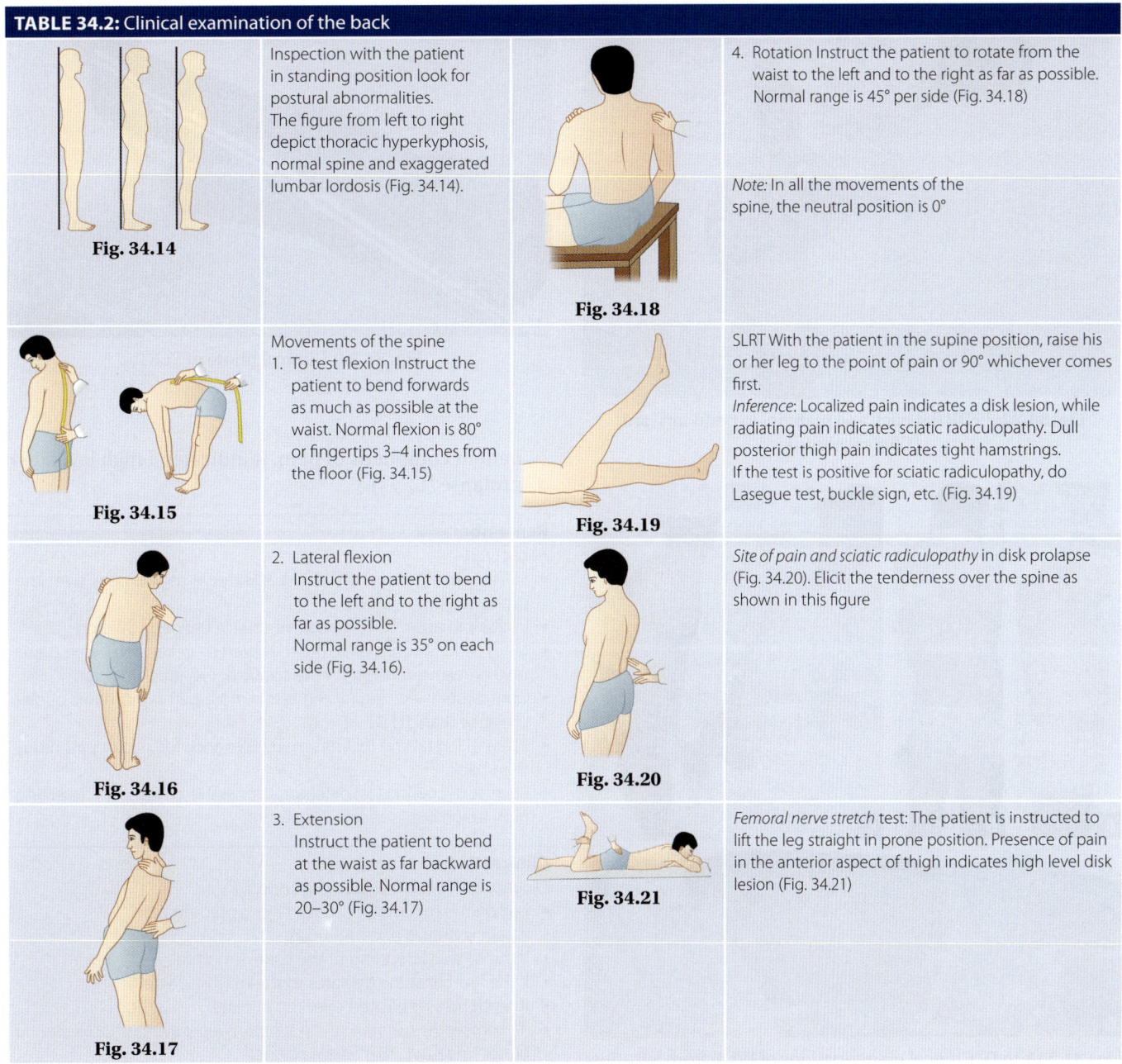

TABLE 34.2: Clinical examination of the back

d. *Straight leg raising test (SLRT):* Patient is in supine position, the examiner raises the leg straight one after the other. Up to 30°, nerve is not put under stretch. Between 30 and 70°, nerve encounters the prolapsed disk and the patient complains of pain. Beyond 70° if the patient complains of pain, it is usually not due to disk prolapse but could be due to sacroiliac joint involvement (Fig. 34.24).

Modifications of SLRT

- Lasègue's test: Here, the hip is flexed, knee is flexed, and the leg is slowly straightened.
- Bückling's sign: Perform an SLRT until the patient complains of pain. Now ask the patient to flex the knee. Pain decreases due to relief of tension on the nerve.
- Sicard's test: After doing SLRT, dorsiflex the great toe. This puts further tension on the sciatic nerve and the patient complains of pain.
- Fajersztajn's test: After doing SLRT, dorsiflex the foot. This tenses the sciatic nerve and the patient complains of pain.
- *Well leg raising test:* Here, the patient is asked to perform SLRT of the normal limb. If the patient complains of pain on the affected side, then it is highly suggestive of disk

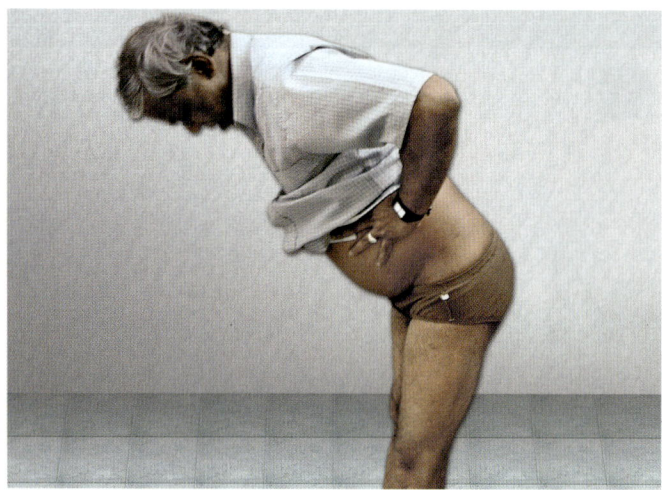

Fig. 34.22: IVDP flat back and inability to bend forward (Clinical photo)

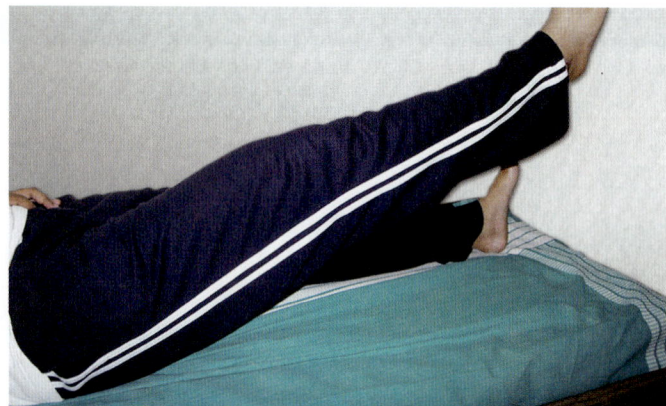

Fig. 34.24: Clinical photo of SLRT

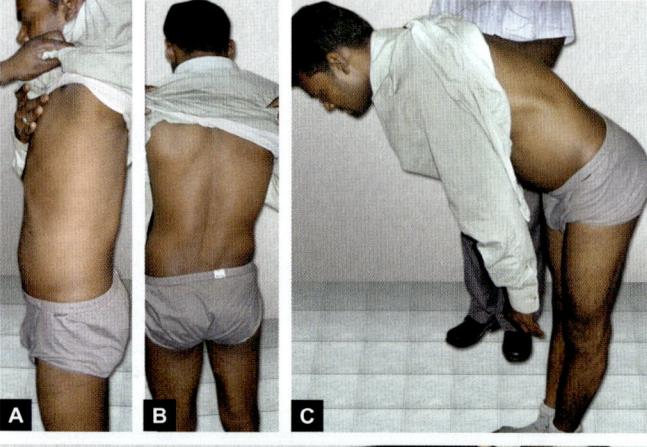
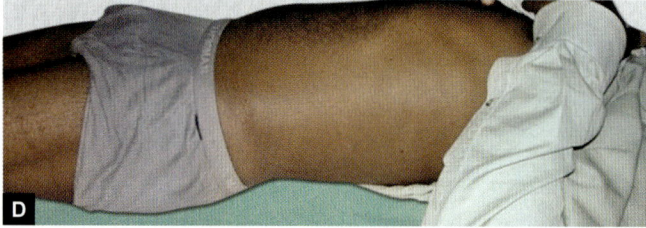

Figs 34.23A to D: Clinical manifestations of IVDP from left—loss of lordosis, scoliosis, movement restricted and flat back

prolapse and this is a pathognomonic test, which has more relevance than the conventional SLRT.
- *Bilateral straight leg raising test:* Here, patient is asked to raise both the legs simultaneously. This is a test for the sacroiliac joint rather than the spine. During the first 70°, stress is on the SI joint, over 70° stress is on the lumbar spine.
- *Femoral nerve stretch test (reverse SLRT):* Here, the patient is in prone position and is asked to lift the leg straight. This puts a stretch on the femoral nerve. If the patient complains of pain, it indicates a high level disk prolapse (L_{1-2-3}).

Remember
About SLRT
- SLRT exerts tension on the sciatic nerve as it passes over the prolapsed disk.
- In disk prolapse, SLRT is positive usually between 30° and 70°.
- Many modifications of SLRT either exert more tension (Fajersztajn's test) or relieve tension on the sciatic nerve. (Buckling sign).
- Contralateral well leg raising test is more pathognomonic of disk prolapse than SLRT.
- Bilateral leg raising test has more relevance for SI joint pathology than back.
- Reverse leg raising test or femoral nerve stretch test is for detecting high lesion like L_1 root involvement.

Clinical Facts
Diagnosis of the disk disease is a suspect, if:
- Leg pain is minimal and back pain is predominant.
- If pain is bizarre or continuous.
- If the forward bending of the spine is normal.
- If the lumbar spine deviates to the opposite side.
- If tenderness is elicited over the midline.
- *Remember the hallmark of disk disease is repetitive low backache and buttock pain, which is relieved by rest.*
- It is important to note that paresthesiae and motor signs are seen in 96 percent of cases of disk prolapse. Sensory signs are seen in 80 percent. They are distributed along the involved nerve roots as explained earlier.

Remember
Diagnostic clues to detect high level disk lesion involving L_1 and L_2 nerve roots
- Pain in the groin or testicles.
- Cauda equina lesion.
- Positive femoral stretch test.
- Atrophy of the involved limb.
- 95 percent of the disk ruptures usually occur at L_4L_5.

Investigations

Radiography of the back is not very reliable as normal findings are observed in 7–46 percent of the cases. Disk space is reduced in old cases; but in acute cases, it is maintained. Oblique view is recommended to rule out spondylolysis. It also helps to detect lumbar spondylosis (Figs 34.25 and 34.26).

Myelography consists of injecting radiopaque dye (Myodil was used earlier now it is the water-soluble Iopamiro 300, which is being used) into the spinal canal and taking radiographs of the back. It is helpful in detecting the intraspinal lesions, spinal stenosis, and cases of previously operated (Fig. 34.27) backs. It is also indicated when the diagnosis is in doubt. It is an invasive procedure and is no longer performed. It is now replaced by noninvasive procedures like CT scan and MRI.

CT scan: It is a very useful noninvasive, painless outpatient procedure. It gives a cross-sectional study of the pathology. It, however, fails to detect intraspinal lesion, arachnoiditis, and scar from disk herniation. It helps to detect the foraminal stenosis and the lateral disk prolapse (Fig. 34.28).

MRI: This is also an extremely useful, painless, noninvasive outpatient procedure. It helps to detect the intraspinal lesion, helps to examine the entire spine, and identifies degenerative disk (Figs 34.29 and 34.30). However, it is expensive and hence prohibitive.

Discography: After identifying the disk correctly, through a needle, a radiopaque dye is injected into the space. This reproduces the pain experienced by the patient previously and is relieved by injecting Xylocaine. This confirms the diagnosis. It is a painful procedure and can introduce infection into the disk. Hence, it is less practiced.

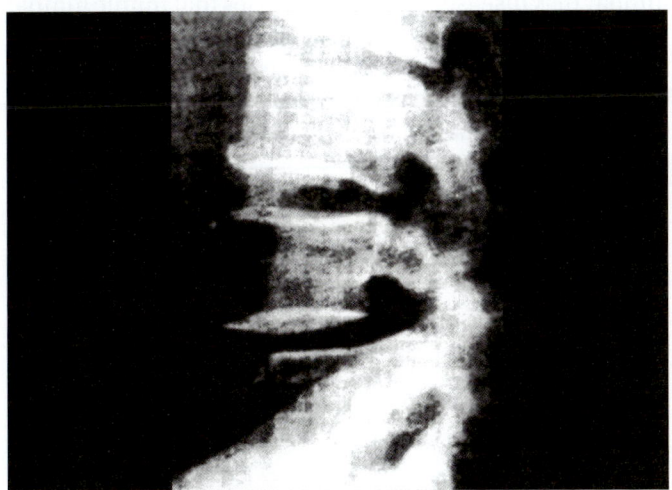

Fig. 34.25: Radiograph showing lumbar spondylosis

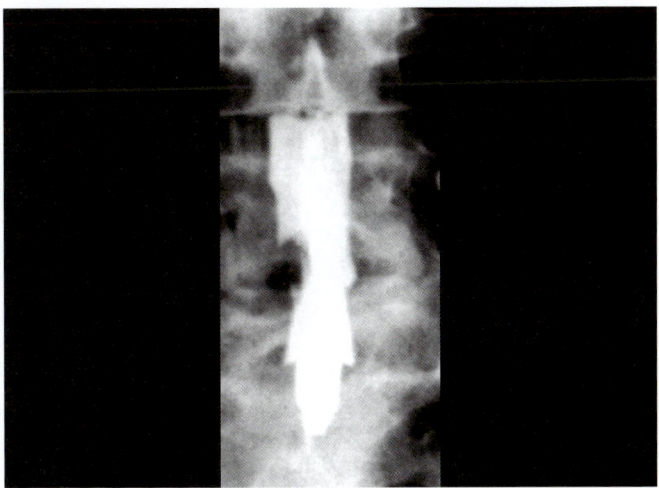

Fig. 34.27: Myelographic study of the lumbar spine

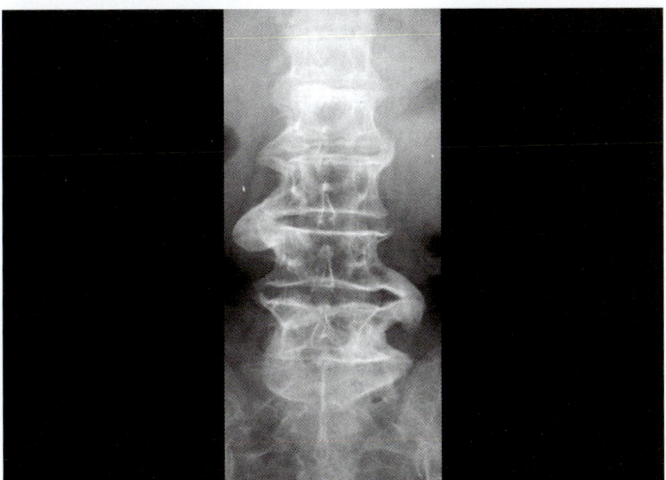

Fig. 34.26: Plain X-ray showing features of lumbar spondylosis (note the bridging osteophytes)

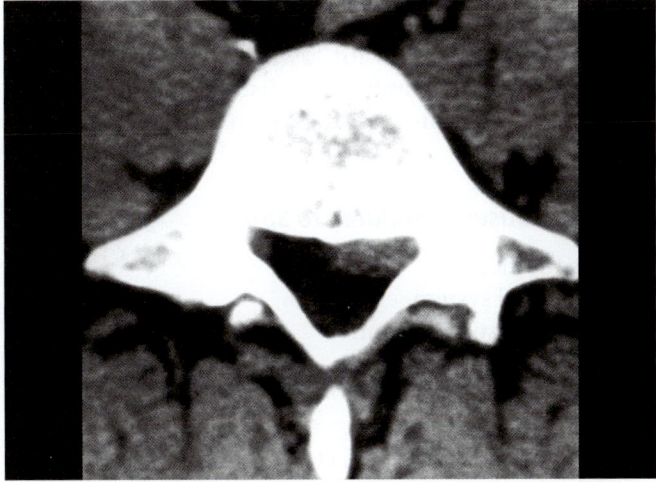

Fig. 34.28: CT scan showing posterolateral disk herniation

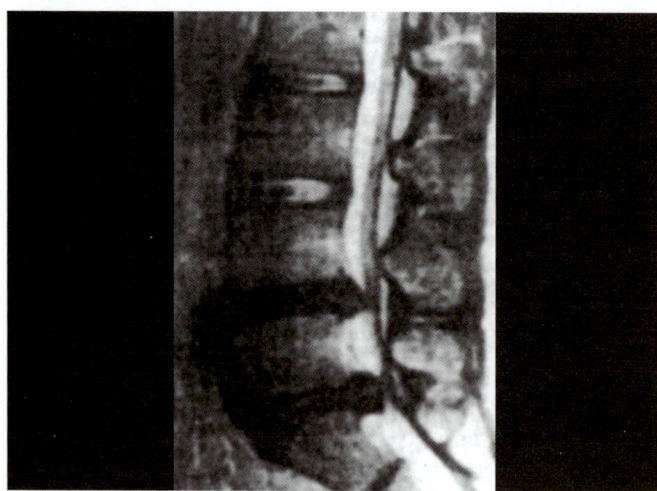

Fig. 34.29: MRI of lumbar spine showing multiple disk prolapse

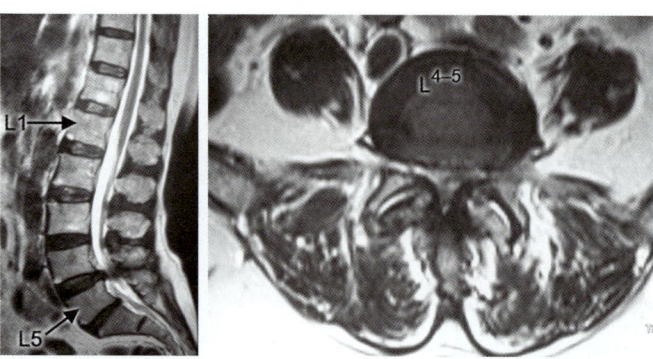

Fig. 34.30: MRI showing L_5–S_1 disk prolapse

Other tests of diagnostic importance are *bone scans, EMG,* routine laboratory studies, injection studies, etc.

Differential Diagnosis

There are many causes for lower backache. The most common one being lumbar disk disease due to abnormal posture and aging process. The differential diagnosis is as follows:

Extrinsic Causes (Unrelated to Spine)

Diseases of the:
- Urogenital system
- Gastrointestinal system
- Vascular system
- Endocrine system
- Nervous system
- Musculoskeletal system, etc.

Intrinsic Causes (Related to Spine)

Important Causes
- Unstable spondylolisthesis
- Osteoporosis and compression of the vertebrae
- Marked loss of disk height at multiple levels
- Severe scoliosis.

Unimportant Causes
- Lumbar spondylosis
- Mild discopathy
- Arthroses of the facet joints
- Disk calcification
- Spina bifida
- Schmorl's nodes
- Mild-to-moderate scoliosis.

Predominant cause of backache as already suggested is lumbar disk disease. Common diseases that mimic lumbar disk disease include ankylosing spondylitis, multiple myeloma, vascular insufficiency, arthritis of the hip joint, osteoporosis with stress fractures, extradural tumors, peripheral neuropathy, herpes zoster, etc.

> **Do You Know the Common Diagnosis of Low Backache?**
> *Well, Here is a List:*
> - Common low backache (disk disease, muscle and ligament strain and sprain of the back)
> - Myofascial pain
> - Spondylosis
> - Spondylolisthesis
> - Facet syndrome
> - Fibromyalgia
> - Lumbar canal stenosis
>
> *Pitfalls:* Only in 15 percent of the cases of low backaches, accurate diagnosis of a specific cause can be made.

Treatment

The principles of treating low backache due to lumbar disk disease are explained by **three R's**:
- **R**elieve pain in acute cases.
- **R**estore normal movements in chronic cases.
- **R**ecurrence is to be prevented.

The following are the treatment modalities in low backache.

Conservative therapy: *Absolute bed rest is the best treatment for acute low backache.* Ice packs, non-steroidal anti-inflammatory drugs (NSAIDs), muscle relaxants, antidepressants are recommended. Bucks extension skin traction and pelvic traction helps to relieve pain. Walking within limits of comfort is also encouraged. Sitting and riding in a car is discouraged. Back braces or belts are recommended in acute stages. They are discarded as soon as symptoms decrease; otherwise, muscles become weak and hasten the degeneration.

Role of exercises: As the pain decreases, isometric abdominal and lower extremity exercises are begun. Choice of exercises is based on the increase or decrease of pain by extension or flexion. *If pain decreases by extension, extension exercises are recommended. On the other hand, if the pain decreases by flexion, flexion exercises are recommended. Improvements in symptoms with extension are indication of a good prognosis with conservative care.* Lower extremity exercises increase the strength and relieve the stress on the back, but they may increase the lower extremity arthritis. Thus, the true benefit of such treatment may be in the promotion of good posture and body mechanics than strength.

Back education and importance of proper posture is taught. See the pictorial display of proper postural habits and back exercises recommended for prevention of low backache (Tables 34.3 and 34.4).

TABLE 34.3: Proper postural habits (Figs 34.31 to 34.36)

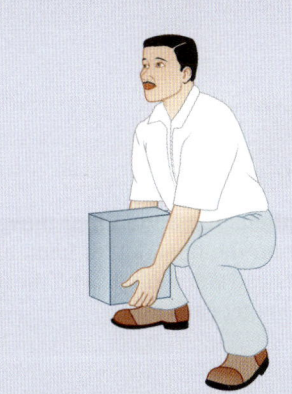

Fig. 34.31: Lifting objects: Bend at your knees and not at your waist. Hold the object you are lifting close to your body, not higher than your chest. It is easier to push rather than pull heavy objects, e.g. furniture, and keep the knees bent while pushing

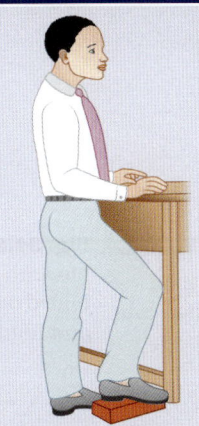

Fig. 34.33: Standing: Keep one foot in front and knees slightly bent while standing upright. If you have to stand for a long time, try keeping one foot higher than the other does, on a low stool. Change your position often

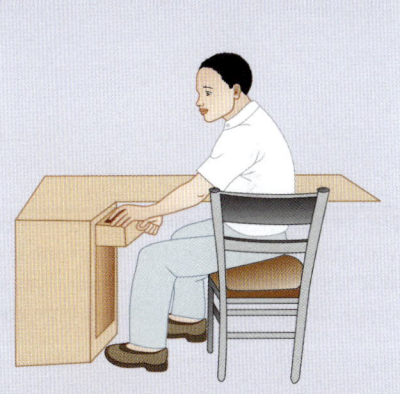

Fig. 34.35: Turning and reaching out: Do not twist your waist. Rather, turn by moving your feet. Keep the phone and such like objects within easy reach; do not strain to reach them. Stand on a stool to reach high objects

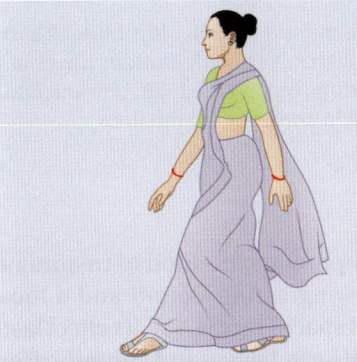

Fig. 34.32: Walking: Walk well with your head high, chin tucked in, toes pointing straight in front. Wear comfortable footwear. Take steps of a natural, comfortable length. Swing the arms naturally

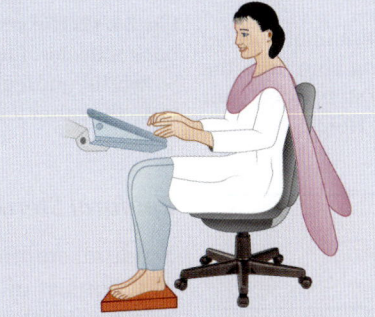

Fig. 34.34: Sitting: Ensure your back is firmly touching the back of the chair. Keep the knees slightly higher than the hips, e.g. by using something to prop up your feet. Sit close to your desk or table to avoid bending forward. Do not sit for too long. In addition, when driving, move the front seat close to the steering wheel and both hands should be kept on the wheel

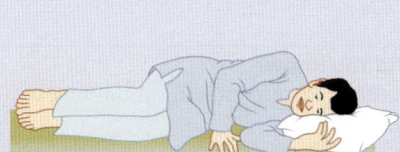

Fig. 34.36: Sleeping: If you sleep on your side, keep knees and lower body bent a little. On your back, put a pillow under your knees. Try not to sleep on your stomach—but if you must, put a pillow under your waist not under your head. Use a firm mattress—neither soft/squashy nor very hard

TABLE 34.4: Exercises for low backache (Figs 34.37 to 34.42)

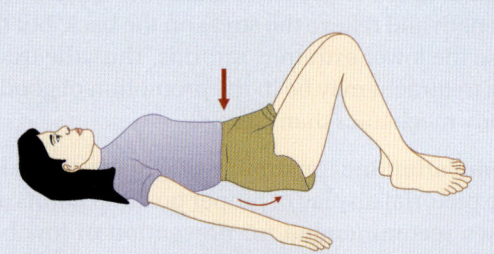

Fig. 34.37: Pelvic tilt: Makes abdominal muscles stronger. Lie on your back, legs bent, and feet flat on the floor with arms to your sides. Push your lower back against the floor— your hips will tilt up. Hold this position for a short while

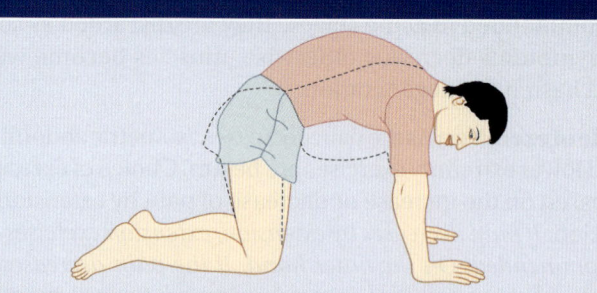

Fig. 34.40: Cat and Camel: Strengthens the back and abdominal muscles. Crouch on hands and knees. Keeping the head parallel to floor, arch your back and then let it gradually sag towards the floor by breathing out. Keep the arms straight

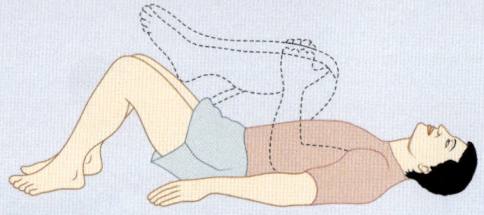

Fig. 34.38: Knees to chest: Lie on your back, knees bent, feet flat, and arms to your sides. Raise first one knee to your chest, then the other, holding them with your hands as shown (or just inside your knee). Bring legs down one at a time and rest. Repeat

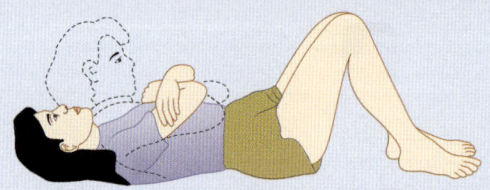

Fig. 34.41: Semi sit-up: Strengthens the abdominal muscles. Lie with your back and feet flat on the floor, knees bent, arms folded on the chest. Lift only your head and shoulders off the floor and hold. Repeat, trying to hold longer each time

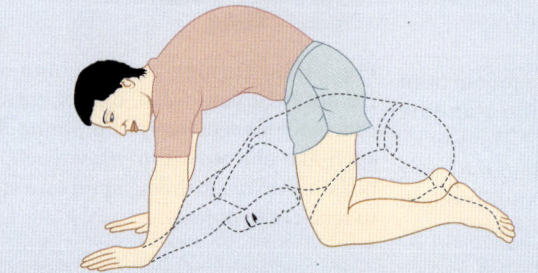

Fig. 34.39: Trunk flex: Stretches the back, abdominal and leg muscles. Crouch on the hands and knees. Bring chin in to the chest, and curve your back upwards. Gradually sit back on your heels, bringing the shoulders down to the floor. Hold

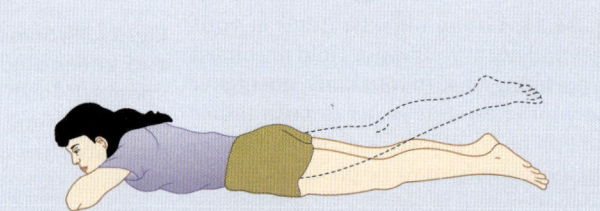

Fig. 34.42: Hip stretch: Strengthens and stretches hip, buttock and back muscles. Lie on the stomach, arms folded under the chin. Slowly lift one leg without bending, but not too high. Lower it and raise the other leg. Keep pelvis in contact with the floor

Did You Know?
Maximal load reduction on the disk with tight corsets is 20–30 percent.

Remember
Contraindications to traction
- Hypertension.
- Peripheral vascular disease.
- Cataracts and glaucoma.
- Labile asthma or COPD.
- Pregnancy, etc.

How traction helps?
- It relieves muscle spasm.
- It may distract the facet joints.
- It may distract the disk space.

Epidural Steroids

Epidural steroids are a symptomatic method of treatment, and consist of injecting a long-acting steroid and a local anesthetic into the epidural space (Fig. 34.43). Its effect lasts for three weeks and is useful for subacute and chronic cases. It also reduces dependence on narcotics in chronic cases.

All About Epidural Steroid Injection
- In vogue since 1950's.
- Effective in approximately 50 percent patients with low backache.
- It decreases inflammation and flushes out inflammatory proteins thereby reducing pain.
- It helps in better back rehabilitation.

CHAPTER 34: Low Backache and Repetitive Stress Injury 459

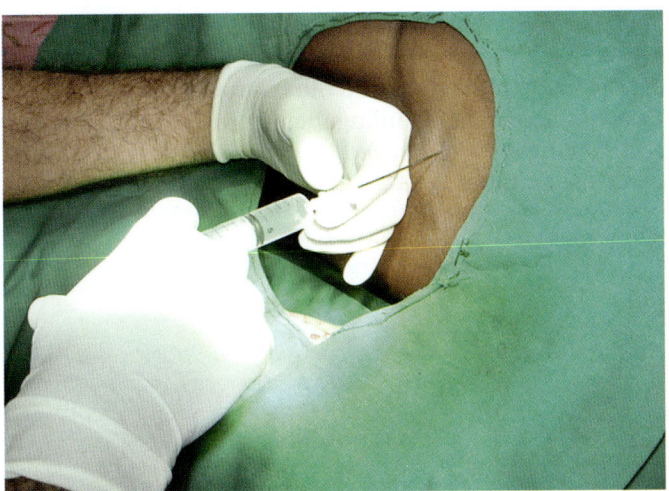

Fig. 34.43: Operative photo showing technique of epidural steroid injection

- Maximum of three injections in a year with a two-week gap is given.
- Adverse features include infection, dural puncture, and arachnoiditis.
- It primarily decreases leg pain.
- After the injection, the patient is advised one-day rest.

Note:
- Each exercise is done one to five times twice daily.
- The number of repetitions should be kept increasing to reach a minimum of ten repetitions twice daily.
- Exercises are to be done slowly and smoothly.

How does Exercise Relieve Low Backache?
- Exercises pump the disk and increase water content.
- Relieves the muscle spasm and increase motion.
- Stretches and mobilizes the facet joints.
- Repetitive motion helps the patient to overcome the fear of movement.
- Decreases the swelling around the nerves.

Surgery

Absolute Indications

- Failed conservative management.
- Marked progressive weakness of muscles.
- Progressive neurological deficit.
- Cauda equina paralysis.

Relative Indications

- Recurrent episodes of incapacitating sciatica.
- Pain unrelieved by complete rest from activity.

Principles of surgery are to see that the pressure on the nerve root is relieved by removing the prolapsed disk. Dissection of muscles and bone removal should be kept at a minimum to prevent weakening of the spine.

Surgical Methods

Laminectomy and disk excision earlier, this was the surgery of choice; but now, it is no longer resorted to as it makes the spine unstable.

Hemilaminectomy: Here, part of the lamina is removed. It is considered by many as extended fenestration approach. If fenestration technique is properly done, hemilaminectomy is not necessary (Fig. 34.44).

Fenestration surgery here, the spine is approached unilaterally and the spine on the opposite side is not exposed. Here, only the contiguous margin of upper and lower laminae is removed and medial facetectomy is done. The disk is now excised. This procedure requires that MRI and radiographic studies correctly locate the affected disk.

Microscopic and Endoscopic lumbar diskectomy (Fig. 34.45) Using an operating microscope or an endoscope, the disk can be excised through a very small incision (<3.5 cm) with minimum damage to the structures and minimal

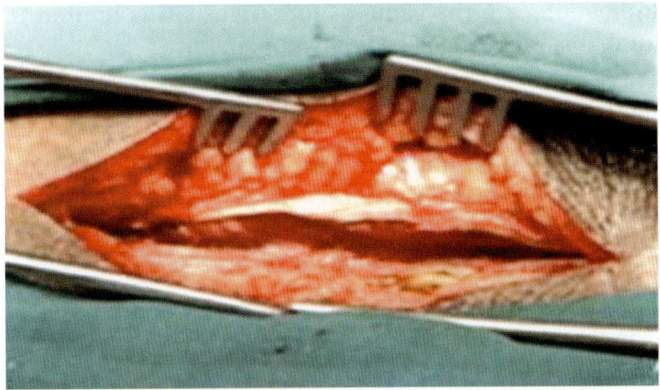

Fig. 34.44: Hemilaminectomy

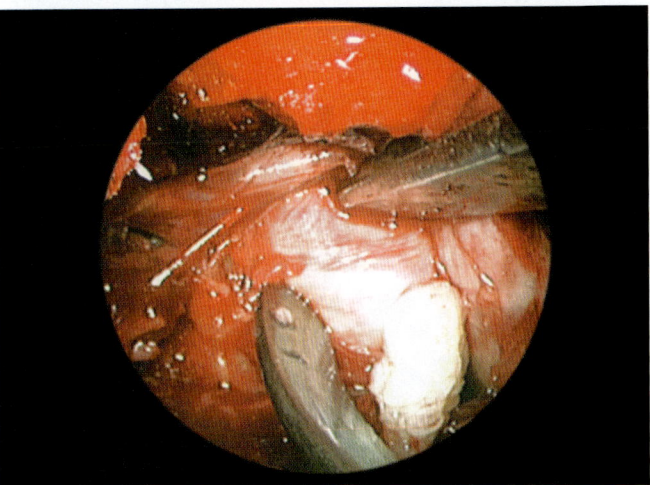

Fig. 34.45: Microscopic lumbar dissectomy (MLD)

blood loss. It is a technically demanding procedure and gives excellent results if done in properly indicated cases like a single level posterolateral disk prolapse. The patient can be discharged home within two days and he or she can return to his or her normal work faster. In short, it can be described as a less invasive, less painful, more specific procedure giving maximum comforts to the patient (Figs 34.46A and B). *Dr PS Ramani calls it as "come today, go tomorrow" surgery!*

What is New in the Treatment of Low Backache?
- MISS-(Minimally invasive spinal surgery), this consists of endoscopic spine surgery diskectomy and was popularized by John Chiu.
- Laser diskectomy.
- Percutaneous diskectomy (manual or automated)
- *Total disk replacement (TDR):* Total or partial disk replacement using a prosthetic disk nucleus for IVDP. It has a hydrogel core and is encased in a polyethylene jacket. It restores disk height and ensures normal range of mobility.

CHEMONUCLEOLYSIS

Indications are the same as for surgery. It is limited to lumbar spine. Drug used is chymopapain.

Ways to Prevent Recurrence

This is the most important aspect of the management of backache. *Like in all other diseases, so in backache prevention is better than cure. Backache can be prevented largely by observing the following measures:*

Adopting proper posture and creating awareness that it is in the erect position that the back can withstand strain the best.

Back education: Stress on the back is less when it is properly used during sitting, walking, etc. These proper habits have to be cultivated with practice.

Back exercises: These aim to strengthen the abdominal, pelvic, back and thigh muscles. Strong healthy muscles reduce load on the disks and other structures.

To avoid All sports including the aerobic ones. Swimming and walking are encouraged.

Treatment Plan of Backache due to Disk Disease

Conservative	- Absolute bed rest
- Traction
- NSAIDs
- Belts
Epidural steroids	- For subacute and chronic cases
- Long-acting steroids + Local anesthetics
- Reduces dependence on narcotics
- Effect lasts for 3 weeks
Surgery	- Done in proper indications
- Open or microscopic or endoscopic lumbar diskectomy
Chemonucleolysis	- Same indications as for surgery
- Limited only to lumbar spine
- Drug used is chymopapain
Physiotherapy	- Active and passive physiotherapy
- Flexion or extension exercises
Recurrence prevention	- Back education
- Proper postural habits
- Back exercises
- Avoid all sports

Remember

Consider serious causes of backache if any one of the following situations is encountered
- Pain in patients less than 10 years of age
- First time backache in patients greater than 60 years
- Unexplained weight loss
- Chronic cough
- Night pains
- Intermenstrual bleeding
- Altered bowel function
- Altered bladder control
- Visual disturbances and balance problems.

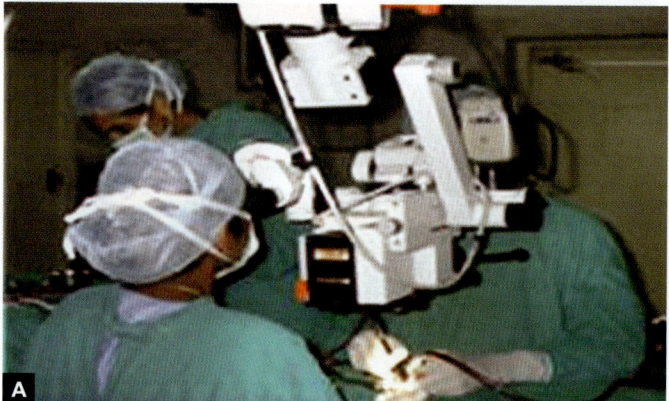 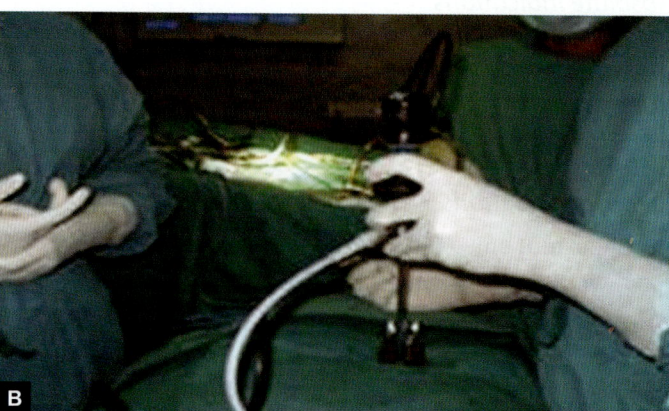

Figs 34.46A and B: Microscopic and endoscopic lumbar dissectomy

Remember the Do's and Don'ts

Do's
- Forward bent attitude.
- Body weight borne on the heels.
- Proper weightlifting as shown earlier.
- Sit with buttocks tucked under.
- While driving, push the seat forwards to raise the knees and decrease the lordosis.
- Flex the knees and hip when lying on the side.
- Turn to the side and then get up.

Don'ts
- Sleep in the prone position.
- Rise from a sitting position suddenly.
- Bend over a washbasin.
- Wear high heels as pelvis is thrust forward and the spine bends backward.
- Use too high a chair.
- Use soft mattress, which increases the lumbosacral extension. A firm mattress encourages lumbar spine to be straight.

Remember B's in Backache
- **B**ad posture
- **B**ed rest
- **B**elts
- **B**ack education
- **B**ack exercises
- **B**ed choice.

APPROACH TO A PATIENT WITH LOW BACKACHE

Low backache is an extremely common malady afflicting the human race across the globe cutting the geographical boundaries, race, culture, etc. Eighty to ninety percent of the human population will suffer from some form of backache, mild or severe in their lifetime. It is of interest to know the historical background regarding low back pain.

Historical Review
- Backache and leg pain are known since beginning of history.
- Primitive culture called it a work of a demon.
- Greeks recognized the symptoms as disease.
- In the 18th century, Cotumis attributed pain to the sciatic nerve.
- In 1881, Lasegue test described a test to distinguish hip disease from sciatica (first described by Frost).
- Virchow Kocher, etc. described acute traumatic ruptures of the disk that resulted in death.
- Goldthwait (1911) first attributed back pain to posterior displacement of disk.
- Dandy (1929) first reported removal of a disk tumor from patients suffering from sciatica.
- Myelography was first described in 1922.
- Barr (1932) finally attributed the source of sciatica to the herniated lumbar disk.
- Barr (1934) suggested surgical treatment for disk excision.
- Layman Smith (1963) suggested enzymatic dissolution of disk.
- Kirkaldy-Willis opines aging as the primary theory in disk disease.
- Nuchenson in 1964, White, and Punjabi in 1982 described biomechanics of spine.
- Schnack in 1983 described clinical anatomy.

CAUSES OF BACKACHE

A variety of conditions related and unrelated to spine cause backache (see the box).

Common Causes of Backache

The common causes of backache are:

Unaccustomed activities: A sedentary person suddenly adopting an active form of life, etc.

Poor posture: Improper posture during sitting, walking, standing, and working places, enormous load on the back and results in backache. This is by far the most common cause of low backache (Figs 34.47 and 34.48).

Occupational backache: Certain occupation places enormous stress on the back, e.g. garbage collectors, porters, etc. (Fig. 34.49).

Obesity: Protruding abdomen places enormous strain on the back (see Fig. 34.2B).

Muscle strain: In 80 percent of the cases, backache is due to sprain of the back muscles during activity, sports, trauma, etc. (Figs 34.50A to C).

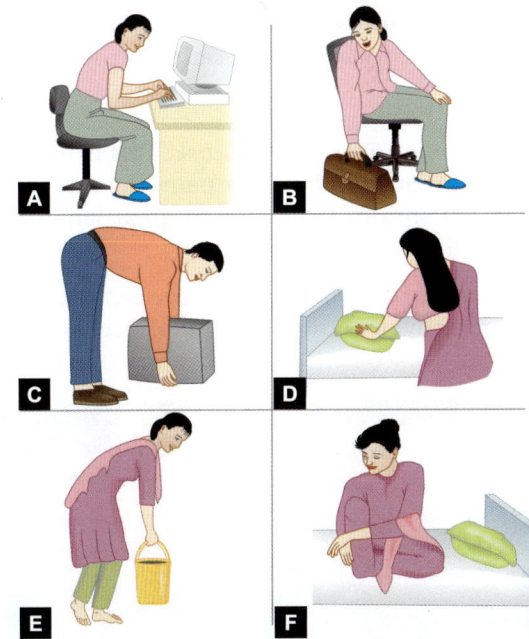

Figs 34.47A to F: Various common mechanisms of acute low backache: (A) Improper posture; (B) Sudden twist; (C) Faulty weightlifting; (D) Bending; (E) Sudden weightlifting; (F) Faulty sitting

462 SECTION 4: Common Back Problems

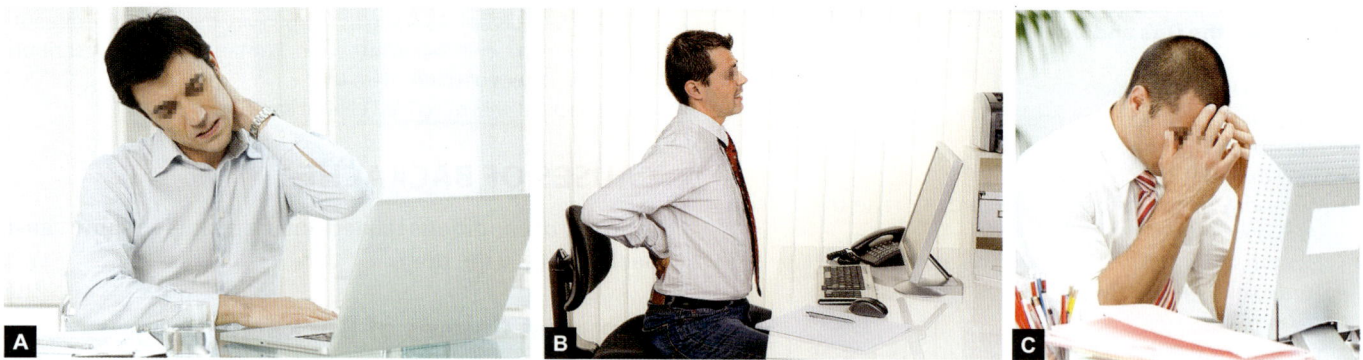

Figs 34.48A to C: Modern day professions are the main cause of today's lifestyle backaches

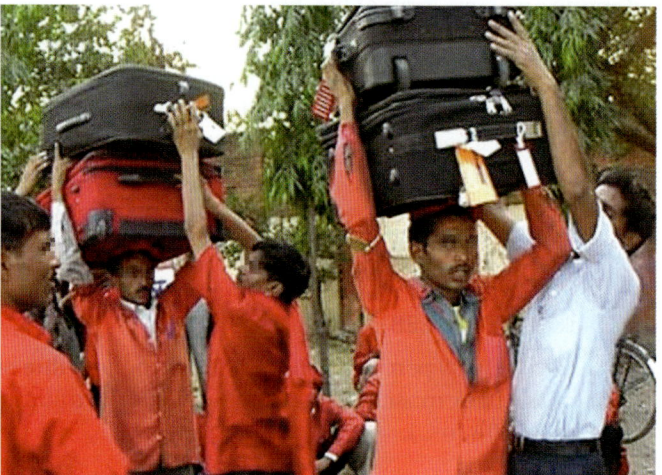

Fig. 34.49: Activities like these can cause backaches

Spinal stenosis: Spinal stenosis due to degenerative process is another common cause.

Uncommon Causes of Backache

Uncommon causes of backache are diseases of the spine, fractures, tumors, inflammatory conditions, etc. (Figs 34.51A to F)

> **Quick Facts: Causes of Low Backache (Fig. 34.52)**
> **Common causes**
> - Back muscle sprain
> - Prolapsed lumbar intervertebral disk
> - Obesity
> - Poor posture
> - Facet joint arthritis
> - Unaccustomed activities
> - Occupational causes
>
> **Uncommon causes**
> *Congenital causes* (4 'S')
> - Scoliosis
> - Spondylolisthesis
> - Spina bifida
> - Spondylolysis
>
> *Infective conditions*
> - Osteomyelitis
> - Tuberculosis

Prolapsed lumbar intervertebral disk: This is the second most common cause for low back pain after muscle strain and ligament sprain. Discussed at great length in the previous section.

The facet joint osteoarthritis due to old age, repeated bending and twisting activities lead to arthritis of facet joints.

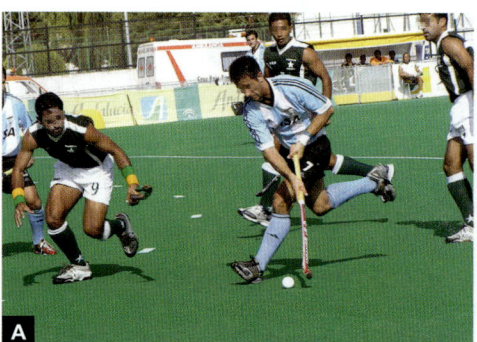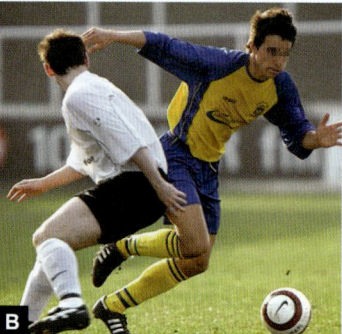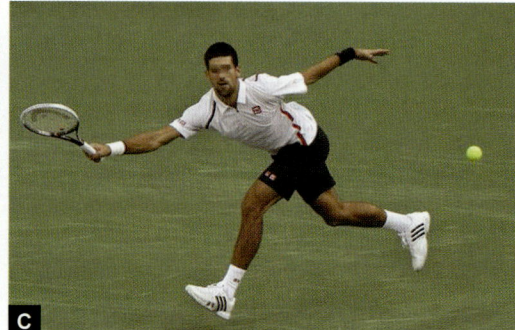

Figs 34.50A to C: Sporting activities like these can cause backaches (Sports injuries)

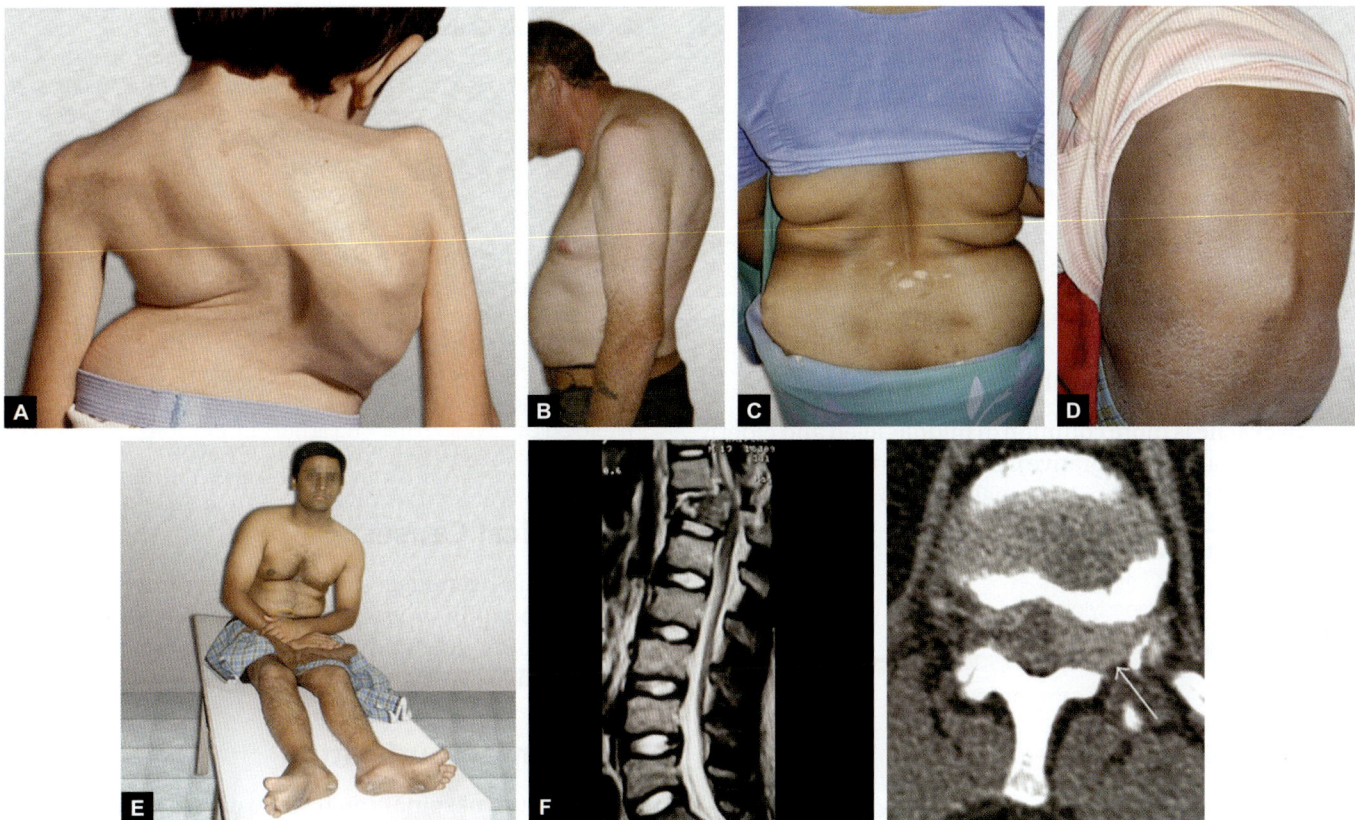

Figs 34.51A to F: Clinical photos showing uncommon causes of backache: (A) Congenital; (B) Inflammatory; (C) Mechanical (Spondylolisthesis); (D) Infective (TB spine); (E) Traumatic; (F) Secondaries

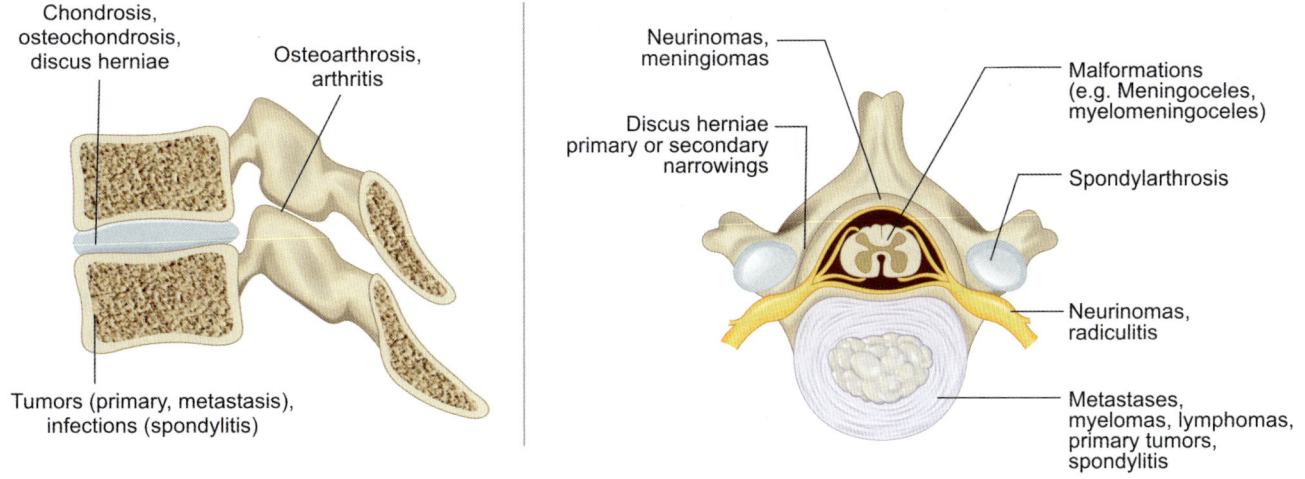

Fig. 34.52: Causes of uncommon low backaches and pathological processes of the spine, which can give rise to local spinal pain syndromes associated with painful muscle spasms

- Brucellosis, etc.

Traumatic causes
- Vertebral body injuries, posterior arch fractures
- Muscle sprain/strain
- Prolapsed disk

Inflammatory causes
- Rheumatoid arthritis
- Ankylosing spondylitis and other SSAs

Neoplasm
- Benign—osteoid osteoma

- Malignant—secondary, multiple myeloma, etc.

Metabolic causes
- Osteoporosis
- Osteomalacia

Degenerative conditions
- Osteoarthritis
- Lumbar spondylosis

Referred pain from
- Gynecological diseases
- Genitourinary diseases
- Gastrointestinal conditions, etc.

Presenting Complaints

Age: Backache is more common in middle-aged and elderly people (usually degenerative). In young adults, it is due to trauma; and in children, it is usually due to organic lesions.

Age Predilection and Low Backache

Age	Common causes
<20 years	Spondylolysis
20–40 years	Disk herniation
>40 years	Spondylosis
	Lumbar canal stenosis

Common to all age groups:
Ligament sprain/muscle strains.

Sex: Osteoporosis, rheumatoid arthritis, etc. are more common in females. Ankylosing spondylitis, trauma, secondary, etc. are more common in males.

Occupation: People with sedentary jobs and heavy manual laborers are frequently prone for backache.

PAIN

Over 90 percent of the patients complain of pain in the lower back. The following points should be enquired:

Nature of pain: Is it sudden (trauma) or gradual (spondylosis)? Did weightlifting, sudden bending, etc. precede it? Is there remissions and exacerbations (disk disease) or is it continuous (tumors)? Is there history of night cries (e.g. TB spine)? Does rest relieve it? Does it radiate to the lower limbs? Etc.

Site: Is the pain in the middle of the spine or para-vertebral muscles. Is it in the dorsolumbar spine (trauma or tumor) or in the lumbar spine (disk disease)?

Sciatic Pain

Here, pain radiates along the course of the sciatic nerve (see causes for sciatica). Common cause is disk prolapse. See Pages 454 to 456 for various tests for sciatica.

Sciatica and its Causes

Sciatica is defined as a radiating pain along the course of the sciatic nerve and is felt in the back, buttocks, posterior of the thigh, legs, and the foot. It is commonly due to disk prolapse. The other causes are:
- Spondylolisthesis.
- Sacroiliac joint arthritis.
- Affliction of the nerve root by herpes simplex virus can cause radicular pain.
- Tuberculoma causing cord compression.
- Lymphomas and pelvic malignancy.
- Incurled thickened ligamentum flavum.
- Cysts of the sacral nerve root.
- Intraspinal neurofibromas and other tumors.
- Hemorrhage in the ependymoma can cause sudden and gross neurological deficit, mimicking acute disk prolapse.
- Diabetic neuropathy, etc.

Biochemical Causes

Recently, it has been suggested but not clearly demonstrated that blood pooling in various blood vessels surrounding the nerve roots may contribute to impaired nerve root formation and sciatica.

Neurogenic Claudication

This is a feature of spinal canal stenosis *(see page 677)*.

Neurological Symptoms

These consist of paresthesia, muscle weakness, disturbance of sphincters, cauda equina syndrome, etc.

Facet Syndromes

Here, the patient complains of chronic backache, early morning stiffness, difficulty in getting out of bed, standing, sitting, or climbing.

Other Complaints

There may be history of stiffness, pain in other joints (e.g. rheumatoid arthritis), constitutional symptoms (e.g. tuberculosis, malignancy, etc.), genitourinary complaints, etc.

Physical Signs

Stance and gait: Does the patient stand with a normal stance or has deformities like scoliosis, kyphosis, lordosis, or pelvic tilt? Is the gait normal or altered? (see Fig. 34.14).

Spasm: This is seen in acute painful conditions of the spine. The patient complains of pain in the paravertebral muscles and painful restriction of all the spine movements (see Fig. 34.9).

Movements: There may be restriction of the spine movements due to the organic lesions affecting the back.

Swelling: Swelling due to cold abscesses may be present.

Tenderness: It may be present over the spinous process, in between the spinous processes, over muscles, ligaments, facet joints, etc.

Neurological Examination

This consists of examinations of the various dermatomes for sensations, myotomes for muscle power and reflexes.

SLRT and Tension Signs

This is to know the effects of disk prolapse on the sciatic nerve (the tests are described on *(refer page* 452).

Other Examinations

Other examinations include examinations of the adjacent joints, peripheral pulses, abdominal, rectal or paravaginal examinations.

Investigations

Blood tests: These are useful in detecting metabolic, hormonal, infective, and malignant conditions.

Radiology: Routine plain radiographs of the lumbar spine are advised. Both anteroposterior and lateral views are usually required. Oblique views are helpful in detecting the fracture of pars. Though X-rays are not very helpful in detecting the disk prolapse, it is of value in diagnosing metabolic, degenerative, inflammatory, malignant conditions affecting the spine (Fig. 34.25).

Myelography: This procedure is not routinely used anymore because of its complications. However, it has a role in demonstrating blocks due to disk prolapse (Fig. 34.27).

CT scan: it is a noninvasive procedure and helps to identify the bone and soft tissue problems with greater accuracy (Fig. 34.28).

MRI scan: This is the gold standard in the investigations of the spine. It is noninvasive and is better than CT scan in diagnosing the bone and soft tissue problems around the spine. However, its high cost is prohibitive and is available only in major cities and centers (Fig. 34.29).

Treatment

The underlying cause has to be detected and managed accordingly. The treatment for backache consists of drugs like NSAIDs, muscle relaxants, physiotherapy, traction, use of belts and corsets (Fig. 34.53). Proper postural habits, back exercises, and back education go a long way in preventing the backache. Surgery is done for specific indications.

Other Important Causes of Backache

- *Spinal stenosis:* This is discussed at length in the Chapter on Regional Disorders of Spine.
- Spondylolisthesis.
- Tuberculosis of spine.
- Spine injuries.
- Lumbar spondylosis.
- Osteomalacia.
- Osteoporosis.
- Ankylosing spondylitis.
- SI joint arthritis.
- Scoliosis.

BACKACHE IN SPECIAL SITUATIONS

BACKACHE IN CHILDREN (School Bag Syndrome)

It is indeed very pathetic that backache is no longer an unknown entity in children. Thanks to the practice of heavy school bags, the tender backs of children are subjected to untold misery.

> **Vital Facts**
> Ideally, a child should not carry a bag of >10 percent of his or her body weight. Nevertheless, the scenario in present-day children's life is very different.

Features

We can call this school bag related problems in a child as "school bag stress syndrome." Its features are:
- Pain in the shoulders, neck, and back.

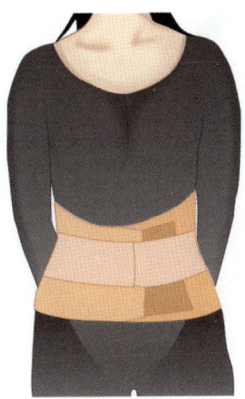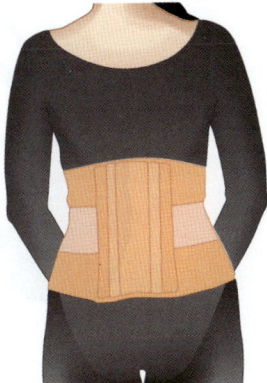

Fig. 34.53: Lumbar sacral belt application in LBA

- Tingling sensation in the arms, wrist, and hands especially at night.
- Head and neck are tilted to one side (postural imbalance).
- Frequent headaches.
- An uncommon gait.

Prevention

Policy Matter

The school administrations and the government should devise strategies to lessen the burden of the books on the children. Providing lockers in the classrooms, reducing the number of books to be carried, giving less homework are some of the options. However, nothing seems to be happening over this front. Hence, the following improvisations can be tried:

- To use ergonomically designed school bags (Orthofix or orthogrip bags) (Fig. 34.54).
- These bags are easy on the shoulder and back.
- They sit against the curve of the back.
- They are provided with good padding for the bag straps, so that it does not burrow the skin (see box for safe school bag instructions).

> **Facts Vital for School Children (Safe School Bag Practice)**
> - Use an ergonomically designed school bag
> - Use both straps to carry the bag
> - The knapsack should have several compartments for equal weight distribution
> - Heavy items are packed at the top, so that weight is borne on the legs instead of the spine
> - Both the straps should be worn across the shoulder and upper back to equalize the weight.

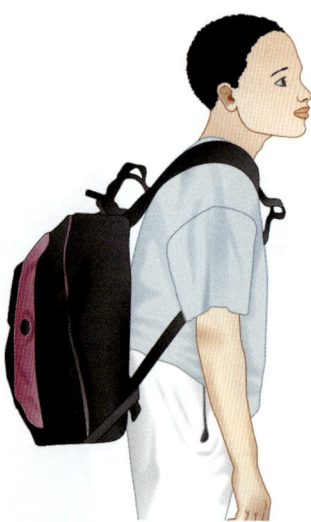

Fig. 34.54: School bag syndrome can be prevented by using ergonomic school bags

REPETITIVE STRESS INJURY (RSI)

Synonyms
- Occupational overuse syndrome (Scandinavia).
- Cumulative trauma disorder (USA).
- Work-related upper limb disorder (WHO).

Thanks to the computer boom in the not-so-distant past, software professionals were catapulted as cynosure of all eyes. However, this euphoria was short-lived when they unsuspectingly became victims of a new computer related health hazard called the RSI. Of late, RSI is hogging all the limelight in the newspapers signifying its increased prevalence in the society. The moral of this story is that every sunny side has its darker shades too!

Definition

It is an overuse injury affecting the soft tissues (muscles, tendons, and nerves) of the neck, shoulder, upper and lower back, arms and hands.

> **Note:**
> In India, it is also called CRI (Computer-related Injury) and is due to improper computer use and improper postures.

Incidence

About 15–25 percent of all the computer users across the globe are affected by RSI. About 75 percent of the IT professionals are affected with RSI at some stage of their career.

> **Did You Know?**
> RSI is not a new entity. It is present since centuries and was widely prevalent in:
> - Musicians
> - Butchers
> - Assembly line centers
> - Barbers
> - Clerks, typists
>
> However, it has seen a sudden boom thanks to the computer and call-center cultures.

> **Who is at Risk? Anyone Who Uses the Computer for More than One Hour Everyday is at Risk and is Seen in:**
> - Software engineers
> - Bank employees
> - Call center staffs
> - Children and elderly.

> **Why does RSI Happen?**
> A look at the list provides the answer (Fig. 34.55):
> - Improper use of the computers.
> - The mouse and the keyboard placed at uncomfortable heights and positions.

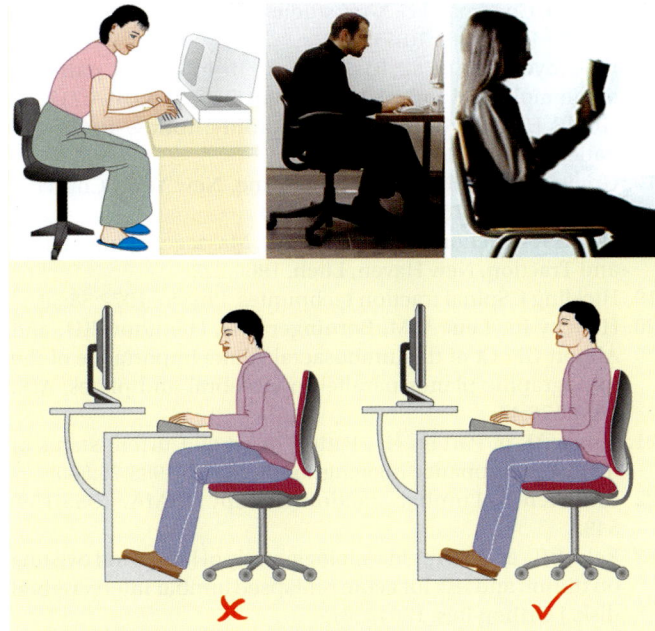

Fig. 34.55: Causes for RSI (Left) and the remedy (Right)

- Very hard keyboards or forceful typing over them.
- Height of the monitors kept at uncomfortable levels.
- Improper postures of the neck and back while working.
- Poorly designed unscientific working chairs.
- Extreme mental and physical stress.

Presentation

RSI is infamous for a varied presentation stumping even a most experienced orthopedician. Hence, a high degree of suspicion is required to diagnose this problem. The presentation could range from (Fig. 34.56):

Neck: It can cause acute and chronic neck pains. In the long run, it may predispose to cervical spondylosis.

Eyes: It may affect the vision and cause irritation and blurring. (It is known as computer eye injury).

Shoulder: Shoulder pain is a very common complaint.

Elbow: It can lead to Tennis elbow, Golfers elbow, pain within the wrist joint, etc.

Forearm: Forearm muscle cramps, fatigue, etc.

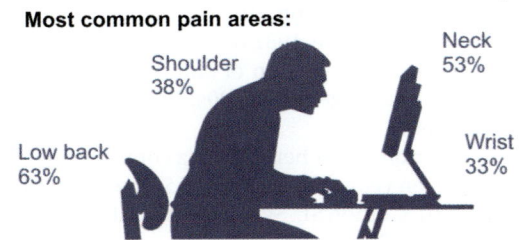

Fig. 34.56: Different sites of pain in modern day computer professionals

*Refer book on Shoulder Pain and Wrist conditions by Dr John Ebnezar.

Wrist: It can lead to Carpal-Tunnel syndrome, wrist pain, etc.

Fingers: It can cause pain in the fingers. There could be a feeling of tingling and numbness of the fingers.

Backache: This is a frequent complaint and can affect the upper, middle, or lower back.

So looking at the long list of complaints makes one weary of this problem and calls for effective preventive and curative measures to tackle this ugly menace.

Stages

Stage I symptoms are seen only while at work and do not persist.
Stage II symptoms persist but disappear with rest.
Stage III symptoms are permanent.

Investigations

Routine investigations like laboratory tests, plain X-ray, CT scan, MRI, etc. are not of much importance in detecting RSI. The diagnosis is mainly clinical.

Treatment

Preventive Measures

In this condition too, prevention is better than cure. The recommended preventive and awareness measures are:
- Awareness about this problem.
- Proper postures during work.
- Using ergonomically designed chairs.
- The neck, elbow, and shoulder should be placed at a comfortable height.
- The height of the computer monitor should be just above the eye level.
- Taking breaks from typing at every five minutes, fifteen and half an hour of typing.
- Taking a short break after every half an hour. Getting up, taking a short walk and sitting against for work is a good practice.
- Neck, shoulder, back, elbow and fingers stretches help to relieve pain and stress.
- Yoga and meditation helps to combat mental and physical stress.
- Keeping realistic goals and philosophical attitude defuses mental tension and prevents burn out.

Curative Measures

Treatment of problems like neck pain, shoulder pain, elbow problems like tennis elbow, wrist problems like compartment syndrome have been dealt in relevant sections.* However in the event of pain, the following general measures are done:

Drugs: Pain killers like NSAIDs are the drugs of choice. The more popular ones belong to nimesulide, rofecoxib, valdecoxib, diclofenac sodium, etc. They are preferably taken for short spells and that too after consultation and recommendation from hour doctor.

Physiotherapy: This consists of gentle massage, heat therapies like hot water packs, TENS, ultrasound, short wave diathermy, etc.

Exercises: Once the pain subsides, patient is instructed to carry out suitable neck, shoulder, elbow, and finger exercises.

Surgery: This is rarely required.

Health Education

This is the most important aspect of tackling this highly preventable problem. The aspects mentioned in the above columns have to be scrupulously enforced to keep this problem at bay.

Role of the Institutions

Institutions should provide good working conditions and facilities to all its workers. Good illumination, recreation facilities, and realistic workloads go a long way in helping the employees cope with this problem.

BIBLIOGRAPHY

1. Anderson GBJ. Epidemiologic aspects of low back pain in industry. Spine. 1981;6:53.
2. Arnaldi CC, et al. Lumbar spinal stenosis and nerve root entrapment syndromes: definition and classification. Clin Orthop. 1976;115:4.
3. Barr JS, et al. Low back pain, and sciatica, results of treatment. J Bone Joint Surg. 1951;33A:633.
4. Basmajian JV. Therapeutic exercises. Baltimore: Williams and Wilkins Co. 1976;410-19.
5. Bell GR, Rothmann RH. The conservative treatment of sciatica. Spine. 1984;9:54.
6. Bradford FK, Spurling RG. The intervertebral disk, Springfield, Charles C Thomas, Publisher; 1945.
7. Breig A, Troup JDG. Biomechanical consideration in the straight leg-raising test. Spine. 1979;4:242.
8. Canthen C. Lumbar spine surgery. Baltimore: Williams and Wilkins; 1983.
9. Christopher R Hyne. Ergonomics and back pain. Physio. 1984;70:9.
10. Cover AB, Curwen IHM. Low back pain treated by manipulation. Br Med J. 1955;19:705.
11. Cuikler JM, et al. The use of epidural steroids in the treatment of lumbar radicular pain. J Bone and Joint Surg. 1985;67A:63.
12. Dankol DK, Pope MH, Lord J, Frymover JW. The relationship between work history, work environment, and low back pain in men. Spine. 1984;9:395.
13. Estridge MN, Routre SA, Johnson WG. The femoral stretching test: a valuable sign in diagnosing upper lumbar disk herniation. J Neurosurg. 1982;57-813.
14. Ford LT, Goodman FG. X-ray studies of the lumbosacral spine. South Med J. 1966;10-1123.
15. Frymoyer JW, et al. Risk factors in low back pain: an epidemiological survey. J Bone Joint Surg. 1983;65A:213.
16. Goald HJ. Micro lumbar discectomy: follow-up of 147 patients. Spine. 1978;3:183.
17. Grieve GP. Mobilization of the spine. New York: Churchill Livingstone; 1975.
18. Harris R. Traction. In: Litchy S (Ed). Massage, Manipulation and Traction. New Haven, Litch. 1960;223.
19. Hickling J. Spinal traction techniques. Physio. 1972;58:58.
20. Hirschy JC, Leue WM, Berninger WH, Hamilton RH, and Abbott GF: Ct of the lumbosacral spine: importance of the tomographic planes parallel to vertebral and plates. AJR. 1981;136:47.
21. James AE Jr, Partain CL, Patton JA, et al. Current status of magnetic resonance imaging south. Med J. 1985;78:580.
22. Judovich B. Lumbar traction therapy. JAMA. 1955;159:549.
23. Kelsey JL, et al. An epidemiologic study of lifting and twisting on the job and risk for acute prolapsed lumbar intervertebral disk. J Orthop Res. 1984;2:61.
24. Kendall PH, Jenkins JM. Exercise for backache: a double blind controlled trial. Physio. 1968;54:154.
25. Lidstrom A, Zachrisson M. Physical therapy on low back pain and sciatica. Scand J Rehab Med. 1970;2:37.
26. Macnab I. Management of low back pain. In: Abstrom JP (Jr) (Ed). Current Practice in Orthopedic Surgery. St. Louis: CV Mosby Co; 1973.
27. Macrae IF, Wright V. Measurement of back movement. Ann Rheum Dis. 1969;28:584.
28. Macre IF, Wright V. Measurement of back movement. Ann Rheum Dis. 1969;28:384.
29. McKenzie RA. Prophylaxis in recurrent low back pain. NZ Med J. 1979;89:22.
30. Nachemson A. Advances in low back pain. Clin Orthop. 1985; 200:266.
31. Nachemson A. Physiotherapy for low back pain patients: a critical look. Scand J Rehab Med. 1969;1:85.
32. Robinson JS. Sciatica and the lumbar disk syndrome: a historic perspective. South Med J. 1983;76:232.
33. Rothman RH. The clinical syndrome of lumbar disk disease. Orthop Clin North Am. 1971;2:463.
34. Steindler A, Luck JV. Differential diagnosis of pain low in the back: allocation of the source of pain by the procaine hydrochloride method. JAMA. 1938;110(2):106.
35. Troup JDG. Straight leg raising (SLR) and the qualifying tests for increased root tension: their predictive value after back and sciatic pain. Spine. 1981;6:526.
36. Wachemson AL. Prevention of chronic low back pain: the orthopedic challenge for the 80s. Bull Hosp J Dis Orthop Inst. 1981;44:1.
37. Weber H. Lumbar disk herniation: a controlled, perspective study with ten years of observation. Spine. 1983;8:131.
38. White AA III, Gordon SL. Synopsis: Workshop on Idiopathic low back pain. Spine. 1982;7:141.
39. Williams RW. Micro lumbar discectomy: a conservative surgical approach to the virgin herniated lumbar disk. Spine. 1978;3:175.

SECTION 5

General Orthopedics

- Congenital Disorders
- Developmental Disorders
- Metabolic Disorders
- Osteomyelitis
- Skeletal Tuberculosis
- Disorders of Joints (Arthritis)
- Rheumatic Diseases
- Neuromuscular Disorders
- Bone Neoplasias

SECTION 5

General Orthopedics

35 CHAPTER

Congenital Disorders

INTRODUCTION

The following congenital disorders of interest are discussed in this chapter (Table 35.1).

Congenital disorders are defined as those *abnormalities of development that are present at the time of birth*. It is quite a common problem exceeded in frequency only by those of CNS and CVS systems.

Congenital Disorders can be Placed in Three Groups

- Those easily noticed by the mother, e.g. clubfoot.
- Those not readily noticed, e.g. congenital dislocation of hip (CDH).
- Those clinically undetected but diagnosed radiologically, e.g. spondylolisthesis.

Congenital disorders are more prevalent in diabetic mothers, multiple pregnancies, older mothers, etc. Male and female have equal predilection.

TABLE 35.1: Congenital disorders

Congenital disorders of trunk and upper extremity
- *Congenital torticollis*
- Congenital elevation of scapula
- Congenital pseudarthrosis of the clavicle
- Congenital radioulnar synostosis

Congenital disorders of hip and pelvis
- *Congenital dislocation of hip*
- Coxa vara

Congenital disorders of the lower limb
- Congenital dislocation of the knee
- Congenital pseudarthrosis of the tibia
- *Congenital talipes equinovarus (CTEV)*

Congenital absence of part or all of long bones
- Radius
- Tibia
- Fibula

Note: The diseases *italicized* are discussed in detail while the rest are merely mentioned.

Causes

The exact cause is not known. Most congenital disorders begin early in the life of the embryo when cell division is most active. Although a few congenital disorders may be due to uterine malposition, most are believed to be due to *genetic defects, environmental influences* or a combination of both.

Genetic Factors

Defects in the chromosomes of sperm and ovum result in specific disorders, which follow Mendel's law.

Embryonic Trauma

Congenital disorders can also result from injury to the developing embryo at the time of differentiation of embryonic tissue into specific tissues by extraneous factors.

> **What is Teratogenesis?**
> *Experimental production of congenital anomalies is teratogenesis.* A teratogenic factor may be metabolic, hormonal, nutritional deficiency, chemicals, X-ray, trauma, infection, mechanical, thermal, anoxia, etc.

Duraiswamy could experimentally produce skeletal defects (Flowchart 35.1) by using the above teratogenic factors.

CONGENITAL DISORDERS OF UPPER LIMB

CONGENITAL TORTICOLLIS (Wryneck)

Congenital torticollis is a condition where the sternocleidomastoid muscle of the neck undergoes contractures pulling it to the same side and turning the face to the opposite side (Fig. 35.1A). The exact cause of this condition is unknown;

Flowchart 35.1: Congenital skeletal problems

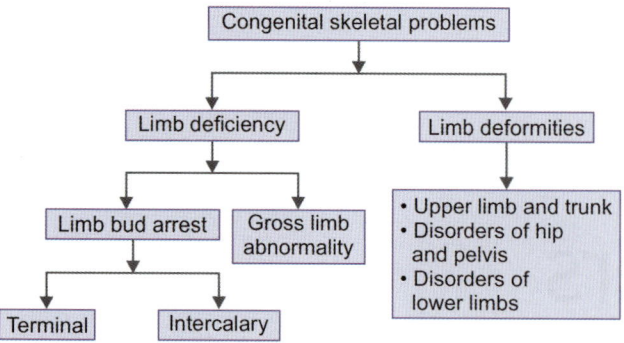

but hypothetically, it may be due to fibromatosis within the sternomastoid muscle.

Features
- Tumor palpable at birth or during the first two weeks of life.
- Common on the right side.
- May include the muscle diffusely but more often, it is localized near the clavicular attachment of the muscle.
- It attains maximum size within 1–2 months; usually it disappears within a year.
- If it fails to disappear, then the muscle becomes permanently fibrotic and contracted and causes torticollis.

Etiology

- Middle part of the sternomastoid is supplied by an end artery, which is a branch of the superior thyroid artery that is blocked due to trauma, etc.
- Birth trauma—Breech delivery, improper application of forceps, etc. may cause injury to the sternomastoid muscle.

The above two reasons can result in sternocleidomastoid muscle ischemia, necrosis and fibrosis later on.

Clinical Features

Deformity is the only complaint initially (Flowchart 35.2). Later, facial changes and macular problems in the retina may develop (Fig. 35.1B).

Flowchart 35.2: Deformities in congenital torticollis

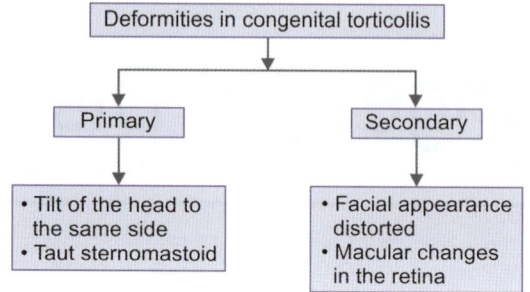

Radiograph

Plain X-ray of the neck AP and lateral views are essential to detect any congenital abnormality of the cervical vertebra that could lead to this condition (Fig. 35.2).

Treatment

Principles

- During infancy, conservative treatment consists of stretching of the sternomastoid by manipulation and physiotherapy. Excision is unjustified in infancy.
- Surgery is delayed until fibroma is well-formed. The muscle may be released at one or both ends and the muscle may be excised as a whole.
- If the muscle is still contracted at the age of 1 year, it should be released.
- If wryneck is persistent for 1 year, it will not resolve spontaneously and needs to be interfered operatively.

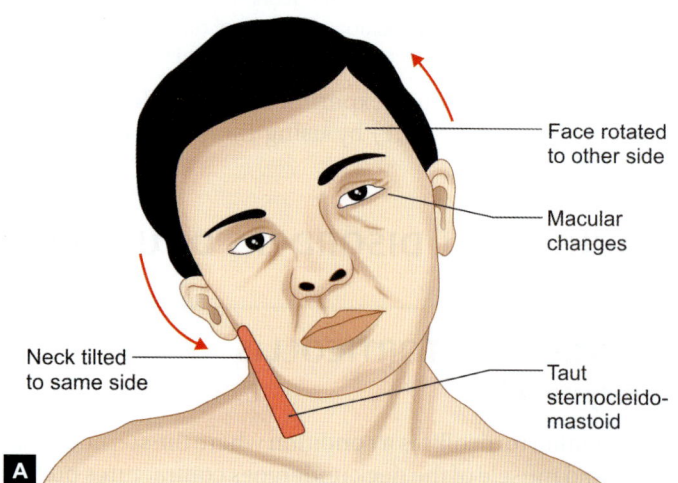
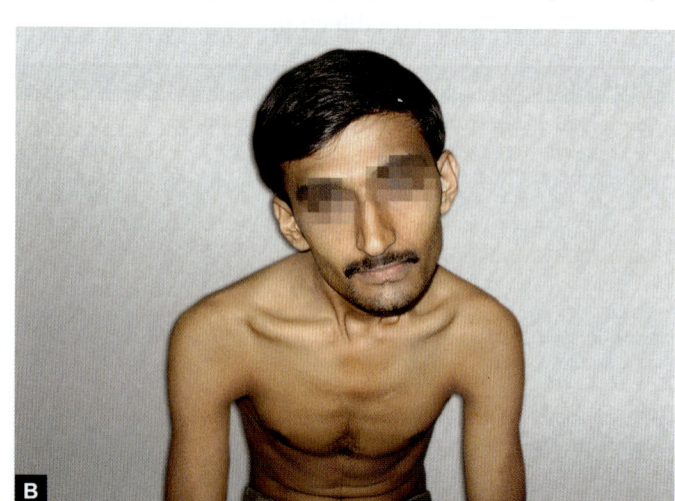

Figs 35.1A and B: Wryneck: (A) Features; (B) Clinical photo

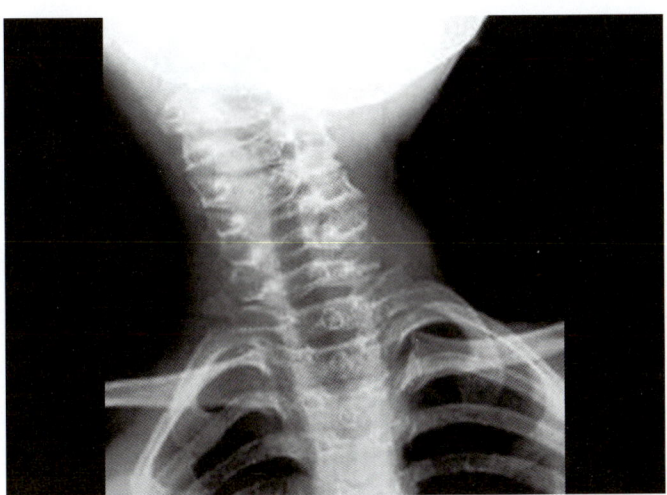

Fig. 35.2: Plain X-ray showing torticollis

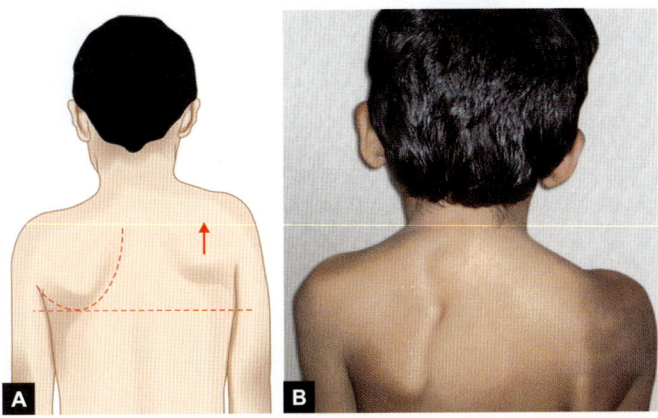

Figs 35.3A and B: (A) Congenital elevation of scapula (Sprengel's shoulder); (B) Sprengel's shoulder deformity (Clinical photo)

- Exercise program is successful:
  – When restriction of motion is less than 30°.
  – When there is no facial asymmetry.
- Nonoperative treatment after 1 year is rarely successful.
- Any permanent torticollis becomes worse during growth. Head is inclined towards the affected side, face is turned towards the opposite side, ipsilateral shoulder is elevated, and the fronto-occipital diameter is increased.

Surgical Methods

The most commonly employed surgical method is subcutaneous tenotomy of the clavicular attachment of the sternomastoid muscle. This procedure is inaccurate and dangerous as there could be an injury to the external jugular vein and phrenic nerve. Hence, release from its attachment on the mastoid process is also tried. Open tenotomy if done before the child is 1 year old, tethering of the scar takes place. If the surgery is done between 1 and 4 years of age, tilt of the head and facial asymmetry are corrected less satisfactorily. If done after 5 years of age, the secondary deformities are less corrected.

For older children or after failed operation, bipolar release of the muscle from both sides, Ferkel's modified bipolar release or Z-plasty of the muscle is tried.

SPRENGEL'S DEFORMITY[1]

In this condition, scapula fails to descend down from its initial high position in the embryo. It is a tale of a disobedient scapula! Here, the scapula lies more superiorly (Fig. 35.3A). It is hypoplastic and improperly shaped. It is associated with other congenital anomalies like cervical rib, etc.

Etiology

This may be due to imperfect descent of the shoulder girdle by third month or a band of muscle from the skull to the scapula, which has failed to grow.

Pathology

The pathological changes are seen in the bones and muscles. The scapula may be normal, broad, or high and there could be other features like hemi vertebra, wedging of vertebra, etc. Among the muscles, the trapezius may be absent, the rhomboids and a thin band represents levator scapulae.

Clinical Features

The scapula is high by 2–10 cm, the deformity is obvious (Fig. 35.3B), there is no functional impairment, all the shoulder girdle movements are normal, torticollis may be present in 10 percent of the cases, crania bifida, and spina bifida may be present (Figs 35.4A to C).

Cavendish's Grading

Group 1: Very mild.
Group 2: Mild, shoulder slightly unaligned.
Group 3: Moderate, shoulder high.
Group 4: Severe, with superior angle of scapula near the occiput (Figs 35.4A to C).

Radiograph

Plain X-ray of the scapula is essential to diagnose this condition (Fig. 35.5).

---

[1] **Otto Sprengel** (1852-1915), a German Orthopedic Surgeon, described in 1891.

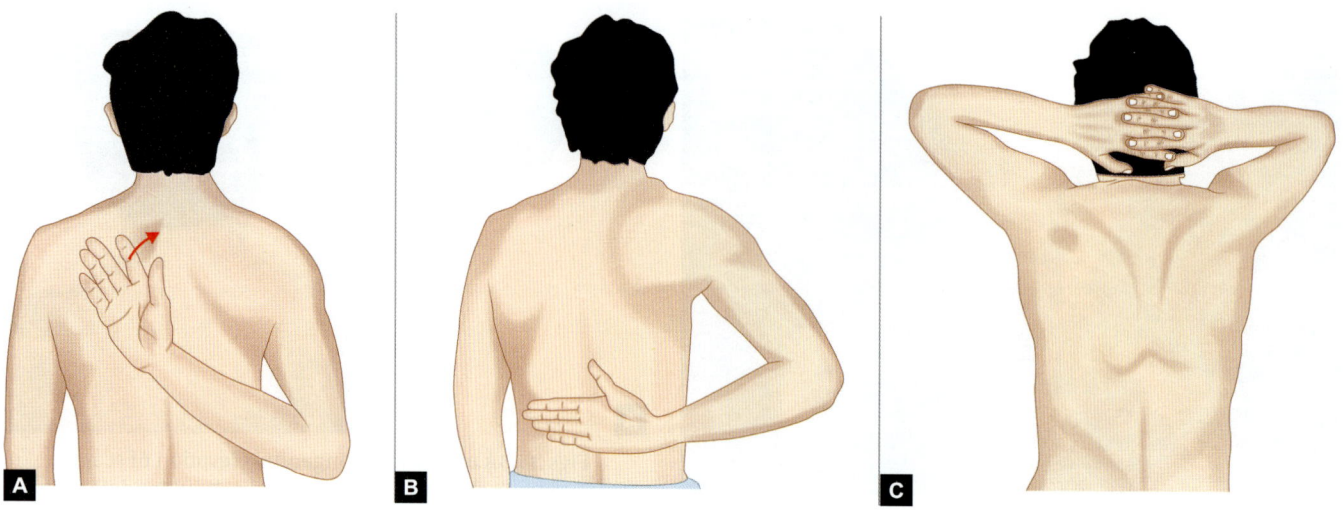

Figs 35.4A to C: Functions in Sprengel's shoulder

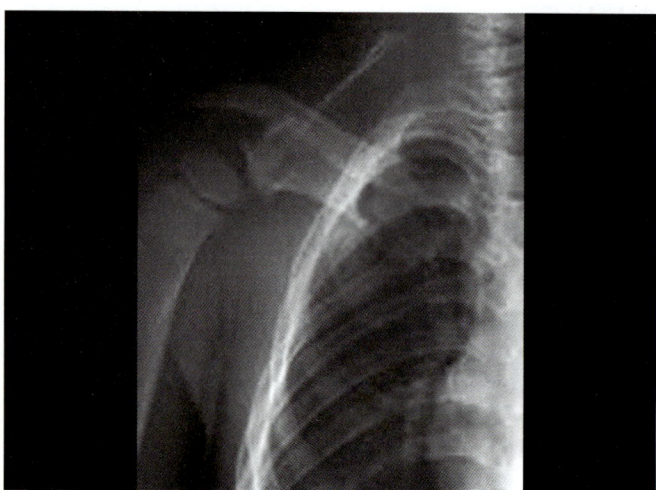

Fig. 35.5: Plain X-ray showing Sprengel's shoulder

Treatment

For cases with mild deformity, no treatment is required and for severe cases, surgery is done after three years, and this consists of release of muscles from the scapula or transfer of origin of the trapezius muscle.

CLEIDOCRANIAL DYSOSTOSIS

For some mysterious reasons, clavicle chooses to remain absent either partially or wholly. It is a rare condition.

Salient Features
- Aplasia of clavicles.
- Exaggerated development of transverse diameter of cranium.
- Delay in closure of clavicles.
- Heredity.
- Equal sex incidence.

Types
- Where ends of the bones are normal, but a pseudarthritic gap is present in between.
- Where there is a partial defect of one end, usually the acromial end.
- Where the whole clavicle is absent.

Deformities of the clavicle are accompanied by variations in the following muscles: Trapezius may be absent, pectoralis major may be maldeveloped, and other congenital malformations may be associated.

Etiology

The exact cause is unknown, but the development of membranous bones may be affected during the first week of embryonic life due to various unknown factors.

Clinical Features

The patient is brought to the surgeon due to accidentally discovered trouble with the shoulder. Features of un-united fracture of the clavicle may be present. It may also present as complete absence of the clavicle. Tips of shoulder can be approximated to each other (Fig. 35.6).

Radiograph

Plain X-ray of the both the clavicles are essential to diagnose this condition (Fig. 35.7).

Treatment

Usually, it does not require any treatment, but if pain is present due to pressure of one or both ends, then removal

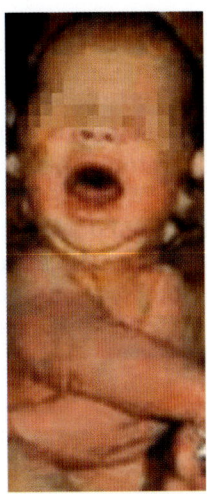

Fig. 35.6: Cleidocranial dysostosis (Clinical photo)

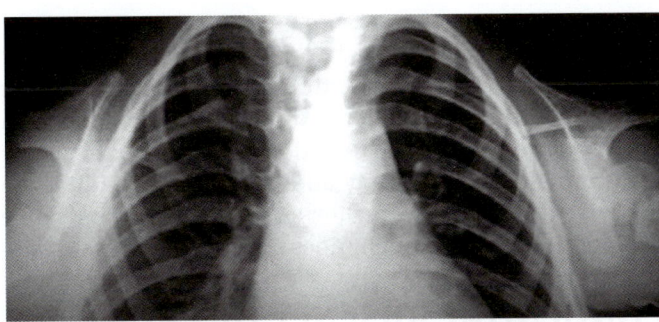

Fig. 35.7: Plain X-ray showing cleidocranial dysostosis

of the part is indicated. As a rule, there is no disability or discomfort and abnormal mobility is not usually a hindrance.

CONGENITAL RADIOULNAR SYNOSTOSIS

I call this an unholy alliance of radius and ulna for their union causes unmitigated hardship to the sufferer.

> **Salient Features**
> - Involves proximal ends of radius and ulna.
> - Bones fix the forearm in pronation.
> - Bilateral.
> - Familial tendency.

Classification

Two types are described, Type I and II and their salient features are depicted in Table 35.2.

TABLE 35.2: Classification of congenital radioulnar synostosis

Type I	Type II
• Medullary canals of the radius and ulna are joined together • Proximal ends of radius is malformed and fused to ulna for a distance of several cm • Radius is longer and larger than ulna and the shaft arches anteriorly	• Radius is normal • Proximal end is dislocated either anteriorly or posteriorly • Fusion to ulna is not as extensive as in type I • Unilateral • Other deformities like syndactyly, etc. are present

Clinical Features

The patient presents with deformity of the upper forearm and the forearm could be fixed in midpronation. There are no pronation and supination movements of the forearm. Elbow flexion could remain unaffected. The patient complains of difficulty in carrying out his day-to-day activities with the affected forearm.

Radiograph

Plain X-ray of the forearm including both elbow and wrist joints are essential to diagnose this condition (Fig. 35.8).

Reasons for difficulty in treatment
- Fascial tissues are short.
- Interosseous membrane is narrow.
- Supinator muscle is abnormal or absent.

Treatment

Treatment is limited to osteotomy, to place the forearm in mid-prone position for better function.

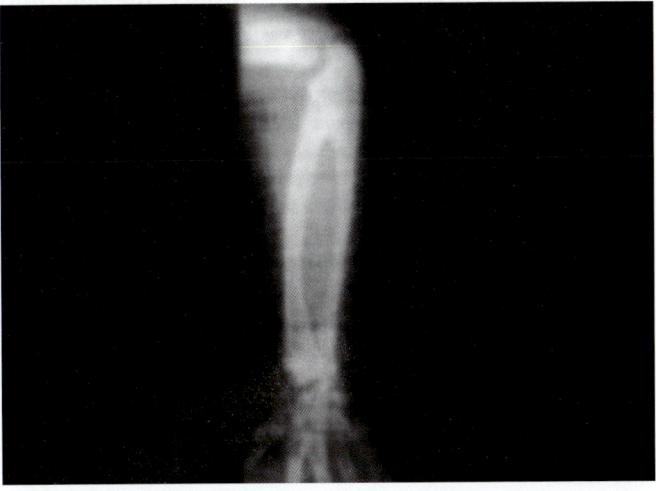

Fig. 35.8: Radiograph showing congenital radioulnar synostosis

Attempts to overcome the synostosis and give rotatory function to the forearm are doomed to failure because of the lack of properly functioning muscles. Fortunately, most patients are not disabled enough to justify an extensive operation.

MADELUNG'S DEFORMITY

It is an abnormality of the *palmar ulnar part of the distal radial epiphysis* in which progressive ulnar and volar tilt develops at the distal radial articular surface, resulting in dorsal subluxation of the distal ulna.

First described by Malgaigne in 1855 and later by [2]Madelung in 1878. Though congenital, it is not obvious until late childhood and adolescence. It is a rare condition, incidence being only 1.7 percent.

Causes

Congenital the causes could be autosomal dominant, dysplastic (diaphysial aclasis), genetic or idiopathic.

Acquired deformities *distinguished by* lack of appropriate physical findings, unilateral, less severe carpal deformities, and history of repetitive injury or stress.

Clinical Features

Madelung's deformity consists of:
- Volar subluxation of hand.
- Prominence of distal ulna.
- Volar and ulnar angulation of distal radius (Fig. 35.9).

Other Features

This condition is commonly bilateral, girls are more affected. There is a positive family history, the deformity manifests in late childhood and adolescents with restricted wrist motion and minimal pain. As growth occurs, deformity worsens and the forearm is short.

Radiographic Abnormalities

Radiographic abnormalities are seen in radius, ulna, and carpal bones. Radius is curved with its convexity dorsal and radial. Distal radial epiphysis is triangular because of the failure of the growth in the ulnar and volar aspects of the epiphysis. Early closure of these aspects of epiphysis is frequent. Ulna is subluxated dorsally, its head is enlarged, and the overall length of ulna is decreased. Carpus appears to have subluxated ulna-ward and palmarwards into the distal radioulnar joint. Carpus appears wedge-shaped with its apex proximal (Fig. 35.10).

Treatment

Conservative Treatment

Children with Madelung's deformity have minimal pain and excellent function. Hence, conservative treatment is given initially.

Surgery

Surgery is considered for severe deformity or persistent pain. In skeletally immature patients, distal radial osteotomy with ulnar shortening is (Milch resection) preferred. In skeletally mature patients, osteotomy and Darrach's procedure are done. Deformity may recur after either procedure and range of motion of forearm usually does not improve after surgery.

CONGENITAL ABSENCE OF RADIUS (Radial Club-Hand)

Failure of the formation of the parts along the preaxial or radial borders of the upper extremity, deficient or absent thenar muscles, short or absent thumb, short or absent radius.

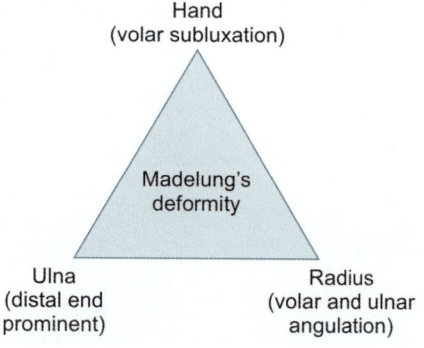

Fig. 35.9: Madelung's deformity

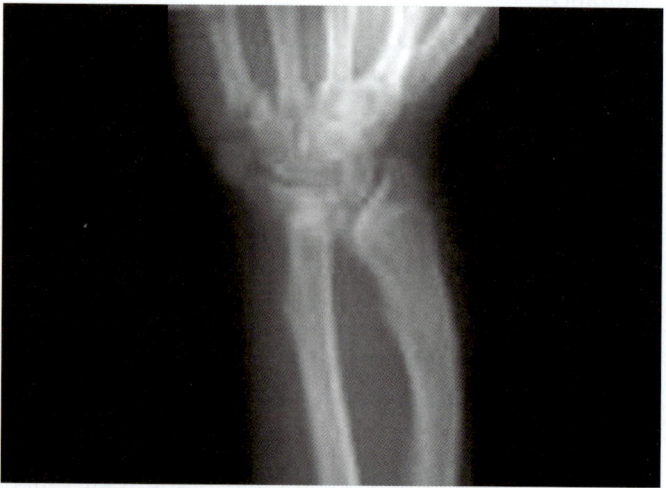

Fig. 35.10: Radiograph of madelung's deformity

---
[2]**Otto Madelung** of Bonn. First described by Malgaigne in 1855 and later by Madelung in 1878.

Quick Facts
- One in one lakh birth.
- Incidence—4.7 percent.
- Bilateral in 50 percent of cases.
- Sexes equal.
- Right side more common.
- Complete absence more common than partial absence.
- Cause unknown/thalidomide/genetic.

Heikel's Classification

Type I: Short distal radius.
Type II: Hypoplastic radius.
Type III: Partial absence of radius.
Type IV: Total absence of radius (most common).

Clinical Features

The patient presents with deformity of the forearm and wrist. The forearm appears short and small and the deformity of the forearm, wrist and hand are quite grotesque (Fig. 35.11A). The forearm and hand functions are severely affected. The patient complains of difficulty in carrying out his day-to-day activities with the affected forearm.

Radiograph

Plain X-ray of the forearm including both elbow and wrist joints are essential to diagnose this condition (Fig. 35.11B).

Treatment

After birth, the deformity is corrected passively and splinted with a short arm plastic splint. Surgical correction, i.e. centralization of hands is usually done at 3–6 months. Pollicization is done at 9–12 months.

CONGENITAL DISLOCATION OF RADIUS

This is uncommon and is often confused with Monteggia fractures.

Clinical Features

A prominent head of the radius is felt in the upper forearm. Forearm function of supination and pronation are affected, but the elbow movements remain normal. Due to long standing dislocation, there could be pain and features of secondary OA of the superoradioulnar joint.

Radiology

Plain X-ray of the elbow and entire forearm is advised to detect this lesion with reasonable accuracy (Fig. 35.12).

Treatment

Consists of excision of the head of radius after skeletal maturity.

CONGENITAL DISORDERS OF LOWER LIMBS

DEVELOPMENTAL DYSPLASIA OF HIP (DDH) [Earlier Known as Congenital Dislocation of Hip (CDH)]

Definition

Developmental dysplasia of hip is defined as partial or complete displacement of the femoral head from the acetabular cavity since birth.

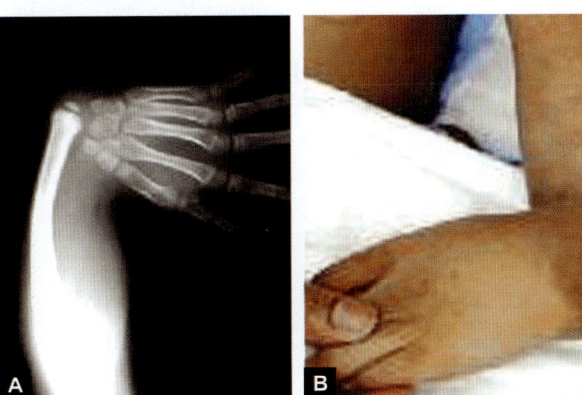

Figs 35.11A and B: (A) Radial club hand (Clinical photo); (B) Radiograph of radial club hand

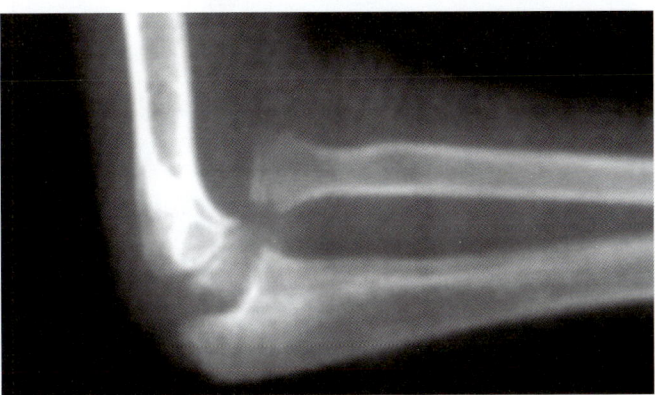

Fig. 35.12: Radiograph showing congenital dislocation of radius

> **Risk Factors (4 F's)**
> - Females
> - First borns
> - Familial
> - Faulty intrauterine position (e.g. breech).

Theories of Etiology

Genetic theory: Dysplastic trait is found in families.
Hormonal theory: Hormone induced joint laxity.
Mechanical theory: Faulty intrauterine positions particularly in the first-born.
Primary: Acetabular dysplasia.

> **Remember**
> *The incidences in DDH*
> - One per 1000 live birth.
> - Left hip affected in 67 percent of cases.
> - Family history present in 20 percent.
> - Incidence of breech 30–50 percent.
> - 1:3 cases are bilateral.
> - Female preponderance.

Pathology

The following pathological changes are observed in DDH (Fig. 35.13) and the severity varies according to the stages of the disease.

Bone

Acetabulum: There could be a primary acetabular dysplasia and the acetabulum is shallow. There could be a gap or groove at posterosuperior aspect. The triangular outer surface of ilium and acetabulum, are in the same line.

Above the acetabulum, there is a depression containing the head of the femur.

Head of femur: The dislocated head of femur at first appears normal, ossification is delayed, and later head is flat on its posterior and medial aspect. Femoral head when present in the ilium is buffer or conical shaped.

Neck of femur: There could be shortening and anteversion.

Pelvis: The pelvis is usually tilted forwards, it is small and atrophied. There is lordosis and it may be more vertical than normal.

Capsule: The capsule could show *hourglass constriction*, one containing head and the other containing the acetabulum. Constriction is produced by iliopsoas, the ligamentum teres passes through this constriction, and it is hypertrophied.

Muscles

Pelvifemoral group: Adductors, sartorius, gracilis, rectus femoris, hamstrings, tensor fascia lata muscles. These muscles are shortened and they prevent reduction of the head.

Pelvitrochanteric group (Obturators, Quadratus femoris, Iliopsoas): These are elongated and the psoas forms an obstacle to reduction.

Glutei muscles: Show little organic change but power is diminished.

> **Remember**
> *Conditions due to packaging problems* (i.e. decreased intrauterine space)
> - DDH
> - Torticollis
> - Metatarsus adductus
> - Increased type III collagen.

Stages of DDH

There are three stages of DDH as shown in Figure 35.14.

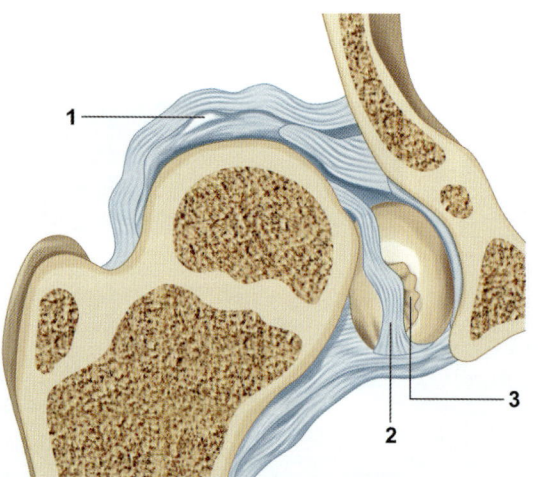

Fig. 35.13: Pathology in DDH: (1) Elongated capsule, (2) Stretched ligamentum teres, (3) Fibro fatty tissue within the acetabulum

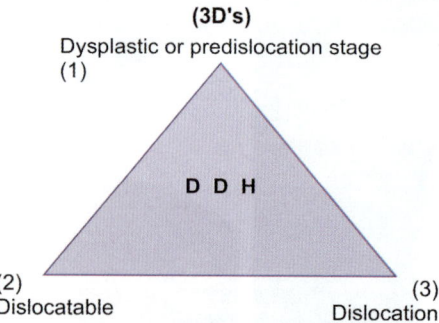

Fig. 35.14: Stages of developmental dysplasia of hip: (1) Dysplastic stage, (2) Dislocatable or subluxation stage, and (3) Dislocation stage

Clinical Features

The clinical features vary in infants, children, and adults (Table 35.3).

In Infants

First a thorough clinical examination is carried out to detect the presence of any other congenital anomalies. If the hip is dislocated, all features of dislocation are present. The glutei and thigh folds are not symmetrical. The perineum is widened and abduction of the hip is decreased by 50 percent while the internal rotation movement is increased. Radiographic examination in infants is of little value, but von Rosen's line (Fig. 35.15) is helpful in making an early radiological diagnosis in this age group.

Children and Adolescents

Here, the patient shows a waddling or sailor's gait. There is an increased lumbar lordosis. The deformity frequently encountered in unilateral cases is shortening. In bilateral cases, the lower limbs are short, perineum is wide, and buttocks are broad and flat. Femoral artery is prominently felt. Abduction and lateral rotation movements of the hip are decreased. Telescopy and Trendelenburg tests are positive. Clinical tests of importance in infants are not of relevance in this age group (Table 35.4).

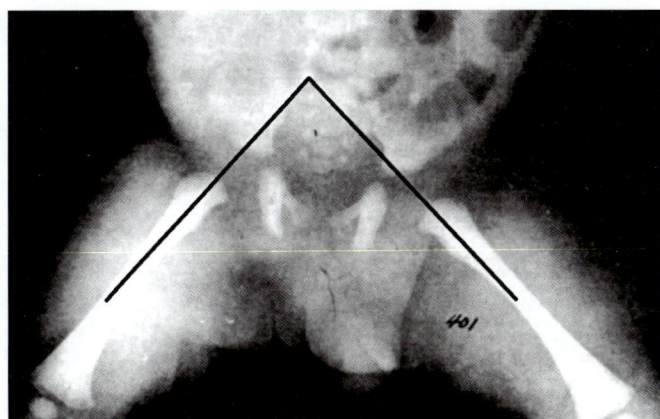

Fig. 35.15: Radiograph showing von Rosen's line

Radiology

Unlike in infants, radiographs of pelvis show important features in this age group (Fig. 35.22A). The following radiological parameters should be noted.

Perkin's line: This is a vertical line drawn at the outer border of the acetabulum (Fig. 35.22C).

Hilgenreiner's line: This is a horizontal line drawn at the level of triradiate cartilage (Fig. 35.22D).

Shenton's line: This is a smooth curve formed by the inferior border of the neck of the femur with the superior margin of the obturator foramen. This line is broken in DDH (Fig. 35.22B).

Acetabular index: Normal value is less than or equal to 30°.

CE angle of Wiberg: The normal value is 15–30°.

The Hilgenreiner's line and the Perkin's line help to assess the position of the femoral head. Normally, the head lies in the lower and inner quadrant formed by these two lines. In DDH, the head lies in the upper and outer quadrant, the continuity of Shenton's line is broken in DDH (Fig. 35.22B). The acetabular index and the CE angle of Wiberg help to assess the acetabulum.

In Adults

DDH in adults shows all the features seen in adolescents. In addition, patient will have features of secondary osteoarthritis of the hip namely—pain, stiffness, limp, crepitus, restricted movements, etc.

Treatment

The aim of treatment in DDH is to achieve and maintain an early concentric reduction to prevent future degenerative joint disease. The methods to obtain reduction of the head into the acetabulum vary according to the age groups (Table 35.5).

TABLE 35.3: Clinical features of DDH in various age groups at a glance

Infants	Childhood and adolescents	Adults
• Look for other Anomalies • If hip are dislocated all signs of dislo-cations present • Thigh and gluteal folds asymmetric • Perineum widened • Abduction decreased by 50% • Internal rotation increased **Tests** • Galeazzi is sign is positive • Ortolani's sign of entry is positive • Barlow's provocative test is positive (2, 3 indicate reducible dislocation) • Delayed walking	• *Gait:* Waddling/sailors • Lordosis • Deformity **Unilateral** shortening of leg **Bilateral** leg shortening with perineum wide, buttocks broad and flat • *Palpation* vascular sign of Narath is positive • Movements: Abduction in addition, lateral rotation is decreased • Telescopy is positive • Measurements • Supratrochanteric shortening is present	• All the signs seen in adolescents • Pain in the hip • All the features of osteoar-thritis hip

480 SECTION 5: General Orthopedics

TABLE 35.4: Clinical tests in DDH

Clinical tests	How to perform?	Inference
[3]Barlow's test (Fig. 35.16) Fig. 35.16	This test is done within 2–3 days of birth. The infant is supine with the knees fully flexed and the hip at 90° of flexion. The hip is slowly abducted to 45° and the head is slowly pushed towards the acetabulum by the fingers	This test is positive when the joint is dislocated and the femoral head returns to the acetabulum with a click or jerk. Reliable and useful up to 6 months after which the greater trochanter cannot be held with tip of the middle finger
[4]Ortolani's test (Fig. 35.17) Fig. 35.17	This test is done between 3 and 9 months. In addition, is not satisfactory in a newborn. Here, the infant is supine, with the hip and knee flexed. The hip is slowly adducted and abducted to detect any reduction of the femoral head into the acetabulum	This test indicates the reduction of the dislocated hip. These two tests are generally reliable and should be performed as a screening tests in all cases of suspected CDH. They are Misleading if abduction is restricted due to adduction contractures
Galeazzi or Allen's sign (Fig. 35.18) Fig. 35.18	The child is in supine position with Both the hip and the knee in flexion. The level of both the knee joints are noted with reference to a horizontal line. This test is useful in assessing unilateral cases of CDH in children between 3 and 8 months	Normally, both the knees should be at the same level. In DDH, the affected knee is seen beneath the horizontal line indicating femoral shortening. The shortening is in the supratrochanteric region and can be assessed by the Bryant's triangle
Skin fold test of thigh (Fig. 35.19) Fig. 35.19	The child is completely stripped and in the vertical position, the levels of the thigh folds studied	Normally, the thigh folds are symmetrical in nature. In DDH, they are no longer symmetrical due to the shortening of the affected limb
Skin fold test of Glutei region (Fig. 35.20) Fig. 35.20	The procedure is similar to the one performed above, but here the Levels of the glutei folds are noted	Normally; the thigh folds are symmetrical in nature. In DDH, they are no longer symmetrical due to the shortening of the affected limb
[5]Trendelenburg test (Fig. 35.21) Normal Positive Fig. 35.21	The patient is made to stand first on the normal limb and then on the Affected limb. The contralateral leg Is then raised from the ground	When standing on the normal limb, the opposite hip is in a higher position, but when the patient or the child stands on the affected limb, the opposite pelvis drops indicating impairment of abductor mechanism due to DDH. This test cannot be performed in infants

[3]Thomas Geoffrey Barlow (1915-1975), Orthopedic Surgeon, England.
[4]Ortolani Marius (1937), Orthopedic Surgeon, Italy.
[5]Trendelenburg Frederick (Berlin). Professor of Surgery of Rostook, Bonn, Liepzig. He first described CDH in 1895.

CHAPTER 35: Congenital Disorders

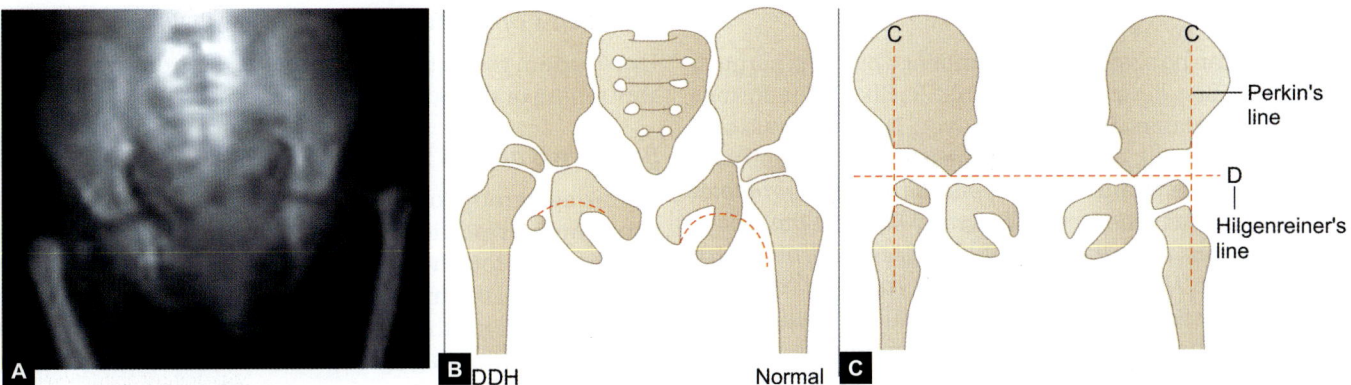

Figs 35.22A to C: (A) Radiograph showing congenital dislocation of hip; (B) Shenton's line is broken in CDH; (C) Perkin's line; (D) Hilgenreiner's line

TABLE 35.5: Treatment divided into five age groups					
Newborn (6 months)	**6–18 months**	**Toddler (18–36 months)**	**Child (3–8 years)**	**Juvenile and young adults (8-18 years)**
Hold if need pull	*Pull and hold*	*Break and hold*	*Open and break*	*Open and replace*
Pavlik harness and von Rosen splint are applied for 2 months. Later wean, by removing it 2 hours/day doubled every 2–4 weeks until device is worn in the night only. Night bracing is continued till X-rays are normal. *X-rays are taken at* 1 month, 6 months, 1 year intervals **If dislocation persists for 6–8 weeks, abandon this program and institute** <ul><li>Traction</li><li>Closed reduction</li><li>Casting</li></ul>	In this age group harness is not successful. The recommended regime as follows: <ul><li>Preoperative traction</li><li>Adductor tenotomy</li><li>Closed reduction and arthrogram.</li><li>Hip spica after confirmation of stable reduction.</li></ul> Desired position of the hip joint is human position (i.e. 95° flexion and 40° abduction at the hip). <ul><li>Open reduction in child less than 18 months is done when closed reduction fails by using the Bikini skin incision</li></ul>	Here open reduction is combined with femoral or pelvic osteotomy or both and is the treatment of choice. *Femoral osteotomy* is tried first for untreated CDH and is useful in less than 8 years of age *Pelvic osteotomy:* The following varieties is described <ul><li>*Salter's:* Uses symphysis pubis as the hinge. Useful between 18 months and 6 years</li><li>*Pemberton:* Uses triradiate cartilage as the hinge. Useful between 1 and 10 years of age.</li><li>*Steel:* (Triple innominate osteotomy) Useful in older children when symphysis pubis and triradiate cartilages are fused</li><li>*Shelf operations:* Here acetabulum is extended anteriorly, laterally and posteriorly. Useful in CDH which have recurred after reduction</li><li>*Chiari's oseotomy:* Here medial displacement of the distal fragment is done usually as a last resort. Useful in children Over 4 years of age</li></ul>	Here open reduction is the treatment of choice and is usually followed with femoral Shortening (Klisic and Jankovic) and if necessary pelvic osteotomy.	Depending on the situation, the following procedures are chosen: <ul><li>Femoral shortening with pelvic osteotomy</li><li>THR when osteoarthritis develops</li><li>Rarely arthrodesis</li></ul>

In Infants

Reduction can be obtained and maintained by Pavlik harness, which was first described by Arnold Pavlik, in the former Czechoslovakia, in the year 1958, von Rosen splints, and other splints. Pavlik harness is the most important appliance useful in this age group. *This is the only harness that promotes spontaneous reduction of a dislocated hip and maintains the reduction, whereas other appliances only maintain the reduction. Hence, Pavlik harness is called as "dynamic flexion abduction orthoses."* This is useful in children less than 6 months of age. Apart from the reduction and the immobilization, it allows active movements in all directions except extension and adduction. Nappies can be changed easily. The success rate of this harness is 85–95 percent. However, as the age advances, soft tissue contractures develop along with secondary changes in the acetabulum, which bring down the success rate of Pavlik harness. Complications include osteonecrosis and failure of reduction.

Between 6 and 18 Months

As mentioned earlier, Pavlik harness has no role in the treatment of DDH in this age group. Here, the treatment of choice is gentle closed reduction and hip spica application. Open reduction is done if this method proves unsuccessful.

> **Remember**
> - Ortolani's test (is a test of entry) relocates a dislocated hip.
> - Barlow's test (test of exit) dislocates a dislocatable hip.
> - Both these tests lose their significance after infancy.

Between 18 and 36 Months

In this age group, open reduction is the treatment of choice as closed reduction is often not successful. Open reduction is to be followed with either pelvic or femoral osteotomy to provide concentric reduction of the femoral head within the acetabulum.

Role of osteotomies: Osteotomies are done for instability, failure of acetabular development or progressive head subluxation after reduction. They are done only if congruent reduction is possible, if there is satisfactory range of movements, and if the femoral head has a reasonable sphericity.

The osteotomies could be femoral or pelvic and the choice is usually left to the surgeons, but there are some guiding principles.

Pelvic osteotomies: These are chosen if there is severe dysplasia and if radiographic changes are seen on the acetabular side. Table 35.5 for different pelvic osteotomies. Femoral osteotomies: This is the procedure of choice if there are changes in the femoral head and if there is increase in ante version of the neck.

Between 3 and 8 Years

Here open reduction is followed either by femoral shortening or pelvic osteotomies.

Between 8 and 18 Years

In this age group, open reduction is followed by femoral shortening or pelvic osteotomies. If osteoarthritis of the hip develops, total hip replacement is the surgery of choice. Arthrodesis of the hip is rarely done.

Table 35.5 for the comparative study of the treatment regimen in various age groups in DDH.

> **Remember**
> *Important radiological parameters in DDH*
> - <6 m: von Rosen's line (see Fig. 35.15).
> - >6 m: Perkin's line, Shenton's line (see Fig. 35.22B), acetabular index and delayed ossification.

> **What is Von Rosen's Line?**
> This is a line, which helps in the diagnosis of DDH radiologically in infants less than 6 months. It is an anteroposterior view of the pelvis taken with the lower limbs in full medial rotation and 45° abduction. When the hip is normal, upward prolongation of the long axis of the shaft of the femur points towards the lateral margin of the acetabulum and crosses the pelvis in the region of the sacroiliac joint. When the hip is dislocated upward, prolongation of this line points towards anterior iliac spine and crosses the midline in the lower lumbar region. This line is not useful after 6 months. Standard anteroposterior views are preferred in a child older than 6 months.

Innominate Osteotomy in DDH

Salter's Osteotomy

This is indicated in patients with instability after reduction or in persistent DDH between 18 months to 6 years. The procedure consists of using the symphysis pubis as a hinge, osteotomizing the acetabulum to cover the head.

Pemberton's Osteotomy (Fig. 35.23)

It is indicated in paralytic dislocation and in postacetabular deficiency between 1 and 10 years. Here, the osteotomy is done through the acetabular roof using triradiate cartilage as the hinge.

Steel's Osteotomy (Fig. 35.24)

This is useful in older children when symphysis pubis and the tri-radiate cartilage are fused. This is a triple innominate osteotomy.

Shelf Operation (Figs 35.25 and 35.26)

It is indicated in CDH with recurrence. Here, the acetabulum is extended laterally and anteriorly by bone graft.

CHAPTER 35: Congenital Disorders

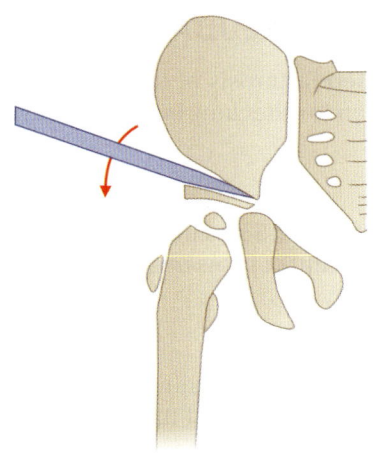

Fig. 35.23: Showing Pemberton's osteotomy

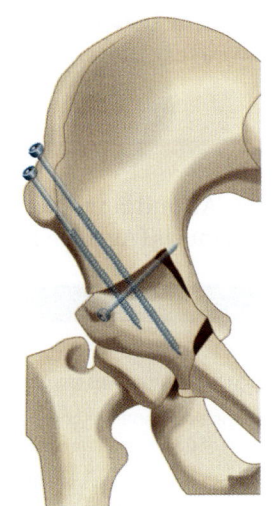

Fig. 35.24: Steel's osteotomy

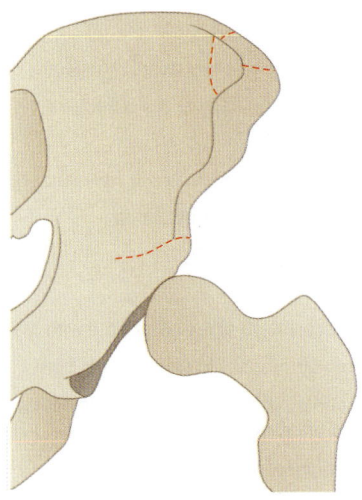

Fig. 35.25: Shelf operation

Chiari's Osteotomy (Fig. 35.27)

This is a salvage procedure and is indicated in children older than 4 years. Here, the osteotomy is done through the ilium above the acetabulum and the distal fragment is pushed medially.

CONGENITAL DISLOCATION OF KNEE

This is uncommon and three types are described:

Traumatic developmental type is the most common, due to malposition in uterus.

A primary embryonic defect is associated with other defects like spina bifida.

Quadriceps contracture or congenital absence or hypoplastic anterior cruciate ligament.

Three degrees
- Congenital hyperextension.
- Congenital hyperextension with anterior subluxation of tibia on femur.
- Congenital hyperextension with anterior dislocation of tibia on femur usually associated with other skeletal abnormalities.

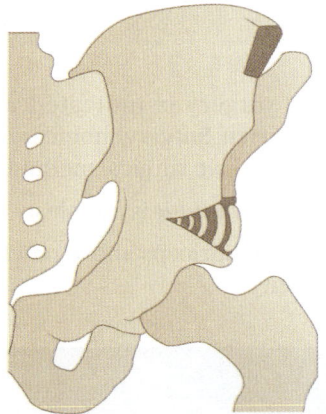

Fig. 35.26: Pictures of shelf osteotomy

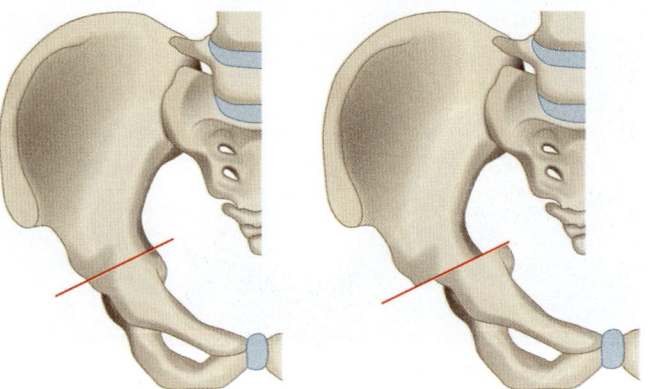

Fig. 35.27: Chiari's osteotomy

Pathology

Varies with severity but anterior capsule and quadriceps are contracted. There are always intra-articular adhesions, hypoplasia, or absence of patella or lateral dislocation of patella, and hypoplastic vastus lateralis.

Clinical Features

The patient presents with hyperextension deformity of the knee and could be quite grotesque. The knee functions are affected. The patient complains of limp and difficulty in carrying out his knee functions.

Radiograph

Plain X-ray of the knee including both AP and lateral views are essential to diagnose this condition (Fig. 35.28).

Treatment

Mild to Moderate

In these cases, conservative methods like Pavlik harness, serial casting, and skeletal traction are the treatment of choice.

Severe

In severe cases, surgery is indicated and is done by anteromedial approach. Surgery should be done before the child is 2 years of age. Two surgical methods are described:

Neibauer and King Technique is a Z-plasty of quadriceps.

Curtis and Fischer Quadriceps above patella is divided by inverted V-incision.

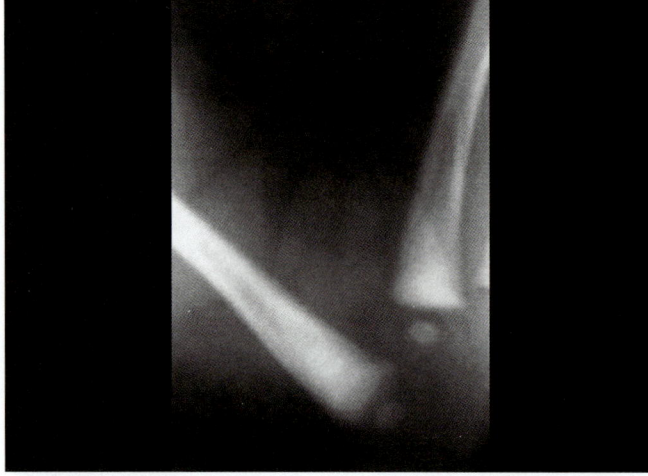

Fig. 35.28: Radiograph of congenital knee dislocation

CONGENITAL PSEUDARTHROSIS OF TIBIA

Congenital pseudarthrosis of tibia is a rare condition. It can also be seen in other long bones like femur (Fig. 35.29).

Incidence

- Incidence is 1 in 2.5 lacs live births.
- In 50–90 percent of cases neurofibromatosis is present.

Classification

[6]Boyd has classified this condition into six types and is the most accepted classification (Table 35.6).

Clinical Features

In this condition, deformity is the chief complaint and the patient develops anterior bowing of the tibia of various severities. In a few cases, there could be pathological fractures.

Radiograph

Radiograph of the leg, AP and lateral views, are sufficient to make an accurate diagnosis (Also see Fig. 36.12).

TABLE 35.6: Boyd's classification	
Type I	• Anterior bowing and a defect in the tibia is present at birth
	• Other congenital anomalies are present
Type II	• Pseudarthrosis with anterior bowing and an hourglass constriction of tibia present at birth
	• Spontaneous fracture occurs before 2 years
	• High-risk tibia
	• Most frequent type
	• Associated with neurofibromatosis
	• Poorest prognosis
Type III	• Pseudarthrosis develops in a congenital cyst
	• Recurrence of fracture is less frequent
	• Good results
Type IV	• Pseudarthrosis originates in a sclerotic segment of bone
	• Medullary canal is obliterated
	• An incomplete or stress fracture develops
	• Prognosis good
Type V	• Pseudarthrosis tibia is associated with dysplastic fibula
	• Pseudarthrosis of fibula or tibia or both
Type VI	• Pseudarthrosis occurs as an intraosseous neurofibromatosis
	• Very rare condition

---

[6]**Boyd HB** (1941) other contributions: (a) Classification of trochanteric fractures, (b) Described nonunion of long bones.

CONGENITAL TALIPES EQUINOVARUS (CTEV)

One may pride in having flatfoot, agile foot, nimble foot, but look at the tale of woes a clubfoot presents to the unfortunate victim affected with this malady!

Interesting Features of CTEV
Talipes: It is a Latin word derived from *Talus* = ankle, *pes* = foot.
Original meaning: A deformity that causes the patient to walk on the ankle.
Present-day meaning is any variety of clubfoot.
Clubfoot: It is so called because severe untreated talipes equinovarus has a club-like appearance. There are various types of foot deformities (Figs 35.30A to I).

This is the most common congenital foot disorder. Incidence is 1.2/1000 live births. Males are more commonly affected than females. How is congenital TEV different from acquired TEV? (Table 35.7)

Types of CTEV (Etiology)	
Osseous type	Clubfoot is associated with absence of tibia and fibula.
Muscular type	Arthrogryposis multiplex congenita or multiple congenital contractures.
Neuropathic type	Due to spina bifida, etc.
Idiopathic type	No apparent cause, commonest variety.

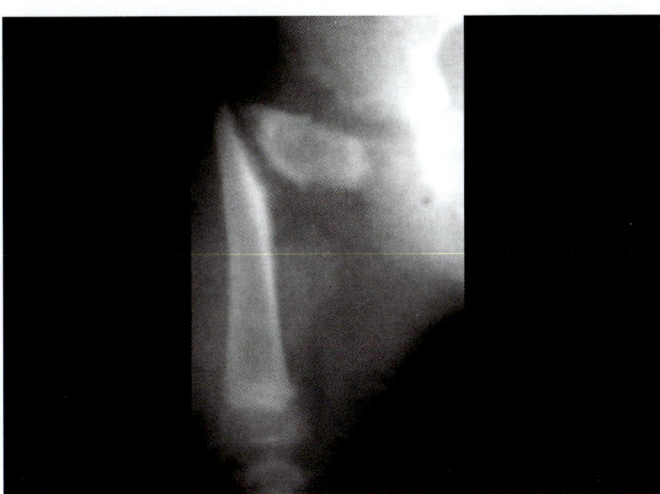

Fig. 35.29: Radiograph showing congenital pseudarthrosis of femur

Treatment

Principles
- It depends on the age and type.
- True pseudarthrosis will not unite with casting alone.
- Tibial cyst curettage and bone grafting is done in small lesions.
- Treatment is usually surgical, once a fracture develops.

Established Pseudarthrosis

Surgery
Boyd dual onlay graft is the treatment of choice in patients with stress fractures.

Osteotomy, intramedullary nailing, bone grafting, and excision of thick tissue is done for more established pseudarthrosis because retraction is common. Bracing is continued until skeletal maturity. Good results. Causes of failure of union in some cases were attributed to distal location of the lateral pseudarthrosis and the concomitant pseudarthrosis.

McFarland's bone grafting for anterior bowing with impending fracture, a single graft is placed posteriorly to span the pseudarthrosis.

Sofield's multiple osteotomies with internal fixation by medullary nails are useful when the distal fragment is too short to be held by a graft.

Other Treatment

- *Pulsed EMF:* This method has been tried and is found to be successful for fracture occurring through a cyst.
- *Free vascularized fibular graft:* This method has also been tried and the results are good.

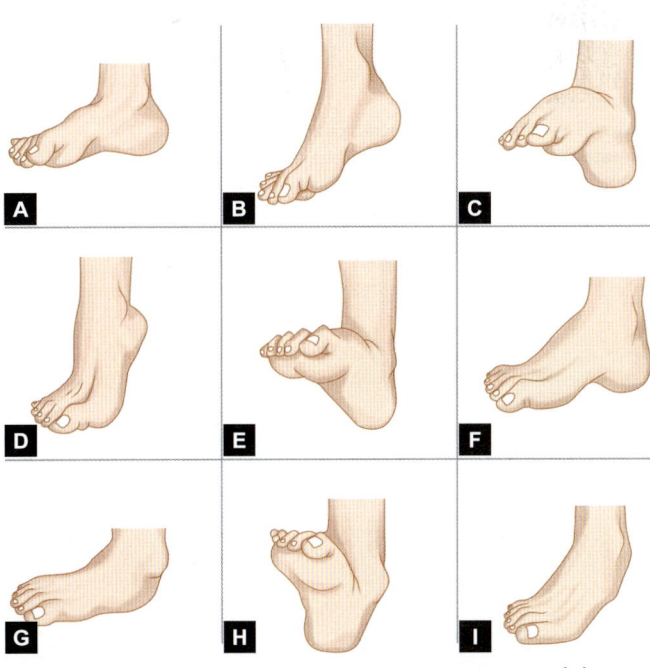

Figs 35.30A to I: Different varieties of foot deformities: (A) Varus; (B) Equinovarus; (C) Calcaneovarus; (D) Equinus; (E) Calcaneus; (F) Cavus; (G) Valgus; (H) Calcaneovalgus; (I) Equinovalgus

Idiopathic CTEV

This is the most common type of CTEV 1 encounters in clinical practice. There is no apparent cause and various theories are proposed (Table 35.8).

Pathology

The pathology in CTEV affects all the bones and joints of the foot with corresponding soft tissue contractures especially of the posteromedial structures. The primary problem usually lies in the bones with secondary soft tissue contractures. However, sometimes the primary pathology may be in the surrounding soft tissues, which brings about secondary changes in the bones; however, the latter event is rare. Table 35.9 shows the bony changes and the structures involved in the posteromedial aspect of the ankle and foot

TABLE 35.7: Differences between CTEV and ATEV (Fig. 35.31)

CTEV	ATEV
• Present since birth • May be associated with spina bifida • Bilateral • Skin, subcutaneous tissue, muscles are normal • Transverse crease is seen across the sole on the medial side • Bones are normal in thickness	• Not present from birth • May be due to polio, cerebral palsy, etc. • Usually unilateral • Tropic changes in the skin, muscles are flaccid (LMN lesion) or spastic (UMN lesion) • No transverse crease • Bones are thinner than normal

TABLE 35.8: Theories of CTEV (Figs 35.21A to I)

Theories	What do they say?
Turco's	Medial displacement of navicular and calcaneus around the talus
Brockman's	Congenital atresia of the talonavicular joint
Mc-Kay's	Three-dimensional bony deformity of the subtalar complex
Intrauterine	Due to compression by malposition of fetus in utero
Genetic	General population 1:800 • In siblings 1:35 • In identical twins 1:3
Germ plasm theory	Primary germ plasm defect in talus with subsequent soft tissue changes.
Soft tissue theory	Primary soft tissue defect with secondary bony changes
Prenatal muscle imbalance theory	Weak pronators and overacting extensors and invertors.

TABLE 35.9: Bony and soft tissue changes in CTEV

Bones and joints (bony)	Muscles, capsules, ligaments (soft tissues)
Calcaneus is in varus position **Talus** displaced medial and plantarwards (Fig. 35.31) **Navicular** medially displaced and rotated **Cuboid** displaced medially and articulates with the non-articular surface of the calcaneus **(Known as cuboid sign or locked cuboid)** **Metatarsals** deviates medially at tarsometatarsal joints **Talocalcaneal articulation** is a ball and socket joint. The anterior and middle articulation of the calcaneum forms the socket and the head of the talus forms the ball which is dislocation in CTEV **Tibia** usually shows medial torsion, rarely lateral torsion In short, all the above bones are displaced down and medial in a case of CTEV	Structures contracted on the medial side (3) — Rule of 3 **3 muscles**: AHL, TP, FHL **3 ligaments**: Deltoid, Spring, Plantar **3 capsules of**: Subtalar, Tarsal, Tarsometatarsal joints Structures contracted on the posterior side (2) — Rule of 2 **2 muscles**: Tibialis posterior, Tendo-Achilles **2 ligaments**: Talofibular, Calcaneofibular **2 capsules**: Ankle joint, Subtalar joint Structures involved on the anterior side (1) — Rule of 1 **1 muscles**: Tibialis anterior inserted abnormally **1 ligaments**: Superior peroneal retinacula **1 capsules**: Calcaneocuboid joint

Abbreviations: AHL, Abductor hallucis longus; TP, Tibialis posterior; FHL, Flexor hallucis longus.

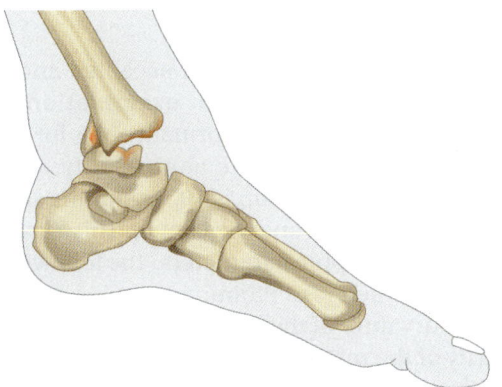

Fig. 35.31: In CTEV the talus is displaced medial and down

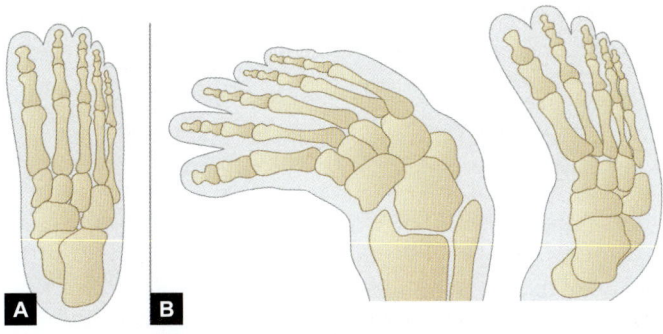

Figs 35.32A and B: (A) Normal foot; (B) Foot in CTEV

in a case of CTEV. All these contracted soft tissue should be released during surgery to bring back the bones to normal alignment (Figs 35.32A and B).

> **Did You Know?**
> Hippocrates first described CTEV.

Clinical Features

Congenital talipes equinovarus is a grotesque looking deformity of the foot. In idiopathic variety, deformity is the only complaint. The diagnosis is fairly simple and straightforward. *Five classical primary deformities are seen and in response to this, secondary deformities develop. These primary and secondary deformities together form the clubfoot complex (Flowchart 35.3).* A detailed examination of the foot is necessary to detect the full spectrum of deformities in CTEV.

With advancing age, the cosmetically unsightly clubfoot (Fig. 35.33) starts posing functional problems like altered gait (stumbling gait), callosities, degeneration and arthritic changes in the ankle and foot joints (Fig. 35.34). Correction is necessary to restore normalcy. In other varieties of CTEV, clinical features peculiar to the etiological factors can be elicited. Three clinical tests are of extreme importance in CTEV and are described below:

Dorsiflexion Test

In a newborn child, it is possible to dorsiflex the foot until its dorsal surface meets the anterior surface of the tibia. This is not possible in CTEV and this can be used as a screening test (Fig. 35.35).

Plumb Line Test

This test helps to detect the tibial torsion. The child is made to sit on a table with both the lower limbs hanging from the edge. A line drawn from the center of the patella to the

Flowchart 35.3: Clubfoot complex

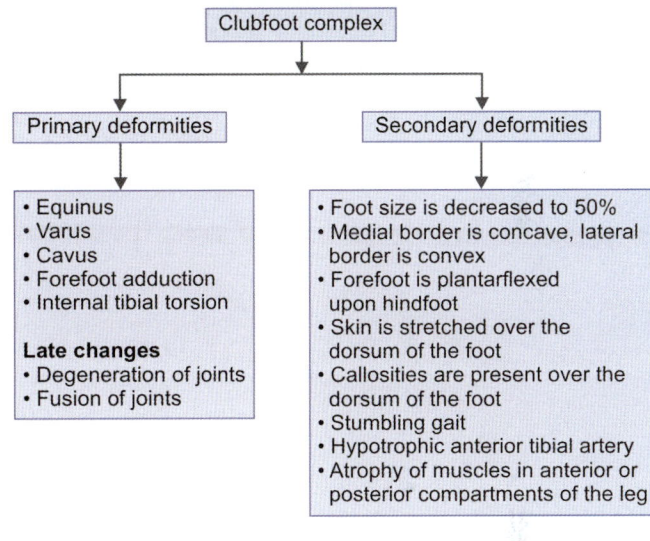

Clubfoot complex
- Primary deformities
  - Equinus
  - Varus
  - Cavus
  - Forefoot adduction
  - Internal tibial torsion
- Late changes
  - Degeneration of joints
  - Fusion of joints
- Secondary deformities
  - Foot size is decreased to 50%
  - Medial border is concave, lateral border is convex
  - Forefoot is plantarflexed upon hindfoot
  - Skin is stretched over the dorsum of the foot
  - Callosities are present over the dorsum of the foot
  - Stumbling gait
  - Hypotrophic anterior tibial artery
  - Atrophy of muscles in anterior or posterior compartments of the leg

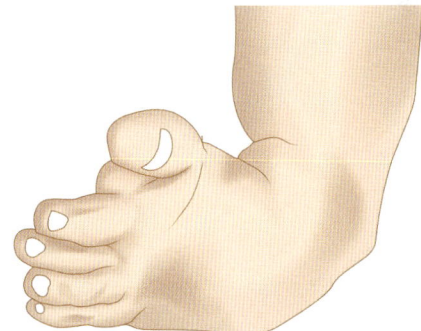

Fig. 35.33: Unilateral clubfoot

tibial tubercle when extended down should cut the foot at the first or second intermetatarsal space normally. This is called the plumb line. In CTEV, with medial rotation of the tibia, it cuts the fourth or fifth intermetatarsal space and vice versa in lateral rotation of the tibia (Fig. 35.36).

Scratch test: This test is performed to detect muscle imbalance in an infant who cannot obey commands.

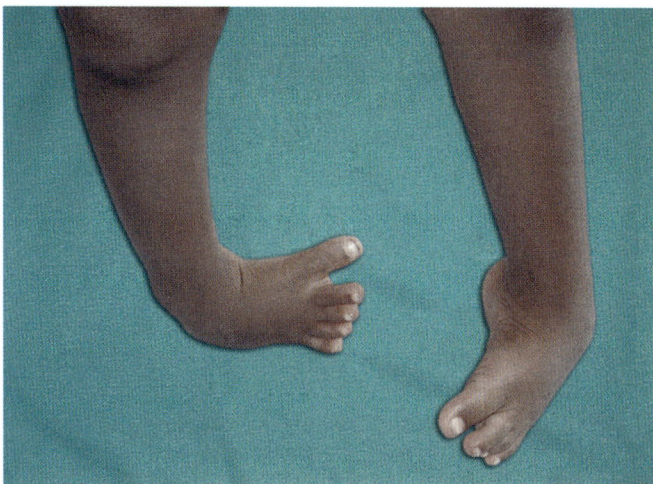

Fig. 35.34: Bilateral CTEV (Clinical photo)

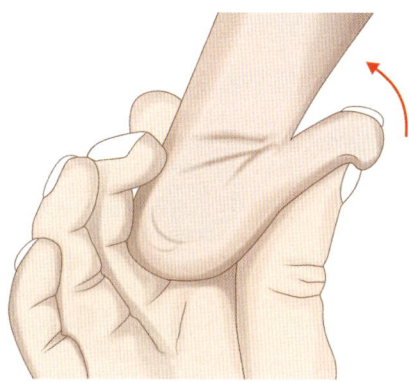

Fig. 35.35: Dorsiflexion test in a newborn

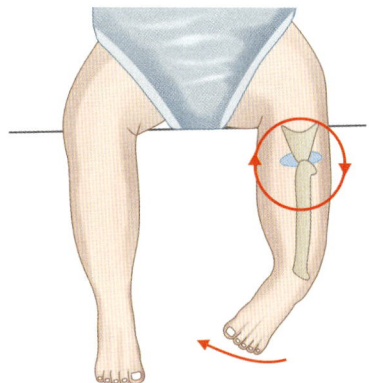

Fig. 35.36: Plumb line test to detect tibial torsion

- *Medial scratch test* in a normal child, when the medial sole is scratched, the foot everts. This tests the peroneals.
- *Lateral scratch test* here, when the lateral sole is scratched, the child inverts the foot. This tests the invertors.

Classification

Pirani's classification is the most accepted and is based purely on 10 different physical examination findings with each scored 0 for no abnormality, 0.5 for moderate abnormality, and 1 for severe abnormality. The points are scored and the maximum is 10, higher the score more severe is the deformity and vice versa. This classification requires no radiographic parameters. The following are the 10 physical parameters of Pirani:
- Lateral curvature of the foot.
- Severity of the medial crease.
- Severity of the posterior crease.
- Medial mallelor navicular interval.
- Palpation of the lateral part of the head of the talus.
- Emptiness of the heel.
- Fibula Achilles interval.
- Rigidity of equines.
- Rigidity of adductus.
- Long flexor contracture.

Dimeglio's classification Another equally effective classification and four parameters are assessed on the basis of their reducibility with gentle manipulation and measurement with a goniometer:
- In the sagittal plane: Equinus deviation.
- In the frontal plane: Varus deviation.
- Horizontal plane: De-rotation.
- Adduction of the forefoot in relative to the hind foot.

Investigation

Since CTEV is a mechanical problem, laboratory investigations are less useful. Radiography is by far the most important investigation. It helps to know the exact angles of each deformity seen clinically in CTEV. In anteroposterior view, the angles formed between the long axis of the talus and the calcaneum (talocalcaneal angles), the talus and the metatarsals (talometatarsal angle) are evaluated. This helps to know the angle of varus and the forefoot adduction. In the lateral view, the angle formed between the talus and the tibia, and talus and calcaneum helps to know the extent of equinus and varus respectively (Table 35.10).

X-ray views are to be taken with feet in the stabilization frames.

AP view is to be taken with tibia vertical.

Lateral view is the stress dorsiflexion view.

In children of older age group, anteroposterior and lateral standing radiographies are preferred. Apart from giving the accurate estimate of the angle of the deformities, radiology helps in confirmation of the correction of the deformities by various treatment modalities. *It is a simple*

CHAPTER 35: Congenital Disorders

TABLE 35.10: Various radiographic angles in CTEV

Anteroposterior	Lateral
• Talocalcaneal angle is reduced (normal is 30–35°)	• Talocalcaneal angle is reduced (normal is 25–50°)
Talocalcaneal Index = TC angle (AP view + TC angle lateral view) should be at least 40°, which is ↓ in CTEV. The study of talocalcaneal angle on the radiographs indicates the extent of varus.	
• Talometatarsal angle • This angle indicates extent of forefoot adduction Normal is 5–15° In CTEV, it is 0° to negative	• Tibiocalcaneal angle • This angle indicates extent of equinus Normal is 5–15° it is negative in CTEV

fact that all angles should be restored back to normal following treatment. *Any residual uncorrected angle is a future pointer to relapse* (Figs 35.37A and B).

Remember
Clinical tests in CTEV
- Scratch test
- Dorsiflexion test
- Plumb line test

Management

Broadly speaking, CTEV can be managed by three methods.
- Conservative management.
- Surgical management.
- Management by external fixators.

Conservative Management

It is the treatment of choice in infants less than 6 months of age. The recommended regime is as follows (after Kite and Lovell) (Flowchart 35.4).

First 6 weeks of life: Weekly serial manipulation of the deformities and above-knee casting for the first 6 weeks of life. Later, it is done every fortnightly until correction is achieved. Manipulation by mother is not usually sufficient (Fig. 35.38). Success rate of serial manipulation and casting ranges from 15–80 percent. If correction is achieved in first 6 months of age, Phelps's brace is used during the daytime and Dennis Browne splint during the nighttime from 6–18 months to prevent recurrence. After 18 months, below-knee walking calipers are given up to 4 years of age. From 4 years to skeletal maturity, regular follow-up is advised.

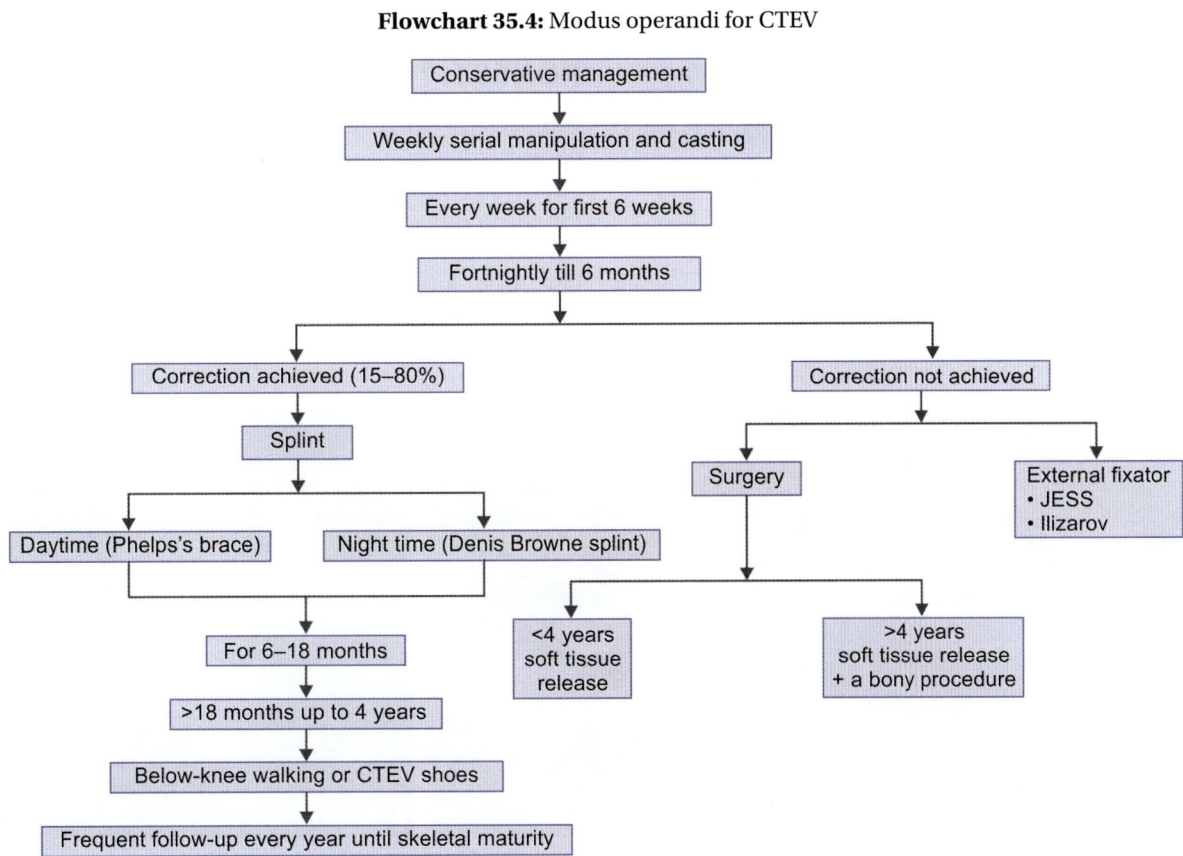

Flowchart 35.4: Modus operandi for CTEV

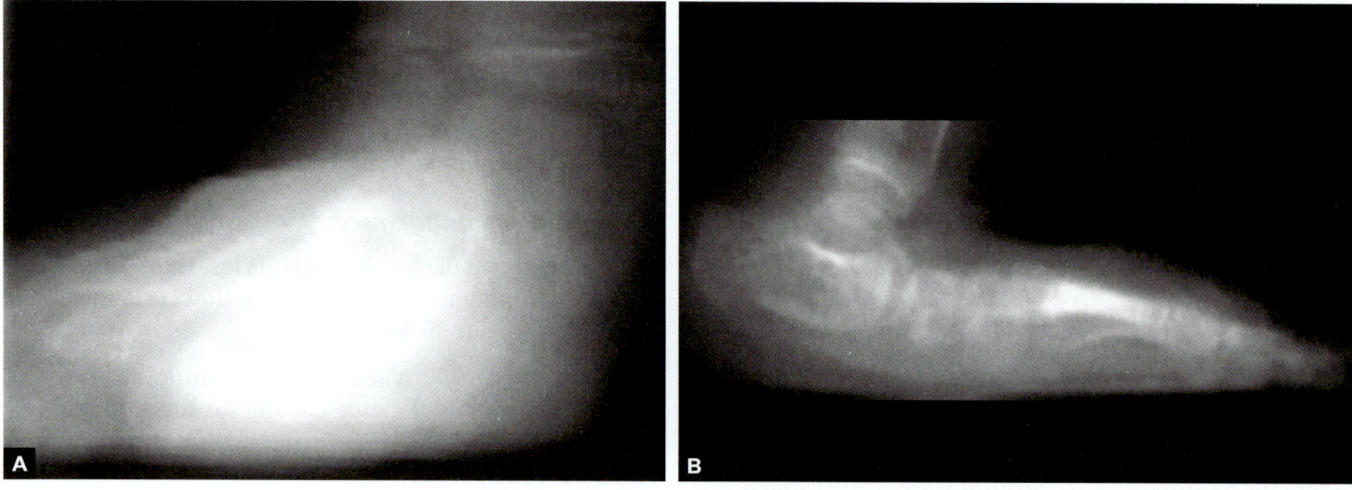

Figs 35.37A and B: (A) Radiograph of clubfoot—AP view; (B) Clubfoot—lateral view

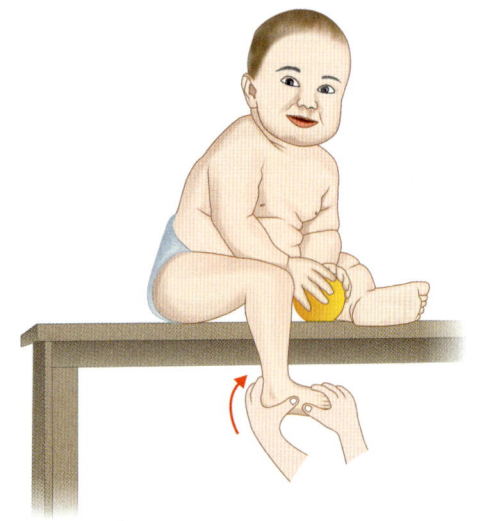

Fig. 35.38: Mother manipulating her child's CTEV foot

> **Remember Order of Correction of Deformity**
> The mnemonic ADVERB helps to remember the order of correction.
> **AD**—Forefoot adduction is corrected first
> **V**—Correction of heel varus next
> **E**—Lastly correction of hind foot equinus
> **RB**—this order is followed to prevent **Rocker Bottom Foot** which develops if foot is dorsiflexed through hind foot rather than midfoot.

PONSETI TECHNIQUE

Ponseti in the year 1950 described a very effective conservative method of treating a clubfeet with very few recurrence rates. There is an extremely high success rate for correcting clubfoot using the Ponseti method for non-surgical cast correction of clubfoot (Figs 35.39A and B). Of late, lot of interest is being revived with this technique of clubfoot management. Here, the success of the reduction is 90–98 percent and is better than the Kite's regime.

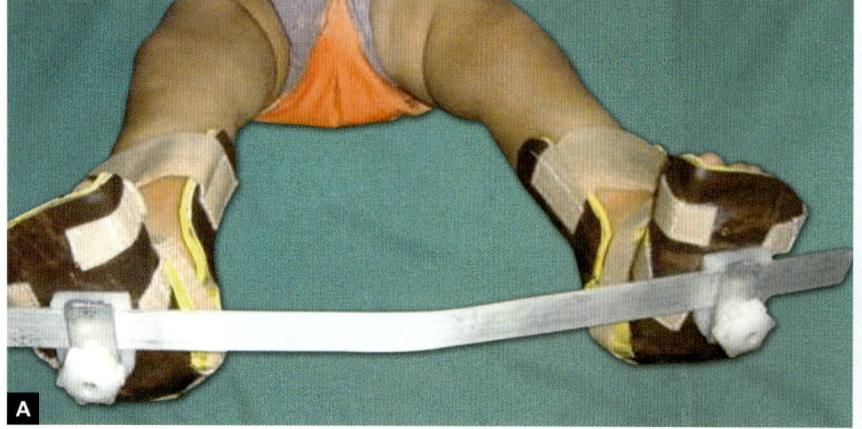 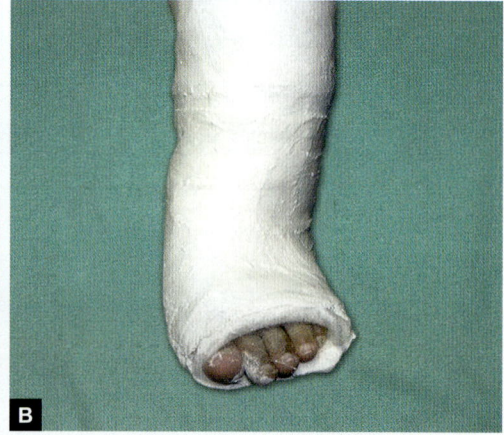

Figs 35.39A and B: Ponseti technique for the non-surgical treatment of clubfoot

It is mooted as a better alternative to the more cumbersome surgical correction. It can be used in older children of 2 years age and also after failed previous nonoperative techniques and thus has a wider application.

Treatment Phase

Ideally, it is begun, as soon as possible after birth. The treatment involves weekly stretching of the foot deformity in the clinic, followed by the application of long leg plaster casts. The cast is changed every 1 or 2 weeks, and a newborn with a congenital clubfoot should expect the deformity corrected in about five to six weeks. Before the application of the final cast, the physician usually performs a tenotomy (Fig. 35.40), an Achilles tendon lengthening using non-invasive surgery. The incision is so small that no stitching is required. The child wears a final cast for three weeks to allow the tendon to heal.

Maintenance Phase

The child then wears a corrective foot orthosis full time (23 hours a day) for three months, followed by night and naptime wear for up to four years to prevent the deformity from recurring.

Benefits of the Ponseti Method

The Ponseti method delivers excellent correction of clubfoot without the associated risks and complications of major foot surgery. Parents, as much as the child, appreciate the fact that clubfoot can be corrected successfully without surgery. Moreover, studies show that patients treated with the Ponseti method enjoy a more flexible foot and ankle than those treated surgically. Long-term studies of the Ponseti method have demonstrated that cast correction of clubfoot not only helps dramatically during childhood, but also in adulthood.

Surgical Management

Indications (5 R's)

- **R**esponse not obtained to conservative treatment after 6 months.
- **R**igid clubfoot (means *forefoot deformities are corrected but hind foot deformities remain uncorrected after conservative treatment*).
- **R**elapsed clubfoot (means deformities are corrected initially, but relapse later, either partial or total).
- **R**ecurrent clubfoot (it is a type of relapse, the cause being muscle imbalance, which was overlooked initially).
- **R**esistant clubfoot (very resistant to correction).

Surgical Methods (Table 35.11)

Soft tissue procedures are advocated for children less than 4 years. Bony procedures are added later on. For mild CTEV with no severe internal rotation deformity of calcaneus, a one-stage posteromedial release of TURCO is preferred.

STRUCTURES RELEASED IN TURCO'S PROCEDURE (Posteromedial Release)

On the posterior side:
- Z-plasty of tendo-Achilles to lengthen it (Fig. 35.41).
- Posterior capsulotomy of the ankle and subtalar joints.
- Release of posterior talofibular and calcaneofibular ligaments.

On the medial side:
- Lengthening of the tibialis posterior, flexor hallucis longus, and flexor digitorum longus muscle.
- Release of talonavicular ligament, spring ligament and the superficial part of deltoid ligament.

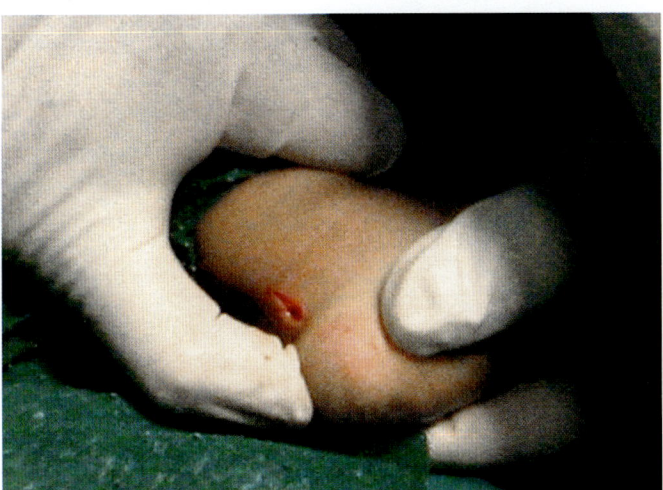

Fig. 35.40: Operative photo showing method of tenotomy

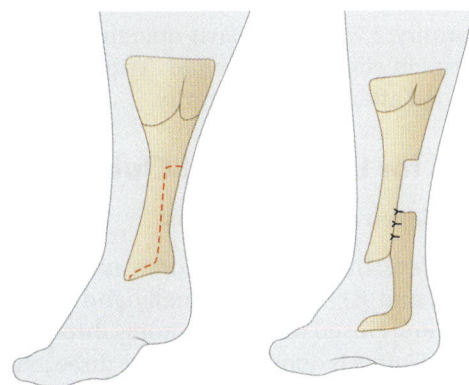

Fig. 35.41: Tendo-Achilles lengthening by Z-plasty for clubfoot

TABLE 35.11: Surgical treatment plan of CTEV			
6–12 months (Turco's)	12–36 months (McKay's)	1–5 years (Gray area)	Older child (untreated or treated with partial or total relapse)

Cincinnati's incision is used
Structures released are:
Medial
• TP/AHL/FHL/FDL muscles
• Capsules of ST/Tarsal/TM joints
Ligaments—deltoid/plantar/spring ligaments
Posterior
• Tendo-Achilles lengthening by Z-plasty (Fig. 35.30)
• Postcapsulotomy of the ankle and subtalar joints
• Calcaneofibular ligaments
Subtalar ligaments
• Talocalcaneal ligaments
• Interosseous ligaments
• Bifurcated Y-ligaments
Postoperative regimen
• Change cast at 2 weeks
• Remove K-wire at 6 weeks
• Long leg cast until 3 months
• Phelps's brace or ankle foot Orthoses for 6–9 months
	Cincinnati's incision
	All the structures on the posteromedial side is released as in Turco.
	In addition, lateral structures released are:
	• Superior peroneal retinaculum
	• Inferior external retinaculum
	• Dorsal calcaneocuboid ligament
	• Origin of extensor digitorum brevis muscle
		Treatment guidelines unclear	**Metatarsus adductus** >5 year metatarsal osteotomy.
			Hindfoot varus >2–3 years modified McKay's procedure.
			3–10 years of age
			    Dwyer's lateral closed wedge osteotomy of calcaneus is done
			    Dillwyn Evan's procedure—resection and arthrodesis of calcaneocuboid joint
			    Davis procedure wedge resection from the midtarsal area
			10–12 years of age
			Triple arthrodesis
			Equinus
			Mild—Tendo-Achilles lengthening and postcapsulotomy of ankle and subtalar joints are done
			Sever-Lambrunidi's triple arthrodesis is done
			All three deformities are present over on years triple arthrodesis is done
			Ilizarov and Joshi's external fixator frames useful in rigid, relapsed and untreated clubfoot

- Release of interosseous talocalcaneal ligament, capsules of naviculocuneiform and first metatarsocuneiform joints.

On the plantar side:
- Plantar fascia.
- Release of abductor hallucis and flexor digitorum brevis.

For severe deformities with severe internal rotation of calcaneum—a one-stage modified Mc-Kay procedure of both posteromedial and posterolateral release is preferred.

Bony procedures: These are added to the soft tissue procedures after 4 years of age. Dwyer's lateral closed wedge osteotomy (Figs 35.42 and 35.43) helps correct the varus deformity; Evan's and Davis operations also help to correct varus in slightly older child. Triple arthrodesis is recommended after skeletal maturity.

Surgeries for Uncorrected Clubfoot

In Older Children and Adolescents:

Triple arthrodesis: Indicated for children more than 10 years (Figs 35.44A and B). It is functionally and cosmetically, superior. Lateral closed wedge osteotomy through subtalar and midtarsal joints is done to fuse all the three joints of the foot namely—the subtalar, talonavicular and calcaneocuboid joints.

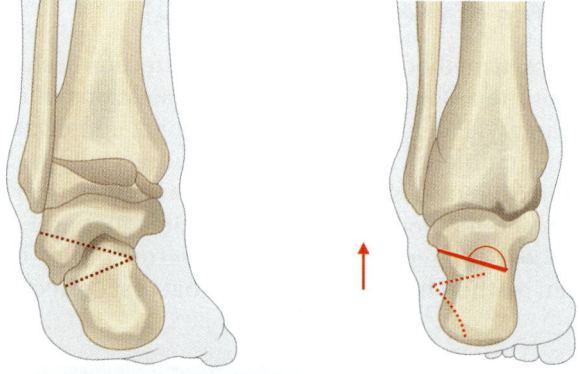

Fig. 35.42: Dwyer's lateral closed wedge osteotomy

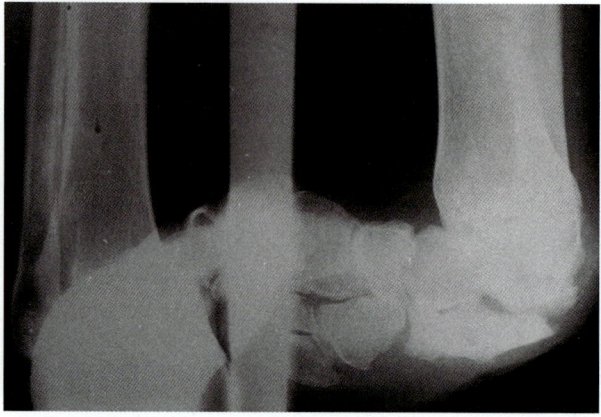

Fig. 35.43: Plain X-ray showing neglected club feet

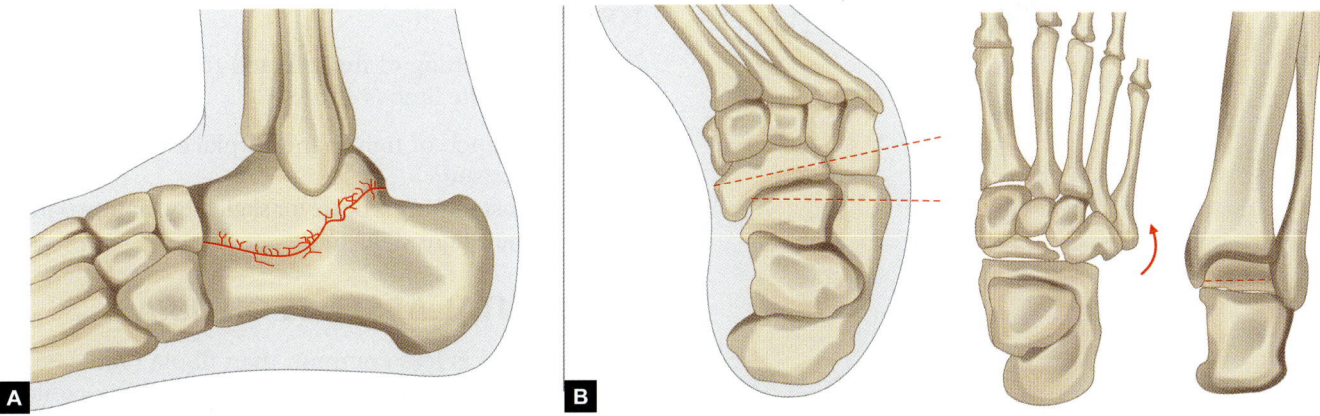

Figs 35.44A and B: (A) Triple arthrodesis in CTEV; (B) Triple arthrodesis in CTEV

Talectomy: It is a salvage procedure and is indicated for severe uncorrected clubfoot. It is also indicated in those cases previously corrected and unsuccessful. For uncorrectable CTEV by any other procedure, talectomy is useful as a salvage procedure.

Surgery for recurrent clubfoot: Recurrence is due to muscle imbalance, here peroneals are weak, and invertors are strong. Surgeries recommended are:

Garceaus method: Transfer of tibialis anterior to middle cuneiform bone.

Modified Garceaus method: Transfer of tibialis anterior to base of fifth metatarsal bone.

Surgery for correction of tibial torsion in clubfoot: (Sell's criteria) more than 15° torsion should be corrected by derotation osteotomy. Otherwise, all deformities will recur due to the pressure of the caliper on the lateral border of the foot.

Caliper is used after the correction to maintain the correction of deformities obtained either by conservative or surgical measures.

Treatment by External Fixators

This is a recent concept in the management of CTEV and is reserved for difficult cases. There are two types of external fixator frames; Ilizarov, a Russian orthopedic surgeon, design one. An Indian orthopedic surgeon, Dr BB Joshi, design the second one. This frame is known as Joshi's external stabilization system popularly called as JESS (Figs 35.45A and B).

When done in properly indicated cases, external fixator produces excellent results. It is a semi-invasive, bloodless surgery and can be done without a tourniquet. Though technically very demanding, it avoids all the complications of surgery and a postoperative scar. It is known to correct all the components of the deformities both bony and soft tissues. The rate of relapse or recurrence is comparatively less; and even if it does occur, the options of surgery are always open.

> **Remember**
> Three I's for relapse
> - Improper and inadequate conservative treatment and surgical release of contracted structures.
> - Imbalance of foot muscles if left uncorrected.
> - Internal torsion of tibia if overlooked.

RETENTION OF CTEV CORRECTION

Whatever may be the methods of correction of CTEV whether conservative, surgical, or external fixators should do retentions of the corrected deformities done by one of the following methods to prevent relapse:
- Denis Browne splint—used usually during the night time (Fig. 35.46).

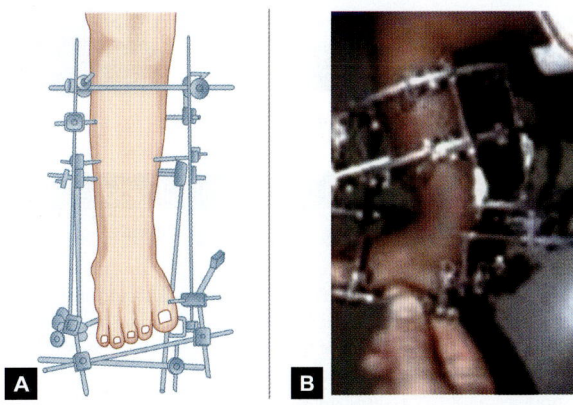

Figs 35.45A and B: External fixators (JESS) for CTEV

494 SECTION 5: General Orthopedics

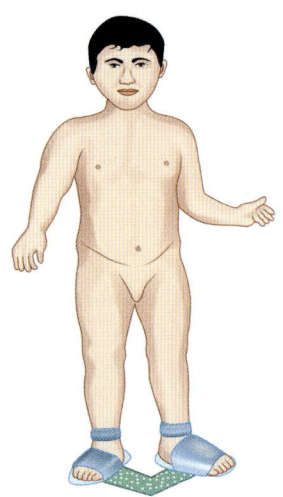

Fig. 35.46: Denis Browne splint

- Phelps's brace—used mainly in the daytime.
- Below-knee walking calipers.
- CTEV shoes—these are mainly used when the child starts walking and up to 5 years of age (Fig. 35.47).

> **Quick Facts**
> *Do you know how does a CTEV shoe differ from an ordinary shoe?*
> - It has a straight inner border, which helps prevent forefoot adduction.
> - It has an outer shoe raise and this helps prevent foot-inversion.
> - There is no heel and this helps prevent equinus.

CONGENITAL ABSENCE OF FIBULA

Fibula is partially or completely absent more often than any other long bones of the body (Table 35.12).

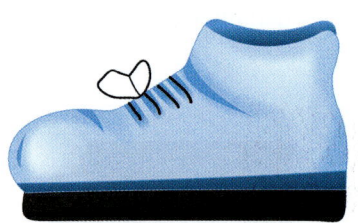 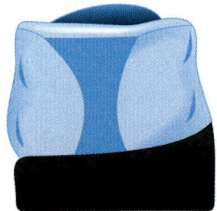

Fig. 35.47: CTEV shoes

TABLE 35.12: Coventry and Johnson's classification

Type I	Type II	Type III
- Fibula is partially absent - Unilateral - Leg is mildly or moderately short	- Unilateral absence of fibula - Anterior bowing with of tibia - Equinovalgus foot - Ipsilateral femur is short	- Unilateral or bilateral - Associated other severe anomalies - Prognosis is poorest

Treatment

Type I: Lengthening of the affected tibia and epiphyseal arrest of opposite limb is done.

Type II: Presence of tight band in place of absent fibula should be excised.

Wiltse's osteotomy is done for skeletally mature patients to correct the valgus deformity.

CONGENITAL ABSENCE OF TIBIA

This condition is less common than fibula (Table 35.13). Deformity may be unilateral or bilateral. Tibia could be aplastic or dysplastic. Leg is short, bowed, and the foot is rigid in varus and the first metatarsal is short.

CONGENITAL VERTICAL TALUS (Syn: Rocker-Bottom Flatfoot, Congenital Rigid Flatfoot)

Though it may appear as an isolated congenital abnormality most often it is associated with other neuromuscular manifestations like AMC, myelomeningocele, etc.

Clinical Presentation

In the initial stages:
- At birth, the rounded appearance of the plantar and the medial surface of the foot is a pointer for the presence of this problem.
- The talus is distorted plantar ward and medially.
- The calcaneus is also in equines position.
- Navicular bone lies on the dorsal aspect of the head of the talus.
- Foot is dorsiflexed at the midtarsal joints.

In the late stages:
- Talus assumes an hour glass shape (Fig. 35.48).
- The longitudinal axis of the talus is almost same as that of tibia.
- Only the posterior third of the superior articular facet of the talus articulates with tibia.
- The anterior part of the calcaneum is rounded.

TABLE 35.13: Types of congenital absence of tibia

Types	Features	Treatment
Type I	Total absence of tibia	Transfer of fibula
Type II	Distal tibial aplasia	Tibiofibular fusion
Type III	Distal tibial aplasia +	- Calcaneofibular fusion
	Diastasis of inferior tibiofibular syndesmosis	- Disarticulation of ankle - Modified Boyd's amputation

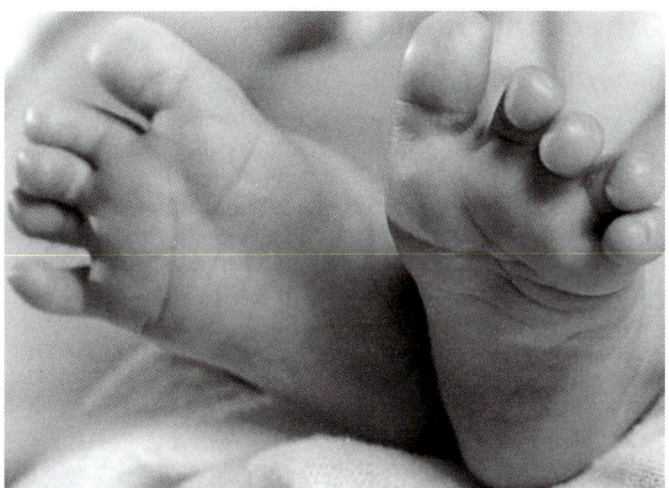

Fig. 35.48: Clinical picture of congenital vertical talus

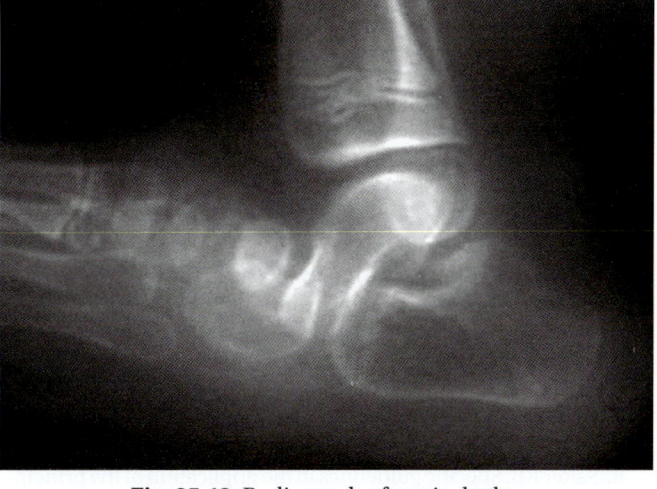

Fig. 35.49: Radiograph of vertical talus

- There could be development of callosities.
- All the soft tissue structures in around the talus become contracted and stiff.

Radiographs

Radiography of the foot including the AP and plantar flexed lateral views help to make a reasonable accurate diagnosis (Fig. 35.49).

Treatment

This is a difficult condition to treat and includes conservative and surgical methods.

Conservative Measures

In the early stages, gentle serial manipulations and immobilization with plaster casts may reduce this deformity.

Surgery

This is reserved for children in whom the conservative treatment fails or if the treatment is begun late.

Children between 1–4 years: Open reduction and realignment of the talonavicular and subtalar joint is done.

In children above 3 years of age: Open reduction and navicular excision.

In children 4–8 years of age: Open reduction, soft tissue release, and extra-articular subtalar arthrodesis.

Children beyond 12 years: Triple arthrodesis.

BIBLIOGRAPHY

Congenital Disorders

Clubfoot

1. Attenborough CG. Severe congenital talipes equinovarus. J Bone Joint Surg. 1966;48-B:31.
2. Barenfeld PA, Wesley MS. Surgical treatment of congenital clubfoot. Clin Orthop. 1972;84:79.
3. Dwyer FC. Osteotomy of the calcaneum for pes cavus. J Bone Joint Surg. 1959;41-B:80.
4. Dwyer FC. The present status of the problem of pes cavus. Clin Orthop. 1975;106:254.
5. Evans D. Relapsed clubfoot. J Bone and Joint Surg. 1961; 43-B:722.
6. Garceau GJ. Recurrent clubfoot. Bull Hosp Joint Dis. 1954; 15:143.
7. Kitc JH. Principles involved in treatment of clubfoot. J Bone and Joint Surg. 1939;21:595.
8. McKay DW. New concept of and approach to clubfoot treatment. Section 111. Evaluation and results. J Paediatr Orthop. 1983;3:141.
9. Turc VJ. Surgical correction of the resistant clubfoot: One stage posteromedial release with internal fixation: A preliminary report. J Bone and Joint Surg. 1971;53-A:477.

Congenital Pseudarthrosis

1. Boyd HB, Sage FP. Congenital pseudarthrosis of the tibia. J Bone and Joint Surg. 1958;40-A:1245.
2. Charnley J. Congenital pseudarthrosis of the tibia treated by an intramedullary nail. J Bone and Joint Surg. 1956;38-A:283.
3. Wall JJ. Congenital pseudarthrosis of the clavicle. J Bone Joint Surg. 1070;52-A:1003.

Congenital Dislocation of Hip

1. Barlow TG. Early diagnosis and treatment of congenital dislocation of the hip. J Bone and Joint Surg. 1962;44-B:292.
2. Chiari K. Medial displacement osteotomy of the pelvis. Clin Orthop. 1974;98:55.
3. Coleman SS. Diagnosis of congenital dysplasia of the hip in the newborn infant. JAMA. 1956;162:548.
4. Colonna PC. Care of the infant with congenital dislocation of the hip. JAMA. 1958;166:715.
5. Ortolani M. Congenital hip dysplasia in the light of early and very early diagnosis. Clin Orthop. 1976;119-26.
6. Pavlik A. Functional treatment with a harness as a principle for the conservative treatment of congenital hip dislocation in infants. Z Orthop. 1957;89:341.
7. Perkins G. Signs by which to diagnose congenital dislocation of the hip. Lancet. 1928;1-648.
8. Salter RB. Specific guidelines in the application of the principle of in nominate osteotomy. Orthop Clin North Am. 1972;3:148.
9. von Rosen S. Diagnosis and treatment of congenital dislocation of the hip joint in the newborn. J Bone Joint Surg. 1962;44-B:284.
10. Wagner H. Osteotomies for congenital hip dislocation. In the hip society. Proceedings of the fourth open scientific meeting of the hip society, 1976. St Louis: CV Mosby Co. 1976.

Other Congenital Disorders

Congenital Wryneck

1. Chandler FA. Muscular torticollis. J Bone Joint Surg. 1948; 30-A:566.
2. Covertry MB, Harris L. Congenital muscular torticollis in infancy: Some observations regarding treatment. J Bone Joint Surg. 1959;41-A:515.
3. Kaplan EB. Anatomical pitfalls in the surgical treatment of torticollis. Bull Hosp Joint Dis. 1954;15:154.

Congenital Elevation of Scapula

1. Cavenelish ME. Congenital elevation of the scapula. J Bone Joint Surg. 1972;54-B:395.
2. Green WT. The surgical correction of congenital elevation of scapula. Personal Communication; 1962.

Congenital Radioulnar Synostosis

1. Cohn BNE. Congenital bilateral radioulnar synostosis. J Bone Joint Surg. 1932;14:404.
2. Wilkin DPD. Congenital radioulnar synostosis. Br J Surg. 1913-1914;1:366.

36 CHAPTER

Developmental Disorders

INTRODUCTION

To understand the developmental disorders of bones, it is very essential to know the basic bone cell types and the method of ossification. The osteogenic or osteoprogenitor cells are the precursors of osteoblasts, chondroblasts, and perhaps osteoclasts also. The osteogenic cells are found in both the periosteum and the endosteum.

The osteoblasts synthesize and secrete the organic intercellular substance called the osteoid tissue. The cells then are trapped within this substance in lacunae or cavity and the cells are now called as osteocytes. The intercellular substance so formed is a mixture of matrix with type-I collagen as its main constituent, inorganic salts consisting mainly of calcium in the form of hydroxyapatite $[Ca_{10}(PO_4)_6(OH)_2]$ and water.

The osteoclasts are multinucleated giant cells, which are concerned with bone resorption and hence take part in bone remodeling. The chondrocytes are the cartilage forming cells.

> **Remember**
> *Bone cell types*
> - Osteoprogenitor cell is a common precursor of osteoblasts, chondroblasts, and osteoclasts.
> - Osteoblasts are bone-forming cells.
> - Chondrocytes are cartilage-forming cells.
> - Osteocytes originate from osteoblasts.
> - Osteoclasts are bone-remodeling cells.

The process of the formation of organic intercellular substance by osteoblasts is known as ossification. This osteoid tissue rapidly is mineralized in normal conditions.

Bone Ossification Methods

In the intrauterine life, bone development starts as a condensation of mesenchymal cells. The gaps in these condensations are future areas of joint development. These mesenchymal cells differentiate into chondrocytes, which form the cartilage. Thus, in embryonic life most of the skeleton is composed of cartilage. The chondrocytes so formed proliferate and secrete intercellular substance. After this, the chondrocytes mature and secrete alkaline phosphatase, which initiates the process of calcification of the cartilaginous matrix. This calcified matrix impairs diffusion of nutrients resulting in death of the chondrocytes. This results in disintegration and dissolution of calcified matrix, paving way for the ingrowths of the vascular and cellular tissue. This brings in osteoblasts, which surround the remnants of calcified cartilage and lay down new bone. Thus, the process of ossification begins. Two centers of ossification are formed, one in the diaphysis which extends to replace the entire diaphysis of the cartilage model with bone and the other in the epiphysis. The growth plate is a condensation of cartilage between these two centers of ossification. It contributes towards longitudinal growth of the bone until skeletal maturity after which it is replaced by bone.

This process of mesenchymal cells changing to chondroblasts, which then become chondrocytes and form cartilage model of bone, which is later converted into bone by the action of osteoblasts is called as *endochondral ossification* and is typically seen in long bones.

When bone is formed directly from the mesenchyme, without intervening stages of cartilage formation, it is called *intramembranous ossification*. This type of ossification is seen in flat bones of the skull.

> **Remember**
> *About bone development*
> - Mesenchymal cells convert into chondroblasts.
> - Chondroblasts change to chondrocytes and forms the cartilage model of the entire skeletal system.

- This cartilage model is replaced by bone due to the action of osteoblasts. This process is known as endochondral ossification.
- Intramembranous ossification refers to a situation wherein the mesenchymal cells directly form bone without the intervening cartilage cells.
- Bone formed by the above two methods undergo constant remodeling.

Thus, the either bone so developed, by intramembranous or endochondral ossification, is constantly being resorbed and reformed by the action of osteoclasts. This process is known as remodeling. Remodeling develops and preserves the structure and size of the bone apart from providing a mechanism for maintaining calcium ionic homeostasis in body fluids. Thus, bone is not a static tissue, as it appears to be. Developmental disorders result if there is any defect in the growth process so far discussed.

Bone dysplasias are generalized disorders of skeleton due to disturbance of growth and development of either bone or the cartilages. There are structural defects in more than one system, with generalized malformations of bone. Genetics has a role in dysplasia, the inheritance being dominant, recessive, X-linked or multifactorial.

Diagnostic Guidelines

Developmental disorders have the following diagnostic guidelines in common.

History

In the patients with developmental disorders usually there is a family history and is associated with multiple fractures.

Clinical Examination

Stature: Many dysplastic patients are dwarfs (less than 1.25 m in height)
Three types of dwarfs are described:
- *Proportionate dwarfs* both trunk and limbs affected
  - Hurler's disease
  - Osteogenesis imperfecta
  - Hypophosphatemia.
- Short-limbed dwarfs with normal spine
  - Achondroplasia
  - Hypochondroplasia.
- Short-limbed dwarfs with considerable spine involvement
  - Spondyloepiphyseal dysplasia
  - Morquio's disease.

Increased joint laxity is seen in:
- Ehlers-Danlos syndrome
- Marfan's syndrome
- Morquio's disease
- Osteogenesis imperfecta.

Distribution
- Generalized in some, familial history is present.
- Not generalized in the rest, affects only one side of the body or one limb, and is not familial.

Remember
Dysplasia hallmarks
- History
  - Familial
  - Multiple fractures
- Examination
  - Dwarfs (Three types)
    - Short-limbed
    - Short-limbed with normal spine
    - Short-limbed with abnormal spine
  - Excessive joint laxity.
- Distribution
  - Usually generalized
  - Rarely localized, e.g. melorheostosis.

CLASSIFICATION OF DEVELOPMENTAL DISORDERS (TABLE 36.1)

Role of Radiographs

It detects lesions even if missed clinically. It also helps to label the lesions as epiphyseal, metaphyseal or diaphyseal

TABLE 36.1: Classification (Aegster's)

Cartilaginous	Bony	Miscellaneous
Disturbed chondroid formation	*Disturbed osteoid formation*	- Cleidocranial dysostosis
Heterotrophic chondroblastic proliferation	**Deficient osteoid formation**	- Nail patella syndrome
- Multiple exostosis	- Osteogenesis imperfecta	- Marfan's syndrome
- Enchondromatosis	**Increased osteoid formation**	- Chromosomal abnormalities producing skeletal dysplasias
Abnormal chondroblast maturation	- Osteopetrosis	
- Achondroplasia	- Osteopoikilosis	
- Metaphyseal dysostosis	**Abnormal osteoid production**	
Abnormal epiphyseal center	- Fibrous dysplasia	
- Multiple epiphyseal dysplasia	- Neurofibromatosis	
- Spondyloepiphyseal dysplasia, etc.	- Pseudarthrosis	
Abnormal mucopolysaccharide metabolism		
- Hurler's disease		
- Morquio's disease		

and shows increase (e.g. osteopetrosis) or decrease (osteogenesis imperfecta) in the bone density. Three films often suffice AP view of the wrist and hands, pelvis and hips and lateral view of the spine.

ACHONDROPLASIA

Achondroplastic is melancholic at heart, as he weeps at his stature but gives the greatest gift to mankind that is laughter, as he dispels the gloom on the weary faces of the people, by his clowning antics at the circus!

Definition

It is a defect in the enchondral ossification of the bone, with the membranous ossification being normal. This is the most common type of dwarfism one encounters in clinical practice. The limbs are short and the head is big; because, along with the growth of the limbs, growth of the base of the skull is affected, but the membranous bones of the vault escape.

Clinical Features

The patient is a short-limbed dwarf (Fig. 36.1). The fingers are short and stumpy and do not reach below the upper one-third of the thigh as he stands (Fig. 36.2). The patient can kiss his toes with the knees straight. Head is large, nose is flattened, but the length of the trunk may be normal and occasionally may show kyphoscoliosis or lordosis. Cervical lordosis and increased lumbar lordosis develop in the later stages of the disease. The intelligence and sexual developments are normal.

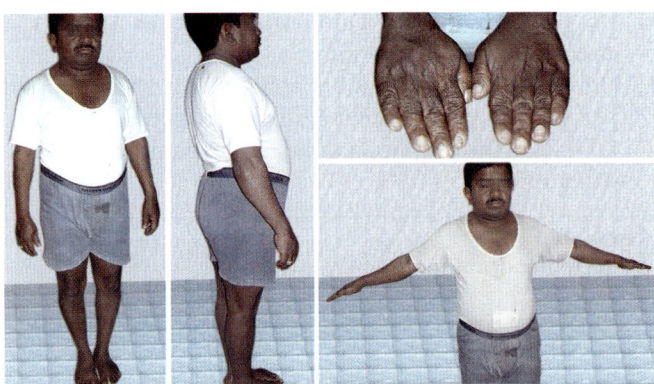

Fig. 36.2: Clinical photos showing features of achondroplasia

Radiograph

Ilium is quadrilateral in shape and there is coxa vara (Fig. 36.3).

> **Quick Facts**
> *Do you know the common causes of dwarfism?*
> - Achondroplasia
> - Cretinism
> - Diaphyseal aclasia
> - Hunter's, Hurler's, and Morquio's disease
> - Malnutrition, etc.

Treatment

Treatment methods consist of limb lengthening procedures to increase the height (Ilizarov's technique). Nevertheless, an achondroplastic is usually reluctant to undergo correction of his height for the following reasons:

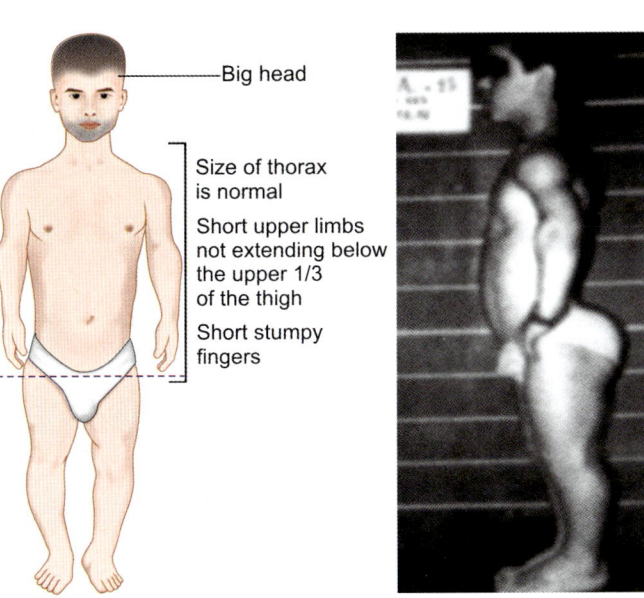

Fig. 36.1: Features of achondroplasia (Clinical photo)

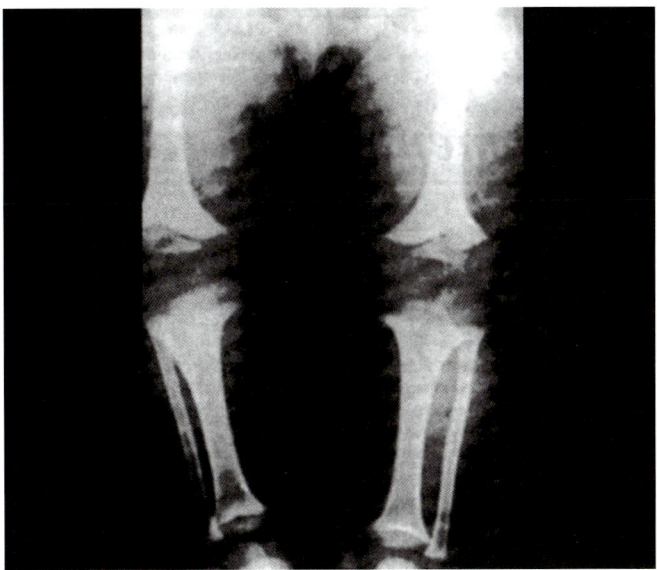

Fig. 36.3: Radiograph showing achondroplasia

- His height helps him gain employment as a clown in circus, movies, and theaters.
- He is entitled for benefits offered to a handicapped person by the government and other agencies.
- Limb lengthening procedures are expensive and time consuming.

Remember
About achondroplasia
- Failure of endochondral ossification
- Commonest type of dwarf
- Normal intelligence
- Usually employed as a clown
- Limb lengthening procedures help.

OSTEOGENESIS IMPERFECTA

To be a blue-eyed boy is great but to virtually have blue eyes is a misery. Read on the story of osteogenesis imperfecta to find out why?

Definition

It is a hereditary condition characterized by *fragility of bones, deafness, blue sclera, laxity of joints and a tendency to improve with age.* It is a disease of the mesodermal tissues with deposition of normal collagen in bone, skin, sclera, and dentine.

Etiology

The etiological factors could be heredity, Mendelian recessive—in prenatal cases, and Mendelian dominant—in postnatal cases.

Pathogenesis and Pathology

Primary defect is failure of osteoblast formation during enchondral ossification; osteoid formation does not take place. Features of bones are:
- Periosteum is thick but the cambium layer is thin (Table 36.2).
- Bone is short and thin and the epiphysis is bulbous.
- Cortex is thin and medullary contents are fatty and fibrous.
- Bones break easily but heal well with abundant callus. Fracture is usually subperiosteal and heals by periosteal bone formation.
- Deformity results from bending and fractures.
- Vertebral bodies are biconcave.
- Scoliosis.
- Skull is thin and globular.

TABLE 36.2: Types of osteogenesis imperfecta

Clinical types	Features
Fetal or prenatal or congenital type	• Multiple fractures are present at birth
	• In severe forms infants may be Stillborn or die within a few Weeks
Infantile form	• Less severe
	• Multiple fractures
	• Skull is thin and globular
Adolescent form	• Normal at birth
	• Fractures due to trivial trauma in childhood

Falvo's Classification

Osteogenesis imperfecta tarda type I: This type has presence of bowing at long bones.

Osteogenesis imperfecta tarda type II: No bowing of long bones in this type.

Fractures may be present in both the types but rare in type II.

Clinical Features

The patient presents with blue sclera, dentinogenesis imperfecta, and generalized osteoporosis (Fig. 36.4A). Blue sclera is seen only in 92 percent of cases, while the other two features are seen in almost all cases. Osteoporosis gives rise to bowing and multiple fractures. Fractures are usually due to trivial trauma but surprisingly heal well (Figs 36.4B). Other features include: Deafness due to otosclerosis, laxity of joints, dwarfism, broad skull, poorly calcified decidual teeth, but permanent teeth are normal and the blood chemistry is normal.

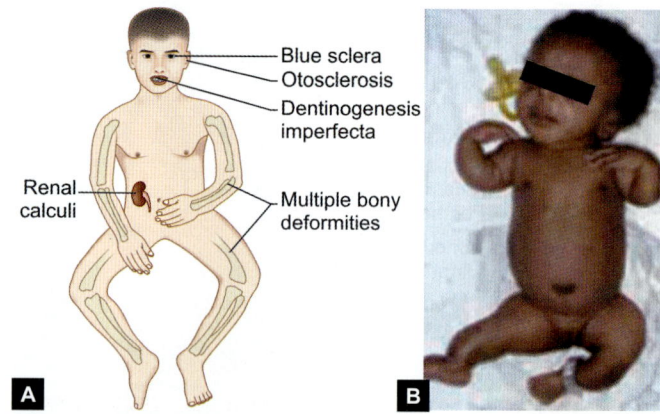

Figs 36.4A and B: (A) Features of osteogenesis imperfecta; (B) Osteogenesis imperfecta (Clinical photo)

> **Remember**
> The mnemonic **BLOOD** in osteogenesis imperfecta.
> **BL**—Blue sclera
> **O**—Otosclerosis
> **O**—Osteoporosis
> **D**—Dentinogenesis imperfecta.

> **Quick Facts**
> *Do you know the 4 O's responsible for easy fractures?*
> - **O**steoporosis
> - **O**steopetrosis
> - **O**steomalacia
> - **O**steogenesis imperfecta.

> **Remember**
> *3F's in osteogenesis imperfecta*
> - **F**ragile bones
> - **F**ractures—multiple and frequent
> - **F**etal variety is fatal.

> **Radiological Types**
> *Thick bone type*
> - Seen only in congenital cases.
> - Shafts of long bones are thicker than normal.
> *Thin bone type*
> - The long bones are thinner and ends are bulbous.
> - Vertebral bones are thin and biconcave.
> - Cortex is thin.
> *Osteogenesis imperfecta cystica*
> Fracture unites promptly with large callus.

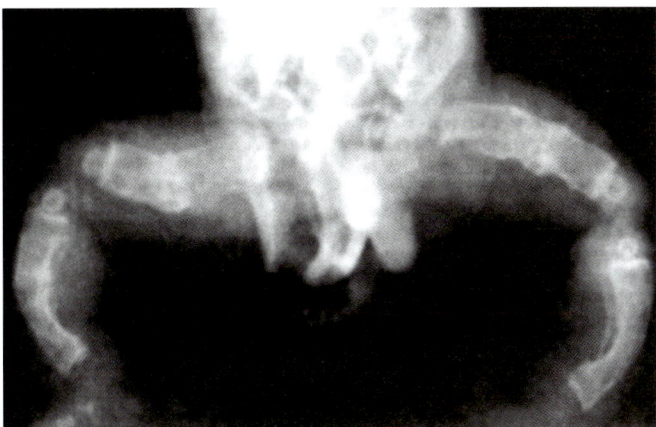

Fig. 36.5: Radiograph showing thick bone type of osteogenesis imperfecta

Investigations

Laboratory tests: There is no specific laboratory test for this disease. Prenatal determination of the probability of osteogenesis imperfecta on the fetus can be achieved by amniocentesis and estimation of *inorganic pyrophosphate*. This compound is elevated 3–4 times the normal value.

X-rays of the affected limbs helps to make a diagnosis.

Three varieties are described—the thick bone type (Fig. 36.5), thin bone type and cystic types (see box).

Treatment

Principles

Protect the child until the tendency of the fracture lessens as age advances.

Administer vitamins, estrogens, and androgens.

Operate in infantile type as the tendency to fracture is much higher and hence the treatment of choice is multiple osteotomies with intramedullary nailing.

Surgical Methods

Sofield's method consists of multiple osteotomies and realignment and IM nail fixation. It is useful for long bones and is indicated for fresh fractures and correction of bowing. There are no growth disturbances in this technique.

Bailey and Duboy's here, telescopic medullary rod is used which elongates as growth occurs.

William's here, retrograde nailing is done by fixing an extension to the distal end of the rod and driving the nail through the heel.

MUCOPOLYSACCHARIDE DISORDERS

The bone has two components—organic and inorganic. The organic component which forms 70 percent of the bone is formed mainly by type-I collagen (90–95%) and the remaining 5–10 percent is formed by the mucopolysaccharides which are protein polysaccharides. The principal mucopolysaccharide is chondroitin IV sulphate. Its role is not clear, but it appears to inhibit mineralization of bone by strongly complexing with calcium ions.

In certain diseases, increased urinary excretion of polysaccharides results in loss of polysaccharides from bone and cartilage causing specific skeletal deformities. These are the inborn errors of mucopolysaccharide metabolism.

MORQUIO-BRAILSFORD DISEASE

The following features are seen, normal development till five years, dwarfism is present, kyphosis is present, manubriosternal angle is more than 96° (pathognomonic), vertebra are too flat with a narrow tongue of bone projecting forwards (platyspondyly), hips are grossly distorted, genu valgum and varum are severe, marked ligamentous laxity, skull and mentality are normal. *Keratin sulfate is found in urine.*

HURLER'S (GARGOYLISM)

The features are coarse skin; wide set eyes with corneal opacity, bloated lips and eyelids, mental retardation, limb deformities are same as in Morquio's. There is no platyspondyly. *Dermatin sulfate and heparin sulfate are found in urine. Cardiopulmonary complications are common unlike in Morquio's.* These patients rarely survive into adults.

HUNTER'S DISEASE

Hunter's disease differs slightly from Hurler's; it is less severe and shows X-linked inheritance. All patients are males.

HEREDITARY MULTIPLE EXOSTOSIS (DIAPHYSEAL ACLASIA)

Diaphyseal aclasia is autosomal dominant and there is a failure of bone remodeling, excess of metaphysis is not resorbed, but forms irregular cartilage capped exostosis.

Clinical Features

Skull and spine are normal, but the patient is slightly short stature and may present with multiple bony lumps in the following areas: Upper humerus, lower end of radius and ulna, around knee, around ankle and flat bones.

Radiology

Plain X-rays of the affected region show the development of outgrowth of bone from the metaphyseal region of the bone (Figs 36.6A to C).

No lumps grow from the epiphysis and rarely an exostosis does migrate as far as middle third of the shaft of long bones. *Deformities* could be bowing of radius, genu valgum, ankle valgum, etc.

Treatment

Usually no treatment is required but if there are complications then surgical excision may be required.

DYSCHONDROPLASIA (Ollier's Disease)

This disease is not familial and the ossification of cartilages at growth plate is defective, with islands of unossified cartilage. It is typically unilateral and the affected limb is short and bent. There is valgus and varus at the knee and ankle. Relative shortening of the ulna with the radius curved and sometimes dislocated is often seen. Malignant change occurs in 1 percent of the cases. Fingers and toes contain multiple enchondromas.

MAFFUCCI'S DISEASE

Dyschondroplasia and multiple hemangiomatas are seen in Maffucci's disease.

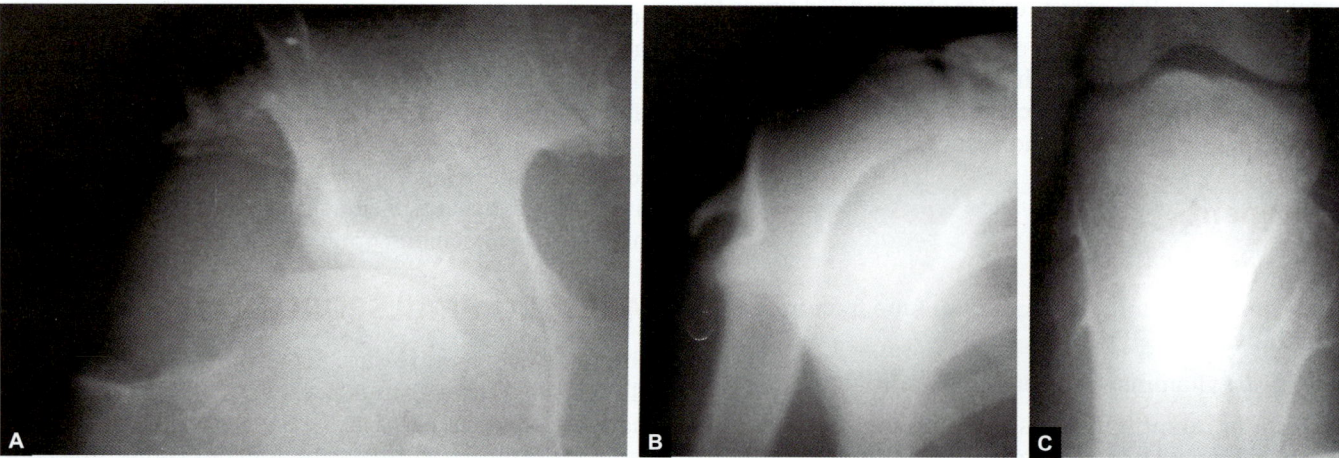

Figs 36.6A to C: (A) Exostosis from pelvis; (B) Exostosis from the proximal humerus; (C) Exostosis around knee

Radiographs

Translucent islands or columns of cartilage are seen in the metaphysis. In addition, there is development of dense irregular spots, shaft is curved but normal, and metaphysis is mottled or streaky.

OSTEOPETROSIS

MARBLE BONE DISEASE, ALBERS-SCHÖNBERG DISEASE

Here, the bone looks excessively dense and structure less on the X-ray. Bone has a marble appearance but breaks easily as it is very brittle.

Note:
Marble bone disease is due to functional deficiency of osteoclasts leading to failure of bone resorption.

Complications

It could be due to insufficient formation of bone marrow, and due to encroachment on cranial foramina, which causes optic atrophy, deafness, and facial palsy.

Pathology

There is continued new bone deposition on unresorbed calcified cartilage and there is failure of remodeling which starts at birth and continues throughout life. Bone is as hard as marble or as brittle as chalk and it is gray or white on section.

Etiology

Etiology is unknown, consanguinity has a role to play, and it is inherited as simple Mendelian recessive or dominant.

Clinical Features

The disease starts during gestation and is progressive until growth stops. The intensity varies; in mild type, formation of dense bones occurs slowly, intermittently and incompletely. Malignant type occurs in consanguineous marriages. Bone is dense and brittle. Fractures are frequent and heal slowly. Anemia, optic atrophy, facial palsy, deafness, hydrocephalus are the other features.

Radiographs

Entire long bone may be dense or dense bone may alternate with normal bone. Metaphysis is club-shaped. The skull

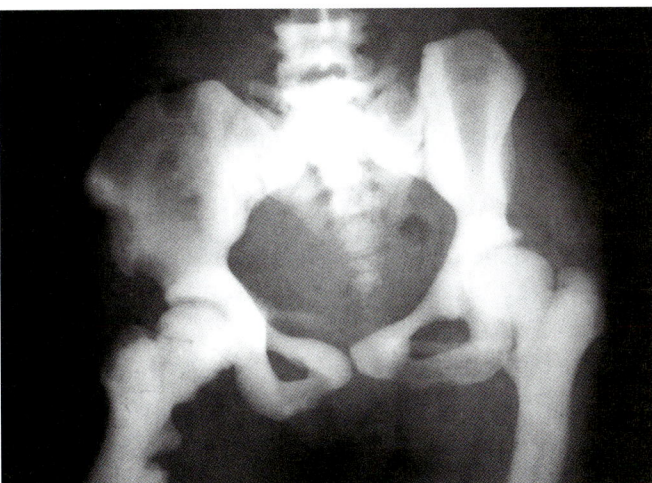

Fig. 36.7: Radiograph showing osteopetrosis

density is maximum at base with a small pituitary fossa and sparing of maxilla and mandible (Fig. 36.7).

Treatment

Conservative Methods

Adult osteopetrosis do not require any treatment. Infantile orthopetrosis requires to be treated with vitamin D which helps to stimulate osteoclasts, gamma interferon improves WBC functions, erythropoietin corrects anemia and corticosteroids help to stimulate bone resorption.

Surgery

Surgery recommended is bone marrow transfusion which is the only curative treatment of this disease but is associated with risks. Surgery may be required for fracture correction of deformities and for functional reasons.

Prognosis

Age at onset and severity determines the outcome. If it appears at birth, it is fatal by the end of two years.

Other Variants

- Candle bones (Melorheostosis, Leri's disease)
- Spotted bones (osteopoikilosis)
- Stripped bones (osteopathia striata).

EPIPHYSEAL DYSPLASIAS

EPIPHYSEAL DYSPLASIA MULTIPLEXA

This is the rarest in this group and is familial. Face, skull, and spine are normal.

Radiographs

Epiphysis appears late and closes early ill formed, irregular, and mottled, shape altered, deformity and stiffness results, and secondary osteoarthritis is common.

EPIPHYSEAL DYSPLASIA PUNCTATA

This is a variation of epiphyseal dysplasia multiplexa. It is more severe and is obvious at birth.

Conradi's Disease

The components are epiphyseal dysplasia, mental retardation, cataract, congenital heart disease, and dwarfism. Mottling disappears with growth.

EPIPHYSEAL DYSPLASIA HEMIMELIA

Epiphyseal dysplasia hemimelia affects epiphysis of ankle, knee, and only one limb is involved. One-half of the epiphysis either medial or lateral is involved. The child presents because of limp or stiffness.

METAPHYSEAL DYSPLASIAS

METAPHYSEAL DYSPLASIA (Pyle's Disease)

It is an autosomal recessive and there is a failure of remodeling of the metaphysis. Erlenmeyer flask deformities of distal femur and proximal tibia may develop. It may also be associated with genu valgum.

CRANIOMETAPHYSEAL DYSPLASIA

It is an autosomal dominant and is confused with Pyle's disease. There is metaphyseal widening, thickening of the skull and mandible.

METAPHYSEAL CHONDRODYSPLASIA

It is autosomal dominant; the metaphysis is irregular and cystic. Varus deformities of the hips and knees may be seen.

DIAPHYSEAL DYSPLASIA

PROGRESSIVE DIAPHYSEAL DYSPLASIA (Canuati or Engelmann's Disease)

This disease shows fusiform widening and sclerosis of shafts of long bones and skull. Femur, tibia, forearm bones are symmetrically affected. Cortical thickening is superficial, bone ends are normal, painful limbs, and waddling gait, weakness, etc. are the other associated findings.

CRANIODIAPHYSEAL DYSPLASIA

Shows expansion of long bone shafts and is associated with gross thickening of skull and face.

FIBROUS DYSPLASIA

Fibrous dysplasia is a rare disease with fibrous replacement of bones. It may be *monostotic or polyostotic*.

Etiology

It is unknown, begins in childhood, progresses beyond puberty, and has equal incidence in both sexes.

Pathology

Gross

Bone is irregular and bent, long bones are shortened, pathological fractures heal readily, *shepherd crook deformity* is seen in upper femur and is the hallmark of this disease (Fig. 36.8) and base of skull becomes hyperostotic (shaft of femur bowed, varus neck).

Microscopy

This shows dense collagen tissue, giant cells are sparse, and islands of cartilage is seen in only 10 percent cases.

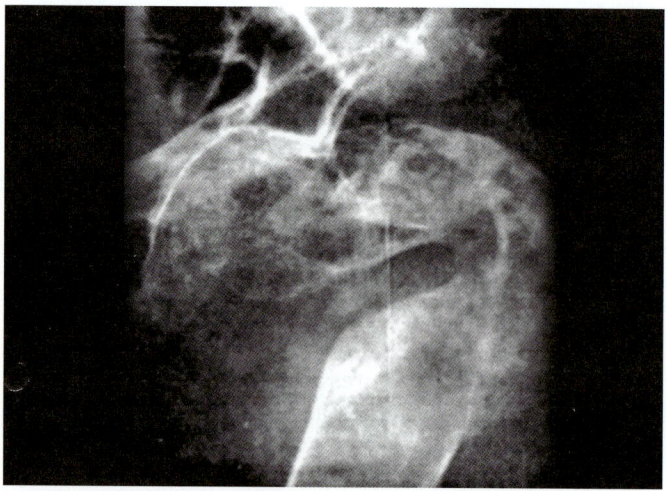

Fig. 36.8: Radiograph showing shepherd crook deformity in fibrous dysplasia

Clinical Features

Clinical features in early childhood are mild and asymptomatic. Onset is seen in less than 10 years of age. The patient may present with limp, pain, and fractures. Females have abnormal vaginal bleeding. Bending deformity and shortening of the bones are common features and lengthening is rare (Fig. 36.9). *Shepherd crook deformity is quite characteristic.* There is asymmetry of head and face and local irregular brown patches if seen are associated with polyostotic types. Sexual precocity is typical in females.

ALBRIGHT'S SYNDROME

It is a unilateral polyostotic fibrous dysplasia with sexual precocity in females.

Laboratory Investigations

Serum calcium, phosphorus, alkaline phosphatase are normal. In severe cases, alkaline phosphatase may increase.

Radiology

Localized lesions are cystic, multilocular, and show ground glass appearance, pathological fracture may occur. Shepherd crook deformity and Harrison's grooves following rib fractures, intrapelvic protrusion of acetabulum, and hyperostosis at the base of the skull, are the other important features (Fig. 36.10).

Treatment

Surgery is the treatment of choice in fibrous dysplasia and varies according to problems:

Problems	Preferred surgery
Long bones fractures	Open reduction + Internal fixation + Bone grafting
Cyst	Curettage + Bone grafting
Coxa vara	Subtrochanteric osteotomy + Internal fixation + Bone grafting
Limb length discrepancy	• Epiphyseal arrest before skeletal maturity • Ilizarov's treatment
Limb severely shortened and deformed	Amputation

> **Remember**
> **4 S's in fibrous dysplasia**
> **S**hepherd crook deformity.
> **S**exual precocity in females.
> **S**erum investigations are normal.
> **S**urgery is the treatment of choice.

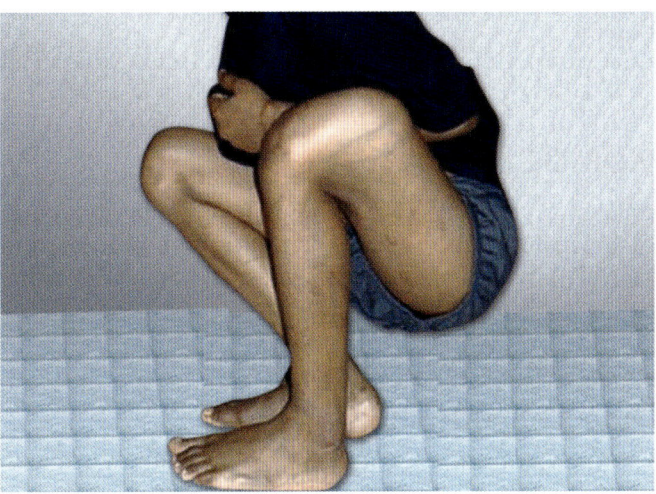

Fig. 36.9: Clinical photo showing deformity in fibrous dysplasia femur

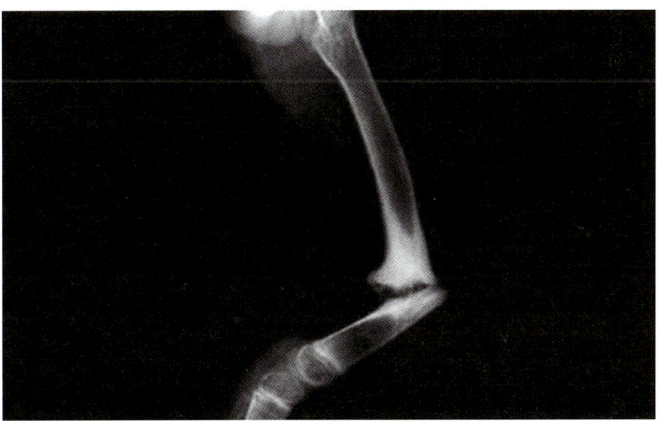

Fig. 36.10: Plain X-ray showing pathological fracture in fibrous dysplasia femur

NAIL-PATELLA SYNDROME (Onycho-osteodysplasia)

The features are autosomal dominant gene, nails are hypoplastic, patella is unduly small or absent, radial head may subluxate laterally, bony excrescences develop on the lateral aspect of the ilium and there could be congenital nephropathy.

[1]MARFAN'S SYNDROME

It is autosomal dominant and there is a defect in elastin collagen. Ocular lens dislocation and aortic aneurysm are seen. The patient is tall with disproportionate legs. Chest deformities, scoliosis, long digits, generalized joint laxity, high arched palate, and hernias may be seen.

---
[1]**Bernard Marfan** (1896), French Pediatrician

> **Note:**
> Marfan's a French pediatrician in 1896, described Marfan's syndrome. Abraham Lincoln was affected with Marfan's syndrome.

HOMOCYSTINURIA

It is autosomal recessive and the patient is prone to lens dislocation. Osteoporosis, widening of epiphysis and metaphysis, mental defect, stickiness of platelets are other associated features.

ACROCEPHALOSYNDACTYLY (Apert's Syndrome)

It is autosomal dominant. Head has a peculiar shape with high broad forehead (tower shaped). Flat occiput, bulging eyes, prominent jaws, and associated syndactyly of fingers and toes are other findings.

CARPENTER'S SYNDROME

Carpenter's syndrome is Apert's syndrome with polydactyly.

CLEIDOCRANIAL DYSPLASIA

See chapter on Congenital Disorders.

CONGENITAL NEUROFIBROMATOSIS (Von Recklinghausen's Disease)

This disease targets the skeletal system with impunity. It is autosomal dominant and development of neurofibromas within ectodermal and mesodermal tissues takes place.

Clinical Features

Clinical features consist of skin lesions—*pigmented cafe-au-lait spots,* multiple neurofibromas that are derived from endoneurium and perineurium, etc.

Locations of the neurofibromas
- *Subcutaneous:* Tender painful palpable nodules.
- *Subperiosteal:* Periosteal reaction or a bone cyst.
- *Endosteal:* Bone cysts, pseudarthrosis, etc.
- *Intraspinal:* Dumb-bell shaped tumor, paraplegia never occurs.

Skeletal changes: Incidence is about 30–50 percent.

Long bones: Show reduced growth rate, periosteal cysts, cortical cysts, osteoporosis, rarely increased density and multiple bone cysts, and congenital pseudarthrosis.

Spine: Scoliosis is the most common skeletal lesion and there could be kyphosis or kyphoscoliosis. This disease is consistently associated with "cafe-au-lait spots" and elephantiasis due to diffuse hypertrophy of all soft tissues. *Less common lesions* are head lesions, macrocranium, optic glioma, bilateral acoustic neuroma, cervical kyphosis, and vascular lesions.

> **Diagnostic Criterion**
> *Any two of the following:*
> - Positive family history
> - Positive biopsy finding
> - Minimum six "café-au-lait spots"
> - Multiple subcutaneous neurofibromas
> - Iris nodules called Lisch nodules.

Radiographs

X-ray features show pseudarthrosis, kyphoscoliosis, lateral scalloping, pencil pointing of vertebral margins, and adjacent twisted *ribbon ribs* (characteristic) (Fig. 36.11).

Treatment

Complete excision is the only treatment and elephantiasis needs repeated resection. Scoliosis needs early correction and fusion. Painful spinal tumors require laminectomy and removal. Kyphosis needs anterior correction and spinal fusion. Anterolateral bowing of tibia should be protected against pathological fracture until skeletal maturity is reached. Surgical intervention is necessary if fracture occurs.

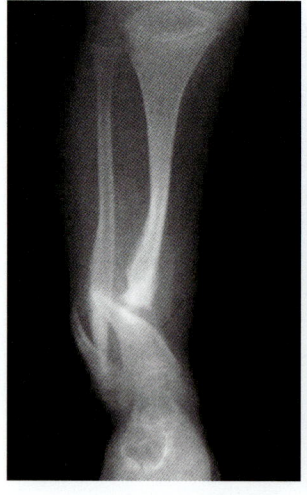 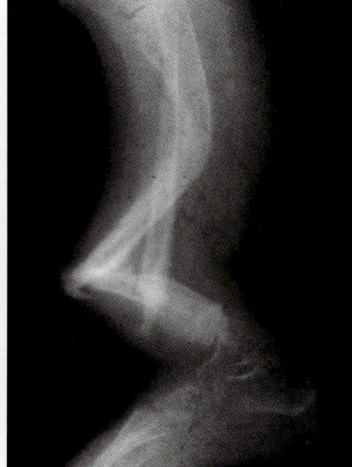

Fig. 36.11: Radiograph of pseudarthrosis tibia

PAGET'S DISEASE

Paget's disease is seen after 40 years of age and is more common in males. There is impairment in the bone resorption and bone formation due to defective osteoclastic functions. Because of this, bone gets thickened and bent more so the tibia. Bone is soft in the initial stages and dense later.

Clinical Features

The affected bones are thickened and bent. The patient complains of dull pain and deformities.

Investigations

Laboratory investigations: Serum alkaline phosphatase is increased.

Radiograph

Radiograph shows multiple lytic areas with intervening new bone formation (Figs 36.12A and B).

Treatment

It is essentially conservative and the drugs of choice are calcitonin or diphosphonate.

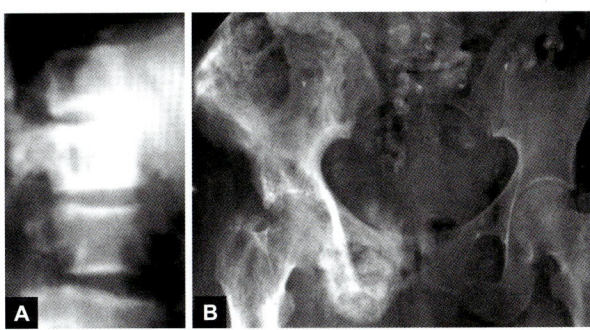

Figs 36.12A and B: Radiograph showing Paget's disease

BIBLIOGRAPHY

1. Albright JA. Management overview of osteogenesis imperfecta. Clin Orthop. 1981;159:80.
2. Albright JA. Systemic treatment of osteogenesis imperfecta. Clin Orthop. 1981;159:88.
3. Bleck EE. Non-operative treatment of osteogenesis imperfecta: Orthotic and mobility management. Clin Orthop. 1981;159:111.
4. Bailey JA. Orthopedic aspects of achondroplasia. J Bone Joint Surg. 1970;52:A;1285.
5. Goldberg MJ. Orthopedic aspects of bone dysplasia. Orthop Clin North Am. 1976;7:445.
6. McKusick VA. Heritable disorders of connective tissue, 4th edn. St Louis: CV Mosby Co, 1972.

CHAPTER 37

Metabolic Disorders

INTRODUCTION

Metabolic bone disease is largely a consequence of an upset in bone remodeling activity and/or mineralization occurring at the periosteal, endosteal, haversian, and trabecular surfaces. The cells involved in remodeling are derived from mesenchymal cells. From these cells, arise multinucleated osteoclasts, which resorb bone, and osteoblasts, which lay down osteoid and initiate mineralization. Some osteoblasts persist as osteocytes and the remainder dies.

Mineralization of osteoid involves the deposition of calcium and phosphate as hydroxyapatite crystals (Flowchart 37.1). These are situated at regular intervals along the collagen fibrils of the osteoid.

Bone Formation and Remodeling

Bone growth starts *in utero* and continues for nearly two decades. Normal bone is formed either *de novo*, by intramembranous ossification from osteoblasts or by endochondral ossification from pre-existing cartilaginous models. The long bones and the vertebrae increase in size by a combination of these two processes.

There is a constant remodeling in such a way that the net bone formation equals net bone resorption. The remodeling takes place by the cells on the periosteum, haversian, endosteal, and trabecular surfaces. This process begins during the fetal period, accelerates during infancy, and continues throughout life.

Flowchart 37.1: Composition and structure of a bone

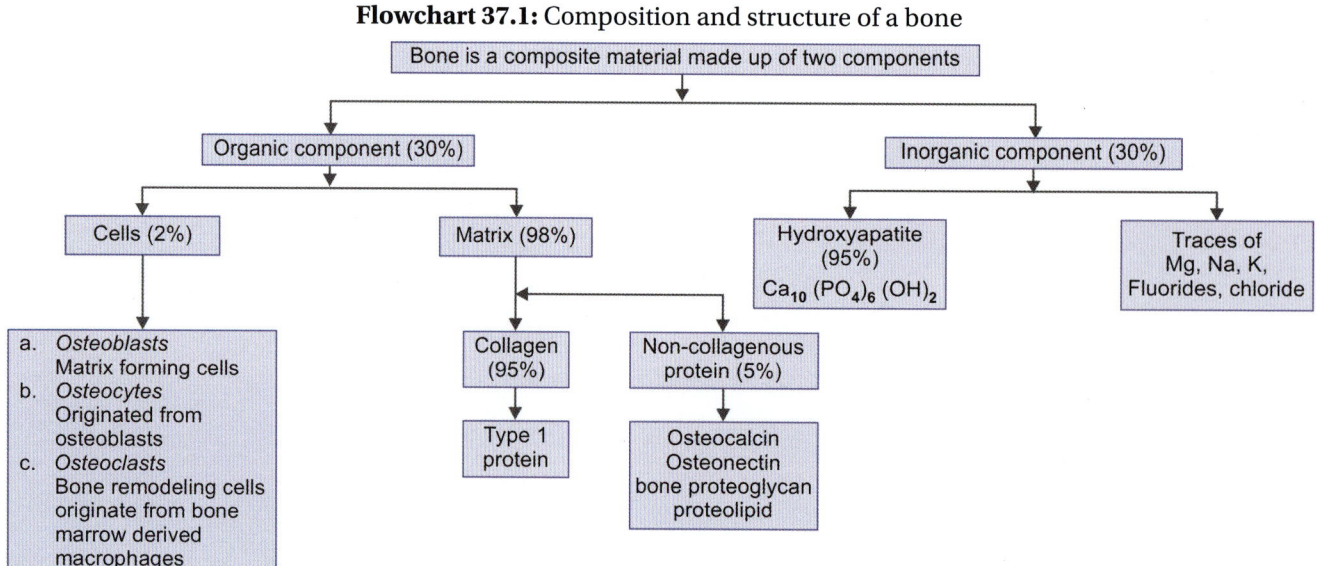

Role of Calcium

The mineral in the bone serves a major structural role and remains metabolically stable under normal circumstances. The main mineral deposited on the organic matrix is calcium in the form of $Ca_{10}(PO_4)_6(OH)_2$. It is deposited in either cortical or trabecular bone. It has a twin role of structural and metabolic importance.

Calcium Metabolism

About 0.6–1.0 g of calcium is ingested and equal amount is excreted every day.

Vitamin D, PTH, bile salts, calcitonin help in the absorption of calcium from the upper small intestine, while the oxalates, citrates, phosphates, phytic acids and fats impair absorption. Calcium so absorbed is deposited mainly into the bone. The remaining is excreted through the kidney and intestine. Hormones regulate this calcium homeostasis (Flowchart 37.2). Hormones, which help calcium to be deposited into the bone, are estrogen, thyroxin, growth hormone, and testosterone, while that which remove the calcium from bone are glucocorticoids, thyroid hormones, PTH and acidosis. Any upset in this delicate balance either results in increase or decrease in serum calcium. These homeostatic mechanisms normally maintain the ratio of calcium and phosphorus ions to 2.5:1 (Table 37.1). The calcium homeostasis and its regulation are displayed in the Flowchart 37.2 and Table 37.1.

> **Remember**
> *About calcium*
> - Indispensable to life.
> - Total calcium content of body is 1 kg.
> - Only one gram is found in ECF and plasma.
> - Remainder is in the skeleton.
> - Normal requirement is 0.6–1.0 g/day.
> - Provides bone its hardness and strength.
> - Helps in blood coagulation, neuromuscular excitability, enzyme actions, etc.
> - Tetany is due to low calcium levels.
> - Sulkowitch test for calcium in urine is important.

> **Remember**
> *Important causes of hypercalcemia*
> - Hyperparathyroidism
> - Chronic renal insufficiency
> - Rickets
> - Osteomalacia
> - Nephrosis
> - Malabsorption syndrome
> - Celiac disease
> - Sprue
>
> *Important causes of hypocalcemia*
> - Hypoparathyroidism
> - Secondaries in the bone
> - Sarcoidosis
> - Multiple myeloma
> - Hyperproteinemia
> - Vitamin D intoxication
> - Production of PTH like hormone by neoplasm of ovary, kidney, lung, etc.

Six important metabolic diseases are discussed in this chapter:
1. Rickets
2. Renal osteodystrophy
3. Osteomalacia
4. Hyperparathyroidism
5. Osteoporosis
6. Conditions causing osteosclerosis.

Flowchart 37.2: Dynamics of bone homeostasis

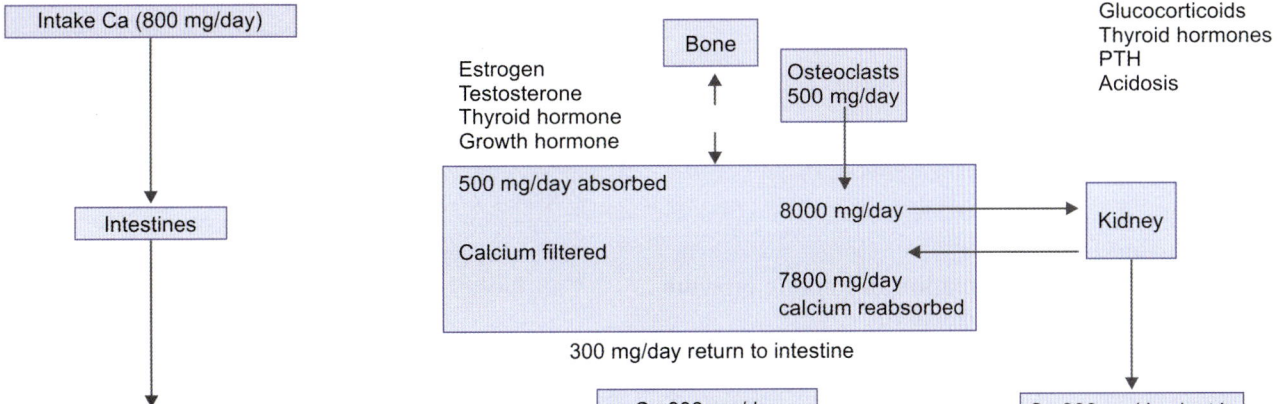

TABLE 37.1: Regulation of calcium and phosphorus metabolism

Hormones	PTH (Parathyroid)	1, 25 (OH)₂ D (Kidney)	Calcitonin (Thyroid)
• Factors ↑	• ↓ Serum calcium	• ↑ PTH • ↓ Serum calcium • ↑ Phosphorus	• ↓ Serum calcium
• Factors ↓	• ↑ Serum calcium • ↑ 1, 25 (OH)₂	• ↓ PTH • ↑ Serum calcium • ↑ Phosphorus	• ↓ Serum calcium
Action on end organs • Intestine	• No direct effect • Acts indirectly on bowel by ↑ 1, 25 (OH)₂	• Strongly stimulates intestinal absorption of calcium and phosphorus	
• Kidney	• Converts 25 (OH) D to 1, 25 (OH)₂ D • ↑ Absorption of Ca • Promotes excretion of phosphorus		
• Bone	• Stimulates osteoclastic resorption of bone • Stimulates recruitment of pro-osteoclasts	• Strongly stimulates osteoclastic resorption of bone	• Inhibits osteoclastic resorption of bone
Net effect on calcium and phosphate in	• ↑ Serum calcium • ↓ Serum phosphate	• ↑ Serum calcium • ↑ Serum phosphate	• ↓ Serum calcium (transient)

Note: The skeletal system consists of 95 percent of calcium and 80 percent of phosphorus in the body.

RICKETS

Definition

It is a metabolic disease of childhood in which, the osteoid, the organic matrix of bone, fails to mineralize due to interference with calcification mechanism. It is usually common between six months and two years.

Causes

Four main causes:

Vitamin D deficiency:
- Reduced dietary intake
- Reduced amount of sunlight
- Pigmented skin.

Malabsorption due to:
- Celiac disease
- Hepatic osteodystrophy.

Renal disease:
- Glomerular failure
- Renal osteodystrophy.

Antiepileptic drugs favor formation of hepatic enzyme, which prevents conversion of calciferol.

> **Remember**
> *About vitamin D*
> - Two principle vitamin Ds nutritionally useful are calciferol D_2 and cholecalciferol D_3.
> - 1,25-dihydroxy vitamin D is formed in the kidney and is the active form.
> - It aids in the absorption of calcium from the gut.
> - It is necessary for calcium deposition in bone.
> - Its lack upsets the calcification of cartilage and mineralization of osteoid.

> **Metabolic Abnormality in Rickets**
> Vitamin D ↓ → ↓ 1, 25 (DH)₂ → D_3 ↑ → ↓ Calcium absorption → Hypocalcemia → ↓ PTH → Ca level ↑ → Bone resorption increased → Compensatory attempts to bone formation → ↑ Alkaline phosphatase → Negative Ca and P level

Ca level is increased by mobilization of bone stock, increased intestinal absorption, decreased renal excretion and decreased phosphate absorption.

> **Quick Facts**
> *Do you know the daily requirements of calcium?*
> | | |
> |---|---|
> | Adult | 50 mg |
> | Child | 700 mg |
> | Adolescent | 1000–1300 mg |
> | Pregnant women | 1500 mg |
> | Lactating women | 2000 mg |
> | Postmenopausal women | 1500 mg |
> | Major fracture | 1500 mg |

TYPES OF RICKETS

Fetal Rickets

This is commonly seen in osteomalacic mothers and will usually lead to achondroplasia.

Infantile Rickets (Nutritional Rickets)

This is rare before 6 months and is the most common form of rickets, seen in 6 months to 3 years of life.

Late Rickets or Rachitis Tarda

This is late onset rickets, familial, and it is vitamin D-resistant rickets.

> **Quick Facts**
> *Varieties of rickets*
> Type I   This is due to dietary deficiency or defects in metabolism of vitamin D.
> Type II This is due to low serum phosphorus due to dietary phosphate deficiency or defective tubular resorption. *Type I dietary deficiency of vitamin D is the most common variety of rickets.*

Clinical Features

Symptoms

Patient complains of bone pain during rest and excessive perspiration in upper half of the body (Fig. 37.1). He or she loathes using the limb and the weakness of proximal muscles of the lower limbs produces waddling gait. There is evidence of catarrh of mucous membranes (recurrent diarrhea, constipation, bronchitis). Irritability of CNS produces convulsions, laryngismus, spasmophilia, Chovstek's sign, opisthotonos, etc.

Signs

Deformities of Rickets (from head to toe)
Skull
- Broadened forehead
- Skull squared (caput quadratum)
- Frontal and parietal bossing—seen after the age of 6 months.
- Craniotabes is a ping-pong sensation on compressing the membranous bones of the skull.

Chest
- Pigeon chest due to prominent sternum (Fig. 37.2).
- Narrow chest.
- Rickety rosary (enlargement of costochondral junction).
- Harrison's sulci due to diaphragmatic pull on the soft ribs.

Bones
- *Enlargement of the metaphyseal segments* of long bones like radius, tibia, costochondral junction, etc. seen in children between 6 and 9 months of age.
- *Vertebral columns* show exaggerated curvature.
- *Pelvis* is trefoil shaped.
- *Coxa vara*
- *Femur* is bent anteriorly and laterally.
- *Knock knee (genu valgum).*
- *Bowed tibia.*

Other Features

Other features encountered in rickets are wizened look, delayed dentition, prominent abdomen, separation of recti, pale and flabby skin, and incomplete fractures, etc.

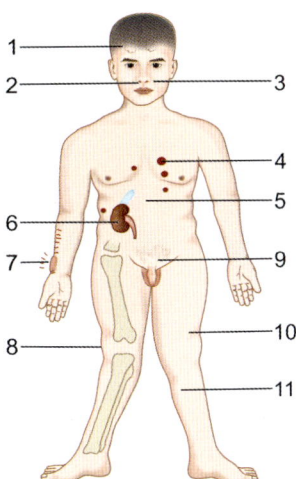

Fig. 37.1: Skeletal changes in rickets: (1) Frontal bossing, (2) Dentition changes, (3) Chovstek's sign, (4) Rickety rosary and pigeon chest, (5) Malabsorption, (6) Aminoaciduria, (7) Expanded wrist, (8) Pelvis deformity, (9) Genu valgum, (10) Myopathy, (11) Skin changes

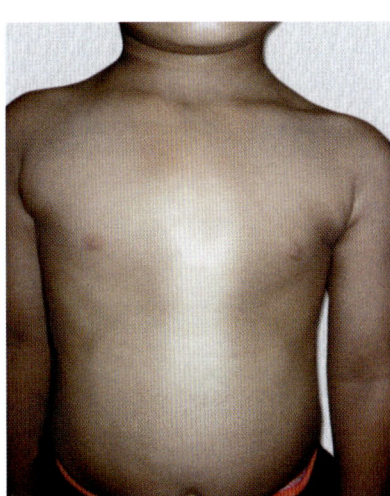

Fig. 37.2: Clinical photo showing prominent sternum

> **Quick Tests**
> *How do renal rickets differ from nutritional rickets?*
> - Less osteoid formation and increased osteoclastic resorption of bone.
> - Osteosclerosis is seen at the base of the skull.
> - Slipped capital femoral epiphysis is more common.
> - Delay in skeletal maturation.

Pathology

Bones of the Skeletal System

Bones are soft and porotic and bend easily. Epiphyseal line of 2 mm is normal but in rickets, it forms a wide irregular band. Metaphysis is broad and irregular.

Bony trabeculae are weak and continued stimulation makes the connective tissue hyperplastic, so that the extremity of bone appears mis-shaped and unmodeled.

These changes are most marked at the actively growing part of the bone and only affect the bone being deposited during the active phase of the disease. Bone formed before and after the active phase is normal.

Investigations

X-ray of the part shows the following Lovette and Jones radiological changes (Table 37.2).

> **Remember**
> *Characteristic X-ray findings (Figs 37.3A and B)*
> - Delayed appearance of epiphysis and widening of the epiphyseal plates.
> - Champagne glass appearance (widening and cupping of the distal ends of long bones) also called 'trumpeting'.
> - Space between diaphysis and epiphysis is increased.
> - Deformity and bowing of the ends of long bones.
> - Thickened epiphysis.
> - Decreased density of cortex (rarefaction).
> - Trabecular pattern is course.

Biochemistry

- Calcium is normal or decreased (due to compensatory hyperparathyroidism).
- Serum phosphorus is low.
- Alkaline phosphatase is normal.
- Urinary calcium is low (excretion less than 5 mg/kg/24 h).
  Importance of biochemical values in this condition is their return to normal upon correct therapy.
- Levels of 2, 5-hydroxyl D if low will indicate effectiveness of treatment.

Treatment

Treatment in Initial Stages

Medical treatment in the initial stages aims to bring about quick healing. A single oral dose of 6 lakh IU of vitamin D is given. A second same dose may be required after 3–4 weeks of treatment if no sclerotic (healing sign) change is seen on the radiograph at the metaphyseal side of the growth plate. A maintenance dose of 4,000 IU of vitamin D may be required if the child responds to the above treatment regimen. Absolute and strict bed rest, rickets splints, etc. can help prevention of deformity.

Treatment of Established Deformity

Correction by splints (Mermaid splint): This is mainly useful when the disease is active and the deformity is slight. It is very effective in children and in preventing deformities concerning the lower limbs. However, it is slow and requires continual supervision (Fig. 37.4).

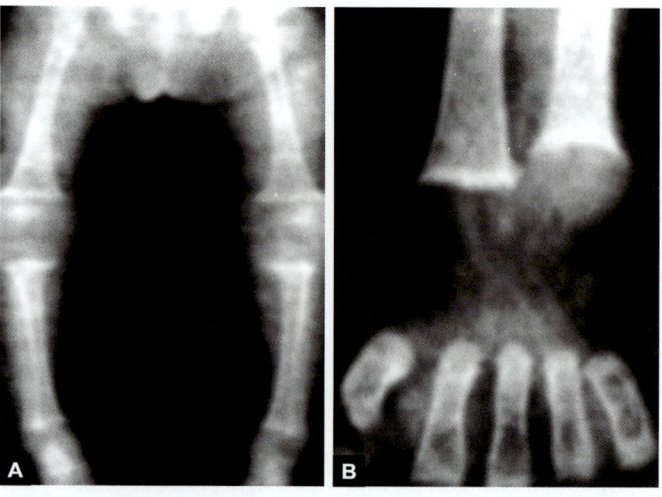

Figs 37.3A and B: (A) Radiograph showing metaphyseal cupping and irregularity of epiphyseal plates seen in rickets; (B) Radiograph showing features in rickets

TABLE 37.2: Radiological changes in rickets

Stages	Epiphysis	Metaphysis	Periosteum	
Acute	Cloudy	Splayed out	Thickened	Fractures of long bones
II	• Mottled • Irregular • Ill-defined	• Ragged broad than normal	Thickening disappears	
III	• Shadow • Denser • Mottled	• Appearance of a dense line	No thickening	
IV		• Increased • Clearly defined Ca^+ (N)		

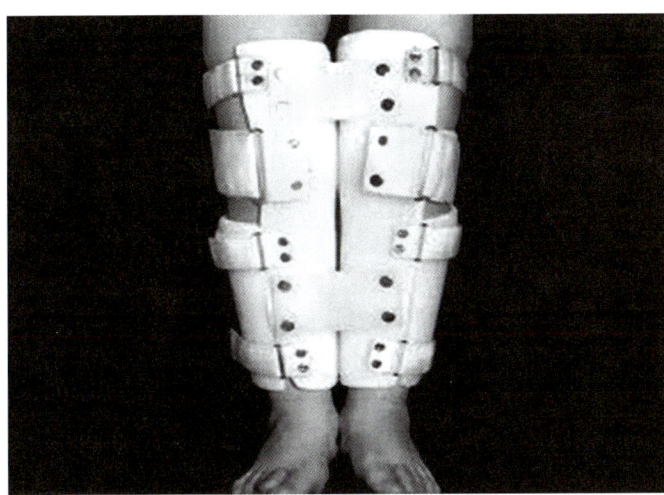

Fig. 37.4: Mermaid splint

Correction by osteotomy is indicated when deformity is near the joint and when the growth stops. It is done during III stage (Lovett's) (nonunion follows if done before).

Differential Diagnosis

Acute poliomyelitis, congenital syphilis, septic arthritis, infantile scurvy, etc.

RENAL OSTEODYSTROPHY

Lucas first described renal osteodystrophy in 1883. In this condition, bone is diseased due to glomerular failure and renal tubular disease.
Three forms are described:
- Renal dwarfism
- Renal pseudorickets
- Renal osteitis fibrosa cystica.

> **Why is Renal Rickets Low-Grade Rickets?**
> Absorption of vitamin D and Ca from GIT is unimpaired. Hence, osteoid tissue is being formed. Therefore, weight-bearing deformities are not as pronounced as in rickets.
> True florid phase of rickets is never seen. Shortness of stature is because enchondral ossification is affected at the growth plate.

Causes

At birth: Congenital polycystic kidney and congenital hydronephrosis, etc.

Later: Chronic glomerulonephritis, chronic interstitial nephritis, chronic pyelonephritis, and nephritis due to heavy metal poisoning, etc.

Clinical Features

In renal rickets (Table 37.3), the clinical features could either be due to renal lesion *per se*, tubular defects (Flowchart 37.3) or due to the growth disturbances and the resultant bony changes. Symptoms are present from early days of life. The child is normal for first few years before the symptoms start appearing. It is considered fewer than three groups. Late onset genu valgum is a common presentation (Figs 37.5A and B).

Parson's Radiological Features

Atrophic Type
- Epiphysis is broad and irregular.
- Metaphysis is broad, uneven, and ragged.
- Bone is osteoporotic and osteomalacic.

Florid Type
Metaphysis has cup-shaped defect due to greater absence of calcium in the central axis of the bone than beneath the periosteum. It is broadened and there is subperiosteal new bone formation.

Wooly Stippled or Honeycomb Type
- Metaphysis is grossly increased and irregularly honeycombed, stippled or wooly.
- Bone is eaten away subperiosteally and has moth-eaten appearance.
- Osteitis fibrosa may develop.

TABLE 37.3: Features in renal rickets

Those due to renal lesion	Due to disturbance of growth	Bone changes

• Thirst
• Polydipsia
• Polyuria
• Urine
  – Low specific gravity
  – Output 1200–3700 mL/day
  – Albumin and Casts++
• CVS symptoms of renal origin
• Kidney failure: Headache, GIT disturbances and drowsiness
• Death due to uremia
	• Stunted growth
	• Body weight small
	• No malnutrition
	• Patient surviving beyond puberty shows infantilism and dwarfism
	• Mental development is normal up to puberty, thereafter mental sluggishness
	• Secondary sexual characters do not appear
		• Genu valgum is the most common manifestation Age of onset is 11–14 years
		• Enlargement of epiphysis
		• Costochondral rosary
		• Bow legs, Harrison's sulci, etc.
		• May be associated with parathyroid hyperplasia

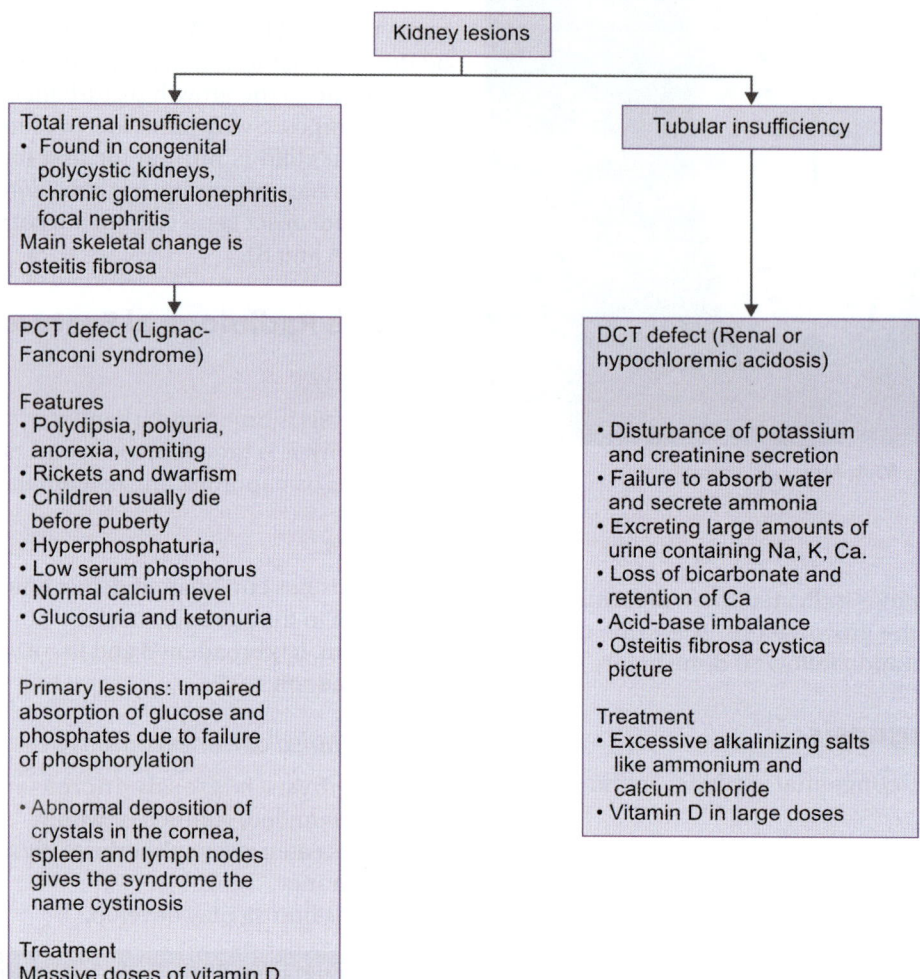

Flowchart 37.3: Tubular defects due to renal rickets

Note: Chronic renal failure causes rickets due to increased PTH level, acidosis and hypocalcemia

Investigations

X-ray demonstrates calcification of kidneys, calculus formation, and osteoporosis and osteitis fibrosa in the bone.

IVP demonstrates irregularities of renal pelvis and ureter.

Treatment

Treat the underlying renal disease (e.g. removal of posturethral valve, etc.). Surgical intervention is done before puberty. Treatment is of little help in congenital polycystic kidney and renal hypoplasia. Good results are seen in hyperchloremic renal acidosis and nephrocalcinosis. Organic acid with sodium citrate helps absorption of calcium from the intestines. Vitamin D in the form of OHD or 1, 25 $(OH)_2$ is to be given in high doses (1 lakh IU). In active stages, weight bearing is prevented and use of splints is recommended. Avascular necrosis of femoral head may appear due to treatment with steroids. Hemodialysis or kidney transplant may help.

VITAMIN D-RESISTANT RICKETS

It develops due to failure of phosphate reabsorption from the kidney. The disease is familial and there is excessive fecal loss of calcium and defect in the formation of 1, 25 $(OH)_2D$

CHAPTER 37: Metabolic Disorders

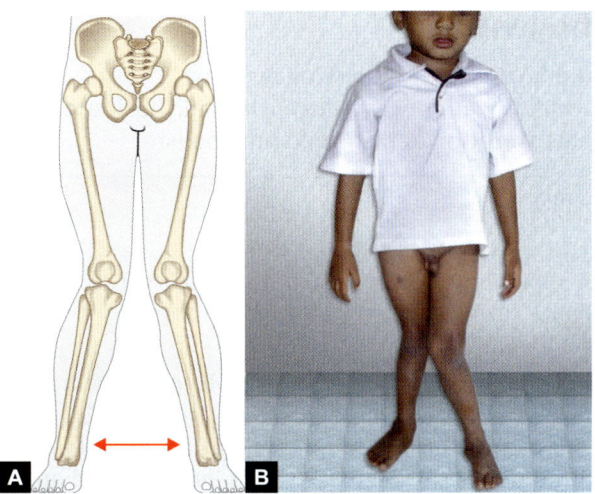

Figs 37.5A and B: (A) Genu valgum deformity with increased intermalleolar distance; (B) Genu valgum in renal rickets (Clinical photo)

TABLE 37.4: Features of rickets: Vitamin D-dependent and vitamin D-resistant

	Vitamin D-dependent rickets	Vitamin D-dependent
Onset	Acquired	Heredity
Muscle wasting	Present	Absent
Hypocalcemic tetany	May occur	Present
Serum phosphorus	Always low, never returns to normal even after large doses of phosphorus	Low or normal, returns to normal with treatment
Growth	Becomes normal with treatment	Will not become normal with treatment. Patient remains dwarfed

by the kidney (Table 37.4). Children tend to survive into adulthood exhibiting features of osteomalacia.

Clinical Features

There is a prominent occipital protuberance and features of dolichocephalism (anteroposterior diameter increases but transverse diameter decreases). The patient has short stature and nose is saddle shaped.

Tackle Deformity

Tackle deformity is the hallmark of this disease (bowleg on one side and knock-knee on the other) (Figs 37.6A and B). There is marked ligamentous instability.

Radiograph

X-ray of both the knees is required to assess the deformities in this condition.

> **Remember**
> The term vitamin D-resistant rickets refers to any condition that requires more than 1 lakh IU of vitamin D to produce healing.

Treatment

The aim of the treatment is to give doses of vitamin D (0.5–1.0 lakh IU/d) and to maintain Sulkowitch test at 1+ or 2+.

Prognosis

Complete cure of skeletal dystrophy may occur if the individual survives more than 16–17 years. Occurrence of

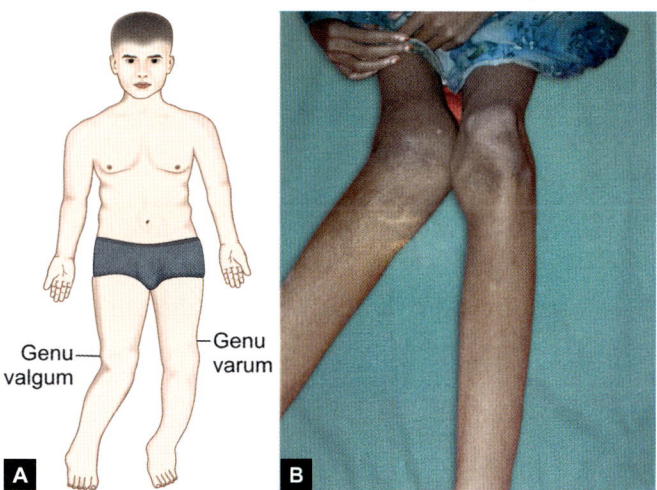

Figs 37.6A and B: (A) Tackle deformity typical of vitamin D-resistant rickets; (B) Tackle deformity (Clinical photo)

bone deformity is a grave omen; average duration of life is less than two years if kidney is untreated.

> **Quick Facts**
> *A quick look at the late deformities seen with vitamin D-resistant rickets*
> - Genu varum/valgum
> - Coxa vara
> - Anterior bowing of femur
> - Anterolateral bowing of tibia
> - Protrusio acetabuli
> - Kyphoscoliosis.

CELIAC RICKETS

GLUTEN-SENSITIVE ENTEROPATHY

This has long escaped notice because celiac disease is characterized in early childhood, while the bone changes are seen after 7 years.

Etiology

It is due to sensitivity to gluten of wheat. Pathology is same as in vitamin D-resistant rickets.

Clinical Features

Onset is during infancy or early childhood. Patient presents with diarrhea, anorexia, and irritability. Pale, foul, bulky stools may be absent but steatorrhea may be seen. Retarded growth and development, wasting of proximal muscles, abdominal protuberance, iron deficiency anemia, rickets, and osteomalacic features are the other clinical findings.

Investigations

Duodenal biopsy shows loss of villi, and fecal examination shows in microscopical smears for fat (quantitative fecal fat normal up to 5 percent of ingested fat).

Treatment

Conservative method consists of gluten-free diet, high potency vitamin D, calcium lactate injections, etc.

Quick tests: Comparative blood picture in the four common varieties of rickets (Table 37.5).

OSTEOMALACIA

It is the adult counterpart of rickets and is characterized by failure of mineralization and an excess of osteoid due to an interference with calcification mechanism. *The osteoid is increased at the cost of mineralized bone.*

Etiology

- Decreased vitamin D absorption from the intestine.
- Derangement of vitamin D and phosphorus metabolism (hereditary or acquired).

TABLE 37.5: Types of rickets

Types of rickets	Calcium	Phosphorus	Creatinine	Alkaline phosphatase
Nutritional	Normal or low	Low	Normal	High
Vitamin D-resistant	Normal	Low	Normal	High
Renal	Normal or low	High	High	High
Hypophos-phatasia	Normal or high	Normal	Normal or high	Very low

Note: Hypophosphatasia is a genetically determined error of metabolism with low alkaline phosphatase activity and increased urinary excretion of phosphoryl ethanolamine.

Pathogenesis

It could be due to the following reasons:
- *Decreased vitamin D metabolism* could be due to dietary malabsorption or disturbed metabolism.

> **Remember**
> Role of vitamin D on
> - Gut—Increase in calcium absorption.
> - Bone—Increase in bone formation and mineralization.
> - Kidney—Decrease in phosphate reabsorption and increase in calcium reabsorption.

- *Inorganic phosphate decreased* Hypophosphatemia impairs function of osteoblasts and thereby affects collagen synthesis and mineralization. It could be due to renal disease, decreased PTH, or increased antacid (non-absorbable).
- *Chronic acidosis* due to renal disease adversely affects the calcium metabolism in the following ways:
  - Bone mineral calcium is used up to buffer excess H^+ ions.
  - Acidosis decreases calcium absorption.
  - Causes hypophosphatemia and vitamin D-resistance.

Pathology

Increased osteoid (due to osteoblastic activity and normal osteoclasis) is deposited in compact and cancellous bone (Figs 37.7A and B). This results in deformities because bone is soft thereby fractures occur easily but heals well.

Clinical Features

Symptoms

The patient complains of generalized skeletal pain and muscle weakness. There may be acute pain due to fracture. Other symptoms related to causative factors like dietary, renal and GIT may be seen.

Signs

The following deformities are encountered; scoliosis, kyphosis, coxa vara, protrusio acetabuli, thighs, and legs are bent, pelvis is trefoil, etc.

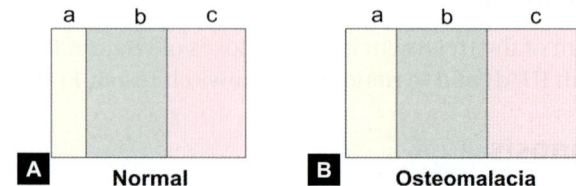

Figs 37.7A and B: Bony densities in osteomalacia: (a) Osteoid, (b) Bone, and (c) Marrow

Radiographs

Radiographic features reveal generalized demineralization, loss of transverse trabeculae, no subperiosteal resorption of bone, etc. Presence of Looser's zones is quite characteristic of osteomalacia (Figs 37.8A and B).

> **Remember**
> *About looser's line*
> - **Looser's line** (Syn: Pseudofracture, Milkman's line) It is transverse, bilaterally symmetrical and incomplete.
> - Fractures healed with defective callus.
> - Sometimes only evidence of osteomalacia in treated cases.
>
> *Sites*
> - Axillary borders of scapula
> - Ramus of pubis or ischium
> - Neck of femur
> - Ribs
>   They heal when osteomalacia is treated.

Spine: The bodies of spine are biconcave and are called "codfish spine."

Hip show protrusio acetabuli and triradiate pelvis.

Laboratory Investigations

The following changes are seen in the blood: Serum calcium is normal or decreased, serum phosphatase is normal or decreased, alkaline phosphatase is slightly increased (rarely exceeds 200 IU), and serum PTH is increased.

Treatment

The following conservative regimen is recommended. Calcium is given at 0.5–3 g/day, vitamin D 10,000 IU/day, and high protein diet. The gastrointestinal tract errors are also corrected simultaneously.

HYPERPARATHYROIDISM

When parathyroid is on the rampage, it out beats its big brother thyroid in ravaging the body but mercifully targets the skeletal system mainly unlike the all system effects of thyroid!

Parathyroid secretes parathyroid hormone, excessive secretion of which results in hyperparathyroidism. It may be *primary* or *secondary*.

PRIMARY HYPERPARATHYROIDISM (Osteitis Fibrosa Cystica, von Recklinghausen's Disease)

In the beginning of the chapter, the role of parathormone has been highlighted. *The net result is it increases serum calcium and decreases serum phosphorus through its action on kidney, bone, and intestines.*

Pathogenesis

Rise in the level of parathormone causes increased osteoclastic activity, which resorbs the bone. Consequently, there is increased osteoblastic activity resulting in fibrous replacement of bone and consequent weakening.

> **Remember**
> *About parathormone*
> - Secreted by principal or chief cells of parathyroid.
> - Maintains serum calcium level.
> - Lowers serum phosphorus level.
> - Increases diuresis of phosphorus.
> - Promotes renal and intestinal reabsorption of calcium.
> - Stimulates action of osteoclasts.
> - It will directly affect dissolution of bone.
> - Inhibits calcifying effect of vitamin D.
> - Increases solubility of calcium and phosphorus.

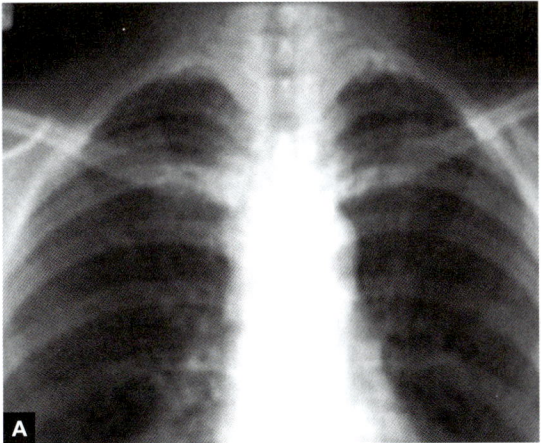 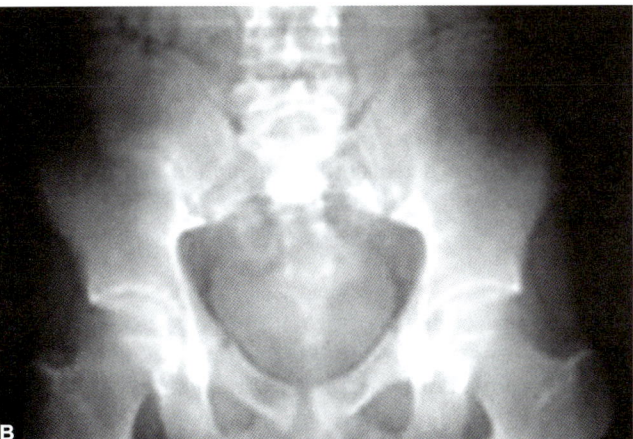

Figs 37.8A and B: Plain X-rays showing Looser's zones in the ribs and pelvis

Pathology

An adenoma in the parathyroid glands is usually seen.

Causes

Adenoma accounts for more than 90 percent of the cases, carcinoma is rare, and hyperplasia of the chief cells is seen in 6 percent of the cases.

Clinical Features

This disease equally affects both sexes. It is common in middle-aged women. The patient complains of severe pain and tenderness over the back and lower limbs, generalized muscle weakness, and hypotonia. Pathological fractures and delayed union may be seen. Deformities of limbs and spine are common features. Hyperphosphaturia, polyuria, polydipsia, renal calculi are some of the urinary complications.

Skeletal Changes

These are diffuse bone resorption due to increased osteoclastic activity, multiple deformities (because bone is soft due to replacement with fibrous tissue), pathological fractures, marrow fibrosis, brown tumor due to cavities filled with blood, multiple bone cysts, etc. Fracture healing is normal.

Radiographs

Radiographic features show generalized rarefaction, trabeculae and cortex are thin, cysts and bending deformities, diffuse osteoporosis of skull, pin head stippling of skull also called salt and pepper appearance, vertebrae are porotic and indented by disks, demineralization of mandible, disappearance of lamina dura in the tooth. Subperiosteal resorption is seen in the fingers (Fig. 37.9).

Laboratory Investigations

Increased calcium levels in the serum, decreased phosphorus levels in the serum, hypercalciuria, hyperphosphaturia, and increased alkaline phosphatase are some of the important laboratory findings (Fig. 37.10).

Treatment

Medical treatment consists of providing large doses of calcium, phosphorus and vitamin D. Treatment of choice is parathyroidectomy. For hyperplasia, three glands and a portion of the fourth are removed. Preoperative calcium is avoided.

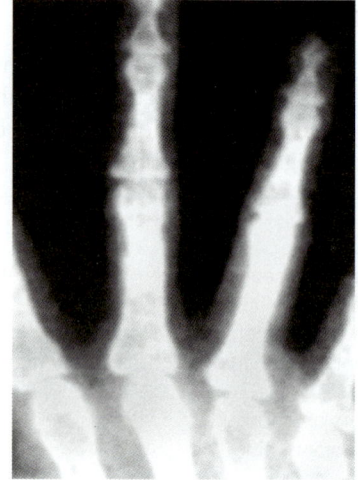

Fig. 37.9: Radiograph showing extensive subperiosteal resorption of bone in hyperparathyroidism

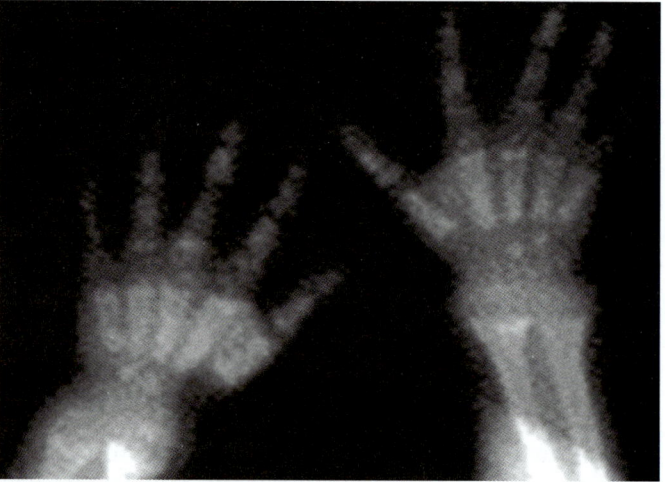

Fig. 37.10: Plain X-ray showing features of secondary hyperparathyroidism

Orthopedic management consists of support by splints and corrective osteotomies for bony deformities.

Differential Diagnosis

- Secondary hyperparathyroidism
- Osteomalacia
- Osteoporosis
- Sarcoidosis
- Vitamin D intoxication.

SECONDARY HYPERPARATHYROIDISM

Normal kidneys eliminate phosphorus easily. When kidney is diseased, phosphorus is not excreted. Increased levels of phosphorus in serum results in increased calcium and phosphorus levels in the serum and the excess is deposited in the tissues. This is the pathogenesis in secondary hyperparathyroidism and is seen in certain diseases of the kidney. Eventual result is renal rickets in a child and renal osteomalacia in adults. This is high phosphorus rickets compared to normal or low phosphorus rickets in vitamin D deficiency.

SCURVY

Definition

It is a nutritional disorder caused by deficiency of vitamin C and is characterized clinically by a generalized hemorrhagic tendency. The severe form of disease is rare and mild varieties are more common. Deficiency targets the cells of skeletal system more often.

Etiology

- Most frequent between 5 and 10 months in artificially fed infants.
- Vitamin C-deficient diet.
- When seen with rickets, it is called Barton's disease.

Pathology

Cohesive property of the matrix of connective tissue and endothelium is impaired resulting in capillary hemorrhage. Gum bleeding is seen. Within the bone, subperiosteal hemorrhage is characteristic. Hemorrhage within the metaphysis interferes with ingrowths of osteoblastic tissue. Thus, ossification is disturbed. This weakens the bone leading to separation of epiphyseo-metaphyseal junction. Bleeding throughout the marrow results in it being replaced by fibrous tissue causing secondary anemia. *Thus, in scurvy osteogenesis is affected while osteoclasts continue normal function.*

Clinical Features

The affected child is restless, pale, and febrile. The affected limb is swollen, tender, and painful, muscles are in spasm, and the child loathes using the limb. This voluntary immobilization of the extremities is called *pseudoparalysis*. The gums display a bluish, spongy swelling, especially around the upper central incisor teeth. Brittle and loose teeth, ecchymosed beneath the skin, hematemesis, hematuria, anemia, weight loss, anorexia, etc. are the other features. Sometimes even death supervenes.

The lower femur, the upper tibia, and the upper humerus are favored sites for epiphyseal fracture separation. Costochondral separation is typical. Mild forms of scurvy are more common. In adults, pain and tenderness over the bone and fracture with mild trauma is suggestive.

> **Did You Know?**
> The combination of rickets and scurvy is known as Barton's disease.

Investigations

Laboratory Tests: Blood ascorbic acid level is normal and is around 0.5 mg/dL (N = 1 g/dL). Anemia is common.

Radiographs

- Characteristic lines (see box) are seen (Fig. 37.10).
- Ground glass appearance of the bone.
- Subperiosteal fractures are seen.
- Epiphyseal fracture separation, etc. results.

> **Remember**
> *The radiological lines in scurvy*
> - *White line of Frankel*—dense line between epiphysis and metaphysis.
> - *Scurvy line*—dense line within the metaphysis.
> - *Weinberger's line*—dense line within the epiphysis.
> - *Pelkan spurs*—a bone spur from the lateral border of the metaphysis.

Differential Diagnosis

- Rickets
- Osteomalacia
- Osteogenesis imperfecta
- Acute poliomyelitis
- Septic arthritis, etc.

Treatment

Treatment is essentially conservative and consists of supplementing vitamin C in the diet and encouraging the child to take foods rich in other vitamins. The painful joints and the fractures needs to be immobilized with plaster splints.

METABOLIC DISORDERS LEADING TO OSTEOSCLEROSIS

Important diseases, which cause osteosclerosis, are fluorosis, secondaries from prostate, osteopetrosis, Paget's disease, renal osteodystrophy, etc. of this fluorosis is of pubic health importance.

FLUOROSIS

Fluorosis is a pubic health problem in our country in states like Andhra Pradesh, Tamil Nadu, etc. It results when the

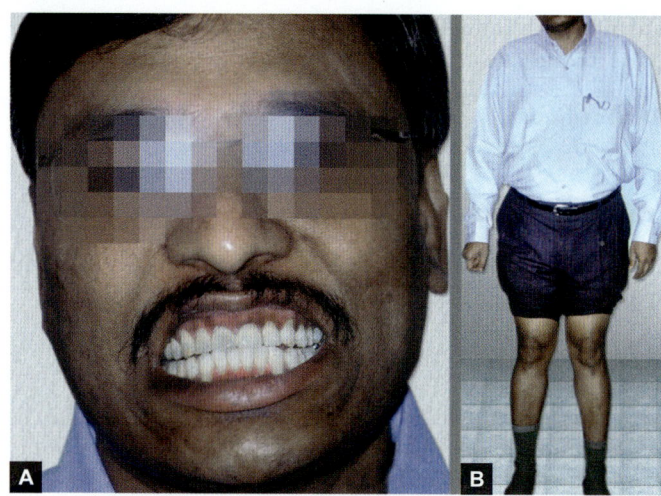

Figs 37.11A and B: Clinical photos of fluorosis, dental and knee changes (genu valgum)

fluoride content of drinking water exceeds 1 PPM. As a result, excess calcium is deposited in bone and soft tissues (Figs 37.11A and B).

Clinical Features

Fluorosis first starts as mottling of the enamel of the upper incisors. Dental fluorosis results in the destruction of the tooth and ultimately its loss. In the skeletal system, spine is more commonly affected. The posterior longitudinal ligament is thickened and may compress the cord. This may lead to spastic paraparesis.

Investigations

Laboratory tests reveal high fluoride levels in blood and urine.

Radiographs show calcification at posterior longitudinal ligament in spine and intraosseous membrane in the leg and forearm. Pelvis, spine, and other bones show increased density.

Bone biopsy clinches the diagnosis.

Treatment

The patient is encouraged to drink defluorinated water. Preventing the disease by defluorination of drinking water is by far the best measure to tackle this menacing problem.

BIBLIOGRAPHY

1. Cartis JA, Kool SW, Fraser D, Greenbery ML. Nutritional rickets in vegetarian children. Can Med Assoc J. 1983;128:150.
2. Doppelt SH. Vitamin D, rickets and osteomalacia. Clin Orthop Clin North Am. 1984;15:671.
3. Klein KL, Maxwell MH. Renal osteodystrophy. Orthop Clin North Am. 1984;15:687.
4. Lavinger RD. Rickets (grand round series). Pediatrics. 1980;66:365.

38 CHAPTER

Osteomyelitis

INTRODUCTION

Osteomyelitis is one of the most difficult and challenging problems encountered in orthopedics. From the life-threatening acute osteomyelitis to the disabling chronic osteomyelitis, it frustrates and thwarts the best efforts of orthopedic surgeons. The ravaging effects of osteomyelitis on a bone and its neighboring joints are a tale of dismay and gloom.

It has been our common clinical experience that the incidence of acute osteomyelitis is definitely on the wane and the incidence of chronic osteomyelitis is on the rise. This is primarily because of the rise in road traffic accidents (RTAs) leaving a bizarre of compound and complex fractures which are the major cause of infection in bone. This is followed next with the rise in infection rate following surgeries on bones and joints. The fall in the incidence of acute osteomyelitis could probably be explained to the frequent and early use of antibiotics in patients presenting with fever. The fall in mortality rate due to acute osteomyelitis is a welcome trend but equally worrying is the high incidence of chronic osteomyelitis, which is a disturbing trend. The fall in mortality rate is compensated by the rise in morbidity rates while the ideal thing would be a fall in both the rates.

Definition

Osteomyelitis is defined as a suppurative process of the bone caused by pyogenic organisms or simply a pyogenic infection of the cancellous portion of the bone.

Classification

Three types are described based on duration of symptoms, route of spread of infection and host response (Table 38.1).

Hematogenous spread with primary infection being elsewhere like tonsillitis, ASOM, pyoderma, etc. is the common mode of spread. Spread from neighboring infective sites like septic arthritis and direct inoculation of infecting organisms by way of penetrating wounds, punctured wounds, trauma, etc. come second.

ACUTE OSTEOMYELITIS

Etiology

The etiological factors causing osteomyelitis can be best understood if discussed under the following heads (Fig. 38.1).

Agent Factors

The following myriad of incriminating organisms is responsible for its causation:

"S" series organisms ("S" denotes severe osteomyelitis and those organisms causing it start with the letter "S")
- *Staphylococcus aureus (60–85%):* This is the most common organism causing acute osteomyelitis.
- *Streptococcus hemolyticus (8–10%)*
- *Salmonella:* Osteomyelitis is relatively rare and presents an interesting picture as most of its features start with "S."
  - Several bones involved

TABLE 38.1: Classification of osteomyelitis

Duration	Route of spread Waldogel's	Host response
Acute (<2 weeks)	Hematogenous (Most common)	Pyogenic
Subacute (2–3 weeks)		Nonpyogenic
Chronic (>3 weeks)	Direct	
Residual	Contiguity	

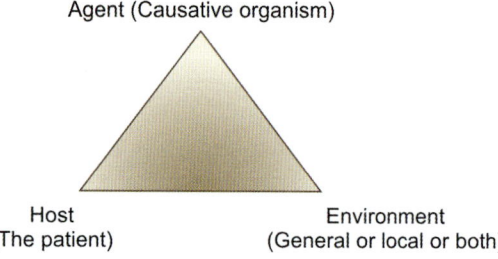

Fig. 38.1: Etiological factors causing osteomyelitis

- Symmetrical involvement of bones
- Severe osteomyelitis
- Spine may be involved
- Sickle cell anemia present
- Stool culture may be positive.

P-series organisms (their mode of entry is through punctured wounds)
- *Pseudomonas*
- *Pneumococcus.*

C-series (C denotes compound fractures)
- *Clostridium welchii*
- *Coliforms (E. coli).*

B-series
- *Brucella bacillus.*

H-series
- *Hemophilus influenzae* (7 months to 4 years)
  This is known to cause osteomyelitis in the age group of 7 months to 4 years.

T-series
- *Treponema pallidum* (syphilitic osteomyelitis)
- Tubercle bacillus (*Mycobacterium*).

Fungal osteomyelitis (ABC)
- Actinomycosis
- Blastomycosis
- Cryptococcosis and coccidioidomycosis
  These usually cause chronic osteomyelitis.

Host Factors

Age

In children: The incidence is 88 percent (because more prone for injury and to fall).

In adults: 12 percent.
 Hence, it is predominantly a disease of childhood.

Sex

Male preponderance (? more playful).

Economic Status

Low socioeconomic groups are more susceptible.

Quick Facts

General factors
- Anemia
- Debility
- Infection
- Poor nutrition
- Poor immune status

Local factors
(Responsible for localization of infection at metaphysis, especially in children)
- Hairpin bend vessels
- Metaphyseal hemorrhage
- Defective phagocytosis
- Rapid growth at metaphysis
- Necrotic tissue acts as a culture media
- Anoxia
- Vasospasm

Environmental Factors

General Factors

All the above-mentioned general factors bring down the resistance of the patient thereby making them susceptible for infection.

Local Factors

These are extremely important in localizing the infection to the metaphysis.

Hairpin bend of the metaphyseal vessels: This slows down the circulation for a moment, which is sufficient for the organisms to escape out (Fig. 38.2).

Metaphyseal hemorrhage: Results from the bleeding due to microscopic trauma. The blood clot so accumulated acts as an excellent culture media for the escaped organisms to grow.

Defective phagocytosis: WBCs here are busy removing the debris of the decalcification due to growth process. Therefore, their function of eliminating the offending organism is slightly impaired.

Rapid growth at the metaphysis: Makes the cells more susceptible to the action of bacterial toxins as the cells are immature.

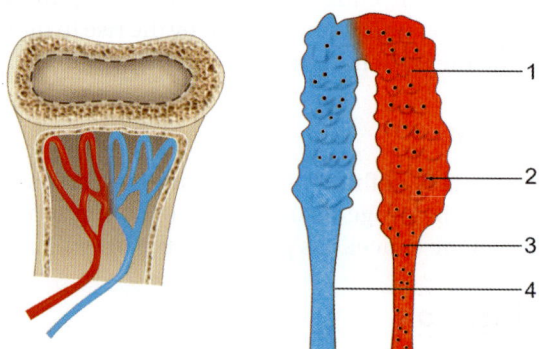

Fig. 38.2: Microanatomy of the hairpin bend vessels: (1) Thrombosed vessel, (2) Bacterial colonies, (3) Artery, and (4) Vein

Vasospasm: Though protective as it arrests further bleeding from the traumatized vessels, it also causes anoxia and failure of antibiotics and other defense cells from reaching the area.

Anoxia: Due to vasospasm, it helps the bacteria grow.

Thus, acute osteomyelitis develops because of the combination of agent, host, and environment factors.

Pathophysiology

The infection results in the formation of abscess at the region of metaphysis. The pus so formed finds its way out through the *area of least resistance*. In children less than 2 years (Figs 38.3A to C), periosteum is loosely attached to the cortex and hence forms a potentially weak point. The subperiosteal abscess so developed will either spread through the soft tissues or drain to the outside by forming a sinus breaking the skin or it will percolate down towards the diaphysis between the periosteum and the cortex and enter the shaft through the widened haversian pores due to anoxia. The growth plate limits spread to the joint. Between 2 and 16 years, periosteum is firmly attached to the cortex, and with the growth plate still present, the pus has to spread towards the diaphysis at a slow pace. Above 16 years, the growth plate has disappeared, the periosteum is firmly adherent, and the pus spreads towards the diaphysis very slowly (Figs 38.4 and 38.5).

Quick Facts
Spread in acute osteomyelitis

<2 years	2–16 years	>16 years
• Subperiosteal (Common)	• Subperiosteal (rare)	• Diaphysis (common but very slow)
• Diaphysis (rare)	• Diaphysis (common but slow)	• Joint space involved
• Joint space (rare)		• Extraperiosteal (rare)

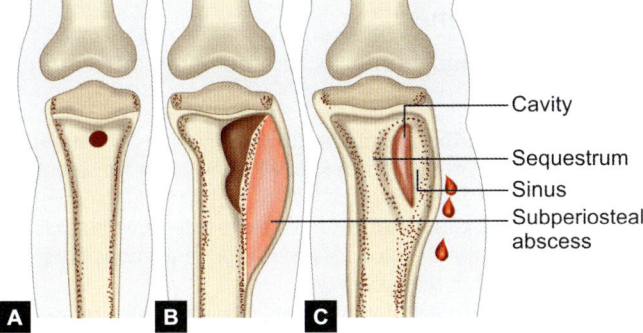

Figs 38.3A to C: Pathological events in acute osteomyelitis in <2 years: (A) Beginning of the infection in the metaphysis; (B) Formation of a subperiosteal abscess; (C) Formation of a discharging sinus and sequestrum

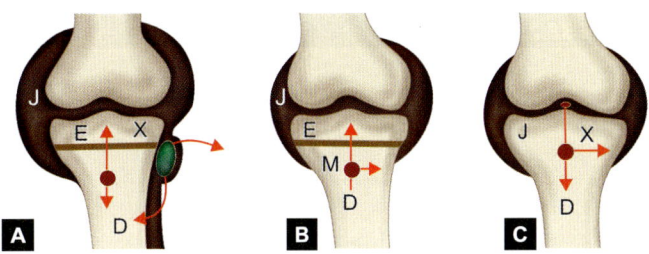

Figs 38.4A to C: (A) Spread of pus from the metaphysis in children of less than 2 years. Subperiosteal common, joint involvement rare but still joint can be involved in two ways: (1) If the capsule encloses the metaphyseal region, (2) Through the common blood supply from the nutrient vessel which gives rise to metaphyseal and epiphyseal vessels; (B) Spread in children between 2 and 16 years. In this age group, diaphyseal spread is common; (C) Spread in patients >16 years. In this age, joint involvement may be direct because the growth plate has disappeared (J—joint, E—epiphysis, M—metaphysis, D—diaphysis, and X—no spread)

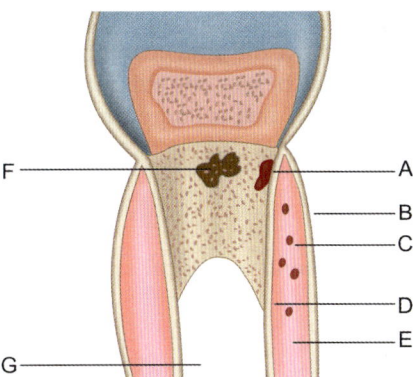

Fig. 38.5: Entire spectrum of pathological changes in osteomyelitis: (A) Sequestrum, (B) Periosteum, (C) Pus, (D) Cortex, (E) Involucrum, (F) Bone abscess, and (G) Medullary cavity

Clinical Features

Acute osteomyelitis is a clinical catastrophe. It presents in the following manner (Table 38.2):

Fever
This is the most common presenting symptom. The child usually has very high fever and is associated with profuse sweating, chills and rigors. Sometimes, the presentation is so acute that the child may be in shock and unconscious.

Swelling
This usually follows the fever and may affect the ends of long bones. The swelling may be acutely painful and the skin may appear red.

TABLE 38.2: Clinical facts

	General	Local
Symptoms	• Fever (95%)	• Local swelling (80%)
	• Sweating	• Limitation of movement (50%)
	• Chills and rigors	
	• Patient is usually in shock	
Signs	• Increased temperature	• Tenderness (80%)
	• Increased pulse rate	• Local erythema (50%)
	• Anemia (?)	• Raised temperature (50%)
	• Signs of dehy-dration and shock	• Fluctuation present (20%)
		• Effusion (10%)
		• Decreased movements (50%)

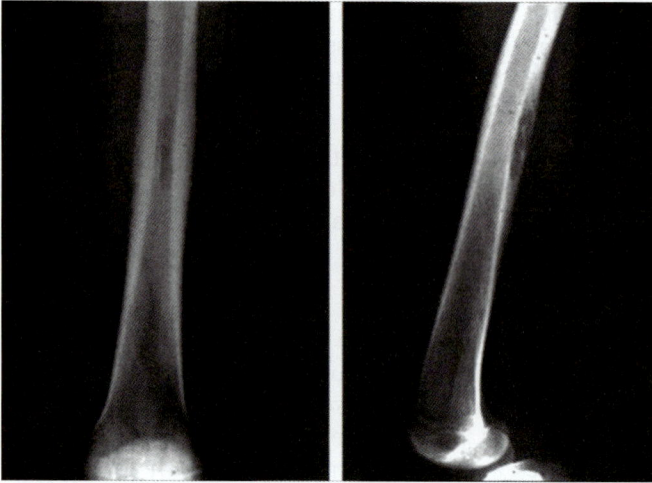

Fig. 38.6: X-ray showing features of acute osteomyelitis

Limitation of Movement

The child may not move the joint near the affected bone due to pain and swelling. In fact, the child may lie still without moving the joint and this is sometimes called a state of pseudoparalysis.

Clinical Signs

This consists of general and local signs and is shown in Table 38.2.

General Features

General features of anemia, dehydration, pyrexia, pulse rate, shock, and toxicity may be present.

Local Features

The local swelling may show increased temperature may be tender to touch, and the skin is stretched. Movements of the neighboring joints are decreased and there may be effusion in them too.

Investigations

The investigations of acute and chronic osteomyelitis is compared for easy remembrance and understanding (Table 38.3 and Fig. 38.6). In general, in acute osteomyelitis, laboratory investigations and bone scan are more useful while radiology is of much help in chronic osteomyelitis (Fig. 38.7).

Management

Acute osteomyelitis is an orthopedic emergency, which needs in patient admission. The management can be discussed as general and local.

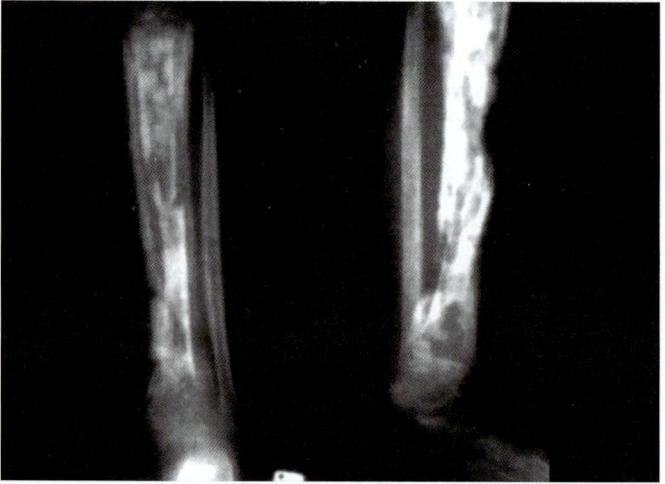

Fig. 38.7: Radiograph showing chronic osteomyelitis with diaphyseal sequestrum of tibia

General Management

Conservative management is the mainstay of treatment (Fig. 38.8).

The mnemonic *RESTS* sums up the conservative line of treatment:
 Rest in bed; protect affected part with splints to alleviate pain and spasm.
 Elevation of the part, warm and moist packs to reduce the swelling.
 Systemic treatment—blood transfusions, intravenous fluids to correct shock and hypovolemia.
 Treatment—with antibiotics discussed below helps to reduce toxicity.
 Surgery—properly indicated and timed to prevent complications.

Principles of antibiotic therapy: This is the mainstay of treatment in acute osteomyelitis. Lack of understanding of the correct principles of antibiotic therapy in acute

TABLE 38.3: Investigations in osteomyelitis

General	Acute osteomyelitis	Chronic osteomyelitis
Hemoglobin (Percentage)	Normal or decreased	Decreased
ESR	Normal or increased	Increased
WBCs	Neutrophils Increased	Lymphocytes are increased
X-rays	<48 hours Few changes • Rarefaction is the earliest sign • Loss of demarcation of line between subcutaneous shadows and muscles • Appearance of transverse lines of increased densities outward from the muscles >2 weeks Periosteal new bone formation is seen • Rarefaction	• Sequestrum identified by the denser X-ray shadow. The density is because of the impermeability for the X-rays. • Involucrum (new bone surrounding the sequestra) • Cloacae (holes through which sequestra is released) • Irregular bone thickening • ? Pathological fracture
Bone scan (Technetium 99m, GA-67, Indium-111-labeled leukocytes)	• Confirms diagnosis as early as 24–48 hours after the onset in 90–95% of cases in early stages • Focal area of early uptake • But it cannot distinguish a tumor from infection (non-specific)	• Useful in detecting sequestrum
Blood culture (Taken at three different times at least two hours apart)	Positive in 60%	—
Gram's staining (Aspirate from infected bones)	Helps choose the appropriate antibiotics	—
Sinograms		• Methylene blue • Radiopaque dyes to identify sinus tract before doing sequestrectomy
Cement beads (Fig. 38.9)	—	• To identify avascular bone from vascular bone

Note: In acute osteomyelitis bone, scan helps in early diagnosis with almost 100 percent accuracy. X-ray has its limitation. Chronic osteomyelitis can reasonably be diagnosed well on X-rays.

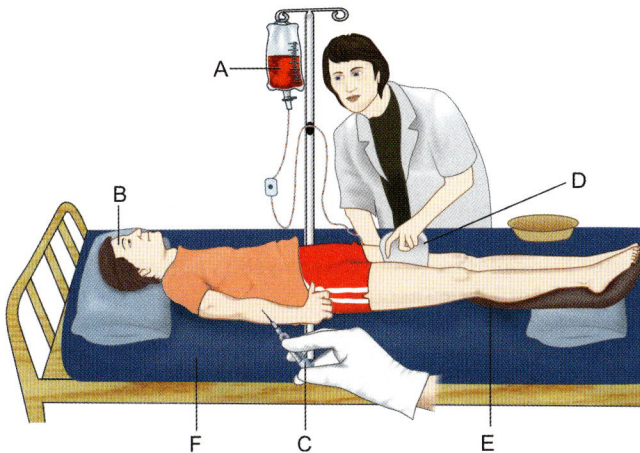

Fig. 38.8: Principles of treatment in acute osteomyelitis: (A) IV fluids and blood transfusion, (B) Tepid sponging, (C) Intravenous antibiotics, (D) Cryotherapy, (E) Splints and elevation of the affected part, (F) Rest in bed and hospitalization

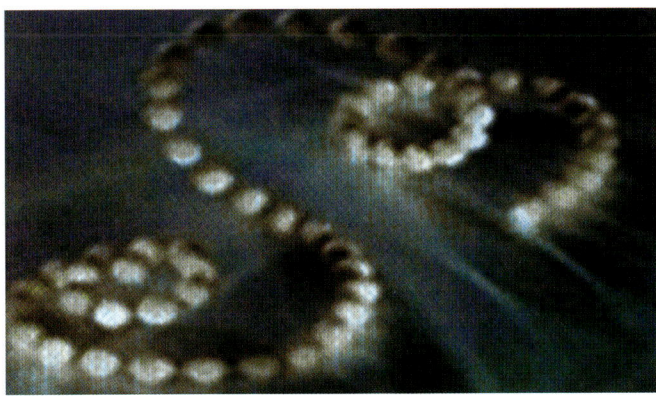

Fig. 38.9: Cement beads in chronic osteomyelitis

osteomyelitis leaves a sequel in the form of chronic osteomyelitis. This underlines the importance of correct antibiotic therapy (all **A's**).

Appropriate drug—usually the drug chosen is a broad-spectrum bactericidal agent.

Appropriate route—intravenous for the first 2 weeks and oral for the next 4 weeks.

Appropriate dose—of the drug depending on the body weight of the patient.

Appropriate time to stop—when the disease is eradicated, controlled or resistance or side effects to the drugs develops.

Appropriate adjunctive measures—a combination of ampicillin and cloxacillin are found to be very effective though penicillin G is still the drug of first choice in our country. Fusidic acid is preferred in the Western countries. *Current trends in antibiotic therapy:* This consists of a short course of intravenous antibiotics for a period of 2 weeks, followed by oral antibiotics for further 4 weeks. Proper monitoring of the serum antibiotic level is very much essential to obtain good results.

> **Nade's Principles for Acute Osteomyelitis Aptly Sums up the Action of Antibiotic Therapy**
> - An appropriate antibiotic is effective before pus forms.
> - Antibiotic cannot sterilize avascular tissue.
> - Antibiotic prevents reformation of pus once removed.
> - Pus removal restores continuity between periosteum and cortex, which restores blood flow.
> - Antibiotics should be continued after surgery.

Local Management

The focus here is on well-timed surgery if any one of the following indications is present.

Nade's indications for surgery
- Abscess formation.
- Severely ill and moribund child.
- Failure to respond to intravenous antibiotics for more than 48 hours.

> **Antibiotics Therapy in Osteomyelitis**
> - Penicillin
> - B-lactamase inhibitors
> - Cephalosporin
> - Ciprofloxacin
>   – Parenteral IV antibiotics for 4–6 weeks.
>   – Oral antibiotics for 2–4 weeks.
>
> *Local antibiotics:* Antibiotics impregnated with cement beads provide high dose of antibiotics locally.

Surgical Methods

Depending upon the situation any one of the following surgical methods could be employed:

Aspiration: it helps in decompression and the material so obtained may be used to identify the organism and check for antibiotic sensitivity.

Incision and drainage helps to drain the subcutaneous abscess.

Multiple drill holes: If the abscess is subperiosteal, this technique helps to drain the pus by making multiple holes in the cortex.

Small bone window: If the multiple drill holes do not drain the pus, a small window of bone is removed from the cortex and the pus is evacuated.

Differential Diagnosis

Acute Septic Arthritis

Here the infection is in the joint, in osteomyelitis, it is in the bone near the joint. Hence, joint movements are severely restricted and more painful in acute septic arthritis.

Scurvy

Features of pseudoparalysis, bleeding gums, tender limbs, etc. are the features.

Acute Anterior Poliomyelitis

Here pain and tenderness are spread throughout the muscle mass, whereas in osteomyelitis tenderness is greatest on direct pressure over the bone.

Cellulitis

It is difficult to differentiate from acute osteomyelitis; however, cellulitis has no edge, no fluctuation, no pus, and no limits.

Other Differential Diagnosis

Erysipelas, erythema nodosum, Ewing's sarcoma, sickle cell anemia, etc.

Complications (Seen in 5% of the Cases)

- Septicemia and pyemia are the common general complications.
- Septic arthritis due to extension of the neighboring foci of infection into the joint.
- Chronic osteomyelitis develops due to improper and inadequate treatment. The incidence rate is 5–10 percent.
- Pathological fractures and growth disturbances are relatively rare.
- Recurrence rate in acute osteomyelitis:
  – Metatarsals more than 50 percent.
  – Around the knee more than 25 percent.
  – Due to late diagnosis more than 25 percent.
- Mortality rate is less than 2 percent due to early antibiotic therapy.

> **Prognosis**
> The following are the bad prognostic factors:
> - *Age:* If children.
> - *Agent:* If S. aureus.
> - *Site:* If nearer to trunk.

Course

- Ninety percent resolve due to early diagnosis and effective antibiotic therapy.

- Eight percent show morbidity.
- Two percent have mortality.

> **Characteristic Points in Acute Osteomyelitis**
> - Disease is common in children.
> - *Staphylococcus aureus* is the common organism.
> - Metaphysis is involved.
> - Fever is the common presenting symptom.
> - Bone scan helps in early diagnosis.
> - Conservative management is the mainstay of treatment. In addition, ninety percent resolve.

Note:
Acute osteomyelitis in epiphysis is taken to be caused by *Staphylococcus aureus* unless proved otherwise.

SUBACUTE OSTEOMYELITIS

Subacute osteomyelitis is caused by *Staphylococcus aureus* (Fig. 38.10). The patient complains of pain without constitutional symptoms. Temperature may be increased or normal. It is not detected until at least two weeks has elapsed. Blood culture is positive in only 60 percent of the cases, and WBC and ESR are raised in only 50 percent of the cases.

Subacute osteomyelitis is due to:
- Increased host resistance.
- Lowered bacterial resistance.
- If antibiotics are administered before symptoms appear.

CHRONIC OSTEOMYELITIS

Any osteomyelitis lasting for more than three weeks is termed as chronic. Chronic osteomyelitis can arise from any one of the following ways:
- Sequel of acute osteomyelitis (5–10%)
- Following compound fractures
- Following surgery on bones and joints
- Chronic from the beginning (e.g. tuberculosis, syphilis, Brodie's abscess)
- Anaerobic organisms (sclerosing osteomyelitis of Garre)
- Fungal osteomyelitis.

> **Quick Facts**
> *Salient features in chronic osteomyelitis*
> - Systemic symptoms would have disappeared.
> - One or more foci in the bone containing pus, sequestra or draining sinuses, etc.
> - Acute exacerbation is due to trauma, lowered resistance, etc.

Clinical Features

Symptoms

Symptoms are very few. Fever, pain, swelling are seen in acute exacerbation of chronic osteomyelitis.

Signs

Irregular thickening of bone develops due to unequal pace of destruction of bone and new bone formation (Fig. 38.11). This is a characteristic feature of chronic osteomyelitis.

Sinuses are usually multiple and are fixed to the underlying bone. The presence of sinuses indicates unabsorbed sequestra, unobliterated cavities, and presence of anaerobic organisms (Figs 38.12A and B). They are immobile and adherent to the bone.

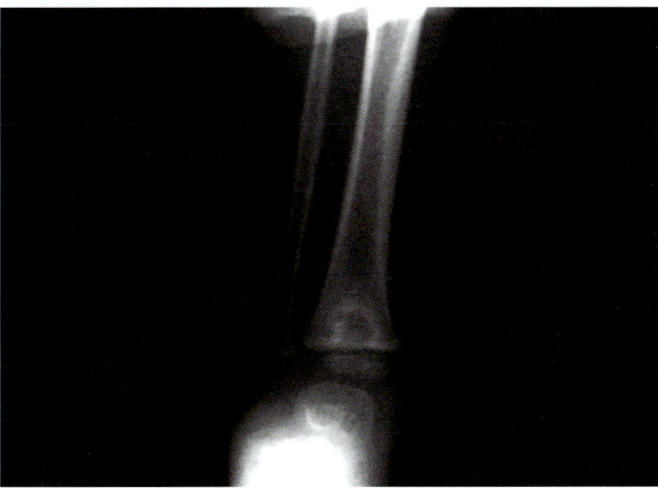

Fig. 38.10: Plain X-ray showing subacute osteomyelitis

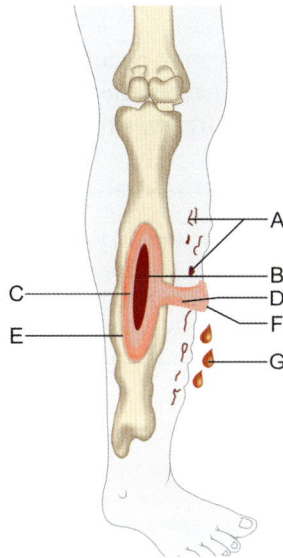

Fig. 38.11: Features in chronic osteomyelitis: (A) Multiple scars and sinuses; (B) Sequestrum; (C) Cavity; (D) Sinus tract, (E) Irregular thickening of bone; (F) Sprouting granulation tissue; and (G) Discharge of bony spicules and pus

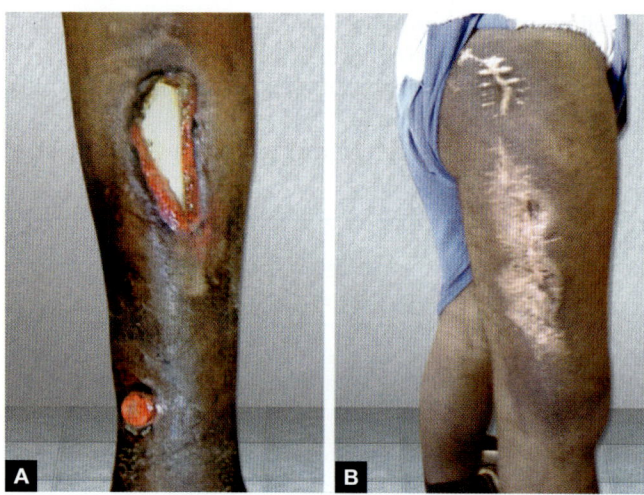

Figs 38.12A and B: Clinical photo showing features of chronic osteomyelitis of tibia and femur

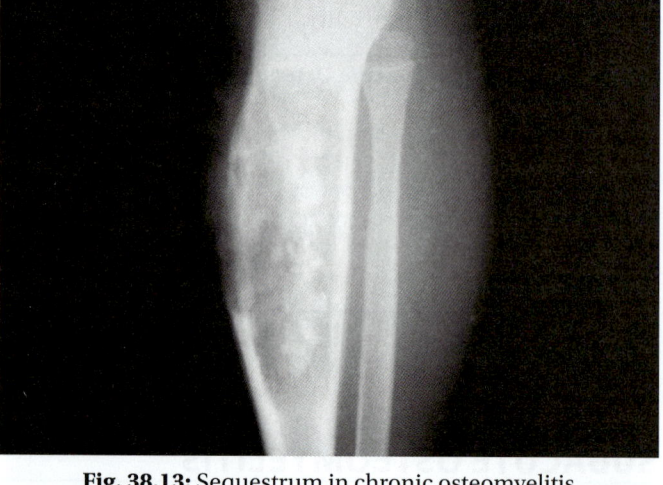

Fig. 38.13: Sequestrum in chronic osteomyelitis

> **Note:**
> History of discharge of tiny bony spicules through the sinus, clinches the diagnosis of chronic osteomyelitis with certainty.

Scars and muscle contractures develop due to the spread of infection from the bones to the muscles and the consequent fibrosis.

Shortening or lengthening of the bones may occur due to the affection or stimulation of the growing epiphysis respectively.

Deformities and decreased movements develop due to scars and contractures.

Pathological fractures may occur either due to chronic osteomyelitis, which weakens the bone, or due to extensive debridement during surgery, which leaves a thin layer of bone.

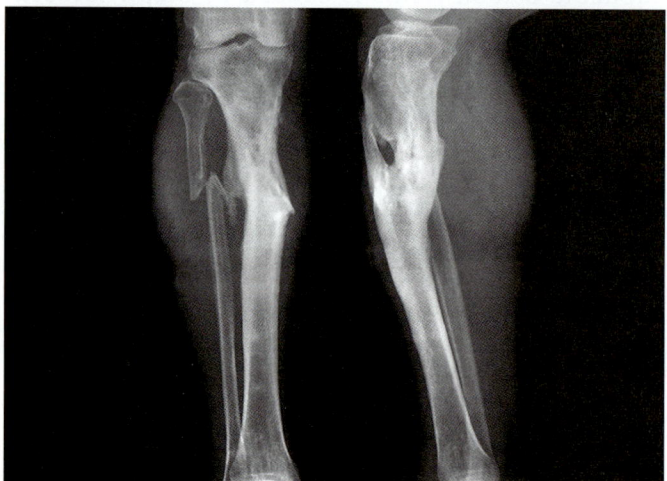

Fig. 38.14: Plain X-ray showing features of chronic osteomyelitis of tibia

> **Note:**
> *Sequestra:* It is a dead bone within a living bone and is defined as an infected granulation tissue. The inflammatory foci are surrounded by sclerotic bone supplied with blood and covered by periosteum, scarred muscle, and subcutaneous tissues.

Quick Facts: Sequestra

Disease	Type of sequestra
TB osteomyelitis	→ Sandy/feathery
Actinomycosis	→ Black
Pin tract infection	→ Ring
Chronic osteomyelitis in children	→ Diaphyseal

Investigations

Sequestra can be identified by X-ray (Figs 38.13 and 38.14), tomography, sinogram, CT scan (Fig. 38.15), gallium-67 and

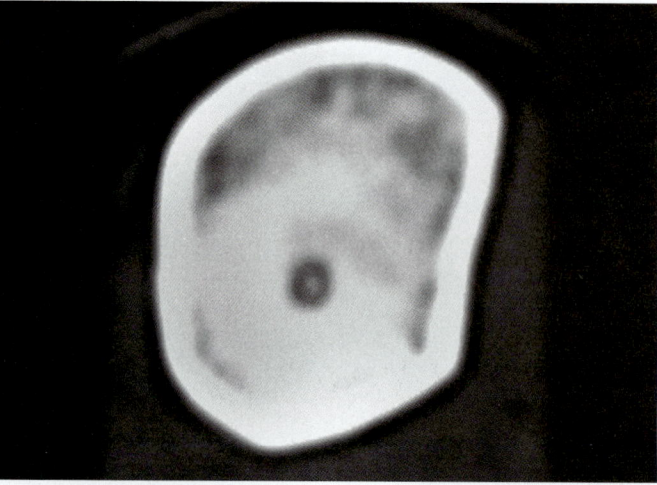

Fig. 38.15: CT Scan showing sequestrum in chronic osteomyelitis

indium-111-labeled leukocyte scan, etc. X-ray changes have been enumerated in Table 38.3.

Classification

As suggested by Cierny and Mader (Fig. 38.16):

Type I: *Medullary osteomyelitis* is due to hematogenically-infected compound fracture or infected intramedullary nails.

Type II: *Surface osteomyelitis* limited to the surface of the bone exposed due to inadequate soft tissue coverage.

Type III: *Localized with full thickness cortical* separation, and is usually common in infected nonunion.

Type IV: *Diffuse* entire bone is involved.

Management

Goal: Eradication of the infection by achieving a viable and vascular environment. This can be done by radical debridement by way of sequestrectomy and resection of scarred and infected bone and soft tissue. Appropriate antibiotic is also required. Finally, reconstruction of both the bone and soft tissue defects may be needed.

Principles of treatment: As is evident from the goal, surgery is the treatment of choice.
- Surgery is to be undertaken only when fever and infection has subsided, living bone can be distinguished from the dead bone and when involucrum appears sufficient to maintain length and contour of the bone after excision of any large sequestra.
- Secondary infection is usually present. When surgery is indicated, culture is done and antibiotics started at least four days before surgery and are continued for two weeks.
- When acute exacerbation fails to respond to conservative treatment, incision and drainage have to be done.

Surgery Methods

Sequestrectomy and saucerization: Sequestrum is identified on the X-ray, as it is denser and lies free in the cavity (Figs 38.17A and B). It takes 2–3 months before it is isolated, separated, and easily seen on the X-ray and only then, sequestrectomy is planned. All the sinus tracts are injected with methylene blue 24 hours before surgery. By making multiple drill holes, the cortex is removed in a rectangular fashion. Sequestrectomy is done next. The cavity is curetted until fresh bleeding occurs and the deep shape of the cavity is converted into a shallow cavity.

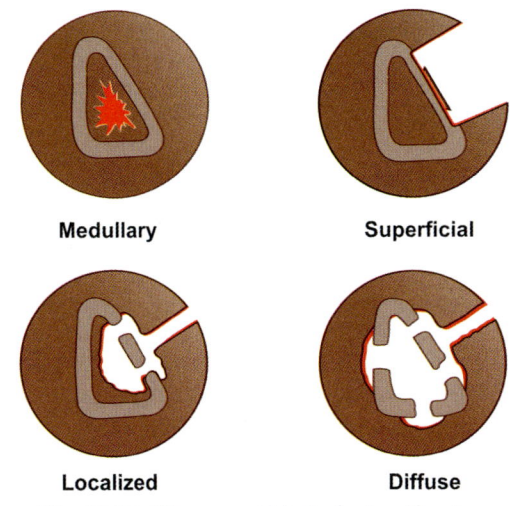

Fig. 38.16: Cierny and Mader's classification

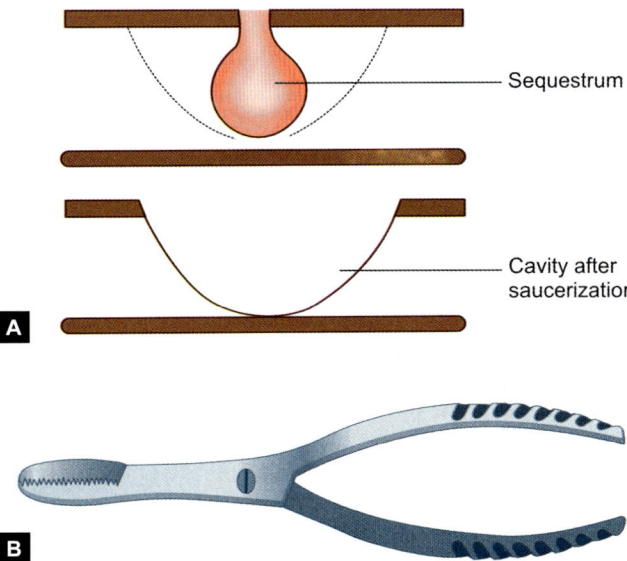

Figs 38.17A and B: (A) Sequestrectomy and saucerization; (B) Sequestrum forceps (19 cm) straight/angular

Note:
Sequestrectomy usually leaves a deep cavity beneath which is potentially a dead space favoring collection of pus and other debris. To prevent this from happening, the deep cavity is made shallow for effective drainage of the collected materials.

After sequestrectomy, there is a huge gap in the bone and there are four basic methods of immediate biological management of dead space so left:
- Local closure if the space left is very small.
- Myoplasty for slightly larger space, surrounding muscles can be packed into the cavity.
- Cancellous bone grafts for a space less than 2.5 cm.
- Free vascularized bone graft for larger areas.

How Much Margin to Resect?
- Marginal resection is less than 5 mm and recurrence is common.
- Wide resection is more than 5 mm and is associated with less recurrence.

Other Methods of Treatment

- *Papineau et al.* described an open grafting technique for chronic osteomyelitis. The operation is divided into three stages:
  - Stage I: Radical excision of all the infected tissue.
  - Stage II: Cancellous autogenous bone grafting.
  - Stage III: Wound coverage by skin grafting and other techniques.
- *Hyperbaric oxygen* therapy.
- *Closed suction drainage:* After sequestrectomy, the wound is closed over a suction drain (Fig. 38.18). Through an inlet tube, an irrigation fluid consisting of saline, antibiotics, and detergent is pushed into the medullary cavity and drained out through an outlet tube to which a slow suction is applied. This enables the wound to be continuously bathed in this antibiotic solution.
- *Amputation* is done rarely in the following circumstances: If the patient's life is endangered by infection or in extensive infection. Lots of circumspection should be used while deciding upon amputation for chronic osteomyelitis. It should be the last choice and not the first. I would like to recall about a patient who had a very bad chronic osteomyelitis following compound fracture of both bones of left leg and was treated with debridement and internal fixation with a medullary nail which also got infected and compounded his problems. He was suggested to undergo a below-knee amputation as he had a very wide-open sinus draining pus for over 3 years. He approached me with a plea to save his limb. Implant was removed, radical debridement was done, a myocutaneous flap was fashioned to close the wound, and the patient was treated with appropriate antibiotics. The results were excellent. Hence, I feel, not to give room for desperation in bad cases of chronic osteomyelitis, but still try to manage it by conventional methods, which is often successful.
- *Ilizarov's method:* It has been found to be a very effective method of managing chronic osteomyelitis of late. Though technically very demanding, if planned and executed properly, it gives very good results in bad cases of chronic osteomyelitis.
- *Excision of bones* can be done, if smaller bones are involved like phalanges, carpal bones, etc.

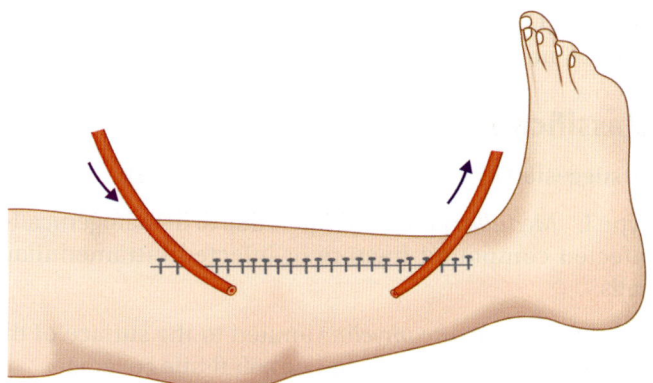

Fig. 38.18: Closed continuous suction irrigation system for chronic osteomyelitis

Complications

Most Common Complications

Pathological fracture is by far the most common complication. The incidence is 5 to 10 percent. It requires Papineau treatment comprising thorough debridement, grafting, and stabilization of fracture fragments by external fixators.

Common Complications

- *Acute exacerbation* of existing chronic disease initiated by a change in bacterial flora or by decrease in the general resistance of the patient, which flares up the dormant infection.
- *Growth disturbances:* Usually, the growth is not affected (64%); more commonly, shortening may be seen (64%) due to the arrest of the growth plate by the neighboring infection and very rarely, there may be stimulation of the growth plate resulting in lengthening (5%) of bones.
- *Deformities* develop due to soft tissue, muscle, and joint contractures and due to growth plate disturbances.

Rare Complications

- *Amyloidosis* due to long-standing infection.
- *Epithelioma* of the sinus tract due to chronic discharging sinus which induces metaplasia and formation of squamous cell carcinoma (incidence <1%).

Residual Osteomyelitis

In residual osteomyelitis, there is complete absence of signs and symptoms. There are no draining sinuses. There is soft tissue scarring, skin is fixed to the bone, and the underlying bone is sclerotic.

OSTEOMYELITIS OF SPECIAL IMPORTANCE

[1]BRODIE'S ABSCESS

Brodie's abscess is a localized form of chronic osteomyelitis, involves metaphyseal and epiphyseal area, and is common in young adults.

Etiology

Causative organism is low virulence *S. aureus* in 50 percent of the cases.

Clinical Presentation

The patient complains of intermittent pain of long duration and local tenderness.

Radiograph

It shows varied appearance. Usually, a cavity with a rim of sclerotic bone is seen at the metaphysio-epiphyseal junction. Frequently requires biopsy for diagnosis (Fig. 38.19).

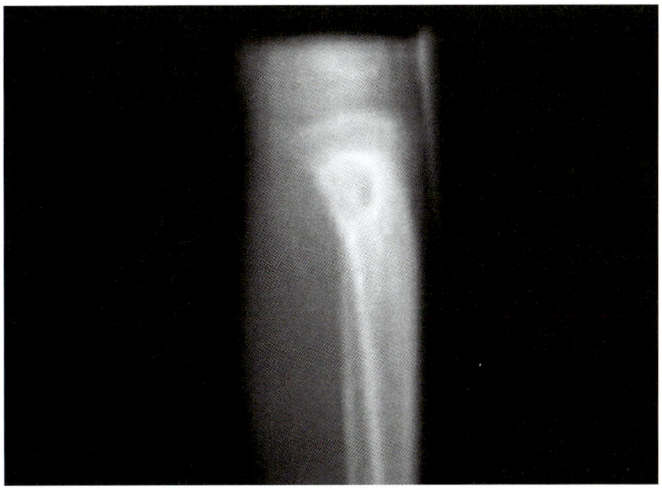

Treatment

Treatment consists of appropriate antibiotics, curettage and bone grafting, and the wound is loosely closed over a drain.

SCLEROTIC OSTEOMYELITIS OF GARRE

This is a chronic or subacute form of chronic osteomyelitis. It is common in children and young adults. It usually affects the subperiosteal region and the bone is thickened. Though the exact cause is not known, it could be due to low-grade anaerobic infection. A secondary infection may occur at a distant site.

Clinical Features

The patient may complain of intermittent pain, swelling, tenderness and low-grade fever, etc.

Investigations

Radiographs show expanded bone with generalized sclerosis.

Fig. 38.19: Radiograph showing Brodies abscess

Laboratory tests—ESR is usually raised.

Biopsy is definitive and confirmatory.

Treatment

Treatment consists of fenestration of sclerotic bone and appropriate antibiotics should be given.

TUBERCULAR OSTEOMYELITIS

Treatment discussed in Chapter on Skeletal Tuberculosis.

BIBLIOGRAPHY

1. Blockey NJ, Watson JT. Acute osteomyelitis in children. J Bone Joint Surg. 1970;52-B:77.
2. Cole WG, Dalziel RE, Leitl S. Treatment of acute osteomyelitis in childhood. J Bone Joint Surg. 1982;64-B:218.
3. Jackson MA, Nelson JD. Etiology and medical management of acute suppurative bone and joint infections in pediatric patients. J Pediatr Orthop. 1982;2:313.
4. Learmonth ID, Dall G, Pallock DJ. Acute osteomyelitis and septic arthritis in children: A simple approach to treatment. S Afr Med J. 1984;65:117.
5. Orr HW. The treatment of acute osteomyelitis by drainage and rest. J Bone Joint Surg. 1927;9:733.
6. Trueta J. Acute haematogenous osteomyelitis: Its pathology and treatment. Bull Hosp Joint Dis. 1993;145.

---

[1]**Sir Benjamin Brodie** (1783-1862), London.

CHAPTER 39

Skeletal Tuberculosis

INTRODUCTION

Though ubiquitous in distribution, tuberculosis has firmly entrenched itself with the Third World, thanks to the illiteracy, poverty, poor hygienic conditions and a host of other favorable factors. India is infamous for hosting nearly one-fifth of the thirty million people suffering from tuberculosis throughout the world. Though largely preventable, tuberculosis can be successfully combated by an effective chemotherapy. The bugbears of treatment being its long duration, poor patient compliance, emergence of drug resistance and others. Skeletal tuberculosis mercifully is not as common as pulmonary tuberculosis and accounts for only 1–3 percent of the cases.

Tuberculosis, being mainly the disease of Third World, it is no wonder that India has produced pioneers like Dr Tuli, Dr Kumar, Dr Shanmugasundaram and others whose work on skeletal tuberculosis has been acknowledged worldwide.

> **History**
> - Hippocrates (460–370 BC) was the first to suggest the relationship between pulmonary disease and spinal deformity.
> - Percival Pott (1714–1788) described the "gibbus" deformity and its sequelae. He did not describe the disease or its tuberculous nature.
> - Laennec (1781–1826) described the basic microscopic lesion, *the tubercle*.
> - Drugs Streptomycin was first used in 1947, PAS in 1949 and INH in 1952.

> **Note:**
> TB is one of the oldest diseases afflicting humankind. It has been found in Egyptian mummies dating back to 3400 BC.

Skeletal tuberculosis is always *secondary*, the primary foci being either in the lungs, lymph nodes or gastrointestinal tract. The incidence of bone and joint tuberculosis is 2–3 percent. Fifty percent of these cases are found in the vertebral column. The other major areas affected in order of predilection are hip, knee, foot, elbow, hand, shoulder, and others.

Skeletal tuberculosis occurs mostly in the first three decades of life but no age is immune.

Etiology

TB bacillus
- Human (more common) *Mycobacterium tuberculosis*.
- Bovine (rare) *M. bovine*.

Route: Always secondary, may spread to the bone through:
- Blood, e.g. through Batson's plexus in tuberculosis of spine.
- Lymphatic spread.
- Direct.

Precipitating factors
- General factors like anemia, debility, etc. help precipitate the infection.
- Local factors like trauma, etc. localize the problem to the bone.

Local trauma causes vascular stasis and intraosseous hemorrhage.

> **Vital Facts**
> *Did you know?*
> A minimum gap of 2–3 years is required between the primary and skeletal TB.

Pathology

Following injury, the vessels rupture and there is hemorrhage. The tubercle bacilli present in the circulation settle and proliferate in the blood clot so formed. A tubercle follicle is formed and it consists of lymphocytes, giant cells, and endothelial cells (Flowchart 39.1). Small such tubercle follicles coalesce to form a larger follicle, which undergoes caseation at the center and fibrosis at the periphery. The

Flowchart 39.1: How does osteoarticular tubercular lesion develop?

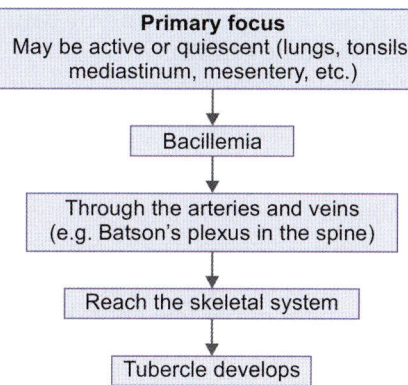

caseation at the center of the shaft breaks down forming pus. It spreads towards the subperiosteal region, breaks the periosteum, and tracks along the lines of least resistance. It reaches the skin and forms the cold abscess (not warm). Later on, it breaches the skin forming the sinus.

Changes in the Marrow

In the early stages, there is increase in the polymorphs. In the later stages, it is replaced by lymphocytes. The marrow is slowly surrounded by fat cells and is replaced by fibrous tissue.

Lamellae

There may be osteoporosis due to the action of osteoclasts or due to metaplasia. Osteosclerosis may also be seen.

Periosteum

Increased vascularity in the periosteum leads to new bone formation and the consequent subperiosteal thickening.

Clinical Features

The diagnostic triad best sums up clinical features (Fig. 39.1).

Insidious

Slow onset.

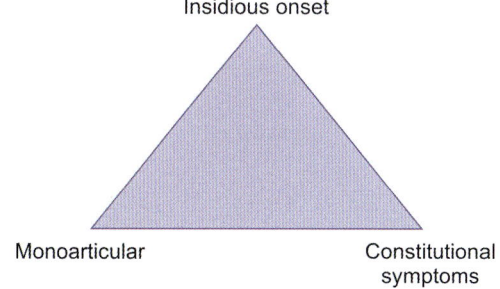

Fig. 39.1: Diagnostic triad of skeletal tuberculosis

Monoarticular

The patient usually complains of pain in one joint, which is dull aching and chronic in nature. He/she may give history of night cries, which is due to the rubbing of inflamed articular surfaces against each other due to the release of muscular spasm at rest. The joint movements are decreased in all directions, initially due to muscle spasm and later due to arthritis. The wasting of the limb muscles is gross and is out of proportion. Regional lymph nodes may be enlarged.

Constitutional Symptoms

This is present in approximately 20 percent of the cases. It consists of low-grade fever, lassitude in the afternoon, loss of appetite and weight, night sweats, anemia, tachycardia and evening rise of temperature.

Investigations

General Investigations

These consists of hemoglobin estimation, total and differential count, raised ESR, urine routine tests, etc.

Other Investigations

- *Positive evidence of the disease*
  - Identification of organism on culture from the joint, histology, etc.
  - Reproduction of disease by inoculating guinea pigs.
- *ZN stains* for acid-fast bacilli in aspirate or excised tissue.
- *Guinea pig test*
- *Mantoux test* is significant only in the first 3–4 years of life, adults are usually positive. Negative test does not rule out tuberculosis.
- *X-ray*
  - No typical finding for tuberculosis.
  - Earliest sign is decalcification of bones (rarefaction).
  - Late signs are joint destruction.
- *Biopsy* of regional lymph nodes may show "tubercles."
- *Exploratory arthrotomy* is the certain way of ascertaining diagnosis. The tissue may be cultured or may be injected into a guinea pig.

Principles of Treatment

General treatment: This includes rich protein diet, hematinics, adequate exposure to sunshine, etc. The general treatment aims at building up the general resistance of the patient.

Chemotherapy is the mainstay of treatment and is discussed in detail below.

Local treatment aims to prevent, correct, or decrease the deformities. If the disease is osseous, aim at ankylosis in functional position by immobilization. If the disease is synovial, aim at mobility by traction.

Operative treatment consists of partial capsulectomy, synovectomy, osteotomy, curettage, arthrodesis, etc. depending on the stage of tuberculosis.

Treatment of tubercular abscess: Conservative treatment is recommended in most of the cases. Aspiration is done if the abscess is tense.

Chemotherapy

The goals of antitubercular chemotherapy are:
- Kill dividing bacilli
- Kill persisting bacilli
- Prevent emergence of resistance.

Drugs used for the treatment of tuberculosis are grouped as follows (Table 39.1).

First line of drugs: These have the greatest level of efficiency and have an acceptable degree of toxicity.

The following are the first line of drugs used in tuberculosis (mnemonic **PRISE**).

P—Pyrazinamide
R—Rifampicin
I—INH
S—Streptomycin
E—Ethambutol.

Second line of drugs: These are useful if the patient develops resistance to the first line of drugs (mnemonic **CAKECAT**). They have either low antitubercular efficacy or high toxicity or both, used in special circumstances as mentioned earlier.

C—Capreomycin
A—Amikacin
K—Kanamycin

TABLE 39.1: Chemotherapeutic drugs in skeletal tuberculosis

Drugs	Antibacterial activity	Mechanism	Absorption	Chemistry	Dose	Untoward effects
INH (primary drug for chemotherapy of tuberculosis)	Bacteriostatic for resting bacilli	Inhibits biosynthesis of mycolic acid, a constituent of the cell walls	Gets rapidly absorbed, diffuses into all body fluids and cells, penetrates the caseous material	Hydroxide of Isonicotinic acids	• Adults 5 mg/kg body wt • Children 10–20 mg/kg body wt	• Rash 2% • Fever 1.2% • Jaundice 0.6% • Peripheral neuritis 0.2%
R-cin (Rifampicin)	Inhibits most of gram positive, gram negative, and myco TB, bactericidal	Inhibits RNA synthesis	Peak action in 2–4 h	Semisynthetic derivative of Rifampicin	10 mg/kg	• Hepatitis • Orange color to urine, etc. Well tolerated
Ethambutol	Bacteriostatic, suppresses growth of most INH and SM-resistant TB bacilli	Inhibits incorporation of mycolic acids	Absorbed well from GIT		15 mg/kg (not used in children <5 years)	• Optic neuritis • Urate concentration increase in blood
Streptomycin	It usually suppresses growth of most INH-resistant TB bacilli	Acts only on extracellular microbes			20–35 mg/kg	• 8.2% incidence, involves auditory and vestibular actions of 8th cranial nerve
Pyrazinamide			Well absorbed	Synthetic analog of Nicotinamide	20–35 mg/kg	Injury to liver hepatitis
Ethionamide	Suppressor	Inhibits acetylation of INH	Rapid and well absorbed	250 mg/BD	Metallic taste 15–20 mg/kg	hepatitis
PAS	Suppressor	Inhibits PABA	Readily absorbed	Structural analogue of PABA	Daily dose of 14–16 gm	Epigastric pain Nausea, anorexia
Cycloserine			Rapidly absorbed		15–20 mg/kg	CNS toxicity
Kanamycin				Amino glycoside	1 g/day	Ototoxic/ Nephrotoxic
Capreomycin Amikacin					15–30 mg/kg	

E—Ethionamide
C—Cycloserine
A—Aminosalicylic acid (PAS)
T—Thiacetazone

The second line of drugs is used only for treatment of the diseases caused by resistant microorganisms or by non-TB mycobacterium. All drugs are given parenterally and are potentially ototoxic and nephrotoxic. Hence, no two drugs from this group should be used simultaneously. These are not used with streptomycin for the same reasons.

Chemotherapy Regimes

Nine-month regime: Nine months of rifampicin and INH are effective for all forms of disease.

Six-month regime: First two months, INH + Rifampicin + Pyrazinamide. Next four months, INH + Rifampicin.

When the primary resistance to INH is high, therapy is usually initiated with four first line drugs.

Third regime: Here three to four drugs are used in the first 4 months, two to three drugs in the second 4 months, one or two drugs in the third 4 months, and one drug (i.e. INH) in the last three to four months of treatment.

The conventional 12-18 month regime has been replaced by more effective and less toxic 6 month regime which is more effective.

Current Trends of Chemotherapy in Musculoskeletal Tuberculosis

- INH is the most potent anti-TB drug currently available.
- 4-drug therapy is the recommended regime and consists of rifampicin, INH, pyrazinamide, and ethambutol. After 3 months, ethambutol is withdrawn and three-drug regime is further continued for nine months. Later, only rifampicin and INH are continued for a further six months. The total duration is thus 18 months.
- Ten mg pyridoxine is given simultaneously to prevent peripheral neuropathy due to INH.

> **Know Tuli's 16-month Chemotherapy Regime:**
> - Rifampicin, INH, and ethambutol for first 4 months.
> - Pyrazinamide replaces rifampicin in the second 4 months.
> - In the next four months, rifampicin is given with INH.
> - In the last four months, INH is the only drug.

Newer drugs: Fluoroquinolones can penetrate; kill mycobacterium lodged in the macrophages. It has good tolerability and is increasingly used in combination regimes against multidrug resistant cases, *M. avium* complex infection in HIV patients.

General Principles of Chemotherapy in Tuberculosis

- Most patients are now treated in ambulatory setting.
- Prolonged bed rest is not necessary.
- The patient is seen at frequent intervals.
- To prevent emergence of drug resistance, treatment must include at least two drugs.
- Standard 6 months regimen preferred for adults and children.
    - Rifampicin—first 2 months.
    - INH and pyrazinamide—next four months.
      Or
    - INH + Rifampicin—for 9 months equally effective.
- Ethambutol is added to the initial treatment for patients when resistance to INH is suspected.
- Treatment is to be continued for at least 6 months and after three negative cultures have been obtained.
- If INH and RMP cannot be used, treatment is continued for 18 months.
- Certain patients should receive initially four drugs to ensure that the microorganisms will be susceptible to at least two drugs.
    - Rifampicin, INH and pyrazinamide (4th drug either ethambutol or streptomycin).
- Ninety percent of the cases who receive optimal treatment will have negative culture within 3–6 months.
- Cultures that remain positive after 6 months indicate emergence of drug resistance and an alternative therapeutic program is then considered.
- The drugs should be continued for an average of 12 months.
- INH must be part of any multidrug therapy.
- In patients on multidrug therapy with neural complications, pyrazinamide should be used for three months.
- Middle path regime was first described in the year 1975 by Tuli and Kumar.

Prognosis

- Ninety five percent of uncomplicated cases of tuberculosis spine heal by conservative regimen.
- In patients with neural complications 50 percent recover with drugs and rest alone, while the other 50 percent recover after surgery.
- After surgery, 70 percent recover completely 15 percent show useful partial recovery, and 15 percent show negligible recovery.

> **Vital Facts**
> The onset of recovery after initiation of chemotherapy may take as long as three months.

Quick Facts
Skeletal Tuberculosis (General)
- Incidence is 2–3 percent.
- Usually monoarticular.
- Always secondary.
- Spine is affected commonly.
- Only 20 percent show constitutional symptoms.
- Cold abscess is a feature.
- Chemotherapy is the mainstay of treatment.

TUBERCULOSIS SPINE

(Known after Sir Percival Pott)

This is the most common form of skeletal tuberculosis constituting about 50 percent of all cases.

Regional Distribution
Cervical—12 percent
Cervicodorsal—5 percent
Dorsal—42 percent
Dorsolumbar—12 percent
Lumbar—26 percent
Lumbosacral—3 percent

As is evident from the above data, spinal tuberculosis commonly affects the lower thoracic and lumbar vertebra accounting for nearly 80 percent of the cases. The reasons cited for this area of predilection are:
- Large amounts of spongy tissues within the vertebral body.
- Degree of weight bearing, which is comparatively more.
- More vertebral mobility is seen here.

Sites of Involvement within the Vertebra

It is observed that spinal tuberculosis could start in any of the part (Fig. 39.2) of the vertebra (95% anterior; 5% posterior elements).

Central Less common. This is known to produce central or *concertina* collapse of the vertebra.

Metaphyseal or intervertebral space (98%): This is the most common area of involvement and is not without reason. Embryological development explains the reasons for this.

Lower half of one vertebra and upper half of the adjacent vertebra with the intervening disk all develop from one sclerotome, which has a common source of blood supply (Fig. 39.3). Hence, bacillemia involves this embryological section more often.

Anterior or periosteal: Here, anterior surface of vertebral body is involved and it may give rise to anterior wedge compression of the vertebra.

Appendiceal occasionally, transverse process, and rarely vertebral arch are affected.

True tubercular arthritis seen in the atlantoaxial and at atlanto-occipital joints.

Sequences of Pathological Events

As mentioned earlier, due to primary foci in the lungs, lymph nodes, or abdomen, bacillemia develops and the organisms reach the spine through the Batson's plexus.

Tuberculous endarteritis, which develops following the infection, results in marrow devitalization. Later on, the tubercular follicle develops. Lamellae are destroyed due to hyperemia causing osteoporosis. Because of this, the vertebral body is easily compressed. In the thoracic vertebrae, because of the normal kyphotic curve, anterior wedge compression is more common. In the lordotic cervical and lumbar vertebra, wedging is minimal.

Two types of vertebral reactions are commonly encountered in skeletal tuberculosis (Table 39.2).

This non-pyogenic infection results in formation of cold abscess, which penetrates the epiphyseal cortex and

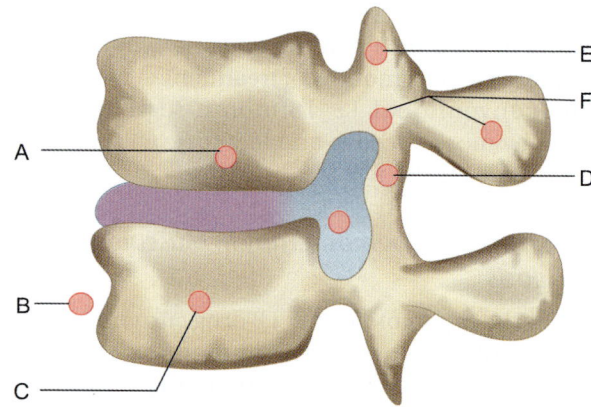

Fig. 39.2: Sites of involvement in TB spine: (A) Metaphyseal, (B) Anterior, (C) Central, (D) True arthritis, (E) Appendiceal, and (F) Posterior spinal elements

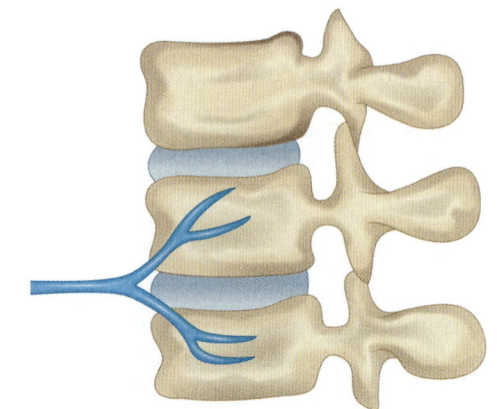

Fig. 39.3: Blood supply of vertebrae

involves the adjacent disk and the vertebra (Fig. 39.4). It may also spread beneath the anterior longitudinal ligament and reach the neighboring vertebra. When it spreads posteriorly, it may cause pressure on the spinal cord, which is more common in the thoracic area as the spinal canal is small here. The posterior longitudinal ligament limits the spread of sequestra and bone fragments into the joints (Fig. 39.5). Sometimes, the cold abscess may penetrate the anterior longitudinal ligament and migrate along the *lines of least resistance* (Fig. 39.4) (i.e. along the fascial planes, blood vessels, nerves).

Note:
Cold abscess consists of serum, WBCs, caseous material, granulation tissue, and tubercle bacilli.

Clinical Features

Tuberculosis of spine is usually insidious in onset although sometimes, it may present acutely. The constitutional symptoms usually antedate local spinal involvement. Weakness, anorexia, night sweats and cries, evening or afternoon rise of temperature, loss of appetite and weight are some of those.

The patient may complain of back pain, which is localized over the site of vertebral involvement or is referred depending on the specific nerve root irritation. Thus, if cervical roots are involved, pain radiates to the arm; if dorsal roots are involved, the patient complains of girdle pain; if lumbar nerve roots are involved; patient complains of radiating pain to the groin; and if sacral roots are involved, the patient complains of sciatica.

Back stiffness is another common earliest complaint given by the patient. The patient is unable to bend and pick-up the objects on the ground. The patient may give history of night cries. If the patient complains of stiffness, weakness, awkwardness of lower extremities, it heralds the onset of paraplegia.

Physical Findings

The patient has a very protective attitude and has a very cautious and careful gait. The muscle spasm straightens out the spine. The spinous process of the involved vertebra is tender to percuss and when an attempt is made to rotate the vertebra. Back movements are decreased in all directions, especially forward, flexion. There is pronounced wasting of the back muscles. The clinical attitude of the patient varies according to the region involved. Cold abscess may be seen as paravertebral swelling or in areas already described (Figs 39.6A and B, and Flowchart 39.2). The patient may develop or present with neurological complications like spastic or flaccid paraplegia. Of the various deformities of spine due to tuberculosis, *kyphotic* deformity is the most common and is seen in over 95 percent of the cases (Figs 39.7 to 39.10).

TABLE 39.2: Types of vertebral reactions

Exudative reaction	Caseative reaction
• Common	• Rarer
• Severe hypergic reaction causes severe osteoporosis	• Mechanism of formation and spread of destruction is similar to exudative type, but is slower
• Rapid spread	
• Abscess is formed frequently	
• Constitutional symptoms are pronounced	

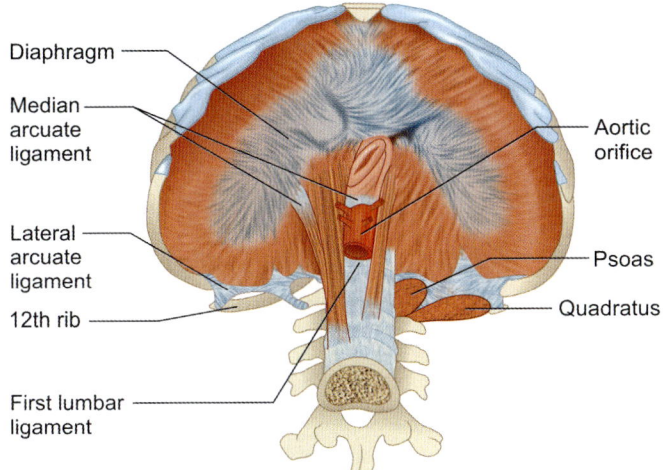

Fig. 39.4: Spread of the cold abscess through the diaphragmatic orifices

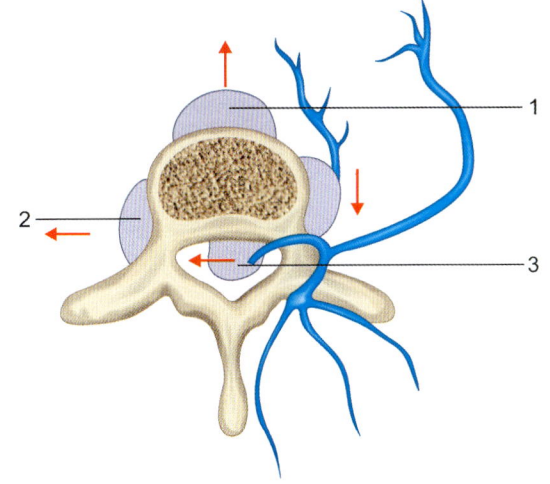

Fig. 39.5: Spread of cold abscess: (1) Anteriorly, (2) Laterally, and (3) Towards spinal canal

538 SECTION 5: General Orthopedics

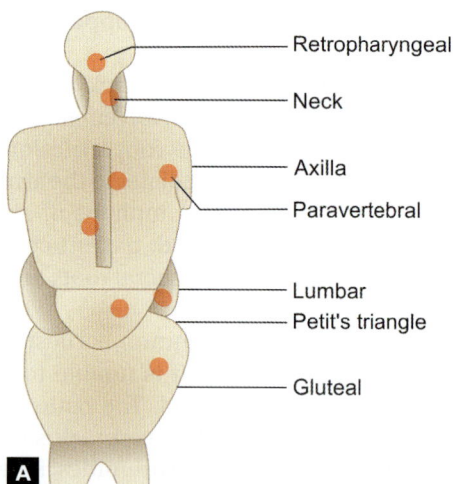

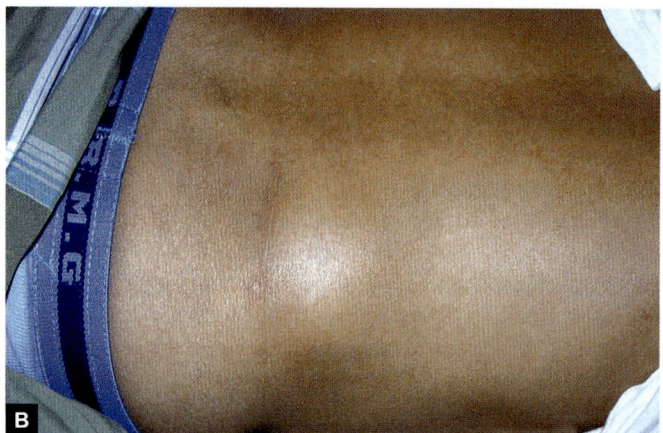

Figs 39.6A and B: (A) Sites of cold abscess in TB spine; (B) Cold abscess in the back (Clinical photo)

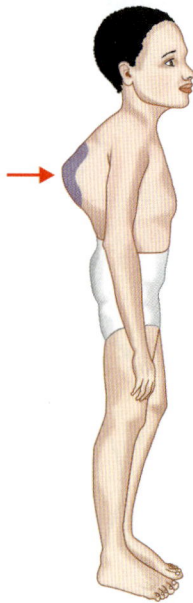

Fig. 39.7: Kyphotic deformity in tuberculosis of spine

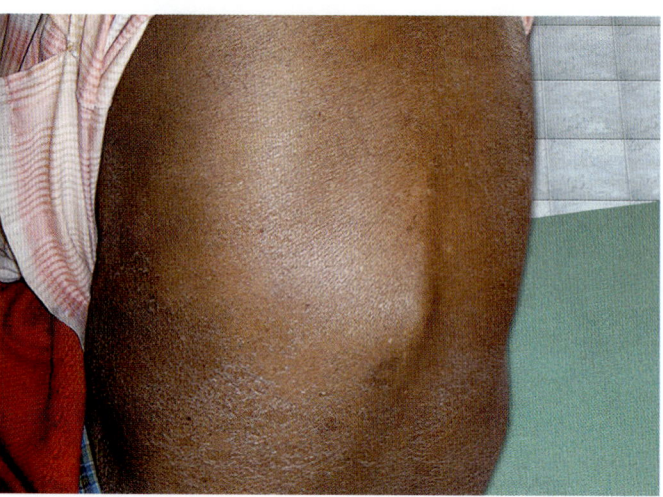

Fig. 39.8: Clinical photo showing kyphotic deformity in TB spine

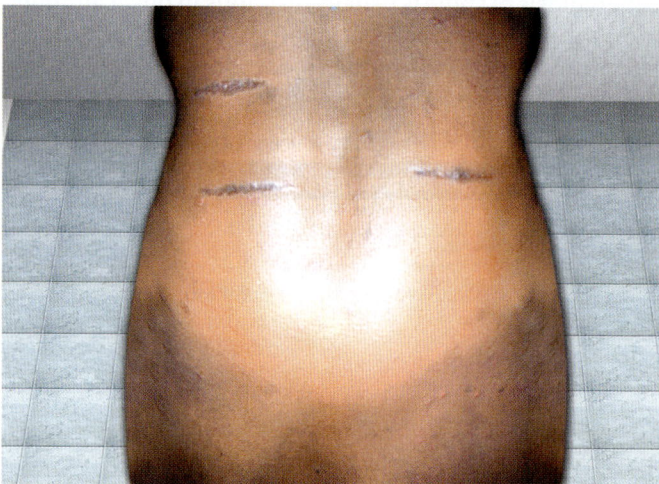

Fig. 39.9: Clinical photo showing cold abscess in the lumbar region TB spine

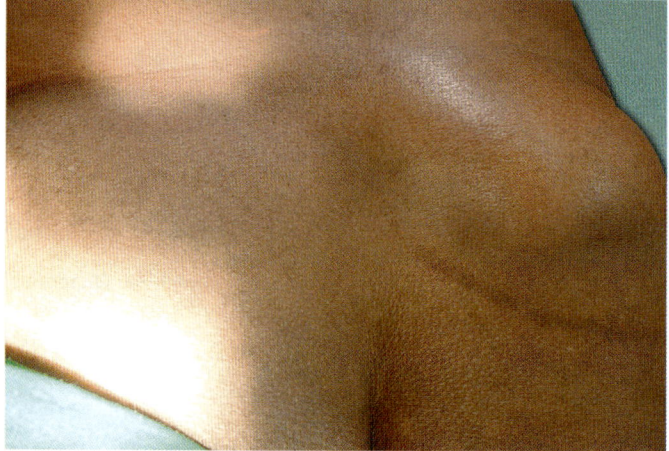

Fig. 39.10: Clinical photo showing cold abscess in the gluteal region in TB spine

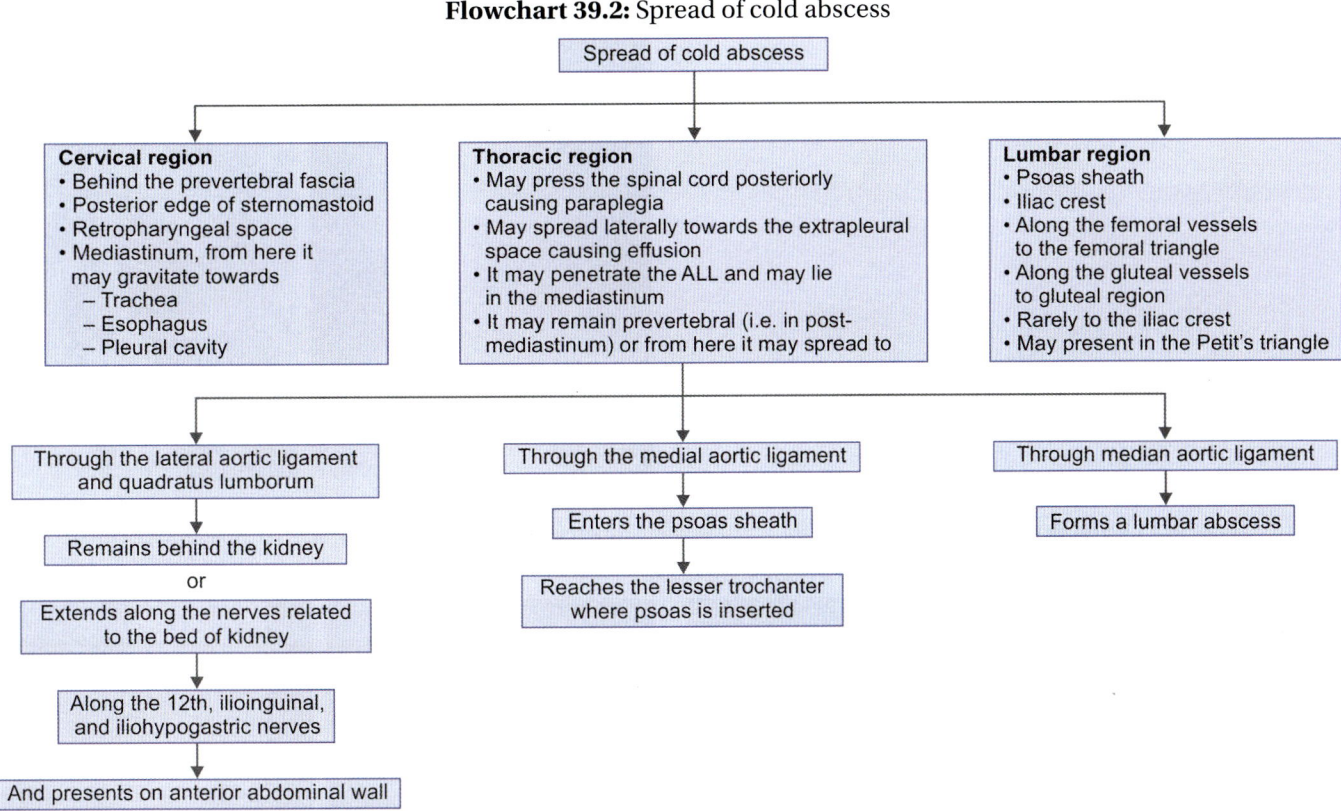

Flowchart 39.2: Spread of cold abscess

Note: Cold abscess is called "cold" because it is not associated with features, like redness, heat, etc. as in pyogenic abscess.

General examination reveals signs of anemia, debility, involvement of lungs, lymph nodes, etc.

Quick Facts

Typical attitudes in skeletal TB
- Upper cervical → Wryneck
- Lower cervical → Military position
- Lower thoracic → Alderman's gait
- Upper lumbar → Prominent abdomen
- Lower lumbar → Increased lordosis

Quick Facts

Spine irregularities in skeletal TB
- Kyphosis (95%)
- Scoliosis (5%)
- Lordosis
- Boarding
- Paravertebral thickening.

Other features
- Muscle spasm
- Wasting of all spinal muscles
- Spastic or flaccid paraplegia (20%)
- Cold abscess (20%)
- Sinuses (13%)
- Complications of skeletal TB.

Investigations

Laboratory Tests

These tests show anemia, lymphocytosis, hypoproteinemia, mild increase in ESR, etc. Mantoux test is helpful, especially in children below 2–3 years but is not diagnostic. The importance of general tests lies in indicating chronic disease.

Radiographs

X-ray of the affected vertebrae is a very important diagnostic test and it is observed that the average number of affected vertebra is usually three. The following changes are seen on the X-ray:

Earliest Change

This consists of disk space narrowing and subsequent loss of disk space in the common paradiskal lesions. The bones look rarefied and osteopenic (about 40% of calcium loss must take place to show a radiolucent sign on the X-ray).

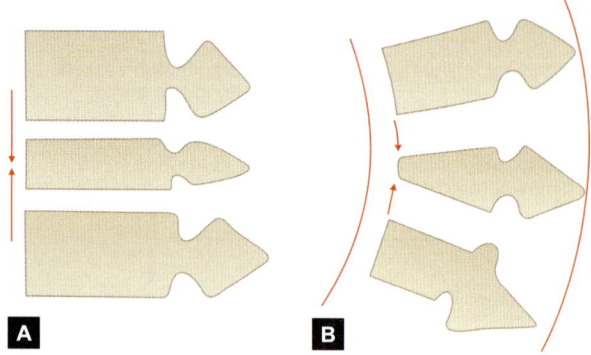

Figs 39.11A and B: (A) Concertina collapse; (B) Anterior wedge compression

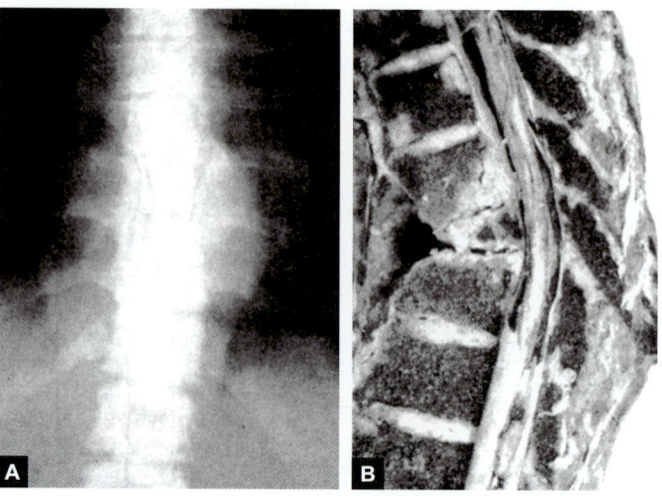

Figs 39.13A and B: (A) Radiograph of tense paravertebral abscess in tuberculosis of lower dorsal spine; (B) Specimen of tuberculosis spine

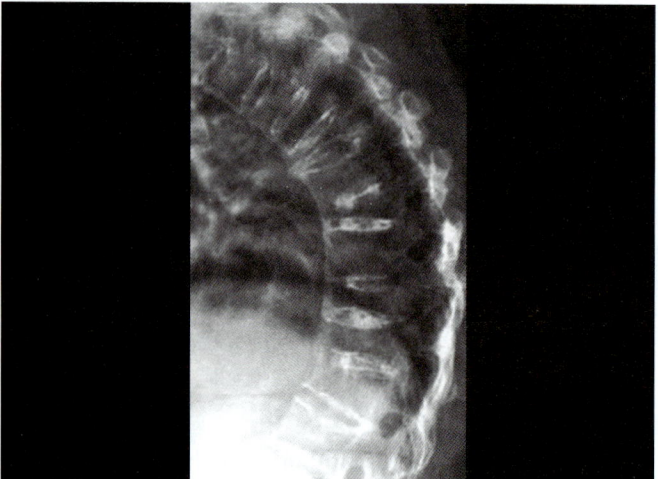

Fig. 39.12: Plain X-ray showing "concertina collapse"

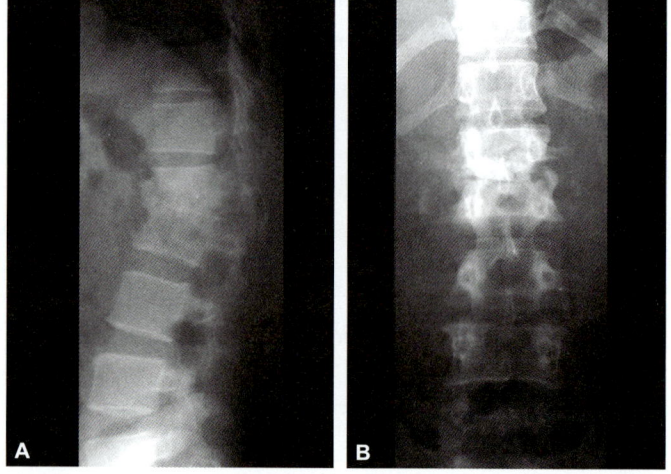

Figs 39.14A and B: Plain X-rays showing features of TB spine

Late Changes

This includes anterior wedge compression in anterior vertebral involvement, central vertebral body collapse also called as "concertina collapse" (Figs 39.11A and B) in central involvement, destruction of the posterior elements in the posterior affection, etc. (Fig. 39.12). Soft tissue swelling and its calcification are highly predictable of tuberculosis. In the healing stages, the vertebral body and the posterior elements may appear denser due to sclerosis.

Paravertebral Shadow

If seen on the X-ray, it indicates cold abscess (Figs 39.13 and 39.14).

Cervical region: In between the vertebral bodies and pharynx (retropharyngeal).

Upper thoracic: V-shaped shadow and widened mediastinum.

Below fourth thoracic vertebra: Fusiform or bird nest shadow appearance.

Psoas abscess: Unilateral or bilateral widening of psoas shadows in the lumbar region.

Aneurysmal phenomenon: Tense thoracic vertebral abscess showing a scalloping effect variety.

> **Note:**
> The most common is paradiskal; rarest is appendiceal involvement in spinal tuberculosis.

CT Scans

Identifies paravertebral soft tissue swelling more readily than X-rays. It helps to assess the degree of neural compromise and helps in better evaluation of the pathologic process. Some prefer CT to X-ray to determine the clinical progress. Findings are similar to X-rays.

> **Note:**
> The only detectable abnormality on plain X-ray and CT scan specifically related to tuberculosis is fine calcification in the paravertebral soft tissue shadow.

MRI

It helps in further delineation of the disease and helps to detect the cord compression. It does not eliminate the need for biopsy. It is 94 percent accurate (Figs 39.15A and B). Small calcifications seen on X-rays are not seen on MRI. *Gallium scanning* is useful in disseminated TB.

Biopsy

No one diagnostic test is 100 percent accurate for definitive diagnosis. Hence, diagnosis is dependent on culture of the organism and requires biopsy by percutaneous technique with CT control.

Ultrasound

It is useful to detect size of cold abscess in lumbar vertebral disease.

CT scan and MRI are also helpful in detecting tubercular affection of posterior spinal elements, craniovertebral and craniodorsal region, sacrum and sacroiliac region.

Treatment

Definitive diagnosis by biopsy and culture is necessary before starting the treatment, because of the toxicity of the chemotherapeutic regime and length of the treatment required.

Nonoperative and operative methods evaluated by the Medical Research Council working party are as follows:

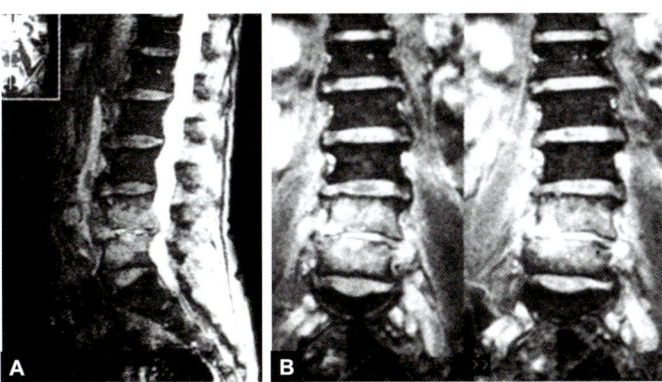

Figs 39.15A and B: Magnetic resonance imaging (MRI) of lumbar spine showing tubercular lesion of L4 and L5 vertebra

- Radical surgery performed under chemotherapeutic coverage gives better results with regard to deformity correction, development of paralysis and resolution.
- Chemotherapy with long-term bed rest with or without cast is ineffective.
- When facilities for radical surgery are not available a*mbulatory chemotherapy* is the treatment of choice. *Chemotherapy* controls 90 percent of tuberculosis spine as already mentioned and has been discussed in detail.

Indications for Surgery

- Neurological symptoms.
- Kyphosis with several vertebral involvement, severe kyphosis, progressive kyphosis, etc.
- Resistance to chemotherapy.
- Recurrence of disease.
- Cord compression.
- Progressive impairment of pulmonary function.
- Spinal instability.

Surgical Procedures

The following surgical procedures are described.

Aspiration: This technique is useful to aspirate the contents of a cold abscess through a thick-bored needle. The needle should be inserted below the abscess to enable the gravity to help drain the contents.

Minimal debridement: This consists of evaluating the cold abscess through costotransversectomy or decompression. Here, the contents are evacuated, the walls thoroughly curetted and bone grafting is done if necessary. Recently, evacuation and debridement of a thoracic cold abscess through a thoracoscope has been successfully tried.

Radical debridement: This is done through the anterior approach and is invariably followed by spinal fusion with a strut graft involving rib or fibula after a thorough debridement. This procedure has to be done before abscess or neurological complications develop. Fusion could be anterior or posterior; but in the former, normal anterior compressive forces are brought into play resulting in a high rate of successful bony fusion. Progression of disease and pseudarthrosis are common in posterior fusion. The only indication for posterior fusion is to add support for the disease at cervicothoracic or dorsolumbar regions.

Objectives of Surgery

Surgery helps to excise the infected tissue, decompress the intraspinal neural elements, reduce the spinal instability, and provide stability by spine fusion techniques.

Complications of Tuberculosis Spine
- Paraplegia
- Cold abscess
- Sinuses
- Secondary infection
- Amyloid disease
- Fatality

Middle Path Regime

Tuli and Kumar advocated triple drug therapy without surgery. In their series, operative treatment was reserved for patients:
- Not responding favorably to drug therapy after six months of treatment.
- Recrudescence of the disease.
- Patients with neural complications.

Operative treatment is combined with 6–12 months of bed rest, followed by 18–24 months of spinal bracing.

Did You Know?
Tuli's middle path regime is the most widely accepted protocol for the management of spinal TB.

TB SPINE WITH PARAPLEGIA

The incidence of this complication is 10–30 percent and it is most often associated with tuberculosis of the dorsal spine.

The Following are the Reasons Cited for this:
- TB is more common in dorsal spine.
- Spinal cord terminates below L_1.
- Spinal cord is smallest in this region.
- Normal curve of the thoracic spine encourages marked kyphosis.
- Anterior longitudinal ligament in the dorsal region loosely confines the abscess.

Pathology

Paraplegia could result due to inflammatory causes, mechanical causes, and intrinsic causes and due to spinal tumor disease (Table 39.3).

TABLE 39.3: Causes of paraplegia

Inflammatory Causes	Mechanical causes	Intrinsic causes	Spinal tumor disease
• Edema • Granulation tissue • Abscess • Caseous tissue This is the most common cause	• Tubercular debris • Sequestra • Stenosis of vertebral canal • Internal gibbus	• Prolonged stretching • Infective endocarditis • Pathological dislocation • Tuberculosis meningomyelitis • Syringomyelia	• Extradural granuloma • Tuberculoma • Peridural fibrosis

[36]**SM Tuli** (1975), Varanasi.

Classification

Seddon's Classification

- Early onset paraplegia is associated with active disease. It is seen within two years of onset of the disease.
- Late onset paraplegia is associated with healed disease. It is seen after two years after the onset of disease.

Clinical Features

Rarely paraplegia may be the presenting symptom. Late onset paraplegia may be associated with clumsiness, twitching, increased reflexes, clonus, positive Babinski's sign, etc. Motor functions are usually affected first. The paralysis usually follows the following stages in order of severity—muscle weakness, spasticity, in coordination, paraplegia in extension, flexor spasms, paraplegia in flexion (severe form), and flaccid paraplegia lastly (see box).

Kumar's Grading of Paraplegia
Grade I : Negligible, patient is unaware, physician detects ankle clonus, and up going plantar.
Grade II : Mild, patient aware but walks with support.
Grade III : Moderate, non-ambulatory, paralysis in extension. Sensory deficit <50 percent.
Grade IV : Severe grade III + severe paraplegia + sensory deficit more than 50 percent.

Clonus is the first most prominent early sign of Pott's disease. Sense of position and vibration are the last to disappear.

Rarely Paraplegia may Develop Suddenly due to:
- Thromboembolism.
- Pathological dislocation.
- Rapid accumulation of infected material.

Principles of Treatment

Three schools of thought are described for management of paraplegia due to tuberculosis.

Bosworth: Immobilization and early posterior arthrodesis.

Hodgson radical: Anterior decompression and arthrodesis.

[36]*Tuli and Kumar's:* Middle path regime. As mentioned earlier, this is the most widely accepted treatment regimen for spinal TB (see box).

What is the Protocol in the Middle Path Regime?
- Admission, rest in bed or plaster of Paris cast.
- Chemotherapy.
- X-ray and ESR once in three months.
- Gradual mobilization in the absence of neurological complications.
- Spinal braces—18 months to 2 years.
- Abscesses are aspirated or drained.

- Sinuses heal within 6–12 weeks.
- If no neural complications develop; if response is obtained within 3–4 weeks of triple drug therapy, surgery is unnecessary.
- Excisional surgery for posterior spinal disease.
- Operative debridement for patients who do not show arrest of disease after 3–6 months of chemotherapy.

Treatment of Pott's Paraplegia

The following measures are adopted in the treatment of Pott's paraplegia.

Conservative Treatment

Chemotherapy is the mainstay of this method and has already been described. Immobilization of the spine to provide rest and thereby promote healing is done by traction (in cervical region) plaster cast or brace (in dorsal region), etc. Management of bedsores, bladder and bowel management is done as already discussed in the management of spinal injury. Physiotherapy and occupational therapy helps in the treatment of the paralyzed lower limbs.

Surgical Treatment

The incidence of surgery has considerably decreased as chemotherapy is found to be successful in treating Pott's paraplegia. Only 5 percent of the cases require surgery in uncomplicated cases and 60 percent of the cases with neurological deficits require surgery.

Main Indications for Surgery
- Failed conservative treatment: If the patient does not respond to conservative treatment even after 3–6 months.
- In doubtful diagnosis.
- Fusion for mechanical instability by some grafts, implants, etc. either by the anterior or posterior approach.
- Recurrence of the disease after treatment.
- In rapid onset paraplegia.
- In disease secondary to cervical disease and cauda equina paralysis.

Other Indications
- Recurrent paraplegia.
- Painful paraplegia—due to root compression, etc.
- Posterior spinal disease—involving the posterior elements of the vertebra.
- Spinal tumor syndrome resulting in cord compression.
- Rapid onset paraplegia due to thrombosis, trauma, etc.
- Severe paraplegia.
- Secondary to cervical disease and cauda equina paralysis.

Surgical Techniques

Costotransversectomy

This is indicated for a tense paravertebral abscess. As the name suggests, excision of the transverse process of the affected vertebra and about an inch of the adjacent rib to facilitate the drainage of abscess is done (Fig. 39.16). If pus is yielded under pressure, one has to wait up to six weeks for improvement. If no improvement occurs, anterolateral decompression is done.

Anterolateral Decompression (ALD)

The structures removed in this procedure are posterior part of the rib, transverse process, pedicle and part of the vertebral body anterior to the cord (Fig. 39.17). This is the surgery of choice for Pott's paraplegia. It helps to effectively remove the solid and liquid debris. ALD is done through an extra pleural mediastinal approach. Bone graft may be inserted if needed (Fig. 39.18).

Anterior Decompression

This is technically more demanding. Here, the affected vertebra is approached through a transplerual or transperitoneal route, diseased tissue is curetted and a bone graft is inserted.

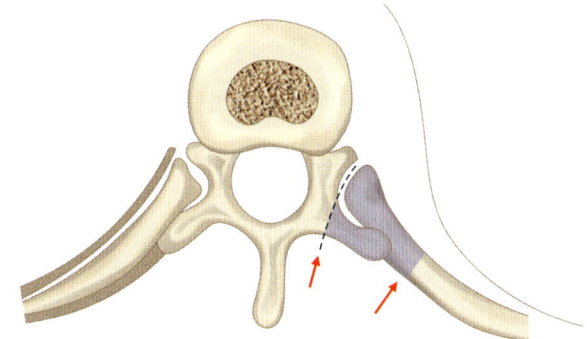

Fig. 39.16: Structures removed in costotransversectomy

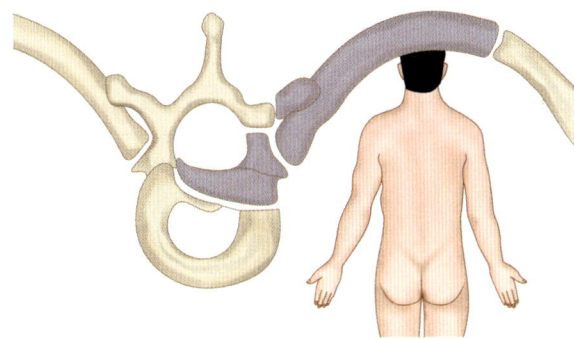

Fig. 39.17: Structures removed in ALD

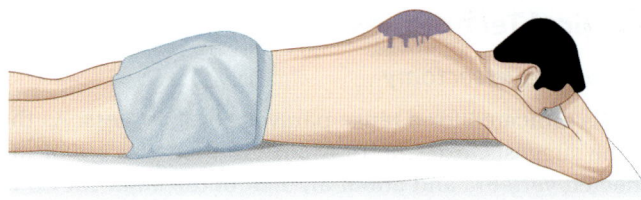

Fig. 39.18: Approach for ALD and costotransversectomy

Laminectomy

In Pott's paraplegia, anterior part of the cord is predominantly affected and laminectomy does not decompress this part of the cord. Moreover, it makes the spine unstable as it removes the healthy areas of the vertebrae. Hence, this procedure is not commonly recommended.

If arthrodesis of the spine is required after the above procedures, anterior arthrodesis is normally preferred. Posterior spinal arthrodesis has limited value and is usually done to stabilize the craniovertebral region. Paralysis secondary to cervical disease is treated by either laminectomy and posterior arthrodesis or radical debridement and anterior arthrodesis. Severe cauda equina paralysis requires lumbar transversectomy.

> **Prognosis in Paraplegia is Better in:**
> - Central cord involvement.
> - Early onset paraplegia.
> - If general conditions are good.

Cold abscess is another complication. It can present as one of the **three P's**:
- **P**alpable tumor in neck, back, thigh, etc.
- **P**ressure symptoms on the cord.
- **P**resent on radiographs of spine.

Treatment

Early aseptic evacuation is indicated. Aspiration if the contents are very fluid, but majority require open surgery for evacuation, e.g. costotransversectomy for tense paravertebral abscess, ALD for less than tense paravertebral abscess.

TUBERCULOSIS OF THE HIP JOINT

Tuberculosis of the hip joint is ranked next to spinal tuberculosis (10:7) and it constitutes 15 percent of all osteoarticular tuberculosis. It is always secondary. The initial focus of infection could be either in the: (i) acetabular roof, (ii) epiphysis, (iii) metaphyseal region, (iv) greater trochanter, (v) synovial membrane (rare), and (vi) trochanteric bursae (Fig. 39.19).

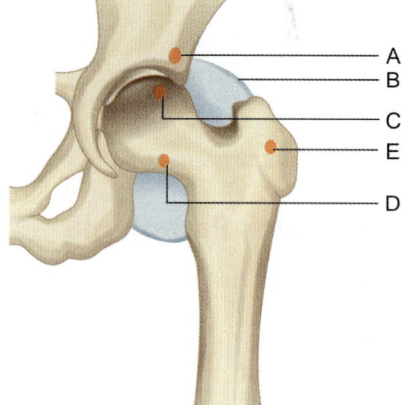

Fig. 39.19: Sites of common tubercular infection of the hip, A—Acetabular roof, B—Synovium, C—Epiphysis, D—Metaphysis, and E—Greater trochanter

Pathogenesis

Tuberculosis elsewhere like lungs, tonsils, GIT, etc. spreads through the hematogenous route, the tubercular infection develops in any one of the six sites already mentioned. Synovial membrane is the one most commonly affected. Here, the tubercle formation causes synovial hypertrophy resulting in pannus formation. This pannus destroys the articular cartilage resulting in the development of fibrous ankylosis of the hip. Bony ankylosis rarely develops.

Microscopy shows tubercle formation, giant cells and lymphocytes. Upper end of the femur is intracapsular and the joint gets rapidly involved. On the contrary, the joint involvement in acetabular lesions is rare.

The smaller tubercles coalesce, undergo caseation, and form a cold abscess. This cold abscess tracks down along the areas of least resistance and may point in any one of following sites: (i) Femoral triangle, (ii) inguinal region, (iii) medial side of the thigh, (iv) greater trochanter, (v) gluteal region, (vi) ischiorectal fossa, (vii) lateral and posterior aspect of the thigh, and (vii) pelvis (Fig. 39.20).

Clinical Features

Symptoms

Tuberculosis of hip is common in the first three decades of life. The patient usually presents with painful limp and is the most common earliest symptom. He or she has an antalgic gait with a short stance phase. Pain is maximum towards the end of the day and there is a history of night cries. There is marked wasting of the thigh and gluteal muscles. There may be presence of scars and sinuses.

Cold abscess: About 8 percent of the patients may develop cold abscess in the regions shown in Figures 39.21A to C above and 10 percent may show pathological sublimation.

Tenderness can be elicited by direct pressure in the femoral triangle or by bitrochanteric compression.

The attitude differs depending upon the stage of the disease, which is discussed later.

Deformities

The following deformities may develop in tuberculosis hip:

Flexion deformity in the initial stages of the disease, patient keeps the hip in flexion, as this is the position of ease and of maximum joint capacity. Soft tissue contractures convert this into a fixed flexion deformity (FFD) making locomotion impossible. *In an effort to bring the limb on the ground and to make locomotion possible, the lumbar spine undergoes exaggerated lordosis and thus conceals the fixed flexion deformity.*

Thomas test: The patient can lie down straight on the bed in the face of this fixed flexion deformity because of the exaggerated lordosis. This is confirmed by the easy passage of the examiner's hand between the bed and the back of the patient. Normally, this is not possible. In order to reveal this FFD, Thomas test is carried out. The unaffected hip of the patient is flexed over the abdomen until the lumbar lordotic curve disappears. The affected hip then assumes a position of flexion and the degree of FFD is calculated by the angle formed between the thigh and the bed (Figs 39.22A and B).

Adduction deformity: Soft tissue contractures convert the adduction position adapted by the patient due to the spasm of the adductor muscles following damage to the articular cartilage, to one of the fixed adduction deformities. *The limb is now brought to the ground by the elevation of the pelvis as evidenced by the anterosuperior iliac spine being at a higher level on the affected site. There is scoliosis of the spine away from the deformity (Figs 39.23A and B).*

The adduction deformity can be revealed by squaring the pelvis. This is done by adducting the affected limb until both the anterosuperior iliac spines lie in the same straight line. The angle formed between the vertical and the adducted limb is the angle of fixed adduction deformity.

Abduction deformity in the initial phases of the disease, because of the increase in the joint space due to effusion, the limb assumes a position of flexion, abduction, and external rotation (Fig. 39.24). If fixed in this position by soft tissue contractures, the patient develops a fixed abduction deformity. *The limb is then brought to the ground by the downward tilt of the pelvis as evidenced by anterosuperior iliac spine (ASIS) lying at a lower level with the corresponding scoliosis of the spine towards the affected side.*

The fixed abduction deformity can be revealed by abducting the affected limb until both the anterosuperior iliac spine lie in the same level. The angle formed between the vertical and the abducted limb is the angle of fixed abduction deformity (Figs 39.25A and B).

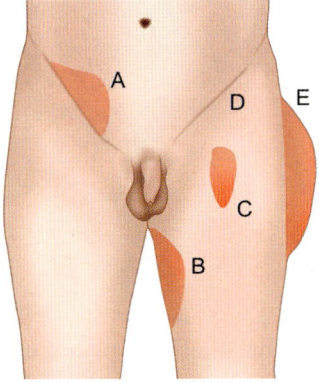

Fig. 39.20: Sites of cold abscess in TB hip (A) Inguinal region, (B) Medial side of thigh, (C) Femoral triangle, (D) Gluteal region, and (E) Lateral aspect of thigh

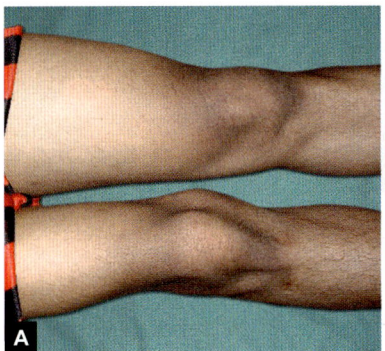 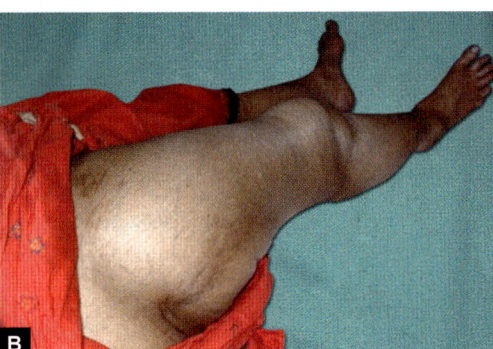 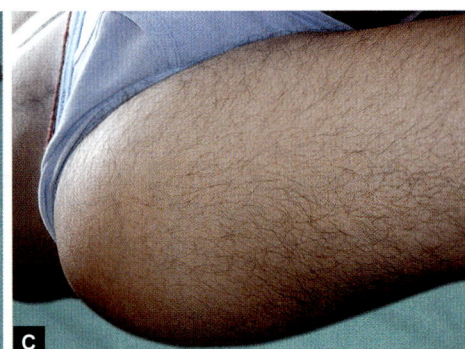

Figs 39.21A to C: (A) Marked wasting of the muscles; (B) Cold abscess in the femoral region; (C) Cold abscess in the trochanteric region

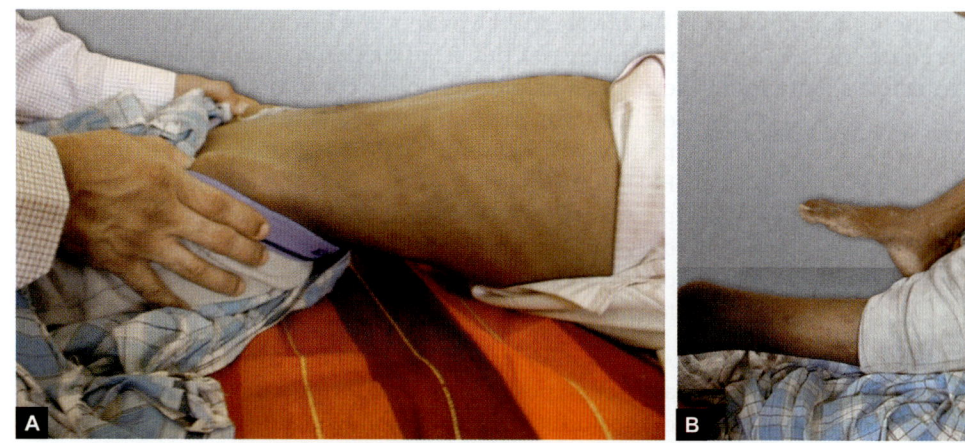
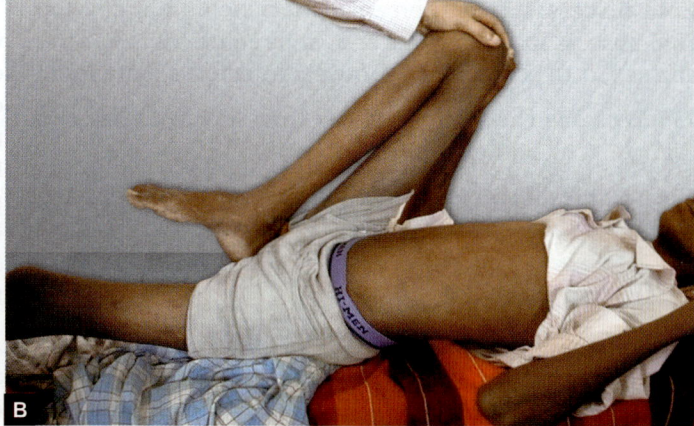

Figs 39.22A and B: Clinical photos showing fixed flexion deformity (Thomas test): (A) Exaggerated lumbar lordosis; (B) Obliteration of the lordosis by Thomas test

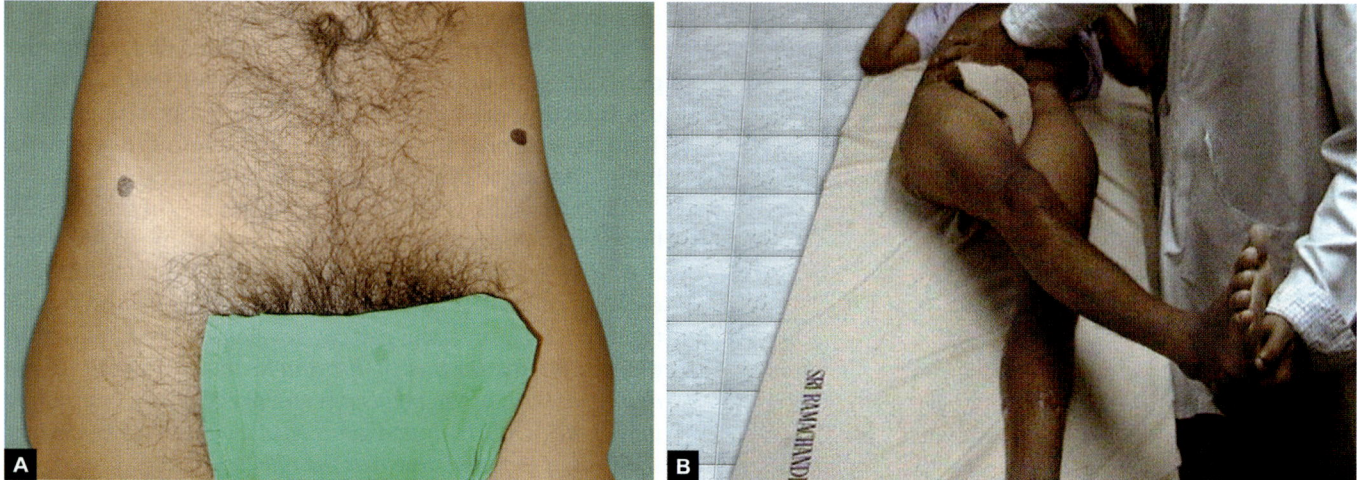

Figs 39.23A and B: Clinical photo showing adduction deformity: (A) ASIS higher level; (B) Squaring of pelvis

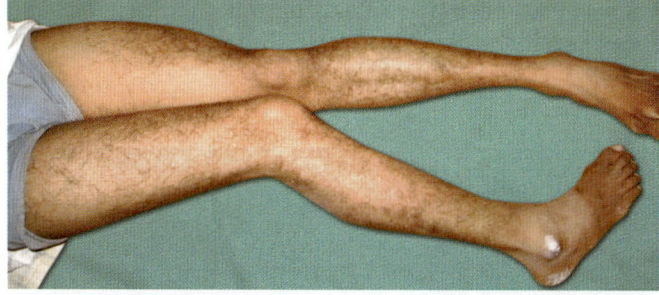

Fig. 39.24: Clinical photo showing adduction deformity

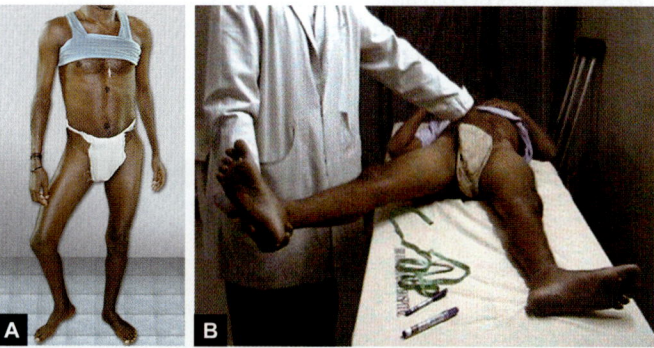

Figs 39.25A and B: Clinical photos showing: (A) Fixed abduction deformity; (B) Squaring of pelvis

Limb Length Discrepancy

In the initial stages, there may be apparent lengthening; but in the advanced stages, the patient develops shortening (Fig. 39.26).

Stages of Tuberculosis Hip

The following stages are described in tuberculosis hip.

Stage I (Stage of synovitis): Here, the disease is synovial with the patient assuming flexed, abducted, and external rotated position of the limb. There is *apparent* lengthening. There is no real shortening and the extremes of movements are decreased and painful (here apparent length more than true length).

Stage II (Stage of early arthritis): The local signs are exaggerated. The spasms of the adductors and flexors result in flexion, adduction, and internal rotation of the affected limb. There is apparent shortening; significant muscle wasting and hip movements are decreased in all directions (Fig. 39.27). True shortening may be less than 1 cm (here apparent length less than true length).

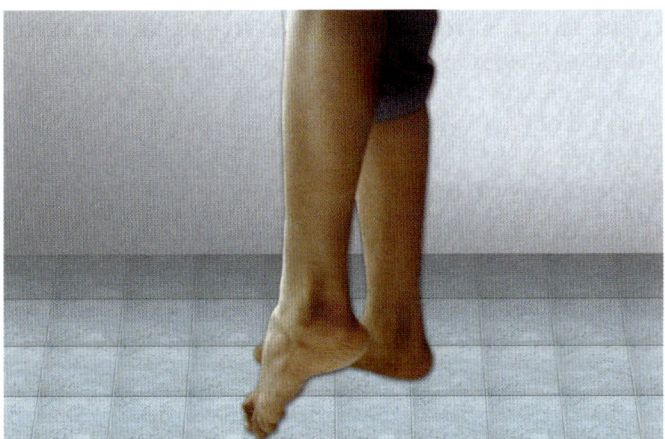

Fig. 39.26: Clinical photo showing limb length discrepancy

Stage III (Advanced arthritis): The flexion, adduction, internal rotation deformity found in Stage II is exaggerated. There is a true shortening with considerable restriction of hip movements and muscle wasting. There is gross destruction of the articular cartilage of the head of the femur and acetabulum (apparent length is less than true length) (Figs 39.28A and B).

Stage IV (Advanced arthritis with subluxation of dislocation): Migrating acetabulum, frank pathological posterior dislocation, mortar and pestle hip, protrusio acetabuli are the features in this stage.

Trendelenburg test is positive in all the above stages (Figs 39.29A and B). When the patient stands on normal limb, pelvis on the opposite side rises and when stands on the affected limb, pelvis on the other side drops.

Investigations

Laboratory Tests

These tests show anemia, lymphocytosis, increased ESR, etc.

Radiograph of the Hip

In the early stages, the radiographs show rarefaction of the bones; and in advanced stages, there may be reduction in the joint space. Depending upon the radiological features, Shanmugasundaram has described seven

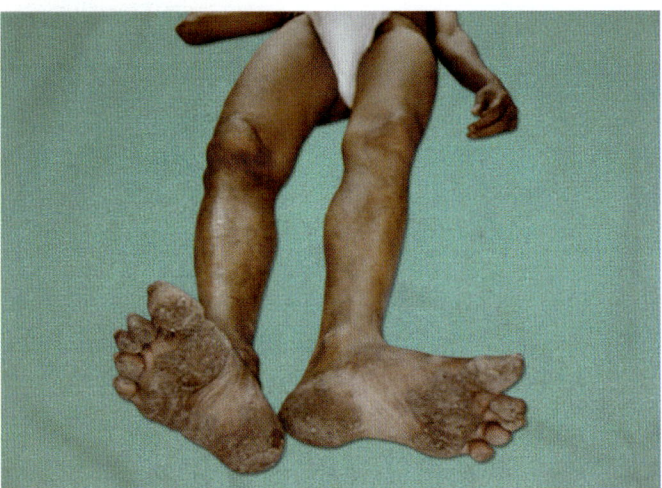

Fig. 39.27: Clinical photo of advanced tuberculosis hip

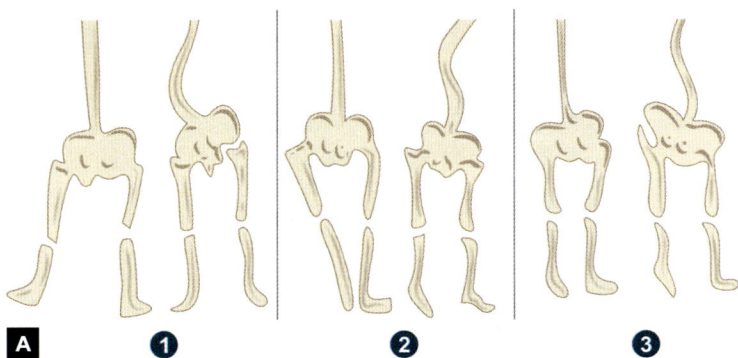 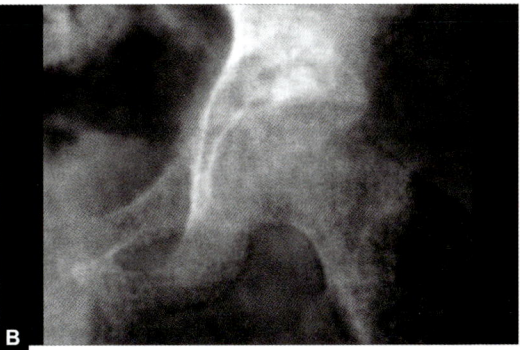

Figs 39.28A and B: (A) Stages of tuberculosis hip: (1) Stage of synovitis, (2) Stage of early arthritis, and (3) Stage of advanced arthritis; (B) Radiograph showing advanced stage of TB hip, sequestra seen in the acetabulum

types of tuberculosis hip in advanced stages of arthritis (Figs 39.30A to E).

- *Normal appearance:* Here the hip almost looks normal but for some rarefaction.
- *Traveling or wandering acetabulum:* Here, because of the destruction of the joint due to arthritis and due to the muscle spasm, the head of the femur comes to lie in the region of the ilium.
- *Dislocated hip:* In this condition, there is pathological dislocation of the hip joint.
- *Perthes' type:* Here, the head of the femur is dense and there could be collapse.
- *Atrophic type:* Here, the head of the femur is small and atrophic.
- *Protrusio acetabuli type:* Here, there is gross reduction of the joint space and head of the femur threatens to protrude through the acetabulum into the pelvic cavity (Figs 39.31 and 39.32).
- *Mortar and pestle type:* In this condition, the head of the femur is small (pestle) and the acetabular cavity (mortar) is wide.

This classification helps to assess the severity of the affection of the hip due to the disease.

Other Investigations

Synovial fluid analysis (estimation of protein, lymphocytes, sugar, etc.), synovial biopsy, Mantoux test, arthrography, etc. may help in the diagnosis.

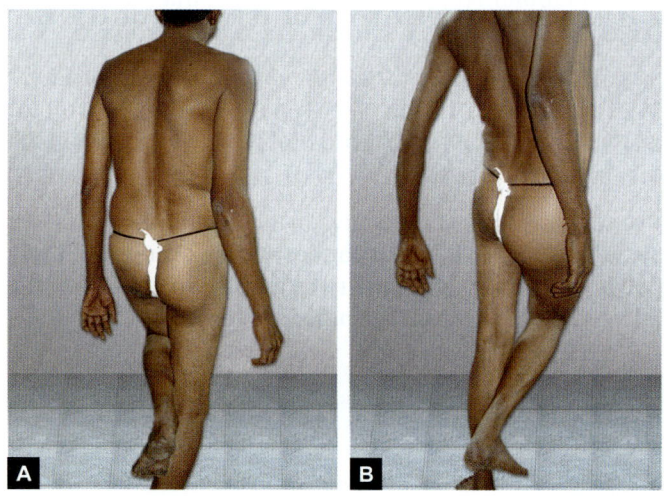

Figs 39.29A and B: Clinical photos showing the Trendelenburg's test

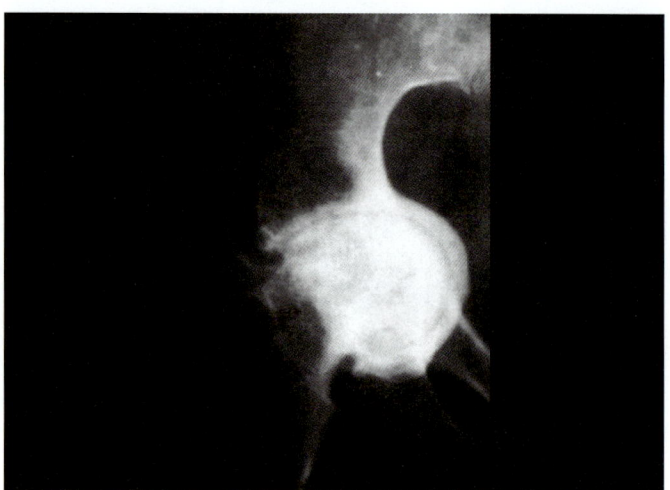

Fig. 39.31: Radiograph showing protrusio acetabuli

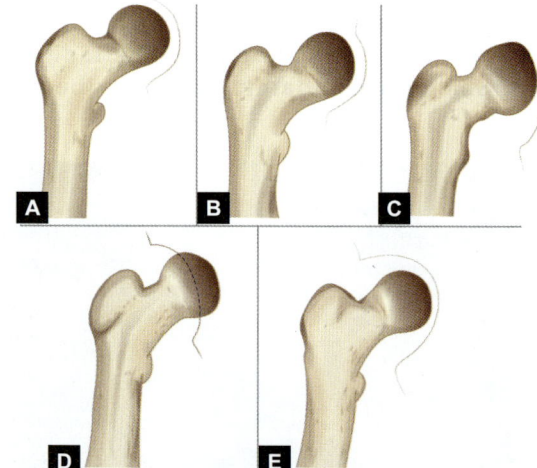

Figs 39.30A and E: Shanmugasundaram's radiological types of TB hip: (A) Normal type; (B) Traveling acetabulum; (C) Dislocated type; (D) Protrusio acetabuli; (E) Mortar and pestle

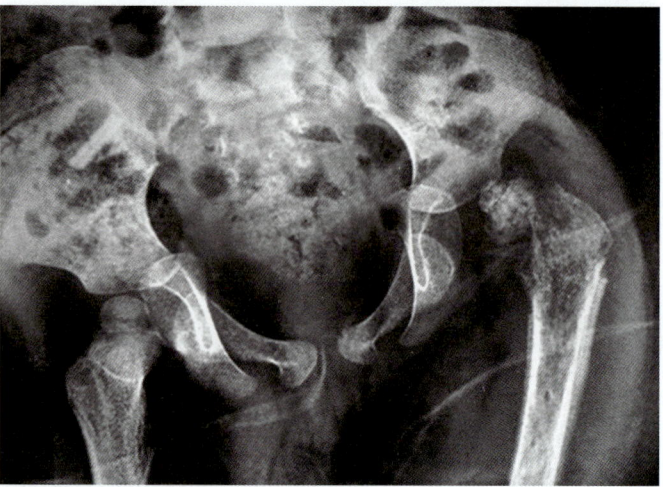

Figs 39.32: Plain X-ray showing pathological dislocation of joint

Treatment

Early stages (synovitis and early arthritis): The patient is put on chemotherapy and traction. Traction reduces the muscle spasm, prevents or corrects the deformity and maintains the joint space. If favorable clinical response is obtained, hip is gradually mobilized. If the disease is not responding favorably, then synovectomy and arthrotomy are carried out in the synovitis stage. Synovectomy and thorough joint debridement is done in cases of early arthritis (Flowchart 39.3).

Late stages (stage of advanced arthritis): The end result of this stage is fibrous ankylosis and the patient is put on chemotherapy and traction. Once gross ankylosis is accepted and if the limb is in proper position (10–30° of flexion, 5–10° of external rotation and neutral between adduction and adduction), the patient is immobilized in plaster of Paris spica for 6–9 months and later the patient is made to bear weight. If the limb is not in functional position, then corrective osteotomy and arthrodesis in proper position are carried out (Flowchart 39.4).

Surgical Treatment in Tuberculosis Hip

Synovectomy and arthrotomy: This is done in synovitis stage when the disease is not responding favorably to conservative treatment. Partial synovectomy and joint drainage and lavage are done (Figs 39.33A and B).

Synovectomy and joint debridement: This is preferred in early arthritis. The joint is exposed through the posterior approach. Thorough debridement of the joint is done by evacuation and the walls are curetted and washed.

Osteotomy: This is an upper femoral corrective osteotomy and is indicated in sound ankylosis in bad position in flexion adduction contractures. This helps to correct the deformity and change the line of weight bearing.

Displacement osteotomy: This is done in fibrous ankylosis with gross deformity.

Arthrodesis: This is indicated in adults with painful fibrous ankylosis with active or healed disease. This procedure converts a painful hip to painless stable hip. The procedure could either be intra-articular or extra-articular or both.

Arthroplasty: Stiff hip is a gross disability and is particularly not acceptable by Indian patients because they cannot use the Indian toilet. Here, girdle stone excision arthroplasty is preferred and it can be done in active or healed disease after the growth stops (Fig. 39.34). This gives a mobile painless hip joint apart from controlling the infection and correcting the deformity. However, it leaves the hip unstable.

Total hip replacement is rarely done in tuberculosis hip. It is suggested after 10 years after the last evidence of active infection.

Amniotic arthroplasty has been tried in tuberculosis hip. Nevertheless, the results are far from satisfactory.

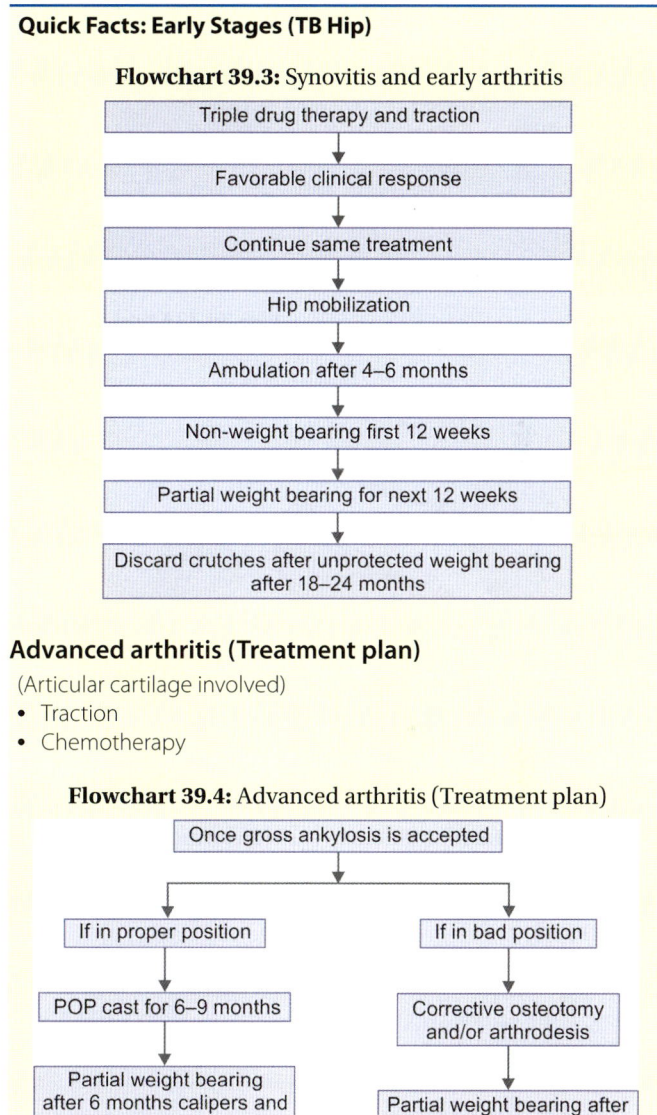

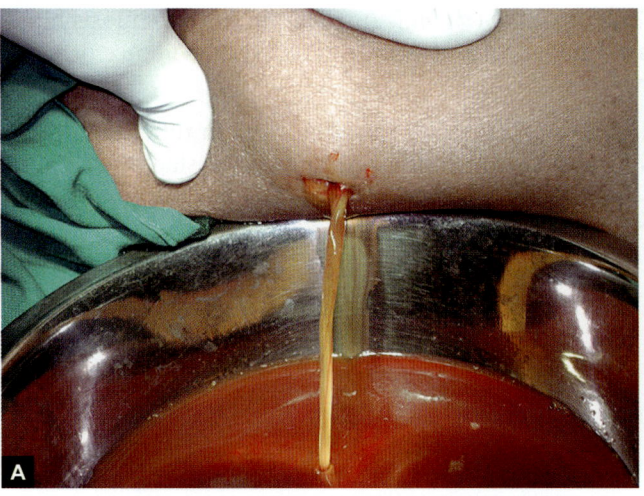

Figs 39.33A and B: (A) Joint lavage; (B) Fluid after lavage

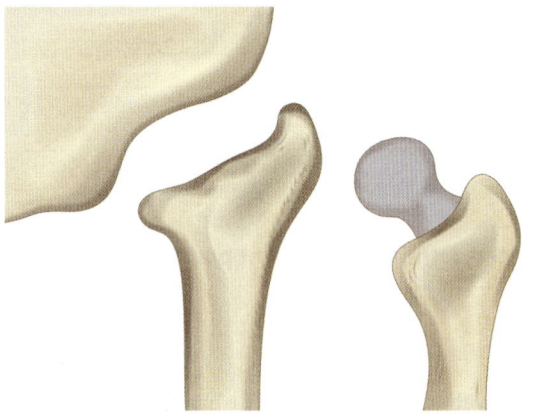

Fig. 39.34: Girdle stone excision arthroplasty

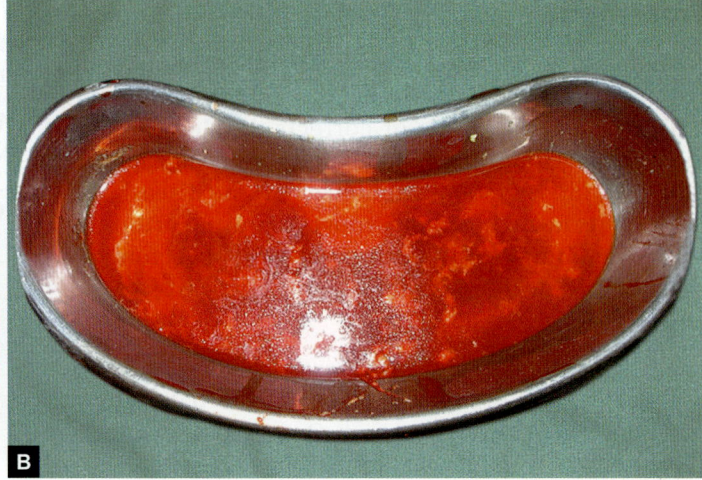

Figs 39.35A to C: Stages of TB knee: (A) Synovitis; (B) Early arthritis; (C) Advanced arthritis fibrous ankylosis

The infection so developed results in tubercle formation and the synovium undergoes hypertrophy forming a pannus, which destroys the articular cartilage of the joint and results in fibrous ankylosis (Figs 39.35A to C).

Remember
Five classical deformities in TB knee
- Flexion
- Posterior subluxation
- Lateral subluxation
- Lateral rotation
- Abduction of tibia
  The above deformities are due to spasm and contractures of the hamstring muscles.

Quick Facts
Tuberculosis hip
- Second in frequency in skeletal tuberculosis.
- Limp is the earliest symptom.
- Three classical deformities.
- Passes through four pathological stages.
- Fibrous ankylosis is the result.

TUBERCULOSIS OF THE KNEE

This is the third common site for skeletal tuberculosis. Incidence is 10 percent. It is also always secondary and may start in any one of the following sites in the knee joint.

Sites
- Synovium (common).
- Subchondral bone (of distal femur, proximal tibia, or patella).
- Juxta-articular osseous foci.

Clinical Features

The disease is insidious in onset, showing systemic and local features of tuberculosis. The joint shows effusion and evidence of synovial hypertrophy. The swelling is white in color (Fig. 39.36). There is tenderness along the joint line and synovial reflections. During the synovial stage, the

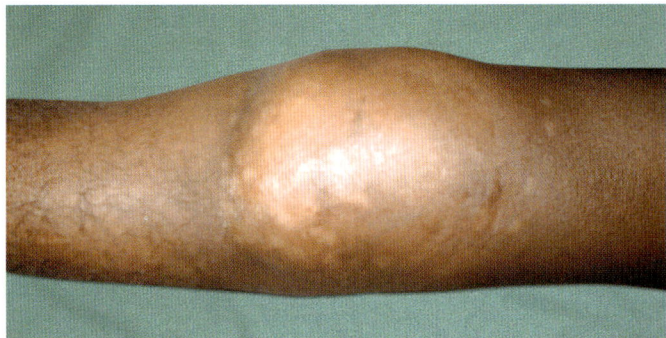

Fig. 39.36: Clinical photo showing swelling of the knee

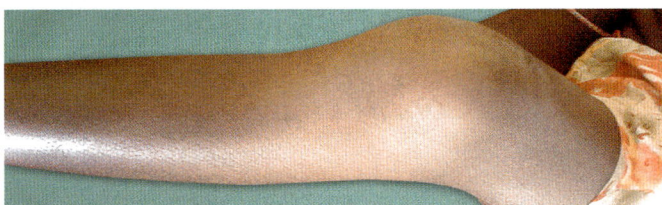

Fig. 39.37: Clinical photo showing fixed flexion deformity of the knee

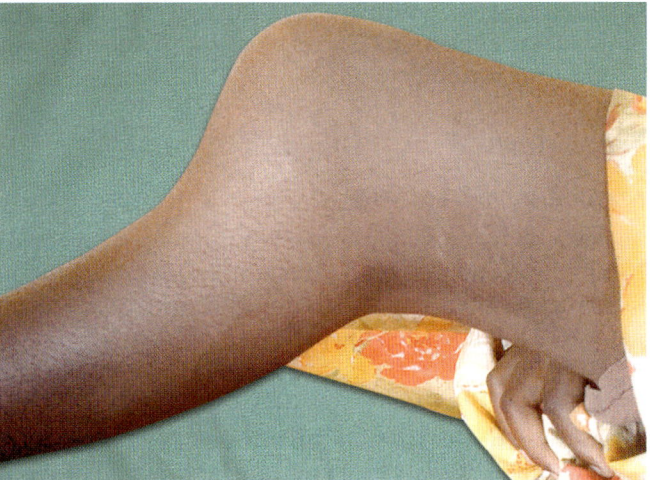

Fig. 39.38: Clinical photo showing triple displacement of the knee

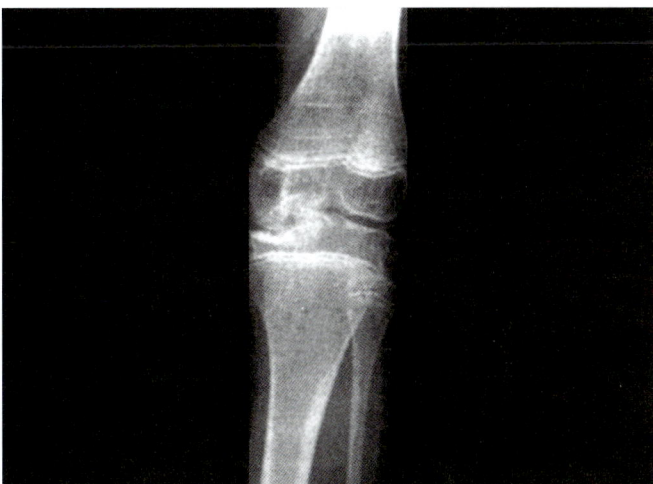

Fig. 39.39: Radiograph showing tuberculosis of the knee

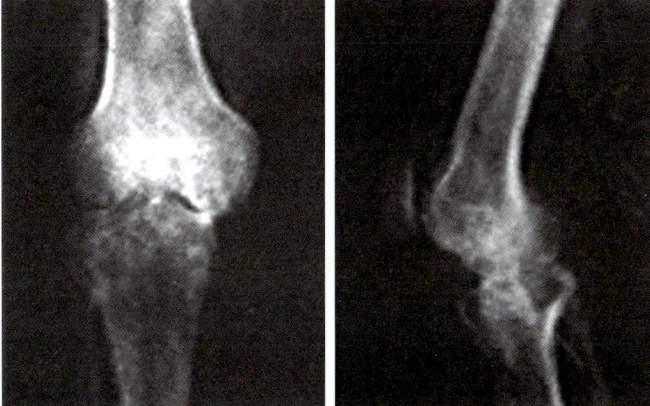

Fig. 39.40: Plain X-rays showing features of TB knee

movements are reduced and painful. In the arthritis stage; the joint movements are grossly restricted with painful spasm. There is gross quadriceps atrophy and lymphadenopathy. In the growing child, transient limb lengthening may be seen due to juxta-epiphyseal hyperemia.

In advanced stages of the disease, triple deformity (actually, it is quadruple deformity) is seen (see box). The pathomechanics of the development of this deformity is interesting:
- To accommodate for the increased swelling due to synovitis, the knee joint assumes the flexion attitude as it is the position of ease and maximum capacity (Fig. 39.37).
- External rotation deformity develops as the patient keeps the lower limb externally rotated from the hip.
- In this position, gravity assisted ITB contracture subluxates the tibiofibular joint.
- Next due to the action of the biceps femoris and ITB, the tibiofibular joint rotates externally.
- The above deforming forces further pull the leg into valgus.

Investigations (Fig. 39.38)

- General investigations reveal the chronicity of the infection.
- Radiographs show osteoporosis in the bones adjacent to the joint. In advanced stages, there is reduction of the joint spaces (Figs 39.39 and 39.40).

- Biopsy gives definitive diagnosis and the material is obtained either by incisional biopsy, aspiration cytology or by needle biopsy.

Treatment

Nonoperative Treatment

This is indicated in children and in the stage of synovitis. It consists of chemotherapy, traction, and joint aspiration. Skin traction helps to prevent triple deformity, corrects the deformities and to keep the joint surfaces distracted.

Surgical Treatment

- In the synovial stage, if the disease is not responding favorably, arthrotomy and partial synovectomy are done.
- In the stage of early arthritis synovectomy, joint debridement and curettage of the juxta-articular foci are carried out.
- In advanced arthritis, arthrodesis is the treatment of choice and the indications being, advanced tuberculosis, triple deformity, gross instability and painful ankylosis after earlier synovectomy.

Supracondylar osteotomy is preferred in varus or valgus deformity. Arthroplasty is also being tried without much success.

Role of Supracondylar Osteotomy

This is indicated in the following situations—where the disease has healed with painless range of movements in an unacceptable position and in valgus or varus deformity.

> **Quick Facts**
> **Treatment of tuberculosis knee**
> *Synovitis*
> - Chemotherapy
> - Traction
> - Joint aspiration
>
> *When active symptoms decrease*
> - Active and assisted exercises
> - Crutch walking after 12 weeks for 6–12 months
> - Protected weight bearing for 18–24 months
> - If disease is not responding favorably, arthrotomy and synovectomy done.
>
> *Early arthritis*
> - Synovectomy
> - Joint debridement
> - Curettage of juxta-articular foci
>
> *Postoperative regimen*
> - Drug therapy
> - Traction
> - Exercises
> - Suitable braces
>
> *Advanced arthritis*
> *Arthrodesis (advantages)*
> - Stable knee
> - Disease foci eliminated
> - Corrects deformity
> - Painless knee
>
> *Charnley's compression arthrodesis*
> - Diseased tissue clearance
> - Compression pin removed at 4 weeks
> - Patient is encouraged to walk after 4 weeks.

TUBERCULOSIS OF THE SHOULDER

This is quite uncommon and accounts for only 2 percent of the cases. It is more common in adults. Incidence of concomitant pulmonary tuberculosis is high. The tuberculosis of the shoulder could start in any one of the following sites:

- Synovium
- Glenoid
- Head of humerus.

Pathology

Same as in other forms of skeletal tuberculosis.

Clinical Features

Tuberculosis of the shoulder rarely presents at the stage of synovitis. Abduction and external rotation movements of the shoulder are grossly decreased. There is wasting of the deltoid and supraspinatus muscles. *Common variety is dry type and is called as caries sicca since there is no effusion into the joint.*

Cold abscess formed could present at:
- Supraspinous fossa
- Deltoid
- Biceps.

Late Stages

In the late stages, destruction of the upper end of humerus and glenoid cavity is seen. Fibrous ankylosis is the result.

Radiographs

Radiographs show generalized rarefaction, articular cartilage erosion, cavities in the head of the humerus and little periosteal reaction. In the advanced cases, there is inferior subluxation of the humeral head (Fig. 39.41).

Treatment

Treatment is essentially same as in other forms of tuberculosis. Chemotherapy is the mainstay of treatment.

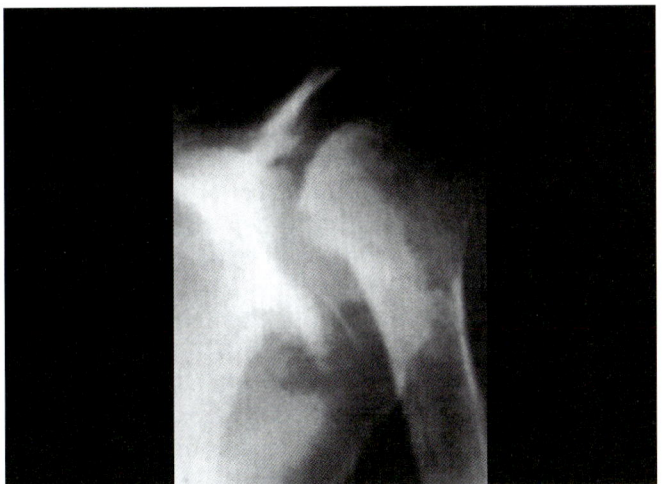

Fig. 39.41: Radiograph showing tuberculosis of the shoulder

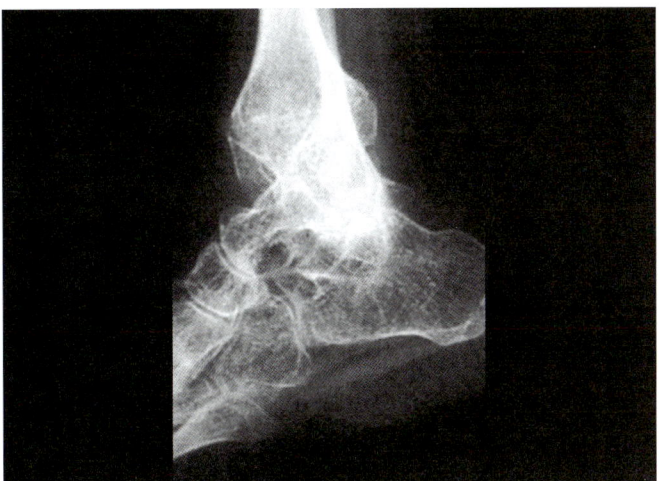

Fig. 39.42: Radiograph showing tuberculosis of the ankle

The shoulder is immobilized in saluting position (70–90° in abduction and 30° in flexion) to encourage ankylosis in functional position. The shoulder is put in abduction frame after 3 months. As a rule, sufficient compensatory movements develop at the scapulothoracic joint. Generally, a sound fibrous ankylosis develops and since this is a nonweight bearing joint, a sound fibrous joint is acceptable.

Indications for arthrodesis are painful ankylosis, uncontrolled disease, recurrence, etc.

TUBERCULOSIS OF THE ANKLE

This is very uncommon, and the incidence is only 5 percent. Sites of involvement could be:
- Synovium
- Distal end of tibia
- Malleoli
- Talus
- Rarely calcaneum.

Clinical Features

Pain in the region of the ankle, limp, swelling over and front of the joint, malleoli and tendo-Achilles. Ankle joint is held in plantar flexion. In the late cases, there is pathological anterior dislocation of the ankle joint. Ankle movements are decreased. There is gross wasting of calf muscles, and evidence of sinus formation.

Radiographs

Radiographs in the early stages show marked osteoporosis of the anklebones and in late stages, there is destruction of ankle joint (Fig. 39.42).

Treatment

Aim

Here, the aim is to achieve painless ankylosis in neutral position of the ankle. This is achieved by observing the following principles. Chemotherapy is as already discussed, immobilization in below-knee plaster cast in neutral position, crutch walking for first 8–12 weeks with plaster on and after 6 months below-knee caliper is worn for 2 years.

Surgery

Indications
- When the conservative treatment fails.
- When the diagnosis is in doubt.

Methods
- *Synovectomy* and joint debridement during the stages of synovitis and early arthritis.
- *Arthrodesis* for advanced and persistent disease.

TUBERCULAR OSTEOMYELITIS

Here, the onset of tuberculosis foci is within the bone. Because of deficient anastomosis of the osseous arteries in the childhood, thrombosis caused by tubercular pathology may lead to sequestration of a major part of the diaphysis.

TUBERCULAR OSTEOMYELITIS WITHOUT JOINT INVOLVEMENT

This can occur in any of the long tubular bones and the incidence is 2–3 percent and 7 percent occurring at multiple sites.

Clinical Features

The patient complains of pain in the affected bone. Swelling is warm and tender. There may be cold abscess or sinus formation or ulcer may be present. Enlargement of regional lymph nodes are seen.

Radiographs

Radiographs of anteroposterior and lateral views of the affected part show irregular cavities, little sclerosis (honeycomb appearance), and soft tissue swelling.

SPINA VENTOSA TYPE

In these cavities, contain soft feathery sequestra. Subperiosteal new bone formation is present. If it is complicated by sinus or secondary infection, intense reactive sclerosis, sequestra, and pathological fractures are seen.

TUBERCULOSIS OF TUBULAR BONES

The incidence is 3 percent and occurs in metaphysio-diaphyseal junction. It may also start as a diaphyseal lesion. *Disseminated skeletal tuberculosis:* This is very rare with 7 percent incidence only. It may be due to hematogenous spread or may be due to repeated impregnations at different sites. Rarely, it may present as multiple cystic lesions called as *osteitis tuberculosa multiplex cystoides.*

Treatment

Chemotherapy is the mainstay of treatment and radiographs are taken once in 6 months (Fig. 39.43).

Short Tubular Bones

Tuberculosis of short tubular bones involves metacarpals and metatarsals. In phalanges, it is uncommon after the age of 5 years. This is called tuberculosis dactylitis (Fig. 39.44). *Hand is more frequently involved than foot.* Due to lavish blood flow through a large nutrient artery entering almost in the middle of the bone.

- The first inoculum of infection is lodged in the center of marrow cavity, which leads to a spindle-shaped expansion of bone called *spina ventosa*.
- There is subperiosteal new bone formation in the X-rays, abscesses and sinus formation is seen clinically (Fig. 39.45).
- Secondary infection causes further thickening of the bones.

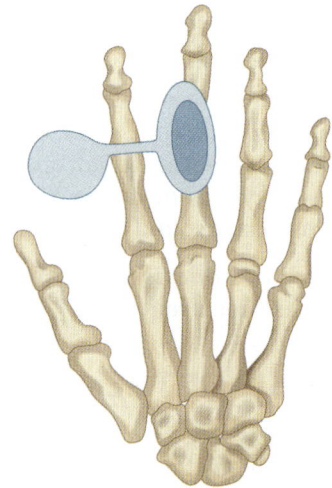

Fig. 39.44: Tubercular dactylitis

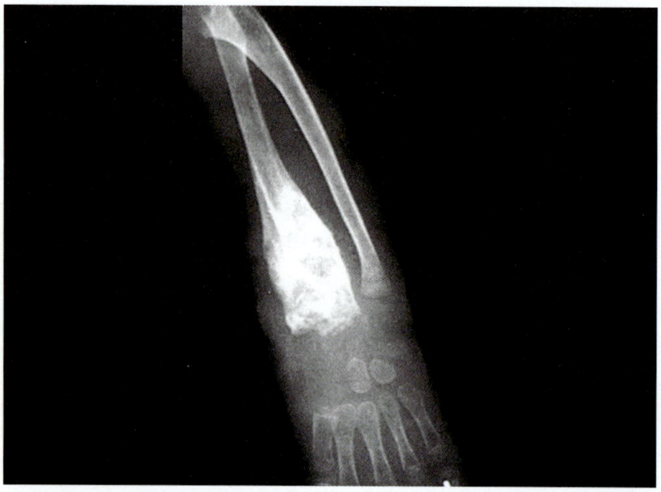

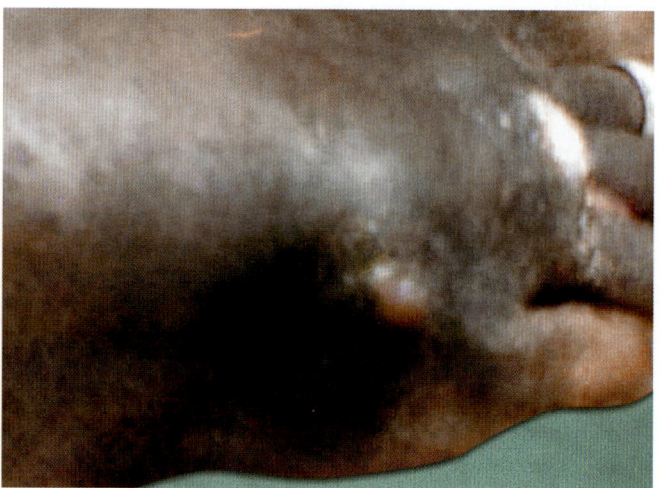

Fig. 39.43: Radiograph showing TB distal third of radius

Fig. 39.45: Tubercular dactylitis (Clinical photo)

Clinical Features

Patient may complain of pain, swelling, skin discoloration, discharging sinuses and scars over the affected parts.

Radiographs

Features are lytic lesions in the middle of the bone; subperiosteal new bone formation is present, soft cork-like sequestra and spina ventosa honeycomb type (Fig. 39.46).

Treatment

Chemotherapy is the mainstay of treatment and has been already discussed. Surgical curettage or bone excision may be required in intractable cases.

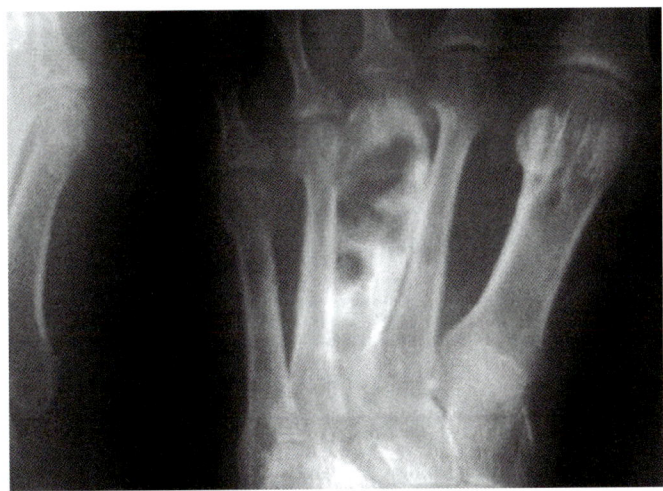

Fig. 39.46: Radiograph of TB dactylitis

BIBLIOGRAPHY

1. Ahm BH. Treatment of Pott's paraplegia. Acta Orthop Scand. 1968;39:145.
2. Allen AR, Stenson AW. The results of combined drug therapy and early fusion in bone tuberculosis. J Bone Tuberculosis, J Bone Joint Surg. 1957;39-A:32.
3. Bickel WH. Tuberculosis of bones and joints. Mayo Clin Proc. 1953;28:370.
4. Bosworth DM. Treatment of tuberculosis of bone and joint. Bull NY Acad Med. 1959;35:167.
5. Freidman B. Chemotherapy of tuberculosis of the spine. J Bone Joint Surg. 1996;48-A:451.
6. Goel MK. Treatment of Pott's paraplegia by operation. J Bone Joint Surg. 1967;49-B:674.
7. Hodgson AR, Skiness OK, Leong CY. The pathogenesis of Pott's paraplegia. J Bone Joint Surg. 1967;49-A:1147.
8. Hodgson AR, Stock FE. Anterior spine fusion for the treatment of tuberculosis of the spine: The operative findings and results of treatment of the first one hundred cases.
9. Konstam PG, Blevosky A. The ambulant treatment of spinal tuberculosis. Br J Surg. 1961-63; 50:26.
10. Longenskiold A, Riska EB. Pott's paraplegia treated by anterolateral decompression in the thoracic and lumbar spine: A report of 27 cases. Acta Orthop Scand. 1967;38:181.
11. Stevenson FH. The chemotherapy of orthopedic tuberculosis. J Bone Joint Surg. 1954;36-B: 5.
12. Tuli SM. Results of treatment of spinal tuberculosis by middle path regime. J Bone and Joint Surg. 1975;57-B:13.
13. Tuli M, Srivastava TP, Verma BP, Sinha GP. Tuberculosis of spine. Acta Orthop Scand. 1967;38:445.
14. Wilkinson MC. The treatment of tuberculosis of the spine by evacuation of the paravertebral abscess and curettage of the vertebral bodies. J Bone Joint Surg. 1955;37-B:382.

40 CHAPTER

Disorders of Joints (Arthritis)

INTRODUCTION

Arthritis is a nonspecific term denoting acute or chronic inflammation of the joint. Clinically, arthritis falls into the following groups:

Osteoarthritis
- Primary
- Secondary

Rheumatoid arthritis
- Adult
- Juvenile

Infective arthritis
- Acute
- Chronic

Metabolic arthritis
- Gout
- Pseudogout

Nonspecific monoarthritis

Neuropathic joint disorders, e.g. Charcot's

Special forms:
- Hemophilic arthritis
- Psoriatic arthritis
- Psychogenic arthritis.

Nearly 10 percent of the population suffers from one form of the arthritis or the other.

INFECTIVE ARTHRITIS (Syn: Pyogenic Infection of Joint or Septic Arthritis)

Definition

Septic arthritis is defined as a bacterial infection of the joint, which causes an intense inflammatory reaction with migration of polymorph nuclear leukocytes, and subsequent release of proteolytic enzymes. This could lead to destruction of the articular cartilage and later the joint.

> **Do You Know?**
> Newer definition of septic arthritis.
> A positive synovial fluid culture or a synovial fluid WBCs count of greater than 50,000 with 75 percent polymorphic neutrophils and a negative lyme titer.

Causative Organisms

The most common offending organisms are *Staphylococcus aureus* (50%), *Streptococcus* (20%), *Pneumococcus* (10%), Gonococcus, E. coli, etc. H. influenzae is very common in children less than 2 years. *Blood culture is positive only in 60 percent of cases.*

> **Routes of Entry for Organisms: 5 P's**
> **P**rimary focus is in RS, GIT, etc.
> **P**yogenic osteomyelitis
> **P**unctured wounds
> **P**neumonia, typhoid, etc.
> **P**rimary focus within the joint, absent in few.

Predisposing Factors

The following act as predisposing factors—trauma, diabetes, steroid therapy, malignancy, etc.

Sites of Involvement of the Joint

In adults
- Knee (53%)
- Hip (20%)
- Elbow (17%)
- Shoulder (10%).

In children
- Knee (39%)
- Hip (32%).

> **Remember**
> Ninety percent of cases of septic arthritis are monoarticular and 10 percent are polyarticular.

Pathology

The following pathological events take place:

Exudation into joint: This could be serous, serofibrinous or purulent depending upon the severity of infection.

Destruction of articular cartilage by plasmin, cathepsin, prostaglandins, etc.

Capsules, ligaments are destroyed by pus.

Clinical Features

Septic arthritis usually presents as monoarticular affection in 90 percent and polyarticular in 10 percent of cases and fever is seen in only 50 percent of the cases (Fig. 40.1). Limp is a common complaint. The severity of clinical manifestation depends upon the severity of disease (Table 40.1). The functions of the joint are securely affected in late cases (Fig. 40.2)

Investigations

Joint Aspirate and Synovial Fluid Analysis

This is the most accurate diagnostic tool for septic arthritis. The synovial fluid is tested for cells, sugars and proteins. Gram staining is positive in 60 percent of the cases for Gram-positive cocci.

Laboratory Investigations

WBCs (polymorphs) are raised to 50,000–1,00,000 (80% of cases), ESR increased more than 20 mm/h (in 50% of cases),

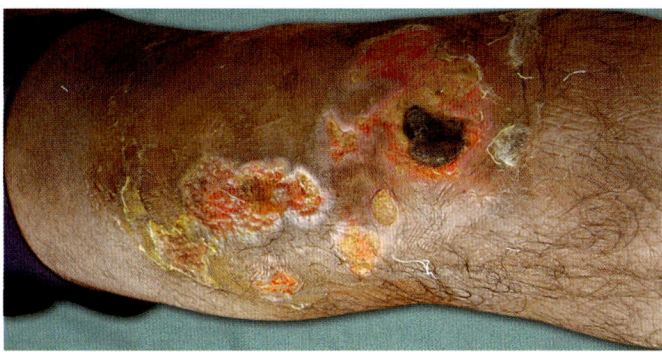

Fig. 40.1: Clinical photo showing septic arthritis of the knee

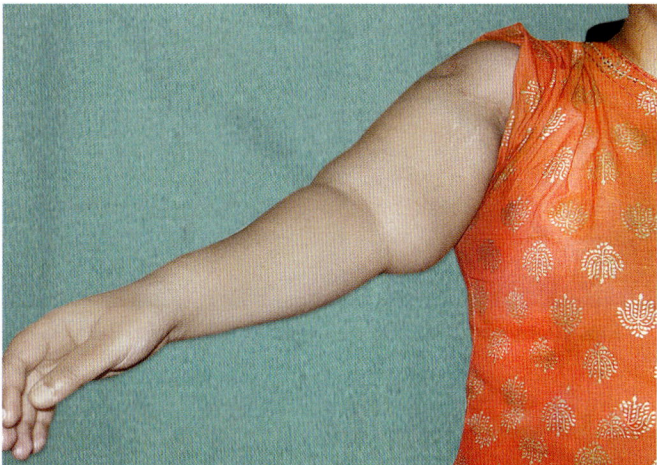

Fig. 40.2: Clinical photo showing septic arthritis of the shoulder

TABLE 40.1: Types of septic arthritis

Serous	Serofibrinous	Purulent
• Pain is less	• Tenderness positive	• Patient is very ill
• Movements of the joint ↓	• Fever positive	• Pain positive
	• Night pains positive	• Wasting positive
• Local temperature ↑		• Temperature ↑
• Flexion deformity		

Note: Nearly one-third of patients affected with bacterial arthritis suffer loss of joint function.

Hb percentage decreases. Blood culture is positive in 35–50 percent of the cases. CRP should be done within 24 hours of presentation.

> **The Importance of C-reactive Protein (Negative Predictor)**
> If the CRP is <10 mg/dL, the probability that the patient does not have septic arthritis is 87 percent.

Radiographs

Early Stages

The earliest findings in the radiographs are soft tissue swelling and periarticular osteoporosis.

Late Stages

In the later stages, cartilage destruction, and loss of joint space, necrosis of bone (Figs 40.3A and B), epiphyseal disturbances, fibrous ankylosis (Fig. 40.4), and bony ankylosis may be seen (Figs 40.5A to C).

Treatment

Arthrotomy or joint drainage the joint is aspirated first, if pus is present, open arthrotomy is indicated. The pus is cultured

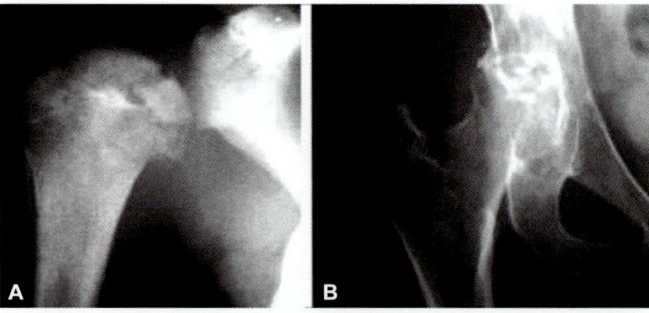

Figs 40.3A and B: Septic arthritis: (A) Shoulder; (B) Bony ankylosis hip

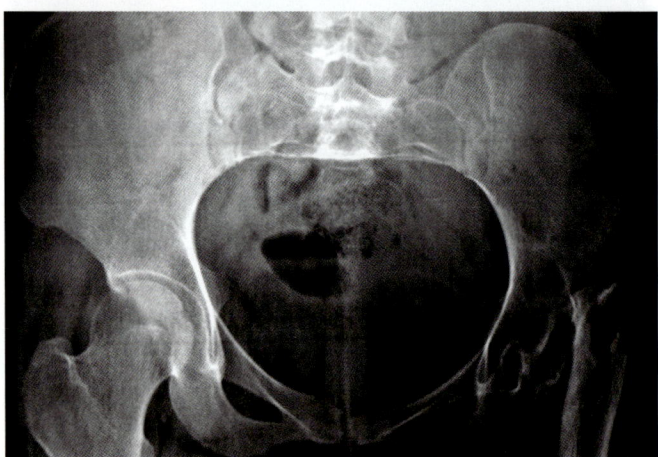

Fig. 40.4: Radiograph showing pathological dislocation

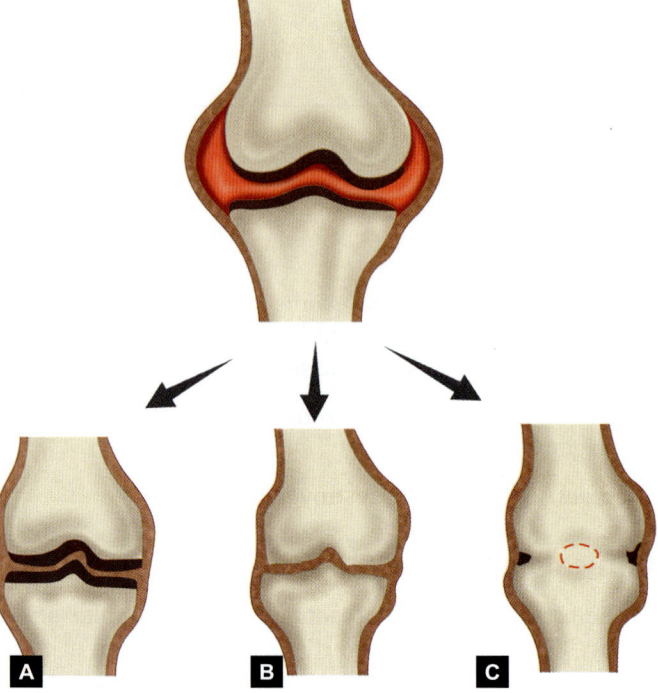

Figs 40.5A to C: Stages of septic arthritis: (A) Synovitis; (B) Arthritis; (C) Bony ankylosis

and is subjected to gram staining. Appropriate antibiotics are then chosen and are given intravenously before surgical drainage. Antibiotics are used for a minimum period of 2–4 weeks.

Immobilization of the joints by using plaster of Paris splints in functional position reduces pain.

Radical treatment is reserved for all except, for very early cases, which do not respond rapidly within 24 hours to antibiotics and immobilization.

If cartilage is destroyed, aim for ankylosis in functional position by plaster casts.

Remember
Tom Smith arthritis is a septic arthritis of the hip joint seen in infants.

Quick Facts
- Sites of septic arthritis in parenteral drug abusers:
  - Sacroiliac joint
  - Sternal articulations
  - Pubic symphysis
- Organisms responsible are:
  - *Staphylococcus aureus*
  - *Pseudomonas aeruginosa*
  - *Serratia marcescens*
- In sickle cell anemia, *Salmonella* is the organism causing septic arthritis.
- In nail pricks *Pseudomonas aeruginosa* is the organism the most common site is the second metatarsophalangeal joint.

Complications

- Joint destruction (Fig. 40.5B).
- Pathological dislocation.
- Osteoarthritis in later years.
- Ankylosis—fibrous or bony (Fig. 40.5C).
- Acute osteomyelitis.
- Amyloidosis very rarely develops.
- Septicemia, pyemia, etc.

GONOCOCCAL ARTHRITIS

The incidence of gonococcal arthritis is less than one percent and it is familiarly known as a three weeks infection. The male to female ratio is 5:1 and the age of predilection is between 20 and 30 years.

It usually results due to lack of treatment for gonorrhea. Forty percent of the cases are monoarticular, knee being the most common.

Pathology

Gonococcal arthritis can present as acute, subacute and chronic. The important pathological features are synovitis, effusion, cartilage erosion, and destruction of cartilage.

Clinical Features

Gonococcal arthritis is usually sudden in onset. The patient presents with chills, fever, pain and swelling of the joint. On examination, there is raised temperature and tenderness. There may be history of urethral discharge. The disease may become chronic due to inadequate and improper treatment.

Treatment

The treatment methods consist of local measures like splints, chemotherapy by intravenous penicillin G, and rest to the part, aspiration with a thick bored needle and arthrotomy to clear the joint debris.

SYPHILIS OF JOINTS

The incidence of syphilis of the joints is definitely on the decline due to the early use of antibiotics. Syphilitic arthritis is caused by *Treponema pallidum* and can be classified as follows.

Clinical Features

This is shown in Table 40.2.

Investigations

- Wassermann's test is positive.
- *Treponema pallidum* immobilization test is positive.

TABLE 40.2: Classification of syphilitic arthritis

Congenital	Acquired

• **Parrot's syphilitic joint**
  Features
  – Epiphysitis
  – Effusion
  – Separation of epiphysis
	Early
	• Arthralgia
	  – Secondary stage of syphilis
	  – Nocturnal pain is present
	  – Spasm of muscles
	• Hydrarthrosis
	  – Serous synovitis
	  – Symmetrical involvement

• **Clutton's joints**
  Features
  – Symmetrical
  – Hydrarthrosis
  – Painless
  – 8–16 years of age
	• Gummatous arthritis
	  – Synovial form
	  – Osseous form usually affects the knee, resembles osteoarthritis, painless polyarthritis, etc.
	• Charcot's joint is a neuropathic joint

- Joint fluid aspiration and synovial fluid analysis—for cell, sugar, protein, etc.

Treatment

Antisyphilitic treatment is done but it is often not successful.

NEUROPATHIC JOINTS ([1]CHARCOT'S)

This causes extensive destruction of the joint, as it is painless. The following are some of the important causes of neuropathic joints.

- Syringomyelia (25%)
- Tabes dorsalis (4–10%)
- Syphilis
- Rheumatoid arthritis
- Intra-articular steroids
- Traumatic division of sciatic nerve
- Chronic liver disease
- Prolonged administration of drugs like indomethacin, etc.

Sites: Knee, ankle, hip, elbow, shoulder, wrist and intervertebral joints in that order. It is rare before 40 years.

Pathology

The following are the pathological changes seen in the joint—gross destruction of the joint, the capsules are thickened, osteophyte formation is seen, joint cavity is distorted and the loose bodies are present.

Pathological stages (Brailsford's stages)
- Stage of hydrarthrosis
- Stage of atrophy
- Stage of hypertrophy.

Clinical Features

In this condition, premonitory signs are rare; onset is usually sudden and unexpected (Fig. 40.6). Gross swelling and lax joint are commonly seen.

In the later stages of the disease, the following features are seen—lax joints, *striking absence of pain,* joint becomes flail and there is a diffuse erythema around the joints.

Radiograph

Gross destruction of the joints is clearly visualized in plain X-rays (Fig. 40.7).

---

[1]**Jean Martin Charcot** (1825-1893) of Paris. He first distinguished between gout and rheumatoid arthritis and Charcot's joints.

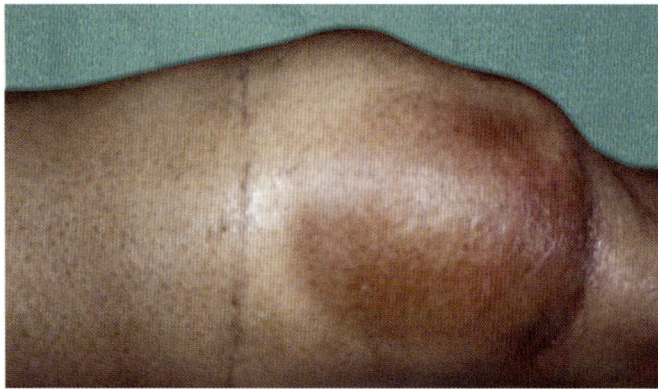

Fig. 40.6: Clinical photo showing gross swelling in neuropathic knee

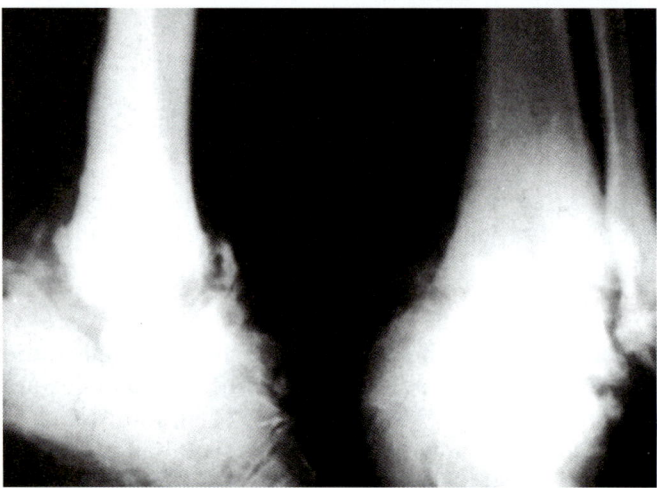

Fig. 40.7: Radiograph showing neuropathic ankle joint (Note the gross destruction)

Treatment

The treatment of choice is Charnley's compression arthrodesis but efficient bracing still has a major role to play (Figs 40.8A and B).

HEMOPHILIC ARTHRITIS (Bleeder's Joints)

Definition

It is a hereditary coagulative disorder characterized by hemorrhages, which is spontaneous and is due to trivial trauma. It is X-linked, carried by female, manifest in male, cause being *prolonged clotting time*. Table 40.3 shows different types of hemophilia.

Incidence is 3–4 per one lakh population.

Severity of factor VIII deficiency and the clinical effects is shown in Table 40.4.

Pathology

The defective blood interacts with the synovial fluid and causes irritation to the synovial membrane. Due to the proliferation of the macrophages, there is synovial

TABLE 40.3: Types of hemophilia	
Hemophilia A	Eighty percent cases due to ↓ factor VIII
Hemophilia B	Fifteen percent due to ↓ factor IX (Christmas disease)
Hemophilia C	Both male and female affected. Autosomal dominant
Von Willebrand's disease	Both platelets and factor VIII are deficient

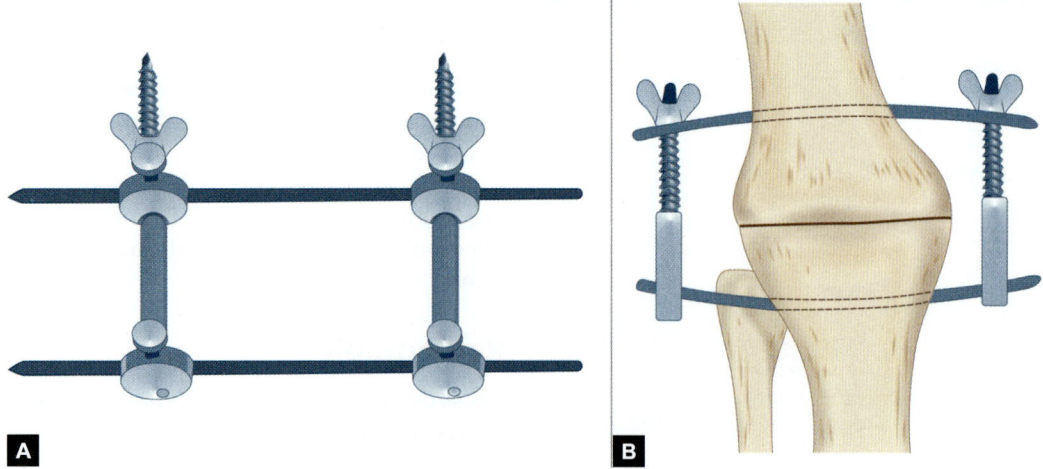

Figs 40.8A and B: (A) Charnley's compression clamp with 2 pins; (B) Charnley's compression arthrodesis

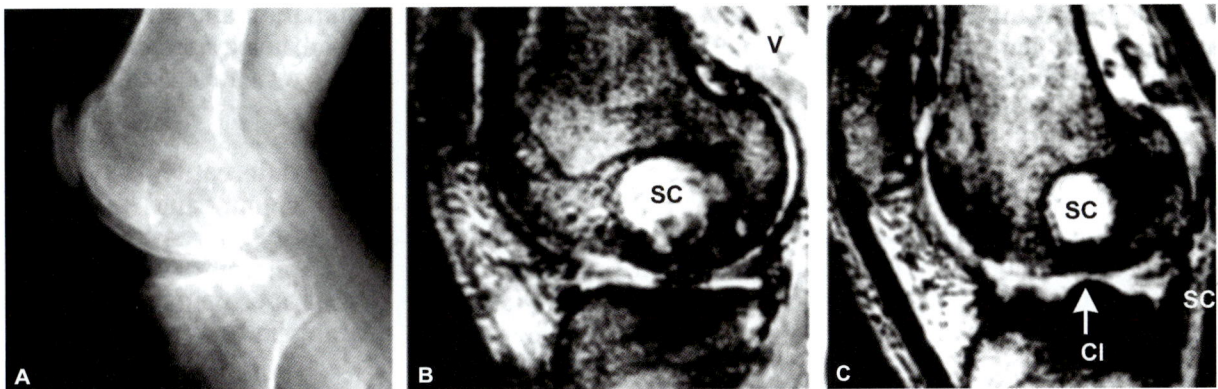

Figs 40.9A to C: Hemophilic arthritis of the knee: (A) Radiograph; (B and C) MRI

TABLE 40.4: Deficiency of factor VIII and its effects	
<1%	Severe bleeding
<5%	Gross bleeding with minor trauma
<5–25%	Severe bleeding after trauma or surgery
<25–50%	Bleeding after excessive trauma or injury

TABLE 40.5: Radiological stages in hemophilia		
Early stage	Intermediate stage	End stage
Distended synovium	• Persistent boggy swelling	• Joint disorganized
No para-articular skeletal abnormality	• Osteoporosis of the epiphysis • Joint interval is normal • Subchondral cysts are present • Squaring of the patella • Intercondylar notch of femur and trochlear notch of ulna widened	• Subchondral cysts are large • Fibrous ankylosis is present

hyperplasia and pannus formation, which ultimately causes destruction of the articular cartilage of the joint (Figs 40.9A to C).

Clinical Features

Bleeding is spontaneous and is usually due to trivial trauma. Acute hemarthrosis occurs within hours. The joint is warm, tender and flexion attitude develops. Acute phase lasts for a few weeks. With each attack joint movement decreases, fixed flexion deformity occurs, degenerative arthritis sets in and results in fibrous ankylosis. There is gross muscle atrophy.

Investigations

Plain X-ray

Based on the radiological findings, hemophilia arthritis can be graded into three stages (Table 40.5 and Fig. 40.10).

MRI

This gives more information about both the soft tissues and bones of the joints than the conventional radiographs.

Laboratory Tests

The classical feature of this disease is bleeding time is normal, but the clotting time is prolonged. Prothrombin

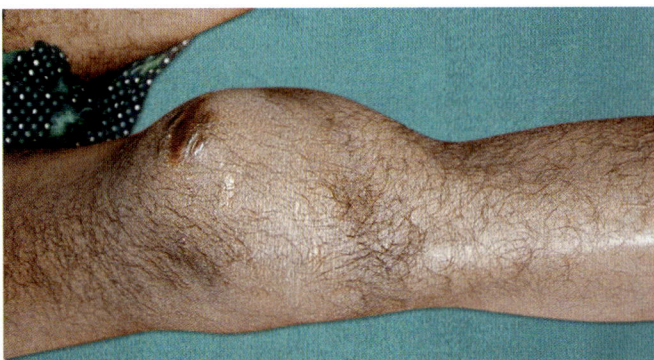

Fig. 40.10: Clinical photo showing hemophilic knee

time and other routine laboratory investigations need to be done.

Treatment

This varies according to the stages of the disease.

Acute Stage

- For injuries of less than four hours, the patient is treated on OPD basis. Factor VIII is replaced and is discharged home on the same day.

- For injuries more than four hours, factor VIII is replaced; joint is aspirated with a thick bored needle and immobilized with splints.

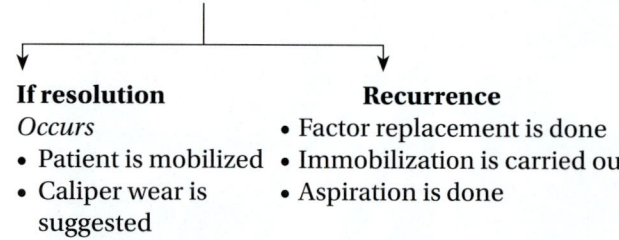

If resolution
Occurs
- Patient is mobilized
- Caliper wear is suggested

Recurrence
- Factor replacement is done
- Immobilization is carried out
- Aspiration is done

Late cases: Treated as in-patient, trial aspiration is done, prolonged immobilization, factor VIII is replaced and later mobilization, caliper and splints are recommended.

Chronic Hemarthropathy

For recent contractures: Plaster immobilization, dynamic traction and physiotherapy.

For postsubluxation of tibia: Dynamic traction.

For painful unstable joints: Orthotic splintage.

Surgery is indicated for painful, stiff joints, stiff contractures, and recurrent bleeding into the joint.

Surgical methods: These include synovectomy and internal fixations for fracture nonunion. Supracondylar osteotomy for severe flexion contractures of knee, arthrodesis for severely disorganized joints, total hip replacement for pain in the hip in advanced stages and tendo-Achilles lengthening for tendo Achilles contractures, etc.

SYNOVIAL CHONDROMATOSIS

Synovial chondromatosis (also called synovial osteochondromatosis) is a rare, benign condition that involves the synovium, which is the thin layer of tissue that lines joints. Although this type of tumor does not spread to other parts of the body, it can cause severe damage to the joint and lead to osteoarthritis. Early treatment is important to relieve painful symptoms and prevent further damage.

What Happens?
In synovial chondromatosis, the synovium grows abnormally and produces nodules made of cartilage. These nodules may break off from the synovium and become loose inside the joint. The loose cartilage bodies in the joint may vary in size from a few millimeters (such as the size of a small pill) to a few centimeters (the size of a quarter). The synovial fluid nourishes the loose bodies and they may grow, calcify, or ossify (turn into bone) (Fig. 40.11). They can then roll around like loose marbles and damage the articular cartilage, causing osteoarthritis. In osteoarthritis, damaged cartilage becomes worn and frayed. Moving the bones along this exposed surface is painful.

In severe cases, the loose bodies may grow large enough to occupy the entire joint space or penetrate into adjacent tissues.

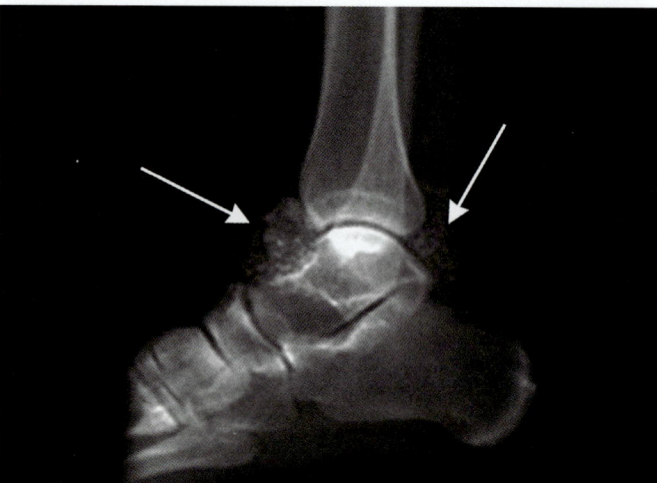

Fig. 40.11: Plain X-ray of an ankle, the calcified loose bodies are clearly visible (arrows)

Synovial chondromatosis most often occurs in the knee, followed by the hip, elbow, and shoulder. In most cases, only one joint in the body is affected.
Most cases of synovial chondromatosis occur in middle-aged people between the ages of 30 and 50. Men are affected twice as often as women.

Causes

Synovial chondromatosis occurs spontaneously. There are no known causes. This condition is not inherited.

Clinical Features

The most common symptoms of synovial chondromatosis are similar to those of osteoarthritis: joint pain, joint swelling, and loss of motion in the joint involved. There also can be fluid in the joint, tenderness, grinding, and popping. The nodules can sometimes be felt in joints close to the skin (knee, ankle, elbow). He or she will ask you to move it in various positions to see if there is pain or restricted motion. Your doctor will also look for creaking or grinding noises (crepitus) that indicate bone-on-bone friction.

Investigations

X-rays: May show the loose bodies, if they are not calcified, however, they may not show up in an X-ray (Fig. 40.12A).

Other imaging tests: Loose bodies typically show up very well on magnetic resonance imaging (MRI), which creates better images of soft tissue (Fig. 40.12B).

Computed tomography (CT): Also provides with a more detailed picture than an X-ray, and loose bodies can usually be seen in these scans.

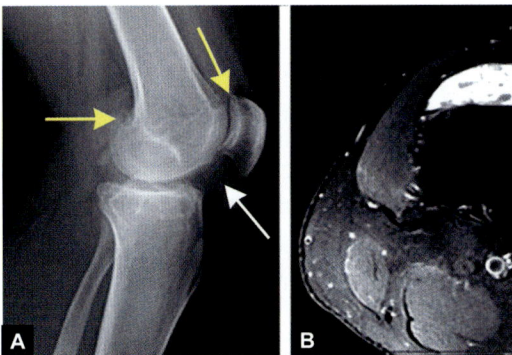

Figs 40.12A and B: (A) Plain X-ray of the knee joint, calcified loose bodies are barely visible (yellow arrows); (B) This MRI shows a cross-section image of the same knee. The loose bodies show up clearly

In addition to the loose bodies, imaging tests can show additional problems, such as fluid in the joint and signs of osteoarthritis.

Treatment

Treatment for synovial chondromatosis involves surgery to remove the loose bodies of cartilage. In some cases, the synovium is also removed. This can be done with an open surgical procedure or an arthroscopic one. A traditional, open surgical procedure involves a single large incision. In arthroscopy, small incisions and miniature surgical tools are used to remove the loose bodies. The end results of traditional and arthroscopic procedures are the same.

41
CHAPTER

Rheumatic Diseases

INTRODUCTION

There is a tendency among the students and most of the clinicians to label all cases of polyarthralgia as rheumatoid arthritis. Though there is no dispute about the fact that the most common cause of polyarthritis is rheumatoid, yet not all cases of polyarthritis is rheumatoid. There is a plethora of conditions with this presentation. Rheumatoid and its variants are infamous in creating diagnostic dilemmas. Difficult to diagnose and difficult to treat, it is indeed a problem which presents a nightmarish experience both to the doctor and the patient.

We are all familiar with the saying regarding rheumatic fever, "It licks the joint but bites the heart." Contrarily, it can be said of rheumatoid arthritis, "It bites the joints, licks all other systems of the body and barks at the treating physicians!"

A chronic scourge, which writes the obituary of the joints, especially those of hands and feet, rheumatoid arthritis, is a problem, which needs to be understood *in toto* to successfully combat it, keep it subdued, and improve the quality of those unfortunate victims afflicted by this malady.

The rheumatic diseases embrace an amazing array of hereditary and acquired disorders with a wide variety of clinical features. As per the present understanding, rheumatic disorders can be classified under three broad headings.

CLASSIFICATION

Diffuse systemic
- Rheumatoid arthritis
- Seronegative spondyloarthritis
- Systemic lupus erythematosus (SLE)
- Polymyositis
- Scleroderma.

Localized articular
- Osteoarthritis
- Crystal-induced arthritis
- Traumatic arthritis.

Nonarticular
- Fibromyalgia
- Low back pain
- Tenosynovitis.

RHEUMATOID ARTHRITIS

Definition

Rheumatoid arthritis is the most common inflammatory disease of the joints. It is a systemic disease of young and middle-aged adults characterized by proliferative and destructive changes in synovial membrane, periarticular structures, skeletal muscles and perineural sheaths. Eventually, joints are destroyed, fibrosed or ankylosed. *It is a widespread vasculitis of the small arterioles.*

Incidence is 3 percent.

Sex: Eighty percent affected are women; Male: Female ratio is 1:3.

Age: No age is exempt, mean age is 40 years.

Etiology

The exact cause is unknown, but malfunction of the cellular and humoral arms of the immune system are cited as the probable cause.

Current Hypothesis

An initiating antigen triggers an aberrant response, which becomes self-perpetuating long after the offending antigen has been cleared.

Antigenic Agents

Antigenic agents, which probably act as predisposing factors, are viruses: rubella, Epstein-Barr, etc. genetic (common in people with HLA DR4 60%), psychological stress, allergic factors, endocrine factors and metabolic factors.

Pathogenic Spectrum

Against unknown exciting antigenic agents, rheumatoid factors are elaborated. Rheumatoid factors are synthesized in rheumatoid synovial tissue and are mainly IgM in 70–90 percent of cases. In the remainder 10–30 percent, it could be IgG, IgA or IgE. This rheumatoid factor along with IgG triggers off a compliment cascade. The WBCs engulf this immune complex and elaborate lysosomes. Neutrophils release procollagenase, which is converted into an active collagenase by the synovial fluid. This splits the collagen of the articular cartilage. The neutral proteases complete the degradation of the collagen fibrils (Fig. 41.1).

Pathology

As explained earlier, due to the synthesis of autoantibodies, against unknown antigenic agents in the synovium, primary synovitis sets in (Fig. 41.2). This primary synovitis gives rise to pannus, which in turn forms the villus. This villus migrates towards the joint causing its destruction and ankylosis, fibrous in the early stages followed by bony ankylosis in the late stages.

Microscopy

It reveals rheumatoid units, which are an area of fibrinoid necrosis surrounded by fibroblasts, arranged radially and it is surrounded by a fibrous capsule. This rheumatoid unit is found in the muscle, vessels, nerves, synovium, etc. Vasculitis is widespread, and commonly affects the arterioles. Muscles show nodular polymyositis.

Subcutaneous nodules (Fig. 41.3) are made-up of central necrotic area, palisade formation by mononuclear cells, round cell infiltration and fibrous capsule. Lymph nodes show hyperplasia. Nerves show perineural necrosis or fibrosis and heart rarely shows changes unlike in rheumatic fever.

> **Recent Diagnostic Criteria for Rheumatoid Arthritis**
> *According to the American College of Rheumatology in 1987 revised criteria, at least 4 out of 7 criteria should be fulfilled to make a diagnosis of rheumatoid arthritis.*
> - Morning stiffness for minimum one hour everyday, at least for six weeks.
> - Arthritis or swelling of three or more joints for >6 weeks.
> - Arthritis or swelling of hand joints (wrist, metacarpal) for more than 6 weeks.
> - Symmetrical swelling (arthritis of same joint areas) more than 6 weeks.
> - Serum rheumatoid factor present.
> - Radiographic features of RA.
> - Rheumatoid nodules.

Clinical Features

Rheumatoid arthritis usually presents in three forms:

Classical Presentation

In this group, the patient is usually a woman in her mid 30s. Pain, swelling, stiffness of the small joints of hands and feet are the common presenting complaints. The patient also gives history of weight loss, lethargy and depression. Joint swelling could be symmetrical and the patient presents with deformities of bones and joints in the late stages. *The patient gives history of remissions and exacerbation of*

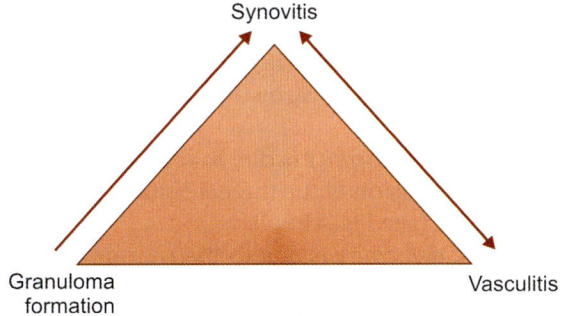

Fig. 41.1: Rheumatoid arthritis = Synovitis + Vasculitis + Granuloma

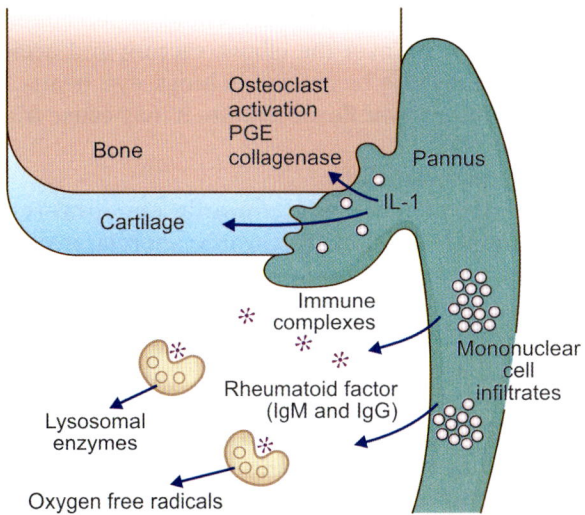

Fig. 41.2: Pathogenesis in rheumatoid arthritis

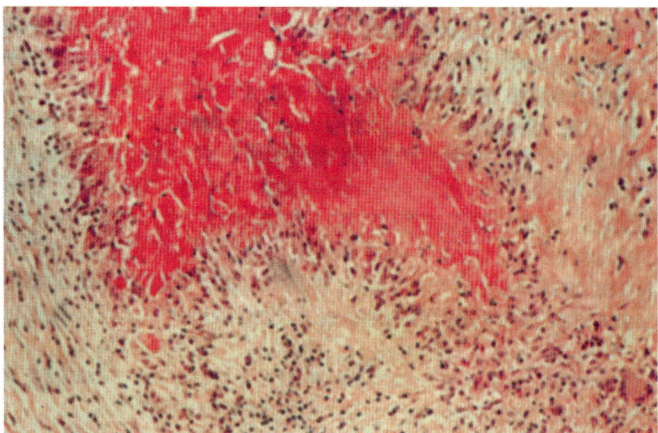

Fig. 41.3: Microscopic features of rheumatoid arthritis subcutaneous nodule

symptoms with seasonal variations. This is a very classical complaint in the absence of which diagnosis of rheumatoid arthritis should be carefully made. Symptoms fluctuate from day-to-day.

Other Presentations

This consists of palindromic presentation involving one or two joints, systemic presentation—usually seen in middle-aged men presenting with pleurisy, pericarditis, etc. It mimics malignancy. It may present as polymyalgia particularly in elderly patients. It may present as monoarthritic swelling. Sometimes, the presentation may be very explosive unlike the usual chronic presentation.

Extra-articular Features

Two or more features are present in 75 percent of the cases. Rheumatoid factor is invariably present and indicates a bad prognosis.
- Subcutaneous nodules are present in 25 percent of the cases. It is seen over the elbow, sacrum and occiput. Nodules may also be present in lungs, eye, hearts, etc. When present over flexor tendon, it may cause trigger finger.
- Widespread vasculitis.
- Blood abnormalities commonly encountered in rheumatoid arthritis are chronic anemia, iron deficiency anemia, vitamin B_{12} and folate deficiency, leukocytopenia, thrombocytosis and marrow hypoplasia.
- Osteoporosis could be generalized or localized in bones around the joints.
- Eye changes seen in rheumatoid arthritis are keratoconjunctivitis sicca or Sjögren's syndrome, episcleritis (common), scleritis (serious problem), secondary glaucoma and scleromalacia perforans.
- Lung affections in rheumatoid arthritis are pleurisy, pleural effusion, Kaplan's syndrome (RA + pneumoconiosis involving the upper lobes) and fibrosing alveolitis in 2 percent.
- Heart affections in rheumatoid arthritis are pericardial friction (10%), pericardial effusion (30%), arrhythmias and heart block.
- Neuromuscular system involvement includes carpal tunnel syndrome, mononeuritis multiplex, muscle wasting, subluxation of C_1 and C_2, etc.
- Reticuloendothelial system affections include splenomegaly (5%), Felty's syndrome in 1% (RA+ splenomegaly + Neutropenia), generalized lymphadenopathy and painless pitting edema of the feet and ankles.

ORTHOPEDIC DEFORMITIES IN RHEUMATOID ARTHRITIS

Rheumatoid arthritis can affect any joint in the body. *It involves the peripheral joints more often and very rarely affects the larger joints.* Of particular importance are the affection of the temporomandibular joint and atlantoaxial joint, which can prove lethal due to the cord compression. Figure 41.4 shows frequency of involvement of various joints in rheumatoid arthritis.

> **Quick Facts**
> *Joints involved in rheumatoid arthritis*
> - Metacarpophalangeal and interphalangeal joints of the hand.
> - Shoulder elbow and wrists.
> - Hip, knee and ankle.
>
> *Others: Temporomandibular joint, atlantoaxial joints and facet joints of the cervical spine.*

Rheumatoid Hand

Orthopedic deformities of the hand (rheumatoid hand) the following are some of the very common deformities seen in the hand (Figs 41.5A to C).
- *Symmetrical peripheral joint swelling* of metacarpophalangeal and interphalangeal joints (Fig. 41.5A).
- *Ulnar deviation* of the hand is due to rupture of the collateral ligaments at the metacarpophalangeal joints, which enables the extensor tendons to slip from their grooves towards the ulnar side (Figs 41.6A and B).
- *Boutonniere's deformity* is due to the rupture of central extensor expansion of the fingers resulting in flexion at the PIP joint (see Fig. 41.5C).
- *Swan neck deformity* is due to the rupture of the volar plate of the PIP joints, which enables the tendons to slip towards the dorsal side. This is also known as *intrinsic*

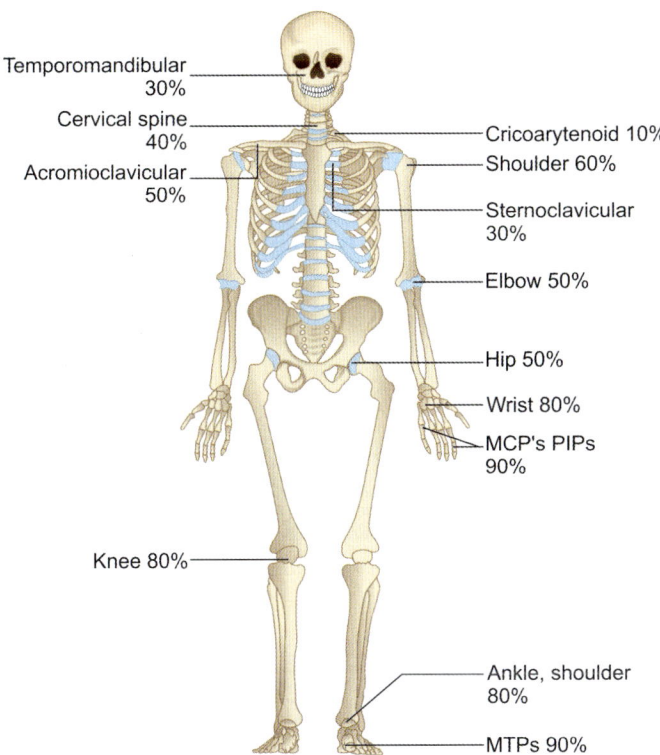

Fig. 41.4: Frequency of involvement of different joint sites in established RA

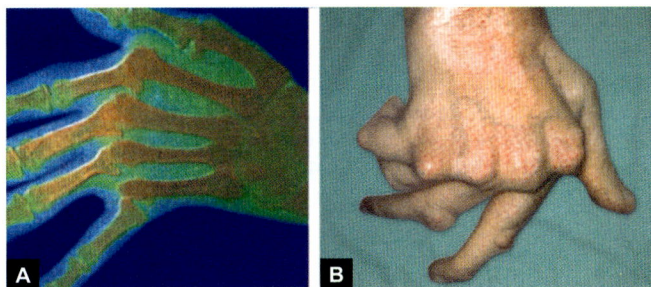

Figs 41.6A and B: Rheumatoid hand (Clinical photo)

plus deformity. Here there is hyperextension of the PIP joint and flexion of the DIP joints.
- *Trigger fingers and trigger thumb are* due to nodules over the tendons.
- Z-deformity of the thumb.
- Subluxation and dislocation of metacarpophalangeal joints.

Rheumatoid Foot

It affects the forefoot, midfoot and hindfoot. In the forefoot, the patient may develop hallux valgus deformity of the great toe, claw toes, callosity over the dorsum and the sole, widening of the forefoot, etc. The heel may show valgus deformity.

Ninety percent of patients with rheumatoid arthritis of long-standing duration have foot deformities (Fig. 41.7). Forefoot is more commonly affected than the hindfoot (Also see box).

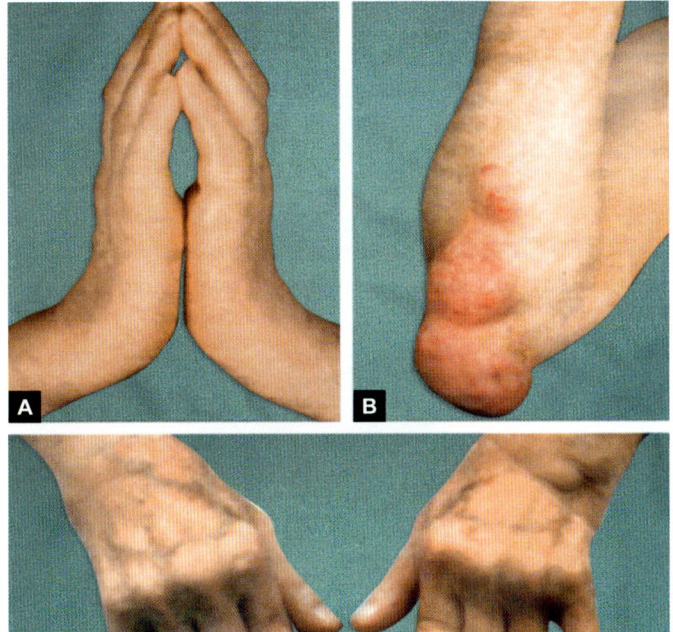

Figs 41.5A to C: Rheumatic features of the hand and the elbow (Clinical photo)

> **Vital Facts**
> *About foot deformities in rheumatoid arthritis:*
> - Callosity under PIP joint
> - Plantar callosity
> - Atrophy of plantar metatarsal fat pad
> - Prominent metatarsal head
> - Excessive plantar tilt of metatarsals
> - Claw toes
> - Hammer toes
> - Rheumatoid nodules
> - Calcaneal erosions
> - Achilles tendinitis
> - Flattening of longitudinal arch
> - Bunion
> - Hallux valgus
> - Over-riding of second and third toes
> - Splaying of forefoot due to divergent metatarsals

Other Joints

In the knee initially, there is a gross soft tissue swelling due to synovitis; and in the later stages, the patient may develop fibrous ankylosis or bony ankylosis due to widespread destruction of the articular cartilage by the pannus. Similarly, other major joints of the body like the hip, ankle, shoulder, and elbow could be involved (Figs 41.8 to 41.12).

> **Do You Know the Frequency of Joint Involvement in Rheumatoid Arthritis? (see Fig. 41.4)**
> - MCP/MTP/PIP joints—90 percent
> - Knee, ankle and wrist—80 percent
> - Shoulder—60 percent
> - Hip, elbow, acromion—50 percent
> - Cervical spine—40 percent
> - Temporomandibular and sternomastoid joints—30 percent
> - Cricoarytenoid joint—10 percent
>
> **Note:**
> Characteristically distal interphalangeal joint and sacroiliac joint are not involved in rheumatoid arthritis.

Investigations

Laboratory Tests

Hb percentage is low and shows normochromic, hypochromic anemia. WBCs are decreased or normal, there are increased lymphocytes and the ESR is raised.

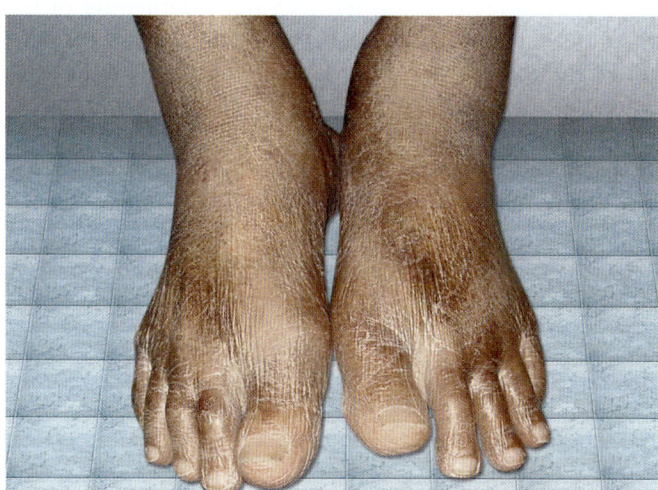

Fig. 41.7: Clinical photo showing rheumatoid foot

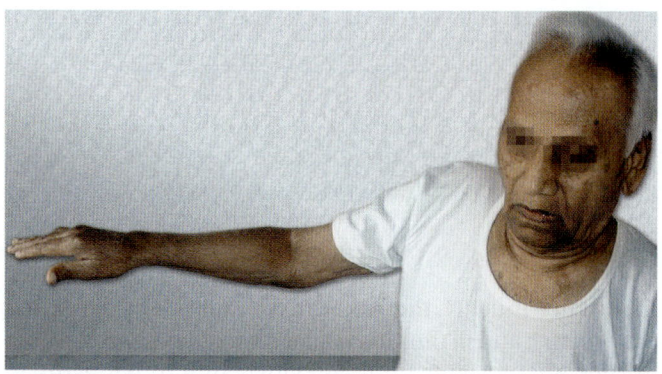

Fig. 41.8: Clinical photo showing rheumatoid shoulder

Serological Tests

Basis rheumatoid patient's serum contains RA factor, which in the presence of g-globulin agglutinates certain strains of streptococci sensitized by sheep cells and latex particles.

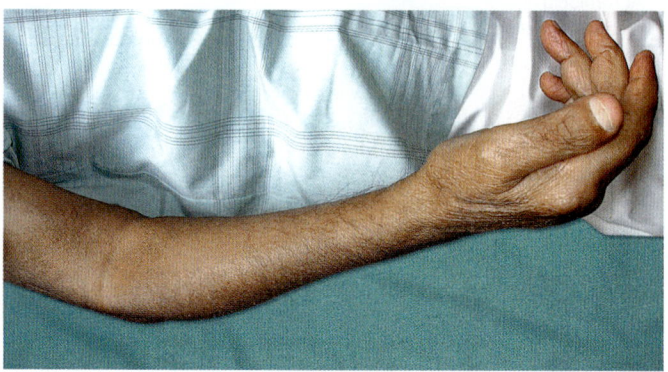

Fig. 41.9: Clinical photo showing rheumatoid elbow

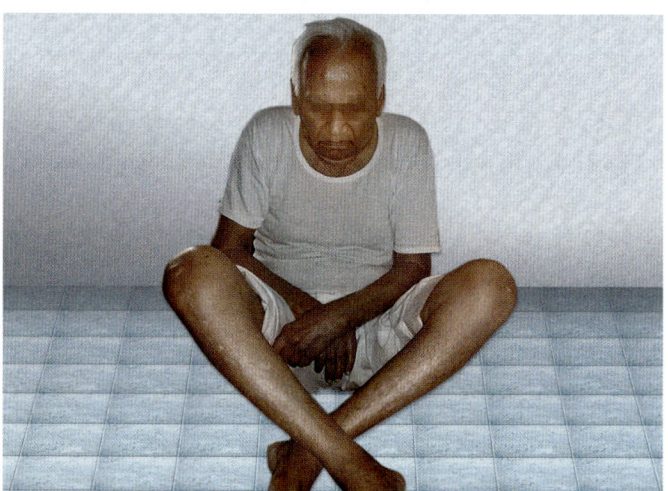

Fig. 41.10: Clinical photo showing rheumatoid hip

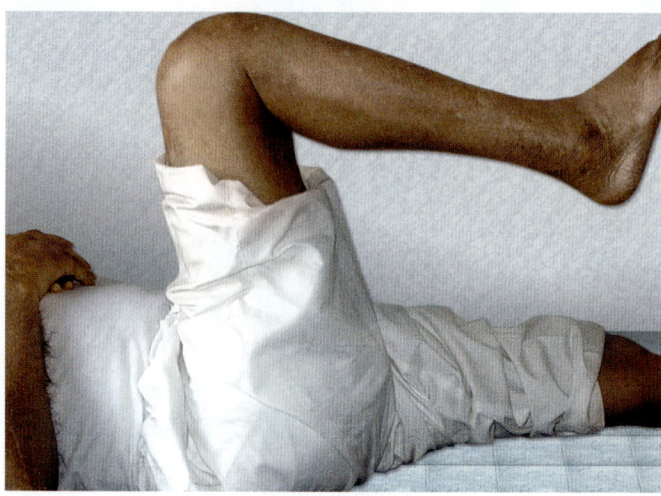

Fig. 41.11: Clinical photo showing rheumatoid knee

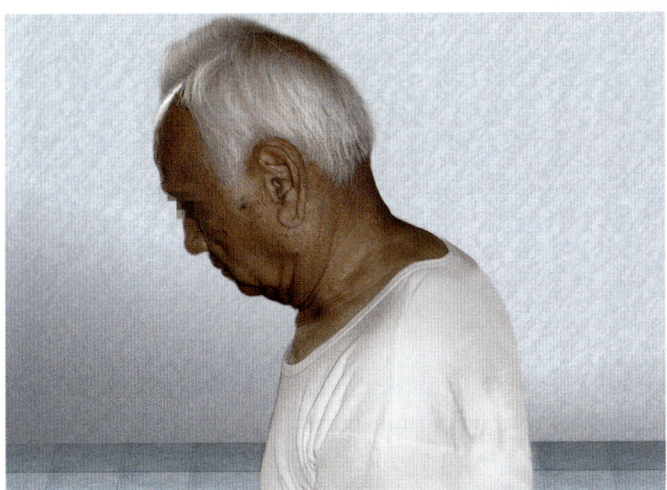

Fig. 41.12: Clinical photo showing rheumatoid neck

- *Latex fixation test (Flowchart 41.1):* Unknown serum + 7-globulin latex suspension
- *Inhibition test (Flowchart 41.2):* This test uses the characteristics of euglobulin from unknown serum. Euglobulin from normal serum neutralizes the rheumatoid factor thereby inhibiting agglutination.

Euglobulin from rheumatoid serum has no effect on the rheumatoid factor and agglutination occurs. *This is the most sensitive test.* Positive even when rheumatoid arthritis factor is present in minute amounts.

Flowchart 41.1: Latex agglutination test

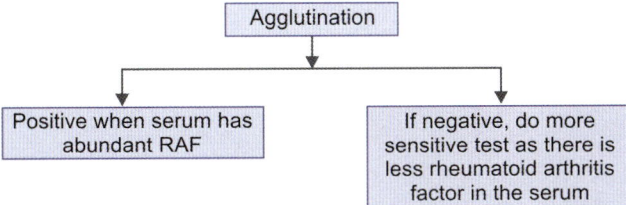

Flowchart 41.2: Inhibition test

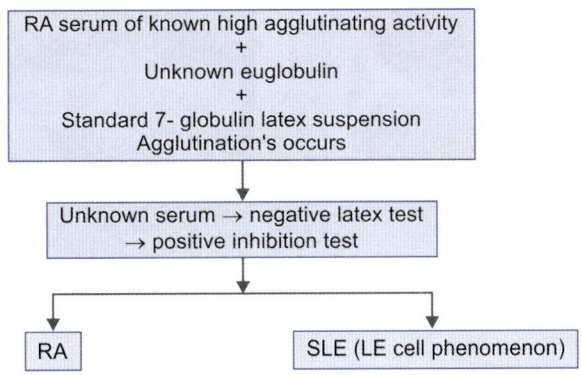

Remember
RA factor is found in:
- 75 percent of rheumatoid arthritis cases
- 10 percent in healthy elderly people
- 10 percent in malaria, etc.

Radiological Features of Rheumatoid Arthritis (Figs 41.13 to 41.15)

Plain X-ray of the affected joints show the following features:
- Soft tissue swelling.
- Juxta-articular osteoporosis.
- Erosion of joint margins.
- Joint spaces are decreased.
- Deformities.
- Atlantoaxial subluxation.
- Subchondral erosions and cyst formation.
- Fibrous and bony ankylosis develops in the late stages.

Other Common Abnormalities
These include increased C-reactive protein (CRP), increased alkaline phosphatase, increased platelets, and decreased serum albumin. Citrulline antibody is present in most cases of early rheumatoid arthritis. Antinuclear antibody (ANA) is also frequently raised in patients with rheumatoid arthritis.

Synovial Fluid Analysis
This is not performed routinely for diagnostic purposes but performed to exclude other causes of inflammation such as infection. Synovial fluid in RA is typically yellow, watery and turbid due to high WBC and has low sugar content.

MRI
This gives valuable information about the various soft tissue damages in rheumatoid with far more greater accuracy (Figs 41.16 and 41.17).

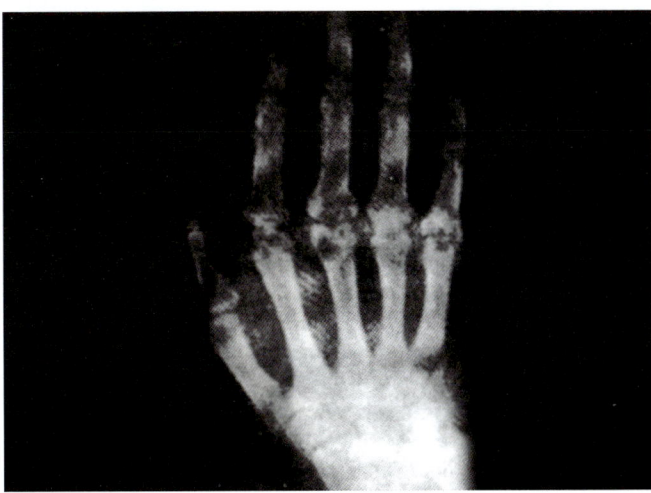

Fig. 41.13: Radiograph showing features of rheumatoid arthritis

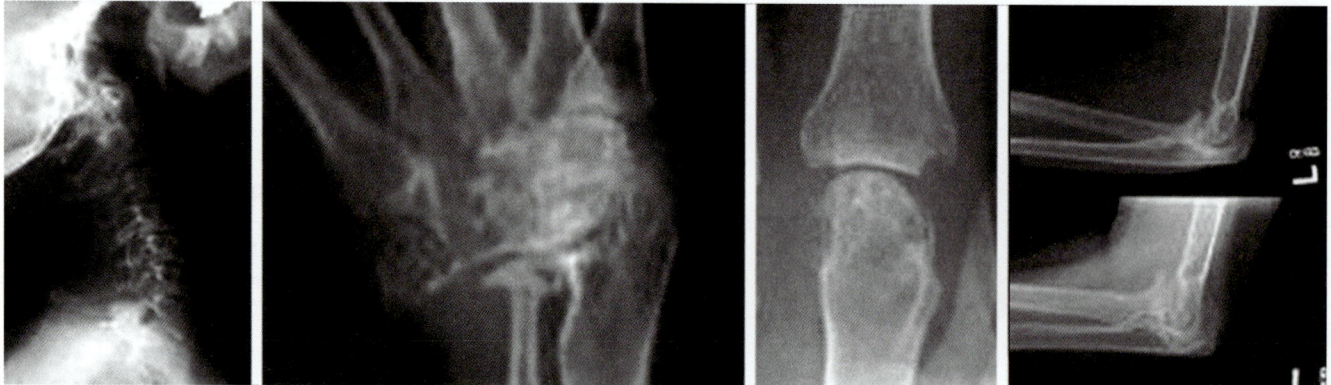

Fig. 41.14: Plain X-rays of the neck, wrist, I MTP and elbow joint in rheumatoid arthritis

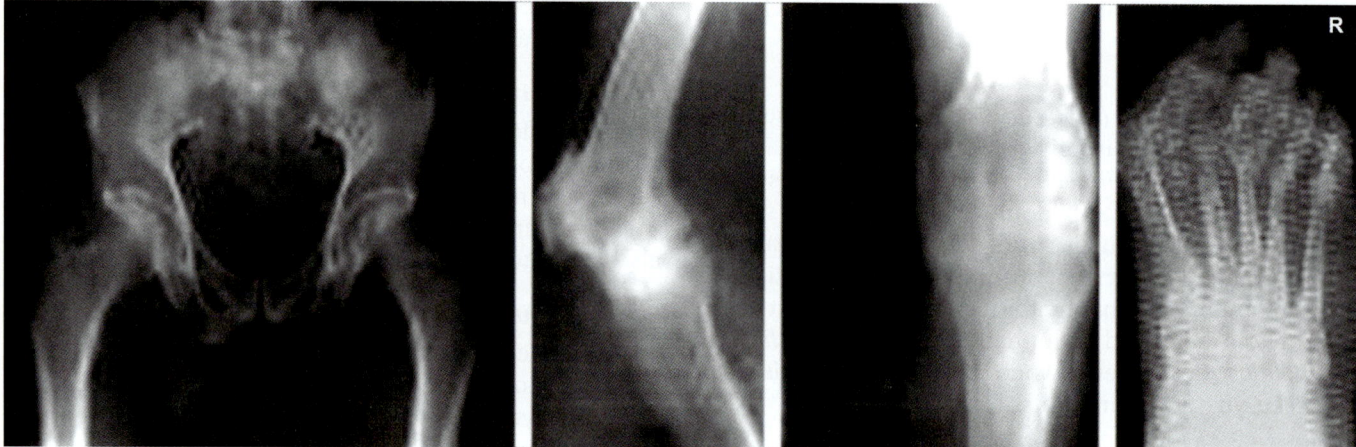

Fig. 41.15: Plain X-rays of the hip, knee and foot in rheumatoid arthritis

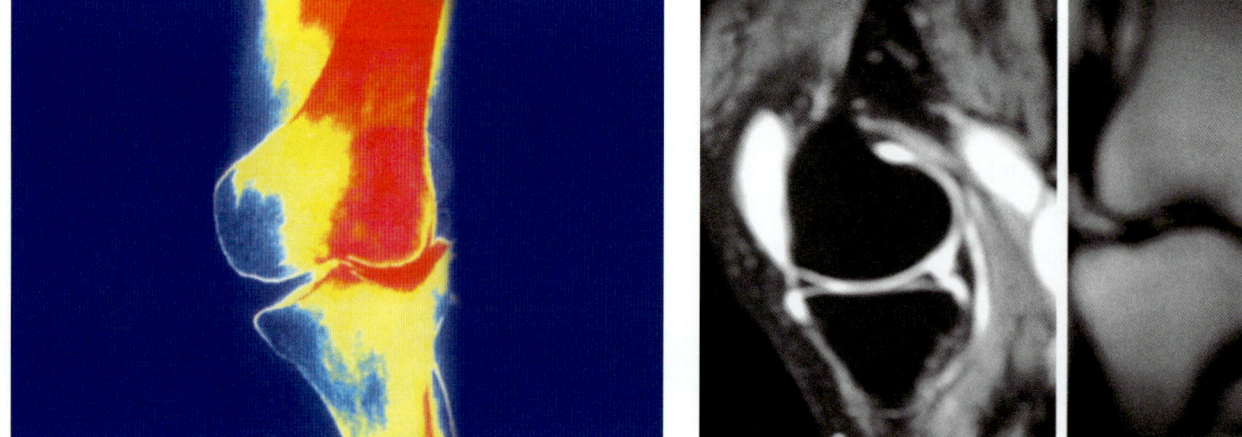

Fig. 41.16: MRI rheumatoid knee

Fig. 41.17: MRI rheumatoid knee

Differential Diagnosis

Differential diagnosis of rheumatoid arthritis with various other conditions is shown in Table 41.1. However, for the differential diagnosis of rheumatoid arthritis with the all-important osteoarthritis (Table 41.2).

Quick Facts of Rheumatoid Arthritis
- Most common chronic inflammatory disorder.
- Eighty percent in women.
- Exact cause is not known.
- Rheumatoid unit is present.
- History of remissions and exacerbations present.
- Symmetrical peripheral joint involvement.
- Rheumatoid arthritis factor is positive in 70 percent.
- Inhibition test is most sensitive.
- Extra-articular features are seen in 75 percent.

Management

Aims of Treatment

- To keep inflammatory process at a minimum, thereby, preserving joint motion, maintaining healthy muscles and preventing secondary joint stiffness and deformity (Fig. 41.18).
- To keep constitutional symptoms at a minimum.
- The possible deformities are anticipated and prevented by appropriate splinting.
- *Finally, surgical measures to correct the deformities, eliminate pain and provide stability are undertaken.*

General Measures

It aims at improving the general condition of the patient and to keep the joints properly splinted in functional position to guard against the ensuing ankylosis.
- Rest in bed.
- Good diet, rich in proteins and minerals.
- Transfusion and hematinics to correct the anemia.
- Hormones combination of estrogen and androgen to improve the bone stock.
- Removal of infective foci.

Splinting in the functional position helps in the event that ankylosis ensues. The splint is removed daily. Hot packs are given or the patient is placed in Hubbard tank at (92.6–102°F) and the joints are put into full range of motion.

While the joints are immobilized, muscle-setting exercises are advocated. After removal of the splints, resistance exercises are begun.

TABLE 41.1: Differential diagnosis of rheumatoid arthritis

Early disease	Established disease
Common	**Common**
• Viral arthropathy • Polymyalgia • Infection • Prodrome of hepatitis • Hypoparathyroidism	• Psoriatic arthritis • Erosive osteoarthritis • Chronic pyrophosphate disease • Chronic tophaceous gout • SLE • Reiter's syndrome • Ankylosing spondylitis
Rare	**Rare**
• Sarcoidosis • Acute leukemia • Coeliac disease • Eosinophilic fasciitis	• Amyloid arthropathy • Multicentric reticulohistiocytosis

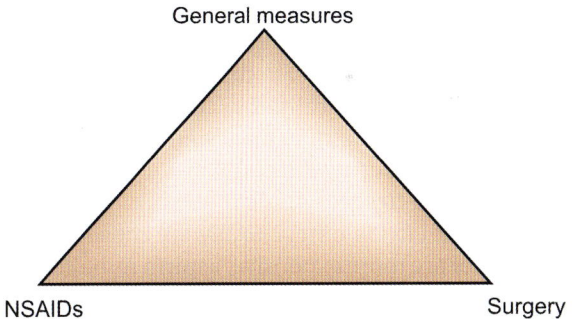

Fig. 41.18: Treatment triad for rheumatoid arthritis

TABLE 41.2: Differences between rheumatoid arthritis and osteoarthritis

Rheumatoid arthritis	Osteoarthritis
• It is an autoimmune disease and often strikes in the prime of life	• It is an age-related disease due to wear and tear of the cartilage
• It is usually seen between the ages of 25 and 50 years of age but can also occur in children and infancy	• It usually affects people after 40 years of age
• It affects joints on both sides of the body and has a bilateral presentation	• It usually affects isolated joints, or joints on only one side of the body at first
• It causes redness, warmth and swelling of the joints	• It usually does not cause redness and warmth of the joints
• It affects many joints usually small joints of the hands and feet, and may affect the elbow, shoulders, wrist, hip, knee and ankles	• It most commonly affects weightbearing joints or joints that are overused (e.g. knees and hip)
• It can affect the entire system, with general feeling of sickness and fatigue, as well as weight loss	• Discomfort is usually related to the affected joint
• There is history of prolonged morning stiffness	• Brief morning stiffness
• It causes major fatigue	• It rarely causes fatigue

Conservative Treatment

Splints

These are known to serve three main functions:
- Rest and relief of pain (*rest splints*).
- Prevention and correction of deformity (*corrective splints*).
- Fixation of damaged joint in a good functional position (*fixation splints*).

Drug Therapy

Three classes of drugs are used regularly.
- Analgesics
- Anti-inflammatory drugs
- Disease modifying drugs.

Steroids especially intra-articular injections have an important role.

No treatment is ideal and it is important to assess the patient's response, so that the most effective regimen is adopted.

Commonly used methods of assessment include; duration of early morning stiffness, number of tender swollen joints. Functional assessment, questionnaires, ESR, radiographs, etc.

First Line of Drugs: NSAIDs

These are aspirin/ibuprofen/ketoprofen/diclofenac sodium/ naproxen/piroxicam, etc. They are the major pharmaceutical agents for pain relief in rheumatic diseases. About 20 percent of patients admitted to the hospital are taking NSAIDs. Though useful, they have significant side effects. Steroids are useful during flare-ups.

Aspirin is the *drug of first choice;* but because of its undesirable side effects, other NSAIDs are chosen. However, since the latter are more expensive, aspirin remains the first choice drug.

Mechanism of action of NSAIDs: They have an inhibitory action on the following pain-mediating agents:
- Prostaglandin synthesis
- Leukotriene synthesis
- Lymphocyte activation
- Oxygen radical generation
- Cytokine production, etc.

Practical Prescribing of NSAIDs: There is no ideal NSAID. It is important to become familiar with a few of these drugs and to find the most appropriate NSAID for one particular patient. *If possible, NSAIDs should be prescribed twice-daily regimen, with a flexible dose to cover the main period of pain.* Initially, clinicians should prescribe NSAIDs with which they are familiar and not necessarily the latest drug.

Only one NSAID should be prescribed at one time and if the patient has not responded to an adequate dose within 2-3 weeks, an alternative NSAID should be given.

It is important to justify the use of NSAID, both in the short- and long-term. Other methods of pain relief should always be considered, such as exercises, heat and cold hydrotherapy.

Quick Facts of NSAIDs
- Drugs of first choice
- Aspirin remains as the first choice
- There are no ideal NSAIDs
- Prescribe NSAID with which clinician is familiar
- Ideal is twice daily regimen
- Only one NSAID at a time
- To be tried for a minimum of 2–3 weeks
- NSAIDs provide only symptomatic relief.

NSAIDs provide only symptomatic relief. Most patients require daily treatment. These drugs probably do not have any influence on the disease process and may, therefore, be regarded as a background therapy with a variable daily dose according to symptoms.

Second Line of Drugs

Second line of drugs are used only if an adequate trial of first line drugs have failed to relieve symptoms satisfactorily or if there is radiological evidence of progressive disease. Second line drugs are alternatively known as *disease-modifying antirheumatic drugs (DMARD)* and are slow acting drugs. It would seem that they have influence on the underlying disease process, and may take several weeks or months to exert this effect.

To get maximum benefit, second line drug therapy should be continued for *at least 6 months;* and in order to sustain the benefit, it needs to be continued indefinitely. They are all toxic.

When second line therapy is introduced, s*ymptomatic NSAIDs need to be continued in parallel.* If the response to the second line drug is good, the dose of NSAID can be reduced.

Commonly prescribed drugs include:
- Injectable gold and oral gold (sodium aurothiomalate). This is no longer preferred.
- Penicillamine
- Sulfasalazine
- Antimalarial drugs (e.g. chloroquine)
- Dapsone and levamisole
- Methotrexate with folic acid.

The choice of the drug to be given first will depend on the experience of the doctor and on the facilities available for monitoring. There is little evidence to suggest which drug should be prescribed first.

If after 6 months of adequate therapy, no response has been observed, an alternative drug may be tried.

At the end of a year of the treatment, 65 percent would have improved, 35 percent will have had to stop therapy because of toxicity or lack of therapeutic effect.

Methotrexate Drug

Currently, gold satts are on the decline due to their side effects. Methotrexate has now emerged as the drug of choice due to its higher efficacy. Early institution and escalation of MTX to its maximum tolerable dose is the latest mantra.

Antimalarial Drugs

They do not require intensive blood monitoring and if these facilities are limited, chloroquine or hydroxy chloroquine can be particularly used.

Other agents known to have second line drug effect include levamisole and dapsone. Levamisole is not freely available in some countries and its toxicity seems to be greater than that of gold and penicillamine. Dapsone has a high toxicity.

Indications of second line drugs: The ideal patient for a second line drug is one who has active synovitis with generalized inflammation in many joints, who is taking the recommended dose of the NSAID which is not producing relief of symptoms.

Quick Facts of Second Line Drugs
- Used only if first line fails.
- Known as DMARD.
- Methotrexate is the drugs of choice
- To be continued for at least 6 months.
- Parallel NSAID is to be used.
- Choice of drugs is based on clinicians' experience.
- Antimalarial drugs are used if proper blood monitoring is not available.
- All drugs are toxic.

Third Line of Drugs

Azathioprine, cyclophosphamide and chlorambucil can exert a second line effect in-patients with rheumatoid arthritis. However, these drugs are considered under third line drugs because in addition to the toxicity, which may arise acutely during their use, *there is also anxiety about late toxicity*. This late toxicity, which may occur after prolonged therapy, is an additional hazard for patients who are suffering from what is essentially a non-fatal condition. These drugs have, therefore, to be treated with respect though in selected cases they may be of benefit.

Corticosteroids: Cyclosporine has been tried in-patients with rheumatoid arthritis. The fact that it does not affect WBC is a theoretical advantage in-patients with Felty's syndrome. Anxieties about long-term nephrotoxicity limit the use of cyclosporine to research programs.

Newer Drugs

Biologicals and biosimilars are the newer drugs which are indicated in resistant cases. They provide good relief of pain but are expensive and has to be given for a longer duration of time (see Box).

Role of Biologicals
Newer drugs for rheumatoid arthritis
- Tumor Necrosis Factor (INF a-blockers)
For example:
- Etanercept (25 mg/subcutaneous, twice a week)
- Infliximab (2 mg/kg at 0, 6, 8 and weekly. IV infusions combined with oral methotrexate).
- Interleukin-1-receptor antagonist (IL-IRA) Dose—100 mg/day by subcutaneous injection.

Indications
Failure of at least two standard DMARD drugs one of which is always methotrexate despite adequate trials (i.e. 6 months).
- Leflunomide (Immunomodulatory drug)
  Indicated dose is 100 mg/day for 3 days than 20 mg/day.

Local Steroids

Role of local corticosteroid treatment is considered when the rheumatoid arthritis affects one or two joints. It is also indicated in tendinitis, capsular or ligament involvement, carpal tunnel and compression syndromes. It is given weekly in acute cases and three monthly in chronic. *If two injections are ineffective, the treatment is discontinued.*

Surgery

Aim of surgery
- Relieve pain.
- Correct the deformity of the joints.
- Reduce joint instability.
- Improve the range of movements of the joints.

Surgical advice should be sought only when the disease is *clearly progressive and conservative measures are failing*, but before the patient starts to lose a significant amount of bone stock. If surgery is delayed, more bone is lost, the soft tissue deteriorates and the deformity increases.

Preoperative Considerations

Before surgery for rheumatoid disease, a number of specific points should be checked. Related conditions such as diabetes, hypertension and anemia should be adequately treated and:
- Steroid dosage should be reduced.
- There should be no active infection.
- A radiograph of the cervical spine should be obtained to exclude instability.

Modus Operandi of Surgical Procedures in Rheumatoid Arthritis	
Synovectomy	• Failed chemotherapy • Joint destruction should be minimal • Useful in knee/ankle
Osteotomy	• Less than 60 years of age • When joint is partially damaged • Commonly done at hip (Intertrochanteric osteotomy and abduction osteotomy)
Arthrodesis	• Long-term relief • Reserved for peripheral joints where arthroplasty results in pain • Causes secondary osteoarthritis in bigger joints
Arthroplasty	• Advanced stages in hip and knee

Surgical Methods

Synovectomy

It may be indicated in patients with rheumatoid arthritis if joint destruction is minimal and if the main cause of pain and swelling is synovitis, which is resistant to medication and physiotherapy. Synovectomy is usually carried out over the knee and ankle, in the elbow with radial head excision if necessary. In the wrist, dorsal synovectomy and resection of the distal end of the ulna can prevent attrition and rupture of extensor tendons. *Synovectomy has to be virtually complete to avoid regrowth with recurrence of symptoms.*

Osteotomy

This should be considered in patients under the age of 60 years with osteoarthritis of the hip or knee due to rheumatoid arthritis. *Osteotomy has the advantage of relieving pain without sacrificing the joint surfaces, which have only been partially damaged.*

At the hip, intertrochanteric osteotomy, which contains the femoral head within the acetabulum, is preferred. At the knee, abduction osteotomy is preferred.

Arthrodesis

Arthrodesis of the joint gives excellent long-term pain relief. Nevertheless, the stress may cause secondary OA in the adjacent joints unless they are able to compensate for the loss of movement. Lack of movement after fusion of the wrist can be absorbed at the elbow and shoulder without significant functional impairment, but fusion of the hip puts considerable strain on the spine and the knee.

Arthrodesis, therefore, tends to be preserved for peripheral joints, such as the wrist, ankle, and IP joints of the hands and feet where the functional loss is less disabling and arthroplasty is less reliable.

Arthroplasties

Arthroplasties of the hip, knee (Figs 41.19A and B), ankle, shoulder, elbow, wrist, and hand (Fig. 41.20) is indicated in advanced diseases causing severe pain and incapacitating disability due to stiffness and instability.

Self-management Techniques for Rheumatoid and Other Forms of Arthritis

Self-management is the most important aspect of the treatment of rheumatoid and other forms of arthritis. People practicing self-management techniques tend to experience less pain and are more active than those who do not practice self-management. In this management, the patient is made aware of the disease and the rationale

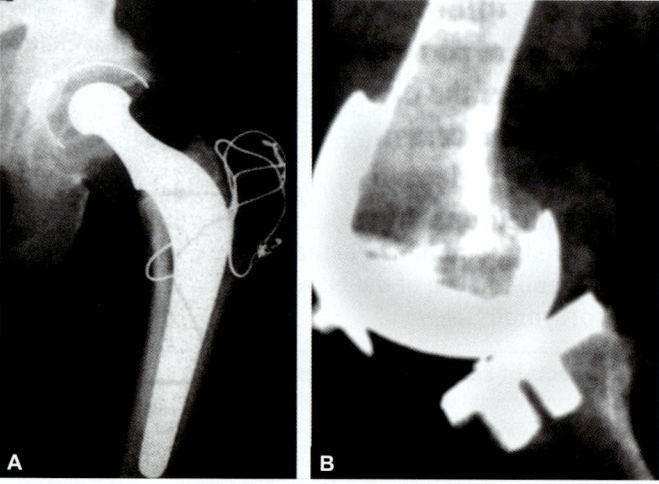

Figs 41.19A and B: Radiographs showing: (A) Total hip replacement; (B) Total knee replacement for rheumatoid arthritis of the hip and knee

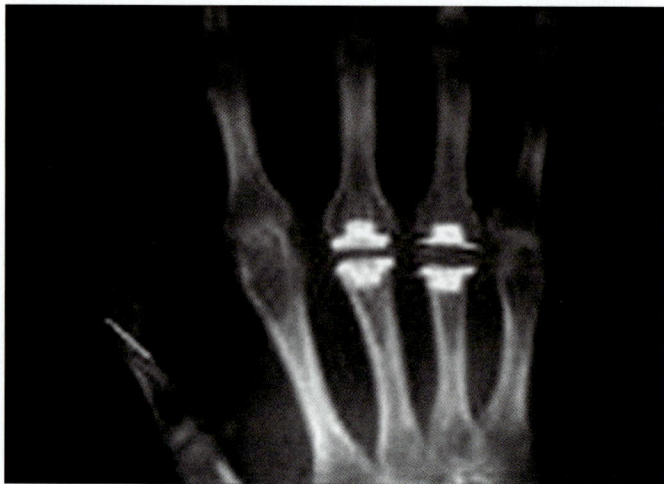

Fig. 41.20: Plain X-ray showing MCP joint replacement in rheumatoid hand

behind the treatment. They are made to realize that the success of the treatment is their ultimate responsibility.

Ten Self-help Techniques

1. *Positive mental attitude*: The patient is told to focus on things other than pain and their own body. They are encouraged to think positively (Fig. 41.21A).
2. *Regular medication*: The patient is told the value of regular and correct medication (Fig. 41.21B).
3. *Regular exercises*: The patient should follow a regular and appropriate exercise program, most suited for them (Fig. 41.21C).
4. *Use of joints*: The patient is told the value of correct posture and the methods of using the joints wisely to reduce stress on the painful joints (Fig. 41.21D).
5. *Energy conservation*: Patients are instructed to listen to the body's "inner signals" for rest. Slowing down and avoiding too many activities reduces the stress on the joints.
6. *Assistive devices*: Devices like splints, braces and walking sticks can help stabilize the joints, provide strength and reduce pain and inflammation (Fig. 41.21F).
7. *Adequate sleep*: A good adequate sleep provides rest to the ailing joints and reduces the pain and swelling (Fig. 41.21G).
8. *Massage*: A good moderate massage brings warmth and relieves pain due to arthritis (Fig. 41.21H).
9. *Relaxation techniques*: Relaxation techniques like yoga, meditation, etc. help to relax the muscles, mind and controls respiration, heart rate, blood pressure. This helps in the control of pain (Fig. 41.21I).
10. *Modification in the daily activities*
    - Using Western toilets (Fig. 41.21J)
    - Bath aids and railings
    - Long handle broomstick and mop to clean the floors (see Fig. 41.21E)
    - Use of walking sticks while walking, climbing, etc.
    - High chairs
    - Avoid squatting on the ground for food, etc. Use of dining table and chairs are recommended
    - To avoid squeezing clothes after washing and just rinse them dry (Fig. 41.21J)
    - To avoid walking on hard and uneven and rough surfaces
    - To sleep on a hard surface.

SERONEGATIVE SPONDYLOARTHROPATHIES

Introduction

Seronegative spondyloarthropathies (SSA) group is gradually emerging as a new entity. These disorders are labeled as *seronegative* to indicate that they have in common the *absence of the rheumatoid factor*. The term spondyloarthropathies is used because in many cases, there is involvement of the s*pine and sacroiliac joints*. Hence, SSA can be defined as an *acute or chronic condition with characteristic involvement of axial joints, absence of RA factor and HLA abnormality*.

The clinical entities, which appear to justify inclusions in the SSA group, are as follows:
- Ankylosing spondylitis
- Reiter's disease
- Psoriatic arthritis
- Ulcerative colitis
- Crohn's disease
- Whipple's disease } Enteropathic arthritis
- Behçet's syndrome

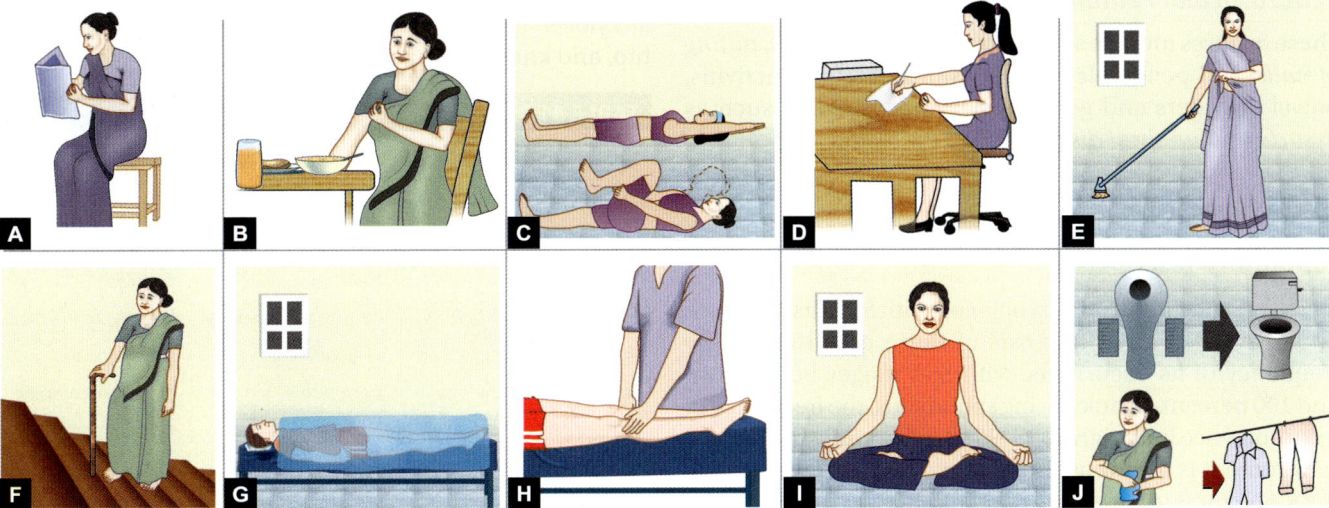

Figs 41.21A to J: Self-management techniques in the treatment of rheumatoid arthritis

Etiology

The exact pathogenic mechanisms involved are not known. However, genetic factors appear to play an important role. The most complete evidence for familial aggregation is that for ankylosing spondylitis. The children of a person with HLA-B_{27} have a 50 percent chance of carrying the same antigen.

There are some postulations regarding the possible mechanism for the association of HLA-B_{27} and SSA.
- HLA-B_{27} is a marker for immune response gene that determines susceptibility to an environmental trigger.
- HLA-B_{27} may act as a receptor site for an infective-agent.
- It may induce tolerance to foreign antigen with which it cross-reacts.

Salmonella, Shigella, Chlamydia, Yersinia and other microorganisms are implicated in the pathogenesis of this group of arthritis.

Clinical Features

The clinical manifestations include *articular* as well as *extra-articular* features.

Articular Features

These include low back pain due to progressive sacroiliitis and spondylitis. The patient complains of morning stiffness and decreasing lumbar lordosis. Diffuse swelling of fingers and toes may occur due to small joint synovitis and tenosynovitis. The manifestation is referred to as *sausage digit*. Enthesopathy, i.e. pain at the site of insertion of ligaments and tendons can occur at Achilles tendon, plantar fascia and ischial tuberosities.

Extra-articular Features

These features include skin lesions such as *psoriasis, pitting of nails*, and penile ulcers, eye lesions like conjunctivitis, bowel disorders and genitourinary disturbances such as *dysuria* and *urethral discharge*.

Investigations

Laboratory Tests

HLA-B_{27} shows a strong association with SSA. Its presence adds weight to the diagnosis of these conditions. The frequency of its occurrence with SSA ranges between 16 and 100 percent. In ankylosing spondylitis, the frequency of its occurrence is as high as 85–90 percent, while in Behçet's syndrome it is as low as 16 percent. *In all patients of SSA, the RA factor is uniformly negative.* ESR, C-reactive protein, ANA tests show increase.

Radiographs

Radiological diagnosis *forms one of the proven diagnostic techniques in diagnosing SSA*. Radiological study of the affected joints will show *punched out areas* exceeding deep into the subchondral bone.

CAT Scan

Computerized axial tomography (CAT) scan is also a very useful method that helps in the diagnosis. *It is indicated when plain X-rays are normal*. Early changes of sclerosis and bone erosion, which are not visible on a plain X-ray, can be clearly demonstrated on CAT scan.

One of the diagnostic pitfalls encountered is a mistaken diagnosis of RA. Hence, at the very outset, it is essential to differentiate between these two conditions (Table 41.3).

ANKYLOSING SPONDYLITIS (Syn: Marie-Strumpell Disease)

Definition

This is a chronic progressive inflammatory disease of the sacroiliac joints and the axial skeleton.

Causes

Causes are unknown. It is found to be strongly associated with HLA-B_{27} genetic marker (about 85 percent).

The infective triggers are certain Gram-negative organisms more so *Klebsiella*.

Age/sex common in young male adults (M : F = 10 : 1).

Pathology

The initial inflammation of the joints is followed by synovitis, arthritis, and cartilage destruction, fibrous and later bony ankylosis. The joints commonly affected are SI joints, spine, hip, and knee and manubrium sterni.

TABLE 41.3: Difference between SSA and RA

	SSA	RA
Age	Young usually less than 40 years	Any age group
Sex	Predominantly Male	Predominantly females
Symmetry	Usually asymmetrical	Usually symmetrical
Number of joints involved	Oligoarticular	Polyarticular
Spine involvement	Common	Only cervical spine
Enthesopathy	Typical	Not a feature
RA factor	Typically negative	Typically positive
HLA-B_{27}	Positive in high Percentage	Negative in normal population

Clinical Features

The patient usually complains of early morning stiffness and pain in the back. On examination, patient has a stiff spine. Tests for sacroiliac joint involvement are positive (Figs 41.22 to 41.24). Cervical spine involvement is tested by asking the patient to touch the wall with the back of the head without raising his or her chin (Fleche's test). If the chest expansion is less than 5 cm, involvement of thoracic spine is suspected (Fig. 41.25). Gradually, a progressive kyphotic deformity of the entire spine develops (Fig. 41.26).

Diagnostic Criteria for Ankylosing Spondylitis
- Insidious onset
- Age <40 years
- Persistence for >3 months
- Morning stiffness
- Improvement with exercise

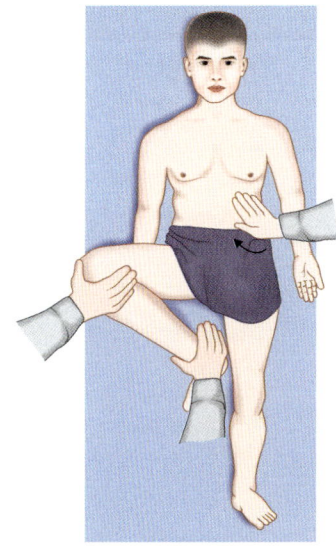

Fig. 41.24: Sacroiliac joint involvement: Fabre's test

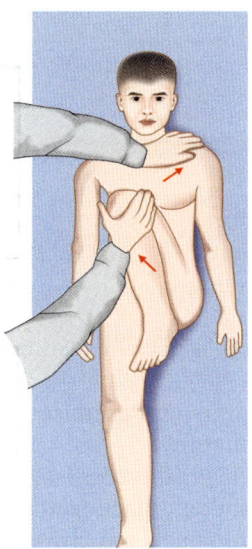

Fig. 41.22: Sacroiliac joint involvement: Pump handle test

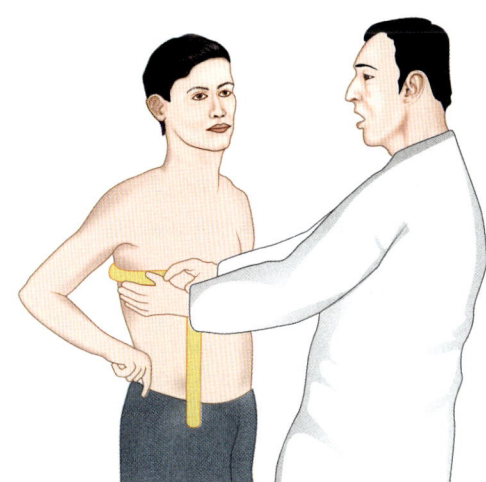

Fig. 41.25: Assessment of chest expansion in ankylosing spondylitis

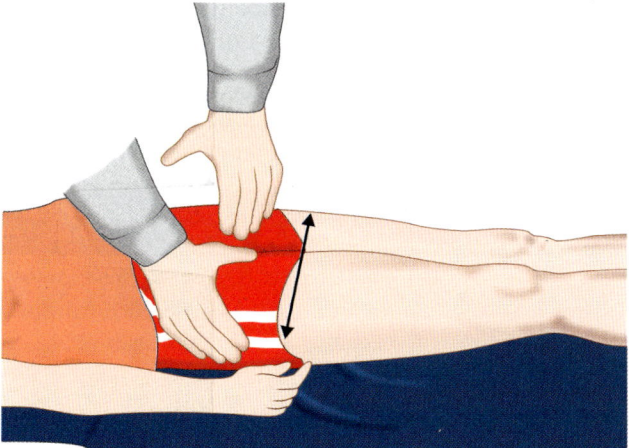

Fig. 41.23: Sacroiliac joint involvement: Tested by the pelvic compression test

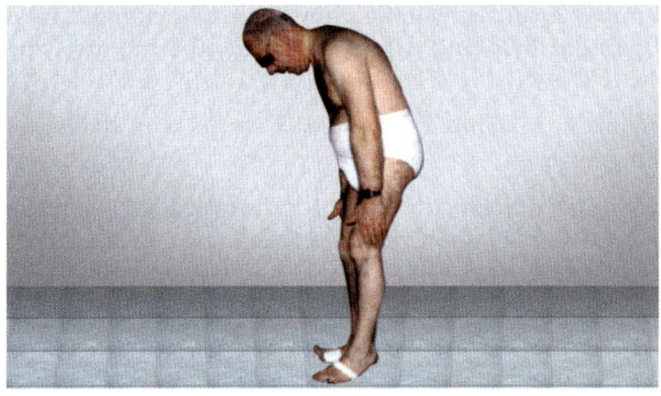

Fig. 41.26: This is how an ankylosing spondylitis patient looks (Clinical photo)

TABLE 41.4: Differential diagnosis SSA

Disease	Sex and age	Onset	Signs and symptoms	Joints involved	Extra-articular lesions	HLA-B$_{27}$
Ankylosing spondylitis	Predominantly males <40 years	Insidious	Low back pain, morning stiffness in heart, CNS disturbances, and pain >3 months	Intervertebral joints	Uveitis, conduction defects pulmonary complications	94%
Psoriatic arthritis	Predominantly females >50 years	Variable	Pain and stiffness on affected joints	Distal and proximal IP joints	Uveitis, conjunctivitis, urethritis, and skin lesions	100%
Reiter's disease	Predominantly females 16–35 years	Sudden	Pain and stiffness of affected joints, diarrhea, dysuria, etc.	Weight bearing joints (knee and ankle)	Conjunctivitis, uveitis, buccal erosions, urethritis	83%
Enteropathic arthropathies males (Crohn's disease, ulcerative colitis, Whipple's disease)	Predominantly Age group is not clear	Variable	Pain and stiffness of the affected joints, weight loss, diarrhea, abdominal pain	Knee, ankle (most common), shoulder wrist, elbow also involved	Aphthous ulcers, uveitis, erythema nodosum	50%
Behçet's syndrome	Predominantly males 15–40 years	Variable	Pain and stiffness of affected joints	Knee, hand, ankle and wrist joints are primarily affected. There is involvement of elbow, shoulder and hip joints	Painful oral ulcers, genital ulcers, ocular lesions, Skin lesions.	16%

Extra-articular Manifestations

These include acute iritis (25%), pericarditis, aortic incompetence, subluxation of atlantoaxial joints, apical lobe fibrosis, generalized osteoporosis, etc.

Differential Diagnosis

For differential diagnosis of various types of SSA, see Table 41.4. For differences between ankylosing spondylitis and backache due to other causes, see Table 41.5.

Investigations

Radiographs of SI joint show haziness, subchondral erosions, sclerosis (Fig. 41.27A) widening of SI joint, etc. Radiographs of spine show squaring of vertebra, loss of lumbar lordosis, calcification of anterior longitudinal ligament bridging osteophytes, bamboo spine (Fig. 41.27B), etc.

Other investigations: This consists of CT scan, MRI, and bone scan, etc.

Laboratory investigations HLA-B$_{27}$ is raised in 95 percent, raised ESR is seen in 50 percent and serum IgA is significantly increased.

Treatment

General measures: This is extremely important and consists of the following measures:

- Patient education
- Family education
- Genetic counseling
- Avoid smoking
- Regular exercises, especially swimming is of tremendous help
- Physiotherapy and joint exercises
- Occupational therapy.

Conservative treatment: This consists of rest, NSAIDs (indomethacin), physiotherapy, back exercises, etc. Radiotherapy may also help. Biologicals are currently being used with good results. They are expensive.

Surgical treatment: Consists of spinal osteotomy to correct spine deformity, total hip replacement and total knee replacement for hip and knee joint ankylosis.

What is new in the Treatment of Ankylosing Spondylitis?
Tumor necrosis factor antagonist etanercept (Enbrel) 25 mg twice weekly is being tried with successful results.

TABLE 41.5: Differential diagnosis of ankylosing spondylitis with other causes of backache

	Ankylosing Spondylitis	Backache due to other causes
Morning stiffness	Present	Nil or minimal
Effect of inactivity	Aggravates pain and stiffness	Relieves pain
Effect of physical activity	Relieves pain	Aggravates pain
Limitation of spine movements	In all directions	Only in some direction

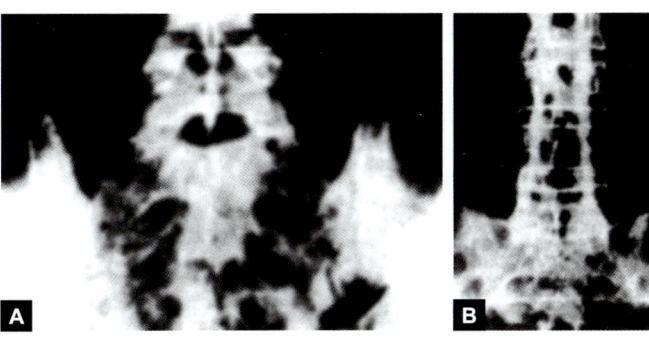

Figs 41.27A and B: (A) Radiograph showing sacroiliac joint sclerosis in ankylosing spondylitis; (B) Radiograph showing bamboo spine in ankylosing spondylitis

Role of Biologicals: This has revolutionized the treatment of ankylosing spondylitis and other chronic inflammatory arthritis like rheumatoid. They give remarkable results, but are expensive and can be used as a last resort when routine drug therapy fails.

FIBROMYALGIA

Introduction

This is a condition where pain is characteristically described as "Charley horses" scattered all over the body. It falls in the gambit of muscular endurance disorders with a widespread musculoskeletal pain involving all the four quadrants of the body namely the right, left, above and below the waist (Fig. 41.28).

Incidence

After osteoarthritis, this is the most common rheumatological disorder. The overall incidence is 2–5 percent with women suffering 8–10 times more than man.

Causative Factors

- In 5–10 percent, it could be hereditary.
- In a majority, any condition that lowers the endurance of the muscles can trigger this condition. Notorious among them are sleep disorders (Loss of Stage IV delta wave sleep), trauma, connective tissue disorders, infections, etc.

Clinical Features

- *Pain:* Its features include widespread gnawing pains, with increased activity, stress or poor sleep.
- Fatigue, stiffness, arthralgia, headache, chest and abdominal pains, etc. are some of the other complaints.

Investigations

Most of the investigations like laboratory tests, X-rays, MRI, etc. are normal.

Diagnostic Criteria

- Widespread pain for at least three months in all the four quadrants of the body
- Pain should be elicited in at least 11/18 established tender points when a digital pressure of 4 kg is applied (Fig. 41.29).

Treatment

A multidisciplinary approach seems to be an effective strategy in tackling this troublesome condition namely:
- *Initial phase*: Treat the underlying cause like sleep disorders, infection, connective tissue disorders, etc.
- *Second phase*: Myofascial release, massage and physical therapy are used to relieve the pain at the tender areas
- *Final phase:* Aerobic exercises are advocated to improve the muscle endurance.

Alternative Therapies

- *Diet therapy*: A diet rich in protein, amino acids and minerals are recommended.

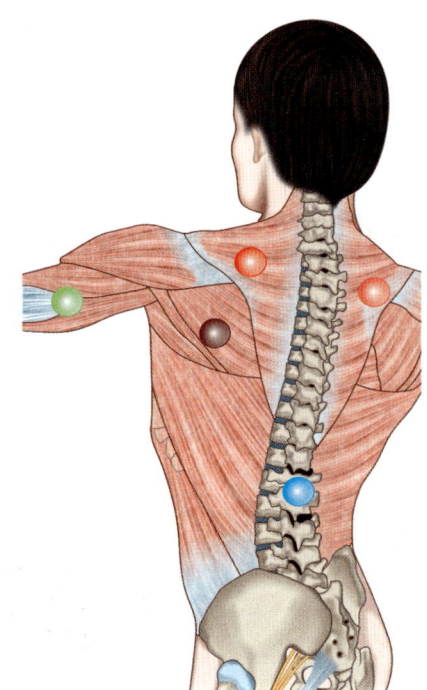

Fig. 41.28: Sites of tenderness in fibromyalgia

- *Injection therapy*: A trigger point injection into the tender area with dry needling or injection, normal saline, local anesthetic and steroid injection helps.
- *Physiotherapy*: Ultrasound, SWD, TENS, manipulations and massage are useful adjunctive measures.
- *Acupressure*: Stimulating the reflex points and specific points helps to lower the pain.

CRYSTALLINE ARTHROPATHIES

This group includes two interesting clinical entities:
1. Monosodium urate arthropathies (gout) (Fig. 41.30).
2. Calcium pyrophosphate deposition disease (CPPD).

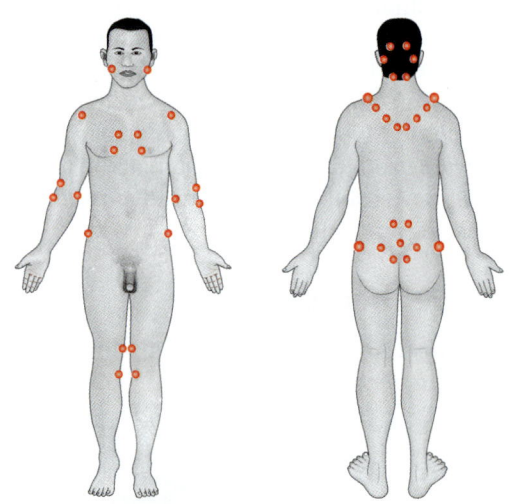

Fig. 41.29: Most common localization of tender points in fibromyalgia.
Source: Adapted from Mau (circles) and Moll (shadowed area).

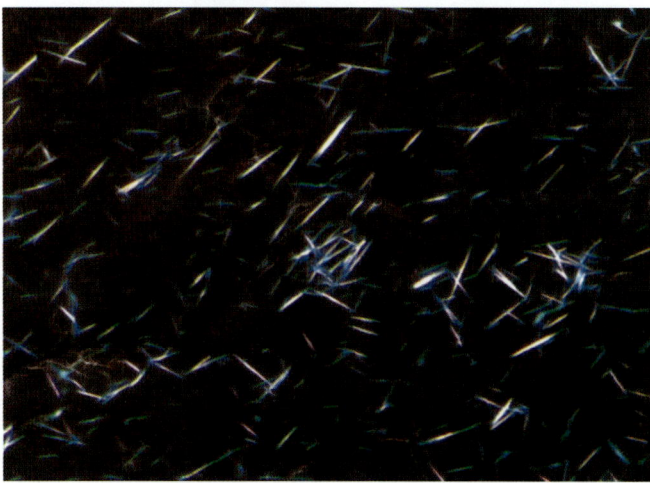

Fig. 41.30: Monosodium urate crystals viewed through a polarizing microscope

MONOSODIUM URATE ARTHROPATHY (GOUT)

This is known as *gout* and may manifest itself as *acute* or *chronic*.

Sites

It is usually monoarticular and the first metatarsophalangeal joint is the most common site of involvement (75%). Ankle, knee, wrist, fingers and elbow are other joints affected (Figs 41.31A and B). *Distal and lower extremity joints are involved more often.*

Role of Hyperuricemia

Gout is usually associated with hyperuricemia and may be associated with hypertension, obesity and atherosclerosis.

> **Did You Know?**
> *Gout is a disease of:*
> - Affluence
> - Alcoholism
> - Obesity
> - Old age
> - Diuretic treatment.

Incidence

It is about 0.3/1000 population.

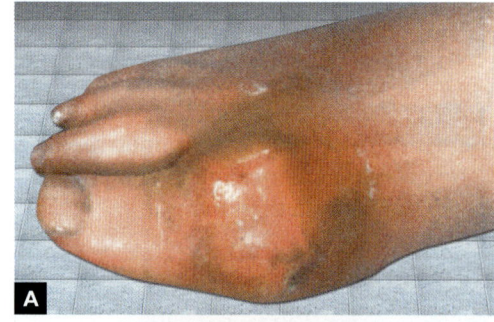
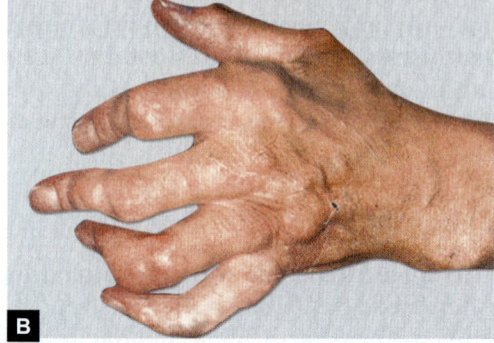

Figs 41.31A and B: (A) Features of acute gout (Clinical photo); (B) Features of chronic gout (Clinical photo)

Age

- Men—after mid-twenties.
- Women—after menopause.

Clinical Features

It has an abrupt onset. The patient may complain of pain, swelling, tenderness and increased temperature of the first metatarsophalangeal joint. Frequent gouty attacks disturb the sleep. Sometimes, the inflammation is so gross that it may resemble cellulitis. Attacks are provoked by surgery, trauma, etc. Mild attacks resolve spontaneously within two days, more severe attacks may last for 7–10 days.

Gout has two extremes. At one end is obese alcoholic with family history of gout and no tophi while at the other extreme is an old, frail, taking thiazide diuretics and with tophi.

TOPHI: These are deposits of monosodium urate crystals over pinnae, elbows Achilles tendon, distal IP joints is elderly patients.

Investigations

Laboratory investigations show leukocytosis and ESR is increased. Synovial fluid study is done under polarized microscopy for the presence of monosodium urate crystals. *This is the most important diagnostic method* (see Fig. 41.30). Raised SUA level may be found.

Radiology

It is usually normal in the initial stages but may provide a helpful clue to detect chondrocalcinosis (Fig. 41.32). However in the late stages it may show erosions, punched out lesions, sclerotic overhanging edges, intraosseous lesions but the joint space is preserved till the last and there will be no periarticular osteopenia unlike rheumatoid arthritis.

Treatment

Conservative method is the mainstay of treatment. The following measures are recommended: Indomethacin 75–100 mg oral initially. Later, it is given as 50 mg every 6 hours. As the attack subsides, the drug may be tapered off. Intra-articular steroid also helps. Recurrent gouty arthritic attacks can be prevented by prophylaxis with colchicines (0.5 mg BD) or indomethacin (25–50 mg everyday). When the above two drugs do not help, Allopurinol is indicated on a long-term basis. Physiotherapy helps to relieve the pain.

Remember the Diagnostic Features of Gout

Attacks (4R's)
- **R**apid onset
- **R**ecurrent
- **R**arely seen >10 days
- **R**emissions

Joints (Remember the Mnemonic FRAME)
- **F**irst MTP joint involved
- **R**ed hot joint
- **A**rticular involvement usually single
- **M**any urate crystals within neutrophils is joint fluid
- **E**xtreme pain.

Non-articular features
- Hyperuricemia
- Tophi (in elderly).

Remember

The drugs used in the prevention and treatment of gout:
- Indomethacin
- Colchicines prevention
- Allopurinol
- Steroids.

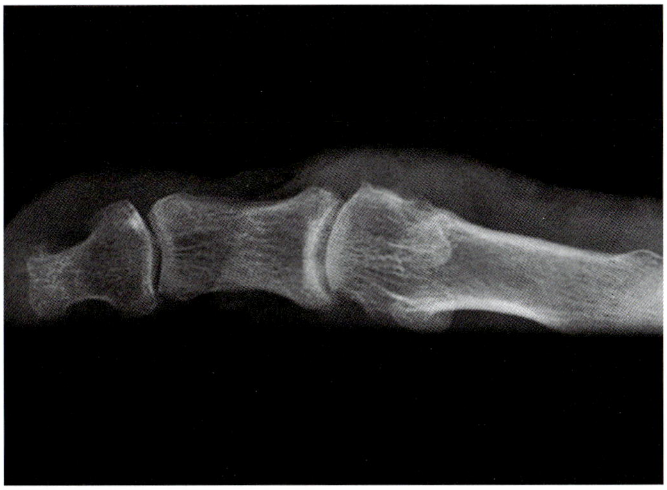

Fig. 41.32: Plain X-ray showing features of gout in 1st MTP joint

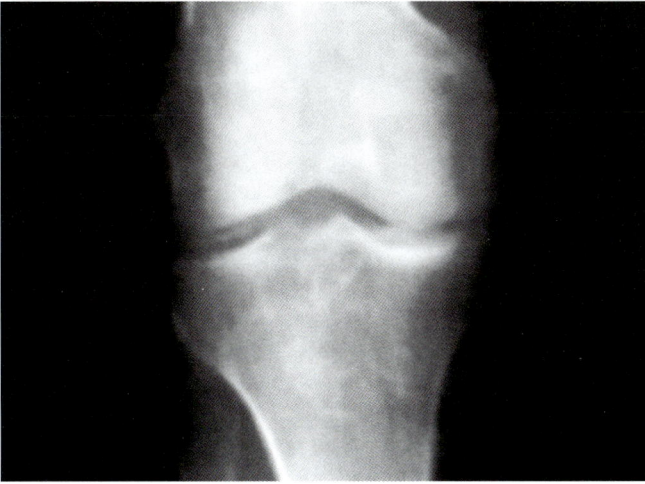

Fig. 41.33: Radiograph showing pseudogout in knee joint

Aspiration of the affected joint and intra-articular steroid injection terminates as acute attack of gout.

PSEUDOGOUT (CPPD)

Pseudogout is due to deposition of calcium pyrophosphate in the joints. Larger joints are more affected and 50 percent involve the knee joints unlike in gout (Fig. 41.33). Other areas commonly involved are elbows, wrists, ankles, shoulder and hip. Synovial fluid study under polarized microscopy reveals CPP crystals. The disease is not as severe as gout and is much rarer.

BIBLIOGRAPHY

1. Cach JE. Cash's Textbook of Orthopedics and Rheumatology for Physiotherapists. In: Downe DA (Ed). London, Boston, Faber and Faber; 1984.
2. Cooper NJ, Mageford M, et al. Secondary Health Service Care and second line drugs, costs of early inflammatory in Nortflok, UK. J Rheumatoid. 2000:27:2115-22.
3. Goldberg VM. Surgery for rheumatoid disease: Part 2: Early management of the rheumatoid joint. In American Academy of Orthopedic Surgeons. Instructional Course Lectures. Vol. 33, St Louis, The CV Mosby Co; 1984.
4. Hill DF, Holbrook WP. Prevention and treatment of deformities in rheumatoid arthritis. JAMA. 1950;142:718.
5. Imaging in rheumatology. Medicine International. 75,3100.
6. Neustadt DH. HLA antigens in rheumatic diseases. Orthop Rev. 1977;6:19.
7. Non-steroidal anti-inflammatory drugs. Medicine International. 75,3105.
8. Principles of the examination of a patient with rheumatic disease. Medicine International. 74,3085.
9. Snne DA. Surgery for rheumatoid arthritis; timing and techniques: general and medical aspects. J Bone and Joint Surg. 1968;50A:576.
10. Verdeck WN, McBeath AA. Knee synovectomy for rheumatoid arthritis. Clin Orthop. 1978;134:168.
11. Wynn Perry CB. Rehabilitation of the Hand, 4th edn. London: Butterworth's.

42 CHAPTER

Neuromuscular Disorders

CEREBRAL PALSY
(Syn: Static Encephalopathy)

Definition

This is a disorder of movement and posture caused by a non-progressive lesion in the immature brain, leading to global dysfunction.

Lesions

In cerebral palsy, the lesion could be in either the brain or the upper cervical cord, and the lesion is static.
Incidence is 0.6–5.9/1000 live birth.

Classification

Cerebral palsy is classified based on various clinical types and based on the degree of severity. This is depicted in Table 42.1.

TABLE 42.1: Classification of cerebral palsy

Based on clinical types (Minear's)	Based on severity
• Spastic (65%) (Commonest type)	• Mild (25%) Independent in daily activities
• Dyskinesia (25%) The following varieties are described: Athetosis Tremor Choreiform Dystonia Rigidity	• Moderate (50%) Needs help in daily activities and ambulation • Severe Patient is bedridden and has a wheelchair existence
• Ataxia	
• Mixed	

Lesions in the Brain

In cerebral palsy, the lesions in the brain can occur in the following four areas:
- Cerebral cortex (spastic type)
- Midbrain (dyskinesia)
- Cerebellum (ataxic)
- Widespread brain involvement (rigidity and mixed).

Causes

In cerebral palsy, the causes are different in prenatal, natal, postnatal and perinatal period and are listed as in Table 42.2.

Clinical Features

This depends on the location of lesions in the brain. Single muscle involvement is rare as in polio and entire portion of the body supplied by that area of brain is involved, the patients show delayed milestones and primitive reflexes are usually preserved (Fig. 42.1). Other clinical features depend on the geographic distribution of cerebral palsy and the associated handicapping situations (Table 42.3).

Orthopedic Deformities

The following are the common orthopedic deformities encountered in cerebral palsy (Figs 42.1A and B).

TABLE 42.2: Causes of cerebral palsy

Prenatal	Natal	Postnatal	Perinatal (0–7 days)
• Rubella infection • Fetal anoxia • Maternal diabetes	• Birth trauma • Anoxia • Prematurity	• Trauma • Encephalitis • Meningitis	• Most lesions causing CP occur during this period

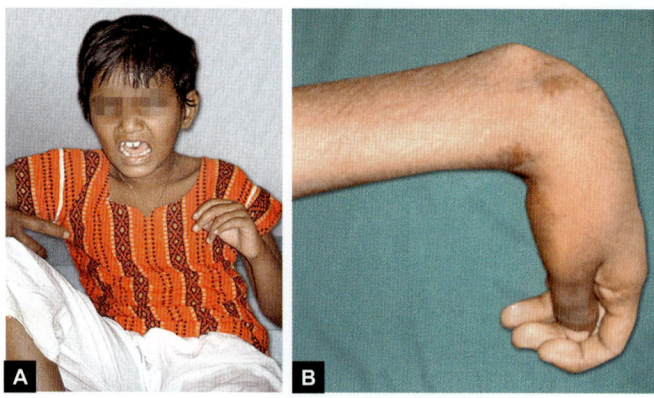

Figs 42.1A and B: Clinical photo of cerebral palsy

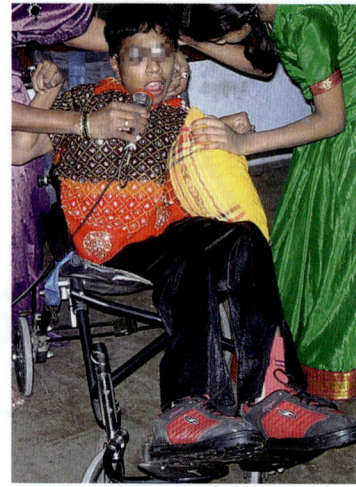

Fig. 42.2: Mental retardation and physical disabilities

TABLE 42.3: Clinical features of cerebral palsy

Geographic distribution of cerebral palsy	Associated handicapping conditions
• Monoplegia (0.3%)	• Sensory deficit in hand (50–60%)
• Hemiplegia (50%)	• Speech problems
• Paraplegia (21%)	• Mental retardation
• Triplegia (3.1%)	• Deafness
• Quadriplegia (25%)	• Visual defects
• Diplegia	• Seizures
• Double hemiplegia	• Perceptual problems
• Tetraplegia	• Emotional problems—most important
• Total body involvement	• Scoliosis

Note: Spasticity is a very common finding and its prominent features are hypertoncity, limp, contractures and hip dislocations.

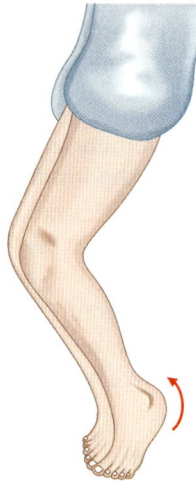

Fig. 42.3: Spastic contracture of the hip, knee and foot in cerebral palsy

Upper Limb
- Pronation contracture of the forearm.
- Flexion deformities of the wrist and fingers.
- Thumb in palm deformity.
- Swan neck deformity.
- Shoulder adduction and internal rotation deformity.

Lower Limb
- Adduction deformity (most common).
- Flexion and internal rotation deformity.
- Dysplastic and subluxated hip.
- Dislocated hip.
- Pelvic obliquity.

Spine
- Scoliosis
- Kyphoscoliosis.

Knee
- Genu recurvatum
- Genu valgum
- Patella alta
- Subluxation or dislocation of patella.
- Knee flexion contracture—(most common) (Fig. 42.2).

Foot
- Equinus deformity (Fig. 42.3)
- Varus or valgus (Fig. 42.4)
- Talipes equinovarus (Fig. 42.5)
- Calcaneus deformity
- Talipes cavus
- Hallux valgus
- Claw toes.

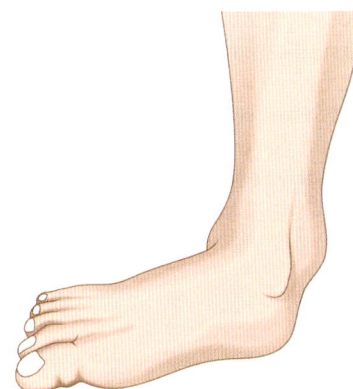

Fig. 42.4: Spastic equinovalgus

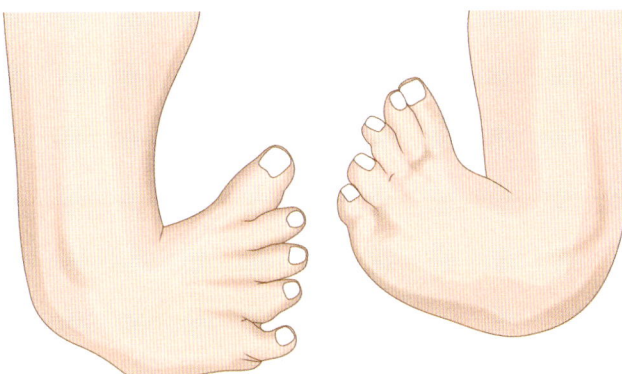

Fig. 42.5: Spastic equinovarus

Quick Facts

Common causes of CP
- Diplegia—seen in premature infants
- Athetoid—kernicterus
- Hemiplegia—trauma, cerebrovascular accidents, infection, etc.
- Quadriplegia—brain anoxia.

Treatment

Unfortunately, there is no cure for cerebral palsy. Hence, the *aim of treatment is to increase the patient's assets as much as possible and minimize his or her defects.*

Order of preference to improve the quality of life in cerebral palsy is as follows:
- Education and communication is the first priority.
- Activities of daily life.
- Mobility
- Ambulation.

The role of orthopedic surgeon starts when the child is 12 months of age and seldom before.

Methods

- *Motor age* test.
- *Physiotherapy*, occupational therapy, speech therapy, etc.

- *Use of braces* to:
  - Improve function.
  - Control unnecessary movements.
  - Prevent and correct deformities.

Drug therapy: The role of drug therapy is disappointing. Muscle relaxants, antiepileptic may have a role.

Surgery

- Not done till the child reaches five years of age.
- Indicated to correct deformity in an ambulatory patient and to make him or her socially more acceptable.
- Commonly indicated in spastic type of cerebral palsy.

Aim of Surgery in Cerebral Palsy is
- To correct the deformity.
- To balance the muscle power.
- To stabilize uncontrollable joints.

Choice of Surgery

Operation on nervous system: Sympathectomy, rhizotomy (see box) (anterior or posterior).

Operation on muscles and tendons:
- Tenotomy, tendon lengthening and tendon transfers.
- Myotomy and muscle transposition.

Operation on bones and joints:
- Bone lengthening or bone shortening to equalize the limb lengths.
- Osteotomies to correct knock knee, and other bone deformities.
- Arthrodesis of wrist, hip and foot to correct deformity, provide stability and to improve functions.

Vital Facts

About rhizotomy
- Popularized by Warwick Peacock of USA in 1980.
- This procedure consists of a selective severing of the distal rootlets of the cauda equina.
- Ideal patient is a spastic diplegic child at 3–8 years of age and who is quite ambulatory.
- This technique decreases the spastic tone without impairing sensation.

Pitfalls: It has no effect on shortened and contracted muscles and it is here that the orthopedic surgery helps.

Prognosis in Cerebral Palsy
- There is no permanent cure.
- Athetoid child is more intelligent than spastic child is.
- Twenty-five percent go to schools.
- Twenty-five percent are mentally retarded.
- Twenty-five percent are not educable.
- All hemiplegics will walk (by 12–16 months).
- Most diplegics will walk (by 4 years).
- Quadriplegics and total body involvement will never walk but can be propped sitters.

POLIOMYELITIS

Definition

This is a viral infection of the anterior horn cell of the spinal cord or nerve cells of brainstem, resulting in temporary or permanent paralysis. Common in children, often attacks young adults.

Viruses

The following Picorna group of viruses is known to cause poliomyelitis:
- Brunhilde (type I)
- Leon (type II)
- Lansing (type III).

Pathogenesis

The virus is transmitted through the feco-oral route, enters the nervous tissue, and destroys the anterior horn nerve cells because of which the peripheral nerve degenerates resulting in muscle and tendon atrophy (Fig. 42.6). The bones become small, the joint capsules and ligaments become lax, as there is no protection by the healthy muscles. All these results in development of various deformities.

Clinical Features

Polio usually affects children less than 12 months. There is a mild episode of fever, headache and diarrhea. On examination, there could be mild neck stiffness and the child may find it difficult to move the affected limb (preparalytic). The lower limbs are more commonly affected and the paralysis could be partial or total (paralytic stage) (Figs 42.7A to C) (Flowchart 42.1).

The paralysis of the muscles whether spinal (75%) or bulbar (25%) usually lasts until two months. Then there may or may not be recovery for a period of two years. Any residual paralysis after two years of affection is permanent with no chance of recovery (Fig. 42.8). Bulbar poliomyelitis is rare and affects the respiratory muscles. It may be fatal.

> **Quick Facts**
> *Features of paralysis due to polio*
> - Lower limb is more commonly affected than the upper limbs.
> - The involvement is asymmetric.
> - Though incomplete most of the times quadriceps are more often affected.
> - Tibialis anterior is most often completely paralyzed.
> - The sensory system is not affected.
> - In the residual stages (postpolio residual stages) the common deformities are (Fig. 42.9)
>   - Hip—Flexion, abduction and external rotation.
>   - Knee—Flexion, triple deformity and genu valgum.
>   - Foot—Talipes equinovarus.

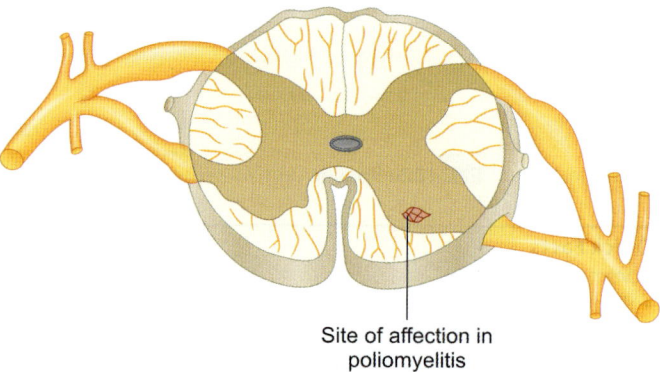

Fig. 42.6: Anterior horn cells are affected in poliomyelitis

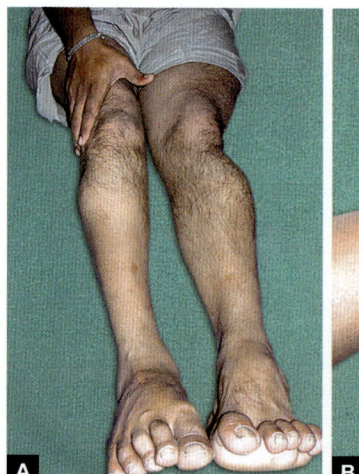
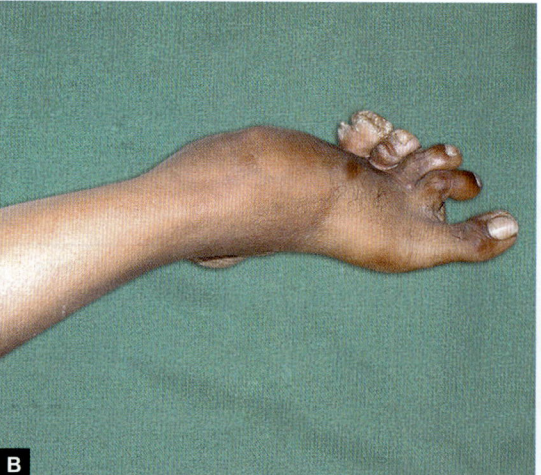
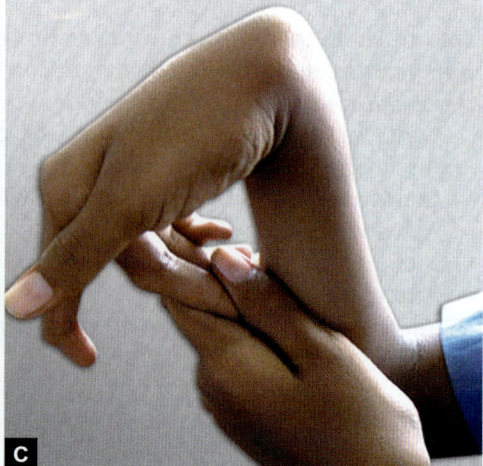

Figs 42.7A to C: Clinical photos of deformities in polio: (A) Lower limb; (B) Foot deformities; (C) Upper limb deformities

CHAPTER 42: Neuromuscular Disorders

Flowchart 42.1: Stages and their corresponding clinical features

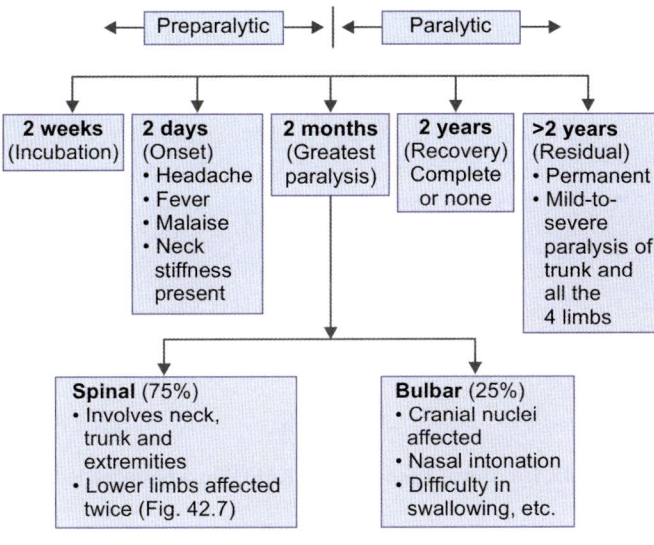

Orthopedic Deformities

Orthopedic deformities encountered in poliomyelitis are listed in Table 42.4.

Differential Diagnosis

Poliomyelitis has to be differentiated in the acute stages from:
- Pyogenic meningitis
- Guillain-Barré syndrome
- Postdiphtheritic paralysis
- Acute osteomyelitis
- Scurvy.

In the late stages from:
- Cerebral palsy
- Spina bifida
- Myopathies
- Muscular dystrophies, etc.

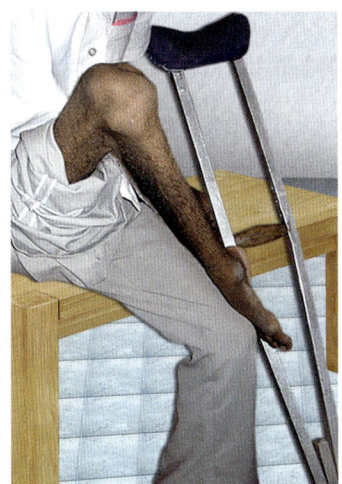

Fig. 42.8: PPRP due to polio

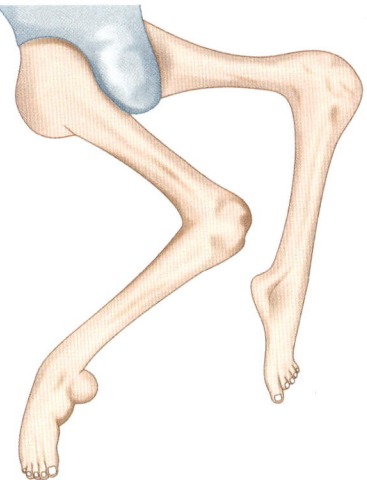

Fig. 42.9: Lower limb deformities in poliomyelitis

TABLE 42.4: Common orthopedic deformities encountered in poliomyelitis	
Foot and ankle	• Claw toes • Claw foot • Talipes equinus • Talipes equinovalgus • Flail foot • Pes cavus • Dorsal bunion • Talipes equinovarus • Talipes calcaneovalgus
Knee	• Flexion contracture of the knee • Quadriceps paralysis • Genu recurvatum • Flail knee
Hip	• Flexion abduction contractures of the hip • Paralysis of gluteus medius, maximus • Paralytic dislocation of hip
Iliotibial band contractures (Results in 9 classical deformities)	• Lumbar scoliosis • Pelvic obliquity • Hip flexed and abducted • External rotation of femur • Flexion and valgus of knee • Posterior and lateral subluxation of tibia • External rotation of tibia • Foot in equinus • Shortening
Spine	• Kyphosis • Scoliosis • Kyphoscoliosis
Upper limbs	• Paralysis of shoulder, elbow, forearm and hand muscles.

Treatment

Broad principles of the treatment
- To prevent deformities from developing.
- To assist returning of muscle power by graduated exercises.
- To reduce disability by appropriate appliance or by operations on joints and muscles.

Treatment Methods

Early stages: During the stages of onset, maximum paralysis and the stages of recovery the following treatment is recommended, the child is admitted into the hospital, and supportive treatment is given. The child is put on a ventilator support if there is respiratory paralysis due to bulbar polio. Warm and moist packs are given to the joints and all intramuscular injections are avoided during this phase. Plaster splints in functional positions immobilize the affected joints.

Recovery stages: In this stage, the joints are properly splinted through various appliances to prevent or correct the deformities (Table 42.5).

> **Quick Facts**
> *Conservative treatment*
> | | |
> |---|---|
> | Stage of onset | • Bed rest |
> | Stage of greatest paralysis | • Splints |
> | | • Artificial respiration, etc. |
> | Stage of recovery | • Physiotherapy |
> | | • Walking aid |
> | | • Crutches, etc. |
> | Stage of residual paralysis | • Can be corrected by provision of suitable |
> | | • Orthotic appliances or by operation |

Role of Appliances

The purpose of external appliances is to support joints that have lost their normal control (Fig. 42.10). They are more often required for lower limbs rather than upper limbs. The commonly prescribed appliances in Table 42.5.

TABLE 42.5: External appliances in poliomyelitis

Spinal brace	To support weak spine
Abdominal support	To check abdominal protrusion when abdominal muscles are weak
Hip, knee, ankle, foot orthosis with or without pelvic support	For deformities of the hip, when ankle
Knee caliper	To hold knee extended in quadriceps palsy
Below knee brace	To stabilize a flail ankle or foot
Single below knee (lateral or medial)	To control varus or valgus
Drop foot appliance	For mobile equinus deformity

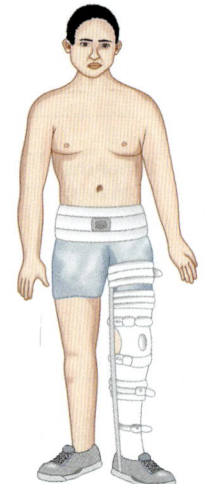

Fig. 42.10: Above knee caliper (KAFO) in a polio patient

Stage of Postpolio Residual Paralysis (PPRP)

During this stage, the role of orthopedic surgeon is predominant and surgery is the treatment of choice.

Goals of Surgery
- To obtain muscle balance.
- To prevent or correct soft tissue contractures.
- To prevent or correct bony deformities.

Surgical Methods

Soft tissue release for soft tissue contractures, e.g.
- *Soutter's release:* Structures arising from anterosuperior iliac spine are released for hip contractures.
- *Ober-Yount's procedure consists* of sectioning the iliotibial band (ITB) contractures.
- *Tendo-Achilles* lengthening for equinus deformity of the foot.
- *Steindler's release* of plantar fascia for cavus foot.

Tendon transfers: This is indicated when dynamic muscle imbalance produces deformity requiring brace protection.

Aims of tendon transfers
- To replace the function of a paralyzed muscle.
- To remove the deforming force.
- To provide stability by improving the muscle balance. Tendon transfers are not limited to any age group.

Arthrodesis: This is done to:
- Stabilize a flail joint.
- Eliminate the need for brace and to improve function.
- For permanent method of joint stabilization.

Osteotomies to correct deformities like genu valgum, etc.
Ilizarov's technique for leg length equalization and deformity corrections.

ARTHROGRYPOSIS MULTIPLEX CONGENITA [Syn: Multiple Congenital Contractures (MCC)]

In the year 1841, Otto first described AMC. Swinyard and Beck gave the name MCC. AMC is a non-progressive syndrome characterized by:
- Rigid and deformed joints.
- Muscle absence or atrophy.
- Cylindrical or ellipsoid joints with skin crease loss and subcutaneous atrophy.
- Contractures of capsules and periarticular structures.
- Dislocation of joints like hip and knee.
- Normal mentality and intact sensation.

Causes

Intrauterine immobilization of joints at various stages of development is due to:
- Myopathic cause seen in 10 percent of cases. Autosomal recessive.
- Neurogenic cause is due to reduced number or improper organization of anterior horn cells, peripheral nerves and motor end plates, weakness of muscles, etc.
- Mechanical causes like breech, twins, oligohydramnios amniotic bands, etc. which reduce the intrauterine space.

Classification (Sharrard, Brown and Robson)

Eight types: Two upper limb and six lower limb deformities are encountered. Common variety is quadriplegic type (Fig. 42.11A). Scoliosis is associated in 20 percent of the cases of AMC; webbing of the knees is seen in some.

Clinical Features

In AMC unlike other congenital anamalies, deformities are the main complaints (Fig. 42.11B). The following are the common orthopedic deformities in AMC:
- *Foot:* Planovalgus and equinovarus.
- *Knee:* Flexion contracture and fixed in extension.
- *Hip:* Extension, abduction, external rotation.
- *Shoulder:* Medial rotation of shoulder.
- *Elbow and wrist* Flexed.

Investigations

- Muscle biopsy.
- Electromyography.
- Nerve conduction studies.

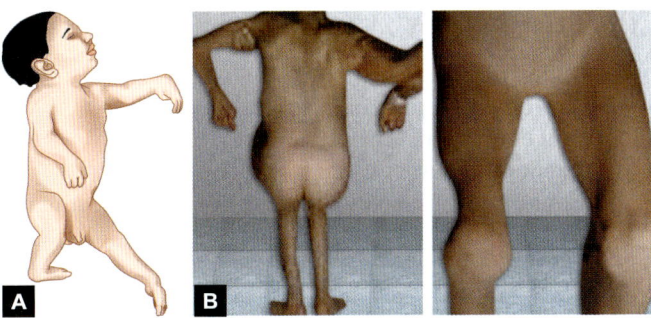

Figs 42.11A and B: (A) Quadriplegic type is the most common variety of arthrogryposis multiplex congenita (AMC); (B) Deformities in AMC (Clinical photo)

- Radiograph for scoliosis, dislocation, etc.
- Chromosomal studies.

Treatment

The treatment consists of passive stretching exercises, serial splinting of the limbs and surgical correction.

Principles of Orthopedic Treatment

- Muscle balance is to be restored if tendons are available for transfers.
- Recurrence is the rule due to tough inelastic capsule and soft tissues.
- Tenotomies should be accompanied by capsulotomy and capsulectomy.
- Osteotomies are to be carried out once skeletal growth is over, otherwise recurrence occurs.
- Maximum correction is to be obtained during the initial surgery. There is no role of wedging, etc.

LEPROSY IN ORTHOPEDICS

Leprosy is a chronic infectious disease caused by *Mycobacterium leprae*. It affects mainly the peripheral nerves and affects the skin, muscles, bones, testes and internal organs.

National Leprosy Eradication Program
It was launched in 1983, with the goal of arresting the disease by the turn of century based on multidrug therapy.

Problem of Leprosy in India
- Four million cases.
- Prevalence rate—5.7/1000.
- Fifteen to twenty percent cases of population are multibacillary.
- Twenty percent result in deformities.

Classification

Three classifications are proposed as given in Table 42.6.

Clinical Features

In early stages
- Hypopigmented patches (Fig. 42.12)
- Loss of cutaneous sensation.
- Thickened nerves.
- Presence of acid-fast bacilli in the skin or nasal smears.

In late stages
- Trophic ulcers.
- Foot-drop/claw toes.
- Claw hand.
- Nasal bridge collapse.
- Loss of fingers or toes.

Investigations

- Bacteriological examination of material obtained from the skin or nasal smears.
- Foot pad culture of mice is 10 times more sensitive than the skin slit smears.
- Histamine test.
- Biopsy.
- Immunological tests.

Tests for detecting CMI
- Lepromin test
- Lymphocyte transformation test.

Tests for detecting humoral antibodies
- Enzyme-linked immunosorbent assay (ELISA) test, etc.

Treatment

General Measures

Primary prevention by vaccine is not possible, so leprosy control is based on effective chemotherapy in Table 42.7. If Clofazimine is not acceptable, Ethionamide—250-375 mg/day.

Duration of treatment is at least for two years until smear is negative.

BCG vaccine showed a high degree of protection in 80 percent and 30 percent in some cases.

ORTHOPEDIC AFFECTIONS IN LEPROSY

Ankle and Foot

Every kind of deformity is seen in the foot. Deformity is gross, because patient continues to use the foot due to loss of sensations. Ankle is rarely affected in this disease (Table 42.8).

In leprosy, due to loss of sensation, there is absence of warning pain because of which, there is injury. Secondary infection following the injury is common.

Classification of Foot Deformities in Leprosy

This classification is shown in Table 42.8.

TABLE 42.6: Classification of leprosy

Indian	Madrid	Ridley and Joppling
Indeterminate	Indeterminate	Tuberculoid
Tuberculoid	Borderline	Borderline tuberculoid
Lepromatous	Tuberculoid	Lepromatous
Borderline	Lepromatous	Borderline both
Neuritic		Lepromatous

TABLE 42.7: Drug treatment in leprosy

Multibacillary	Paucibacillary
Ripampicin 600 mg/month	R-cin 600 mg/month for 6 months
Dapsone 100 mg/day	+
Clofazimine 300 mg/month	Dapsone 100 mg/day for 6 months

TABLE 42.8: Classification of foot deformities in leprosy

Forefoot	Midfoot	Hind foot
• Plantar ulcers • Toe deformities • Chronic osteomyelitis of metatarsals • MTP joints destruction	• Aseptic necrosis of talus, etc. • Infective arthritis and osteomyelitis • Degenerative arthrolysis • Proliferative ankylosing arthropathy	• Chronic osteomyelitis of calcaneum • Plantar ulcers • Calcaneal spur • Gross destruction

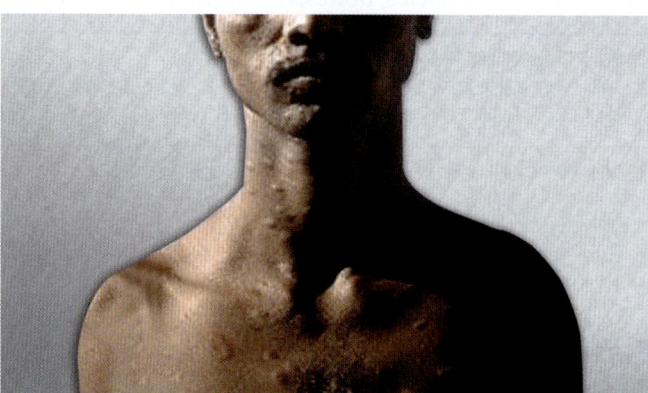

Fig. 42.12: Patches on the body (Clinical photo)

FOOT-DROP

This is one of the very common complications encountered in leprosy. It is seen in 2 percent of the cases.
- Common peroneal nerve is more commonly involved.
- Usually, it is completely damaged, sometimes only deep peroneal or superficial branch is involved.
- Occasionally, only external hallucis longus muscle is involved.

Consequence of Paralysis

- Foot-drop, drop toes, inversion and plantar flexion of the foot is decreased (Refer page 334).
- High stepping gait.
- Instability of gait.
- Deformity due to contractures of tendo calcaneus and capsules of subtalar and ankle joints.
- Fixed equinovarus deformity.
- Destruction of foot.

Plain X-ray of the foot-shows destruction and deformities (Fig. 42.13).

Treatment

Conservative Methods

For recent or incomplete drop foot: Toe raising spring, physiotherapy, short wave diathermy, ultrasound, local steroids, etc. are the recommended forms of treatment.

Surgery

If more than one year after affection or if the lesion is complete, surgical correction is needed.
Before the surgical correction, ensure the following:
- Noninvolvement of medial plantar nerve.
- No contractures of tendo-Achilles.
- At least 20° of dorsiflexion should be present. Tendo-Achilles shortening requires physiotherapy in the early stages and in the later stages tendo-Achilles lengthening.

Surgical Methods

- When there is no contracture and if the foot is mobile, tibialis posterior transfer is indicated.
- Triple arthrodesis of Lambrinudi for fixed equinovarus deformity of the foot.

PLANTAR ULCERS

This is the other important foot complication in leprosy. It is also known as trophic ulcers due to neurological deficit. It has a spontaneous onset, it is painless, persists, and recurs. Healing process is not defective. Recurrent ulceration causes progressive destruction of the skeleton.

Sites: Plantar ulcers are commonly seen over the ball of feet, especially the first metatarsal, and heel (Fig. 42.14).

Treatment

Aims

- To get the ulcer healed.
- To prevent its recurrence.

Treatment Methods

Various methods of treating the plantar ulcers are mentioned in Table 42.9.

AFFECTIONS OF THE HAND IN LEPROSY

The following are the common hand deformities encountered in leprosy (Fig. 42.15).

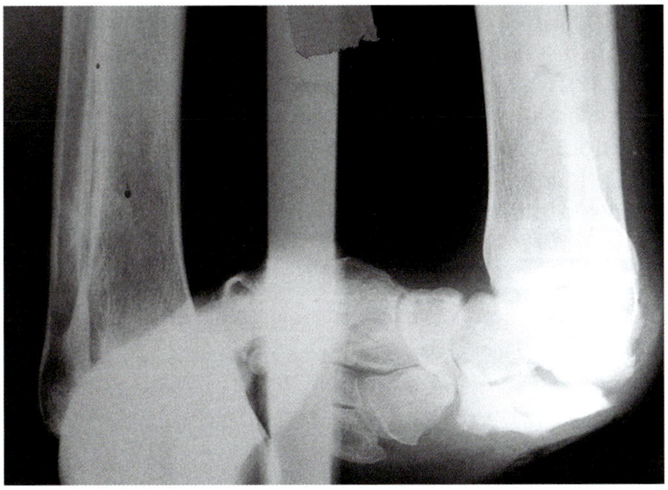

Fig. 42.13 : Radiograph of the foot in leprosy

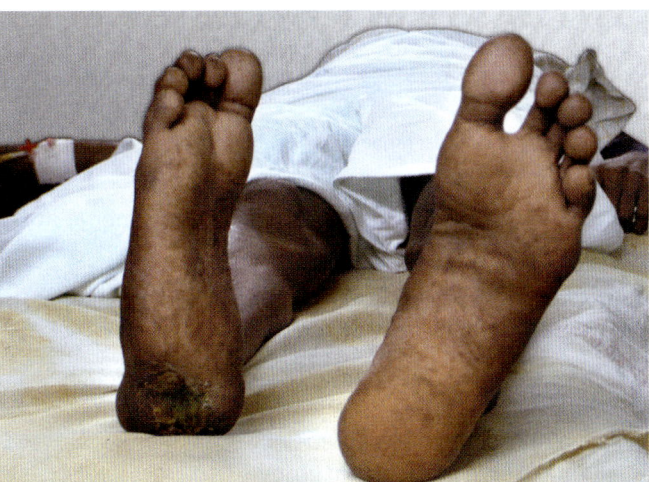

Fig. 42.14: Plantar ulcers in leprosy (Clinical photo)

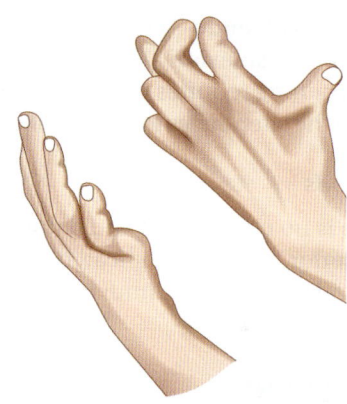

Fig. 42.15: Hand deformities in leprosy

TABLE 42.9: Treatment plan in plantar ulcers

I. To heal the ulcer	II. To prevent recurrence
Principles Provide rest Control infection Promote healing	1. Nonsurgical measures • Healthy instructions • Protective footwear – To protect skin from injury—use tough outer sole
State of ulcer 1. If acute • Rest, elevation • Eusol applications • Antibiotics • Incision and drainage • Dressing	– To reduce stress of walking—use MCR in sole – To relieve vulnerable sites from pressure modification of footwear or use orthosis
2. If chronic: • Rest • Below knee caliper • Below knee plaster cast	**Methods to relieve pressure** – Metatarsal bar (20%) – Arch support (30%) – moulded insole (40%) – PTB cast rest
3. Complicated ulcer: When it spreads to deeper structures like bone, joints, tendon, etc. • Ulcer debridement • Once infection is controlled treat it later as chronic ulcer as mentioned above • Protective footwear later	2. **Surgical measures** Supplements and not substitutes for non-surgical measures **Methods** • Scar excision • Osteotomies • Arthrodesis • Resection, etc. depending on indications

Note: MCR—microcellular rubber.

Ulnar claw hand is due to affection of ulnar nerve at the elbow.

Total claw hand is due to the affection of ulnar nerve at the elbow and median nerve at the wrist.

Triple nerve palsy: The following nerves are affected:
- Ulnar nerve at the elbow.
- Median nerve at the wrist.
- Radial nerve at the spiral groove.

See page 325 for more details on claw hand.

Surgery for Hand

Brand's many tailed tendon transfer operation (EF_4T): Developed by Paul Brand at the Christian Medical College, Vellore, Tamil Nadu, India.

Extensor carpi radialis longus is released from its insertion and brought into the flexor aspect of the forearm. Free graft from palmaris longus tendon is taken and is split into four strips, which are then attached to the extensor expansion of the respective fingers (EF_4T).

Restoration for opponens palsy: Flexor digitorum superficialis is detached from its insertion rooted through the palm and attached to the lateral margin of the extensor expansion.

Ulnar claw hand S. Bunnel's operation (refer Chapter on Peripheral Nerve Injuries).

Triple nerve palsy this is difficult to correct surgically.

MUSCULAR DYSTROPHIES

These are difficult problems to treat and the cause is usually not known.

Classification

Three types namely sex-linked recessive, autosomal dominant and autosomal recessive, are described. This is shown in Table 42.10.

[1]DUCHENNE MUSCULAR DYSTROPHY

This is the most common type of muscular dystrophy encountered in clinical practice.

Clinical Features

This consists of delayed walking, abnormal gait and multiple falls (in less than 3 years child does). Gower's sign is positive (Fig. 42.16), hypertrophy of calf muscles, waddling gait, increased lumbar lordosis, weakness of shoulder muscles around 5–6 years, serrati, pectorals, deltoid, latissimus dorsi, biceps, triceps and brachialis muscles are weak. In lower limbs weakness of hip flexors, evertors of feet,

TABLE 42.10: Classification of muscular dystrophies

Sex-linked recessive	Autosomal dominant	Autosomal recessive
• Duchene's	• Facioscapulohumeral	• Limb girdle
• Becker's	• Scapuloperoneal	• Childhood variety
• Emery and Dreifus	• Distal	• Congenital dystrophy
	• Oculopharyngeal	• Limited to quadriceps

---
[1]**Guillaume BA Duchenne** (1806–1875), a French Neurologist, described muscular dystrophy.

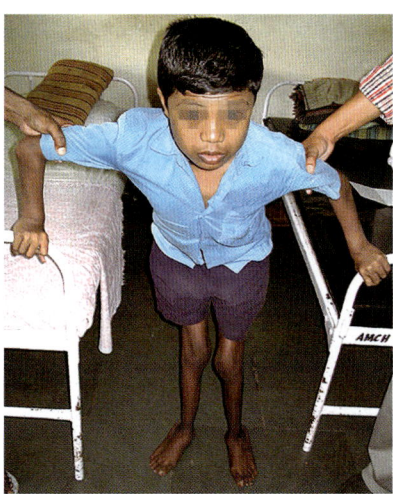

Fig. 42.16: Posture and gait in Duchenne dystrophy (Clinical photo)

tibialis anterior are seen, ocular; pharyngeal and masticator muscles are never involved. Knee jerk is absent earlier than ankle jerk. Tendo-Achilles contractures appear first, later hamstrings, hip flexors and elbow follow. Intellectual impairment is present. Death below 16 years is due to respiratory infection or cardiac failure.

Investigations

- Serum glutamic oxaloacetic tranzminase (SGOT), serum glutamate pyruvate transaminase (SGPT), lactate dehydrogenase$_5$ (LDH$_5$) aldolase and creatine phosphokinste (CPK) levels are raised.
- Muscle biopsy and electromyography (EMG) helps.
- Electrocardiogram (ECG) shows biventricular hypertrophy.

FACIOSCAPULOHUMERAL MUSCULAR DYSTROPHY

This is seen in second decade of life and the fascial musculature is involved early. The patient complains of inability to close the eyes, slurred speech, etc. Elevation of the scapula on abduction is characteristic. In the upper limbs, deltoid and wrist flexors are spared. In the lower limbs, anterior tibial muscle is involved earlier. Majority of the patient suffering from this dystrophy have a normal life span.

LIMB GIRDLE MUSCULAR DYSTROPHY

It is seen in the second or third decade. Lower limb girdle weakness appears first followed by upper limb. Muscular hypertrophy is rare. Winging of the scapula is seen. There is no involvement of cardia.

Treatment for Muscular Dystrophies

This consists of physiotherapy, mental and physical support, speech therapy, and mechanical aids like splints, walking aids, etc.

NEURAL TUBE DEFECTS (DYSTROPHISM)

SPINA BIFIDA

Definition

Neural tube defects are due to failure of neutralization of the primitive neural tube between the 3rd and 4th week *in utero*.

This is due to the failure of the fusion of the two vertebral arches in the embryological stages of development usually during the 17th to 35th day after conception. The failure of fusion could be limited, only to the spinous process resulting in spina bifida occulta, the most common variety or the entire vertebral arch including the neural elements may fail to fuse giving rise to the rare variety of spina bifida aperta.

> **Note:**
> Spina bifida is a Latin term, which means, "split or open spine".

SPINA BIFIDA OCCULTA

This is the most common variety and is generally mild. Lumbosacral spine and the first sacral vertebra are commonly affected.

Clinical Features

The overlying skin may be normal or there may be presence of a tuft of hair, pigmentation, lipoma, dimple, etc.

There may be muscle imbalance in the lower limbs resulting in equinovarus or cavus deformity of the foot due to tethering of the cord by a membrane either to the skin or filum terminale. Rarely, there could be a bifid cord.

Treatment

Asymptomatic cases require no treatment except physiotherapy and back exercises. Surgical correction of foot deformities is as discussed in earlier chapters.

SPINA BIFIDA APERTA OF MANIFESTA

> **A Must Know Facts**
> - About 80–90 percent infants born with NTDs survive.
> - In India, about 107,814 children are born with NTDs every year.

Causes

The actual cause is still unknown. However, the likely causes are:
- Poor economic status
- Alcohol use
- Vitamin A deficiency
- Folic acid deficiency
- Familial
- Maternal use of valproic acid.

Note:
Incidence of spina bifida is 1/1000 live births.

Here the defect involves the vertebral arches, skin, meninges and cord. The following varieties are described (Figs 42.17A to D):

Meningocele in which there is protrusion of the meninges (4%).

Myelomeningocele in which there is protrusion of meninges and cord (96%) (Fig. 42.18).

Syringomyelocele in which the central canal of the cord is dilated and the cord is protruded.

Myelocele in which the central cord remains unfused and exposed.

Next to spina bifida occulta, myelocele is the next common variety. Most of the cases of spina bifida aperta either are still born or die within a few days of birth. The surviving children may suffer from paralysis and complex severe orthopedic deformities, bladder and bowel incontinence and foot deformities (Figs 42.19A and B).

Do You Know What Orthopedic Problems are Encountered in Myelomeningocele?
- Kyphosis (10–20%)
- Scoliosis (42–90%)
- Hip dislocations
- Congenital clubfeet.

Moreover, what about associated CNS defects:
- Congenital hydrocephalus (most common)
- Acquired hydrocephalus
- Tethered cord syndrome leading to traction injury of the cord and cauda equina
- Syringomyelia (40%).

Investigations

Early Diagnostic Tools to Detect Neural Tube Defects (Dysraphism)

- *Ultrasound scanning*: Sensitivity is 96–100 percent
- Specificity is 30–80 percent.
- *Amniotic fluid examinations*: This is to detect the presence of α-fetoprotein (AFP) and acetyl cholinesterase levels by 15–16 weeks.
- Estimation of AFP in maternal serum.

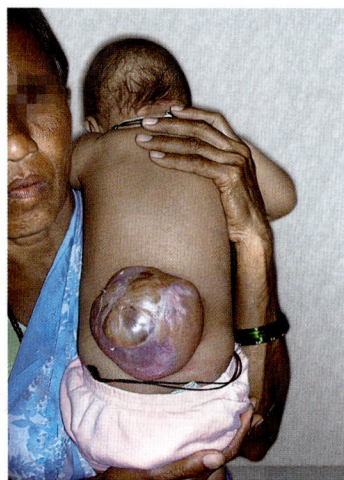

Fig. 42.18: Myelomeningocele (Clinical photo)

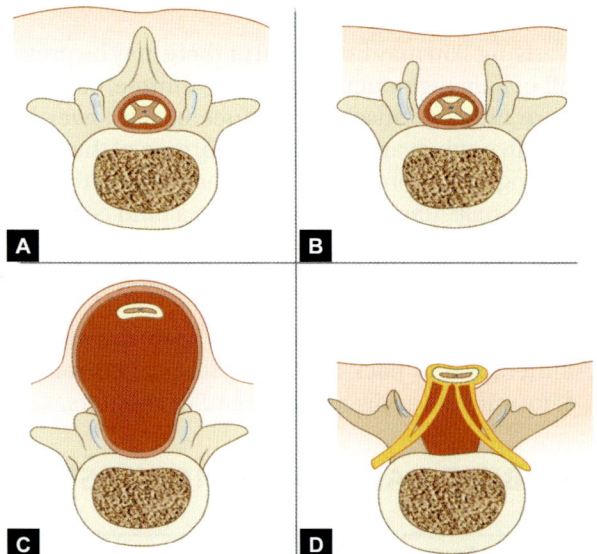

Figs 42.17A to D: Different types of spina bifida: (A) Spina bifida occulta; (B) Spina bifida aperta (meningocele); (C) Myelomeningocele; (D) Myelocele

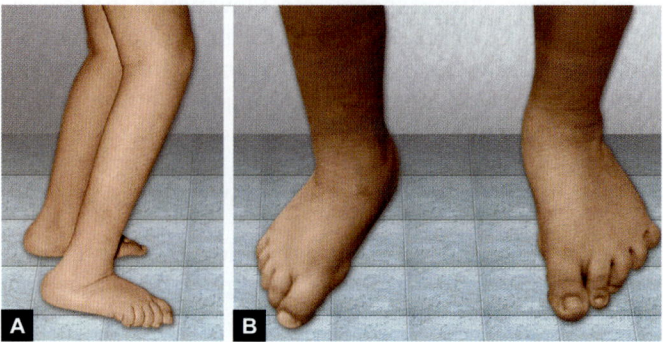

Figs 42.19A and B: Orthopedic deformities due to spina bifida

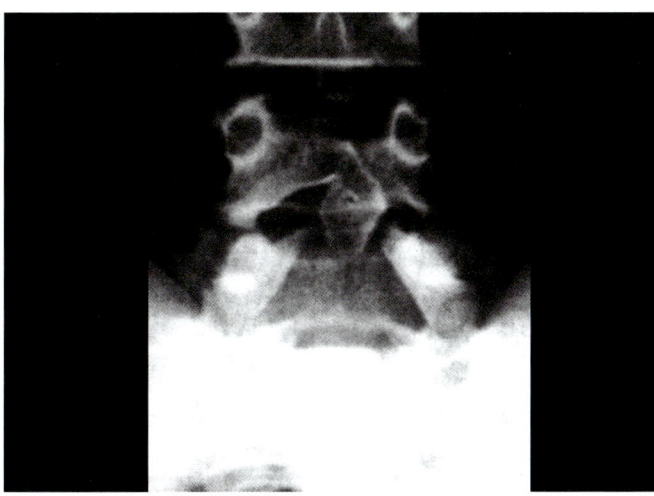

Fig. 42.20: Radiograph showing spina bifida

Other Investigations

- *Radiology:* X-ray of the LS spine (AP/Lat/Oblique) helps to detect this abnormality (Fig. 42.20).
- CT scan and MRI are extremely useful in studying the entire spectrum of this problem.

Treatment

Preventive Measures

Needless to say, that this is the most easiest and effective way of tackling this menace. Instead of trampling the head of this unkind problem, it is better to see that it does not raise its ugly head in the first place. Some of the recommended measures are:
- All pregnant women should take folic acid or fortified folic acids during the period of pregnancy.
- Dose of folic acid:
  - In all women — about 400 mcg/day
  - In high-risk and those with familial history, previous history of NTD's birth, etc.
  - 4000 mcg/day for 3–4 months before conception.

Curative Measures

Surgery are the treatment of choice to close the neural tube defects or correct the orthopedic deformities. Surgery to close NTDs should be done within 24 hours after birth to preserve the function of the spinal cord and minimize infection. Shunting operation is performed to tackle the associated hydrocephalus.

Treatment is aimed to surgically correct the spina bifida, foot deformities and other orthopedic deformities. Bladder incontinence may require urological treatment.

BIBLIOGRAPHY

Cerebral Palsy

1. Baker LD. A rationale approach to the surgical needs of the cerebral palsy patient. J Bone Joint Surg. 1956;38-A: 313.
2. Bax MCO. Terminology and classification of cerebral palsy. Dev Med Child Neurol. 1964;6:295.
3. Bleck EE. Orthopedic management of cerebral palsy. Philadelphia: WB Saunders; 1979.
4. Bost FC, Ashley RK, Kelly WJ. Role of the orthopedic surgeon in the treatment of cerebral palsy. JAMMA. 1956;160-256.
5. Lord J. Cerebral palsy: A clinical approach. Arch Phys Med Rehabil. 1984;65:542.
6. Person P, Williams CE. Physical Therapy Services in the Developmental Disabilities. Springfield III, Charles C Thomas; 1980.
7. Steindler A. Orthopedic operations Springfield, III, Charles C Thomas, Publisher; 1940.

Poliomyelitis

1. Barr JS. The management of poliomyelitis: The late stage: In poliomyelitis. First International Poliomyelitis Congress, Philadelphia: JB Lippincott Co; 1949.
2. Goldner JL, Irwin CE. Paralytic deformities of the foot. In American Academy of Orthopedic Surgeons: Instructional Course Lectures, Vol 5, Ann Arbor, and JW Edwards; 1948.
3. Perry J, Barmes G. The postpolio syndrome. Clin Orthop. 1988;233:145.
4. Shar WJ. Muscle recovery in poliomyelitis. J Bone J Surg 1955;37-B:163.
5. Steindler A. Orthopedic operations: Indications, techniques and results. Springfield III, Charles C Thomas, Publisher; 1940.

Spina Bifida

1. Allan JH. The challenge of spina bifida cystica. In: Adams JP (Ed), Current Practice in Orthopedic Surgery. St Louis. CV Mosby Co, Vol II; 1963.
2. Sharard WJW. The orthopedic management of spina bifida. Acta Orthop Scand. 1975;46:356.

43 CHAPTER

Bone Neoplasias

INTRODUCTION

Like other systems in the body, musculoskeletal system may also develop tumors, either as a primary from this system itself or as a secondary from a distant primary location. The *latter appears to be more common.* Some of the tumors are benign and others are malignant. The accurate diagnosis of a neoplasm is necessary before planning the treatment strategy. Diagnosis is best established by history, a proper physical examination and investigations like histological examination, biochemical assays, X-ray, CT scan, MRI, bone scans, arteriography, ultrasound, biopsy (both frozen section and permanent paraffin section), etc.

Primary bone tumors may be benign or malignant. Here is a quick review of the differences between benign and malignant tumors (Table 43.1).

Since the cells of the skeletal system are derived from the mesoderm, primary malignant bone tumors are called *sarcomas.*

Tumors spreading secondarily to the bone are generally primary carcinomas of breast, kidney, thyroid and lung. These tumors are called *metastatic carcinomas* because the tissue of origin is ectoderm.

Tumor cells may produce either tumor bone or osteoid (e.g. osteogenic sarcoma) or may cause reactive bone formation. Periosteal response may also be seen (e.g. Codman's triangle or onion peel appearance, etc.).

Treatment of benign tumors is usually by excision and if the defect is large, it is packed with bone grafts. Malignant tumors require a multipronged approach in the form of surgery, radiation, chemotherapy, immunotherapy, etc. With a combination of the above modalities of treatment, the recurrence rate has dropped considerably.

Knowledge of the origin, biologic behavior and treatment of bone tumors is quite incomplete now and much of the information is conflicting and controversial.

GENERAL PRINCIPLES OF TUMORS

A proper understanding of the general principles of tumors enables one to make a correct diagnosis, choose the correct line of treatment, which helps to minimize the recurrence rate and improve the survival rate.

The following are the parameters of general principles of tumors.

History

Salient features are:
- Pain, mass, disability is the usual presenting symptoms.
- Anorexia, weight loss and fever are more pronounced in malignant tumors.
- Onset—it is acute in malignant tumors and insidious in benign tumors.
- Age—certain tumors have predilection for certain age groups, e.g. Ewing's sarcoma has a predilection for children.

TABLE 43.1: Differences between benign and malignant tumors

Benign tumors	Malignant tumors
• Slow growing	• Rapidly growing
• Well circumscribed	• Not well circumscribed
• Non-invading	• Invading
• No or few symptoms	• Associated with pain and disability
• Does not metastasise	• Metastasises
• X-ray shows lesions bone	• X-ray shows ill-defined borders, mottled appearance, cortex may be broken
• Does not cause death of the patient	• May cause death of the patient

Clinical Examination

General examination for evidence of anemia, cachexia, lymphadenopathy, etc.

Local examination to know the extent, plane of the tumor, presence of pathological fractures, etc.

Joint examination to know the involvement of the joint, mechanical effects, etc.

Neurological examination to assess the damage to the peripheral nerves due to the spread of tumor.

Assessment of the status of arterial and/or venous circulation.

Investigations

Routine Laboratory Investigation

Hb percentage is decreased, total WBC count and differential count is increased or decreased, ESR is increased, urinalysis. Serum calcium and phosphorous is increased, serum alkaline phosphatase is increased in tumors like osteogenic sarcoma, serum acid phosphatase is increased in metastatic tumors, etc.

Special Investigations

Radiological examination of the part is done in two planes anteroposterior and lateral.

Chest radiographs for evidence of secondaries.

CT scan detects pulmonary metastasis at the earliest. It picks up the metastasis of the size of 2 mm compared to X-ray, which does so at 2 cm size. It also helps in cross-sectional study of the tumor.

Arteriography: This helps to determine the spread of the tumor to the vessel.

Ultrasonography: This helps in some situations, though it has a very limited role.

MRI: This is the most accurate method of assessing the bone and soft tissue involvement. It also helps in assessing the medullary spread of the tumor.

Bone scans help to detect the extent of spread of bone tumor to other areas of skeletal system and to detect occult bone metastasis.

Biopsy: This is an ultimate diagnostic technique in diagnosing bone tumors (Flowchart 43.1).

Usually, closed biopsies are preferred in malignant tumors. Needle biopsy has an accuracy rate of over 90 percent in malignant tumors. If incisional biopsy is chosen, the incision should be placed longitudinally and should not exceed more than 2 cm.

Types

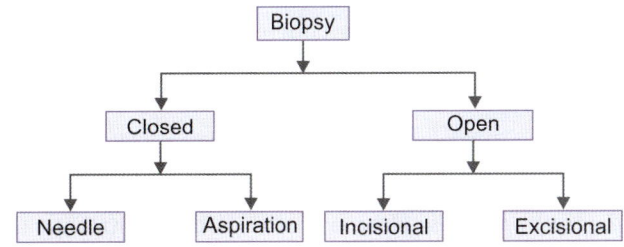

Flowchart 43.1: Types of biopsy

Remember
Tumor biopsy rules
- In malignant tumors, remove the tumor *en bloc*.
- No transverse incisions.
- No important neurovascular structures should be exposed.
- It should traverse only one compartment.
- Collect the sample from periphery of the tumor.
- If bone sample is to be taken, make a small circular or oval hole in the bone to prevent pathological fracture.

All the above investigations help to stage the bone tumor. Staging helps in detecting the type of surgical procedures needed for local control of the tumor.

Enneking's Staging

Enneking's staging is based on three criteria, histological grading, anatomical site, presence or absence of regional or distant metastasis.

IA   *Low-grade:* Intracompartmental (lesion confined to single anatomical plane).

IB   *Low-grade:* Extracompartmental (beyond a single compartment).

IIA *High-grade:* Intracompartmental.

IIB *High-grade:* Extracompartmental.

III   *Lesion high- or low-grade:* Intra- or extracompartmental with distant or regional metastasis.

The high- or low-grade is a histological grading done based on changes within the cells like pleomorphism, anaplasia, multicellularity, etc. due to malignancy.

0 = benign; 1 = low-grade malignancy; 2 = high-grade malignancy.

Surgical Techniques

Curettage

Many benign bone tumors and locally malignant tumors are treated this way, but it leaves microscopic remnants. It gives good results if combined with cryosurgery, bone cement, or allograft, etc. If the lesion is diaphyseal, bone grafting is rarely necessary but if it is epiphyseal or metaphyseal, allografting is necessary. Since curettage alone is associated with a high rate of recurrence, its role is limited.

Resection or Excision

Tumor removing procedures not involving amputation are called as local (limb sparing) excision or resection. It may be any one of the following.

Debulking or intralesional excision: Here excision is done within the lesion.

Marginal margins: Here excision is done through the pseudocapsule, which is a thin rim of fibrous tissue formed by the surrounding tissues due to the compression, by the tumor mass.

Wide margin: Here the excision is carried out through the surrounding normal tissues. It is not useful in high-grade tumors because here the spread is along the fascial planes and this method still leaves some metastasis.

Radical resection: Here all normal tissues of one or more compartments involved are removed from the origin to the insertion.

Radical amputation: Here amputation is done at a high level.

Extracorporeal irradiated and reimplantation (ECIR) with composite arthroplasty: Here autogenous bone graft is either autoclaved or irradiated and reimplanted back combined with conventional arthroplasty which is fast emerging as an alternative to limb salvage surgery.

Choice of the Surgical Procedures

Surgery is usually advocated for local control of the tumor. Enneking's staging of the tumor decides the choice of surgery as suggested below.

Grade IA	:	Requires local procedure
Grade IB	:	Wide excision
Grade IIA	:	Radical excision
Grade IIB	:	Radical amputation
Grade III	:	Multipronged approach likes surgery + chemotherapy + radiotherapy

Adjunctive Therapy

Radiotherapy

It should not be used for benign tumors (exception, pigmented villonodular synovitis) for the fear of inducing malignant changes within the cells. Its role is mainly *palliative* in non-resectable malignant tumors; but sometimes, it has a *definitive role* in shrinking the size of the tumor making the surgery less traumatic, and it is also known to make the cells *non-viable* and thereby minimize the chances of metastasis elsewhere, when these cells get into the circulation during the surgical procedure.

Chemotherapy

This is the treatment of choice for micrometastasis with almost 100 percent cure rate. If it is given early, it prevents the formation of metastasis. If given late, it shrinks the size of the tumor and thereby facilitates excision. It is highly effective against small tumors when given in combinations. Dosage, sequence, schedule and proper monitoring are matter of extreme importance.

Frequently, a combination of treatment modalities like radiotherapy, chemotherapy, etc. is used along with surgery. In these cases, less radical surgery are used to achieve local control. Limb sparing procedures are preferred over amputations.

Newer Modalities of Treatment

Hyperthermia: This is usually tried in combinations with radiotherapy or chemotherapy.

Therapeutic embolization: Embolizing agents like gelfoam, PVA particles, pure alcohol, etc when introduced through a selective catheter placed in an arterial or venous vessel helps achieve thrombus formation and occlusion leading to ischemia and necrosis in the center of bone tumor.

Immunotherapy: Bacille-Calmette-Guérin (BCG) vaccines are found to be of use in control of certain tumors. The above three treatment modalities are at an experimental stage and are outside the scope of discussion here.

CLASSIFICATION OF BONE TUMORS

Various classifications have been proposed for bone tumors like Dahlin's classification, Mercer's classification, Turek's classification, etc. The ABC classification of *Bristol Bone Tumor Registry* proposed by *Charles Price* is by far the easiest to understand and remember (Table 43.2).

BONE TUMORS OF CARTILAGINOUS ORIGIN

OSTEOCHONDROMA (Exostosis)

This is the most common benign bone tumor. It is an offshoot from the spongy bone tissue covered with a cartilaginous cap (size of the cap may vary from 1–40 cm).

Age: It is common during the growth period.

Sex: It has a male preponderance.

TABLE 43.2: Classification of bone tumors

Section	Benign	Malignant
Section A Angioid tumors	• Angioma • Aneurysmal bone cyst • Glomus tumor	• Angiosarcoma
Section B Bone forming tumor	• Osteoma • Osteoblastoma	• Osteosarcoma • Parosteal osteosarcoma
Section C Cartilage forming tissue	• Osteoid osteoma • Chondroma • Osteochondroma • Chondroblastoma	• Chondrosarcoma
Section D Dental and allied structure	• Odontogenic cyst • Ameloblastoma	• Malignant odontoma
Section E Embryonic vestigial tissue		• Chordoma
Section F Fibroblastic	• Fibroma	• Fibrosarcoma
Section H Heterotropic tissue	• Dermoid	• Adamantinoma of long bones
Section N Nonosseus connective tissue	• Lipoma • Neurofibroma • Neurilemmoma	• Liposarcoma • Reticulum cell sarcoma • Myeloma • Leukemia • Hodgkin's • Ewing's
Section S Synovial tissue	• Synovioma	• Leiomyosarcoma
Section U Undifferentiated connective tissue	• Chondroma • Osteoclastoma	• Synovial sarcoma • Malignant osteoclastoma
Section X	• Undiagnosed primary bone tumors	• Undiagnosed primary bone tumors

Area: Location favors the sites of *tendinous attachments,* which are usually around the metaphysis of long bones in the region of knee, ankle, hip, shoulder and elbow.

Theory of Histogenesis

- Though the exact cause is not known various theories have been postulated suggesting the possible mechanism of origin of this tumor. The cambium layer of the periosteum retains throughout life its ability to form cartilage and bone. It may be due to perverted activity of the periosteum that it reverts to its role as the "perichondrium".
- At points of tendinous insertion, there is focal accumulation of embryonic connective tissue.

Clinical Features

Symptoms

Usually, it is symptom less, but the patient may complain of pain, swelling, etc. once complications like bursitis, malignant change, fracture, etc. have developed (Fig. 43.1A).

Signs

A firm nontender swelling fixed to the bone around the joints is the most common clinical finding (Figs 43.2A and B). A bursa if inflamed will give rise to tenderness and local warmth. Joint movements may be decreased because of the tumor causing a mechanical block rather than the extension of the tumor into the joint.

Radiographs

This consists of an outgrowth of bone at the metaphysis. This attachment is sessile or pedunculated. The tumor is composed of cortical and medullary portions, which are *continuous with the main bone.* The cartilage and capsules are not seen *unless it calcifies* (Figs 43.1B to D).

Treatment

Usually, it requires no treatment, but complete surgical excision is indicated in the following situations (Fig. 43.3):

Joint interference: If the tumor is large and obstructing the joint movements, it needs excision of the tumor along with its periosteal cover to prevent recurrence of the tumor.

Painful bursitis: A bursa usually develops because of the constant friction between the tumor and the surrounding soft tissues. If inflammation develops within this bursa, it gives rise to pain necessitating its excision.

Fracture of the bony stalk may occur due to trauma.

Malignant change (1–2%): Local irradiation may convert this benign tumor into malignant. It grows rapidly and has to be excised.

Pressure on the neighboring vessels and nerves may give rise to neurovascular complications.

CHONDROMA (Enchondroma, Hondromyxoma)

This is a benign cartilaginous tumor centrally located when it occurs in phalanges and humerus (Fig. 43.4). It causes destruction of the cancellous bone and has a potential for undergoing malignant change, especially when it is situated in the long bones.

- *Age:* 10–50 years.
- *Site:* Metaphysis is usually involved. It is common in the phalanges of hand (little finger common) and feet. Innominate and large long bones may also be involved.

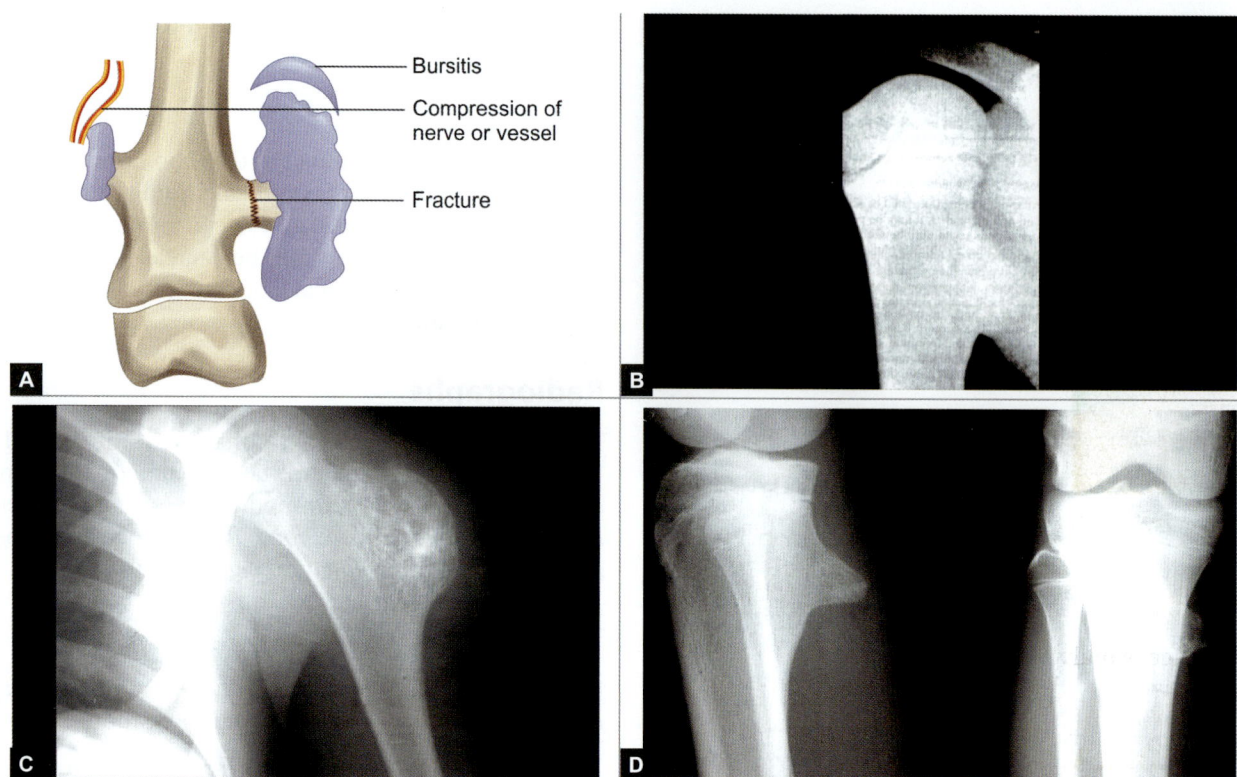

Figs 43.1A to D: (A) Osteochondroma and some of its complications; (B) Radiograph showing osteochondroma of upper end of humerus; (C) Exostosis humerus; (D) Exostosis upper end of tibia

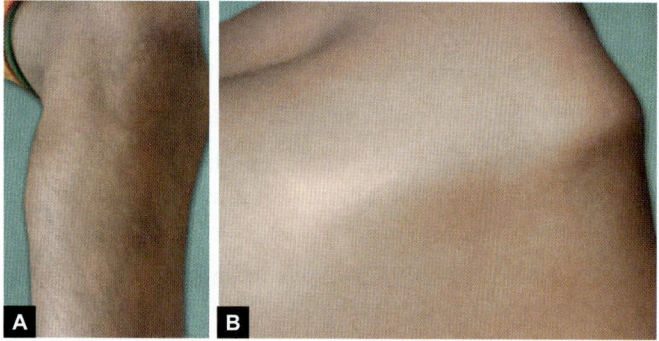

Figs 43.2A and B: Clinical photo showing osteoclastoma proximal tibia and fibula and shoulder

Fig. 43.3: Clinical photo showing excised osteoclastoma

Clinical Features

Symptoms are practically none. There may be slight pain and the phalanx may be enlarged (Fig. 43.5A). The course of the tumor is very slow.

Radiographs

The tumor appears cystic (loculated or non-loculated), cortex is thin and expanded, it may be perforated; and at the center, fibrous septa may be seen interspersing the central cavity (Fig. 43.5B). Stippling or calcification may be present. There is *no reactive bone formation*. There could be pathological fracture (Fig. 43.5C).

Treatment

Curettage is done and the wall is cauterized if the tumor is small. The surgery done in cases of large tumors is excision and removal of the capsule to prevent recurrence. Radical resection is done for tumors of long bones and pelvis. *Recurrence is common with chondromas of the long bones.*

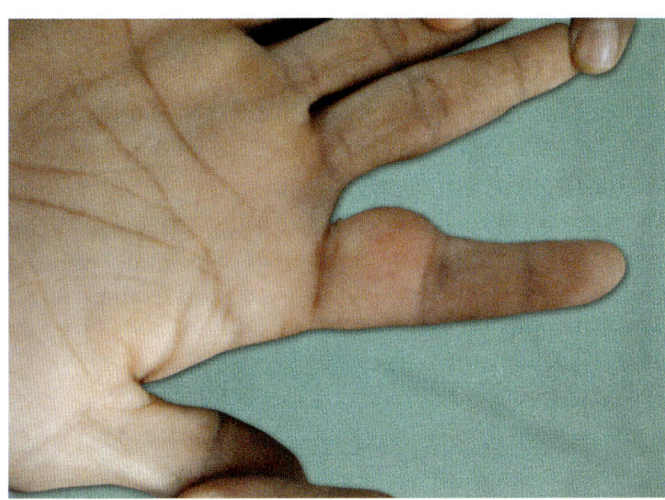

Fig. 43.4: Clinical photo showing enchondroma

Symptoms: The patient may present with pain, swelling, joint effusion, etc.

Radiographs

Radiographic features of the tumor are areas of rarefaction at epiphysis, eccentric position of the tumor, thin cortex and mottled areas of calcification.

Treatment

This consists of curettage and bone grafting if the lesion is small, excision in bigger tumors. If it is accidentally irradiated, it may turn malignant. Recurrence rate after excision is 25 percent.

Prognosis

The incidence of malignant change is 25 percent, especially in the pelvis.

CHONDROBLASTOMA

This is a highly cellular, vascular, and cartilaginous benign bone tumor of the cancellous bone. Here the cancellous bone is destroyed and multiple calcium deposits are usually found within the tumor.

Age: 10–20 years.

Sex: Male preponderance.

Sites: Epiphyseal ends of long bones are commonly affected.

CHONDROSARCOMA

This is s*econd* in frequency to osteosarcoma. It arises from the cartilage cells. It is a malignant but *slow* growing tumor. It has a long history and a better prognosis. Unlike osteogenic sarcoma, there is *no neoplastic osteoid formation and alkaline phosphatase is usually not raised.* It ranges from being locally aggressive to high-grade malignancy.

Classification

Primary/secondary: Secondary tumors develop when benign cartilaginous tumors are irradiated.

Peripheral/central/juxtacortical: Depending on the situation of the tumor within the bone.

Low-medium- and high-grade malignancy depending on the cellularity.

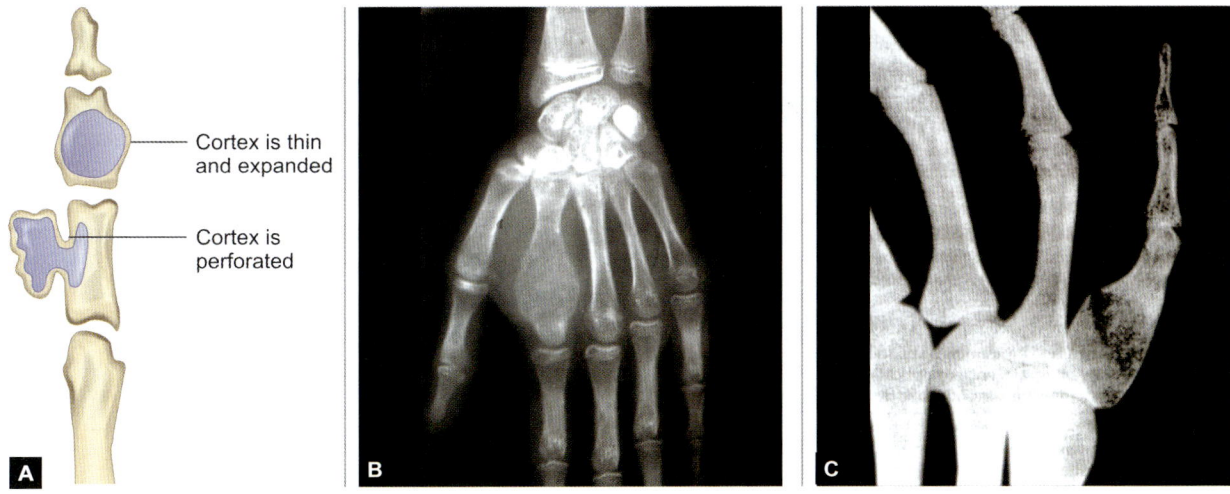

Figs 43.5A to C: (A) Enchondroma and its features; (B) Radiograph showing enchondroma of the proximal phalanx; (C) Enchondroma with pathological fracture

Antecedent Lesions

- Multiple enchondroma (Ollier's disease)
- Osteochondroma, etc.

Location: It is common at the sites of proximal femur, humerus, ribs, scapula, innominate bones, rare in hands and feet except in calcaneus, occur in pelvis or upper femora.

Sex: Males are more commonly affected than females.

Age: Twenty to sixty years, rare below 20 years, peak in the sixth decade.

Clinical Features

The duration of symptoms are usually less than 2 years in 75 percent of the cases and less than 5 years in the remaining 25 percent. Pain is usually not a prominent feature unlike osteogenic sarcoma. The central tumor remains entirely asymptomatic until it has eroded and penetrated the cortex or caused a pathological fracture. A palpable firm mass attached to the bone is the common physical sign. The tumor may assume large proportion (Fig. 43.6A).

Radiographs

Central tumors Central lytic lesion with calcification gives a fluffy, cotton wool, popcorn or breadcrumb appearance (Fig. 43.6B). Metaphysis or diaphysis of the long tubular bone is usually affected. Very rarely epiphysis may be involved. Greater degree of calcification is observed in slow growing tumors. It invades the soft tissue, there is little or no periosteal reaction seen.

Peripheral tumors: These are very large tumors and the central part is heavily calcified.

Juxtacortical tumors are seen adjacent to the cortex.

Diagnosis

Biopsy is the only criterion to establish a diagnosis with certainty. This tumor is notorious for soft tissue seeding during biopsy. Hence, the biopsy scar should be small and within the area of resection.

Treatment

Surgery is the treatment of choice.

Low- and medium- grade lesions: Require wide excision, e.g. Forequarter amputation (Thikor-Lindberg) for the shoulder girdle; hindquarter amputation for the pelvic girdle.

High-grade lesions: Require radical marginal excision, role of systemic chemotherapy in chondrosarcoma is controversial.

Palliative radiotherapy is indicated when the tumor cannot be resected because of its enormous size or if the tumor is present in inaccessible region.

Prognostic Factors

The following factors indicate poor prognosis:

Location: Axial skeleton and proximal portions of the long bones.

Age: More aggressive in childhood and young adults.

Cytological features: Suggesting high-grade malignancy are:
- Increased water and calcium (85%).
- DNA more than 5.5 µg/mg.
- Excess protein more than 350 µg/mg.
- Increased $Ch\text{-}4\text{-}SO_4$ decreased $Ch\text{-}6\text{-}SO_4$ (ratio > 1).
- Decreased keratin sulfate.
- Galactosamine/xylose ratio more than 10.
- Hexosamine concentration less than 75 µg/mg.

Size: Larger the tumor, greater is the chance of malignancy.

Secondary chondrosarcomas are more malignant. Survival time after treatment is 10 years. The comparative statistics are as follows after treatment:
- Low-grade tumors have 70 percent survival rate.
- Medium-grade tumors have 50 percent survival rate.
- High-grade tumors have 30 percent survival rate.

> **Quick Facts in Chondrosarcoma**
> - Second in frequency to osteosarcoma.
> - No neoplastic osteoid.
> - Long history.

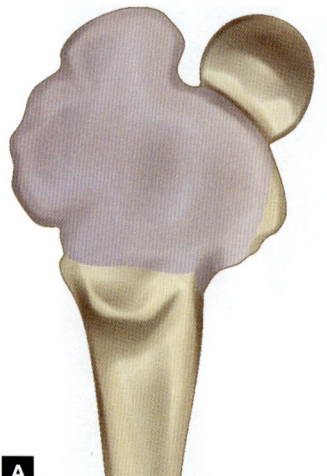 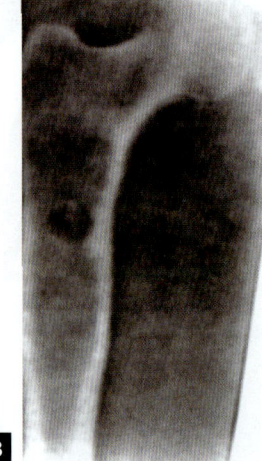

Figs 43.6A and B: (A) Chondrosarcoma affecting the upper end of the femur; (B) Radiograph showing chondrosarcoma

- Pain is not a prominent feature.
- X-ray—*popcorn* appearance.
- Wide excision is the treatment of choice.
- Better survival rate.

CHONDROMYXOID FIBROMA

This is the least common benign cartilaginous bone tumor.

Age: Young adults in the 2nd and 3rd decade are commonly affected.

Sex: Equal incidence.

Location: Metaphyseal ends of the long bones are commonly involved.

Clinical Features

Usually, the patient does not give a history of pain but complains of increasing swelling. A tender tumor mass may be palpable. Symptoms are more severe if the tumor develops in patients less than 10 years of age. Usually, it does not show sarcomatous change or metastasis.

Radiographs

Radiographic features show eccentrically located tumor in the metaphysis. Cortex is expanded, thin and interrupted (Fig. 43.7). Medullary margins are scalloped and sclerosed; the base of the tumor shows triangular periosteal bone formation.

Treatment

The treatment of choice is local excision and bone grafting for small tumors, wide *en bloc* excision for large tumors.

OSSEOUS ORIGIN BONE TUMORS

OSTEOMA

Osteoma is a benign bone tumor, occurs in membranous bones of skull and face. Usually, there are very few complaints, the history is long and the finding is a diffuse bony hard tumor. It rarely requires treatment.

[1]OSTEOID OSTEOMA

This is a benign osteoblastic tumor with a well-demarcated nidus of less than one cm surrounded by a distinct reactive bone (Fig. 43.8).

This tumor presents very interesting clinical features. It is a tumor of young adults, benign in nature and occurs in enchondral bones.

Age: It is common in young adults between 10 and 25 years of age.

Sex: Male preponderance (M : F = 2 : 1).

Sites: Long bones usually tibia and femur are more commonly affected.

Clinical Features

The patient complains of vague and intermittent pain, which is more at night. The pain dramatically decreases after giving aspirin so much so that this is called the *therapeutic test*. The patient also complains of limp due to pain. There is a mild swelling, the local area may be tender, temperature is not raised, and the skin is not stretched, shiny or warm. When the lesion occurs in the spine, the patient presents with acute low backache.

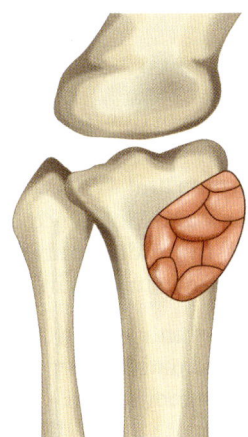

Fig. 43.7: Chondromyxoid fibroma, characteristic findings, lytic lesion, trabecular pattern and cortex slightly expanded

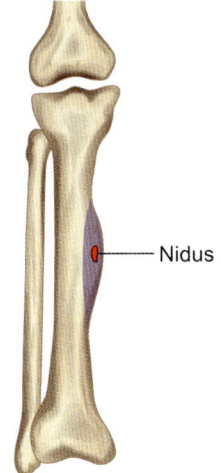

Fig. 43.8: Osteoid osteoma in tibia

---

[1]**Osteoid osteoma.** Jattle HL of USA described this in the year 1935.

Radiographs

It usually shows small-rarefied lesion <2 cm in diameter found in either the cortex, subcortical or subperiosteal regions. A thick sclerotic bone surrounds it. A small dense center of ossification seen in the center as the *nidus* (Figs 43.9A and B). Five percent of the cases of sciatica are due to osteoid osteoma.

CT scan and MRI also help in diagnosing this tumor.

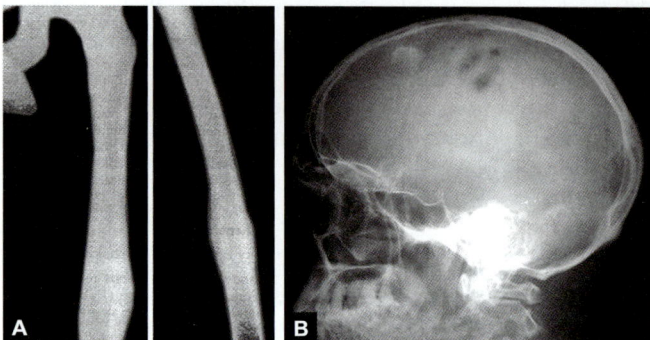

Figs 43.9A and B: (A) Radiographs showing osteoid osteoma of the femur; (B) Osteoid osteoma of the skull

Treatment

Conservative line of treatment consists of rest to the part and analgesics. If the tumor is too troublesome, complete excision of the cortex, containing the nidus is sufficient.

> **Do You Know What is New in the Management of Osteoid Osteoma?**
> - For the rare intra-articular situation, arthroscopically assisted excision is done.
> - CT-guided endoscopic removal.
> - Percutaneous excision.
> - MRI-guided cryotreatment.
> - CT-guided biopsy and thermocoagulation.

OSTEOGENIC SARCOMA

Osteogenic sarcoma is a highly malignant bone tumor (Fig. 43.10). Here tumor cells invariably form a neoplastic osteoid, bone, or both. It arises from a common multifactorial mesenchymal tissue; and hence, the tumor could be either *fibroblastic, osteoblastic* or *chondroblastic*.

This is the most frequent primary bone tumor next only to multiple myeloma.

Age: It is common in the second decade, rare below 10 years of age, 75 percent of the cases are seen below the age of 25 years.

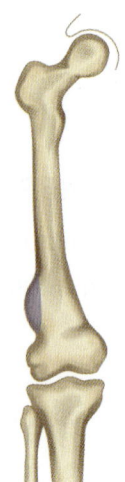

Fig. 43.10: Osteogenic sarcoma lower end of femur

Sex: Male preponderance. When found in females, it starts at an early age.

Incidence: It is 1/75,000 population.

Site: Ninety percent of the tumor occurs in the metaphysial region of the ends of long bones. It has a predilection around the knee and upper humerus. It may affect the jaws in the aged.

Location
- Fifty-two percent of the cases occur in the femur (9% in greater trochanter).
- Twenty percent of cases are seen in the tibia (90% in upper medial aspect).
- Nine percent are seen in the humerus. It is common in the upper end but rare below the deltoid tubercle.

Exciting Factors

The predisposing factors of this tumor are:
Virus
- DNA virus—Polyoma and SV 40 virus.
- RNA virus—Harvey and Moloney mouse sarcoma virus. These are known to produce tumors in experimental animals but not known in humans.

Radiation: If a dose of more than 2000 rads is given to osteoprogenitor cells situated in areas of active growth at the metaphysis, malignancy sets in.

Chemicals: 20-methylcholanthrene, beryllium compounds are known to induce malignancy changes.

Pathology

The tumor could be either osteoblastic, chondroblastic or fibroblastic. Consequently, the tumor may be osteosclerotic or osteolytic. Most common tumor is both a combination of osteosclerotic and osteolytic variety.

Gross: The tumor is more commonly situated in metaphysis of a large long bone. It is a large tumor with areas of destruction (Fig. 43.11) gives an appearance of *leg of mutton*. The consistency ranges from stony hard to soft. The color of the tumor could be *white* if the tumor is *fibroblastic*, y*ellowish white* if *osteoblastic; bluish white;* if the tumor is *cartilaginous*. At the areas of rapid growth, there are necrotic foci, cavitation and hemorrhage. *Sunray* appearance is seen in the subperiosteal space due to bone deposition along the vessels. *Codman's triangle* is a reactive bone formation parallel to the bone and is triangular.

Histology

Small spindle cells with hyper chromatic nuclei are seen. The shape may be round, cuboidal or columnar. Cells are pleomorphic in nature. Large spindle-shaped cells are rare. Giant cells are often present. Matrix may be myxomatous, cartilaginous or osseous. Areas of hemorrhage may be present. Normally, when the bone forms an osteoid tissue, it is preceded by the stage of chondrification. *Neoplastic or tumor osteoid formed from the primitive malignant cells skip the stage of chondrification and form the ossified tissue directly without any intervening stage of chondrification.*

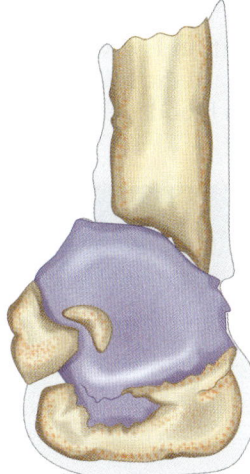

Fig. 43.11: Osteogenic sarcoma showing widespread destruction of the metaphysis, extension into the soft tissue and epiphysis. The growth plate limits spread to the joint

Classification

Primary and secondary.
Dahlin's (prognostic) classification:
- *Osteoblastic:* Poor five-year survival rate.
- *Chondroblastic:* Five-year survival rate is three times more than that of osteoblastic variety.
- *Fibroblastic:* Five-year survival rate is two times more of osteoblastic variety.

Geschickter and Copeland classification:
- Sclerosing type.
- Osteolytic type.
- Mixed type of both osteoblastic and osteolytic varieties.
- Telangiectatic type.

Secondary Osteosarcoma

This is less malignant than the primary, develops in bones affected with Paget's disease, diaphyseal aclasia, enchondromas, irradiation, etc. It is more common in older age groups and is treated on the same lines as the primary.

> **Lichtenstein's Criteria to Identify Osteogenic Sarcoma Include the Presence of the Following:**
> - Sarcomatous stroma
> - Spindle cells
> - Direct formation of neoplastic osteoid and bone.

Clinical Features

The patient usually presents with pain as the first symptom. It precedes the tumor, is seen first at night and is intermittent in nature. History of trauma is a common feature. The patient complains of tired feeling and limp. General condition is good until the late stages. Pyrexia is seen with increased WBCs. the patient is usually anemic than cachetic. Skin over the tumor is stretched, shiny and mobile (Fig. 43.12). Local temperature is increased, consistency of the tumor is variable, dilated veins are present (and is evident at an early stage).

Investigations

Laboratory Tests

This shows low Hb percent, raised ESR, lymphocytosis, etc.

Plain X-ray

This shows sclerosis or destruction of the bone at the metaphysis (Figs 43.13A to C). Other radiological features are *Sunrays* appearance is seen in the subperiosteal space

606 SECTION 5: General Orthopedics

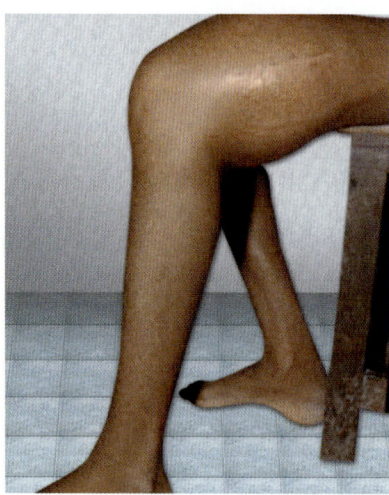

Fig. 43.12: Clinical photo showing skin over tumor becomes stretched and shiny

due to bone deposition along the vessels. *Codman's triangle* is a reactive bone formation parallel to the bone and is triangular. Plain X-ray of the chest helps to know the chest metastasis.

CT Scan and MRI

These reveal more information and helps to study the extent of spread of the tumor within the bone and outside.

Frozen Biopsy

This helps to identify the histopathological changes in the tumor.

Bone Scan

Bone isotope studies help to detect the metastasis in different bones.

Treatment

General Principles

- Early radical amputation is done to remove the primary tumor.
- An attempt is made to prevent metastasis or control it if it has already formed by preoperative irradiation, chemotherapy or both.
- Resection of large pulmonary metastasis is carried out.

Surgery

Early and radical ablation is the surgical procedure of choice. Having first established the diagnosis by biopsy, the level of amputation is determined after carrying out the various investigations mentioned above. Surgery is done at the *earliest* possible time.

> **Quick Facts**
> *Osteosarcoma: Levels of amputation*
> - Upper end of humerus: Forequarter amputation.
> - Upper end of tibia: Midthigh amputation.
> - Upper end of femur: Hindquarter amputation and hip disarticulation.
> - Lower end of femur: Midthigh amputation and hip disarticulation.

Newer Techniques

- *Limb salvage with tumor endoprosthesis:* This is showing a better final clinical outcome in recent times.
- In juxta-articular osteogenic sarcoma, intraepiphyseal excision and biological reconstruction to give excellent functional results.

Megavoltage Radiotherapy

Megavoltage irradiation is given preoperatively before amputation to decrease the *viability* of the cells that may be disseminated into bloodstream by surgical trauma. It is

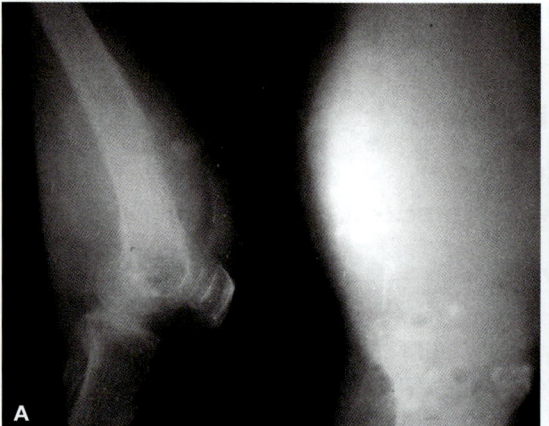 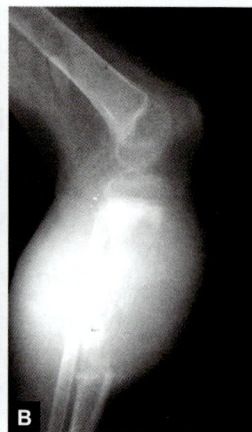 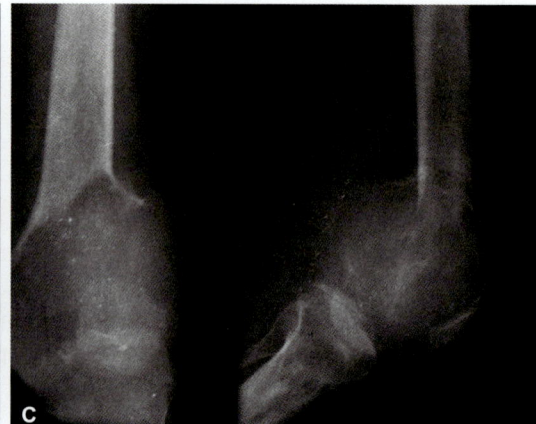

Figs 43.13A to C: Radiograph showing (A) Osteogenic sarcoma lower end of femur; (B) Osteogenic sarcoma upper end of tibia; (C) Osteogenic sarcoma lower end of femur (osteolytic type)

a useful adjunct in the treatment of resectable tumors. Its efficacy is doubtful in the non-resectable tumors, e.g. vertebra. Irradiation destroys tumor cells with minimal effect on the uninvolved parts.

> **Preliminaries before Irradiation**
> - Bone scans are done to detect the skip lesions.
> - Biopsy scar is limited to <2 cm size to avoid skin necrosis.
> - Chemotherapy is given to increase the susceptibility of tissues to irradiation.
> - Dose—Total dose of irradiation is 6,000–8,000 rads, 230 rads/day, or 1000 rads/week.

Chemotherapy (CT)

Role of chemotherapy is as follows:
- After ablation of the primary tumor, it produces a disease-free state for many months.
- If given before the metastasis is apparent, it improves the 5-year survival rate by 60 percent.
- Chemotherapy approach assumes that at least 80 percent of the patients have microscopic foci in the lungs at the time of initial diagnosis.
- Chemotherapy started early after the diagnosis destroys the microscopic foci at a stage when they are most susceptible to the action of chemotherapy drugs.
- It prevents metastasis in 60 percent of the cases. The remaining 40 percent become disease free due to aggressive attack on the metastasis. After metastasis has occurred, chemotherapy decreases the tumor size and enables easy surgical removal.
- When the patient refuses amputation, but accepts local resection and implant, chemotherapy decreases the size of the tumor.

Earlier osteogenic sarcoma was refractory to chemotherapy. Nevertheless, it has now been found that high doses of Methotrexate, Citrovorum factor rescue (CFR) and Adriamycin are effective. By using the above drugs in short cyclical courses, toxic effects can be held to a minimum. Addition of an alkylating agent, like cyclophosphamide, has increased the interval between the administrations of individual drugs. This has markedly reduced the toxicity of the drugs. The treatment triad in order of sequence is shown in Figure 43.14.

In summary, after having established the diagnosis of osteogenic sarcoma with certainty, the patient is initially put on chemotherapy. The role of chemotherapy has already been discussed. Local irradiation of the tumor is done next. Early radical surgical ablation is then carried out at the appropriate time.

Treatment of Pulmonary Metastasis

Pulmonary microemboli are best managed by chemotherapy. Large lesions require removal by wide resection or lobectomy after giving chemotherapy.

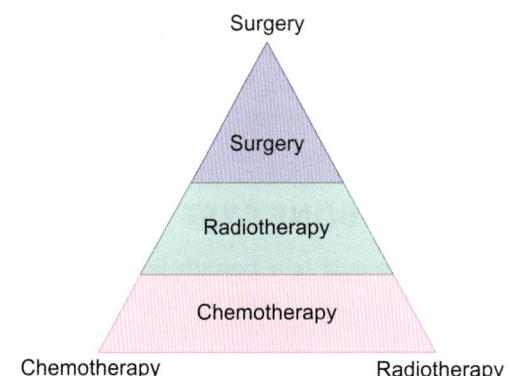

Fig. 43.14: Triad of treatment in osteogenic sarcoma

Another experimental approach to manage the lethal metastasis is the immunological approach. The immunological status is increased by giving specific antibiotics, BCG vaccine, and allergenic sarcoma tumor cell vaccine for two years, interferon therapy, etc.

Prognosis

Prognosis of osteogenic sarcoma has dramatically improved by the combined approach of ablation, megavoltage irradiation and chemotherapy.

In untreated cases, survival time after pulmonary metastasis has developed (around 2.9%).

With the combined approach of chemotherapy, radiotherapy and pulmonary resection, the five-year survival rate has increased by 60 percent.

Osteogenic sarcoma is curable and warrants intensive treatment with chemotherapy and surgical resection.

> **Remember**
> *Characteristic facts of osteogenic sarcoma*
> - Highly malignant bone tumor.
> - Arises from multipotent cells.
> - Most frequent primary bone tumor next only to multiple myeloma.
> - Seventy-five percent are below 25 years of age.
> - Ninety percent occur in the metaphysis.
> - Neoplastic osteoid is always present.
> - Both osteosclerotic and osteolytic variety is the most common.
> - Leg of mutton appearance.
> - Spindle cells.
> - No giant cells.
> - Pain is the first symptom.
> - Skin is stretched shiny, dilated veins are present.
> - Pathological fractures are not common.
> - Eighty percent has blood spread.
> - Sunray appearance and Codman's triangle are special X-ray features.
> - Multipronged approach gives better survival rate.

RESORPTIVE BONE TUMORS

These are not true tumors but tumor-like conditions (hamartoma). These are benign and may cause pathological fractures.

ANEURYSMAL BONE CYST

Aneurysmal bone cyst is a benign lesion eccentrically situated in the metaphyseal ends of the long bones. It grows outwards and is located subperiosteally.

Age: 10–30 years.

Sex: Males are more commonly affected than females.

Pathology

It is a thin shell of bone enclosing cystic blood-filled spaces. Partially organized clots remain in the center of the tumor. Microscopy shows blood-filled spaces. Giant cells are seen.

Clinical Features

The patient usually gives history of mild trauma. Pain and swelling are the main complaints. Joint movements may be decreased.

Radiographs

Radiographic features of the tumor consist of radiolucent area situated at the metaphysis. It extends outwards eccentrically, periosteal new bone formation is seen, and pathological fractures may be present (Figs 44.15A and B).

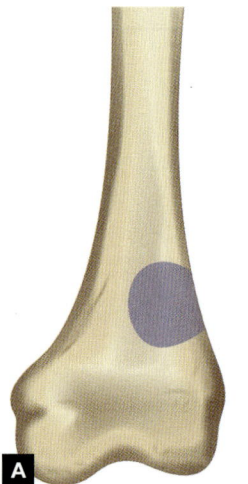 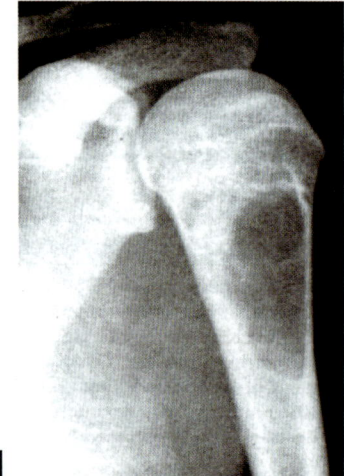

Figs 43.15A and B: (A) Aneurysmal bone cyst; (B) Radiograph showing aneurysmal bone cyst upper end of humerus

Treatment

Surgery is the treatment of choice. Curettage and bone grafting is the procedure commonly followed.

UNICAMERAL BONE CYST

Jaffe and Lichtenstein first described unicameral bone cyst in the year 1942.

It is an uncommon, non-neoplastic lesion commonly seen in the first two decades of life. It is situated in the metaphysis of the long bones and its proximity towards the epiphysis may affect the growth plate. Pathological fracture is a common entity. The cyst will not disappear on its own and remains so unless obliterated by surgery.

Age: Fifty percent lesions are seen in less than 10 years of age, forty percent between 10 and 20 years.

Sex: The male to female ratio is 2:1.

Location: Upper end of humerus in 55 percent, upper end of femur in 26 percent.

Pathology

Gross: It is a fusiform swelling, occupying the metaphyseal region of the bone. The underlying bone is thin with areas of hemorrhage present.

Microscopy: The cells are flat and vascular tissue is present. It has characteristic *giant cells*.

Types of Cyst

There are two types of bone cysts:

Active cyst is so called if the cyst is situated close to the epiphyseal plate.

Latent cyst is so called if the cyst moves away from the growth plate.

Clinical Features

The tumor is asymptomatic until fracture occurs through the cyst wall, which causes pain and draws the attention of the patient towards the problem. In most cases, the cyst is juxtaepiphyseal. Due to its proximity to the growth plate, the cysts may cause shortening, lengthening, coxa vara or coxa valga deformities. The tumor weakens the bone and the patient is susceptible to pathological fractures. Spontaneous obliteration of the cyst is seen in 15 percent of the cases and in 30 percent of the cases, cyst is displaced down the shaft due to continuous bone growth.

Radiographs

Radiographic examination of the tumor shows lytic lesion in the juxtaepiphyseal portion of the metaphysis, the lesion is expansive, the regional cortex is attenuated and pathological fractures may be seen (Figs 43.16A and B).

Treatment

Surgical excision is the treatment of choice. The following are some of the surgical procedures.

Types of Surgery

Curettage and bone grafting: This procedure is associated with high rate of recurrence.

Subtotal resection and bone grafting here: One cm of the normal bone above and below the lesion is excised.

Total resection and bone grafting is the other method of treatment.

Intracystic injection of corticosteroids: Steroids injected into the cysts are known to cause obliteration of the cyst 40–80 mg of prednisolone for smaller cysts recommended, larger cysts may require 200 mg of prednisolone.

Complications

Since the tumor is situated in the juxtaepiphyseal region, complications like shortening, coxa vara, coxa valga and bone overgrowth may develop.

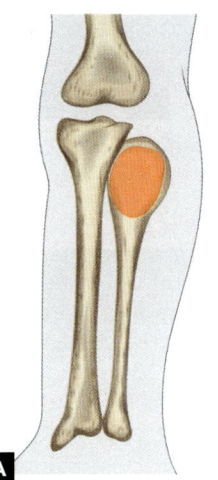 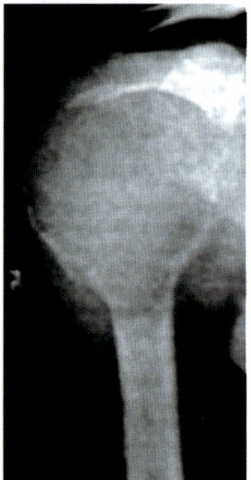

Figs 43.16A and B: (A) Features of unicameral bone cyst; (B) Radiograph showing unicameral bone cyst of upper end of humerus

GIANT CELL TUMOR (GCT) (Syn: Osteoclastoma)

BENIGN GIANT CELL TUMOR

Benign giant cell tumor (GCT) is an osteolytic tumor arising from the *epiphysis* and is common in young adults. Though it is benign, it is *locally* malignant. The presence of *tumor giant cells* is the hallmark of this tumor.

Sex: The male : female ratio is 1.5 : 1.

Age: It is common between 15 and 35 years (80% occur in more than 20 years of age and the average age group is 35 years).

Areas affected are asymmetric portions of the epiphysis of long bones. About 75 percent of GCT occurs in lower end of femur, upper end of tibia, fibula and the distal end of radius.

Pathology

Gross

The tumor consists of ragged, friable, bleeding tissue filled with old or fresh blood clots with various sized cysts and cavities. Color varies from red to brown. Epiphyseal end of the bone is distorted. Tumor extension into the joint cavity is usually not seen and there is no evidence of periosteal reaction.

Microscopy

The tumor is encompassed by a fibrous capsule at the periphery. Presence of abundant tumor giant cells is quite characteristic. These cells are characterized by their larger size, multiple nuclei more than 150 in number which are distributed throughout the cell. Appearance of spindle cells indicates *malignant* potential.

Histological Grading (Jaffe's Criterion)	
Grade I	• Presence of characteristic stromal cells • Little intercellular collagen • Spindle cells are adjacent to the necrotic tissue
Grade II	• Random distribution of giant cells are seen among the stromal cells
Grade III	• Nuclei of giant cells are identical to those of the stromal cells

Clinical Features

The course of the tumor is chronic. Unlike osteogenic sarcoma, pain is not the presenting feature but trauma is, the patient complains of swelling which is situated on one side of the bone. Skin over the tumor is stretched, but there are no dilated veins. Tenderness is moderate or absent, *eggshell-crackling* sensation may be present or absent. Limitation of joint movements is not seen until the late stages (Fig. 43.17).

There is no increase in joint fluid and the joint is rarely invaded. Pathological fracture is a late feature.

Radiographs

- An osteolytic area is seen near the epiphysis.
- The cortex is expanded and thin.

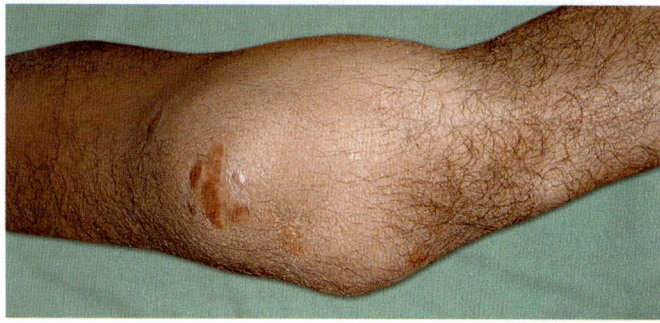

Fig. 43.17: Clinical photo showing benign GCT lower end of femur

- There is no periosteal new bone formation.
- Thin septa of bone traverse the interior and produce a *soap-bubble appearance* (Figs 44.18A and B).
- The cortex may be disrupted in late stages.
- Joint extension is rare.

Campanacci's radiographic grading:
Grade 1: Cystic lesion.
Grade 2: Cortex is thin but not perforated.
Grade 3: Cortex is perforated with extension into soft tissues.
MRI reveals more accurate information and shows the intramedullary spread and soft tissue involvement.

MALIGNANT GIANT CELL TUMOR

Primary

This develops as a frank sarcomatous lesion. The swelling is quite gross and show other features of malignancy. The X-rays show gross destruction of the epiphyseal region of the affected bone (Figs 43.19A to C).

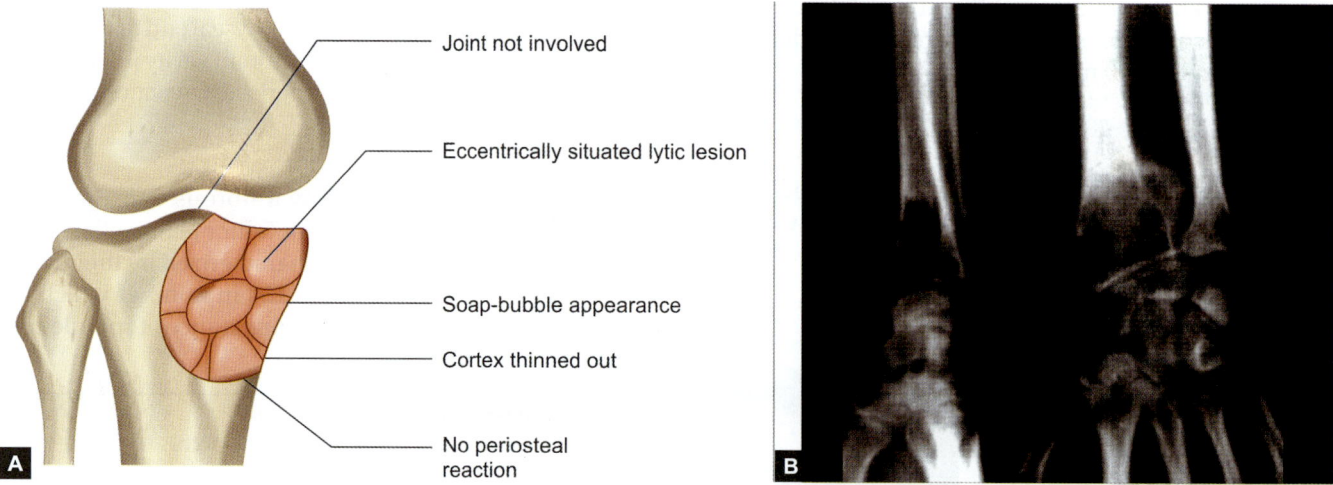

Figs 43.18A and B: (A) Features of giant cell tumor; (B) Radiographs showing the giant cell tumor of the lower end of radius showing the soap-bubble appearance

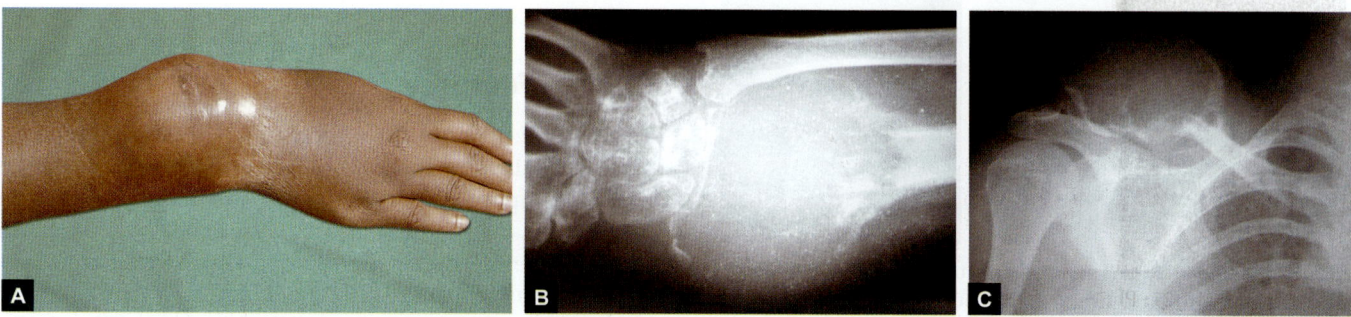

Figs 43.19A to C: (A) Malignant GCT (Clinical photo); (B) Radiograph showing gross destruction in GCT; (C) Osteoclastoma—lateral end of clavicle

Secondary

This develops at the site of previously treated GCT (Figs 43.20 and 43.21).

Enneking's Staging of Benign GCT

Stage I (Latent)	• Incidence is 10–15 percent. • Discovered accidentally, no symptoms. • Pathological fracture may be present.
Stage II (Active)	• Incidence is 70 percent. • Symptomatic, pathological fracture may be present. • Benign.
Stage III (Aggressive)	• Incidence is 10–15 percent. • Symptomatic, rapidly growing. • Benign. • Cortex is perforated.

Treatment of GCT

Principles of tumor treatment:
- The tumor is invasive and aggressive.
- It commonly recurs, may become malignant after unsuccessful removal.

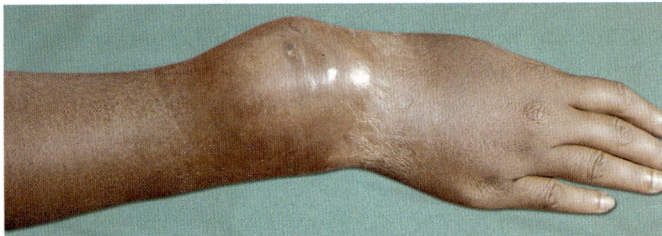

Fig. 43.20: Clinical photo showing malignant GCT lower end of radius

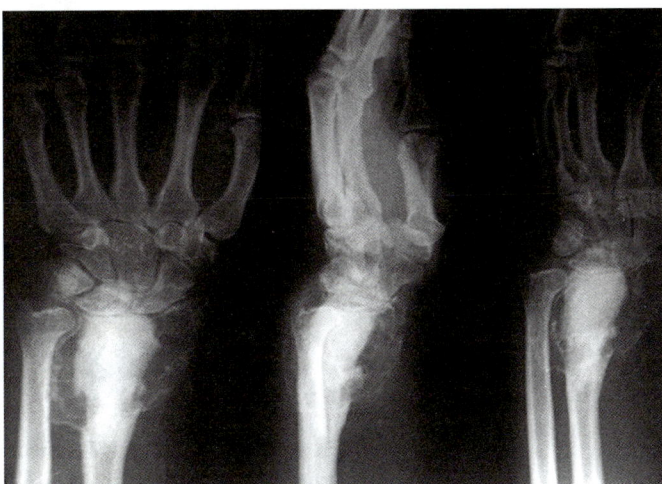

Fig. 43.21: Plain X-ray showing recurrent GCT

- Recurrence is treated with *en bloc* excision.
- *En bloc* excision is also indicated if the tumor has eroded the cortex and extended into the soft tissues.

Surgical Methods

Approach that is more aggressive is adopted for lesions that are more aggressive and the surgical methods described are:

Curettage and bone grafting: It is a simple technique but is associated with high recurrence rate (about 30%).

En bloc excision: This is the initial procedure of choice and here 2 cm of normal tissue is also excised. Defects are filled with cancellous bone grafts, freeze-dried allograft or prosthesis. This technique has low recurrence rate.

Curettage and acrylic bone cementation: This has a low rate of recurrence and the heat of polymerization destroys residual stromal and giant cells (0.5 cm).

Curettage and cryosurgery: This destroys the residual tumor at its margin of curettage by repetitive freezing and thawing by liquid nitrogen. Malignancy change rate decreases from 15–1.9 percent.

Excision and reconstruction: This procedure can be followed for GCT affecting the lower end of femur or upper end of tibia. After *en bloc* excision, one of the following methods can do reconstruction.
- *Turn-o-plasty technique:* Here after excision of the tumor in the lower end of femur, the required length of the proximal tibia is chosen, split into two halves and one-half of it is turned upside down and fixed with the left over stump of the femur. If the lesion is in the tibia, the procedure is done by taking half of the femur.
- Arthrodesis is done by using the fibula from both the sides to bridge the excised gap.
- *Arthroplasty:* After tumor excision, arthroplasty is done either by using an autograft, allograft or prosthesis.

Irradiation therapy induces malignant change if it is given to the benign lesion. Megavoltage therapy is permissible only for inaccessible lesions located in the spine, sacrum, pelvis, etc. The recommended dosage is 1,500–5,000 rads for 5–6 weeks.

Other Methods

Marginal resection with curettage: This is done using power burrs with copious irrigation of 5 percent phenol and 70 percent alcohol.

Resection of distal radius and using ipsilateral proximal fibula to reconstruct the wrist joint.

Amputation is done for widespread aggressive tumor as a last resort.

Treatment Facts of GCT

Site	Surgical option
• Upper limb	
– Lower end of ulna	Excision
– Lower end of radius	Excision with reconstruction by ipsilateral fibula
• Lower limbs	
– Lower end of femur	Excision with turn-o-graft
– Upper end of tibia	Excision with turn-o-graft

Quick Facts of GCT
- Locally malignant.
- Affects young adults.
- Arises from the epiphysis.
- Giant cells are characteristic.
- Egg shell crackling may be present.
- Soap-bubble appearance is characteristic.
- *En bloc* excision and reconstruction is the surgical method of choice.
- One-third are benign, one-third is locally malignant and one-third is malignant.

Quick Facts: Differential Diagnosis of GCT
Benign chondroblastoma.
Localized osteitis fibrosa.
Unicameral bone cyst.
Nonossifying fibroma.
Aneurysmal bone cyst
Chondromyxoid fibroma.
Hyperparathyroidism.

Note:
Mnemonic BLUNACH denotes lesion with giant cells (Differential diagnosis of GCT).

TUMORS OF NONOSSEOUS ORIGIN

²EWING'S SARCOMA

Ewing's sarcoma was first described by Ewing in the year 1928. This is a rare primary malignant bone tumor (10–14% of all malignant bone tumors) affecting children. It is a lethal tumor with a poor 5-year survival rate.

Age: Persons commonly affected are 4–25 years of age group (about 80%).

Sex: More common in males.

Site: Long bones affected are femur, tibia, fibula and humerus in that order. About 20 percent of tumors are seen in flat bones.

Location: Diaphysis of the long bones is commonly affected.

Pathology

Gross: It is a grayish white tumor encapsulated by fibrous tissue. It may contain hemorrhagic foci and areas of cystic formation. From the medulla, it reaches to the surface through the haversian canals.

Histology

The tumor is very *cellular*. The cells may be small, round or polyhedral in shape and may be arranged as cords or sheets. Intercellular substance is minimal. Necrosis is common. Cells are arranged round the vessels justifying the term *perithelioma*. Many tumors show *Rosette* formation with central fibril. *Pseudorosettes* are more common (no central fibril). Giant cells are not found and there is no new bone formation.

Differential diagnosis is between reticulum cell sarcoma and Ewing's sarcoma:
- Ewing's stains for *glycogen positivity* by PAS.
- In reticulum cell sarcoma *silver stain* is positive.

Clinical Features

The patient presents with pain, which is intermittent in nature. The pain is worse at night. The tumor is diaphyseal and fixed to the bone, skin is red, dilated veins may be present (Fig. 43.22A). Sometimes the tumor may present with constitutional symptoms like fever, sweating, chills, leukocytosis, and anemia. This may create confusion as it mimics acute osteomyelitis (Fig. 43.23).

Course
- Exacerbation and remission is characteristic.
- Blood and lymphatic spread is common.

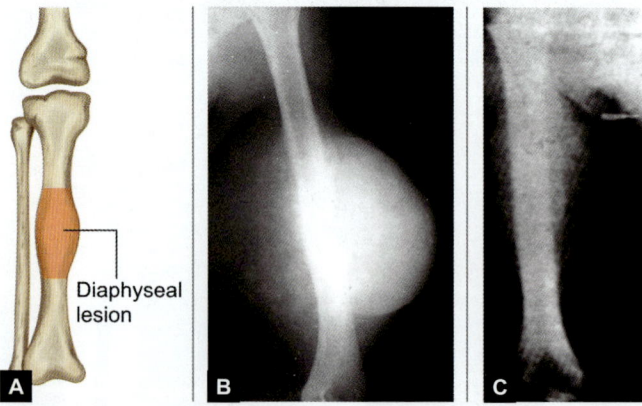

Figs 43.22A to C: (A) Features of Ewing's sarcoma; (B) Radiograph showing Ewing's sarcoma of femur; (C) Ewing's sarcoma of humerus

---

²**James Ewing** (1866–1943), Oncologist, USA. It was first described by Ewing in the year 1928.

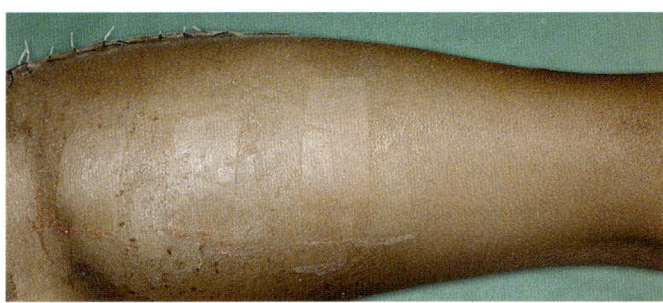

Fig. 43.23: Clinical photo showing Ewing's sarcoma femur

- Metastasis to other bones like skull, vertebrae, ribs, lungs, etc. may occur.

Investigations

Radiographic Features

- The lesion could be lytic, sclerotic or mixed.
- Diaphyseal lesion with irregular destruction (moth-eaten appearance or cracked ice appearance) (Fig. 43.22B).
- Periosteal reaction is deposited in layers giving an *onion peel* appearance (Fig. 43.22C).
- Permeative margin.

Biopsy

Biopsy is necessary for diagnosis.

Other Tests

- *Urine* for vanillylmandelic acid (VMA).
- *Tissue* for glycogen stain.
- Immunohistochemical markers.
- *Electron microscopy study.*

> **Note:**
> Onion peel appearance is also seen in:
> - Osteomyelitis
> - Osteosarcoma
> - Malignant lymphoma

Recommended Treatment

This tumor is highly radiosensitive, disappears with radiation only to recur (melts like snow). Hence, a combination of local radiotherapy with systemic chemotherapy brings down the recurrence rate dramatically. Nevertheless, even this treatment has a recurrence rate of 20–30 percent and because of the possibility of radiation-induced sarcomas; surgical resection for the control of the primary lesion is being used. The surgery planned is conservative in nature and aims at limb preservation.

Effective Chemotherapy

Effective chemotherapy is given using newer chemotherapeutic drugs like Ifosfamide, cisplatinum, epipodophyllin toxin for a short period.

Radiation

Radiation is the mainstay of local treatment, especially in axial skeleton. Dose required is high 4,000 rads for the entire limb and 1000 rads as boost to the tumor.

Surgery

Conservative surgery like debulking of the tumor or limb preservation surgery has a role.

Unfavorable prognostic features are:
- Male patients.
- Humerus if involved.
- Pelvic bones if involved.
- Distant metastasis.

Primary irradiation followed by amputation has a two-year survival rate of 15 percent. A combination of chemotherapy, radiotherapy with surgery improves the survival rate to 50–75 percent for 3–5 years.

> **Quick Facts of Ewing's Sarcoma**
> - Rare primary malignant tumor.
> - Common between 5 and 15 years.
> - Tumor of the diaphysis.
> - Clinically may mimic acute osteomyelitis.
> - X-ray shows moth-eaten appearance and onion peel appearance.
> - Tumor is highly cellular.
> - Highly radiosensitive (melts like snow).
> - High rate of recurrence.
> - Combination of radiotherapy, chemotherapy and surgery has improved 2-year survival rate.

MULTIPLE MYELOMA (PLASMACYTOMA)

This is the most common bone tumor in adults. It accounts for 50 percent of all bone tumors. Here plasma cells replace the bone. It affects elderly persons between 40 and 60 years of age.

Sex: Males and females are equally affected.

Pathology

Gross: The tumor is dark red in color, soft in consistency and lies within the medulla. The cortex is thin and broken.

Microscopy: It consists of round cells with eccentrically placed nucleus with nucleolus. The chromatin is sparse and is arranged in *"spokes of wheel fashion".* Perinuclear halo typical of plasma cells is not seen in multiple myeloma.

Associated pathology
- Interstitial fibrosis in the kidney.
- Nodules in the lungs.
- Amyloidosis may occur (in 10–15%).

Clinical Features

Tumor runs a chronic course. It is silent at first; later on, the patient complains of vague pain, which is mild and intermittent in the beginning. It also affects lumbar spine, sacral region, chest and ribs. Severe attacks of sharp pain, superimposed at intervals may develop. Often, the patient may complain of a diffuse, persistent, backache.

Findings

In the early stages, there are hardly any clinical findings. Later on, the patient may complain of soft tissue swelling in about 10 percent of cases. Signs of pathological fracture are present in about 20 percent of cases. The sternum and ribs may be tender and there may be signs of vertebral collapse.

Course: The tumor is chronic, later the marrow replacement causes anemia, thrombocytopenia and hemorrhages. Renal failure due to tubular block by protein casts may also be seen (myeloma kidney).

Investigations

Laboratory Findings

- *Bence Jones protein* is found in only 30 percent of the cases. On boiling, a white precipitate appears at 50°C, dissolves at boiling point after acidifying the urine; on cooling, the precipitate reappears.
- Serum globulin is increased.
- Hypercalcemia.
- ESR is increased (sludged blood).
- *Low alkaline phosphatase* is seen despite extensive bone destruction or it may be normal.
- *Marrow biopsy* reveals anemia, is refractory to iron, B_{12}, folic acid, etc.

Radiographs

The affected bones show diffuse osteoporosis or lytic lesions. *Biconcave* vertebral bodies and collapse of vertebra. *Punched-out* lesions in skull and pelvis are the characteristic findings in the X-rays (Figs 43.24 and 43.25).

Typical Lesions

- Osteolytic lesion penetrates the cortex, but there is no periosteal reaction.

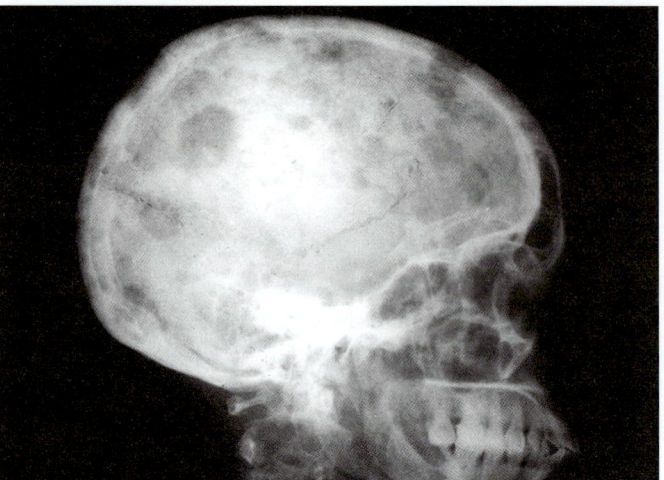

Fig. 43.24: Radiograph showing multiple myeloma (Punched out skull)

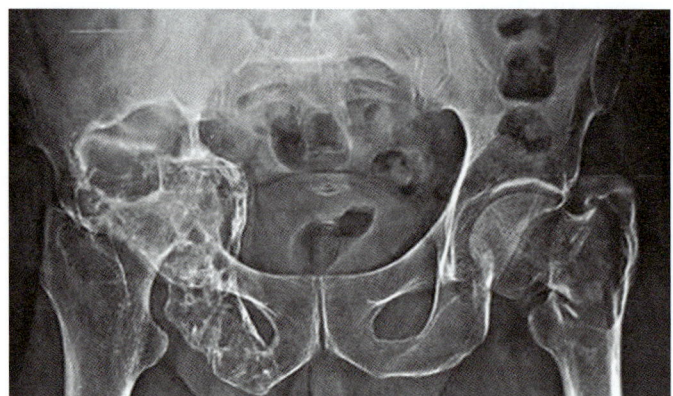

Fig. 43.25: Plain X-ray showing features of plasmacytoma

- Rarefaction of vertebrae may be extensive (disappearing vertebrae), vertebral pedicle involvement is more common, when involved it is called as the "pedicle sign" (common in secondaries).

MRI

MRI helps in more accurate assessment of the extent and spread of the tumor.

Treatment

When the tumor is widespread, it is usually fatal and then treatment is only palliative. The tumor is radiosensitive.

Chemotherapy

Agents like steroids, cyclophosphamide, urethane and melphalan (SCUM) are found to be effective.

> **What is New?**
> High dose VDD (vincristine, doxorubicin, and dexamethasone) with stem cell infusion is emerging as a better alternative to the conventional chemotherapy.

Surgery

- Laminectomy is done when there is evidence of compression of spinal nerves.
- Intramedullary fixation is done for pathological fractures of long bones.

Prognosis

- The disease is widespread and fatal.
- Death occurs within three years in majority of cases and in all by five years.

Complications

- Pathological fracture of the ribs.
- Spinal cord or nerve root compression.
- Anemia, leukopenia, thrombocytopenia.
- Renal failure.
- Severe infection.
- Amyloidosis.

METASTATIC TUMORS OF BONE

Definition

These are cancerous tumors originating in other organs and involving the skeletal structures of the body.
Bones may be involved by:
- Direct invasion.
- Blood-borne metastasis (most common route).
- Very-rarely through the lymphatic.

Blood-borne metastases to the bone greatly outnumber the primary bone tumors.
Incidence is 27–70 percent.

Tendency Percentagewise	
Ca Breast	73 percent
Ca Lungs	32 percent
Ca Kidneys	24 percent
Ca Rectum	13 percent
Ca Stomach	11 percent

Sites: The secondary bone tumors commonly involve vertebrae (Fig. 43.26), ribs, pelvis, sternum, skull and proximal ends of femur and humerus. It is unusual for metastatic neoplasm is to involve bones distal to the elbows or knees.

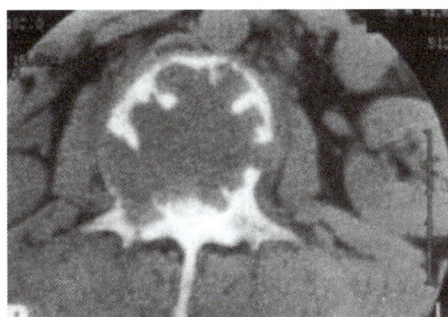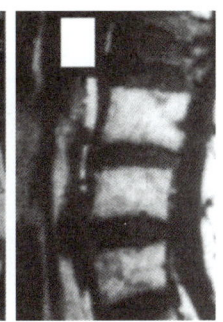

Fig. 43.26: CT scan showing metastasis in a vertebral body

Occurs in Three Clinical Settings

- Pain in the spine or extremity without a known history of primary tumor (rare).
- Pathological fracture with or without known primary.
- The third and most common is a patient with a known primary tumor with a painful lesion in the spine or extremities.

Clinical Features

The patient is usually an adult, in the middle or late life, and may present with pain, pathological fracture or anemia. The patient complains of headache if the skull is involved. Spine involvement causes girdle pains, spastic paralysis, etc. Pathological fractures are frequent in femur. Collapse of vertebrae may be present.

Laboratory Diagnosis

- Blood picture may be normal or bizarre showing features of anemia, thrombocytopenia or thrombocytosis, leukocytosis or leukopenia, eosinophilia, etc.
- Sometimes, anemia is associated with leukoerythroblastic reaction.
- Sometimes, a syndrome of hemolytic anemia, thrombocytopenia, and fibrinogenopenia can be seen with cancer of stomach and pancreas, etc.
- Alkaline phosphatase is increased normally, but acid phosphatase increases in cancer of prostate.

Other Investigations

Radiographs

Radiographs fail to detect secondary in the bone in 20–25 percent of the cases.

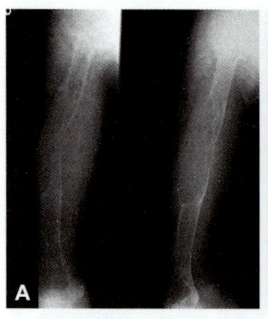 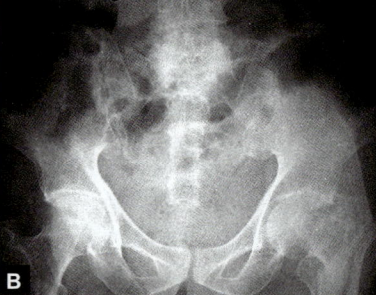

Figs 43.27A and B: (A) Secondaries in long bones with pathologic fracture; (B) Osteoblastic lesion

Two types are recognized:
- Osteolytic variety is frequent (Fig. 43.27A).
- Osteoblastic variety shows increased density (cancer prostate) (Fig. 43.27B).

Periosteal reaction and mottled or marble appearance are the other radiographic features.

Bone Scan

This is the most sensitive method of investigation. MRI, PET scan helps to assess the extent and spread of the metastasis.

Biopsy

Fine needle biopsy is accurate in over 90 percent of the cases.

Treatment

The following are the various modalities of treatment.

Radiotherapy is by ^{60}Co 3000–4000 rads for 3–4 weeks.

Surgery: If the patient has developed pathological fracture, internal fixation with acrylic cement is done. Decompressive laminectomy is done for secondary in the spine. Endocrine surgery for cancer breast, cancer prostate, etc.

Hormone therapy
- For prostatic cancer, estrogen.
- For breast cancer, diethylstilbestrol.
- For thyroid cancer, T_3 and ^{131}I.

Radioisotope therapy is by using
- Radioactive phosphorus.
- Radioactive ^{131}I.

Chemotherapy is by using drugs like alkylating agents, antimetabolites, etc.

Treatment of hypercalcemia is by using cortisone, mithramycin, etc.

Amputation is indicated for intractable pain and as a last resort.

Prophylactic nailing is considered for those cases with more than 50 percent destruction of the cortex.

> **What is New?**
> *Radiofrequency ablation (RFA)*
> In failed or poor candidates for conventional radiation or chemotherapy, RFA has emerged as an effective alternative palliative treatment of osteolytic metastatic lesion. However, ablation has to be done right up to the bone and not just in the center of the tumor.

INCLUSION TUMORS

SYNOVIOMA (SYNOVIAL SARCOMA)

Definition

Synovioma is a slowly growing malignant tumor occurring in juxtaposition to and attached to the synovial tissue but almost invariably lies outside the joint.

Pathology

It is difficult to find the synovial attachment of the tumor. The tumor may be circumscribed, rounded, lobulated, and may be surrounded by a pseudocapsule. The tumor lies closely to the tendons, bursa and joint capsules.

Microscopy

Three basic patterns indicate synovial origin: (i) formation of tissue spaces, (ii) formation of cell tufts, and (iii) the presence of epithelial cell tufts. Evidence of malignancy is seen in fibrosarcomatous stroma.

Clinical Features

This is a tumor of young adults, rare in people more than 40 years of age, common in the lower extremity, around the knee. Soft tissue outside the joint is involved, painful swelling, slowly increasing in size, firm or soft and tender. Restriction of joint movements may be seen.

Course: The course is very slow, metastasis is eventually into the lungs.

Radiographs

Soft tissue shadows are seen. Stippling is observed if the tumor contains small areas of calcification.

Treatment

Synovioma is a slow growing tumor. It metastasizes late. Surgery is the treatment of choice and includes local excision. Radical amputation is preferred if the tumor has a widespread involvement.

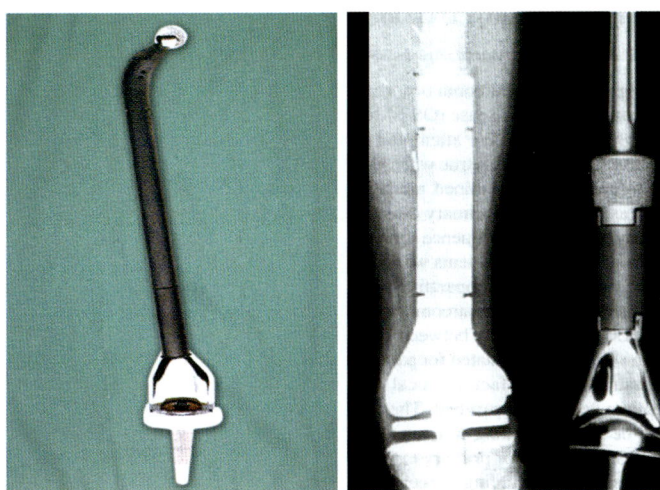

Fig. 43.28: Custom prosthesis

RECENT TRENDS IN LIMB SALVAGE SURGERY

Mercifully, gone are the days when amputation was an inevitable and inescapable event in the surgical management of bone tumors. Due to improvement in tumor control due to modern chemotherapy, limb salvage operation is gaining prominence.

The principles of limb salvage in bone tumor management are to eradicate the tumor, retain the integrity of the skeletal system and preserve the limb with useful function. After the resection, skeletal reconstruction can be done by bone grafting (auto- or allograft) or by endoprosthesis (modular or custom made) (Fig. 43.28). Prosthetic reconstruction is found to be more effective from a functional point of view than other alternatives.

When compared to the radical amputation and external prosthetic fitting or limb sparing surgery with bone grafting, this method of treatment is found to be more effective in early mobilization of the patient, limb function that is satisfactory and a better emotional acceptance by the patient.

BIBLIOGRAPHY

1. Baker DM. Benign unicameral bone cyst: A study of 45 cases with long-term follow-up. Clin Orthop. 1970;71:140.
2. Bhansali SK, Desai PP. Ewing's sarcoma: Observations in 107 cases. J Bone and Joint Surg. 1963;45-A:541.
3. Bhulla SK. Metastatic disease of the spine. Clin Orthop. 1970; 73-152.
4. Biesecker JL, et al. Aneurysmal bone cysts: A clinico-pathologic study of 66 cases. Cancer. 1970;26:615.
5. Brostrom LA. On the natural history of osteosarcoma: Aspects in diagnosis, prognosis and endocrinology. Acta Orthop Scand Suppl. 1984;53(Suppl):183.
6. Campanacci M, Bacci G, Pagani P, Giunti A. Multiple drug chemotherapy for the primary treatment of osteosarcoma of the extremities. J Bone Joint Surg. 1980;62-B:93.
7. Campanacci M, Guinti A, Ohm R. Giant cell tumors of bone. A study of 209 cases with long-term follow-up in 130. Ital J Orthop Traumatol. 1975;1:249.
8. Coventry MB, Dahlin DC. Osteogenic sarcoma: A critical analysis of 430 cases. J Bone Joint Surg. 1957;39-A:741.
9. Craig FS. Metastasis and primary lesions of bone. Clin Orthop. 1970;73-133.
10. Dias LS, Frost HM. Osteoid osteoma: Osteoblastoma. Cancer. 1974;33:1075.
11. Enneking WF, Spanier SS, Goodman MA. A system for the surgical staging of musculoskeletal sarcoma. Clin Orthop. 1980;153:106.
12. Erickson AL, Schiller A, Mankin HJ. The management of chondrosarcoma of bone. Clin Orthop. 1980;153:44.
13. Grimmer RJ, Cannon SR, et al. Royal Orthopedic Hospital, London.
14. Jaffe HL, Lichtenstein L, Portis RB. Giant cell tumor of bone: Its pathologic appearance, grading supposed variant and treatment. Arch Pathol. 1940; 30:993.
15. Johnston JO. Local resection in primary malignant bone tumors. Clin Orthop. 1980;153:75.
16. Lichtenstein L. Bone tumors, 5th edn. St Louis: CV Mosby Co; 1977.
17. Mizuta H, Yamasaki M. Nuclear magnetic resonance studies on human bone and soft tissue tumors. J Jpn. Orthop Assoc. 1984;58:97.
18. Murray JA. Multiple myeloma. Curr Pract Orthop Surg. 1975; 6:145.
19. Onolenghi CE. Diagnosis of orthopedic lesions by aspiration biopsy: Results in 1,063 punctures. J Bone Joint Surg. 1955; 37-A:443.
20. P Sonneveld, et al. Dept. of Clinical Oncology, Leiden, Netherlands.
21. Radiofrequency ablation (RFA). Source Orthonet. 2003; 63:5.
22. Treatment of osteoid osteoma, recent trends. Source: Orthonet India. April, 2002.
23. W Piotz, et al. Clinical orthopedics and related research. Dec, 2002.

SECTION 6
Geriatric Orthopedics

- Distal Forearm Fractures
- Fracture Neck of Femur
- Osteoporosis
- Osteoarthritis
- Cervical Disk Syndromes
- Degenerative Lumbar Disk Disease and Canal Stenosis

Section 6

Geriatric Orthopedics

44
CHAPTER

Distal Forearm Fractures

COLLES' FRACTURE

This is also called as **Poutteau's** fracture in many parts of the world. Abraham Colles first described it in the year 1814.

Definition

It is not just fracture lower end of radius but a fracture dislocation of the inferior radioulnar joint. The fracture occurs about 1½" (about 2.5 cm) above the carpal extremity of the radius (Fig. 44.1).

Following this fracture, some deformity will remain throughout the life, but pain decreases and movements increase gradually.

Mechanism of Injury

The common mode of injury is fall on an outstretched hand with dorsiflexion ranging from 40–90° (average 60°) (Fig. 44.2).

The force required to cause this fracture is 192 kg in women and 282 kg in men.

Fracture pattern: It is usually sharp on the palmar aspect and comminution on the dorsal surface of the lower end of radius.

Clinical Features

Usually, the patient is an elderly female in her 60s and the history given is a trivial fall on an outstretched hand.

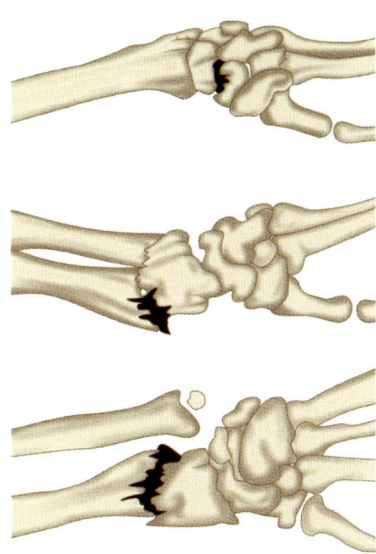

Fig. 44.1: Colles' fracture

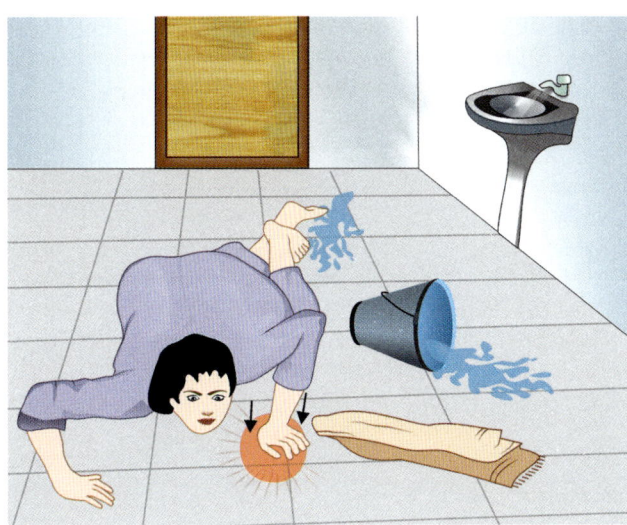

Fig. 44.2: Colles' fracture is usually due to a slip and fall on the outstretched hands in elderly females

The patient complains of pain, swelling, deformity and other usual features of fracture at the lower end of radius. Though *dinner fork* deformity is a classical deformity in a Colles' fracture, however, it is not found in all cases but seen only if there is a dorsal tilt or rotation of the distal fragment (Figs 44.1 and 44.3). However, the styloid process test is more reliable. There are six classical displacements in a Colles' fracture (Table 44.1).

Did You Know?
Dinner fork deformity is also called:
- Silver fork deformity.
- Spoon-shaped deformity.

Styloid Process Test

Normally, the radial styloid process is lower by 1.3 cm when compared to the ulnar styloid process. In Colles' both radial and ulnar styloid processes are at the same level and are found in all displacements of Colles' fracture. *Hence, this is a more reliable sign than dinner fork deformity* (Figs 44.4A and B).

Note: Dinner fork deformity is seen only in *d*orsal displacement and *D*orsal tilt in a Colles' fracture (note the *d*'s).

Radiology

Radiographs of the wrist (Figs 44.5A and B) both AP and lateral views of the affected wrist and lower end of the radius are taken. The points noted in the AP view are metaphyseal comminution, fracture line extending into the radiocarpal or inferior radioulnar joint and fracture of the ulnar styloid process (seen in about 60% of the cases). In the lateral

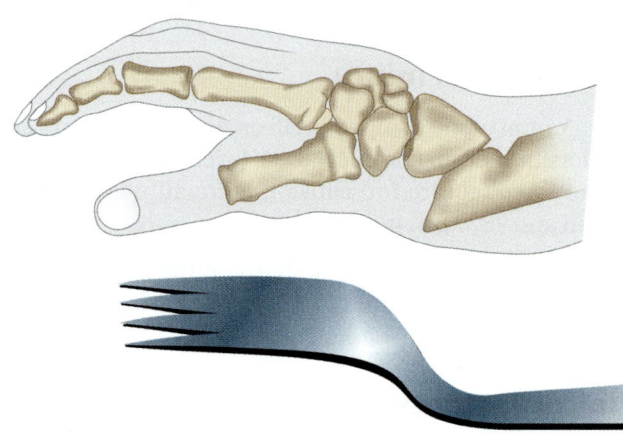

Fig. 44.3: Colles' fracture (A dinner fork deformity)

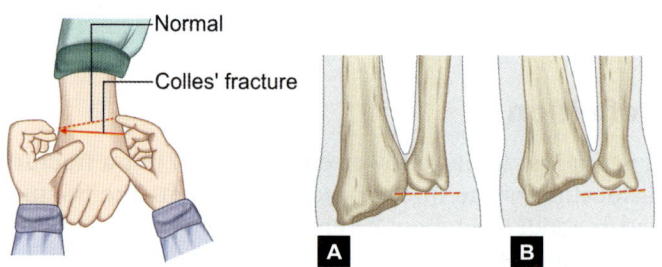

Figs 44.4A and B: Styloid process test: (A) Normal; (B) In Colles' fractures

TABLE 44.1: Colles'"A Fracture of 8"			
6 Displacements	6 Immobilization methods	6 Complications	
		Early complications	Late complications
1. Dorsal displacement	1. Below elbow cast (10–20° palmar flexion, 15–20° ulnar deviation) Colles' cast (see Figs 44.7A and B)	1. Unstable reduction	1. Malunion
2. Dorsal rotation	2. Above elbow cast in supination	2. Median or ulnar nerve stretched	2. Rupture of extensor pollicis tendon
3. Lateral displacement	3. Above elbow cast in pronation	3. Post-reduction-swelling	3. Sudeck's osteodystrophy
4. Lateral rotation	4. Above elbow cast in midpronation is the best (tension on interosseous membrane is less because brachioradialis muscle is relaxed in this position)	4. Compartmental syndrome	4. Frozen shoulder
5. Impaction	5. Cotton loder's position (wristfully flexed, useful in markedly displaced fractures)	5. Anesthesia problems	5. Carpal tunnel syndrome
6. Supination	6. External fixators. Immobilized for 6 weeks	6. Injury to proximal segment of the bone during reduction	6. Nonunion
Principal displacements			
1. Dorsal displacement			
2. Dorsal angulation			

view, the points noted are dorsal displacement and dorsal tilt of the distal fragment, sharp palmar surface and dorsal comminution of the lower end of radius, distal radioulnar joint subluxation, etc.

Classification

Contrary to popular belief, Colles' fracture is both intra-articular and extra-articular and not only extra-articular. Frykmann's classification takes into consideration both and the fracture of ulna (Fig. 44.6 and Table 44.2).

Treatment Methods

Aim: The aim of treatment is to restore fully functional hand with no residual deformity. The treatment methods include conservative methods, operative methods and external fixators (Figs 44.7 to 44.9).

Conservative Methods

Here fracture reduction is carried out by closed methods under general anesthesia (GA) or local anesthesia (LA).

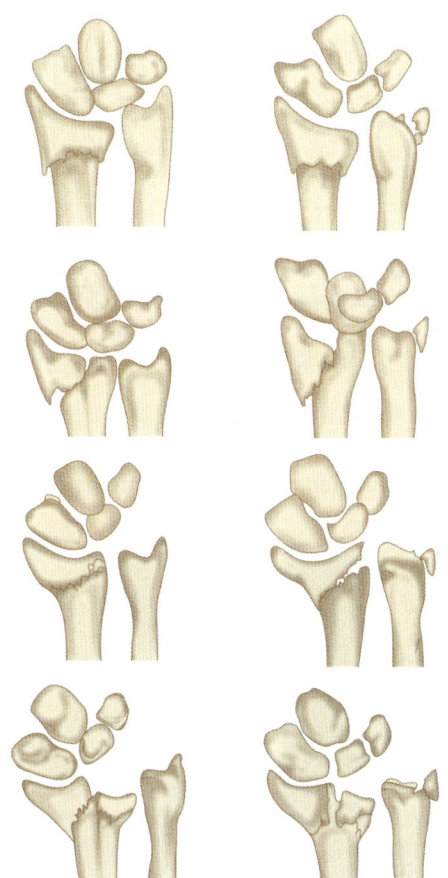

Fig. 44.6: Frykmann's varieties of Colles' fracture

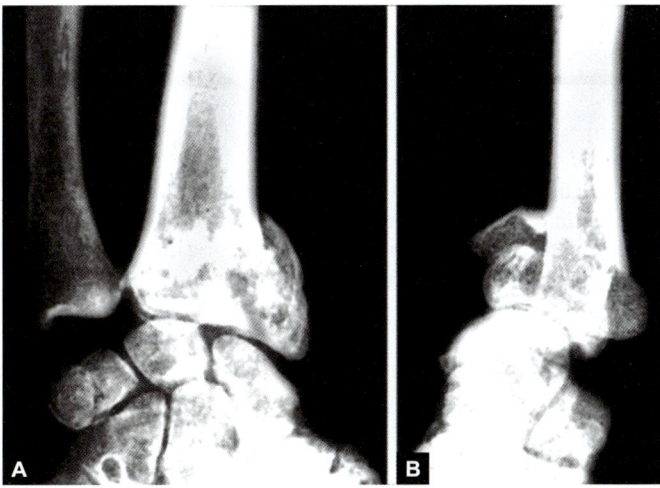

Figs 44.5A and B: Radiographs showing Colles' fracture: (A) AP view; (B) lateral view

TABLE 44.2: Frykmann's classification		
Fracture line	Distal ulnar fractures	
	Absent	Present
I. Extra-articular	I	II
II. Intra-articular (involvin gradiocarpal joint only)	III	IV
III. Intra-articular (involving distal RU joint only)	V	VI
IV. Intra-articular (both RC + inferior RU joints)	VII	VIII

Abbreviations: RC, radiocarpal; RU, radioulnar.

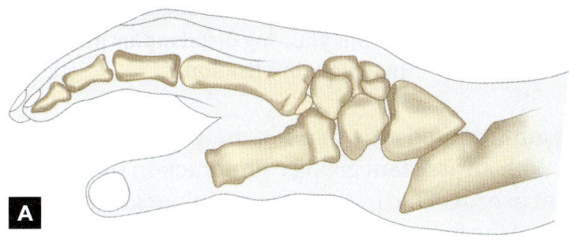
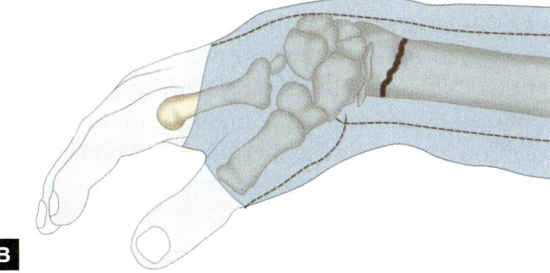

Figs 44.7A and B: (A) A typical Colles' fracture; (B) A typical Colles' cast

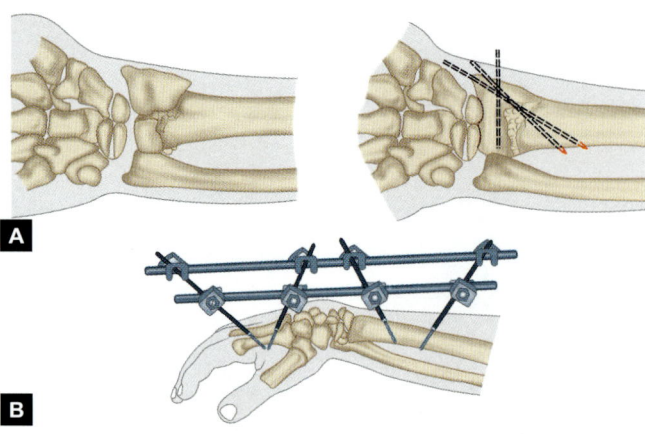

Figs 44.8A and B: Treatment method of Colles' fracture by: (A) Percutaneous fixation; (B) External fixation

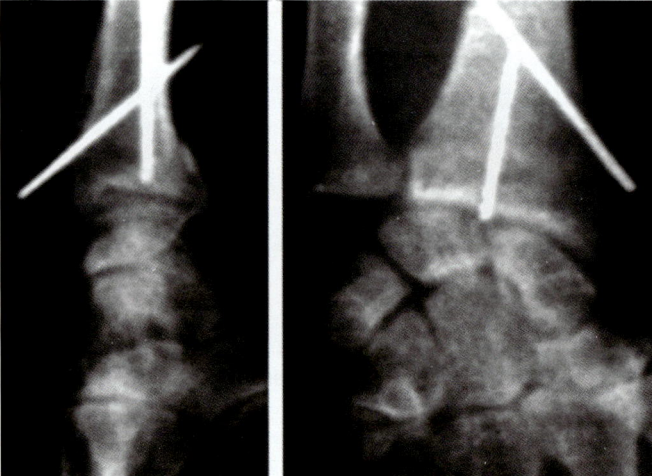

Fig. 44.9: Radiographs showing distal radius fracture percutaneous fixation

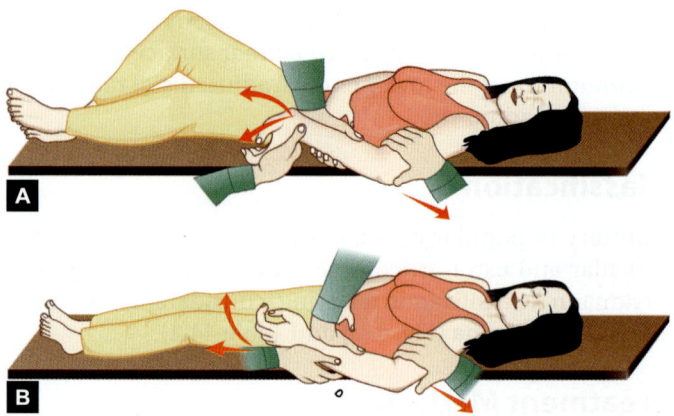

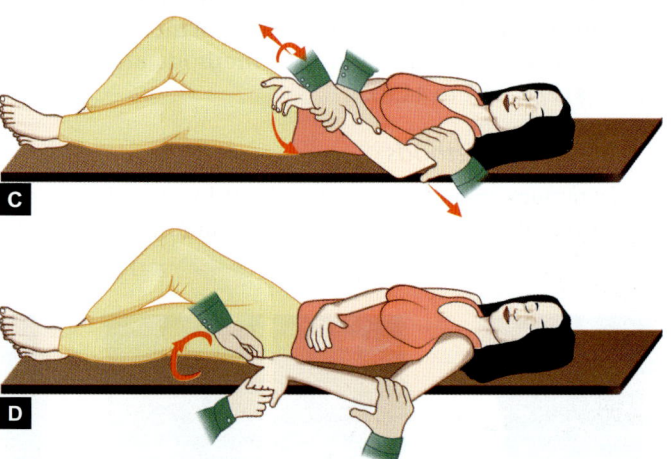

Figs 44.10A to D: Step by step closed reduction methods of Colles' fracture in an elderly woman: (A) Disimpaction; (B) Correcting anteroposterior displacements; (C) Correcting medial and lateral displacements; (D) Final manipulation

The examiner holds the hand of the patient as if to shake hand. With an assistant giving counteraction by holding the forearm or arm of the patient, the examiner gives traction in the line of the forearm. This disimpacts the fracture and the examiner corrects the other displacements of the fracture. At the end of the procedure, styloid process test is carried out to check the accuracy of reduction. If the level of the styloid processes is restored back to normal, it indicates that the reduction has been achieved satisfactorily. Then the limb is immobilized by any one of the methods in the table above (mainly Colles' cast) and a check radiograph is taken. The plaster cast is removed after 6–8 weeks and physiotherapy is begun (Figs 44.10 and 44.11).

Colles' Cast
It is a below elbow cast in supination and ideally, it has to meet the following four criteria:

- Firm fit at the dorsum.
- Firm fit at the volar fracture apex.
- Just snuggly fitting at the forearm.
- Metacarpophalangeal joints should be free to move.

What is New?
Sonographically guided closed reduction is an accurate, radiation free, simple tool that is as accurate as the conventional radiographic techniques.

The common causes for failure of reduction are incomplete reduction of the palmar fracture line and dorsal comminution of the lower end of radius.

Vital Facts
Do you know the acceptable limits of Colles' fracture after reduction?
- A dorsal tilt of less than 10 degrees.
- A radial shortening of less than 5 mm.

Technique of Closed Reduction and Application of a Colles' Cast Under Local Anesthesia (Figs 44.11A to I)*

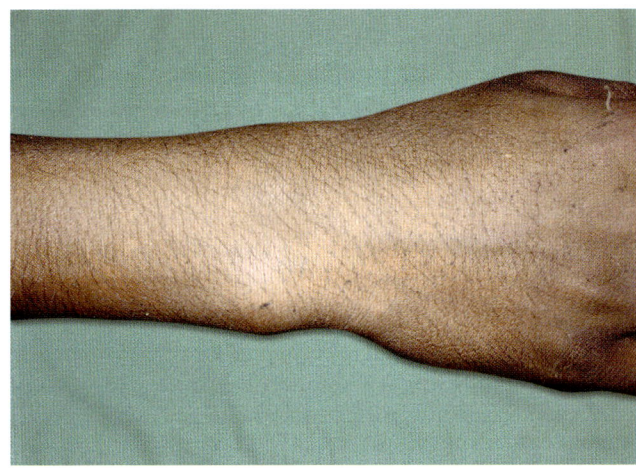

Fig. 44.11A: Dinner fork deformity

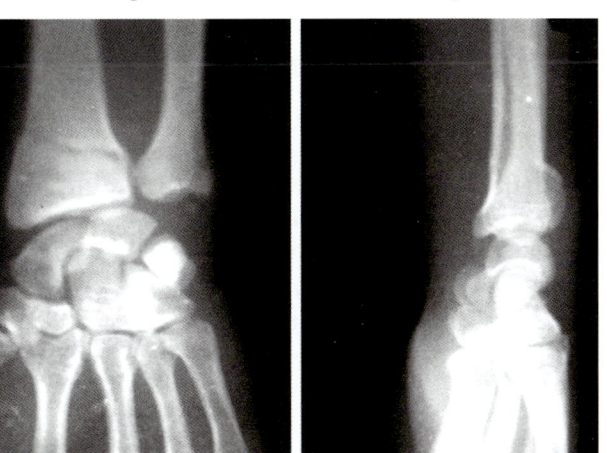

Fig. 44.11B: Radiograph showing AP and lateral views

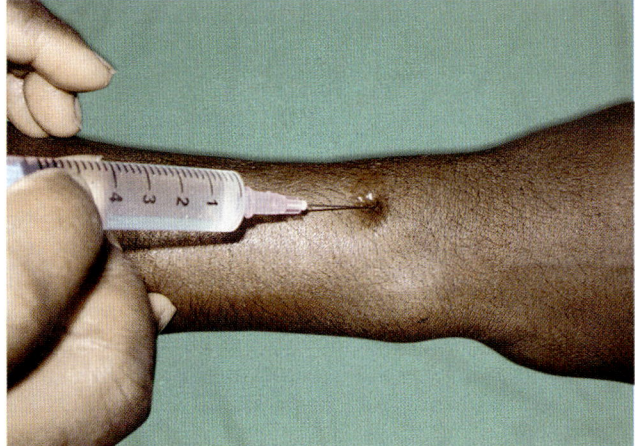

Fig. 44.11C: Injecting local anesthetic into the fracture site

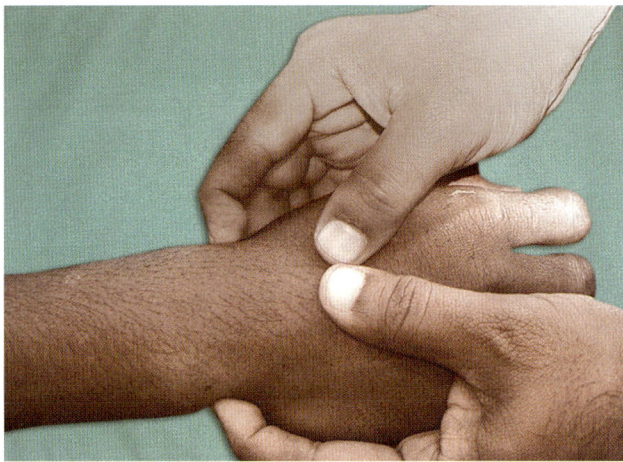

Fig. 44.11D: The styloid process test

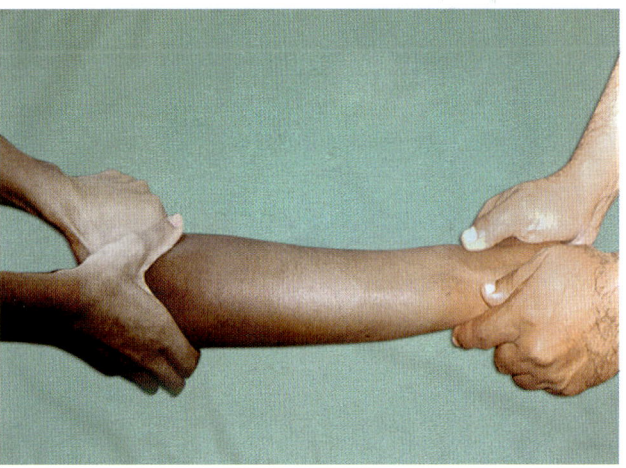

Fig. 44.11E: Reduction by traction and counter traction

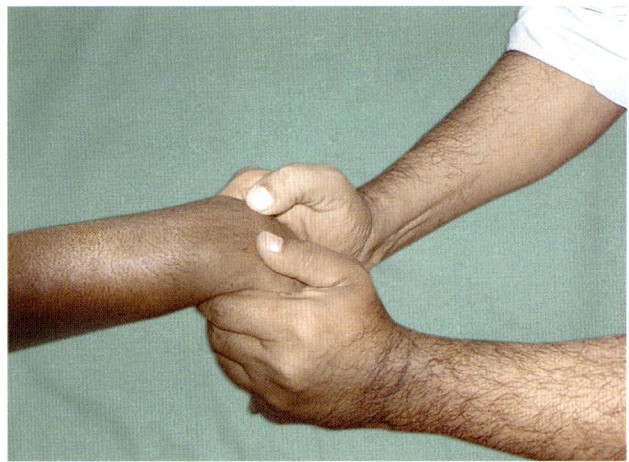

Fig. 44.11F: Manipulation of the fracture

*From "Step by Step Fracture Treatment" by Dr John Ebnezar.

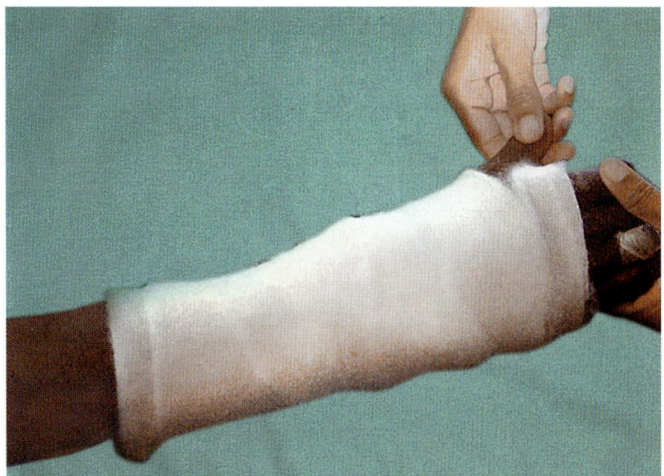

Fig. 44.11G: Application of soff ban

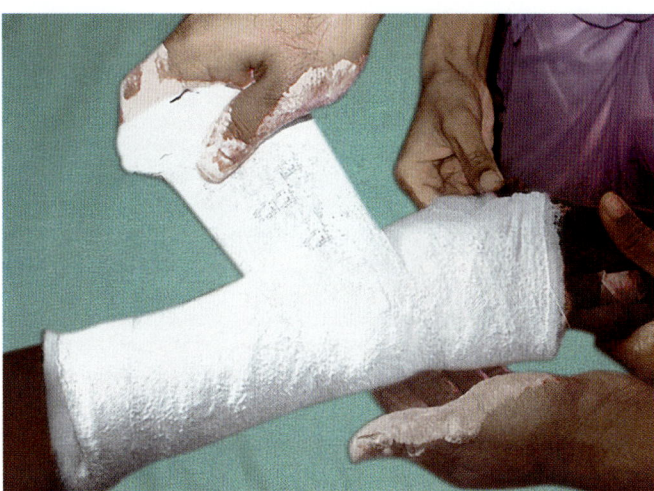

Fig. 44.11H: Application of the cast

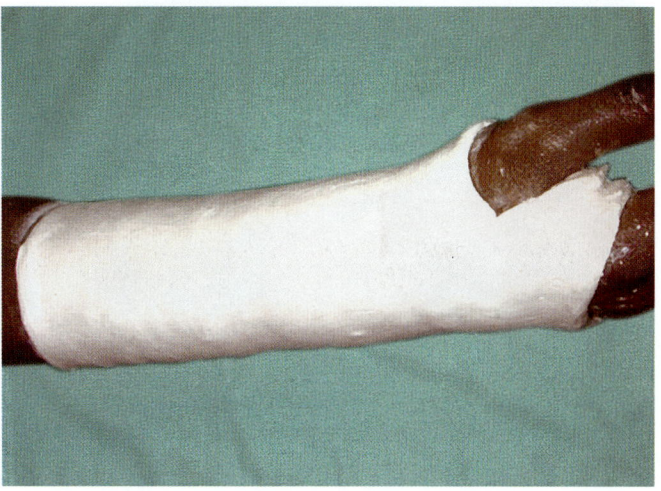

Fig. 44.11I: Colles cast final presentation

Operative Methods

Operative treatment is rarely required for Colles' fracture and may be required in the following situations:

Indications: Extensive comminution, impaction, median nerve entrapment and associated injuries in adults.

Modalities of operative treatment: Depending upon the degree of comminution and the intra-articular extensions, one of the following surgical methods is chosen:

Closed reduction and percutaneous pinning with K-wires: Here, after closed reduction by the usual methods, the fracture fragments are held together by percutaneous pinning by one or two K-wires.

Arm control: This method is known to prevent collapse and gives good results in a few select cases.

Salient Features of Percutaneous Fixation
- It is becoming popular, as it is simple.
- It prevents redisplacement.
- Always needs an external support.
- One of the cortexes should not be comminuted.
- Preferably two pins are used (one radial and other dorsal).
- Care should be taken not to injure the radial sensory branch, the tendons, etc.

Open reduction in certain fractures involving the rim of the distal articular surfaces (Barton's variety), open reduction and plate fixation (Ellis' plate) is advocated (*see* Fig. 44.13).

Indications: Same as for external fixation and for marginal volar or dorsal Barton's fractures.

Advantages
- Provides buttress
- Resists compression
- Load sharing
- Early mobilization.

What is New?
Arthroscopically assisted internal fixation.

External fixators (Fig. 44.13): These are found to be extremely useful in highly comminuted fractures, unstable fractures, compound fractures and bilateral Colles' fracture. Through a lightweight UMEX frames, two pins are placed in the forearm bones and two pins in the metacarpal bones of the hand. These pins are then fixed to an external frame and the fracture fragments are held in position by ligamentotaxis. The frame should be applied after obtaining closed reduction by the usual method (Figs 44.14A and B).

What is New?
Closed reduction and finger-trap traction is found to ensure better reduction and a lower rate of redisplacement than just manual manipulation (Fig. 44.15).

CHAPTER 44: Distal Forearm Fractures

Technique of Closed Reduction and Percutaneous Fixation with K-wires Under GA (Figs 44.12A to P)*

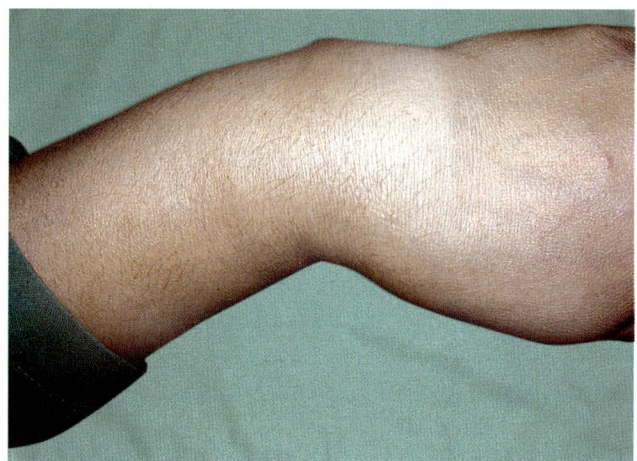

Fig. 44.12A: Gross deformity as viewed from the radial side

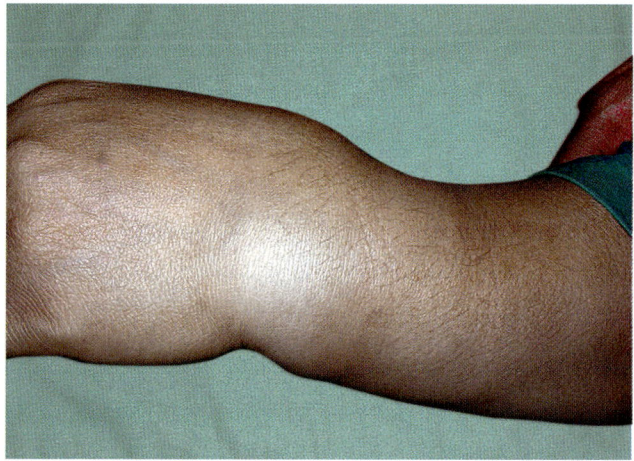

Fig. 44.12B: Deformity as viewed from the ulnar side

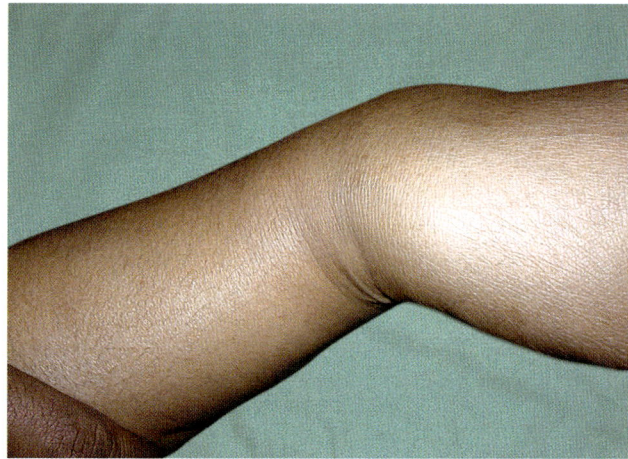

Fig. 44.12C: Deformity as viewed from the sides

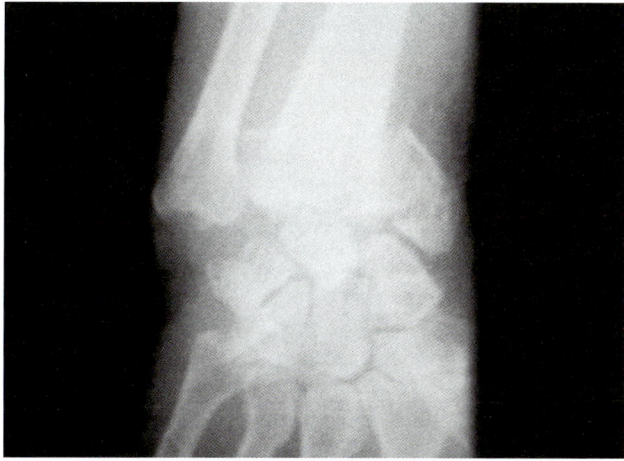

Fig. 44.12D: Radiograph showing comminuted intra-articular fracture of radius and subluxation of inferior radioulnar joint

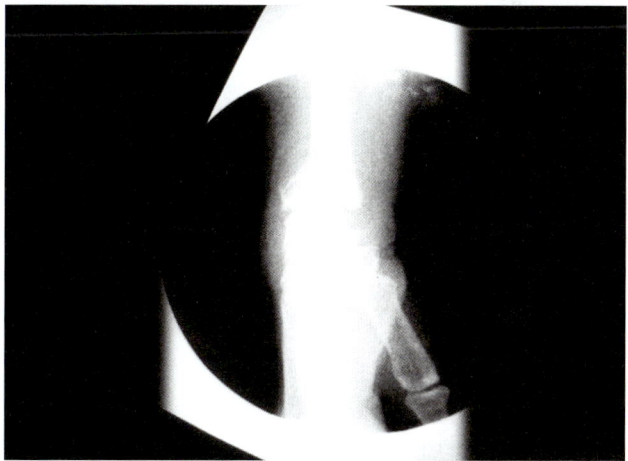

Fig. 44.12E: Radiograph showing lateral view

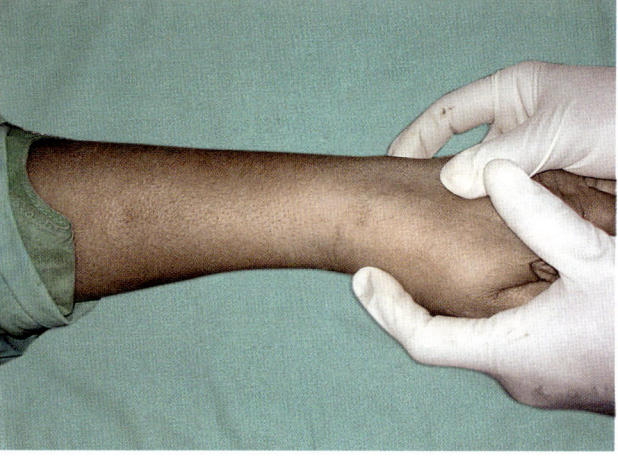

Fig. 44.12F: The styloid process test before closed reduction

*From "Step by Step Fracture Treatment" by Dr John Ebnezar.

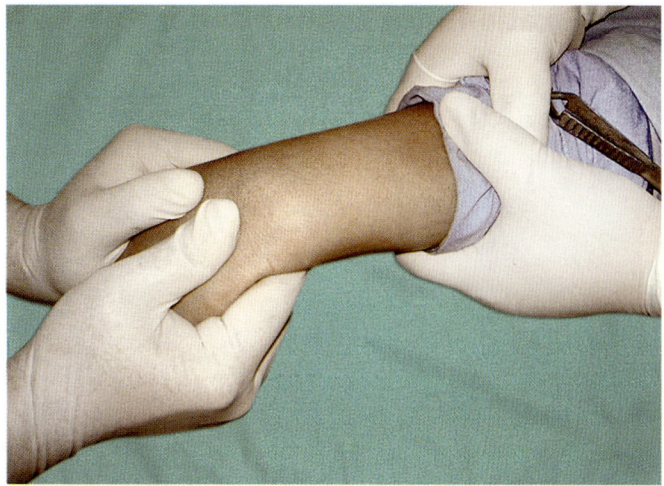

Fig. 44.12G: Reduction by traction and counter traction

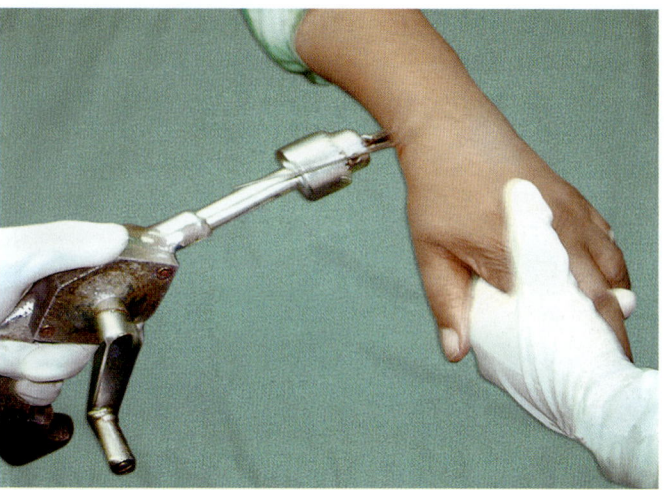

Fig. 44.12J: Placement of second pin

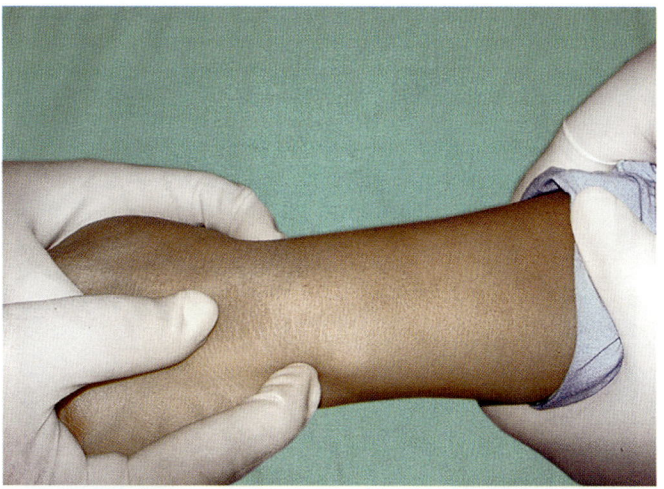

Fig. 44.12H: Checking for the satisfactory reduction

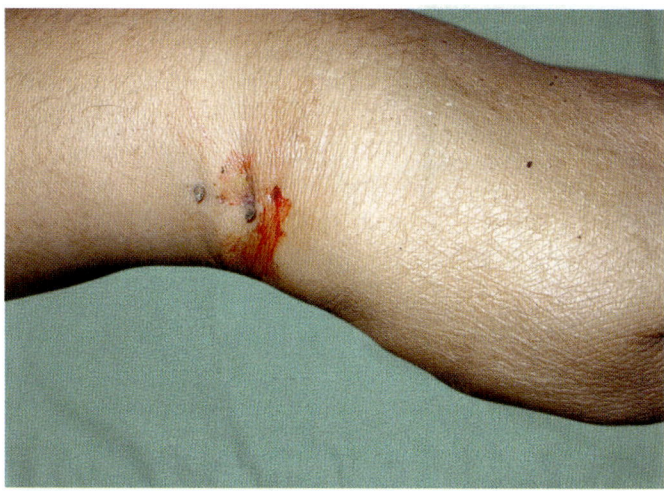

Fig. 44.12K: Pins cut flush to the skin

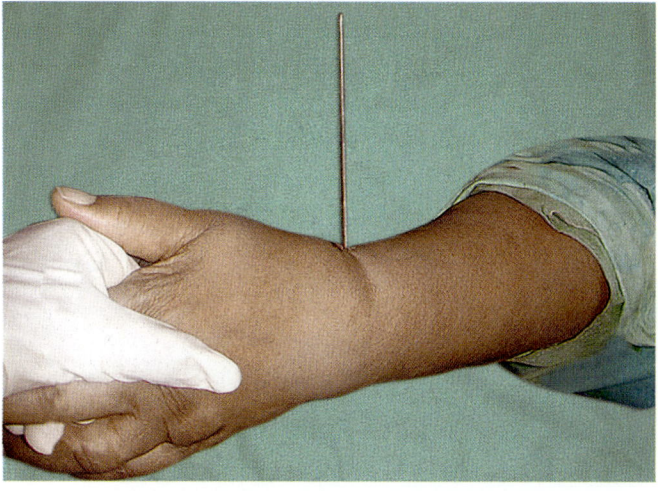

Fig. 44.12I: Percutaneous K wire fixation

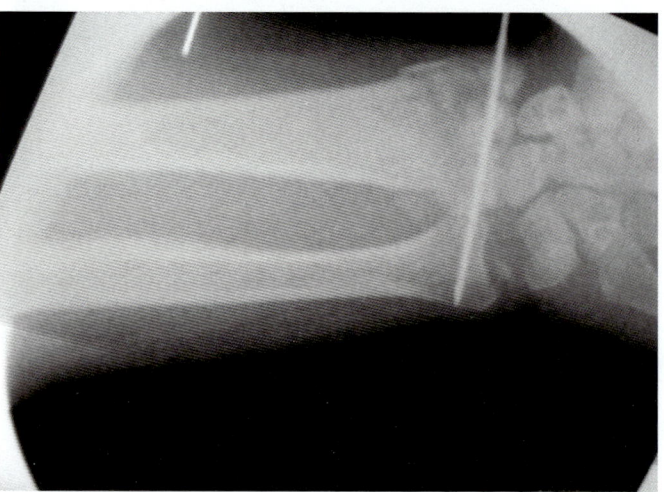

Fig. 44.12L: C-arm view after the first pin

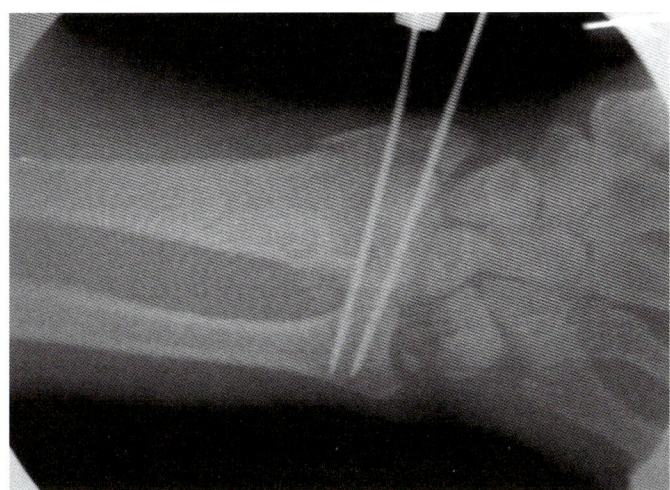

Fig. 44.12M: C-arm view after the second pin

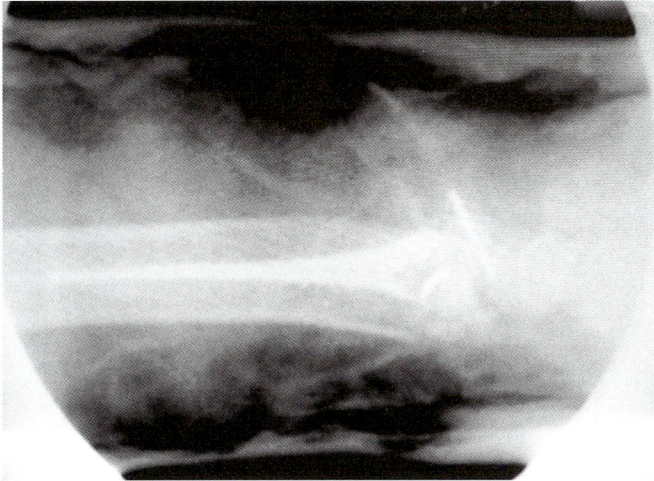

Fig. 44.12P: Lateral view

Complications

The important complications of Colles' fracture are listed in Table 44.1. Few significant complications are discussed here.

Malunion: This is the most common complication of Colles' fracture. Six important causes are responsible for it (Figs 44.16A to D).

- *Improper reduction:* If the fracture is not reduced properly, in the initial stages it may result in malunion later.
- *Improper and inadequate immobilization:* This fracture needs to be immobilized at least for a period of six weeks failing which malunion results.
- *Comminuted dorsal surface:* Due to extensive comminution, the fracture collapses and recurs after reduction and casting.

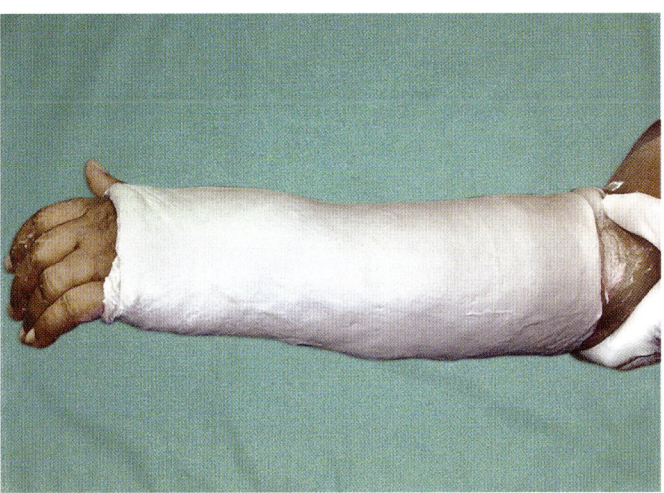

Fig. 44.12N: Colles cast applied

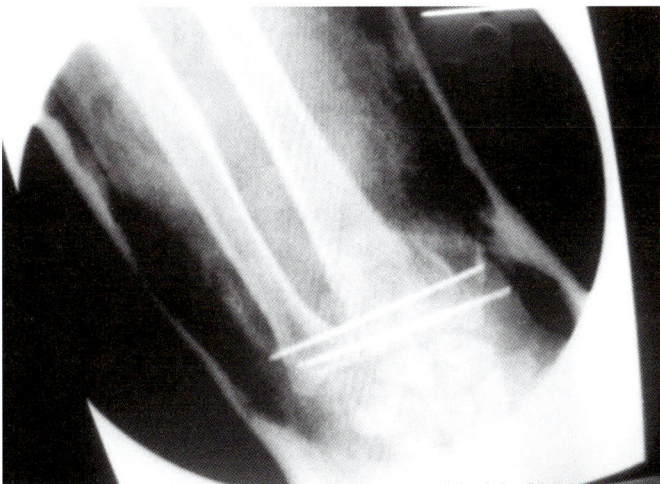

Fig. 44.12O: C-arm view after the pins and plaster

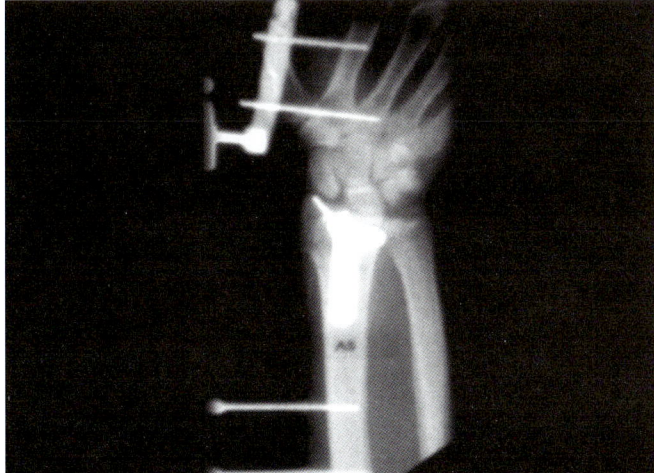

Fig. 44.13: Radiograph showing distal radius fracture being treated by both external fixator and plate screws

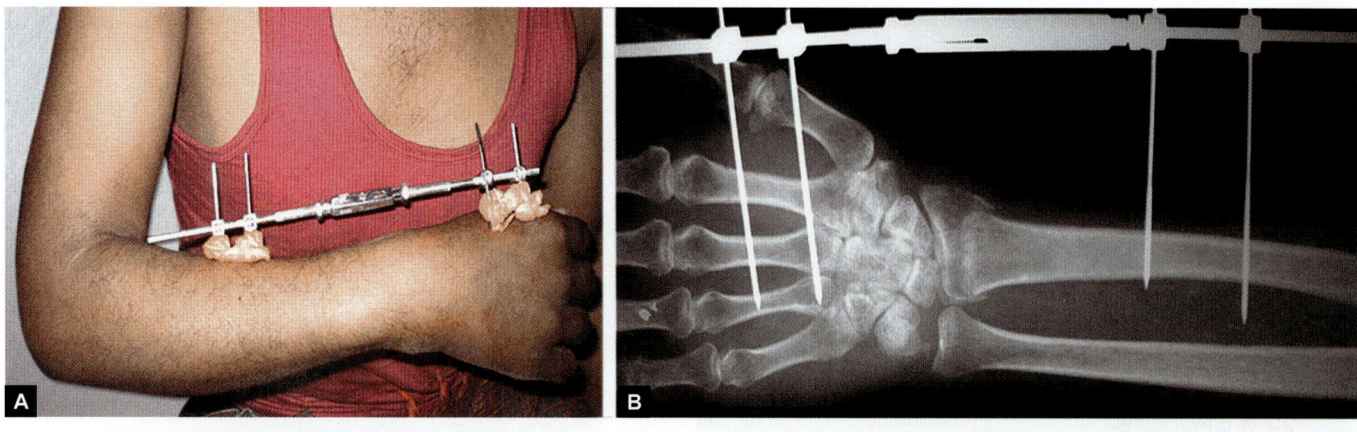

Figs 44.14A and B: (A) Clinical photo and (B) plain X-ray showing external fixation in distal radius fracture

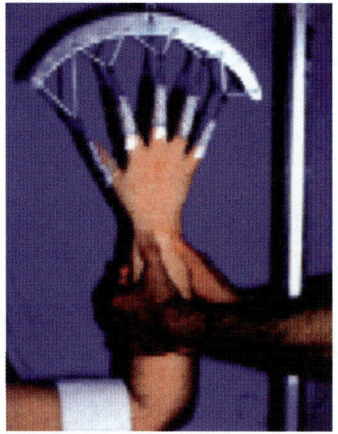

Fig. 44.15: Finger-trap traction for fracture reduction

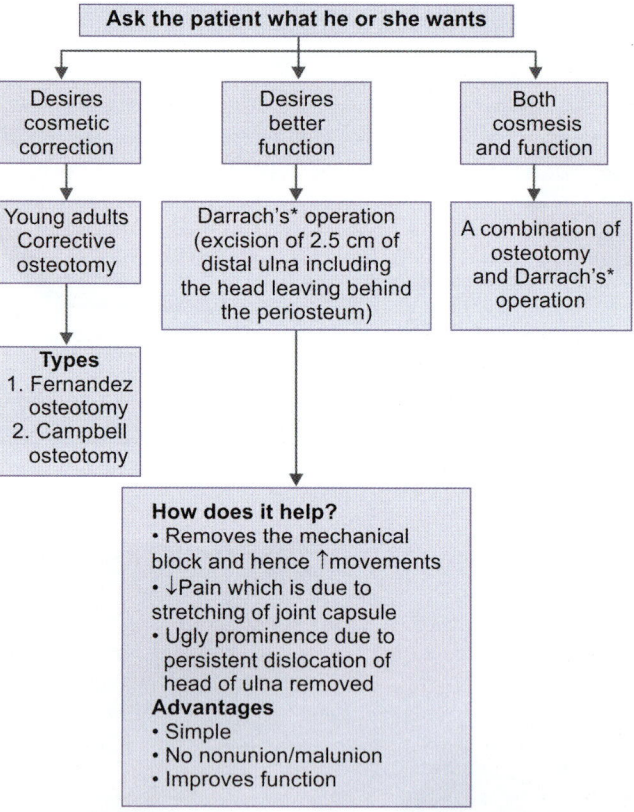

Flowchart 44.1: Approach to a patient with malunited Colles' fracture

*Darrach's is the most common surgery done for malunited Colles' fracture. It improves the function more than cosmesis, but still, it is preferred because Colles' fracture usually occurs in elderly women for whom function is important rather than cosmesis. If cosmesis is the priority, corrective osteotomy done at the radial fracture site gives good results.

- Osteoporosis may lead to collapse and recurrence.
- *Recurrence:* This is due to extensive comminution and osteoporosis.
- *Rupture of the distal radioulnar ligament:* This usually goes undetected in the initial stages of treatment and is responsible for the later recurrence.

Treatment

There are six options of treatment in a malunited Colles' fracture (Flowchart 44.1).
- No treatment is required if the patient has no functional abnormality.
- Remanipulation is attempted if fracture is less than 2 weeks old.
- Darrach's operation is more often indicated if the patient complains of functional disability.

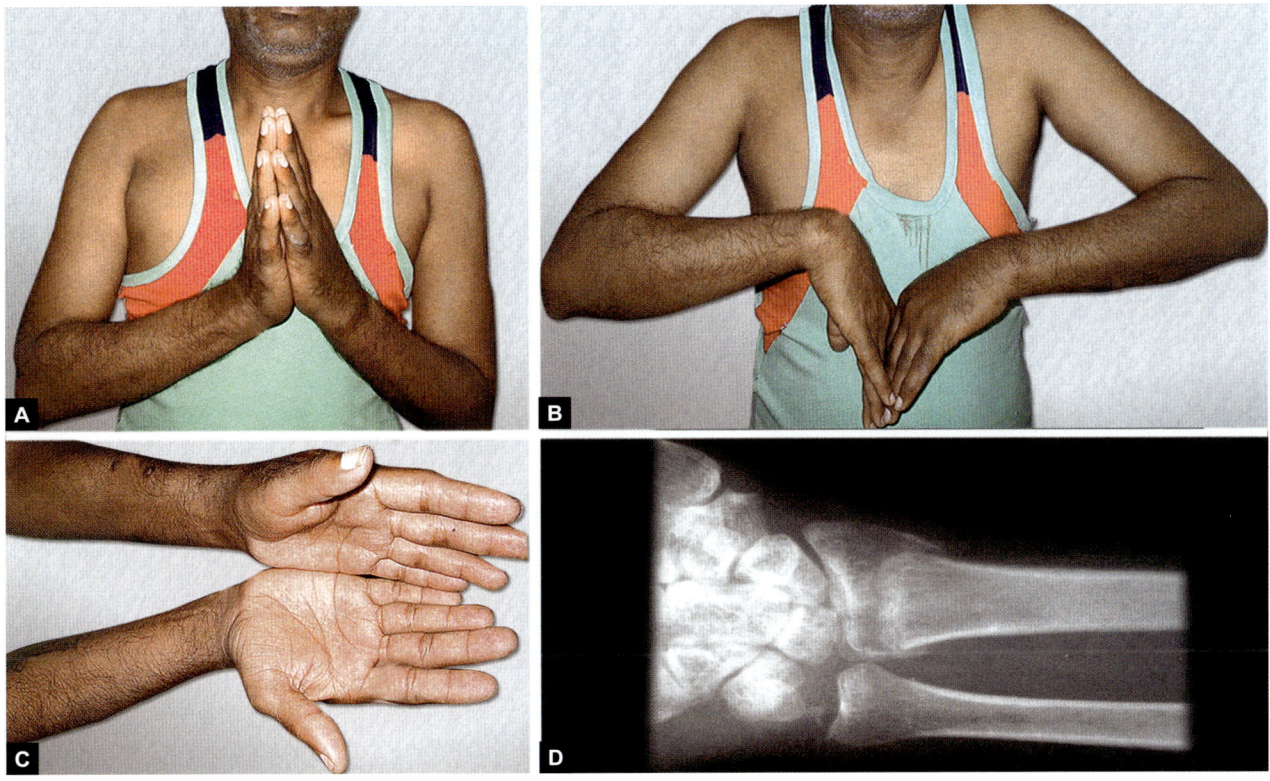

Figs 44.16A to D: Clinical photos and plain X-rays showing loss of dorsiflexion, palmar flexion and rotations of the forearm in malunion Colles fracture

- Corrective osteotomy and grafting if the patient wants cosmetic correction and if the patient is young (Fernandez and Campbell).
- Fernandez is a dorsal wedge osteotomy and Campbell is a lateral wedge osteotomy.
- *Arthrodesis (for intra-articular fracture):* The patient complains of pain in the wrist joint due to traumatic osteoarthritis following an intra-articular fracture. In these patients, arthrodesis of the wrist in functional position is the surgery of choice.
- Combination of these like Darrach's operation with osteotomy, etc. is also tried in some situations.

Rupture of extensor pollicis tendon: This occurs due to the attrition of the tendon as it glides over the sharp fracture surfaces. This usually occurs after 4–6 weeks and may be repaired or left alone with no residual disability.

Sudeck's osteodystrophy: This is due to abnormal sympathetic response, which causes vasodilatation and osteoporosis at the fracture site (Fig. 44.17). The patient complains of pain, swelling, painful wrist movements and red-stretched shiny skin (Fig. 44.18). Treatment consists of immobilization of the affected part with plaster splints, injection of local anesthetics near the sympathetic ganglion in the axilla or cervical sympathectomy in extreme cases.

Frozen hand shoulder syndrome: This is a troublesome complication, which develops due to unnecessary voluntary

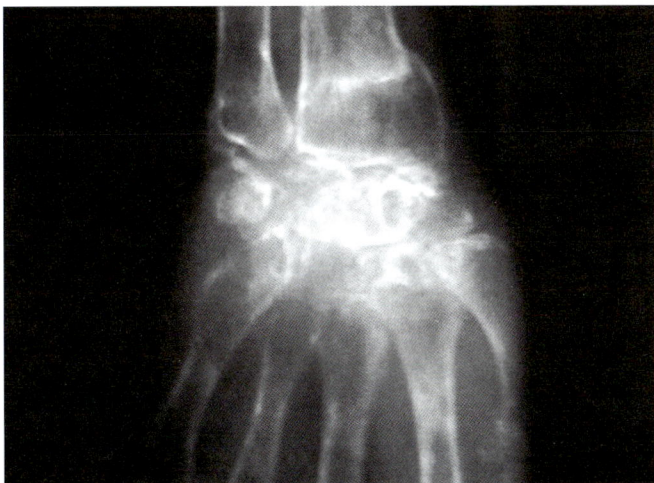

Fig. 44.17: Plain X-ray showing Sudeck's osteodystrophy

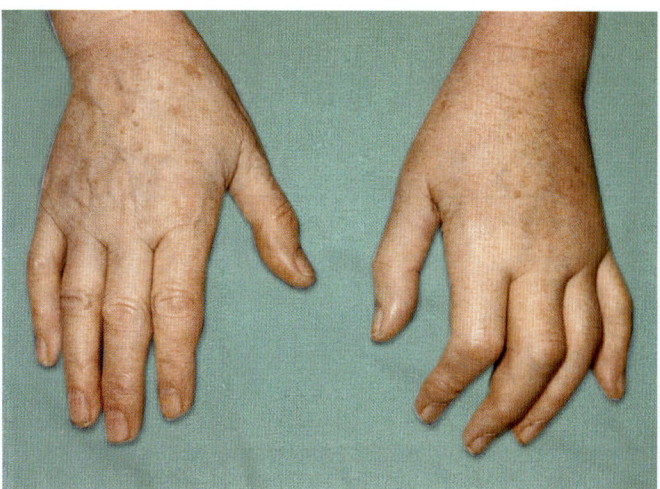

Fig. 44.18: Sudeck's osteodystrophy (Clinical photo)

shoulder immobilization by the patient on the affected side for fear of fracture displacements. It is said that the patient has performed a *mental amputation* and kept the limb still. (Fig. 44.19)

Carpal tunnel syndrome: Malunion of Colles' fracture crowds the carpal tunnel and compresses the median nerve.

Nonunion: This is extremely rare in Colles' fracture because of the cancellous nature of the bone, which enables the fracture to unite well. However, soft tissue interposition may cause this problem. The treatment consists of open reduction, rigid internal fixation and bone grafting.

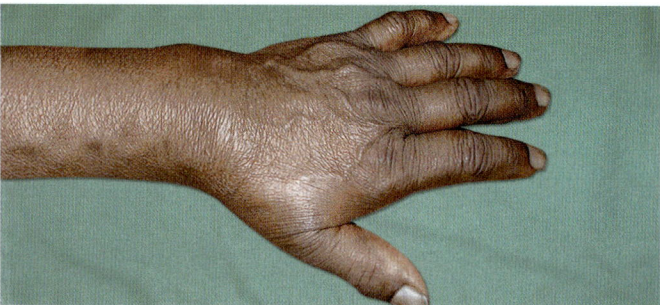
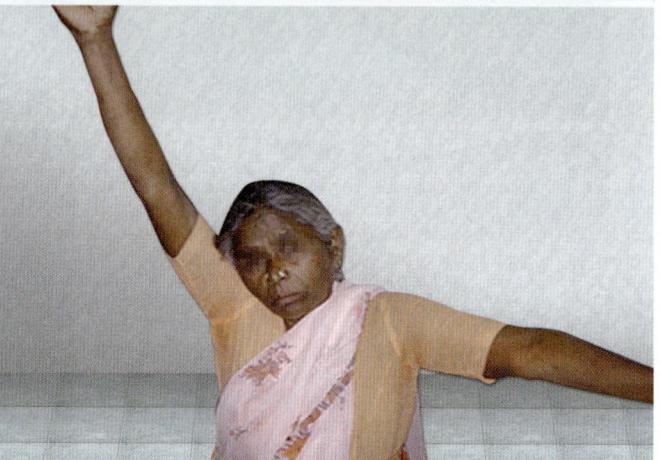

Fig. 44.19: Clinical photos showing frozen hand shoulder syndrome in Colles fracture

Quick Facts
Colles' fracture—why is it called fracture of 6?
- Common at 60 years.
- Force required to cause Colles' fracture are multiples of 6.
- 6 classical displacements.
- 6 methods of fracture immobilization.
- 6 weeks immobilization.
- 6 important early and late complications.
- 6 causes for malunion.
- 6 methods of managing malunion.
- 60 percent cases have fracture ulnar styloid.

45 CHAPTER

Fracture Neck of Femur

BRIEF ANATOMY

The Hip Joint Speaks
- I am an articulation between the femoral head and the acetabulum. I am a ball and socket variety of joint with a high degree of stability and an excellent range of movements exceeded only by my counterpart the shoulder joint. The head of the femur, which has a small fovea in the center, form the ball. This gives attachment to the ligamentum teres, which carries a small artery to the head. The deep socket of mine is formed by the acetabulum, which is lined by a horse shoe-shaped articular cartilage. The acetabular notch forms its inferior aspect, which is devoid of hyaline cartilage. The transverse ligament completes the socket inferiorly.
- The neck of femur is placed at an angle of 135° to the shaft and it projects 10-12° anteriorly to the coronal plane. My inherent strength depends upon the trabecular pattern (Fig. 45.1) which consists of primary and secondary compression and tensile trabeculae. These trabeculae are continuous with the trabeculae of the acetabulum. The degree of movements include flexion 0-140°, extension 0-15°, adduction 0-25° and abduction 0-30°.

FRACTURE NECK OF FEMUR

Quotation: We come to the world under the brim of pelvis and go out of the world through the fracture neck of femur.

Fracture neck femur could be intracapsular or extracapsular (see Figs 45.12A to C). Intracapsular fracture neck femur is notoriously known as an orthopedic enigma, since a permanent solution for its treatment still eludes the orthopedic surgeon. Hence, it is infamously termed as an unsolved problem. Fracture neck of femur does not unite readily and this makes it a difficult problem to tackle (see box for the reasons).

Problems of Healing, Why?
- No cambium layer in the intracapsular area, so no peripheral callus. Healing is only by endosteal callus.
- Synovial fluid lyses blood clot at the fracture site and thereby destroys another mode of secondary healing.
- Displaced fracture leads to avascularity.

Clinical Significance of Vascular Anatomy

Avascular necrosis of femoral head and nonunion fracture neck femur are the two very important and common complications of intracapsular fracture neck femur.

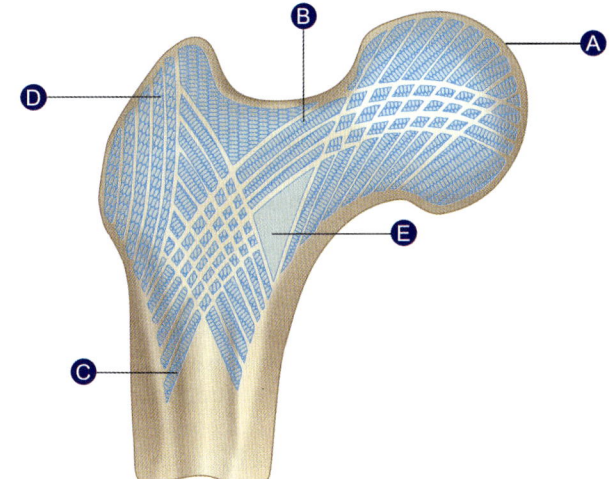

Fig. 45.1: Trabecular pattern or proximal femur: (A) Primary compressive trabeculae; (B) Primary tensile trabeculae; (C) Secondary tensile; (D) Secondary compressive trabeculae; (E) Ward's triangle

Flowchart 45.1: Blood supply of femoral head

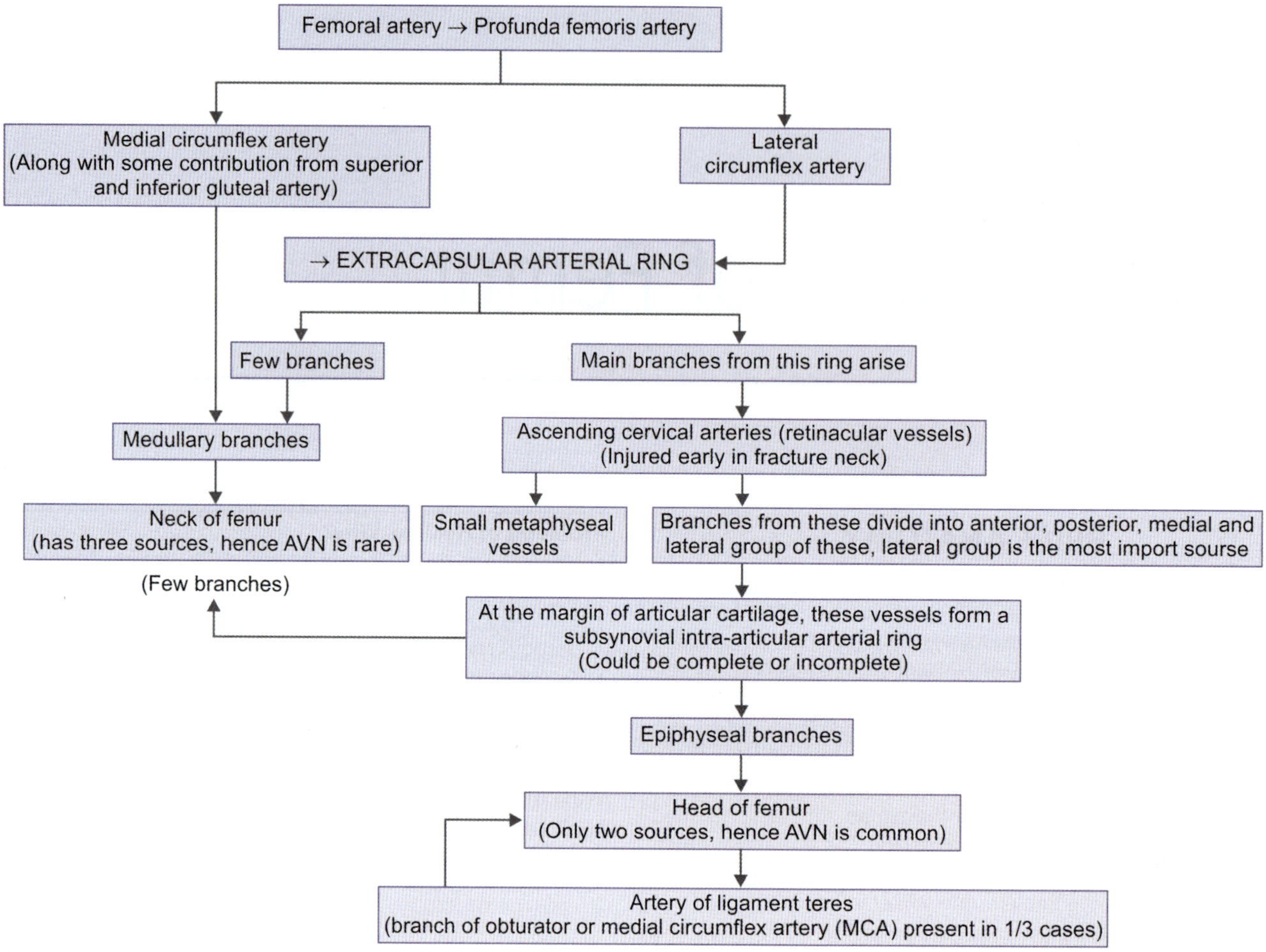

```
Femoral artery → Profunda femoris artery
         │
    ┌────┴────┐
    ↓         ↓
Medial circumflex artery        Lateral circumflex artery
(Along with some contribution
from superior and inferior
gluteal artery)
         │
         ↓
→ EXTRACAPSULAR ARTERIAL RING ←
         │
    ┌────┴────┐
    ↓         ↓
Few branches    Main branches from this ring arise
    │              │
    ↓              ↓
Medullary     Ascending cervical arteries (retinacular vessels)
branches      (Injured early in fracture neck)
    │              │
    ↓         Small metaphyseal    Branches from these divide into anterior,
Neck of femur  vessels             posterior, medial and lateral group of
(has three                         these, lateral group is the most import source
sources, hence
AVN is rare)
(Few branches)
              At the margin of articular cartilage, these vessels form a
              subsynovial intra-articular arterial ring
              (Could be complete or incomplete)
                         │
                         ↓
                 Epiphyseal branches
                         │
                         ↓
                 Head of femur
                 (Only two sources, hence AVN is common)
                         │
                         ↓
                 Artery of ligament teres
                 (branch of obturator or medial circumflex artery (MCA) present in 1/3 cases)
```

A thorough knowledge of the vascular anatomy (Fig. 45.2) is necessary to understand the reasons behind. Femoral head circulation is through three sources:
- Intraosseous cervical vessels.
- Artery of ligamentum teres.
- Retinacular vessels.

In fracture neck femur, intraosseous cervical vessels are disrupted and blood supply is dependent on artery of ligamentum teres and retinacular vessels only (Flowchart 45.1). Artery of ligamentum teres supplies only a small portion of head, hence, avascular necrosis of the head of the femur occurs if retinacular vessels, the only main source, are damaged in fracture neck femur. There are two sources of viability of femoral head after a displaced femoral neck fracture:
1. Residual uninjured vascular supply.
2. Revascularization of neck of femur from surrounding soft tissue before late segmental collapse.

"Therefore, the aim of treatment is early anatomical reduction, impaction and rigid internal fixation to protect

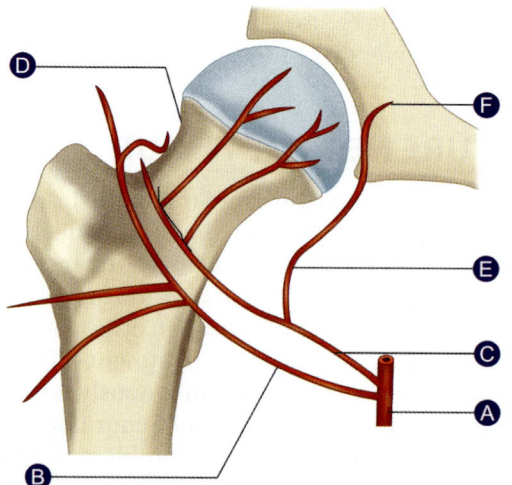

Fig. 45.2: Vascular anatomy of femoral head: (A) Profunda femoris artery; (B) Lateral circumflex artery; (C) Medial circumflex artery; (D) Ascending retinacular vessels; (E) Obturator branch of medial circumflex artery; (F) Artery of the ligamentum teres

the existing circulation and to allow revascularization to take place before late segmental collapse can occur."

Etiology

- It is common in older patients with osteoporosis or osteomalacia (12%) and in them; usually it is fracture through a pathological bone.
- It is common in elderly women secondary to senile osteoporosis. It also causes marked comminution of the posterior cortex and thus decreases the quality of reduction.

Mechanism of Injury

- Majority are due to trivial fall, because of direct blow over the greater trochanter (Fig. 45.3).
- Second mechanism is mainly due to lateral rotation of the extremity, which causes marked posterior comminution of the neck.
- Recent suggested mechanism is cyclical loading due to muscle force and torsion.
- Major trauma in young adults like road traffic accident (RTA), fall, etc.

Classification

Many classifications are proposed for fracture neck femur. Few important ones are mentioned here.

Broad Classification

- Intracapsular—from subcapital area to the middle of the neck.
- Extracapsular—from base of the neck to the pertrochanteric region (Fig. 45.4).

Structural Classification

- Impacted—here the fragments are telescoped into each other.
- Undisplaced.
- Displaced.

Causatively

- Stress fractures (seen in soldiers, athletes, etc.)
- Pathologic fractures (seen in osteoporosis, etc.)
- Postirradiation fractures.

Based on Fracture Character

- *Anatomical location:*
  - Sub capital—beneath the neck.
  - Transcervical—in the middle of the neck.
  - Basal—at the base of the neck.
    * Bank's subclassification
      - Classical subcapital
      - Wedge subcapital (common)
      - Inferior beak appearance.
- *Fracture angle:*
  - Pauwel's (Angle the fracture line forms with respect to horizontal line—Fig. 45.5).
    More the angle more is it likely to be unstable.
    - I 30°
    - II 50°
    - III 70°
  - Perlington's (Angle the fracture line forms with respect to the vertical line)
    - I 70°
    - II 50°
    - III 30°

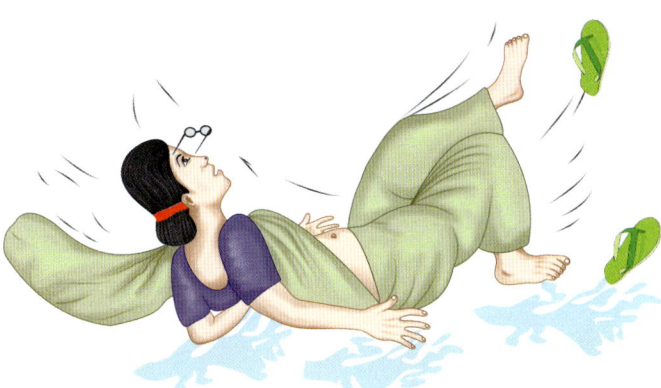

Fig. 45.3: Fracture neck femur is common in elderly females due to trivial fall like a slip and fall in the bathroom

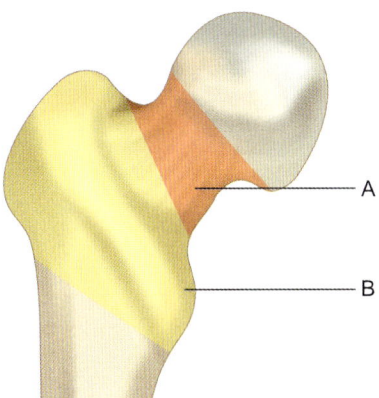

Fig. 45.4: Fracture neck femur types: (A) Intracapsular region; (B) Extracapsular region

- [1]Garden's classification (Fig. 45.6) This is the most accepted classification and is based on the pattern of fracture line and the displacement of the fracture:
  - Incomplete fracture
  - Complete fracture but undisplaced
  - Complete fracture with partial displacement
  - Complete fracture with total displacement.

Delbet's Classification (Fig. 45.7) in Children

- Transepiphyseal—at the junction of the head and neck.
- Transcervical—through the middle of the neck.
- Cervicotrochanteric (basal) at the junction of neck and shaft.
- Intertrochanteric in between the greater and lesser trochanters.
- Pertrochanteric—at the level of the trochanter.

> **Note:**
> Garden and Pauwel's classification in adults and Delbet's classification in children are widely used while the others are mentioned for student's information.

Clinical Features

Usually, the patient is an elderly female and gives history of trivial trauma like slip and fall in the bathroom (see Fig. 45.3). The patient complains of pain and restriction of movements of the affected hip. On examination, there is tenderness over the anterior hip joint line. There is minimal shortening and external rotational deformity of the affected limb due to the fracture being intracapsular. The capsule prevents the muscular forces from displacing the fracture fragments grossly. Active straight leg rising is difficult. In impacted fracture neck of femur, the patient complains of groin pain, antalgic gait and restriction of hip movements.

Investigations

Radiography

Consists of routine AP and lateral views of the hip joint. The following points are noted (Fig. 45.8).
- The extent of fracture line whether complete or incomplete
- The fracture angle
- Break in the *Shenton's line* (Fig. 45.9)

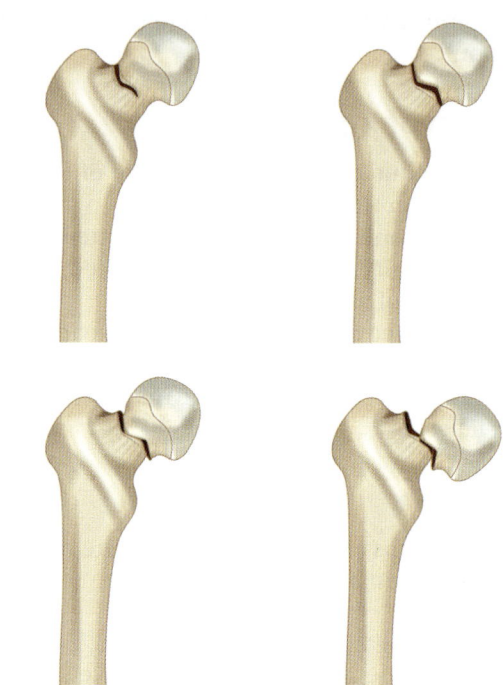

Fig. 45.6: Garden's classification

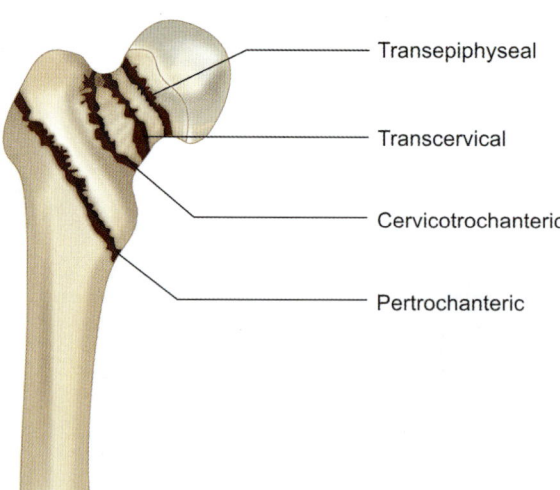

Fig. 45.7: Delbet's classification for fracture neck of femur in children

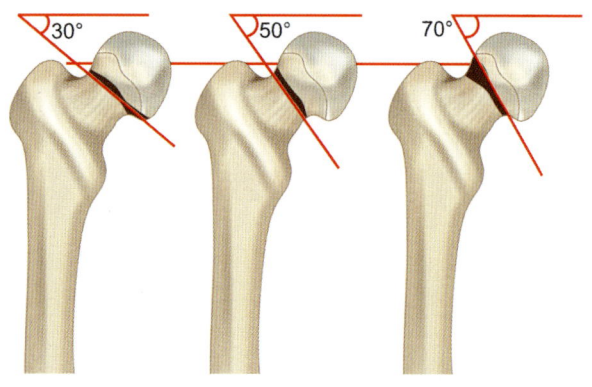

Type I 30° Type II 50° Type III 70°
Fig. 45.5: Pauwel's classification of fracture neck femur

---

[1]**RS Garden**. Orthopaedic Surgeon, Preston, England, described this classification in 1961.

CHAPTER 45: Fracture Neck of Femur

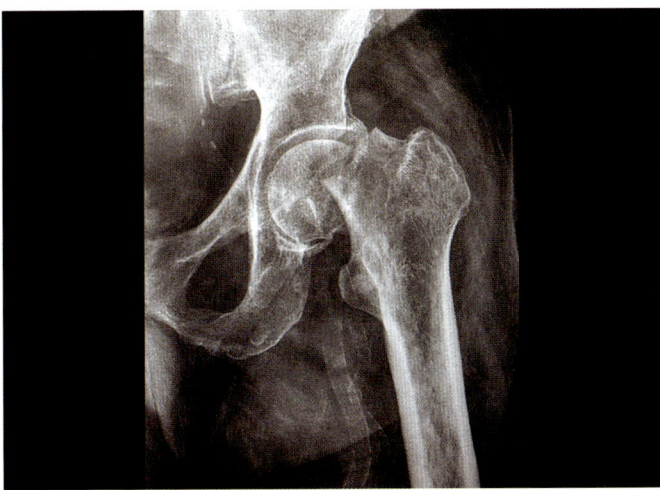

Fig. 45.8: Radiograph showing intracapsular fracture neck femur

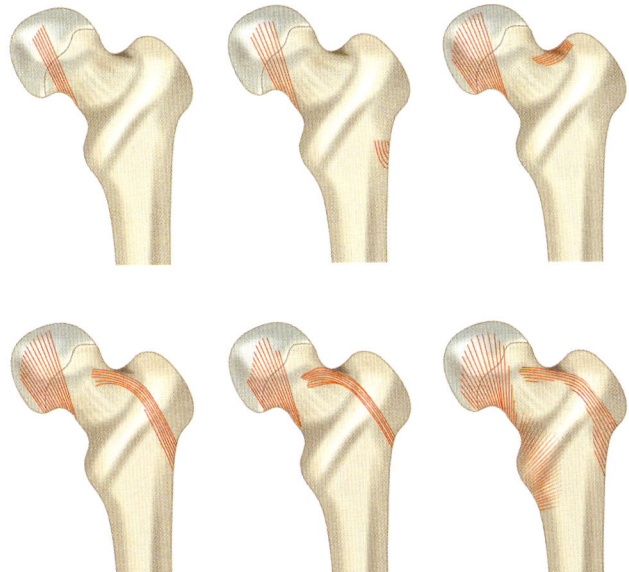

Fig. 45.10: Singh's index

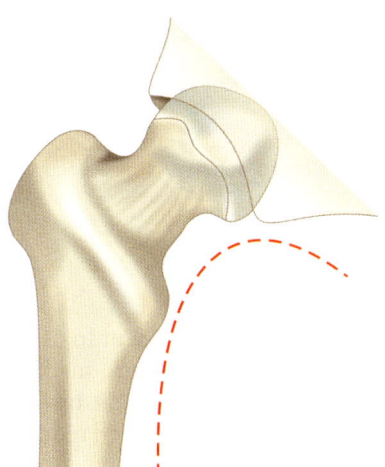

Fig. 45.9: Shenton's line

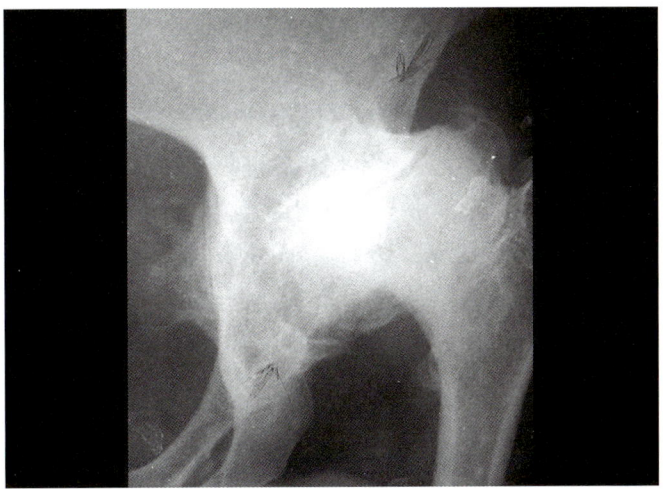

Fig. 45.11: Radiograph showing avascular necrosis of femoral head

- Posterior wall comminution of the neck is best seen in the lateral view
- Prominent lesser trochanter
- The degree of osteoporosis (Singh's index)
- *Shenton's line* is a line drawn from the superior margin of the obturator foramen to the margin of the neck
- *Singh's Index:* This classification system measures the degree of osteoporosis in the proximal femur based on radiographic evaluation of the trabecular pattern (Fig. 45.10). This helps to decide the choice of implants.

Other Investigations

Radiography has limited value in assessing the vascular status of the femoral head. The time required for a radiograph to show avascular changes is 3-6 months (Fig. 45.11). Hence, viability and vascularization of femoral head at the time of surgery is determined by:

- Oxygen tension measurement
- Venography
- Intraosseous pressure recording
- Isotope scanning
- Bone scan with technetium-99m, sulphur colloid, etc.

Treatment

Fracture neck femur is an orthopedic emergency, which needs to be reduced and fixed within 24 hours to get an optimum result. Hence, *speed is the watchword* in managing fracture neck femur and invariably needs to be operated because of the small proximal fragment accurate reduction is required, which is usually not possible by conservative methods.

Aims of Treatment

- Early anatomical reduction, which helps and prevents further vascular damage.
- Impaction of the fracture fragments.
- *Rigid internal fixation:* Enables revascularization from the surrounding soft tissues and uninjured bones, which helps in early callus formation.

Broad Treatment Guidelines (Earlier)

Age group	Undisplaced	Displaced
>70 years	• Dynamic hip Screws (DHS)	• Prosthesis • Total hip replacement (THR)
Young adults	• DHS • Cannulated screws (ASNIS)	• DHS • Later osteotomy or prosthesis
Children	• HIP spica • Multiple Moore's pinning	• Multiple Moore's pinning • Osteotomy • Arthrodesis

Broad Treatment Guidelines for Displaced Neck Fracture (Now)

- < 65 years—CRIF/Or ORIF if necessary
- 65-75 years—CRIF and if closed reduction is unsuccessful then cemented bipolar arthroplasty.
- >75 years—Cemented bipolar arthroplasty
- >75 years (and poor home ambulator)—cemented unipolar arthroplasty
- >75 years (bedridden)—Percutaneous CRIF under local or sedation
- Persistent arthritis—Total hip replacement
- Bed ridden and not mobile—Non operative or CRIF

Treatment Plans as per Garden's Classification

Garden I:
- Conservative Hip spica is applied if fracture is several weeks old and if the patient is unfit for surgery.
- Surgical Multiple pins by Moore, Knowles cannulated screws, etc.

Garden II: Here the fracture is complete and may be displaced. Hence, it is fixed with either DHS or multiple cannulated AO screws.

Garden III/IV: Conservative treatment is rarely indicated except in severely ill patients and mentally ill patients, e.g. hip spica and well leg traction. Surgery is the treatment of choice.

Surgery

Goal of surgery is anatomical reduction, impaction and stable internal fixation.

Closed reduction with hip in extension	Closed reduction with hip in flexion
Whitman's method Extension + internal rotation + abduction Movements of the hip	**Lead better method** Flexion of hip, traction along long axis of femur, thigh internally rotated and abducted. Evaluate reduction by *"heel palm test".
Massie Forceful internal rotation of the limb	**Smith Peterson** Slight hip flexion + then internal rotation + abduction + extension
Mc Elevenny	**Flynn** Flexion, traction along the femoral neck
Extension + external Rotation + Internal Rotation + adduction movements	
Deyerle Traction with extension + foot is internally rotated + Force applied on greater trochanter from anterior to posterior direction	

*Note: What is 'heel palm' test?
It is a clinical test to assess the accuracy of reduction of fracture neck femur. The heel of the affected limb should remain neutral in the palm of the clinician's hand and not lie externally rotated after reduction.

Reduction Techniques

Acceptable reduction is the key factor in decreasing risk of avascular necrosis following fracture neck femur. Closed reduction is tried first failing which open reduction is resorted to. The following are the closed reduction methods:

Radiograph

Radiographic evaluation of the accuracy of reduction of the fracture neck femur, obtained by any one of the methods employed above is done. It is mandatory before proceeding with internal fixation. The following are some of the parameters:

- Head and neck always form an S-shaped curve. If the radiograph reveals an unbroken C-shaped curve the fracture is not reduced.
- *Garden's criteria:* In AP view, normal alignment index between proximal and distal fragments post-reduction is 155-180°.
- In lateral view, it is 160-180°. If the angle is less than 155° or more than 180° in of the views, then the reduction is not acceptable.
- *Lateral view* helps to detect the posterior wall comminution. Stability of reduction depends on posterior wall comminution, which causes nonunion in 60 percent of the cases.

- Slight valgus with 2-3 mm separation of the fracture site at the medial calcar is not acceptable. However, varus is not accepted at all.

If two attempts at closed reduction fail, then open reduction is resorted to. Probably, there is no other fracture, which needs such an accurate reduction before proceeding for internal fixation. Hence, the reduction should be accurately assessed to get good results.

Techniques of Internal Fixation

However, there are many choices for internal fixation in fracture neck femur, the principles of preoperative preparation, reduction of the fracture, C-arm or radiographic control, surgical approaches and methods of insertion of fixations are the same.

Procedure

The patient is fixed to the fracture table after anesthesia. Closed reduction of the fracture is done under radiograph or C-arm control. If the reduction is satisfactory, the greater trochanter and upper end of femur is exposed through a lateral incision. Midway between the anterior and posterior cortices of the lateral femur and about 2 cm distal to the edge of the greater trochanter drill a hole, insert a guidepin at an angle of 45° to the shaft, and parallel to the ground. Check the positions of the guide-wires by lateral radiographs or C-arm. If satisfactory, insert the cannulated screws or Moore's pins parallel to the guide-wire and if Richard's screw is used through the guide-wire. Confirm the position of all the pins as mentioned above and close the wound in layers. Postoperatively, the patient is mobilized early.

Choices of Implants for Internal Fixation

After having accurately reduced the fracture and ascertained the accuracy, the fracture neck femur can be fixed by any one of the methods mentioned below. However, no ideal internal fixation methods are available (Figs 45.12A to C).
- *Multiple Pins (Knowles, Moore)* for impacted fracture, percutaneously for medically unfit persons, and for fractures in children (Fig. 45.12D).
- *ASNIS:* This is a system of cannulated screws that provide improved pullout and bending and torque strengths as compared to Knowles pins. These are the commonly preferred screws for the intracapsular variety (Fig. 45.12E).
- *Fixed angle nail* has fallen into disrepute because the nail is rigid and may penetrate the joint (Fig. 45.12B).
- *Sliding or telescoping nails (dynamic hip screws):* It has replaced the fixed angle nail. The nail offers collapsibility which ensures continuous impaction at the fracture site and which lessens the chance of nail penetration through the femoral head. This is the most commonly employed fixation method for fracture neck femur, especially the extracapsular variety (Fig. 45.12C).

Cardinal Points in Internal Fixation

- Guidepins should be inserted at an angle of 45° to the shaft and parallel to the ground.
- Guidepin should be in the center and stop short of the head by 1.3 cm.
- The internal fixation screws or pins should be in the midcenter of the neck or below and posterior to prevent damage to the retinacular vessels.
- The guidepin should be inserted slowly and should pass smoothly without any resistance.
- The screws or pins should be 0.6 cm shorter when placed above and 0.6 cm longer when placed below the guidepin.

Complications of Internal Fixation

Infection: This is due to poor aseptic measures during surgery. The infection may be superficial or deep and is a troublesome problem to treat.

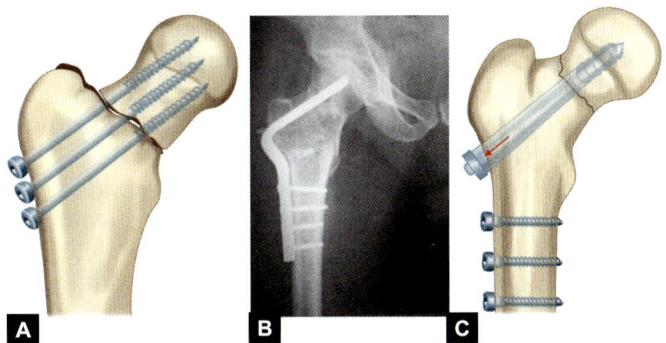

Figs 45.12A to C: Methods of internal fixation of intracapsular fracture neck of femur: (A) Multiple pins; (B) Blade plate fixation; (C) Dynamic hip screw

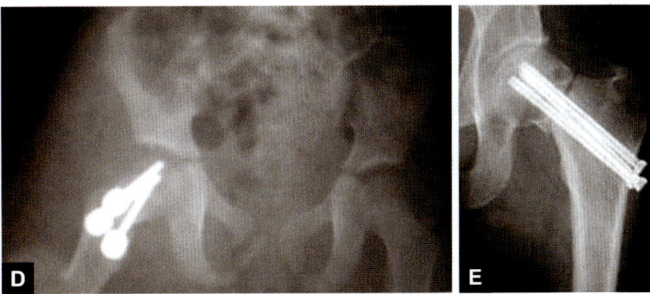

Figs 45.12D and E: Fixation with multiple Moore's pin in children; (E) Fixation with multiple cannulated screws

Nonunion results if the fixation methods are not rigid.

Avascular necrosis: This is due to faulty position of the pins in the superior part of the neck, which may damage the retinacular vessels leading to avascularity.

Loss of fixation: This could occur due to osteoporosis, loosening, etc.

Meyer's Muscle Pedicle Graft

A mention has to be made about the posterior muscle pedicle grafting technique. Muscle pedicle graft from the gluteus maximus or quadratus femoris (Meyer's technique), is particularly useful in posterior wall comminution. Dr Bakshi of Kolkata has popularized this technique.

Other Treatment Options

These include hemireplacement arthroplasty, osteotomy and very rarely THR. However, they are not recommended as the primary modality of treatment in fresh fracture neck of femur. They are indicated in special situations like nonunion, AVN, etc. and are discussed below.

But however, Hemireplacement arthroplasty as a primary treatment in displaced intracapsular fracture neck of femur over 70 years is a better option than internal fixation except in very frail patients where internal fixation seem to do better. When compared to fixation techniques, primary prosthetic replacement preferably with a bipolar prosthesis allows for immediate weight bearing, eliminates the chances of AVN and nonunion and has reduced chances of resurgery later.

Now *bipolar arthroplasty* has largely replaced the unipolar arthroplasty of yesteryears with the Austin and Thompson's prosthesis as this eliminates the complication of protrusio acetabuli which may be associated with unipolar prosthesis.

However, after 70 years, in displaced fracture of femoral neck, amongst the treatment options of internal fixation, hemireplacement arthroplasty and THR, THR seems to be the best bet with lower complications.

COMPLICATIONS OF FEMORAL NECK FRACTURE

THROMBOEMBOLISM

Thromboembolism is a leading cause of death within first 7 days. Incidence is 40 percent.

NONUNION

Only one-third of the fracture neck femur are known to heal with OR + IF. Nonunion rate is 85-95 percent. If there is no evidence of radiological healing taking place between 6 and 12 months at treatment on a radiograph, it is declared as nonunion.

Causes

a. Inaccurate reduction.
b. Poor internal fixation.
c. Lack of cambium layer in the periosteum of the neck.
d. Avascularity of femoral head.
e. Posterior wall comminution.

Clinical Features

The patient is unable to bear the weight on the affected side. Trendelenburg test, telescopic test will be positive. Wasting of the muscles and minimal shortening of the affected lower limb are the other features.

Radiograph

Radiographs of the hip reveal ununited fracture neck of femur and there may be avascular changes in the head (Fig. 45.13).

Treatment

Surgery is the treatment of choice. The method chosen takes into account the viability of the head (Flowchart 45.2).

OSTEOTOMY

To treat nonunion of fracture neck femur, two types of osteotomies and their modifications have been described and they are as follows:

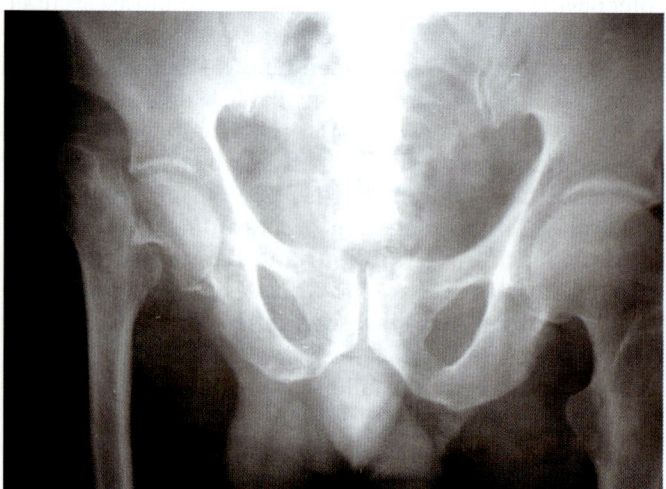

Fig. 45.13: Radiograph showing nonunion fracture neck of femur

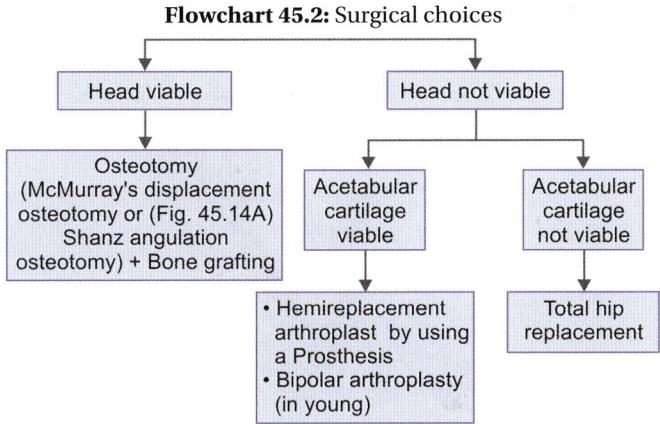

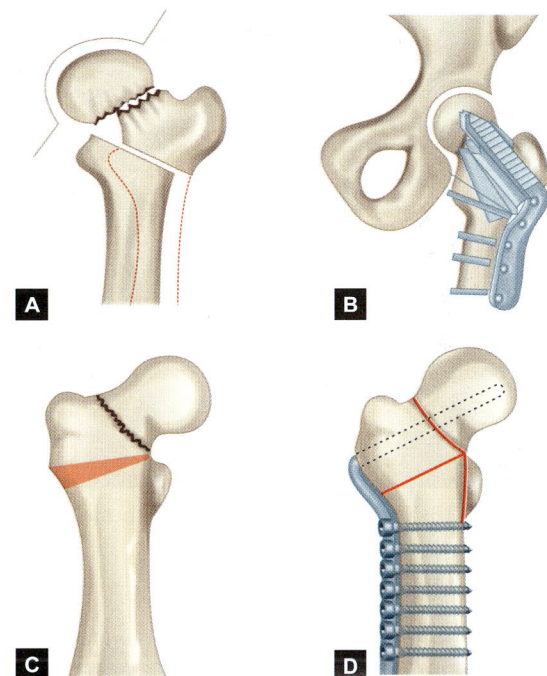

Figs 45.14A to D: Different types of osteotomies (A) McMurray's osteotomy; (B) Shanz angulation osteotomy; (C) Angulation osteotomy; (D) Pauwel's osteotomy

McMurray's displacement osteotomy: In this, the osteotomy is made just proximal to the lesser trochanter and the distal fragment is pushed medially and fixed internally (Fig. 45.14A).

Shanz angulation osteotomy: In this, the osteotomy is made through or just distal to the lesser trochanter. A laterally based wedge of bone is removed and the varus angulation is corrected and fixed with plate and screws (Fig. 45.14B).

Role of Osteotomy

Displacement or angulation osteotomy helps to convert the shearing force at the fracture site into compression force by changing the line of weightbearing and thereby enhances the chances of fracture union (Figs 45.14C and D).

Among the two, angulation osteotomy is preferable because the position of greater trochanter is more satisfactory, function of the abductor muscles is re-established more effectively, there is no further shortening and internal fixation is maintained more satisfactorily.

Osteotomy as a treatment for nonunion fracture neck femur has a role only if the head of the femur is viable otherwise, hemiarthroplasty is preferable.

Hemireplacement Arthroplasty

As mentioned earlier, if the head is not viable but the acetabular cartilage is viable, and if the patient is over 60 years of age, hemireplacement arthroplasty is the treatment of choice. However, the choice of prosthesis depends upon the existing calcar femori. If sufficiently present (at least 1–3 cm), [2]**Austin Moore's** prosthesis (Figs 45.15) is the choice and if it is inadequate, [3]**Thompson** prosthesis is preferred (ref. to section on instruments for details). Bipolar hip replacement is another option (Fig. 45.16).

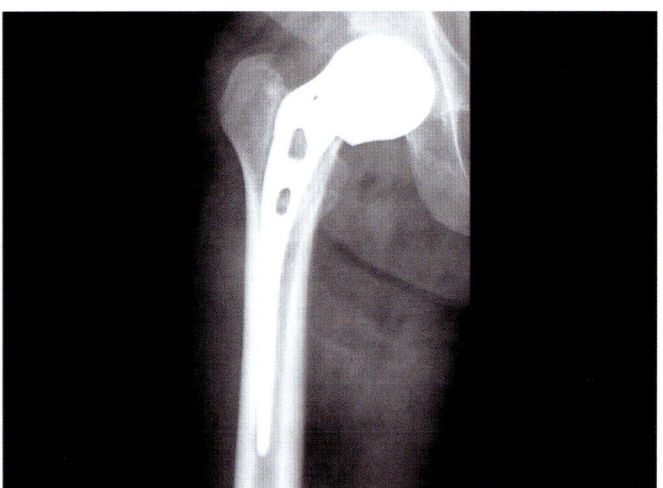

Fig. 45.15: X-ray Image of AMP

Total Hip Replacement

If both the femoral head and the acetabular cartilage is not viable and if the patient is more than 60 years old total hip replacement is the surgery of choice (see Fig. 47.16).

---

[2]**Austin Moore** (1957), USA. He described: (a) Self-locking hip prosthesis, (b) A new low posterior approach for hip (Southern approach).
[3]**Frederick and Thompson** (1955), USA.

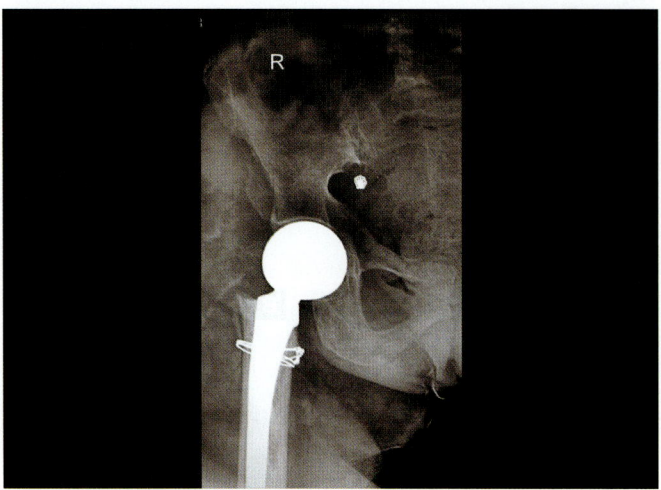

Fig. 45.16: X-ray image of bipolar prosthesis hip

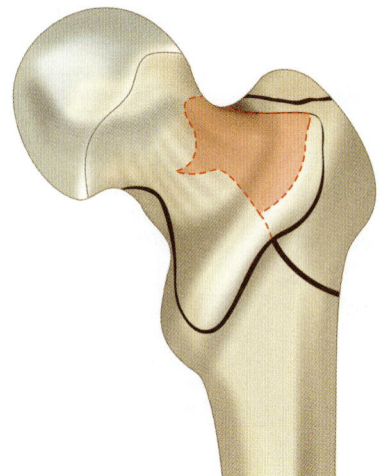

Fig. 45.17: Comminuted intertrochanteric fracture

AVASCULAR NECROSIS

It is the next important complication. Two types are described:
- *Due to actual AVN:* This is secondary to ischemia and is an early phenomenon. It shows characteristic microscopic appearance.
- *Late segmental collapse:* It is due to collapse of subchondral and articular cartilage that overlies infarcted bone. It occurs late.

Incidence

- *Aseptic necrosis*—66–84 percent.
- *Late segmental collapse*—7–27 percent.

In displaced femoral neck fracture, femoral head survival is dependent on vessels of ligamentum teres which is absent in one-third cases and subfoveal artery anastomosis which is variable and incomplete. All vessels within femoral neck and most of the retinacular vessels are disrupted in displaced fracture. Hence, survival of head depends on:
- Uninjured vascular supply
- Revascularization.
- Vascular injury occurs:
  a. At the time of fracture commonly.
  b. During reduction or internal fixation.

Hence, good anatomical reduction and stable internal fixation is required to preserve the remaining blood supply, which helps in revascularization.

Investigations

Radiograph shows increased density of the femoral head, and this may take 6 months to 2 years to be seen on radiograph (see Fig. 45.11).

Bone scan Early and accurate determination of avascularity can be made, but it is not 100 percent accurate.

Treatment

- Symptomatic treatment like bed rest, nonsteroidal anti-inflammatory drugs (NSAIDs), etc.
- Displacement or angulation osteotomy in early stages.
- If acetabular cartilage is viable, hemireplacement prosthesis is preferred.
- Total hip replacement if acetabular cartilage is not viable.

> **Fracture Neck of Femur at a Glance**
> - An unsolved problem.
> - Fracture of the elderly.
> - Majority due to trivial fall.
> - Garden's classification widely accepted.
> - It is an orthopedic emergency.
> - Speed is the watchword in management.
> - Early anatomical reduction, impaction, and rigid internal fixation are the aim of treatment.
> - DHS and multiple cannulated cancellous screws is the currently accepted method of fixation.
> - Nonunion and AVN are very common.

TROCHANTERIC FRACTURE

> **Salient Features**
> - An intertrochanteric fracture occurs along a line between greater trochanter and lesser trochanter with variable comminution (Fig. 45.17).
> - Totally extracapsular.
> - Internal rotators of the hip remain attached to the distal fragment; short external rotators are attached to proximal head and neck. Hence, limb has to be kept in external rotation after reduction to align the distal fragment with proximal one.
> - Cancellous bone heals well by 8-12 weeks.
> - Four times more common than intracapsular fracture.

Age Seen in elderly patients 10-12 years older than intracapsular fracture neck femur.

Sex More common in females (2.8 : 1).

Mechanism

Direct trauma as in RTA, fall, etc.

Indirect due to muscle pull, etc.

Clinical Features

The patient will have pain, marked shortening of the lower limb, complete external rotation deformity, swelling, ecchymosis and tenderness over the greater trochanter.

Radiograph

A true anteroposterior view in internal rotation and a lateral view help to study the fracture pattern (Fig. 45.18).

Treatment

Conservative treatment: There is 10 percent mortality associated with conservative treatment.

Indications

- Poor medical and surgical risk patients.
- Terminally ill patients.
- Very old patients.

Methods

- Simple support with pillows
- Buck's traction
- Plaster spica
- Skeletal traction through distal femur or tibia for 10-12 weeks (Fig. 45.19).

Surgical: Though not an emergency, there is an urgent need for surgery as there is a 10-fold increase in mortality if surgery is delayed for more than 48 hours.

Advantages of surgery include increased comfort, good nursing care and hospitalization stay is considerably reduced.

Goal is to fix a stably reduced fracture internally.

Methods of Reduction

Closed reduction is by traction, slight abduction and external rotation. If reduction is not obtained, open reduction is done.

Open Reduction

Indications:
- Failed closed reduction.
- Large spike on proximal fragment with lesser trochanter intact.
- Reverse oblique fracture.

Choice of an Implant

Once stable reduction has been obtained either anatomically or by any one of the non-anatomical means (e.g. by osteotomy, etc.), implants are chosen. For stable fractures, choice of an implant does not matter. For unstable fractures, sliding hip screw (DHS) is most suitable and the 135-150° angle side plates are most commonly used. Placement of the DHS screw in the neck should be either central or posteroinferior (Fig. 45.20).

Dynamic hip screw (DHS) allows to secure fixation of the fracture and permits controlled impaction at the fracture site thereby reducing the risk of fixation failure seen in rigid nail-plate like SP nail, etc. (Fig. 45.21A). PFN is being preferred over DHS in recent times (See box).

> **What is New in the Treatment of Trochanteric Fractures?**
> Proximal femoral nails (PFN) are emerging as an effective internal fixation device.

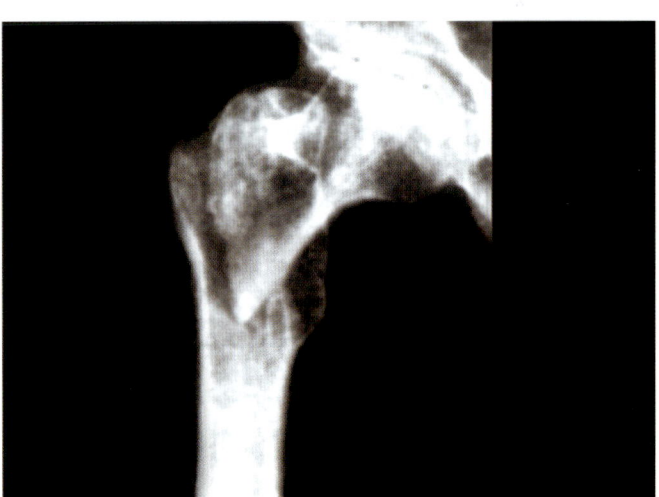

Fig. 45.18: Radiograph showing comminuted trochanteric fracture femur

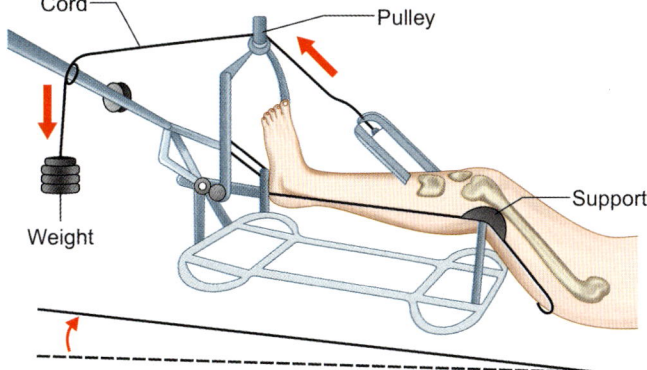

Fig. 45.19: Skeletal traction through Böhler-Braun frame for trochanteric fracture

Comparison of Fracture Neck Femur and Trochanteric Fracture

Features	Fracture neck femur	Trochanteric fracture
Age	Elderly	More elderly
Incidence	Common	Four times more common
Blood loss	Less	More
Mechanism	Trivial fall	Major trauma
Signs:		
Shortening	Minimum	Gross
Deformity	Minimum external rotation	Gross external rotation
Site of tenderness	Anterior hip joint line	Over greater trochanter
Conservative treatment	Not successful	Successful
Surgery	Absolutely indicated	Indicated for early mobilization
Complications		
Nonunion	Very common	Rare (1%)
Malunion	Unheard	Very common

Fig. 45.20: Radiograph showing trochanteric fracture fixation with DHS

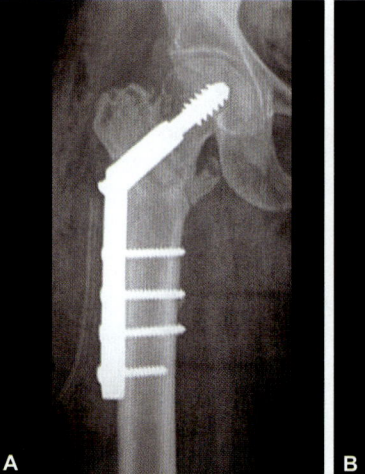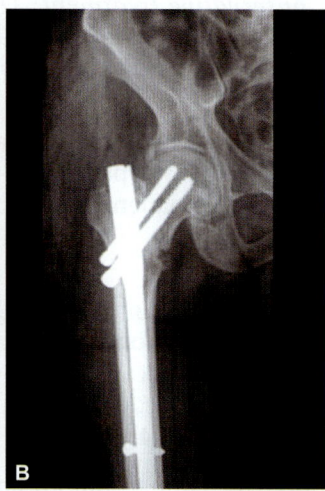

Figs 45.21A and B: Internal fixation methods for trochanteric fractures (A) DHS; (B) PFN

Complications

Due to the cancellous nature of bone, these fractures unite well unlike fracture neck femur but malunion is quite common. Coxa vara, nonunion (Fig. 45.22) is less than 2 percent (rare) and traumatic osteoarthritis is seen. These fractures also carry a higher incidence of mortality (more than 10%). Avascular necrosis is very rare (0.8%).

Quick Facts

In intertrochanteric fracture, the success of fracture implant fixation depends upon:
- Degree of osteoporosis (Singh's index).
- Fracture pattern.
- Accurate reduction.
- Implant designs.
- Placement of the implant.

Vital Facts

Treatment of Proximal Femoral Fractures
- Stable trochanteric fractures are fixed with DHS
- Unstable trochanteric fractures cannot be fixed with DHS as it cuts through due to comminution. Hence, the choice of implants in these situations is:
  a. Medoff plate or trochanteric stabilization plate (TSP, AO).
  b. **Condylocephalic nails:** These could be proximal femoral nails, Ender's nail or Gamma nail.
  c. 95° condylar blade plate or dynamic condylar screw.
  d. Proximal femoral nails (PFN) (Fig. 45.21B).

In comminuted unstable trochanteric fractures, IM nails are better suited to resist the deforming muscle forces. Hence, proximal femoral nailing is superior to DHS.

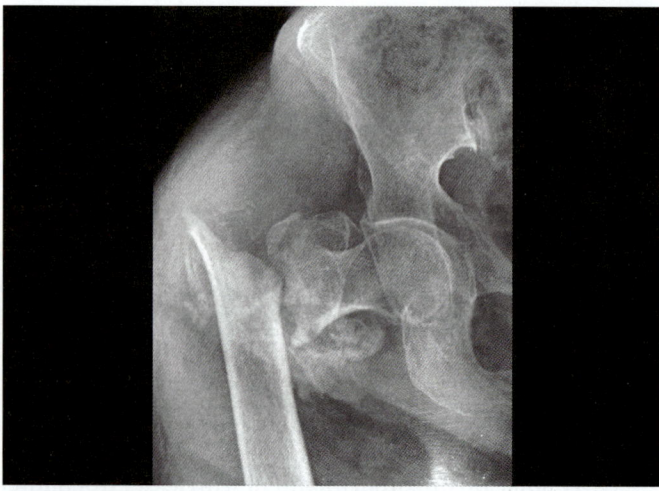

Fig. 45.22: Nonunion trochanteric fracture—rare complication

Advantages of PFN
- It can be inserted quickly
- Less blood loss
- Early ambulation
- Sliding and limb shortening is less
- It is more successful in reverse oblique fractures.

Features of PFN
- Standard length is 24 cm
- Long PFN is available in > 36 cm length (for low subtrochanteric fractures or two level fractures).
- *Proximal wide portion:* Here a long screw and hip-pin can pass through the head and neck.
- Distal part has a dynamic and static locking holes.

Problems with PFN
- Entry point has to be chosen carefully (preferably pyriformis fossa).
- Excessively curved femur is a central indication.
- Postoperative thigh pain is seen
- It cannot be used if fracture line extends into pyriformis fossa (Here DCS or condylar blade plate is better).

CHAPTER 46

Osteoporosis

DEFINITION

It is a generic term referring to a state of decreased mass per unit volume of a normally mineralized bone due to loss of bone proteins. It is called as silent epidemic and usually remains undetected till the patient sustains a hip, rib or spine fracture.

> **Remember**
> *About osteoporosis*
> It is the most common skeletal disorder in the world, next only to arthritis. In osteoporosis, there is a long latent period before clinical symptoms develop. Most prevalent complications are fractures of vertebral bodies, ribs, proximal femur, humerus, distal radius with minimal trauma.

Most common cause is involutional bone loss in perimenopausal age group (Fig. 46.1).

Dexa criteria for osteoporosis as determined by WHO, are BMD of spine and hip of 2–5 SD's or more below the mean for healthy young women (T-score of –2.5 or below) and osteopenia between 1 to 2.5 SD's or more below the mean.

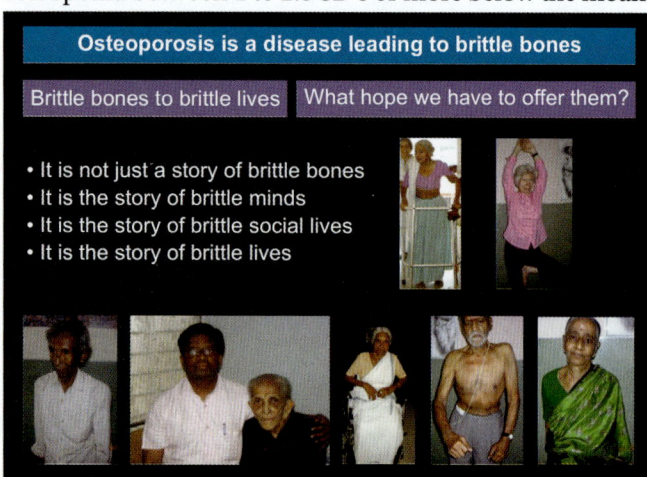

Fig. 46.1: Osteoporosis

Causes

Disuse

- Prolonged bed rest or inactivity.
- Prolonged casting or splinting.
- Paralysis, space travel, etc.

Diet

- Calcium, protein, vitamin C low in the diet.
- Chronic alcoholism.
- Anorexia nervosa.

Drugs: Whose prolonged use causes osteoporosis are heparin, methotrexate, ethanol, glucocorticoids, etc.

Idiopathic variety is seen in adolescent and middle-aged male population.

Genetic role is seen in osteogenesis imperfecta.

Chronic illness like rheumatoid arthritis, cirrhosis, sarcoidosis, renal tubular acidosis, etc.

Neoplasm like bone marrow tumors (myeloma, lymphoma, leukemia).

Endocrine abnormalities: Hyperparathyroidism, increased levels of glucocorticoids, estrogens, etc.

Risk Factors for Osteoporosis (Fig. 46.2)

> **Remember**
> *In osteoporosis*
> - Decreased density is due to deficiency of protein matrix in which calcium is laid down.
> - Here rate of bone resorption is greater than bone formation.
> - Most commonly, it is due to ageing process.
> - But the most common cause is involutional bone loss in perimenopausal women.

Criteria for screening: The following group of people need to be screened:
- All women >65 years of age
- All men >70 years of age
- Selected post-menopausal men and women who are 50–69 years with risk factors for fractures.

Types

There are two types of osteoporosis. Type 1 is postmenopausal and type 2 age related. Table 46.1 shows the features in these two types of osteoporosis.

Clinical Features

Early symptoms: The patient complains of acute pain in middle or low thoracic or high lumbar region (Fig. 46.3A). Sudden movement, sitting, sneezing, cough, etc. increases pain. Rest relieves it.

Most common symptom of osteoporosis is back pain secondary to vertebral compression. However, in some cases, fractures of axial skeleton may be seen with trivial trauma. Round type of gibbus due to compression of thoracic vertebrae is commonly seen (Fig. 46.3B). Other features of osteoporosis are shown in Figure 46.4.

> **Did You Know?**
> - Osteoporosis was officially recognized as a disease by WHO in 1994.
> - 1 in every 2 women, 1 in every 4 men suffer an osteoporosis related fracture once in their lifetime.
> - It is a silent epidemic and killer.
> - Osteoporosis is usually first detected following a fracture.

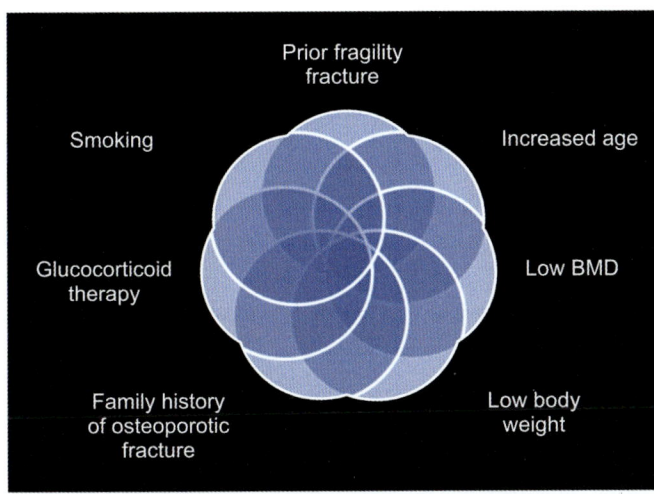

Fig. 46.2: Major risk factors for osteoporosis

TABLE 46.1: Types of osteoporosis		
Classification Epidemiological factor	Type I: Postmenopausal	Type II: Age related
Age	55–75 years	Seventy years (Female) 50 years (Male)
Sex (Female : Male)	6:1	2:1
Bone metabolism		
• Pathogenesis	Osteoclast activity	Osteoblastic activity
• Net bone loss	Mainly trabecular.	Cortical and trabecular
• Rate of bone loss	Rapid/short duration	Slow/long duration
• Bone density	2 SD below normal	Low or normal
Clinical signs Sites	Pain and stress fracture of Vertebra (rush) Distal forearm	Pain and stress fracture of: Vertebra (multiple wedge) Proximal hip and tibia. Hip (extracapsular) Dorsal kyphosis
Other sites	Hip (intracapsular) Tooth loss	
Laboratory values		
• Serum calcium	N	N
• Serum phosphorus	N	N
• Alk phosphatase	N	N
• Urine calcium	↑	N
• PTH function	↓	↑
• Renal conversion of 25 (OH)2 D to 1,25 (OH)D • GIT calcium absorption	Secondary ↓ due to ↓ PTH ↓	Primary ↓ due to ↓ responsiveness
Prevention • High-risk patients	Estrogen, calcitonin and calcium supplementation; adequate vitamin D is given; Adequate weight bearing activity; minimization of associated risk factors are recommended.	Calcium supplementation, Adequate vitamin D, Adequate weight bearing activity and Minimization of risk factors.

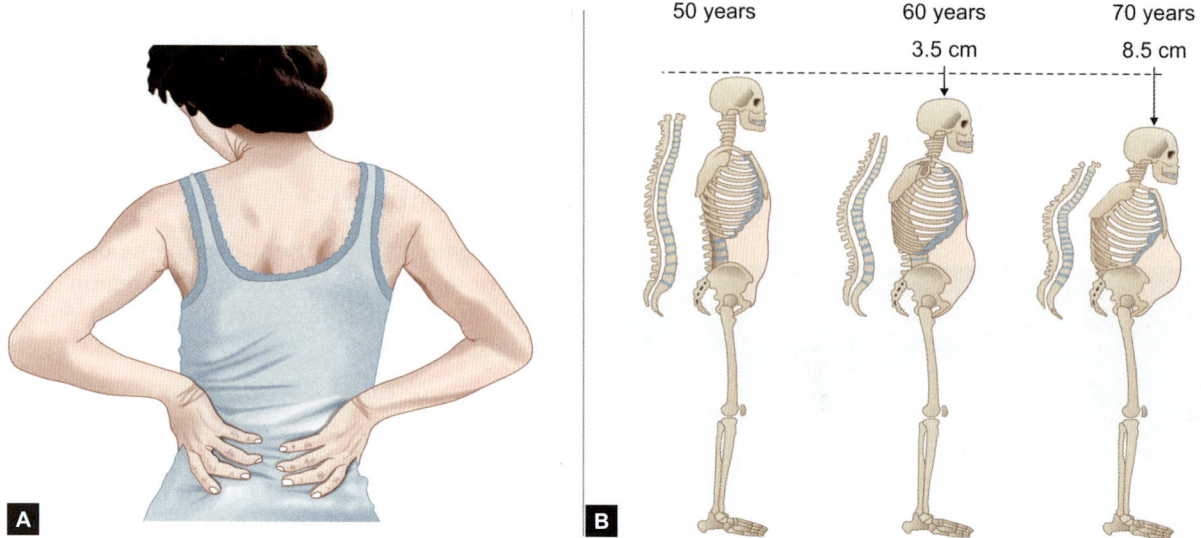

Figs 46.3A and B: Common presentation in osteoporosis: (A) Backache; (B) Progressive loss of height

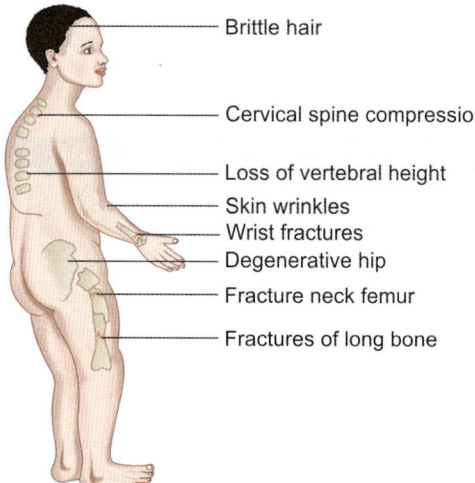

Fig. 46.4: Features of osteoporosis

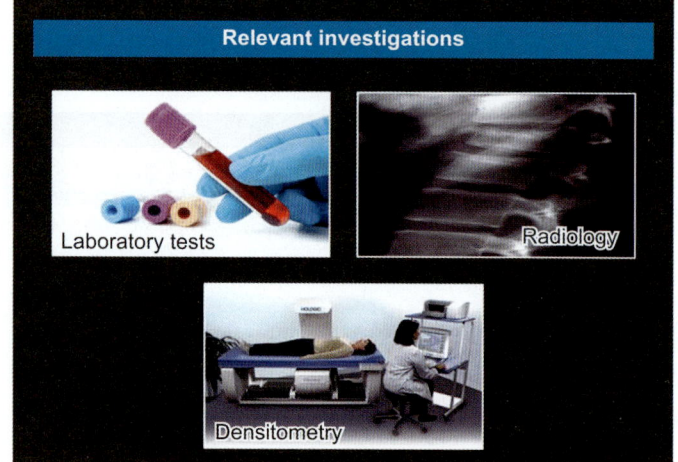

Fig. 46.5: Method of investigations for osteoporosis

Investigations (Fig. 46.5)

Radiographs

Radiographs changes seen in the spine are:
- Loss of vertebral height due to symmetric transverse compression.
- Biconcave central compression (Codfish spine) due to the pressure of the bulging disk into the bodies.
- Anterior wedge compression (Fig. 46.6A).
- The bone density of the vertebra is reduced (Figs 46.6B and C, and 46.7).

Other bones
- Ground glass appearance due to generalized rarefaction.
- *Singh's index* is the grading of the trabecular pattern of the neck of femur from 1–6 (see Fig. 45.10).
- Metacarpal index, etc.
- Pathological fractures.

Densitometry

Techniques for bone mass measurement:
- Single photon absorptiometry is used to assess the amount of cortical bone mineral in appendicular skeleton.
- Mineral status of axial skeleton is assessed by dual photon absorptiometry (DEXA) and quantitative CT scan (Fig. 46.8).

- Total body neutron activation analysis to determine calcium content of the entire body.

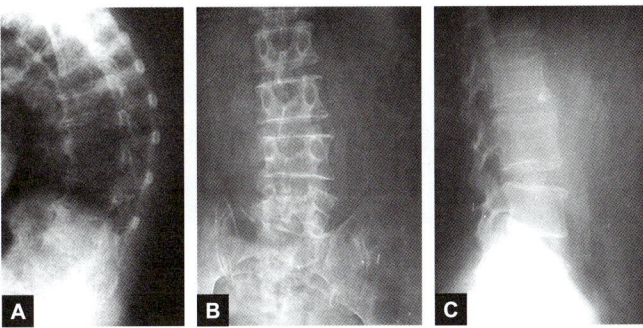

Figs 46.6A to C: Radiographs showing: (A) Kyphotic deformity in osteoporosis; (B and C) Reduced density of the spine AP and lateral views due to osteoporosis

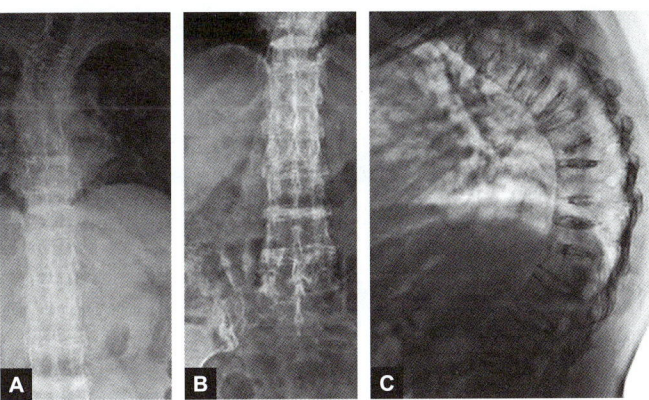

Figs 46.7A to C: Plain X-rays showing decreased bone mineral density

Transiliac bone biopsy: It is an important diagnostic tool in patients of more than 50 years in postmenopausal diseases.

Laboratory tests: Serum calcium, phosphorus and alkaline phosphatase levels are usually normal. Osteoblastic and osteoclastic blood and urine markers help us to diagnose and monitor the treatment for osteoporosis (Fig. 46.9).

Management of Osteoporosis

Preventing osteoporosis is lot easier than treating it. The treatment plan consists of general measures exercises, diet and drug therapy.

General Measures

- High protein and calcium rich diet (Fig. 46.10).
- Rest that is adequate.

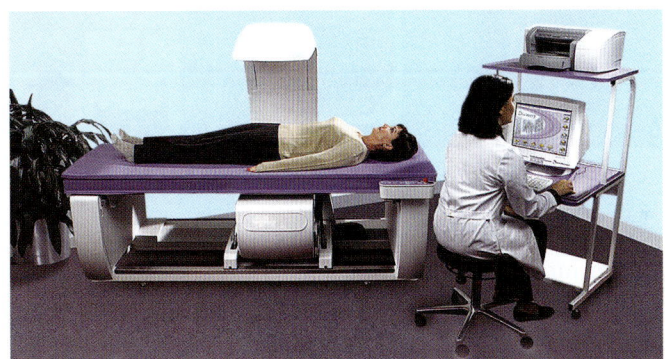

Fig. 46.8: DEXA to evaluate bone mineral density (BMD)

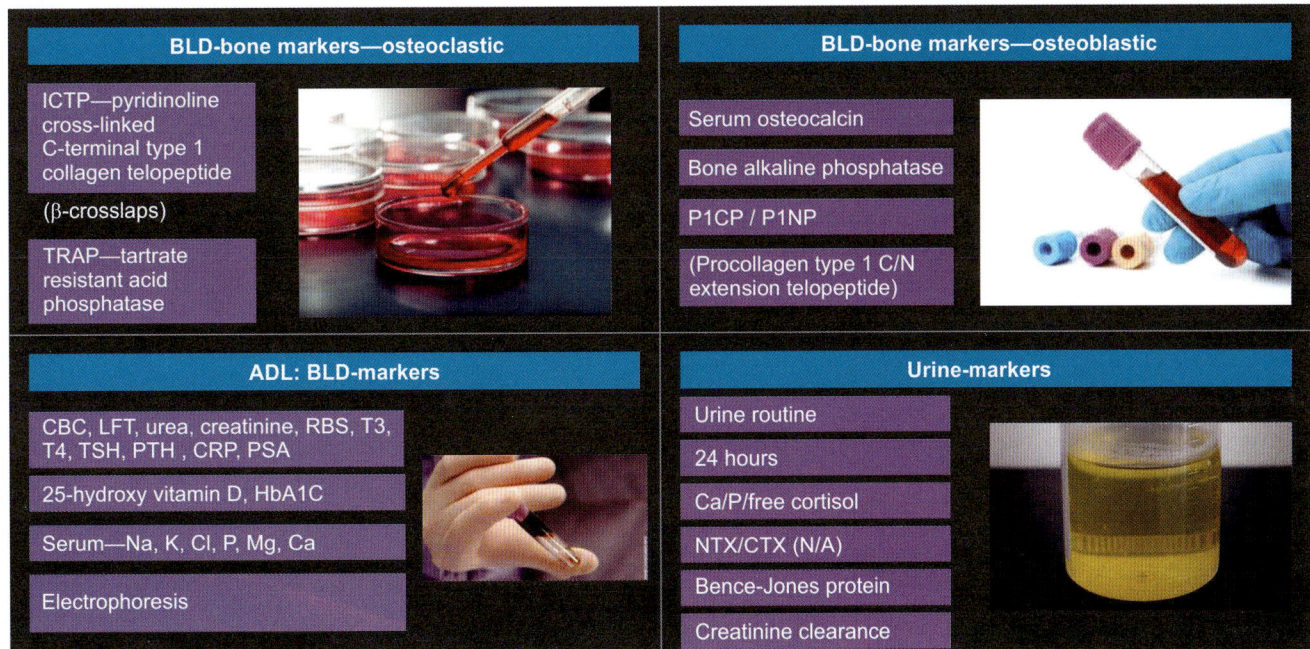

Fig. 46.9: Laboratory tests for osteoporosis

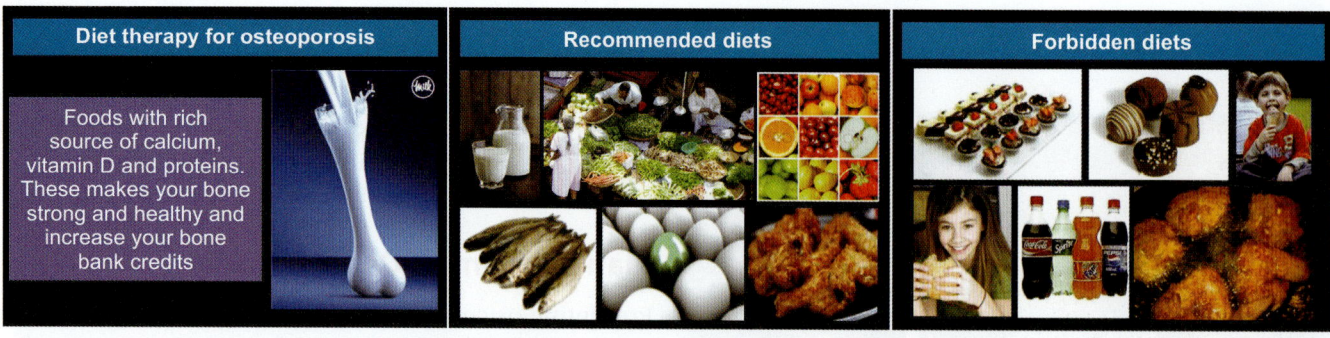

Fig. 46.10: Diet therapy for osteoporosis

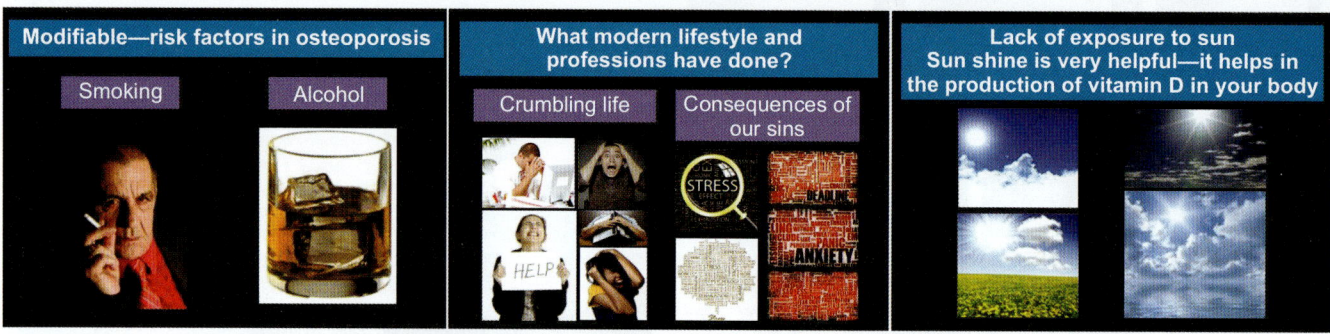

Fig. 46.11: Important mesures to prevent osteoporosis

- NSAIDs muscle relaxants and supports like belt, collar, etc. for symptomatic relief of pain.
- Spinal orthosis when patient is erect and mobile.

Improvement in the Lifestyle

Smoking and alcohol are two biggest culprits in osteoporosis and needs to be stopped to prevent fragility fractures. Modern day stress is also contributory and needs to be avoided (Fig. 46.11).

Exercises

Exercises like walking and light aerobics are beneficial (Fig. 46.12). Here are the three popular choices of exercises in osteoporosis (Fig. 46.13).

Posture exercises: Wall arch, back bending and wall sliding postural exercises help to improve posture and overcome hunched back (Figs 46.14A to C).

Fall prevention is of utmost importance. These are extrinsic and intrinsic measures (Figs 46.15A and B). The following measures helps prevent falls in the elderly:

Drug Therapy in Osteoporosis

Drugs form the mainstay of treatment of osteoporosis. The various combinations suggested are as confusing as

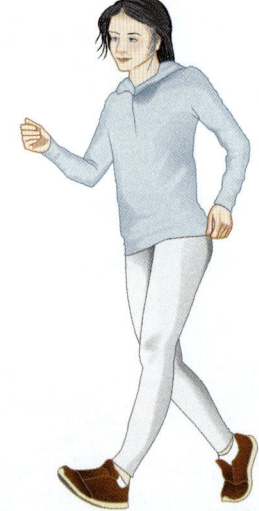

Fig. 46.12: Regular exercises like walking is of great help in elderly patients suffering from osteoporosis

the disease. However, an effort is made here to provide a simplistic analysis of the drugs commonly used in osteoporosis.

Anti-resorptive Drugs (Fig. 46.16)

Calcium and vitamin D: For those patients diagnosed by DEXA as osteoporosis, 1,200 mg of calcium and 700–800

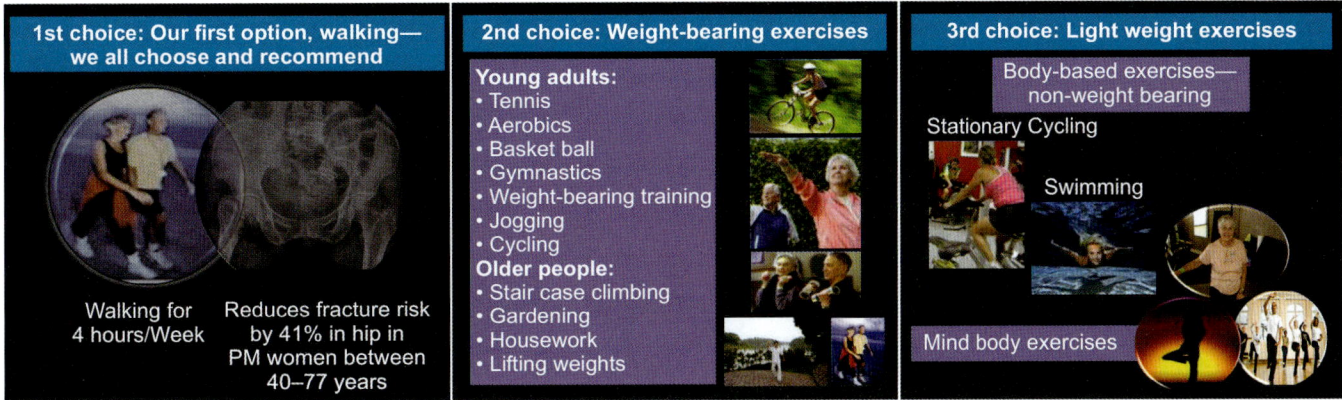

Fig. 46.13: Three popular choices of exercises in osteoporosis

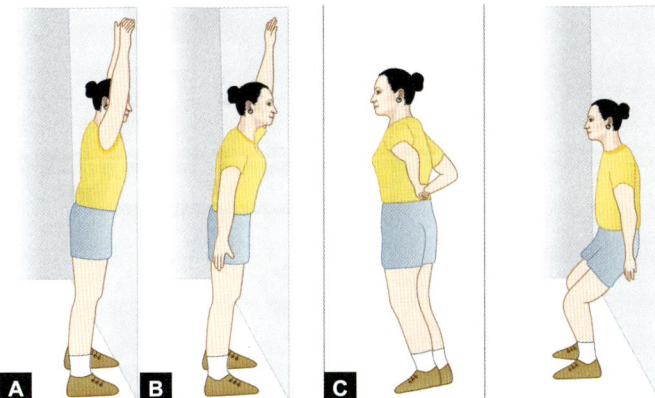

Figs 46.14A to C: Various posture correction exercises in osteoporosis patients: (A) Wall arching; (B) Back bending; (C) Wall sliding exercises

IU of vitamin D per day is recommended as the first line of therapy.

Hormone Replacement Therapy (Fig. 46.17)

The role of estrogen and progestogens in preventing and treating osteoporosis has been well documented. Estrogens are the most effective treatment for osteoporosis in perimenopausal and early menopausal women. Estrogens dose is 0.625 mg daily or 0.3 mg if combined with calcium. HRT is known to reduce the rate of fractures by 75 percent in the estrogen group. Birth control pills are also known to prevent osteoporosis. The role of progesterone is still not well-documented.

Biphosphonates

These drugs inhibit the action of the osteoclast bone cells, which are responsible for removing the bone mass by binding themselves to the inner linings of the bones. The dose of alendronate is 10 mg/day. Etidronate is another commonly used biphosphonate. Tiludronate, risedronate, and ibandronate are some of the newer drugs.

Calcitonin

Salmon calcitonin has been used for treating osteoporosis. Calcitonin can be given in the form of injections (Dose 50–100 IU/day) or in the form of nasal spray (dose 200 IU). It is used for the treatment of osteoporosis in women who are at least five years postmenopausal and in some cases of men. It is known to slow down bone loss, as it is a powerful inhibitor of osteoclastic activity, increase bone density and reduce the risk of fractures. It is also known to reduce the pain.

Alfacalcidol

This is a synthetic analogue of calcitriol, an active metabolite of vitamin D. It changes to calcitriol in the liver. It decreases bone resorption, increases bone mineralization and formation. It also reduces the rate of fractures and improves the bone quality. Recommended dose is 0.5 mcg/day. It is sometimes given along with calcium.

Role of Fluorides in the Treatment of Osteoporosis

Fluorides are known to increase the bone mass. Lower dose of 25 mg slow release fluorides twice daily along with 400 mg of calcium twice daily is recommended. The side effects are gastrointestinal upsets and increased risk of cortical bone fractures.

A Quick Recap of the Drugs Used in Osteoporosis:
- Calcium and vitamin D
- HRT
- Biphosphonates
- Calcitonin
- Alfacalcidol

SECTION 6: Geriatric Orthopedics

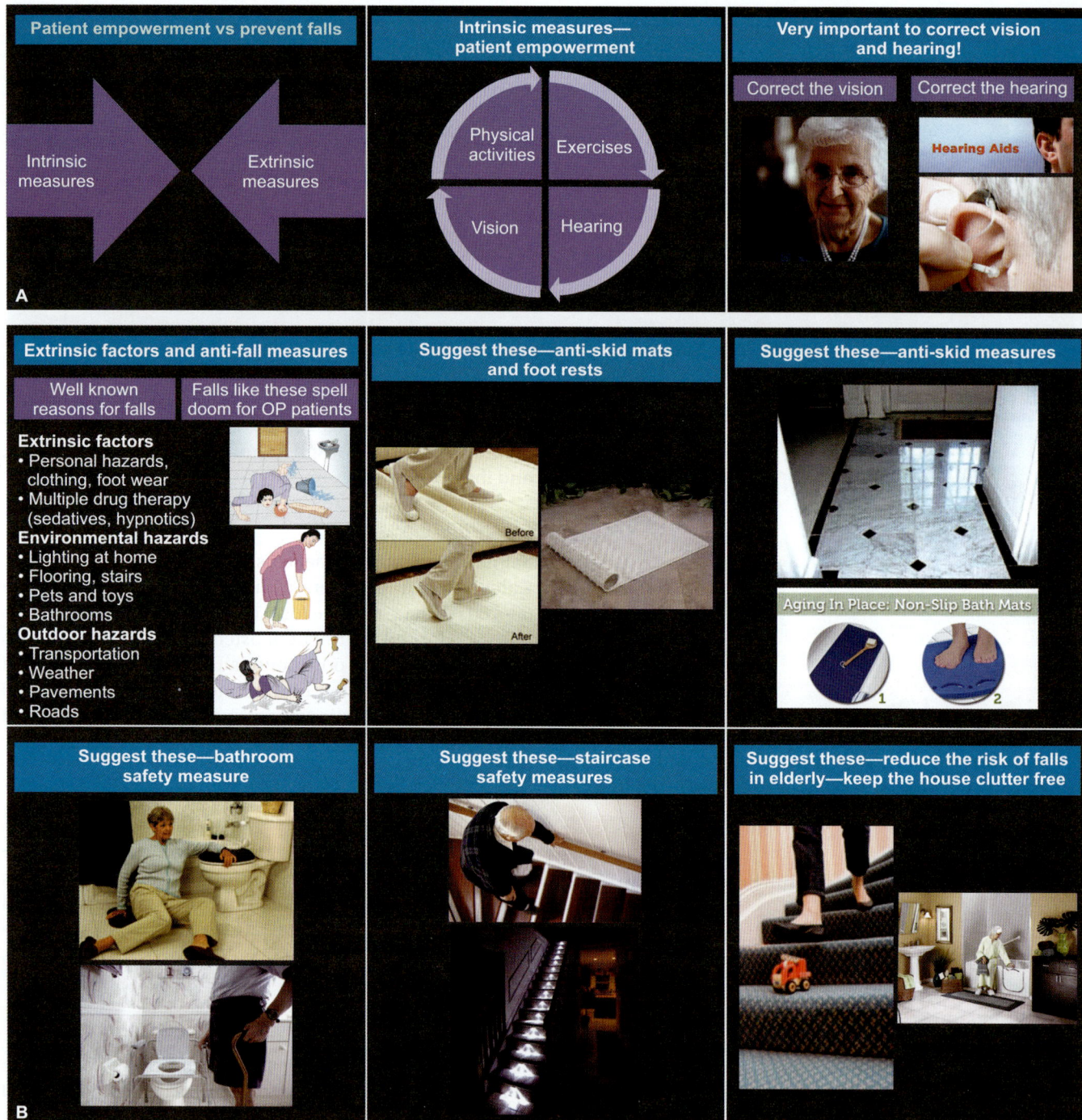

Figs 46.15A and B: Anti-fall measures: (A) Intrinsic measures; (B) Extrinsic measures

- Fluorides
- SERMS
- Phytoestrogens
- Painkillers
- Anxiolytics and antidepressants.

Drug Options in the Treatment of Osteoporosis (Fig. 46.18)

Treatment of osteoporosis with the drugs is as confusing as the disease itself. Many drugs are now available in the market with many permutations and combinations. Though the initial choice of the drugs depends on various factors like sex, age, presence or absence of uterus in women, tolerability, etc.; most of the times, it is the treating physician who makes the choice based on his experience.

An effort is made here to present the more appropriate of the drug options in the order of preference.

ANTI-RESORPTIVE DRUGS

First Preference

Perimenopausal and early postmenopausal (first 5 years) estrogen replacement therapy (0.625 mg/day).

Second Preference

For the next ten years, selective estrogen receptor modulators (SERMs) (e.g. Raloxifene). They are known to decrease the estrogens dreaded side effects (like causing increased incidence of uterine or breast cancers), while maintaining their beneficial effects (like increasing bone mineral density), decreasing menopausal symptoms, cardioprotective activity, etc. SERMS are known to act by selectively blocking certain estrogen receptor sites, hence their name (FIg. 46.19).

Third Preference—Bisphosponates Types (Fig. 46.20)

Fourth Preference

Calcitonin 200 IU puff/day intranasal or 100 IU subcutaneously (Fig. 46.21). This is found to be very effective to reduce the pain due to crush fractures of the vertebra.

Fifth Preference

Combination of the above drugs. However, despite of the several options, the final choice is of the treating physician, weighing all the necessary factors.

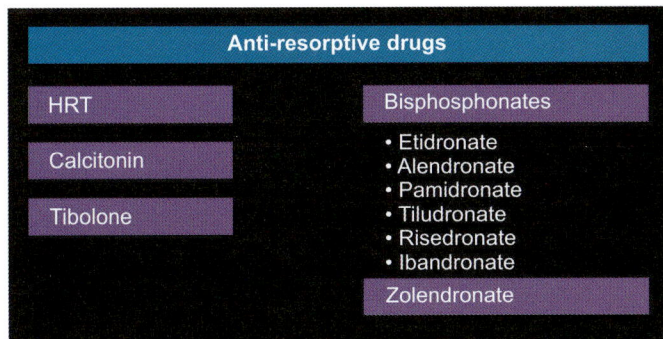

Fig. 46.16: Anti-resorptive drugs for the treatment of osteoporosis

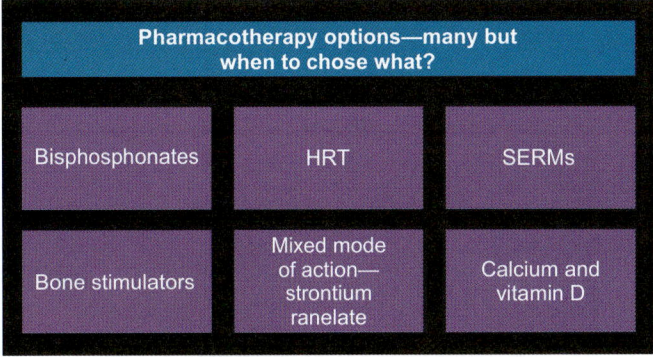

Fig. 46.18: Drug options in osteoporosis

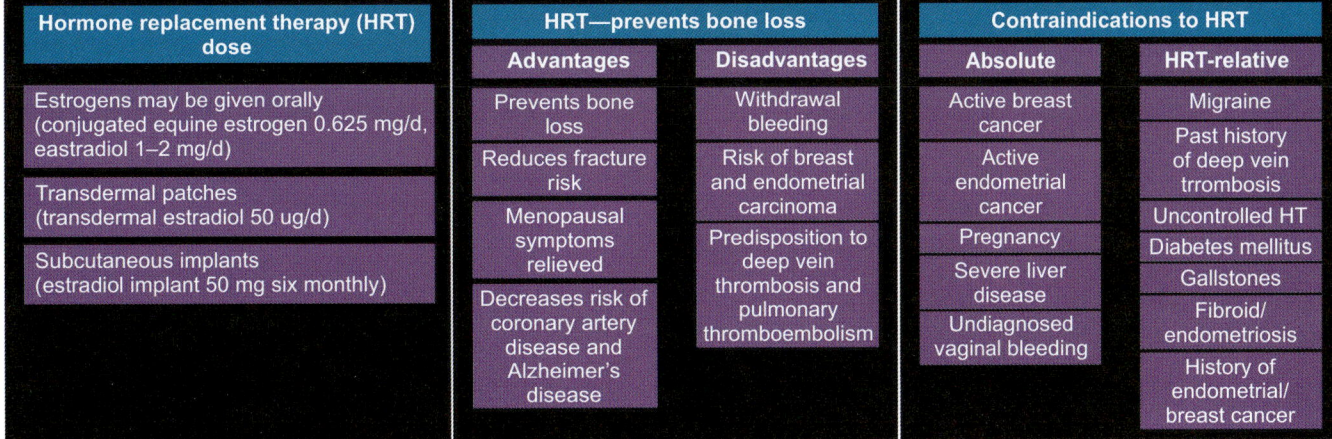

Fig. 46.17: Process of hormone replacement therapy and its contraindications

Common Preference

Calcium supplements in the dose of 1000–1500 mg/day and vitamin D analogue (0.25 mg BD or vitamin D in the dose of 600–2800 IU/day) (Fig. 46.22).

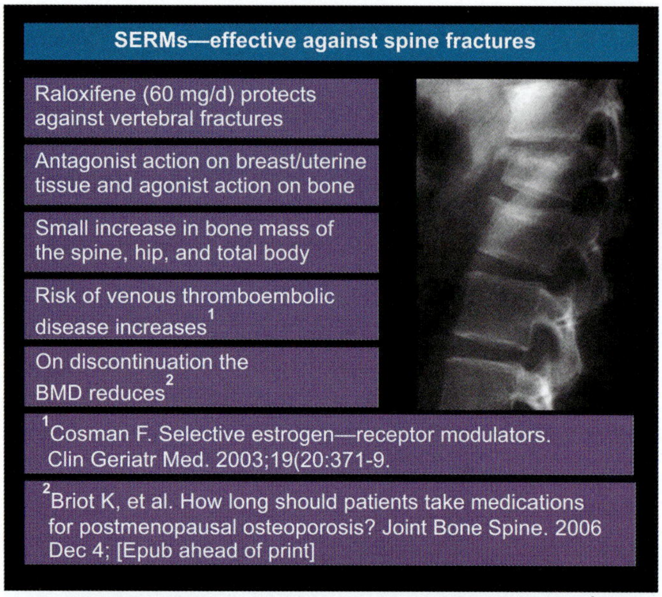

Fig. 46.19: Selective estrogen receptor modulator

Role of Teriparatide (Parathormone) in Management of Osteoporosis

Teriparatide is the only osteoblastic agent which stimulates bone formation and is used to prevent recurrence of fractures after the patient suffers a fracture (Fig. 46.23).

Drugs Preferences in Osteoporosis in Order of Importance
- In all age groups: Calcium and vitamin D.
- Perimenopausal and early menopause: HRT.
- Next 10 years: SERMs.
- After 65 years preferably: Alendronate.
- For severe pain due to vertebral fractures: Calcitonin.
- Combination of the above drugs.

Note:
Choice of the drugs varies according to the treating physicians. This is only a guideline and can be tailor-made to suit the individual patient.

Fragility Fractures and Their Management

Fractures in old age are due to trivial fall and is due to extensive weakening of the bones due to osteoporosis. They lead to morbidity and mortality in old age and is best prevented as the treatment of these fractures is complex and difficult. Fragility fractures and their treatment is shown in Figures 46.24 to 46.26.

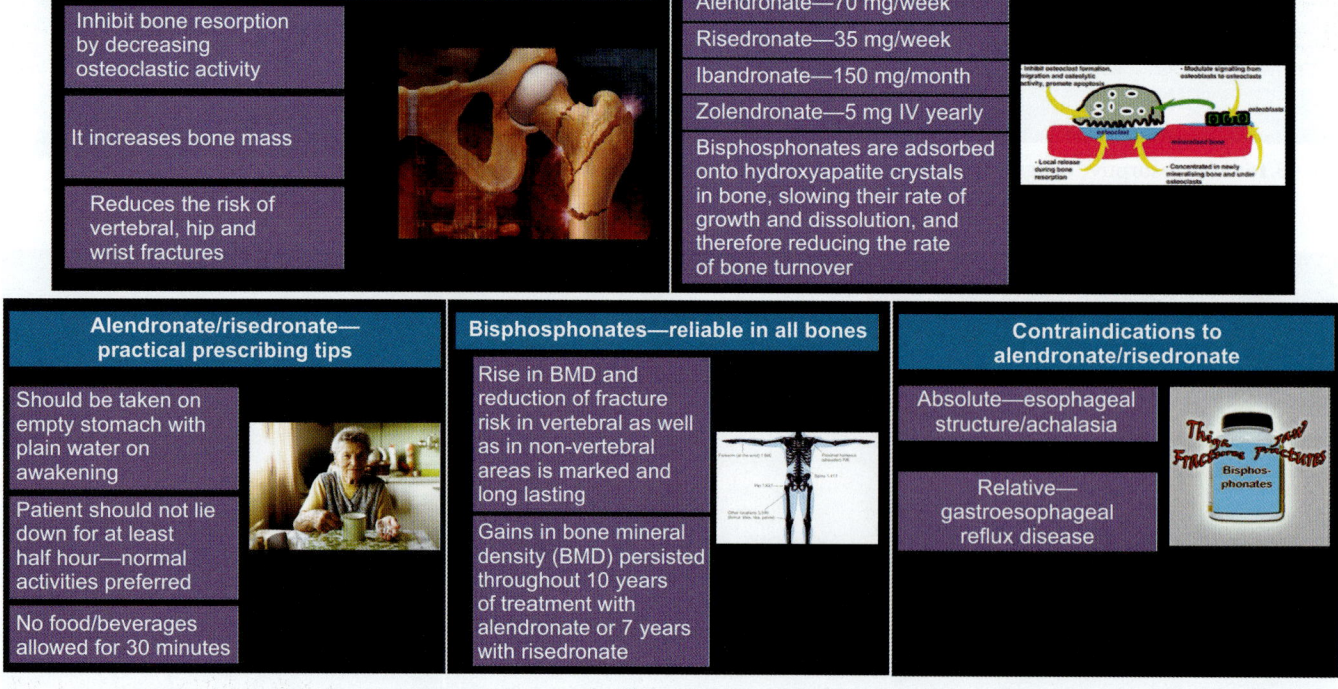

Fig. 46.20: Use of bisphosphonates in osteoporosis

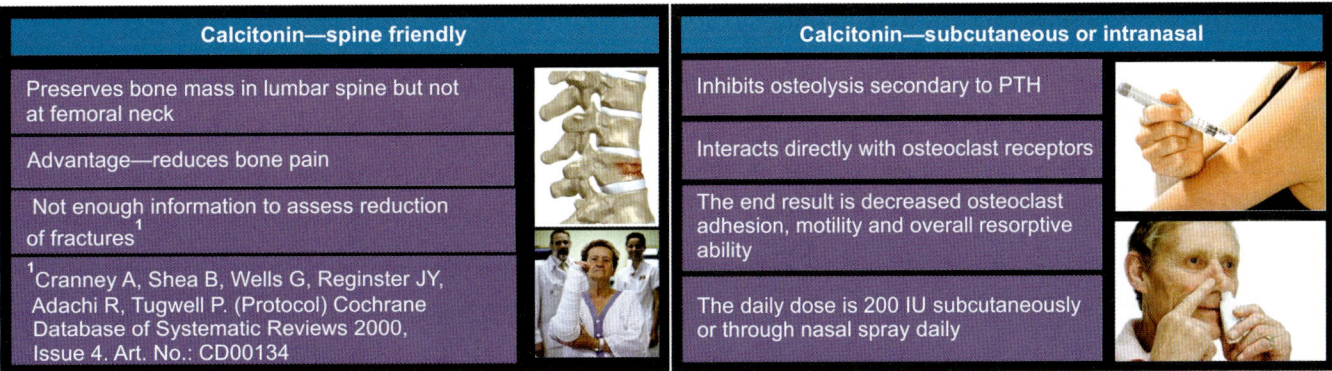

Fig. 46.21: Use of calcitonin in osteoporosis

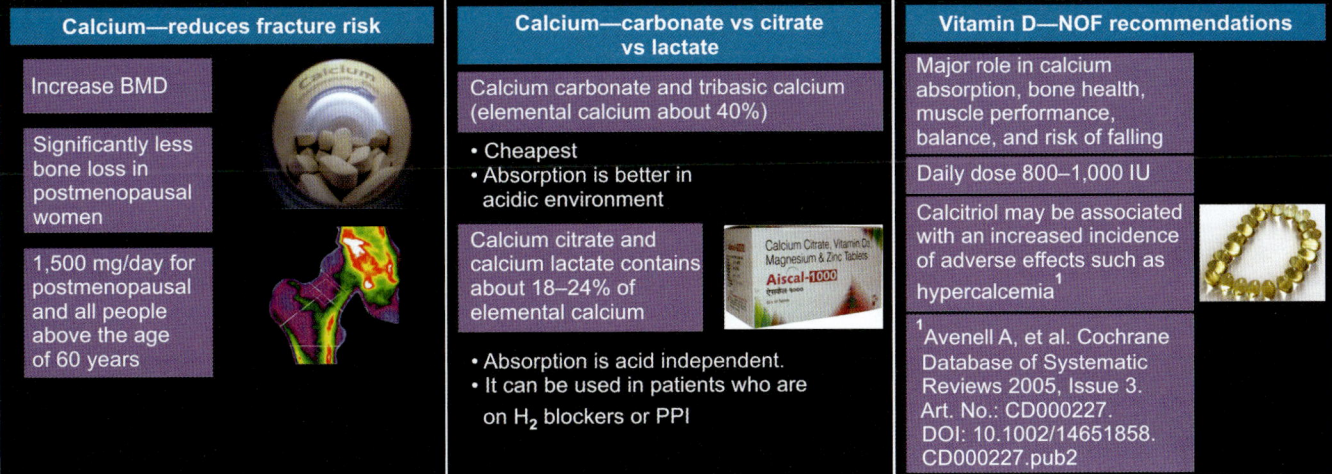

Fig. 46.22: Use of calcium supplement in osteoporosis

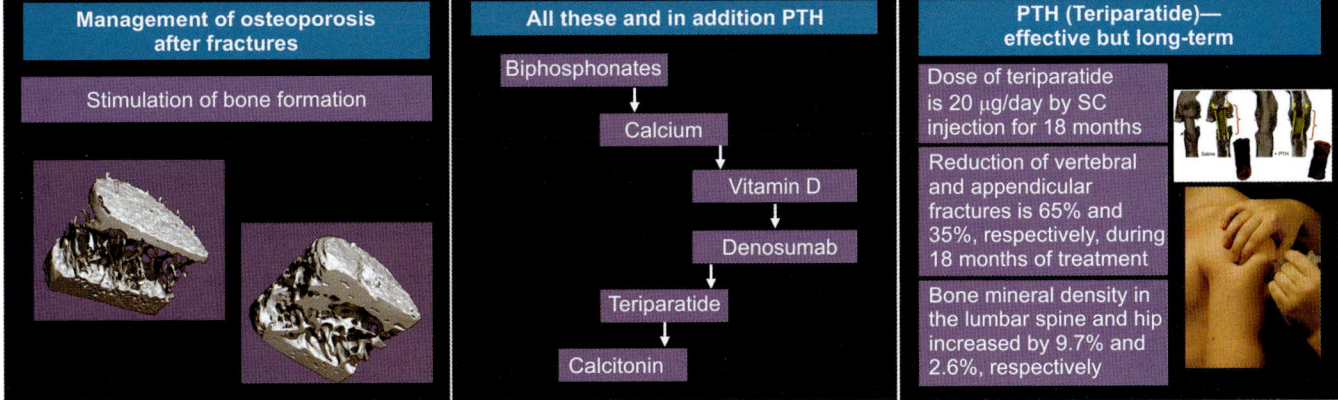

Fig. 46.23: Use of parathormone in osteoporosis

Prevention of Osteoporotic Fractures

The following measures help prevent osteoporotic fractures:

- Anti-fall measures for old persons at home by evaluating and correcting home hazards and encouraging exercises and other physical activities (Fig. 46.15).
- Vitamin D (700–800 IU) with or without calcium (1200 mg/day) daily doses for all persons >60 years of age.
- To prevent hip, spine and non-vertebral fractures biphosphonates in varying doses (e.g. Alendronate 70 mg/week, Ibandronate 150 mg/month, Risedronate 35 mg/week) are recommended.
- In postmenopausal women with osteoporosis, raloxifene is used.
- Calcitonin can be used to prevent recurrent vertebral fractures.
- Table 46.2 shows anti-fracture efficacy of drugs used in osteoporosis.

TABLE 46.2: Anti-fracture efficacy of the most frequently used drugs for postmenopausal osteoporosis as derived from placebo controlled randomized trials

Drug	Vertebral fractures	Non-vertebral fracture (hip)
Alendronate	+++	++
Calcitonin (nasal)	+	0
Etidronate	+	0
HRT	++	+
PTH	+++	++
Raloxifene	+++	0
Risedronate	+++	++
Strontium ranelate	+++	+

Source: Adapted from Delmas PD, Lancet. 2002;359:2018-26.

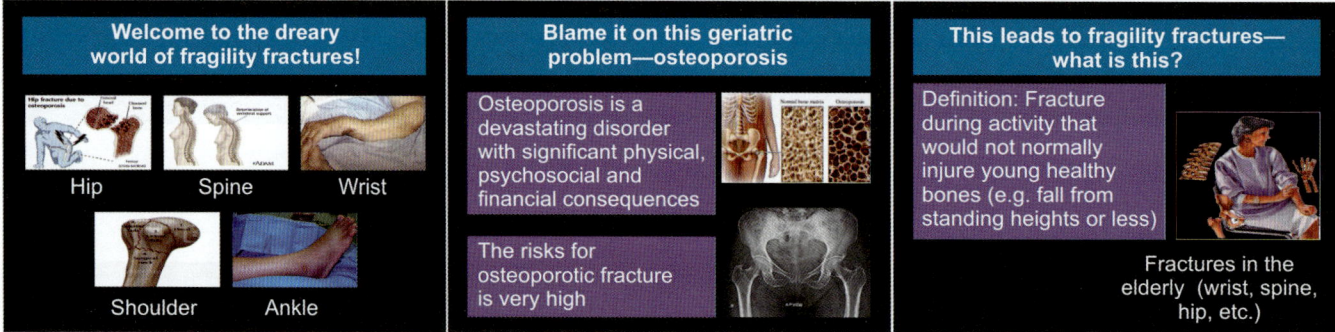

Fig. 46.24: Fragility fractures and their management

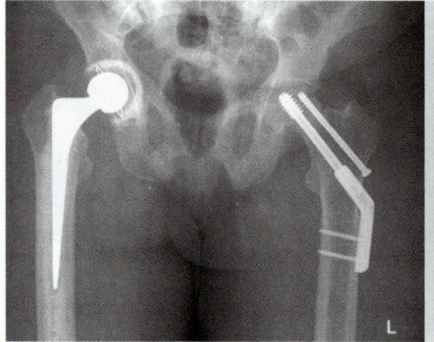
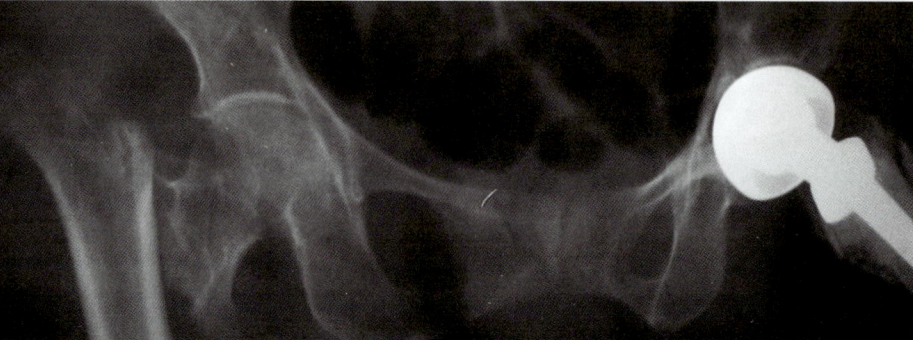

Fig. 46.25: Plain X-rays showing recurrence of fractures in fragility fractures (Once a fracture always a fracture)

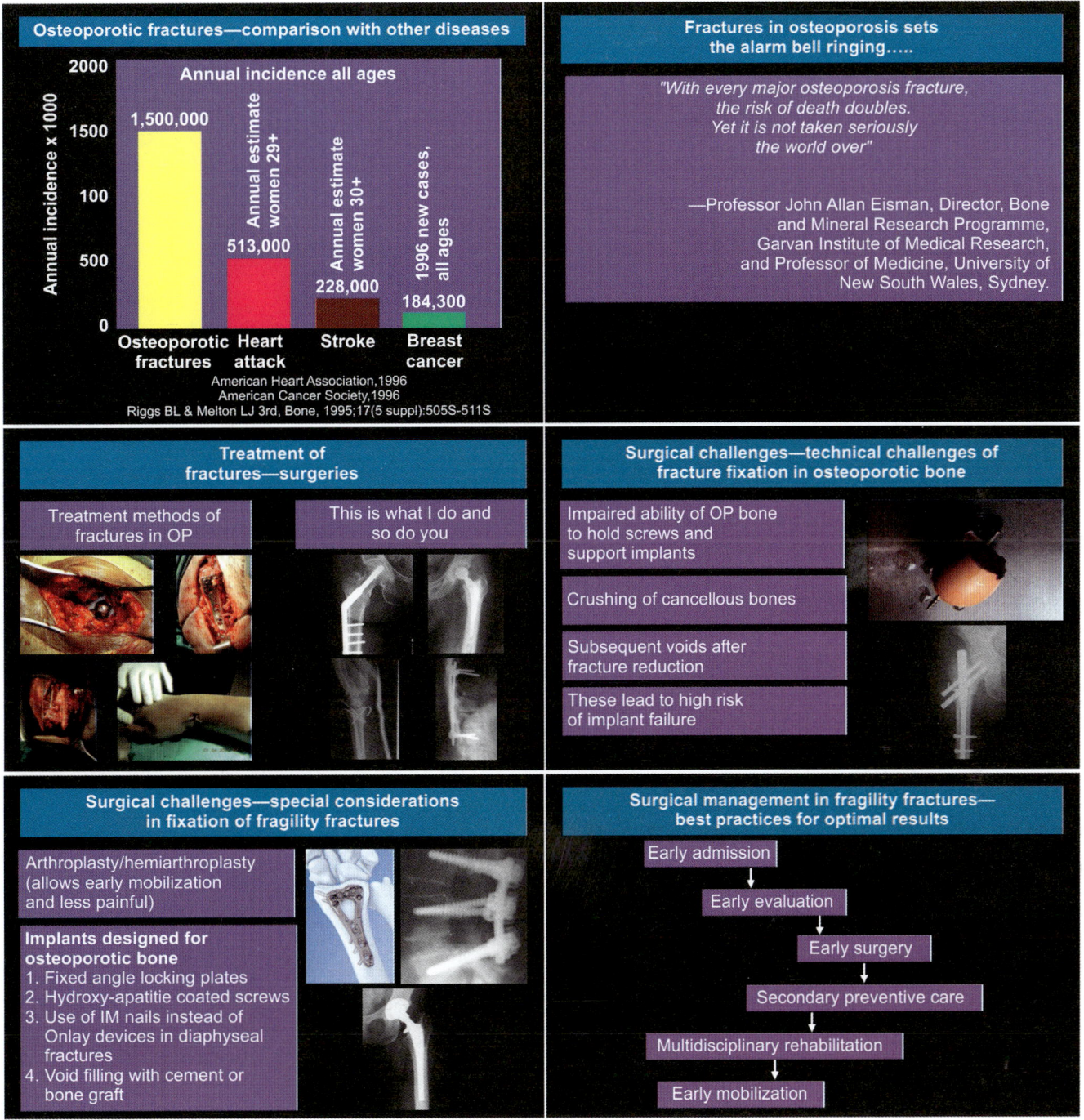

Fig. 46.26: Prevention and management of fragility fractures

47 CHAPTER

Osteoarthritis

Definition

It is defined as a degenerative, non-inflammatory joint disease characterized by destruction of articular cartilage and formation of new bone at the joint surfaces and margins.

The term osteoarthritis was coined by *John Spendon*. However, it is a misnomer and the right term is osteoarthrosis or degenerative joint disease. It could be primary or secondary and the former is more common.

Osteoarthritis affects the synovial joints, though it can affect any joint, it is more common in the weight bearing joints like the hip, knee, spine, etc. (Fig. 47.1).

OSTEOARTHRITIS OF THE KNEE

PRIMARY OSTEOARTHRITIS OF THE KNEE (Also Called Idiopathic)

Etiological causes for primary osteoarthritis: Though exact cause is not known, the following factors are suspected to play an important role in the causation of primary osteoarthritis—obesity, genetics and heredity, occupation involving prolonged standing, sports, multiple endocrine disorders and multiple metabolic disorders.

Note:
Genetic tendency in OA knee is twice as strong as OA hip.

Risk Factors
There are many risk factors that predispose to the development of this condition. The important ones are listed in the box on the page 659. They could be modifiable or non-modifiable.

Features

- It commonly affects the knee joint.
- All races are susceptible.
- Common in older age groups.
- Eighty percent of people are affected by 65 years, but only 40 percent show symptoms.
- It causes varus deformity of the knee in the late stages.
- More than 50 percent have bilateral OA knee.

Quick Facts: Osteoarthritis
Who is prone to get osteoarthritis?
- Middle-aged patients
- Women have a greater tendency than men do
- One in three people over 60 years are affected and more than three in four persons over the age of seventy show some radiographic evidence of the condition
- Very rarely it can be seen in younger people.

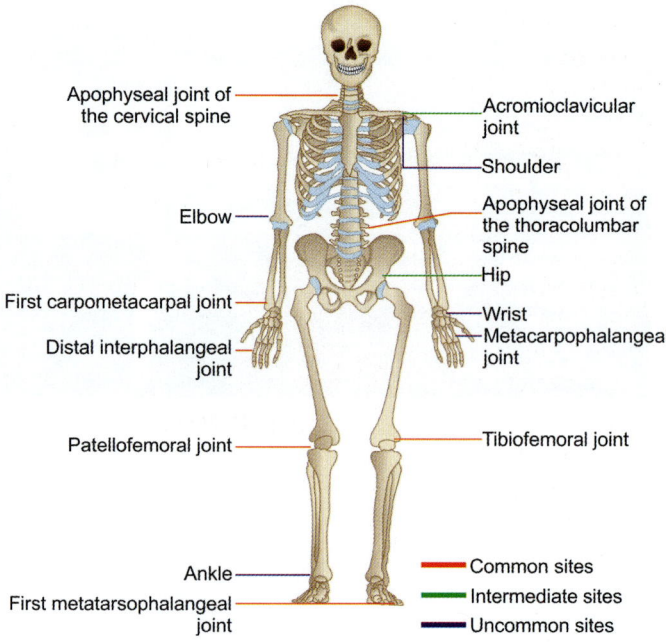

Fig. 47.1: Sites of primary osteoarthritis

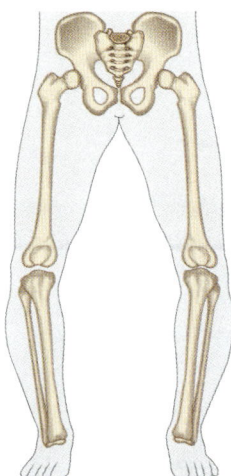

Fig. 47.2: Genu varum deformity in advanced osteoarthritis of knee

What are the typical symptoms of osteoarthritis?
- Pain
- Early morning stiffness
- Restricted range of joint movements
- Swelling of the joints.

What joints are usually affected?
- Weight bearing joints like hip, knee, ankle, etc.
- Spine
- Fingers.

What causes osteoarthritis?
- Age more than 40 years
- Female
- Hereditary conditions
- Previous joint injuries
- Obesity
- Diseases of the joints
- Poor posture
- Occupational stress
- A combination of the above factors.

Note: The only factor, which can be modified, is obesity.

How to make a diagnosis?
- Physical examination
- Symptomatology
- Radiography
- Blood tests
- CT scan and MRI.

Remember the Risk Factors
- O – Obesity
- S – Senility or old age
- T – Trauma
- E – Emotional stress
- O – Osteoporosis
- A – Alcohol
- R – Rigorous lifestyles
- T – Taxing professions
- H – Hormonal imbalances
- R – Repetitive injuries
- I – Indian cultural habits
- T – Axing sports
- I – Improper postural habits
- S – Smoking

Sequence of pathological events in osteoarthritis: The disease process usually begins in the anteromedial compartment of the knee joint.

Fibrillation due to loss of water of the weight bearing articular cartilage is seen in early stages of the disease followed by complete loss of articular cartilage. This puts enormous pressure on the underlying bone, which causes sclerosis and later eburnation. Cysts may develop in the subchondral area due to microfractures that degenerate. New bone formation takes place and results in osteophyte formation (Figs 47.3A to C).

Note:
OA is characterized by architectural deterioration of articular cartilage and formation of new bone at the joint surfaces.

Clinical Features

Predominant symptom is pain which increases on walking. The pain is poorly localized and is dull aching in nature. The patient has mild swelling of the knee joint and complains of early morning stiffness. Minimal tenderness and coarse crepitus can be elicited. If there are loose bodies in a joint, the patient gives history of locking or giving way. Terminal movements of the knee are restricted (Fig. 47.4A). The patient complains of early morning stiffness, which subsides over the day after some activity. Genu varum deformity may be seen in very advanced cases (Figs 47.2 and 47.4B). Minimal effusion may be present. In some cases, osteophytes may be palpable.

Do You Know the Sources of Pain in OA Knee?
Well, it could be from
- Inflamed synovium
- Microfracture of subchondral bone
- Periosteum stretching by osteophytes
- Venous congestion in intraosseous compartment
- Joint distension
- Muscle spasm
- Bursal inflammations
- Affered joint mechanics
- Mental depression.

Quick Facts: About Complaints in OA Knee (Flowchart 47.1)
- Pain limits walking distance and capacity to work
- Limp
- Difficulty to knee, get up from the chairs, getting in and out of the car
- Descend and ascend the stairs
- Limits capacity to work, even housework.

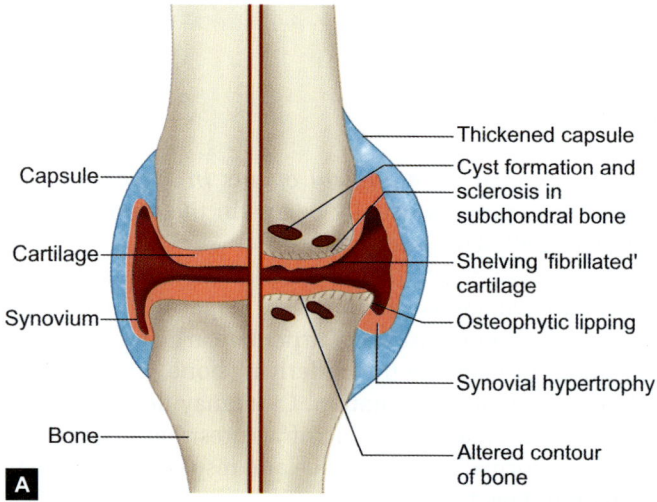

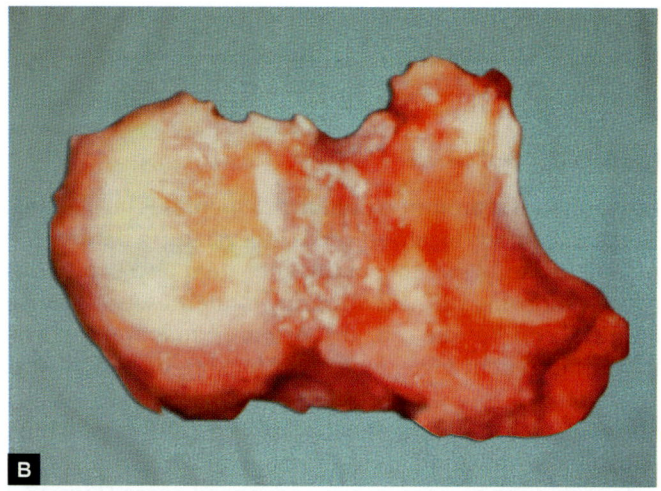

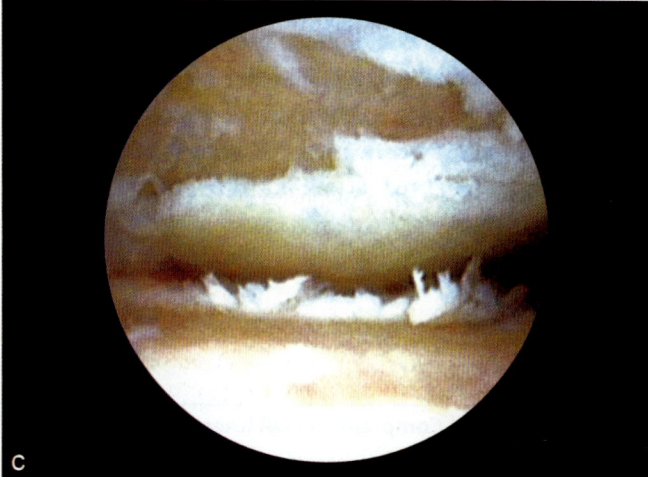

Figs 47.3A to C: (A) Pathological features of osteoarthritis knee; (B) Pathological specimen showing destruction of articular cartilage in OA knee; (C) Arthroscopic view of degenerated cartilage in OA knee

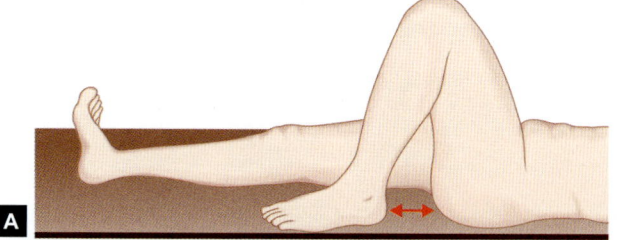

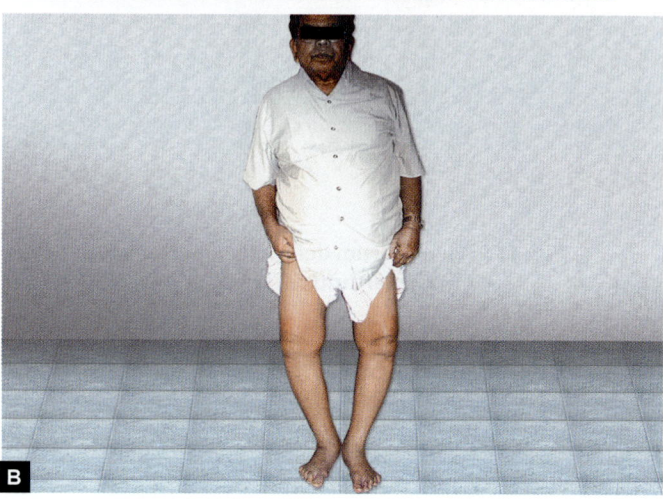

Figs 47.4A and B: (A) Loss of terminal flexion in osteoarthritis knee; (B) Genu varum deformity (Clinical photo)

Flowchart 47.1: Examination of the patient in OA knee

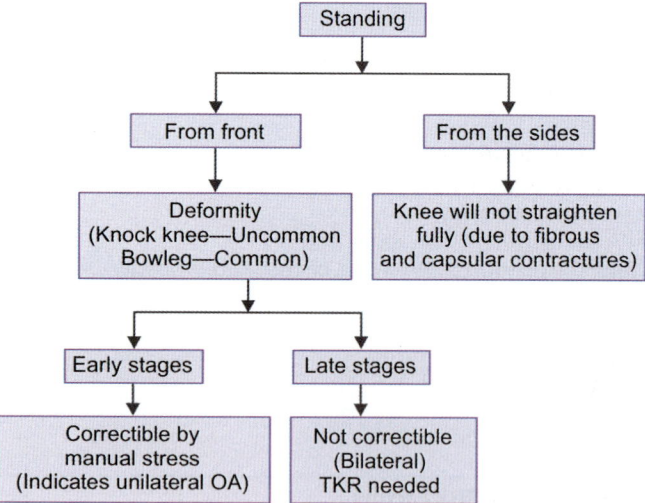

Criteria and Classification of OA Knee (American College of Rheumatology—ACR)

Clinical

- Knee pain for most days of prior month.
- Crepitus on active joint motion.

- Morning stiffness equal and not more than 30 minutes in duration.
- Age equal to more than 38 years.
- Bony enlargement of the knee on examination.

Clinical and Radiological

- Knee pain for most days of the prior month.
- Osteophytes at joint margins.
- Synovial fluid typical of OA knee.
- Age—40 years.
- Morning stiffness equal and not more than 30 minutes.
- Crepitus on active joint motion.

OA is Present (Clinical)

1, 2, 3, 4 or 1, 2, 5 or 1, 4, 5
OA present (Clinical and radiological)
1, 2 or 1, 3, 5, 6 or 1, 4, 5, 6. Modified from Attman (1986) and Atman (1991).

Investigations

Laboratory investigations are usually within normal limits. *Radiological examination* of the knee joint is the most important diagnostic tool. The following are the radiological features seen in osteoarthritis (Figs 47.5A and B) of the knee.

- Loss of joint space (due to destruction of articular cartilage).
- Sclerosis (due to increase cellularity and bone deposition).
- Subchondral cysts (due to synovial fluid intrusion into the bone).
- Osteophytes (due to revascularization of remaining cartilage and capsular traction).
- Bony collapse (due to compression of weakened bone).
- Loose bodies (due to fragmentation of osteochondral surface).
- Deformity and malalignment (due to destruction of capsules and ligaments).

Kellegren and Lawrence Radiological Grading

Grade I: Doubtful narrowing of joint space and possible osteophyte lipping.

Grade II: Definite osteophytes and possible narrowing of the joint space.

Grade III: Moderate multiple osteophytes, definite narrowing of joint space and some sclerosis and possible deformity of the bone ends.

Grade IV: Large osteophytes, marked narrowing of joint space, severe sclerosis and definite deformity of the bone ends.

Pitfalls of X-rays in OA Knee
- Not reliable in about 15 percent of the cases.
- Weight bearing AP and lateral views are desired.
- Only 40 percent of the people with severe X-ray changes experience pain.

Radiological Classification of OA Knee (Ahlbach) AP Weight Bearing and Lateral Views
Type I : Joint space narrowing.
Type II : Total loss of joint space.
Type III : <5 mm tibial erosion but posterior part of the plateau intact.
Type IV : >5 mm tibial erosion and erosion of posterior plateau.
Type V : Subluxation.
Note: Grades IV and V: TKR is the line of treatment.

Other Investigations

- *Arthroscopic examination:* This allows direct inspection and visualization of the damaged joint surfaces. But arthroscopy alone for diagnostic purposes is rarely used. (Fig. 47.3C)
- Synovial fluid analysis shows non-inflammatory picture. Bone scan shows increased uptake of technetium-99m, MRI and CT scan also helps to diagnose, subchondral cysts, osteophytes, etc. (Fig. 47.6).

Treatment

- Before beginning the treatment, the diagnosis of OA is a must. ACR diagnostic criteria for OA knee to be followed.
- Treatment to be individualized and tailored to severity.
- Multiple strategies may be required in most of the cases.

ACR Guidelines: Traditional Format

- Knee pain.
- Radiographic osteophytes.

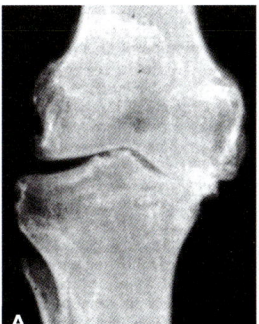 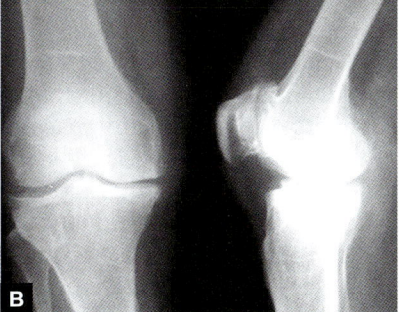

Figs 47.5A and B: (A) Radiograph showing knee joint showing loss of joint space, osteophytes, subchondral sclerosis and varus deformity; (B) Radiograph showing tri-compartmental OA knee

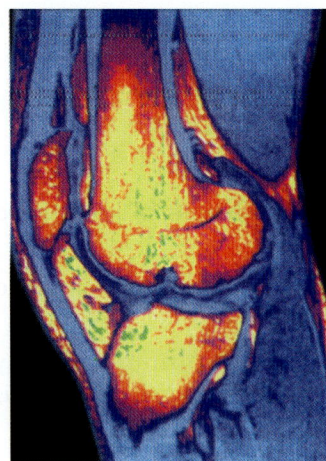

Fig. 47.6: MRI OA knee

- At least one of the following three:
  - Age greater than 50 years.
  - Morning stiffness less than or equal to 30 minutes.
  - Crepitus on motion.

Aims of Treatment of OA Knee
It can be best illustrated by 4 R's: • Relieve pain. • Restore function. • Reduce disability if any • Rehabilitation.

Conservative Methods

This forms the mainstay of management in osteoarthritis of the knee. About 50 percent of patients respond to conservative treatment, which consists of the following measures.

Nonpharmacological Treatment

This is the initial and main stay of treatment in OA knees. The important recommendations of ACR are:
- Self education—Educating the patient and his relatives measures about the disease is the most important aspect of the non-pharmacological treatment and should be done first.
- Health professional social support
- Weight loss
- Physiotherapy
- Therapeutic exercises
- Assistive devices
- Occupational therapy
- Aerobic exercise program
- Strengthening of the quadriceps
- Supervised fitness walking program
- Swimming/hydrotherapy
- Modifications of activity of daily living.

Mechanical Aids

- Cane in the contralateral hand
- Mechanical aids
- Medial taping of the patella in PF diseases
- Light weight knee braces in TF diseases. Now let us analyze the treatment methods:

Components of Therapeutic Exercise

- *Range of motion and flexibility:* Soft tissue flexibility of both contractile (muscle, tendon) and noncontractile tissues (capsule, ligaments) is affected by arthritis and inactivity. Joint stiffness and soft tissue shortening can be reduced with appropriate range of motion (ROM) and stretching exercises.
- *Muscle strengthening:* All aspects of muscle strength (strength, endurance, power) can be impacted as a result of intra-articular and extra-articular inflammatory processes, disuse, reflex inhibition in response to pain and joint effusion, decreased protective muscular reflexes, loss of mechanical integrity around the joint, and even medication side effects. Muscle strengthening exercises helps to overcome these problems.

  Quadriceps exercises strengthening of quadriceps musculature with either isometric or isotonic, resistive exercises was associated with significant improvement in quadriceps strength, knee pain, and function.
- *Aerobic (Cardiovascular) exercise:* Persons with arthritis tend to be less fit than noninvolved peers. However, there is strong evidence for the role of regular and vigorous exercise to improve all components of physical fitness, including cardiovascular fitness and endurance even in people with arthritis. Most studies have limited their interventions to walking, stationary bicycling, aerobic dancing, aquatic exercise, and circuit training at moderate intensity levels.
- *Body awareness exercise:* Body awareness exercises address posture, core stability, balance, proprioception, coordination, and relaxation. Benefits of these exercises include decreased risks for falls and musculoskeletal injury.
- *Recreational and community-based exercise:* The advantages of community-based exercise include a focus on wellness, increased socialization, and peer support. As well, the greater variety in exercise facilities, classes, and equipment may enhance motivation and ongoing adherence. Aquatic exercises are a good choice for individuals with arthritis, particularly those with lower extremity involvement.

Physiotherapy

Physical modalities that may contribute to pain relief include the application of superficial heat (hot packs, heating pads, hot water bottles, or paraffin) and/or cold (cold packs or ice packs).

Weight Loss

Obesity is a risk factor for the development of OA, and is associated with radiological progression of the disease, and disability. When people walk, 3–6 times their body weight is transferred across the knee joint; any excess weight should be multiplied by this factor to estimate the excess force across the knee joint of overweight people.

In managing OA, weight reduction should be a key goal. Exercise plays a role, but pain and disability can make it difficult for patients to exercise sufficiently to lose weight. Weight loss can be achieved with regular sessions with a dietitian who can provide instruction on reducing caloric intake and the use of food diaries, and cognitive-behavioral modification to change dietary habits.

Pharmacologic Drugs

- *Nonopioid analgesics*—e.g. Acetaminophen: This is the drug of first choice. Up to 4 g/day can be given.
- *NSAIDs:* If patients fail to respond to paracetamol or other oral or topical analgesics, then the use of an NSAID is indicated.
- *Opioid analgesics:* These can be tried if patients fail to respond to paracetamol and NSAIDs.
- *Food supplementation—Glucosamine and chondroitin sulfate:* Can reduce 20–25 percent pain in mild to moderate OA. Over-the-counter food supplements, 1500 mg/day for at least 3 months.
- *Intra-articular steroids:* This is indicated if there is effusion and there are signs of inflammation.
- *Viscosupplementation:* Injection of hyaluronic acid into the joint. Once a week for 3 weeks. Adverse reactions in 2–3 percent.
- *Topical analgesics:* These are indicated in the following situations:
  - If patients do not respond to oral analgesics.
  - If patients do not wish to take systemic drugs.
  - Can be used as a monotherapy or adjunct.
  - Capsaicin cream—4 times a day.

> **Viscosupplementation in OA Knee?**
> *Viscosupplementation* (Intra-articular hyaluronan therapy): This procedure consists of removal of pathologic osteoarthritis synovial fluid and replacement of hyaluronan-based products that restore the molecular weight and concentration of hyaluronan to normal values that is reduced in OA knee.
> Hyaluronan helps in joint lubrication, buffers load transmission, imparts anti-inflammatory properties to synovial fluid.

> **Indications for Intra-articular Hyaluronic Acid Injection**
> - Failed conservative treatment
> - If there are major risk factors for surgery
> - Failed intra-articular steroid injections
> - Advanced osteoarthritis.

By combining steroid injection with joint lavage, OA patients get more effective pain relief than with either therapy alone and pain could reduce for as long as 24 weeks.

Mechanical Aids

They reduce the load on the knee joint and provides support to the weak knees. The following are used in OA knees:
- Cane
- Shoe inserts
- Shoe supplements: Good shock absorber, good mediolateral support, adequate arch support, calcaneal cushion.
- Lateral heel wedges: To reduce pain of medial tibiofemoral joint OA.
- Knee brace and support in varus knees.

Alternative Therapies

- Acupuncture
- Biofeedback
- Naturopathy
- Aquatic physical therapy
- Massage
- Acupressure
- Tai Chi
- Balneotherapy
- Yoga.

The proponents of alternative therapies claim good results from their respective interventions. The results are good in the hands of experts.

Surgery

Indications for Surgery

- Pain refractory to conservative measures.
- History of frequent locking episodes.
- Hemarthrosis due to loose bodies or osteochondral fractures.
- Deformity, usually genu varum.
- Joint instability.
- Progressive limitation of knee motion.

Surgical Methods

- *Excision of osteophytes* is rarely done alone.
- *Excision of loose bodies, meniscectomy, synovectomy,* and *reconstruction or joint debridement* are best done by arthroscopy.

664 SECTION 6: Geriatric Orthopedics

- *Proximal tibial osteotomy (Slocum's):* Indicated for unicompartmental osteoarthritis of knee with pain and also to correct varus (less than 15°) or valgus deformity (less than 12°). Pain is decreased in 80 percent of the cases following surgery as osteotomy changes the line of weight-bearing and brings the more normal surface to carry out the function of load transmission (Fig. 47.7). Mean failure rate is 40 percent at 4 years.
- *Distal femoral osteotomy* is indicated when varus or valgus deformity of the knee is more than 12–15°.
- *Chondral resurfacing procedure*
  - *Autologous chondrocyte grafting*: Autologous chondrocytes from the patient's knee are cultured for two weeks, reinserted under a patch of periosteum.
  - *Mosaic plasty*: Spare autologous hyaline cartilage from other areas of knee is inserted into the defect.
- *Arthroscopic debridement:* This is a successful palliative, temporizing treatment of OA knee.
- *Total knee arthroplasty:* This is indicated when both the compartments of the knee joint are destroyed or if valgus or varus deformity is more than 15°. It is also indicated in failed conservative treatment (Fig. 47.9).

Limitations of TKR
- Only 1 in 6-gain normal knee function after TKR, and the rest have residual symptoms.
- Full flexion not regained.
- Anterior wound prevents kneeling.

- *Arthrodesis* is indicated less commonly than arthroplasty. If the patient is young and involved in heavy occupation, arthrodesis is indicated to give him a stable and strong knee. However, arthrodesis results in a stiff knee, which is a severe disability.
- *Patellectomy:* It is rarely done except as a last resort. Contemplated in osteoarthritis present for several years.

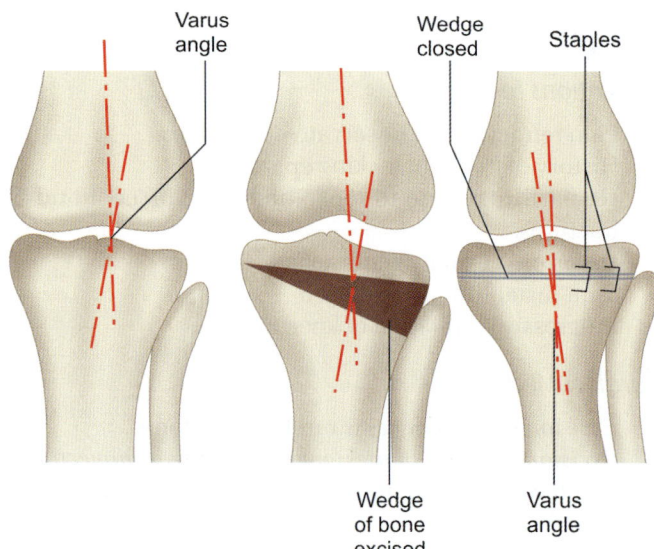

Fig. 47.7: Valgus high tibial osteotomy

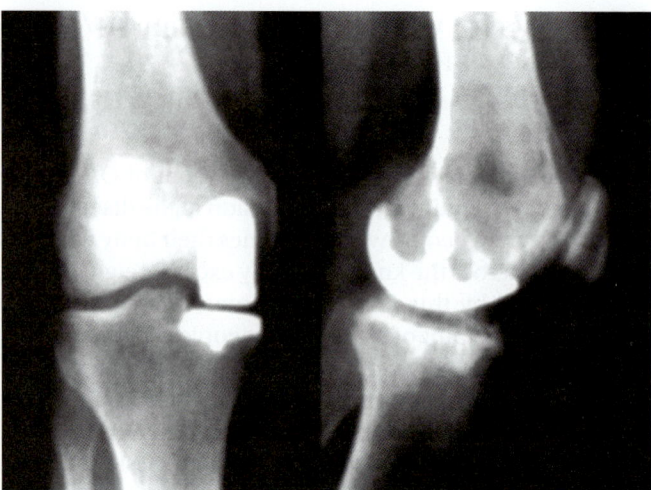

Fig. 47.8: Radiographs showing unicondylar knee replacement

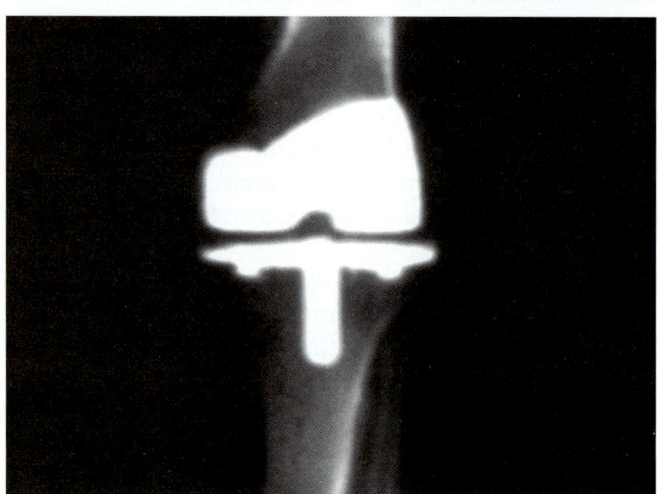

Fig. 47.9: Radiograph showing total knee replacement

- *Unicompartmental knee arthroplasty (UKA):* This is again regaining its popularity over tibial osteotomy in treating unicompartmental OA, as it helps in early postoperative rehabilitation (Fig. 47.8).

Macquet's HTO (High Tibial Osteotomy) this is Another Useful Procedure
Did You Know?
Steindler described osteotomy for OA knee in 1940.

What does the Evidence Say About Various Non-arthroplasty Treatments in OA Knees?

There are various modalities of treating OA knees. Of these which is the best? Which are the ones that have strong recommendations and can be safely applied and which are the ones that are less than strong recommendations and not applied routinely. Here is the recent AAOS guidelines practiced worldwide (Table 47.1).

2013 AAOS Recommendations—Treatment of OA Knees (Nonarthroplasty)

The **AAOS**, with inputs from representatives of the **American College of Rheumatology, the American Academy of Family Practice, and the American Physical Therapy Association**, recently published a collaborative clinical practice guideline (CPG) on the *Treatment of Osteoarthritis (OA) of the Knee (Non-arthroplasty)—2nd Edition.* www.aaos.org/guidelines

TABEL 47.1: Conservative treatment—Recommendations 1-11

Recommendations	What is It	Quality of Recommendations	Strength of evidence
Recommendation 1	Self management program, light impact exercises, strengthening exercises, neuromuscular education, physical activity	Strongly recommended practitioners should follow	Strong (Based on 7 high strength studies, out of which 3 studies are by Dr John Ebnezar)
Recommendation 2	Weight loss	Practitioners can follow/Be alert/Patient preference	Moderate
Recommendation 3A	Acupuncture	Cannot be recommended	Strong
Recommendation 3B	Physiotherapy	Practitioners can follow/Be alert/Patient preference	Mixed
Recommendation 3C	Manual therapy	Unable to recommend	Strong
Recommendation 4	Braces	Practitioners can follow/Be alert/Patient preference	Inconclusive (Unable to recommend for or against)
Recommendation 5	Lateral wedge Insole	Practitioners can follow/Be alert/Patient preference	Moderate
Recommendation 6	Glucosamine, chondroitin sulfate	Not recommended	Strong
Recommendation 7A	NSAID'S	Recommended	Strong
Recommendation 7B	Paracetamol/Opiaids/ Pain patches	Practitioners can follow/Be alert/Patient preference	Mixed—Inconclusive (Unable to recommend for or against)
Recommendation – 8	I A steroids	Practitioners can follow/Be alert/Patient preference	Mixed—Inconclusive (Unable to recommend for or against)
Recommendation – 9	Hyaluronic acid	Not recommended	Strong
Recommendation – 10	Growth factor injections/PRP	Practitioners can follow/Be alert/Patient preference	Mixed
Recommendation – 11	Needle lavage	Not recommended	Moderate
Surgery – Recommendations 12–15			
Recommendation – 12	Arthroscopy (Lavage)	Not recommended	Strong
Recommendation – 13	Arthroscopy–Partial Meniscectomy	Practitioners can follow/Be alert/Patient preference	Inconclusive (Unable to recommend for or against)
Recommendation – 14	Valgus osteotomy	Practitioners can follow/Be alert/Patient preference	Limited
Recommendation – 15	Free floating (unfixed IA device)	Flexible/Patient preferences	Consensus

- More than 10,000 separate pieces of literature were reviewed during the evidence analysis phase. The AAOS used a "best-evidence synthesis" form of evidence analysis, meaning that only higher quality evidence is used in meta-analysis and network meta-analysis.
- A total of 137 research publications have been used in the preparation of these guidelines.
- All my 3 research publications of OA Knees have been accepted by these august bodies.
- Only Indian and only Orthopedic Surgeon to have his research publications on Yoga accepted in toto by AAOS.
- The CPG on the Treatment of Osteoarthritis of the Knee (Nonarthroplasty)—2nd Edition—including the full guideline document, along with all supporting documentation and workgroup disclosures—is available on the AAOS website, at www.aaos.org/guidelines
- Strong positive (2): Recommended—1,7A
- Strong Negative (4): Not recommended—3C,6,9,12
- Moderate (2): 5,11
- Inconclusive(Mixed)-5: 4,7B,8,11,13
- Limited (1): 14
- Consensus (1):15

Atkins D, Best D, Briss PA, et al. Grading quality of evidence and strength of recommendations. BMJ. 2004;328:1490.
Grade A/High/Strong: Further research is very unlikely to change our confidence in the estimate of effect
Grade B/Moderate: Further research is likely to have an important impact on our confidence in the estimate of effect and may change the estimate.
Grade C/Low: Further research is very likely to have an important impact on our confidence in the estimate of effect and is likely to change the estimate
Ebnezar J. Nagarathna R. Bali Y. Nagendra HR. Effect of an integrated approach of youga therapy on quality of life in osteoarthritis of the knee joint: A randomized control study. Int J Yoga 2011;4(2):55-63. PM:22022123
Ebnezar J. Nagarathna R. Yogitha B. Nagendra HR. Effects of an integrated approach of hatha yoga therapy on functional disability, pain, and flexibility in osteoarthritis of the knee joint: a randomized controlled study. J Altern Complement Med 2012:18(5):463-472. PM:22537508
Ebnezar J. Nagarathna R. Yogitha B. Nagendra HR. Effect of integrated yoga therapy on pain, morning stiffness and anxiety in osteoarthritis of the knee joint: A randomized control study. Int J Yoga 2012:5(1):28-36. PM:223460063

So, my concept of blending modern orthopedic treatment with our own traditional Yoga in the treatment of OA knees through research has received the approval and acceptance of the highest academic bodies in the world and my research publications on OA knees has been accepted as high strength studies and is the basis for the **STRONG*** recommendations by the **American Academy of Orthopedic Surgeons (AAOS)** recent 2013 guidelines in the nonarthroplasty conservative management of OA knees.

AAOS, with inputs from representatives of the **American College of Rheumatology, the American Academy of Family Practice, and the American Physical Therapy Association**, has formed guidelines for the treatment of OA knees, that are accepted worldwide and out of 10,000 research publications very few were selected after high level scrutiny by a highly specialized research committee. AAOS accepting all my three research studies out of the seven studies used to formulate recommendation 1 of the CT guidelines speaks volumes about my high quality research work which had earlier fetched me the Best Research Award in 2012 by S-VYASA Yoga University, Banglauru.

Out of the 11 modalities of conservative treatment mentioned by AAOS, only 2 have been strongly recommended, one is mine and the other is drug therapy through NSAIDs. The same body has not recommended the Chinese method of acupuncture, hyaluronic acid injections, glucosamine and chondoitin combinations and none of the non-TKR surgeries have received strong recommendations. Now what this does is that it opens up a huge opportunity for the Indian-based Yoga into modern orthopedics.

SECONDARY OSTEOARTHRITIS OF THE KNEE (FIG. 47.10)

It is generally observed that secondary osteoarthritis occurs in the younger age groups and is more severe than the primary. Apart from all the features of osteoarthritis, secondary osteoarthritis has the features of the corresponding etiological condition.

The causes for secondary osteoarthritis of the knee are as follows:
- Obesity.
- Valgus and varus deformities of the knee.
- Intra-articular fractures of the knee, etc.
- Rheumatoid arthritis, infection, trauma, TB, etc.
- Hyperparathyroidism.
- Hemophilia.
- Syringomyelia.

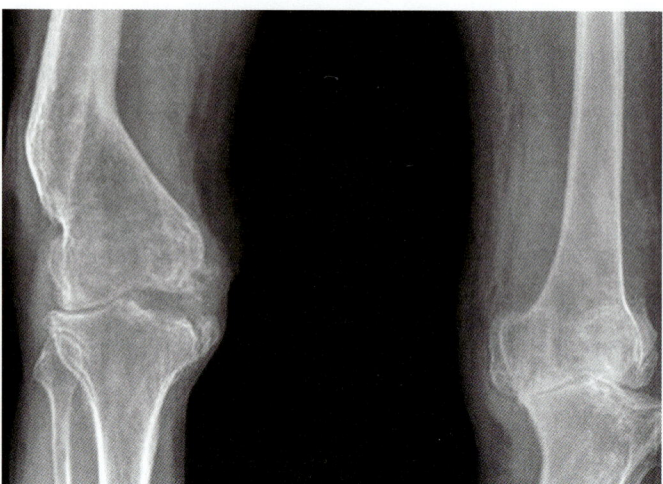

Fig. 47.10: Plain X-ray of the knees showing secondary OA knees due to femur malunion fracture

- Neurological disease like diabetes.
- Overuse of intra-articular steroid therapy.

Remember
Major complications of osteoarthritis of knee
- Joint deformities
- Subluxation
- Ankylosis
- Intra-articular loose bodies.

Remember
O's in osteoarthritis of the knee
- **O**besity
- **O**ccupation
- **O**ver 40 years of age
- **O**ther predisposing joint diseases
- **O**steophytes main characteristic feature of osteoarthritis
- **O**utward deviation of knee
- **O**steotomy required correcting bone deformities.

OSTEOARTHRITIS OF THE HIP (Familiarly Called as Malum Coxae Senilis)

This is second in frequency to knee joint, and it could be primary or secondary.

PRIMARY OSTEOARTHRITIS OF THE HIP

This is idiopathic and forms 50 percent of the osteoarthritis of the hip. In this variety, the exact cause is not known and

---

*Strong recommendation means—Practitioners must follow and further research is very unlikely to change our confidence in the estimate of effect. Atkins D, Best D, Briss PA, et al. Grading quality of evidence and strength of recommendations. BMJ 2004; 328:1490.

the causative factors suspected are increased anteversion, and trabecular microfracture causing stiffening of the subchondral bone.

SECONDARY OSTEOARTHRITIS OF THE HIP (FIG. 47.11)

The following factors are responsible for the development of secondary osteoarthritis of the hip joint.
- *Incongruity of the articular surface,* e.g. trauma, Perthe's, CDH, slipped epiphysis, etc.
- *Instability of the hip,* e.g. subluxation.
- *Concentration of pressure load,* e.g. coxa vara, anteversion.
- *Direct injury,* e.g. infection, trauma, etc.
- *Constitutional causes,* e.g. obesity, hyperthyroidism, etc.
- Bone diseases like AVN, rheumatoid arthritis, etc.

Remember
About secondary osteoarthritis
- Progress is relentless.
- Occurs in younger age group.
- Nonsurgical treatment is futile.
- If surgery is prolonged for long, the optimal time for surgery is missed.

Pathology

The changes in the articular cartilage vary from fibrillation to complete destruction depending on the severity of osteoarthritis. The synovium is thick and congested. The subchondral bone shows sclerosis and cyst formation. The capsule is thick and fibrosed. New bone growth results in osteophyte formation in areas not under pressure.

Clinical Features

In osteoarthritis of the hip joint, the patient is asymptomatic in the early stages, later patient may complain of slight pain in the hip lasting for 1–2 days (Figs 47.12A to D). Stiffness of the hip, muscle spasm, limp, restriction of terminal hip movements is the other complaints. As the disease advances, pain decreases, but the hip becomes more and more stiff. A mild flexion, adduction and external rotation deformity may be seen.

Radiographs

Primary Osteoarthritis
In the early stages, no changes are seen. In the later, stages joint space is reduced, subchondral sclerosis, cysts, osteophytes, etc. may be seen (Figs 47.13A and B).

Secondary osteoarthritis: Apart from features of osteoarthritis, features of the predisposing causes are also seen.

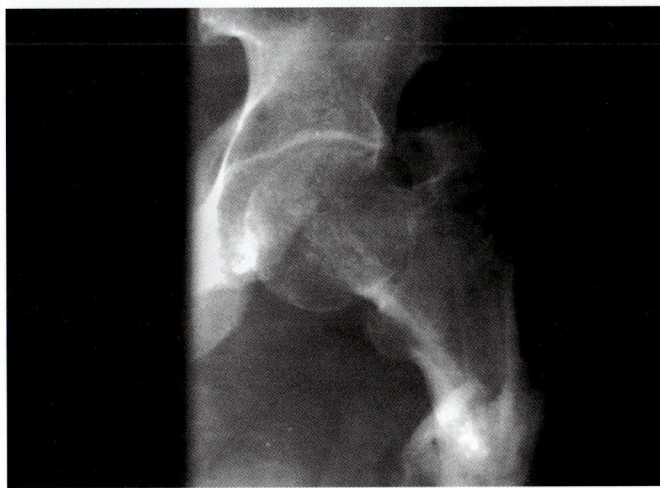

Fig. 47.11: Plain X-ray showing secondary OA hip due to malunited femur fracture

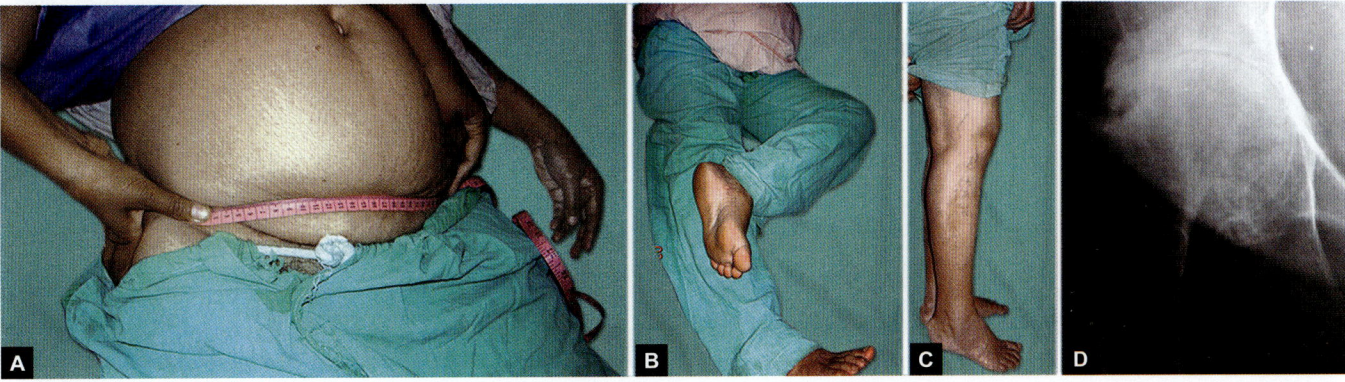

Figs 47.12A to D: Clinical photos and plain X-ray showing features of OA hip: (A) Hip deformity; (B) Restricted hip movements; (C) Minor flexion deformity; (D) Plain X-ray of hip

Treatment

Conservative Measures

Consist of rest, heat, NSAIDs, DMARD's muscle relaxant, massage, traction, manipulation, intra-articular steroids, physiotherapy, exercises, etc.

Surgical

Careful selection of the cases is done. Primary aim of surgery is relief of pain, while secondary aim is to restore movements, increase stability and deformity correction.

In the early stages of the disease when a fair amount of hip movements is still present, osteotomy helps.

Choice of Osteotomy

Pauwell's varus osteotomy: It is done if osteoarthritis is due to coxa valga.

Valgus osteotomy: This is more common and is done in adduction deformity of the hip.

Displacement osteotomy (Mc Murray's): This is indicated in severe osteoarthritis of hip with large osteophytes.

Osteotomy helps by changing the line of weight bearing and bringing the normal surface into the line of weight transmission (Figs 47.14A and B).

Hip arthroplasties: In the late stages of osteoarthritis, in elderly and in restriction of flexion less than 70°, osteotomy is of no value. The choice is then between cup arthroplasty, arthrodesis, hemireplacement arthroplasty and total hip replacement (Figs 47.15 and 47.16).

Resurfacement arthroplasty: Birmingham hip resurfacing arthroplasty is emerging as an effective alternative to the conventional THR. Here only the diseased head is resurfaced and not resected. It preserves unaffected portion of the head and neck. It is indicated in slightly younger patient.

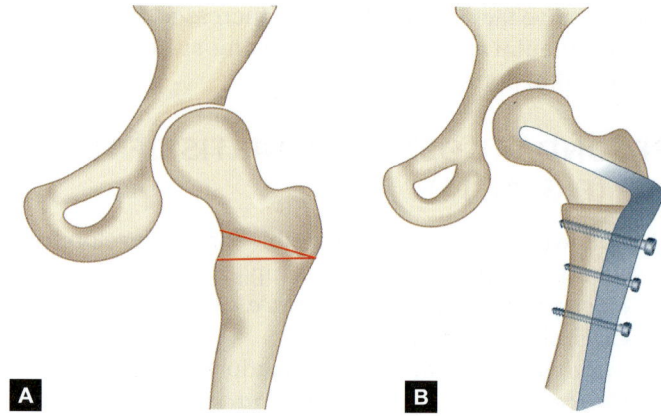

Figs 47.14A and B: Osteotomy for hip in osteoarthritis: (A) Before operation; (B) After operation

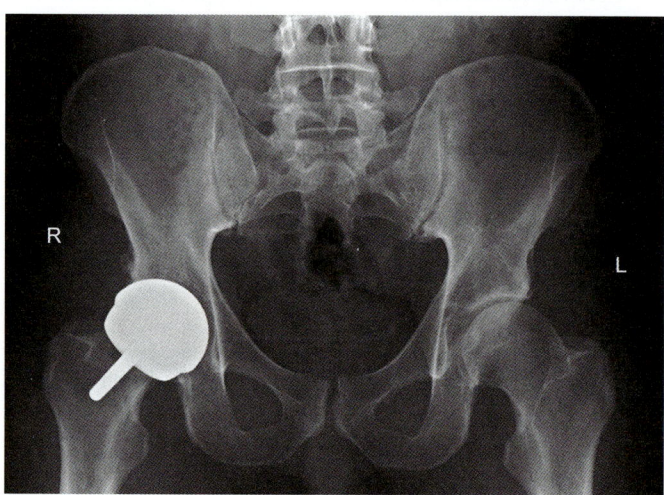

Fig. 47.15: Birmingham hip resurfacing (BHR) for osteoarthritis of hip

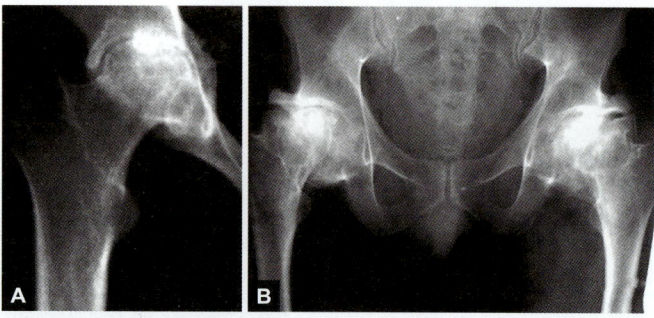

Figs 47.13A and B: (A) Radiograph showing osteoarthritis of hip; (B) Bilateral OA hip

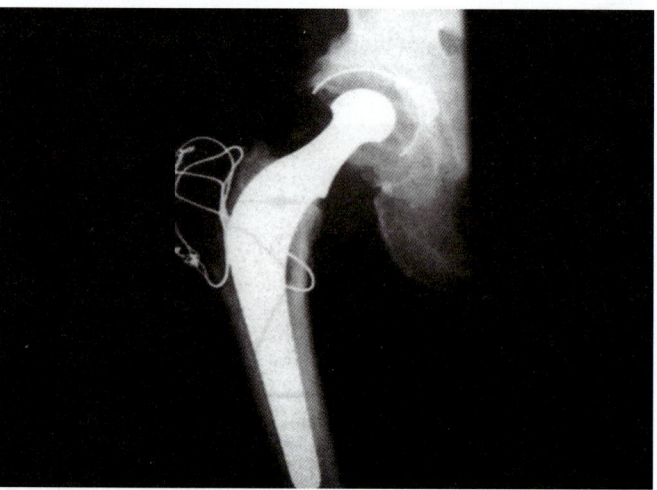

Fig. 47.16: Radiograph showing THR

Modifications of Activity of Daily Living in the Management of Osteoarthritis of Hip and Knee Joints

Simple changes around the home and daily activities causes dramatic improvement in the symptomatology of osteoarthritis. The following are some of the measures:
- Use of higher chair, which require less effort to get in and get out, should be considered (Fig. 47.17A).
- Changes to be made in the bathroom:
  - Use of Western toilets and avoiding the Indian types.
  - To fit the bath aids to facilitate easy getting in getting out of a bath.
  - To fit railings next to the toilet and bath to facilitate ease of movement.
- Patients are advised to *climb* the stairs leading the *good leg* taking one stair at a time and to *descend* the stairs leading with the *bad leg*, again taking one stair at a time (Fig. 47.17B).
- To reduce the force acting across the injured joint, the patient is advised to use a walking stick, which acts as a *third limb*. The stick should be held in the hand opposite to the affected hip or knee. Initially, it should be used around the home. The top of the stick should come up to the wrist when the patient stands and the tip should be provided with a firm rubber to avoid slipping. A walking stick, by providing a third limb through which forces can be transmitted, enables the reduction of force across the injured joint from peak values of 5–1.5 times the body weight (Fig. 47.17C).
- Footwear with hard soles and high heels should be avoided.

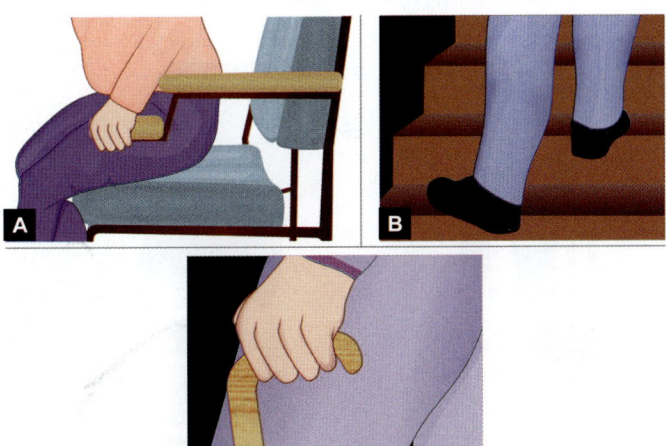

Figs 47.17A to C: Modification of living habits in the management of osteoarthritis of hip and knee: (A) Higher chairs, less effort; (B) Stairs often present a problem; (C) Walking sticks of the right height

- Cars with raised platforms and seats, which facilitate easy getting in and getting out, should be used.
- If the patients are overweight, reduction in the weight helps to reduce the load on the joints.
- General advice when standing:
  - Keep as upright as possible as this helps to put equal weight on both the legs.
  - Avoid sitting on a low or soft chair.
  - Avoid curling up in bed.
  - To stretch the front of the thigh and hip, lie on the stomach at least once a day for 5–30 minutes.
  - To use a walking stick when walking inside or outside the house (cane reduces load by 40–50%).
  - To avoid uneven and rough ground or surfaces while walking.
  - To wear comfortable footwears.

Role of Exercises in the Management of Osteoarthritis of the Hip and Knee

Exercises from the mainstay of the patients own contribution in the treatment of osteoarthritis of the hip and knee.

> **Quick Facts**
> Aims of the exercises in osteoarthritis hip and knee
> - To increase the range of movements.
> - To increase stability and shock absorption.
> - To prevent deformity.
> - To improve posture.
> - To reduce pain and stiffness.
>
> **Rules of the Exercises**
> - Build-up the exercises gradually.
> - Avoid rough ground while exercising.
> - To take warm baths before starting the exercises.
> - To perform the exercises 20 times each twice a day and later four times a day.

Types of Exercises in Osteoarthritis of Hip

Exercises lying on the back (Figs 47.18A to D)
- *Pelvic tilt:* Tighten the thigh and buttock muscles, pushing the knees flat, hold for a count of five and relax (Fig. 47.18A).
- *Pelvic lift:* Bend both the knees up, push on the feet and lift, hold for a count of five and relax (Fig. 47.18B).
- *Leg stretch:* Push one leg along the floor as though you are trying to make it longer than the other. Hold for a count of five and then repeat with the other leg (Fig. 47.18C).
- *Alternate leg rising:* Keeping the knees straight, lift alternate legs six inches from the ground (Fig. 47.18D).

Exercises lying on your side, with the painful hip up (Figs 47.19A to C)

- *Side leg rising:* Keep the top leg straight and lift it up as high as possible, hold for a count of five and relax (Figs 47.19B and C).
- *Knee and hip flexion:* Bend the hip and knee of the top leg forwards, and hold for a count of five. Then straighten the leg and stretch backwards as far as it will go, hold for a count of five, then relax (Fig. 47.19A).

Exercises in sitting posture (Figs 47.20A and B)
- *Knees together, feet apart:* Keep the knees together and move the feet apart, hold for a count of five then relax (Fig. 47.20A).
- *Feet together, knees apart:* Keep the ankles together and move the knees apart, then relax (Fig. 47.20B).

Exercises in standing Posture (Figs 47.21A and B)
- *Standing leg swing:* Hold into a table or chair with one hand, swing one leg forward and backward. Try to get the backwards swing as wide as possible (Fig. 47.21A).
- *Standing side leg swing:* Hold on to a chair with both hands. Swing bad leg out as far as it will go and then in. The outward swing is the hardest part and the leg should be allowed to fall back under muscular control (Fig. 47.21B).

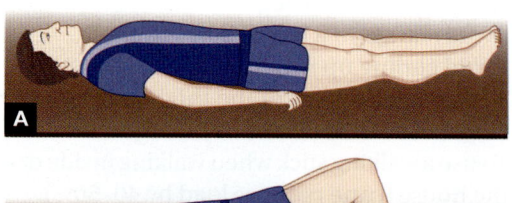
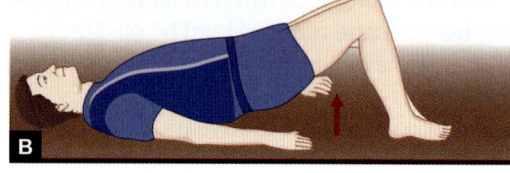
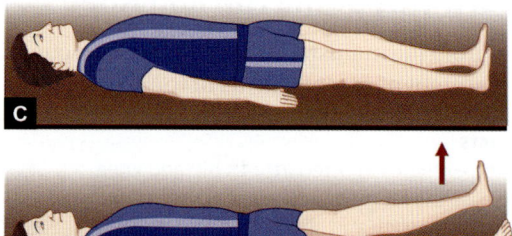

Figs 47.18A to D: Exercises on lying back: (A) Pelvic tilt; (B) Pelvic lift; (C) Leg stretch; (D) Alternate leg raising

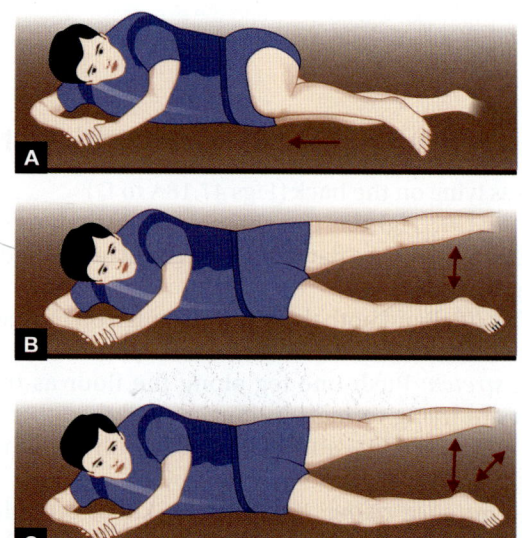

Figs 47.19A to C: Exercises lying on side: (A) Knee and hip flexion; (B and C) Side leg raising

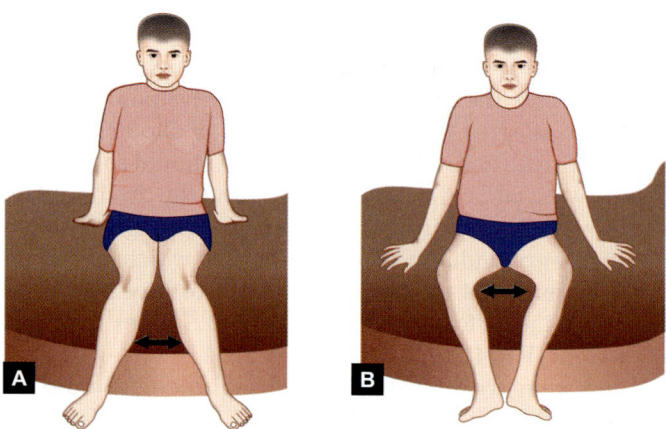

Figs 47.20A and B: Exercises while sitting: (A) Knees together, feet apart; (B) Feet together, knees apart

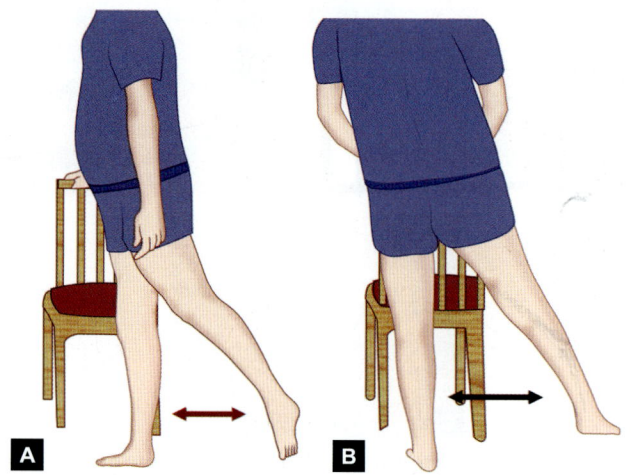

Figs 47.21A and B: (A) Standing swing; (B) Standing side leg swing

OSTEOARTHRITIS OF OTHER REGIONS

Osteoarthritis spine (cervical and lumbar spondylosis): It is usually seen in the elderly age group and the patient presents with low backache. Osteophytes may compress the nerve roots at their exit at the intervertebral foramen and may cause neurological disturbances. Conservative treatment usually helps, but surgery may be required for prolonged pain and neurological deficits (Figs 47.22A and B). See Chapters 48 and 49 for details.

Osteoarthritis of the small joints: Osteoarthritis may affect the peripheral joints of the hand and foot. It may cause ankylosis at an increased rate in these joints (Figs 47.23 and 47.24).

> **Remember in Osteoarthritis of Other Joints**
> - Heberden's node—osteophytes around distal interphalangeal joints of the hand.
> - Bouchard's node—osteophytes along proximal interphalangeal joints (Fig. 47.24).
> - Mucinous cysts—cysts containing degenerative myxomatous fibrous tissue at the distal or proximal interphalangeal joints.
> - Bunion is a combination of osteoarthritis and valgus angulation of the first metatarsophalangeal joint of foot.
> - Erosive osteoarthritis: It is a hereditary severe osteoarthritis involving distal and proximal interphalangeal joints. Joint deformities and ankylosis result more often.
> - Osteoarthritis of the first carpometacarpal joint of the thumb—seen in women more than 50 years (Fig. 47.23). They complain of pain and loss of grip.
> - Osteoarthritis of the wrist—seen in Kienbock's disease, trauma, gout, nonunion scaphoid, etc.
> - Osteoarthritis of the acromioclavicular joint—this is quite common.
> - Osteoarthritis of the ankle joint though not as common as OA knee but is increasingly being seen of late and leads to troublesome pain and limp (Fig. 47.25).
> - Osteoarthritis of the shoulder joint is rare and is not as common as OA hip joint (Fig. 47.26).

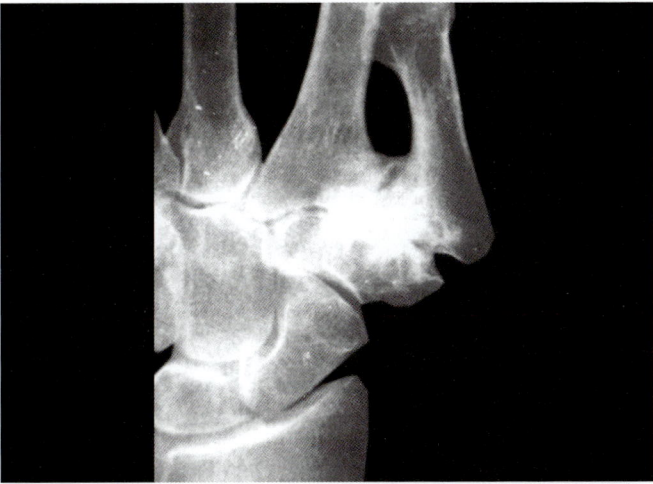

Fig. 47.23: Radiograph showing carpometacarpal joint of the thumb: Loss of joint space and sclerosis

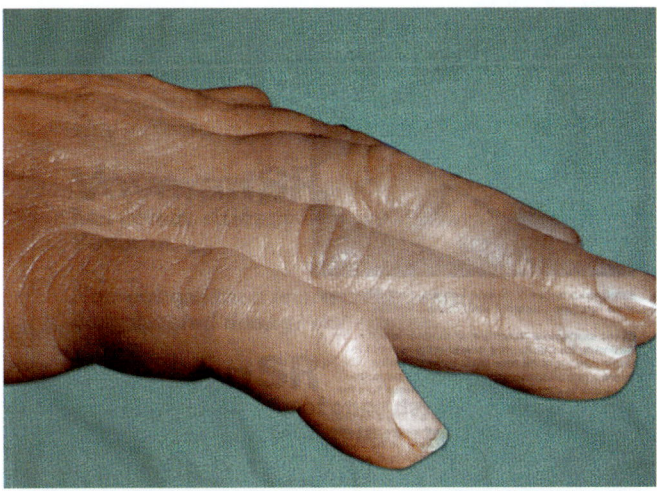

Fig. 47.24: Clinical photograph of OA hand

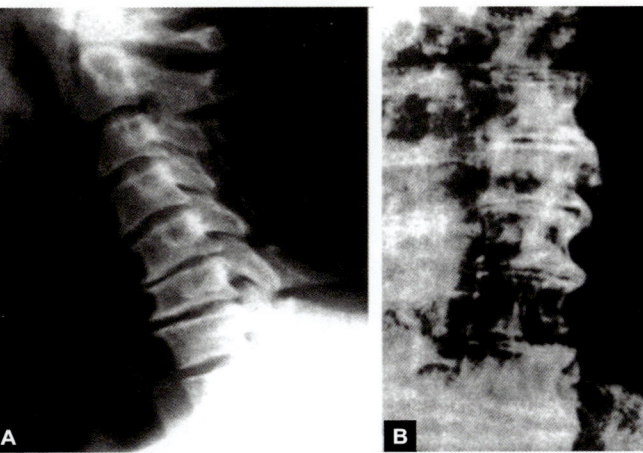

Figs 47.22A and B: (A) Radiograph showing cervical spondylosis; (B) Radiograph showing narrowing of disk space and osteophyte formation in lumbar spondylosis

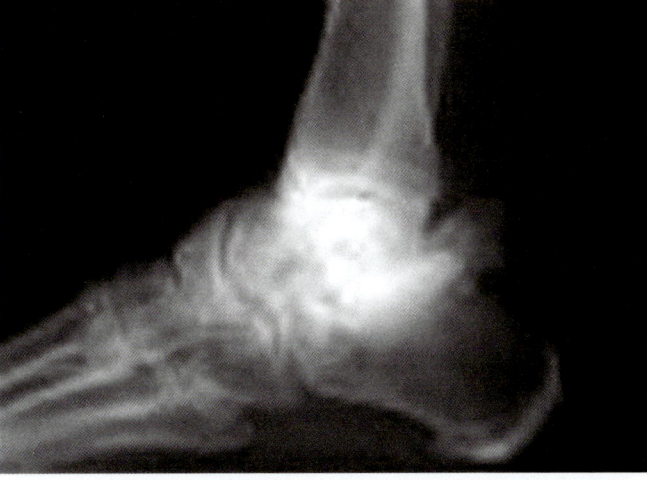

Fig. 47.25: Radiograph showing OA ankle

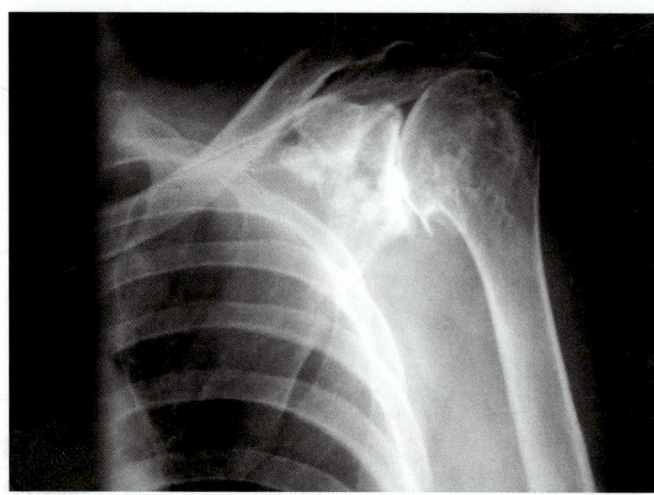

Fig. 47.26: Radiograph showing OA shoulder

BIBLIOGRAPHY

1. Ahlbach S. OA knee, a radiologic investigation. Acta Radiology. 1968;277:7-72.
2. Appel H, Freiberg S. The effect of high tibial osteotomy on pain of osteoarthritis of the knee joint. Acta Orthop Scand. 1972; 43:558.
3. Bomboelli R. Osteoarthritis of the hip, 2nd edn. Berlin: Springer Verlag; 1983.
4. Broughton NS, Newman JH, Baily RA. Unicompartmental replacement and high TO for OA knee. JBJS. 1986;68-B: 447-512.
5. Bryan RS. In: Abstrom JP Jr (Ed): Management of arthritis of the knee joint. Current Vol 5, St Louis: CV Mosby Co; 1973.
6. Chamberlain MA, Care G, Harfield B. Physiotherapy in osteoarthritis of knee. Annls Rh Disc. 23:389.
7. Harrison MHM, Schajowicz, Traueta J. Osteoarthritis of hip; a study of the nature and evolution of the disease. J Bone Joint Surg. 1953;35-B:598.
8. K Wayne Marshal. Current Opinion Rheumatology, Sept 2000.
9. Leach RE, Baungard S, Broom J. Obesity: Its relationship to osteoarthritis of the knee. Clin Orthop. 1973;93:271.
10. Parish LC. A historical approach to nomenclature of rheumatoid arthritis. Arthritis Rheum. 1963;6:136-58.
11. Pridie KH. A method of re-surfacing osteoarthritis knee joint. J Bone Joint Surg. 1959;41-B:618.
12. Riggins RS, Kraus JP, Lipscomb PR. Osteoarthritis of the hip, a survey of treatments. Clin Orthop. 1975;106:56.
13. Rodis EL. Osteoarthritis, what is known about prevention? Clin Orthop. 1987;222:60.
14. Sheila CO Reilly, American Rheumatic Association, Jan 1999.
15. Steven E Harwim. Arthroscopy, March 1999.

Cervical Disk Syndromes

INTRODUCTION

The cervical region consists of seven cervical vertebrae with their intervening disks. The disk is made-up of central nucleus pulposus and annulus fibrosus at the periphery. The disk functions as an effective shock absorber and gives the cervical spine more mobility. If the disk material herniates (Fig. 48.1) because of trauma or old age, it gives rise to the cervical disk syndrome.

More than 90 percent of the disk lesions in the cervical spine occur at the C_5 and C_6 levels as these are the most mobile segments. About 70 percent of the people are affected with these changes by the age of 70 years.

Types

- *Soft disk lesions:* It is common in young adults and is usually following trauma. In this, there is only a nuclear herniation through the wide annulus fibrosus of the disk.
- *Hard disk lesions:* This is more common than the first, seen in older age group, gradual in onset and is usually due to cervical spondylosis. Rarely large posterior osteophytes may cause pressure on the anterior portion of the spinal cord and produce mixed symptoms of the upper limb nerve root pain and lower extremity weakness (cervical spondylosis with myelopathy).

Clinical Features

Symptoms

The patient complains of pain in the neck, which is gradual or acute in onset. There is history of morning stiffness. Extension of the neck increases the pain. *Tingling* and *numbness* develop if the nerve root is compressed, but it does not follow the dermatomal pattern. Patients may also complain of radiating pain along the neck, shoulder, upper arm, forearm and hand (Fig. 48.2).

Signs

Movements of the neck are decreased due to pain. Pain increases on hyperextension. There is localized tenderness over the spinous process. Trigger point tenderness at the scapular region is present. Pressure against the top of the head increases pain (Fig. 48.3). If the nerve root is compressed by the disk herniation sensory, motor and reflex changes occur and follow the dermatomal pattern (Table 48.1 and Fig. 48.4). Rarely symptoms referable to the lower limbs develop due to pressure of posterior osteophytes on the anterior portion of the cervical cord. This symptom complex appears as a combination of cervical roots and cord symptoms [LMN upper limbs + UMN lower limbs].

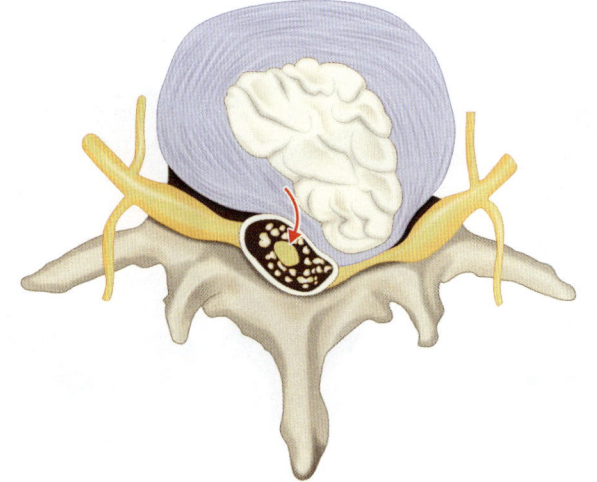

Fig. 48.1: Cervical disk herniation compressing the nerve root

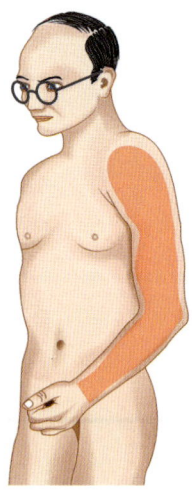

Fig. 48.2: Distribution of radiating pain in cervical syondylosis

TABLE 48.1: Dermatomal and myotomal pattern			
Root	Motor	Reflex	Sensation
C_5 (C_{4-5} lesion)	Deltoid ↓	Biceps reflex ↓	Numbness in the deltoid region
C_6 (C_{5-6} lesion)	Wrist extension ↓	Brachioradialis reflex ↓	Dorsolateral aspect of the thumb and index finger
C_7 (C_{5-6} lesion)	Wrist flexion ↓	Triceps reflex ↓	Index, middle and dorsum of the hand
C_8	Finger flexion ↓	None	Ring, little finger, medial border of forearm

Do You Know?
At what levels does cervical spondylosis most typically occur? Well it is:
$C_{5-6} > C_{6-7} > C_{3-5} > C_7T_1$

Investigations

X-ray
Normal in soft lesions but in hard lesions it shows, narrowing of disk space, anterior and posterior osteophyte formation, and narrowing of IV foramen (Figs 48.5 and 48.6).

Myelography
It helps in localizing the lesion but is invasive.

MRI
This is useful, as it is non-invasive, and helps localize the lesion, but its high cost is prohibitive (Fig. 48.7).

CT Scan
It is more useful in evaluating traumatic conditions of the neck than degenerative conditions. *EMG, diskography, thermography* is occasionally used.

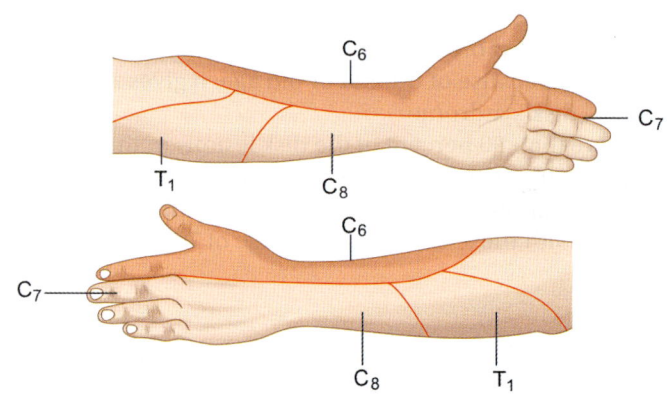

Fig. 48.4: Dermatomal pattern of upper limb

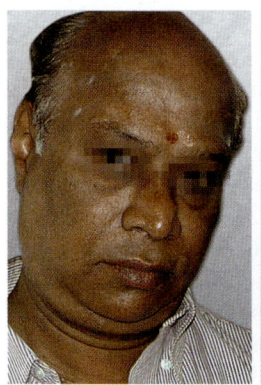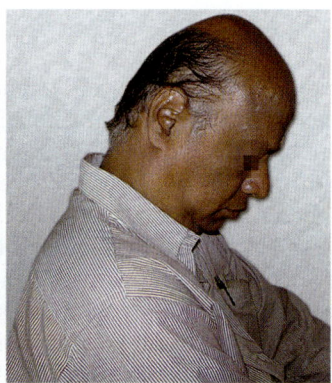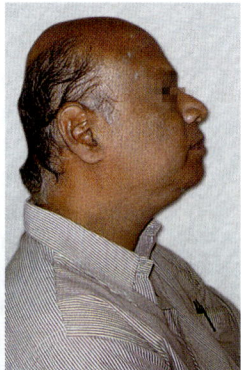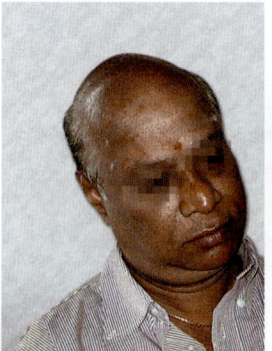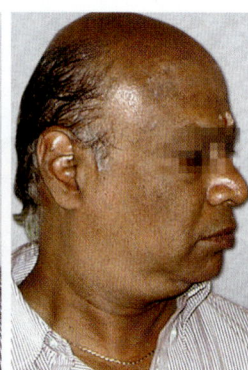

Fig. 48.3: Clinical photos of cervical spondylosis from left to right—deformity, loss of flexion, extension, lateral flexion and side rotations

CHAPTER 48: Cervical Disk Syndromes

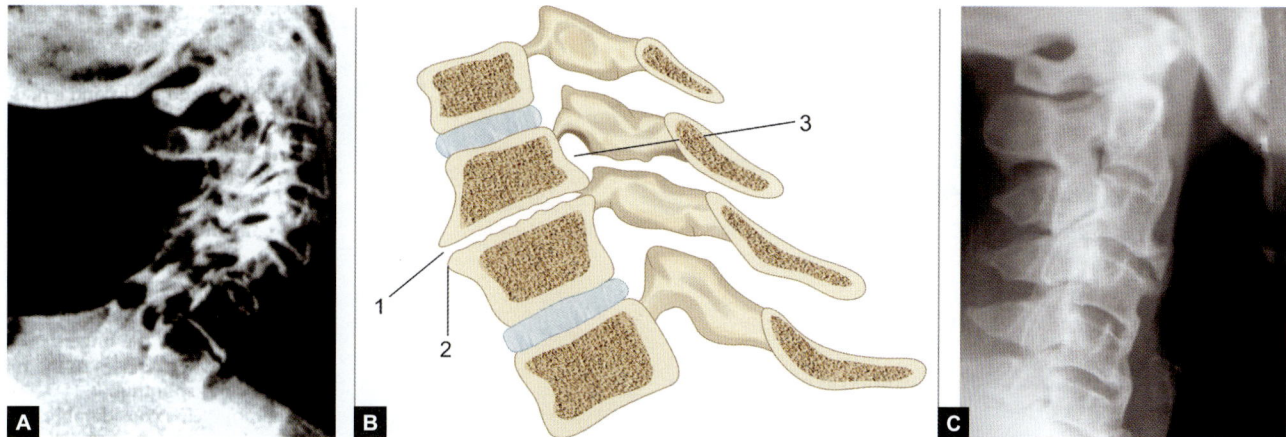

Figs 48.5A to C: Radiograph showing cervical spine: (A) Loss of intervertebral disk space and osteophyte formation seen in cervical spondylosis; (B) Pictorial display of a radiograph in cervical disk syndrome: (1) disk space narrowing, (2) osteophyte formation, and (3) narrowing of intervertebral foramina; (C) Cervical spondylosis showing anterior bridging osteophytes (severe cases)

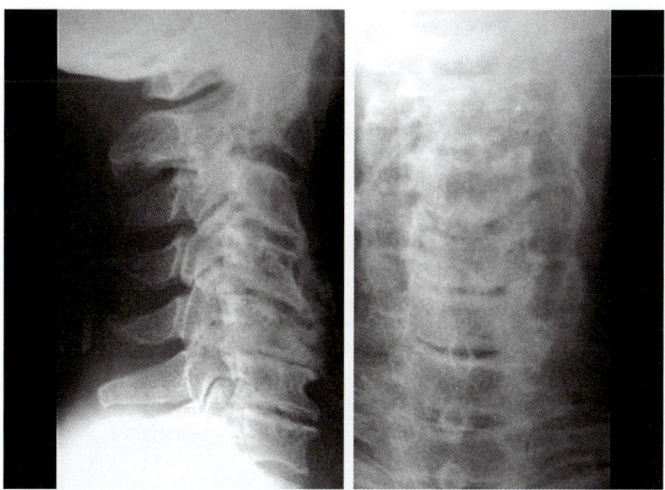

Fig. 48.6: Plain X-rays showing features of cervical spondylosis

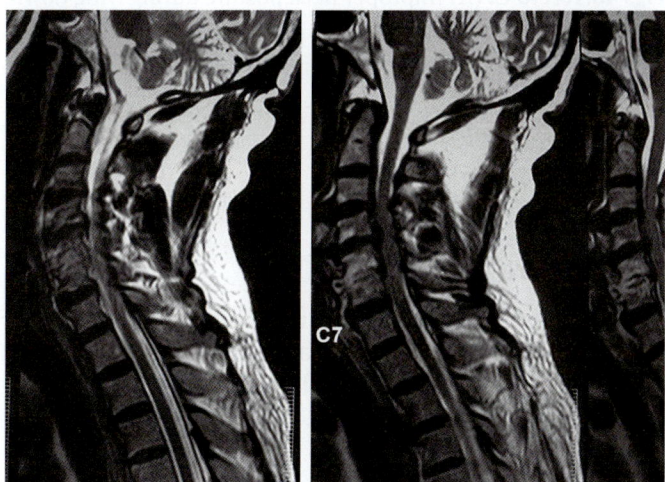

FIg. 48.7: MRI scans neck showing degenerative conditions

Treatment

Conservative Treatment

It is the more accepted form of treatment in cervical disk syndrome. It consists of rest, which is the cornerstone of the treatment as it allows soft parts to heal by reducing the inflammation. Cervical traction could be continuous or intermittent depending on the severity of the symptoms. Traction helps by reducing the muscle spasm, increasing the disk space and reducing the tension on the nerve roots. Physiotherapy like short-wave diathermy, ultrasound, and infrared rays are useful. NSAIDs once a day are usually preferred. After the pain decreases, patients are encouraged to perform gradual graded isometric neck exercises.

NECK EXERCISES

Neck exercises aim to improve the mobility of the stiff neck and strengthen the weakened neck muscles. Hence, the following two sets of exercises are recommended:
- *Mobilization* exercises this consists of gradual active mobilization of the neck by performing all the movements of the neck.
- *Strengthening exercises* here the patient is instructed to offer resistance by the other hand to all the active movements of the neck. These self-resistance exercises strengthen the neck muscles.

Both these exercises should be done for 15–20 minutes everyday (Figs 48.8A to E).

CERVICAL COLLAR

I hope you are all familiar with the scene of some elderly people walking around like a stiff robot wearing a neck

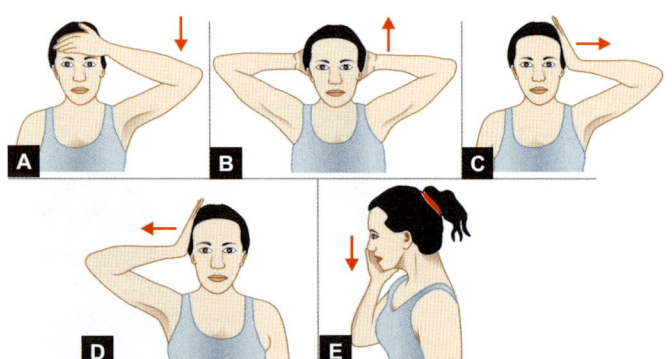

Figs 48.8A to E: Different self-resistive isometric neck exercises (A) Neck flexion; (B) Neck extension; (C) Lateral flexion; (D) Neck rotation; (E) Neck flexion

collar. People immediately surmise that such a person could be a case of cervical spondylosis and well they are more or less correct. There is a lot of misconception among the people about collars. They presume it to be a definitive form of treatment, while it is only supportive (Fig. 48.9).

It is indicated during acute exacerbation of chronic spondylosis and should be worn only for a short duration. If used for long, it weakens the neck muscles, thereby nullifying the beneficial effects of neck exercises.

> **Did You Know?**
> HO Thomas discovered cervical collar.

Surgical Treatment

Less than 5 percent of the cases of cervical spondylosis require surgery and is usually indicated in cases of chronic pain, failed conservative treatment and neurological deficits due to root or cord compressions.

The surgical procedure usually consists of removal of the cervical disk through an anterior approach and cervical interbody fusion by placing an autologous iliac bone graft. Excision of large osteophytes can also be done through this route. Excision of one or two cervical bodies (corpectomy) may be justified in multiple level disk pathology. Laminectomy usually does not produce the desired results.

> **Quick Facts**
> *Surgical treatment of cervical spondylosis*
> - Anterior cervical discectomy with interbody fusion for single or 2 level disk involvement.
> - Corpectomy and strut graft or cages for multiple level disk involvement.

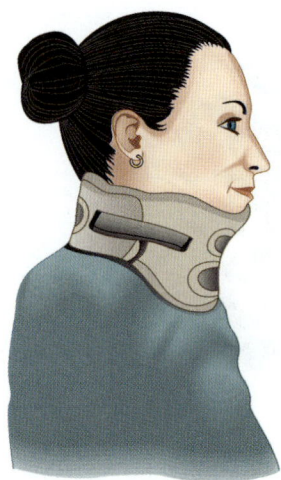

Fig. 48.9: Wearing a cervical collar is a popular method of treatment of cervical spondylosis

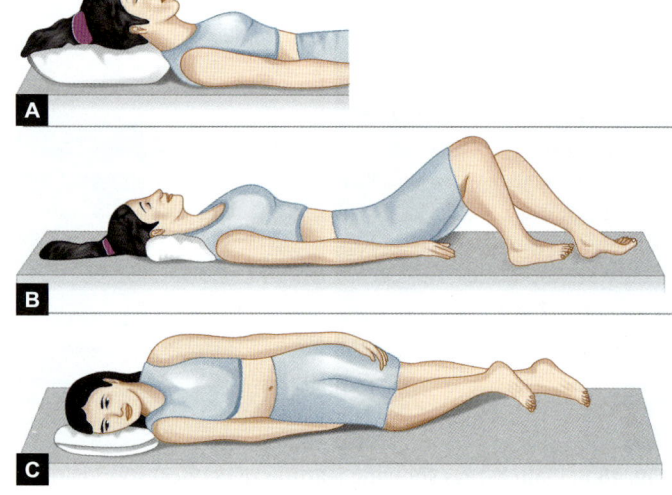

Figs 48.10A to C: (A) Improper neck posture during lying down. Correct neck posture; (B) During supine position; (C) During side-lying

> - Cervical disk replacement (CDR) is now being done in few advanced cases.
> - Laminectomy has a doubtful role.
> - Surgery is required in less than 5 percent of cases.

Preventive Measures

This can be done by good postural habits and using proper sized pillows of 7.5–10 cm thickness and should be placed under the neck rather than the head (Figs 48.10A to C).

49 CHAPTER

Degenerative Lumbar Disk Disease and Canal Stenosis

Lumbar disk disease is dealt in the chapter on low backache.

CANAL STENOSIS

Introduction

Spinal canal stenosis is narrowing of the spinal canal and the consequent compression of the cord and the nerve roots. It may affect the cervical thoracic or lumbar spine.

Canal stenosis is common in lumbar vertebrae. One or more roots of the cauda equina may be affected due to the constriction in spinal canal before it exits through the foramen. This condition was first described by Portal in 1803.

Definition

Lumbar canal stenosis is a cauda equina compression in which the lateral or anteroposterior diameter of the spinal canal is narrow with or without a change in the cross-sectional area (Fig. 49.1). The nerve root canals and the IV foramen may also be narrowed.

Patient may present with low backache, neurological symptoms in the lower limbs and bladder, bowel dysfunctions in extreme cases.

Classification

- Generalized/localized.
- Segmental (local area of each vertebral spinal segment is affected):
  - Central
  - Lateral recesses
  - Foraminal
  - Far out
- Anatomical area:
  - Cervical (seen)
  - Thoracic (rare)
  - Lumbar (most common).

Causes

- Pathological (Arnold's classification):
  - Congenital, e.g. achondroplasia
  - Acquired—degenerative, iatrogenic, and spondylitic.
- Other causes:
  - Paget's disease
  - Fluorosis
  - Kyphosis
  - Scoliosis
  - Fracture spine

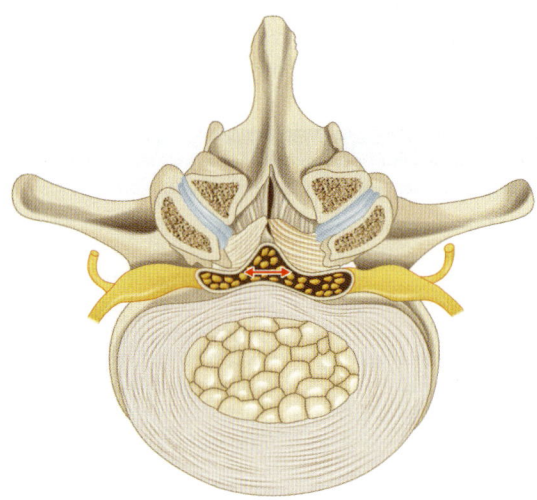

Fig. 49.1: Lumbar canal stenosis (AP diameter <10 mm)

- DISH (Diffuse idiopathic skeletal hyperostosis) syndrome.
- Iatrogenic causes, e.g. hypertrophy of posterior bone graft, incomplete treatment of stenotic condition, etc.

Degenerative lumbar disk disease leading to thickening and narrowing of the spinal canal is the most common cause.

Clinical Features

Lumbar canal stenosis is common in males above 50 years. Usually, the symptoms are fewer in number, but the patient may complain of low backache.

Cauda equina claudication is the common symptom. Here, the patient complains of pain in the buttocks and legs after walking, which decreases on sitting, rest and forward bending. Patient may complain of hypoesthesia and paresthesia. Usually, the patient finds no problem walking uphill or riding a bicycle. Nerve root entrapment in the lateral recess causes claudication and sciatica. Stoop test is positive (see Box).

Difference between ischemic claudication and cauda equina claudication (neurogenic claudication) is mentioned (Table 49.1).

Stoop test: It is positive in lumbar canal stenosis.
Ask the patient to walk briskly → pain develops → continues to walk → patient assumes a stooped posture → symptoms disappear. The pain decreases by forward bending because the canal length increases by 2.2 mm.

Other Important Tests
- *Bicycle Test of Van Gelderen:* The patient is made to pedal a stationary bicycle first in an upright position and later in a forward flexed position. If he pedals more during the latter event, the test is positive.
- *Walking Test:* The patient is made to walk on a level surface first in an upright position and then in a flexed position. If he walks more during the latter event, the test is positive.

TABLE 49.1: Features of different types of claudications

Cauda equina claudication	Ischemic claudication
• Pain in the buttocks and lower extremities after walking • Relieved by sitting forward for 20 minutes • Hypoesthesia, paresthesia precipitated by walking, walking uphill, cycling, etc. • Pulses are felt • No trophic changes • Walking downhill worse • Walking uphill better	• Pain in the legs appears on walking • Appears and diappears fast • Decreases in standing • No neurological deficit • Absent pulses • Trophic changes in foot and toes • Walking downhill unchanged or better • Walking uphill unchanged or worse

Investigations

Radiographs of the lumbar spine consisting of AP, lateral and oblique views are recommended (Figs 49.2 and 49.3). However, radiology may not show stenosis. The following points are looked for:
- Reduced interpedicle distance.
- AP or midsagittal diameter of the affected vertebra (Normal—15 mm), absolute midsagittal diameter of the canal is decreased.
- Measurement of the lateral sagittal diameter.
- Hypertrophy and sclerosis of the facet joints.
- Reduced interlaminar space and short, stout spinous process.
- Associated features like presence of listhesis, prolapsed disk, osteophytes, etc. (Figs 49.4A to C).

Quick Facts: Radiological Stenotic Facts AP or Midsagittal Diameter:
- Normal—>13 mm
- Relative stenosis—10–13 mm
- Absolute stenosis—<10 mm

Myelographic findings consist of waist-like narrowing of the dural sac at the level of facet joint and indentation of the dural tube due to disk prolapse, etc. (Fig. 49.5).

MRI and CT scan: These are more useful and help to diagnose lateral recess stenosis, facet hypertrophy, midsagittal distance, etc. (Figs 49.6A and B).

Note:
Trefoil canal — It resembles a triangular shape in extreme cases.

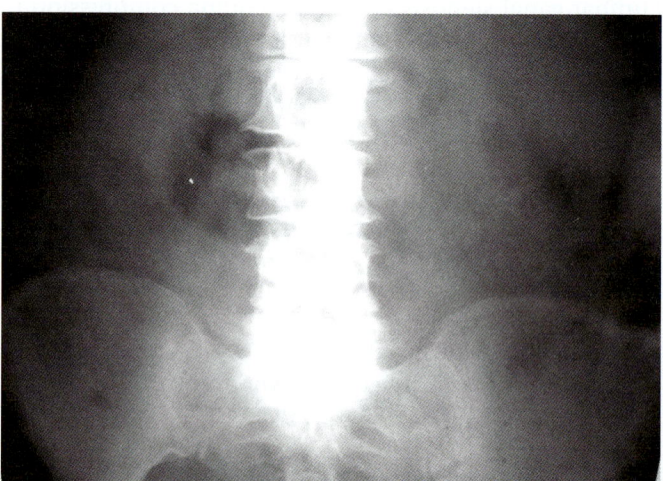

Fig. 49.2: Radiograph showing lumbar spondylosis changes that can lead to canal stenosis (Degenerative) (AP view)

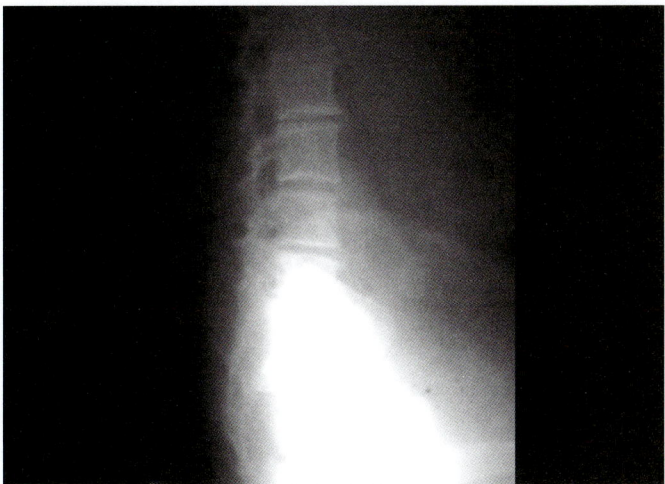

Fig. 49.3: Radiograph showing lateral view of LCS

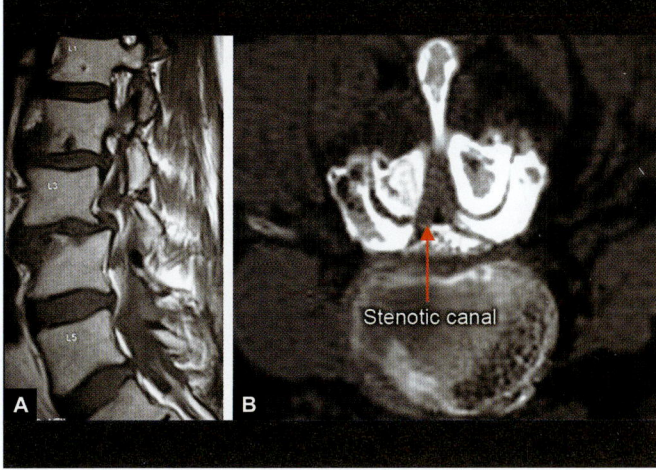

Figs 49.6A and B: MRI showing degenerative lumbar spine leading to lumbar canal stenosis

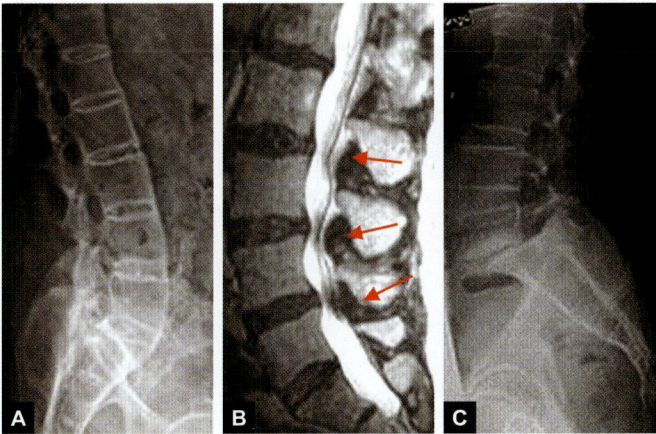

Figs 49.4A to C: Causes of LCS: (A) Ankylosing spondylitis; (B) Intervertebral disk prolapse (IVDP); (C) Listhesis

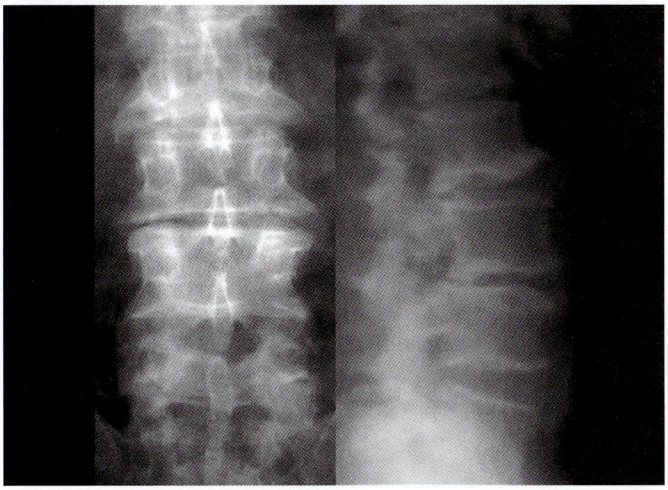

Fig. 49.5: Plain X-ray showing LCS

Treatment

Conservative Methods

This aims at symptomatic relief of pain.
- Drug therapy like the NSAIDs, etc.
- Epidural steroids may help in some cases.
- Physiotherapy with heating modalities helps.
- Pelvic traction may help relieve compression.
- *Exercises:* General conditioning exercises like walking, swimming and flexion-oriented exercises are useful.
- *Deweighted Treadmill ambulation:* This consists of applying vertical traction with a harness while doing the treadmill exercises. This offers twin benefits of both exercises and traction.
- *Belts and corsets (soft):* These may offer some relief.

Surgical Methods

Most of the surgical methods described for lumbar canal stenosis aim at decompressing the constricted lumbar canal. Laminectomy is useful in central canal stenosis. Diskectomy and osteotomy of inferior articular process to remove the hypertrophic elements help.

For lateral canal stenosis laminotomy, disk excision, partial medial facetectomy and foraminotomy help. Spinal fusion to stabilize the lumbar spine is usually not required as instability is less commonly seen in lumbar canal stenosis.

It should be noted that neurogenic claudication responds poorly to the conservative treatment but responds well to surgical decompression.

> **Did You Know?**
> That lumbar canal stenosis is the most common reason for undergoing spinal surgery after the age of 65 years.

SECTION 7
Common Surgical Techniques

- Common Surgeries of the Humerus
- Common Forearm Surgeries
- Common Hip Surgeries
- Common Surgery of the Femur
- Common Surgery of the Patella
- Common Surgery of the Tibia
- Turco's One Stage Posteromedial Release for Congenital Talipes Equinovarus
- Common Surgery of the Spine
- Common Finger and Toe Surgery (Percutaneous Fixations)
- External Fixation

50 CHAPTER

Common Surgeries of the Humerus

This section on Common Surgical Techniques deals with those common surgeries in orthopedics that are usually asked in the practical examinations. Students are advised to refer major books on operative orthopedics for details. Here only a few common surgeries of the upper limbs, lower limbs and spine are covered in addition to arthroplasty and arthroscopy.

- DCP plating for fracture shaft of humerus
- Interlocking humerus
- Supracondylar fracture humerus—percutaneous fixation
- Intercondylar fracture humerus—reconstructions.

DCP PLATING FOR FRACTURE SHAFT OF HUMERUS

Indications
Fracture shaft of humerus in adults.

Approach
Anterolateral approach or the Thompson and Henry approach.

Surgical Steps (Figs 50.1 to 50.17)

- Incise the skin in line with the anterior border of the deltoid muscle from a point midway between its origin and insertion.
- Proceed in line with the anterior border of the biceps muscle up to 7.5 cm of the elbow.
- Divide the superficial and deep fascia.
- Ligate the cephalic vein.
- If the fracture is in the proximal part, expose it by retracting the deltoid and biceps muscles.
- If the fracture in the middle part exposes the brachialis muscle, split it vertically and retract it subperiosteally and expose the shaft.

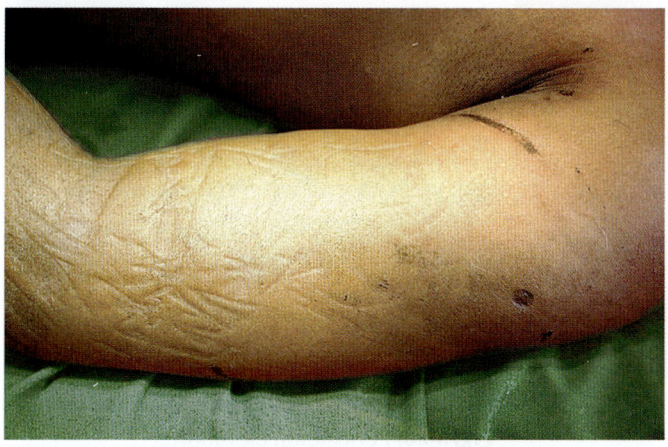

Fig. 50.1: Painting and draping

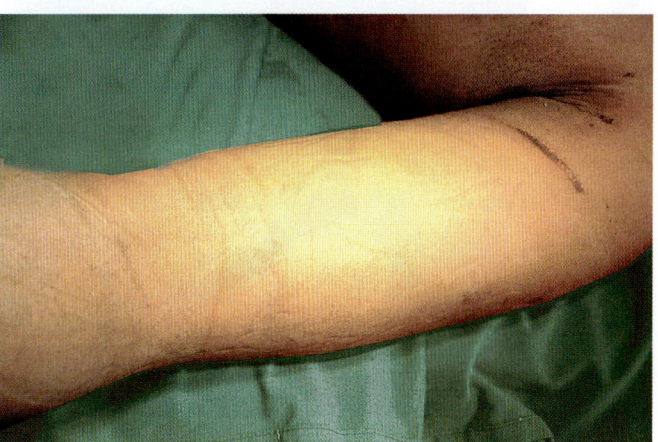

Fig. 50.2: View of the deformity

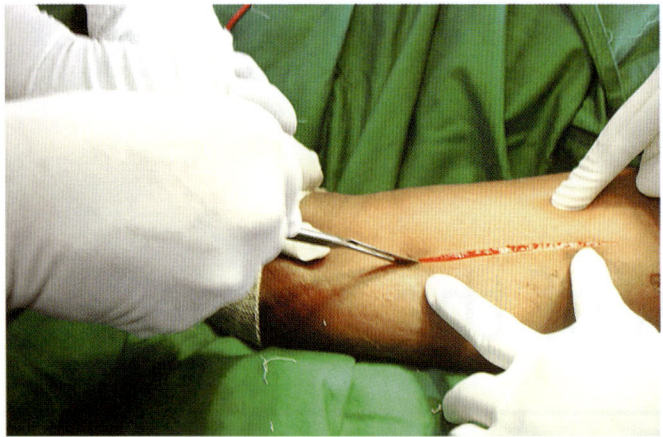

Fig. 50.3: Incision through the anterolateral approach

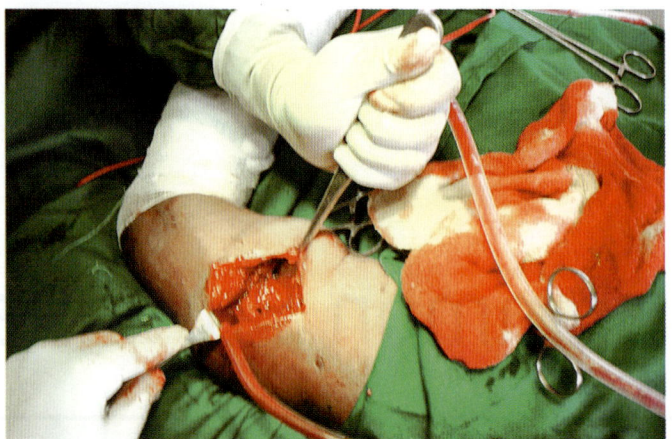

Fig. 50.6: Deep surgical dissection

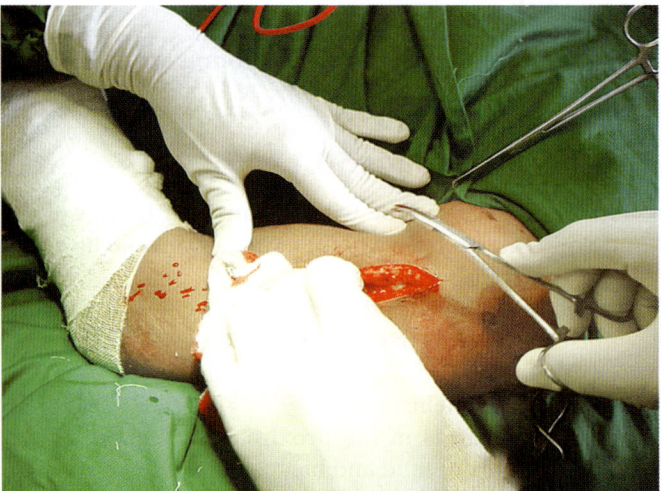

Fig. 50.4: Exposure of the soft tissue

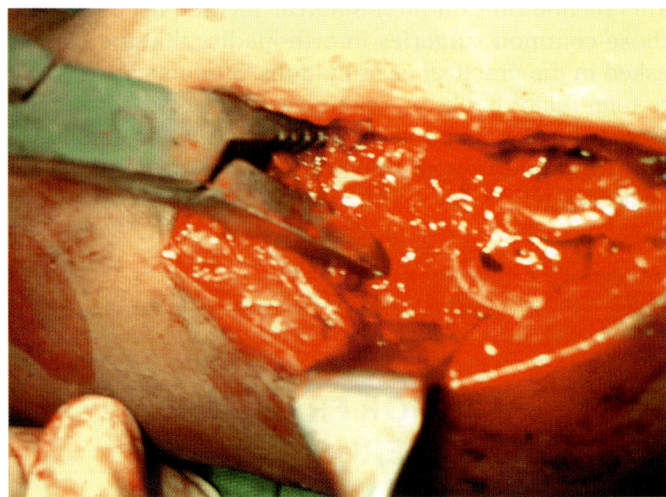

Fig. 50.7: Exposure of fracture fragments

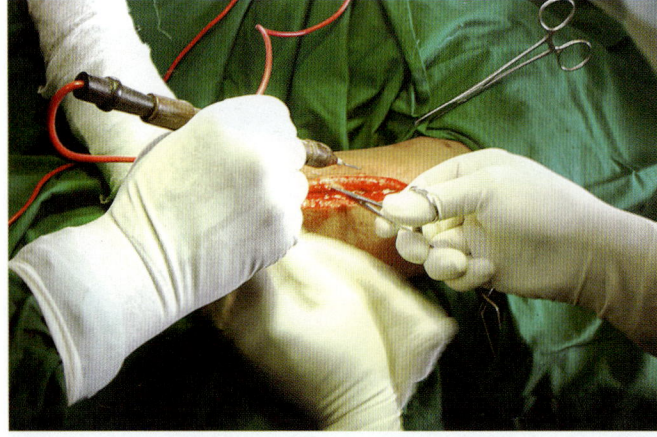

Fig. 50.5: Cauterizing the bleeders

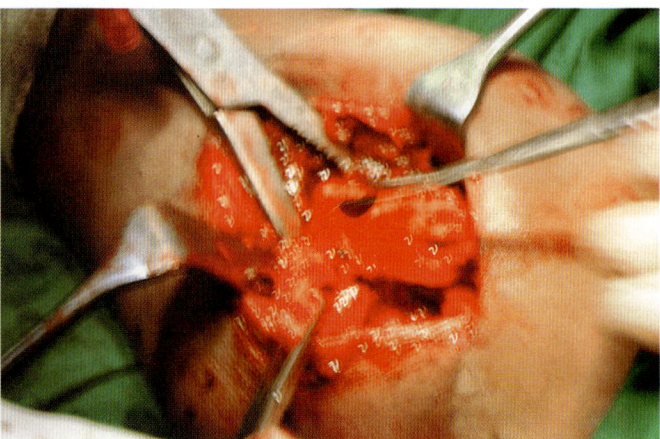

Fig. 50.8: Periosteum elevation

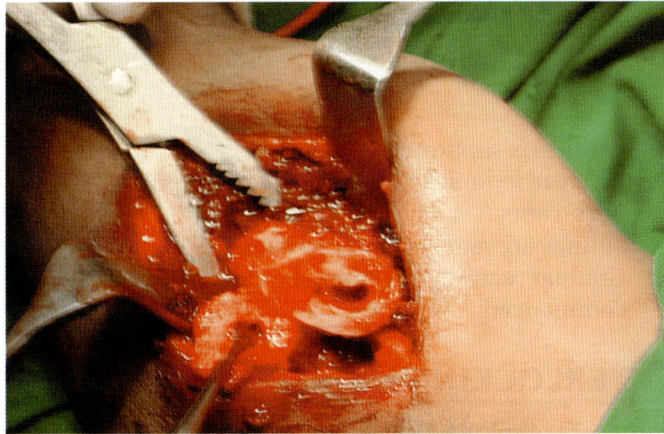

Fig. 50.9: Exposing the butterfly fragment

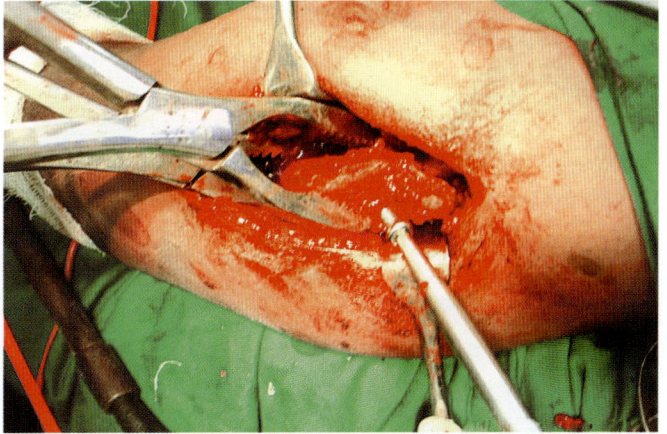

Fig. 50.12: Fixing the butterfly fragment with an interfragmentary screw

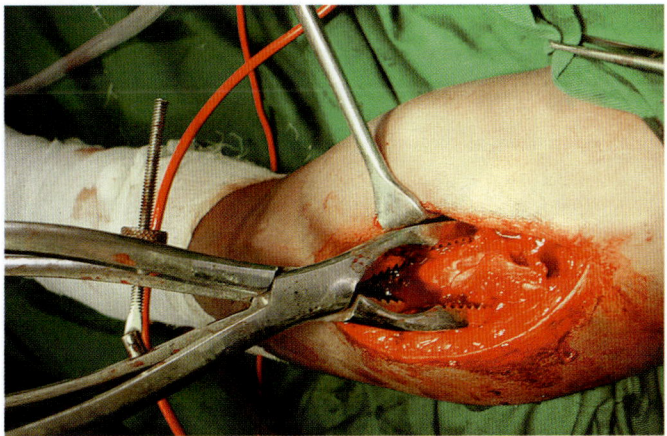

Fig. 50.10: Reducing the butterfly fragment

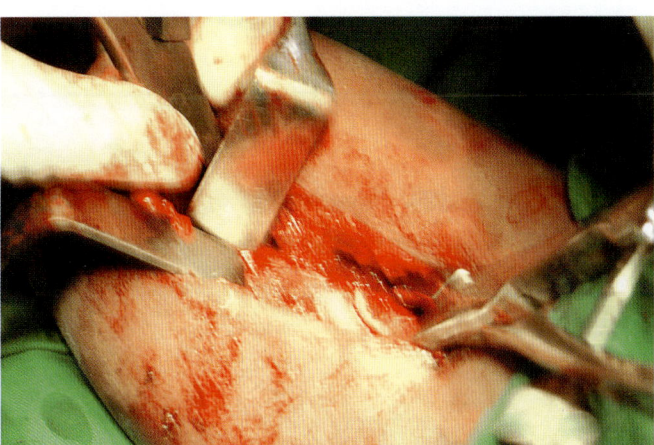

Fig. 50.13: Reduction of the fracture fragments

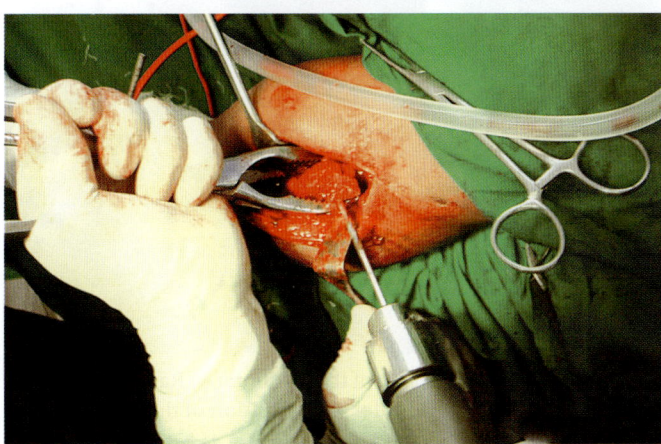

Fig. 50.11: Drilling the butterfly fragment

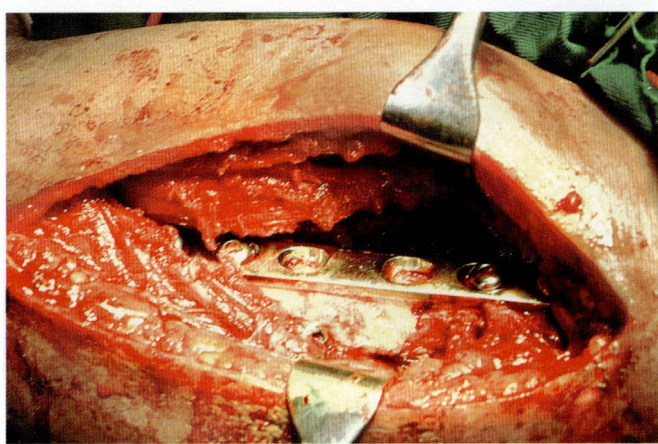

Fig. 50.14: Placement of the DCP plate

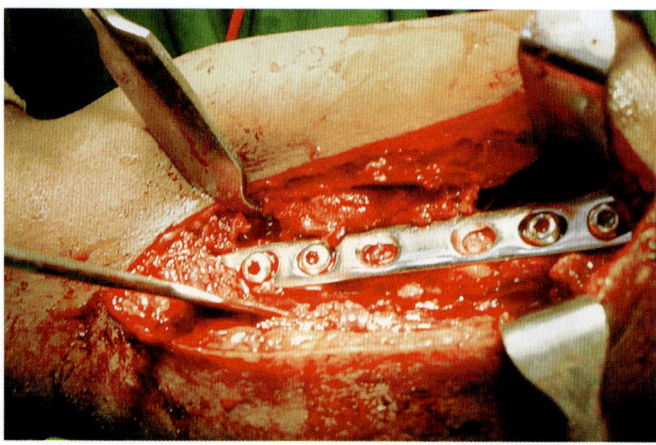

Fig. 50.15: Fixation of the plate with screws

- The technique of DCP plating is the same as described for tibia and radius.

Aftercare

- The arm is supported in a sling.
- Range of motion active and active assisted exercises are begun after 3–4 days.
- Sutures are removed after 14 days.
- Gradual actively of the shoulder and elbow are commenced.

INTERLOCKING HUMERUS*

Surgical technique of interlocking nailing (Figs 50.18 to 50.33).

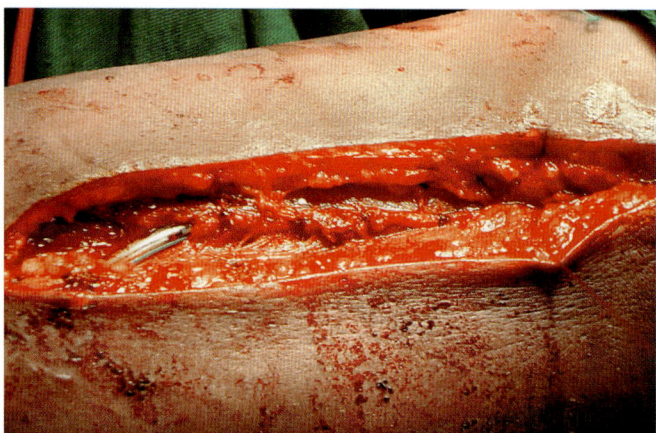

Fig. 50.16: Closure of the wound over a drain

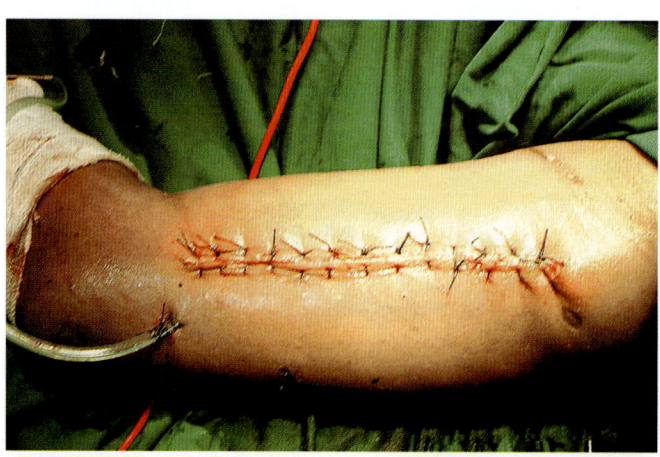

Fig. 50.17: Final skin closure

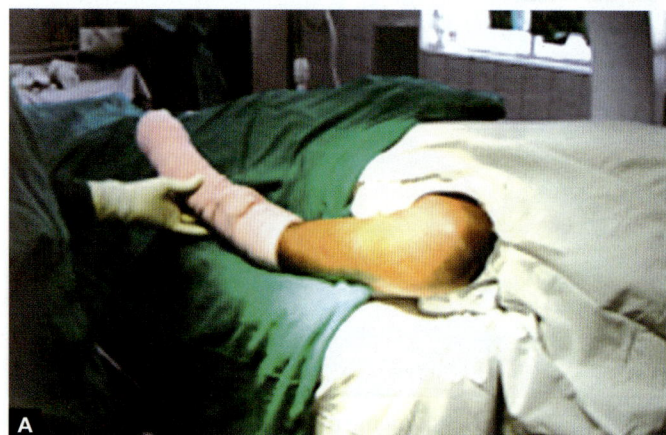

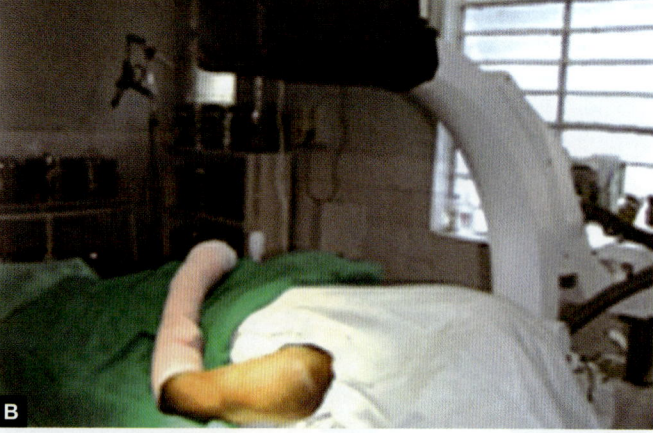

Figs 50.18A and B: Position of the patient: (A) Radiolucent table (slight extension of shoulder); (B) Position of the C-arm IITV

---

*From "Step by Step Operative Orthopedics" by Dr *John Ebnezar*.

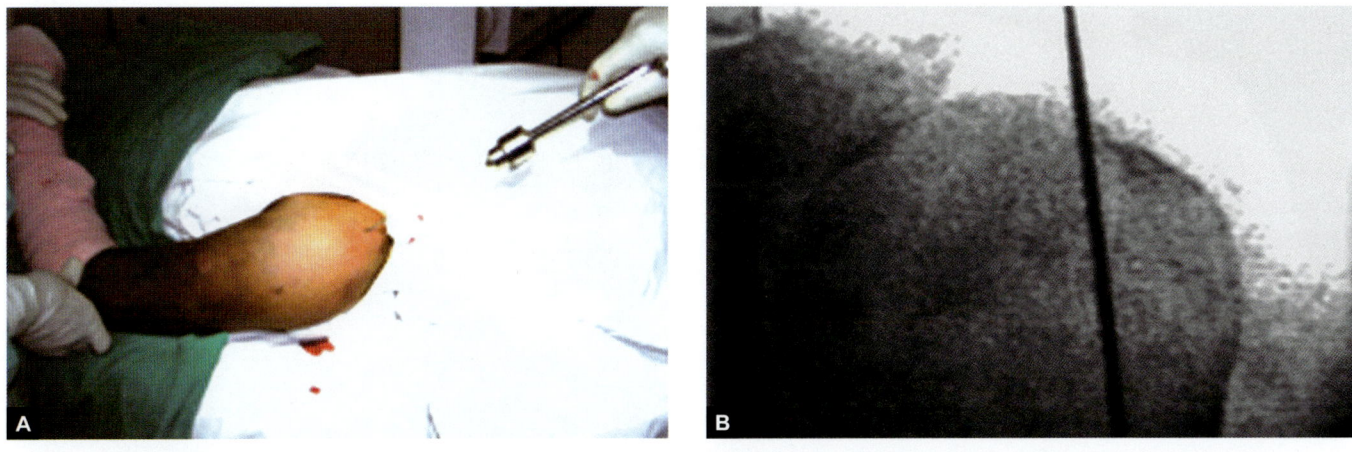

Figs 50.19A and B: K-wire introduced under C-arm control between the articular surface and the greater tuberosity

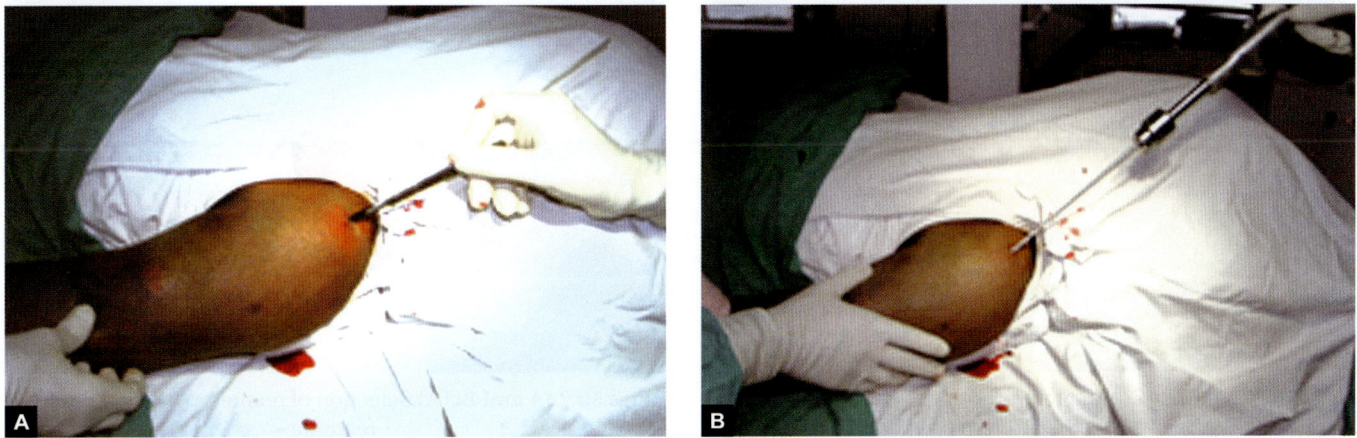

Figs 50.20A and B: (A) 2 cm incision on the K-wire; (B) Cannulated drill over K-wire: to be rotated, not to be drilled

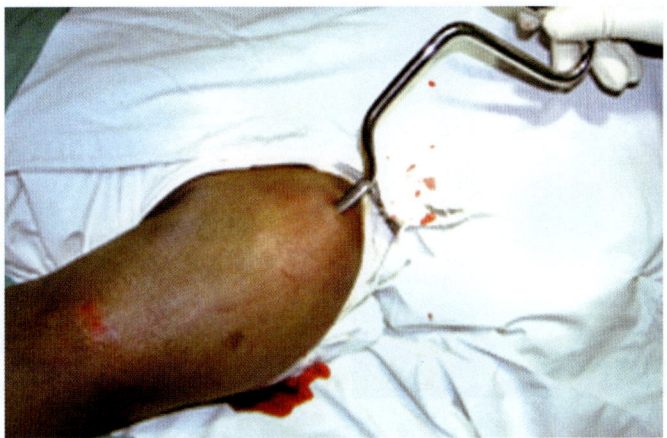

Fig. 50.21: Entry of guidewire

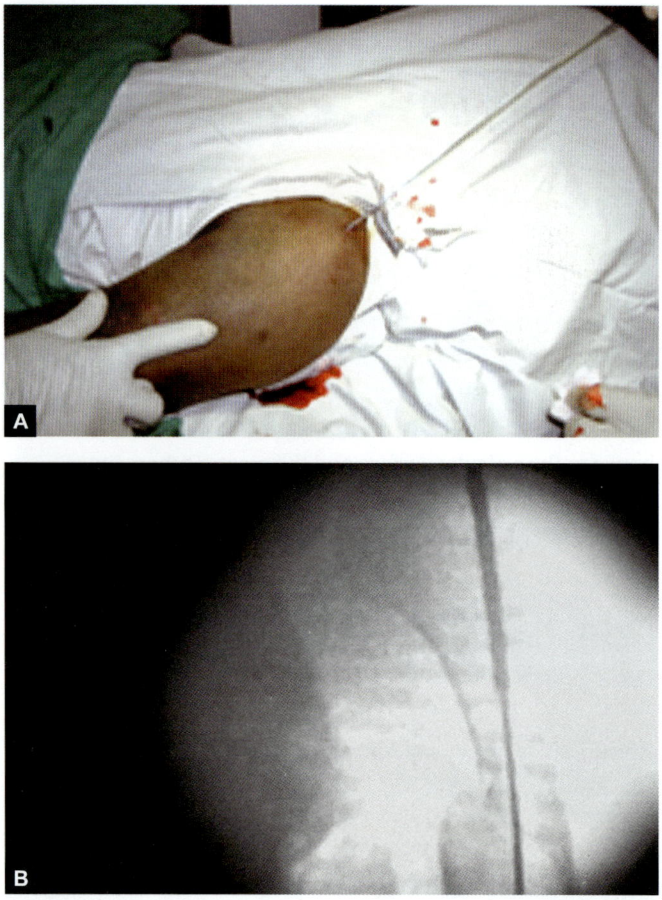

Figs 50.22A and B: C-arm picture, both views, of the guidewire in the humerus

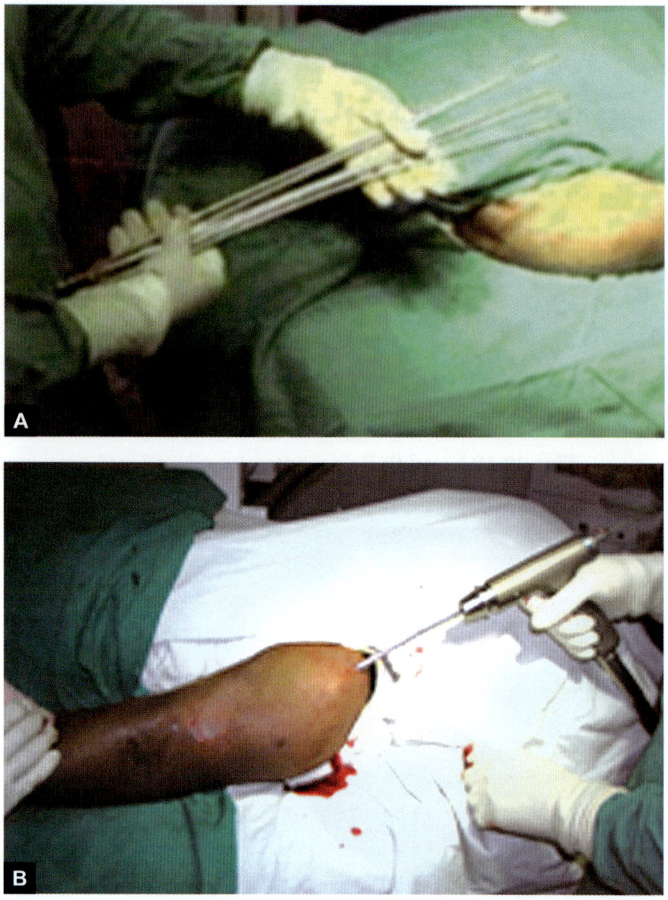

Figs 50.24A and B: (A) Selection of reamers; (B) Technique of reaming

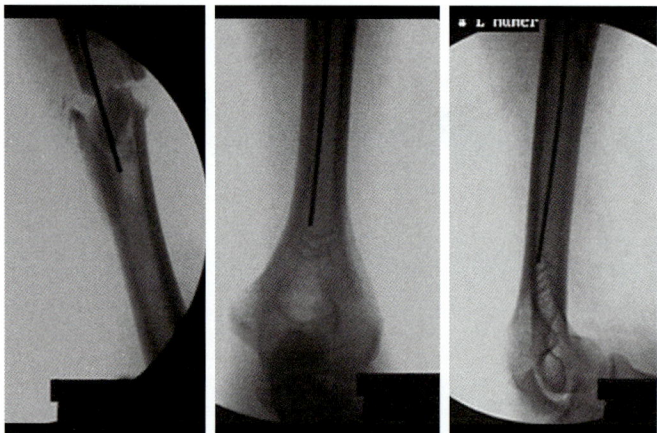

Fig. 50.23: Negotiation of guidewire

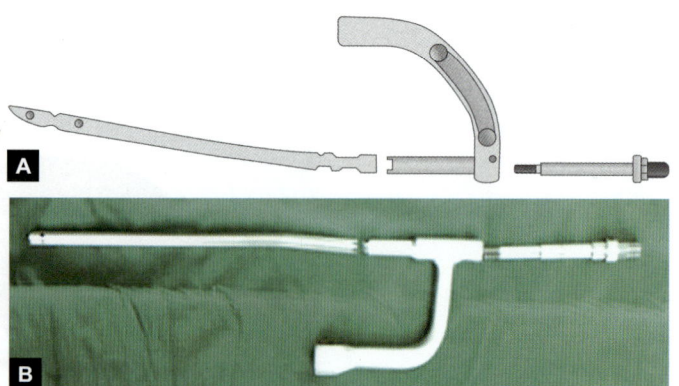

Figs 50.25A and B: Nail jig assembly

- Drill the nearest screw first, tap and seat the proper sized screw.
- Next drill the eccentric hole, tap it and put the screw in an eccentric fashion. As the screw is being tightened the fracture fragments will be impacted and compression occurs.
- Using the neutral guide insert the remainder screws one-by-one.
- Close the deep fascia loosely to prevent compartment syndromes.
- Close the wound and skin lairs over a suction drain.

Aftercare
- An above elbow plaster slap is applied for 3–4 days.
- Remove the suction drain after 2–3 days.
- Instruct the patient to perform active and active-assisted range of motion exercises for the shoulder, elbow and hand muscles.
- After removal of the splint begin the pronation and supination range of motion exercises.

MEDULLARY FIXATION FOR FRACTURE OF RADIUS AND ULNA

Indications
Both bones fractures of the forearm or isolated fracture radius and ulna in adults.

Some Principles According to Stage
- If ulna is to be nailed, place the forearm across the chest.
- If radius or if both the radius and ulna are to be nailed, keep the arm on a side table or on a arm board.
- Nail the ulna first, if both bones have to be nailed.

Surgical Steps

For Ulna
- Through a direct short longitudinal incision over the subcutaneous border of the ulna expose the ulna fracture first.
- Reduce the fracture by traction and bone clamps.
- See that there is no rotatory misalignment.
- Bring the proximal fragment of the ulna out of the wound and clear the medullary canal and the fracture ends of clots.
- Pass a nail into the canal for test fit.
- Now progressively ream the medullar canal of the ulna till the smallest diameter of the canal is overcome and the reamer is felt through the skin at the olecranon tip.
- Select the correct length nail by strapping it along the ulna outside.
- In a retrograde fashion drive this nail through the proximal fragment till the skin over the olecranon is stretched.
- Now make an incision over the stretched skin and drive the nail further till its distal end is near the fracture end.
- Reduce the fracture now and drive the nail back into the distal fragment till the proximal end is flush with the olecranon.
- Check for the stability of the fixation before proceeding to nail the radius.

Nailing of Radius
- The radius needs to be exposed through an anterior Henry approach for distal half and Thompson's posterior approach for proximal half.
- After exposure, reduce the fracture taking care to avoid rotatory misalignment.
- Ream the proximal and distal medullary canals progressively.
- Select the correct sized nail. The nail should extend from the radial styloid to within 1.3 cm of the radial head or to within 3.8 cm of the lateral epicondyle of the humerus.
- To make the radial styloid process prominent, flex and deviate the wrist ulna ward.
- Make a 2.5 cm incision over the radial styloid.
- Using a drill (3.2–4.8 mm) drill a hole through the exposed cortex of the radial styloid process.
- Begin drilling vertically and slowly angle it directing it towards the lateral epicondyle of the humerus.
- As you advance the drill for 5–6 cm, the hole becomes oval and a channel is created that is parallel for the medullary canal.
- Insert the nail such that its dorsal or long bow parallels the long arc of the radius.
- Holding the fracture reduced, drive the nail gently proximally till the distal end is flush with the radial styloid process.
- Check the stability of the fracture under direct vision.
- Place some autologous cancellous bone grafts around the fracture fragments.

Aftercare
- With elbow in 90 degrees flexion and forearm in neutral rotation, apply an above elbow plaster slab.
- Sutures are removed after 2 weeks.
- Continue the external support for 8–12 weeks.
- Begin active and active-assisted range of motion exercises after 3–4 weeks.

DARRACH'S OPERATION

Indication
Malunited Colles fracture with functional impairment.

Approach
Dorsal approach.

Surgical Steps
- Expose the distal ulna through a medial longitudinal incision.
- Incise and lift the periosteum taking care not to damage it.
- Drill transverse holes through the ulna about 2.5 cm proximal to its distal end.
- Complete the osteotomy with a bone cutter and lift the distal fragment outside the wound.
- Cut the capsule of the joint close to the articular cartilage.
- Divide the styloid process at its base and leave it attached to the ulnar collateral ligament.
- Repair the periosteal sleeve and ligament to the bone ends.

Aftercare
- No immobilization is required.
- Suture removal after 12 days.
- Active and active-assisted range of motion exercises can be commenced the next day.

CHAPTER 52

Common Hip Surgeries

HEMIREPLACEMENT ARTHROPLASTY

Indications

Nonunion fracture neck of femur in patients between 50–60 years of age (Less than 50 years of age, it is internal fixation and above 60 years, it is THR).

Approaches

There are three approaches
- *Anterior or Smith Peterson approach:* This is preferred if there is fixed flexion deformity of the hip. FFD can be corrected by osteotomizing the iliac crest and division of the iliopsoas tendon.
- *Lateral or Gibson's approach.*
- *Posterior or Moore's approach:* This is the most preferred method and is described here in detail.

Advantages

- Bleeding is less.
- Natural external rotation of the limb relieves the tension on the wound and decreases the chances of postoperative dislocation.

Disadvantages

Proximity to the perineum increases the chances of infection.

Surgical Steps (Figs 52.1 to 52.36)

- After exposure dislocate the hip posterior.
- Remove the head from the acetabulum.
- Rotate the stump of the neck.
- Open and reshape the medullary canal of the neck and upper shaft with a rasp.
- Cut a notch in the proximal end of the greater trochanter with a starter.
- Measure the femoral head removed from the acetabulum and select a prosthesis of the same size.
- Check the size of the prosthesis directly by inserting it into the acetabulum before inserting the stem into the medullary canal.
- Using a saw shape the ends of the femoral neck.
- Take care to leave enough calcar to support the medial aspect of the prosthesis.
- Insert the prosthesis into the canal and remove any obstructing bone pieces.
- Reduce the prosthesis into the acetabulum and check for the stability.
- Close the wound in layers over a drain.

Aftercare

- Keep the limb in a splint for 1–2 weeks.
- Start early active and passive motions on the first day after surgery.
- By 10–14 days, commence more vigorous active and passive exercises.
- Parallel bar walking may be commenced by 2 weeks.

Complications

Common Ones

- Infection
- Dislocation of prosthesis
- Fractures of the femoral shaft

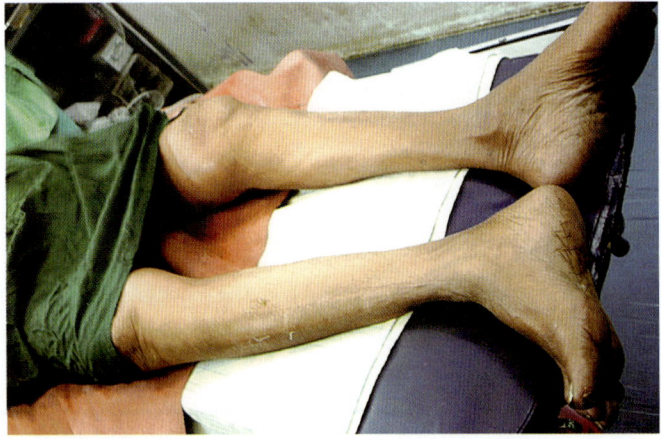

Fig. 52.1: External rotation deformity of the lower limb

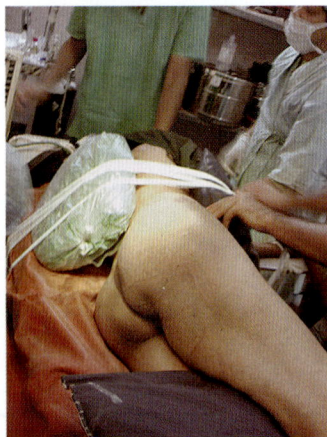

Fig. 52.4: Positioning of the patient

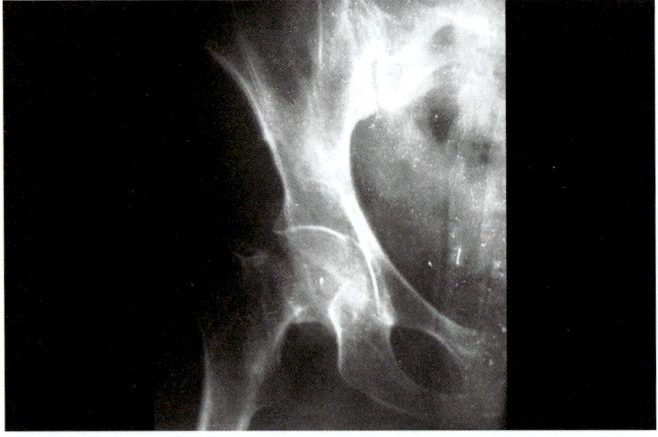

Fig. 52.2: Radiograph of the right hip showing intracapsular fracture

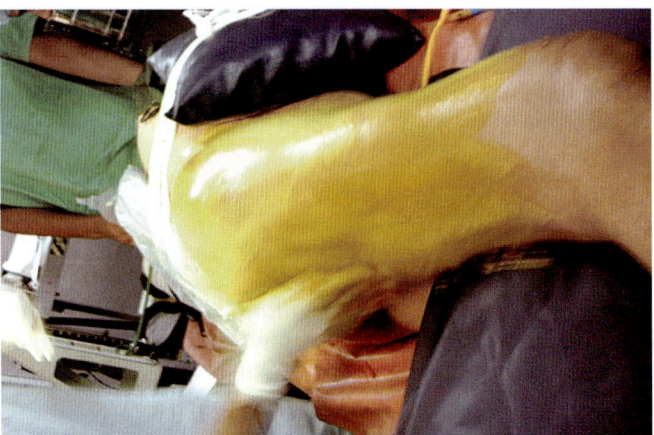

Fig. 52.5: Preparation of the right hip

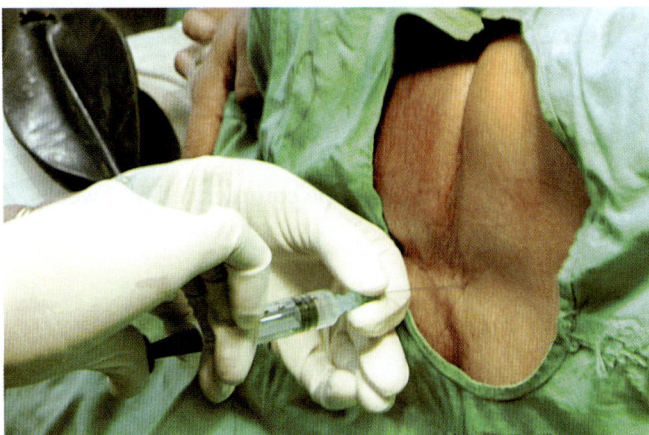

Fig. 52.3: Giving spinal anesthesia

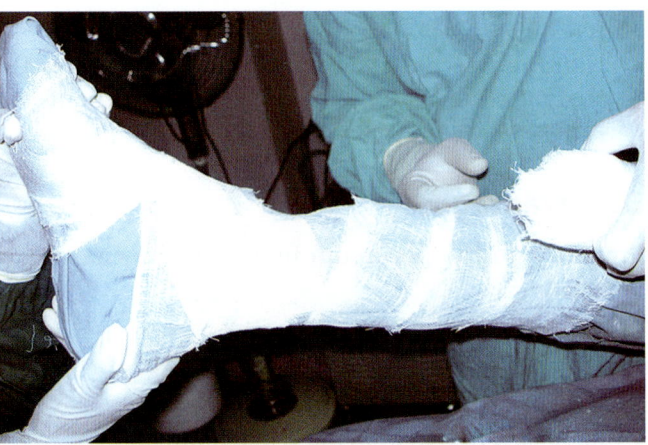

Fig. 52.6: Draping of the right lower limb

CHAPTER 52: Common Hip Surgeries **709**

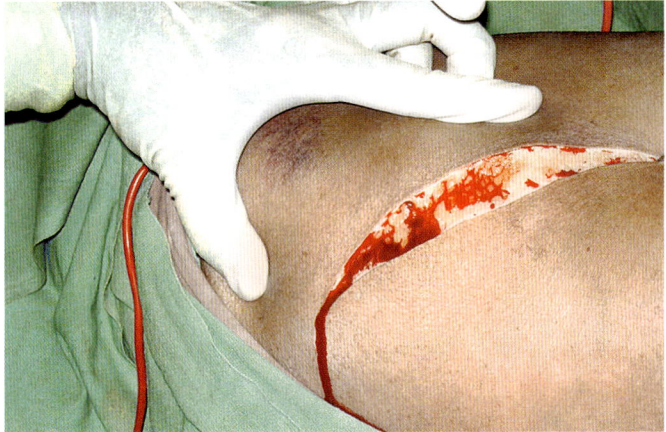

Fig. 52.7: Moore's approach

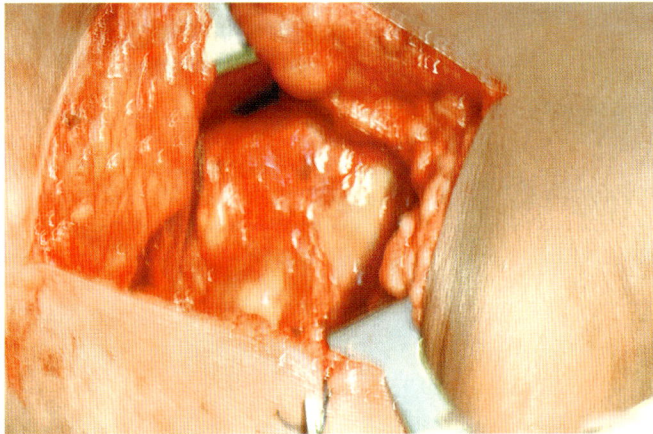

Fig. 52.10: Deep dissection

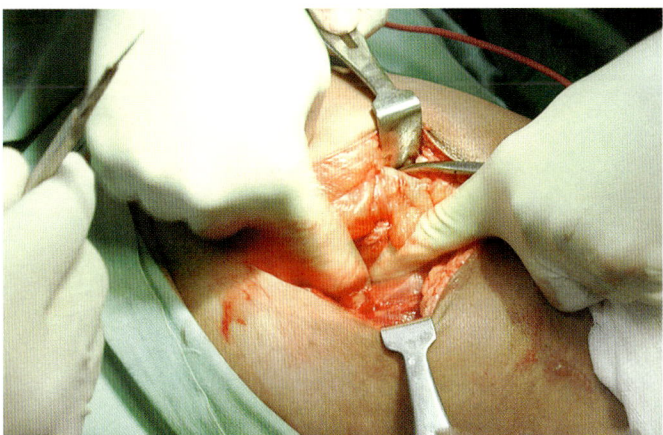

Fig. 52.8: Exposing the subcutaneous tissue and fat

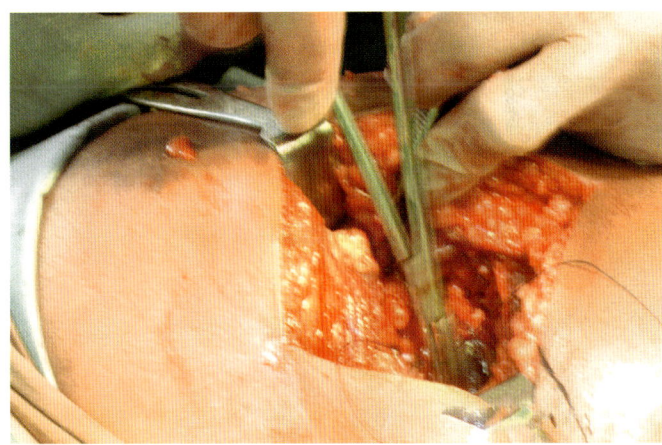

Fig. 52.11: Tying the external rotator muscles

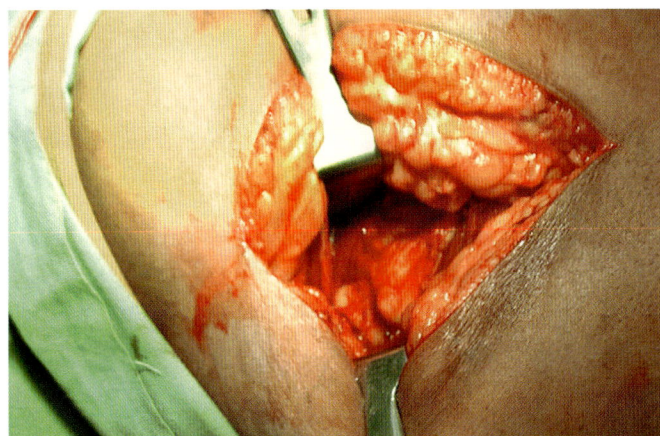

Fig. 52.9: Exposing the muscles

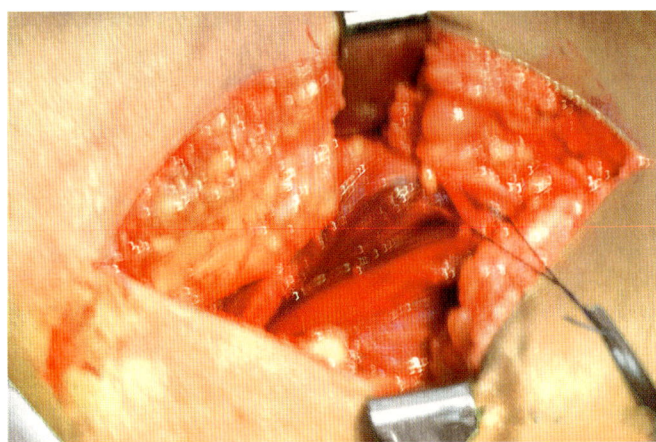

Fig. 52.12: Dissecting the external rotator muscles

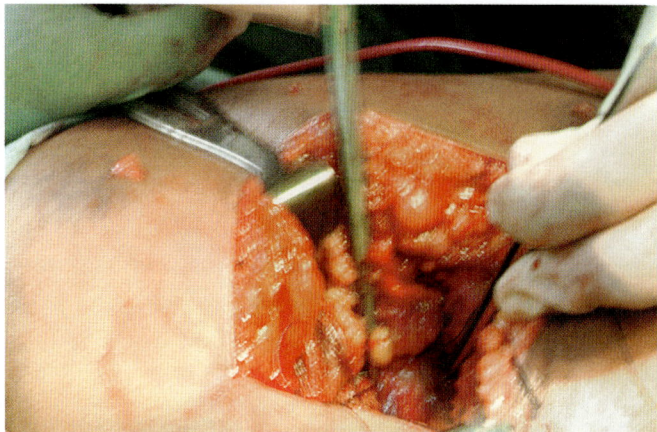

Fig. 52.13: The hip capsule exposed

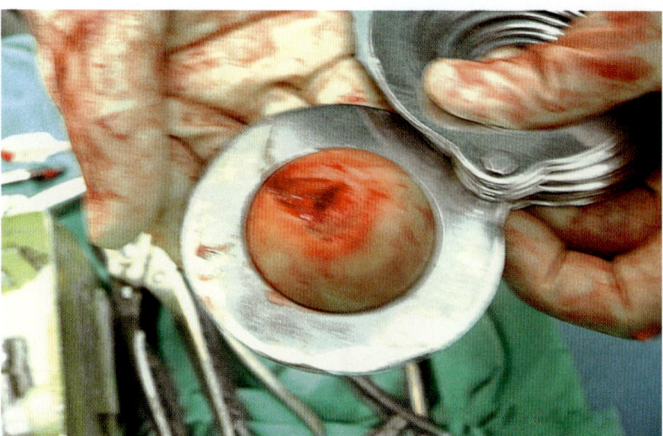

Fig. 52.16: Measuring the size of the excised femoral head

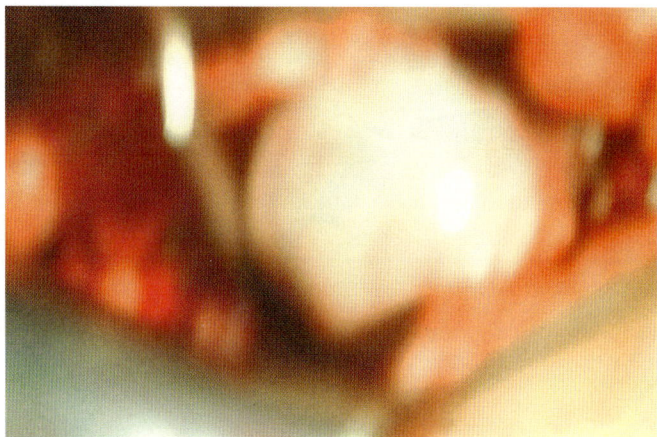

Fig. 52.14: Delivering the head of femur

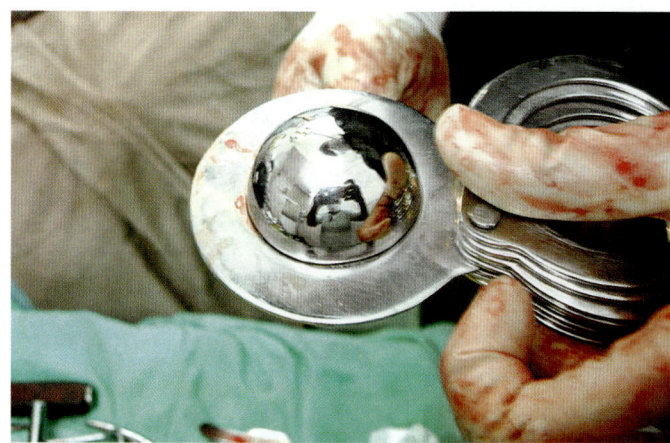

Fig. 52.17: Measuring the size of head of the prosthesis

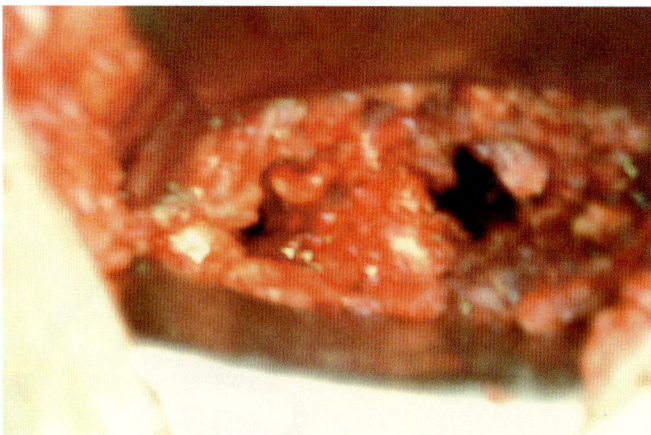

Fig. 52.15: The acetabular cavity exposed

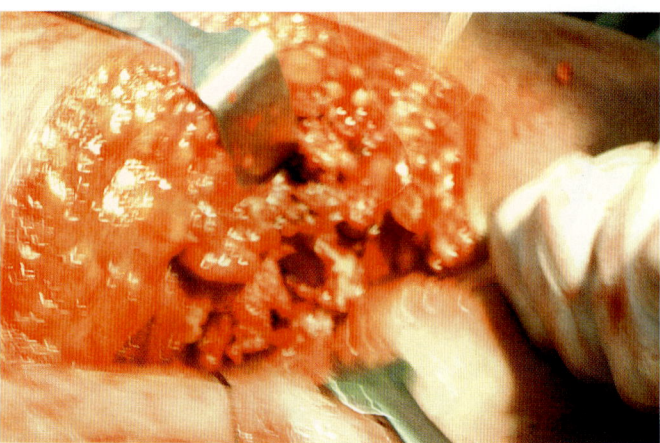

Fig. 52.18: The femoral neck being exposed

CHAPTER 52: Common Hip Surgeries

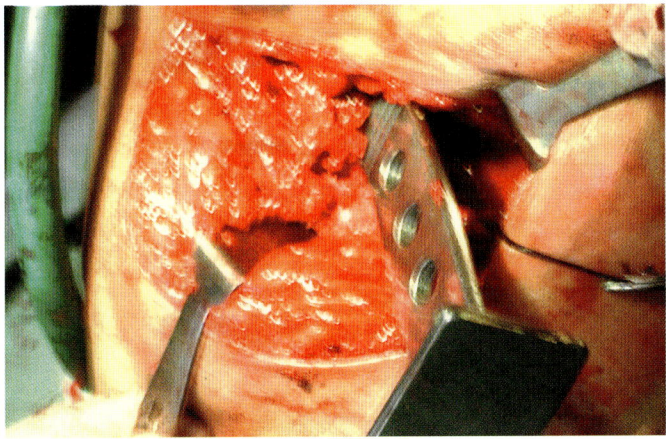

Fig. 52.19: Reaming of the medullary canal of the femoral neck

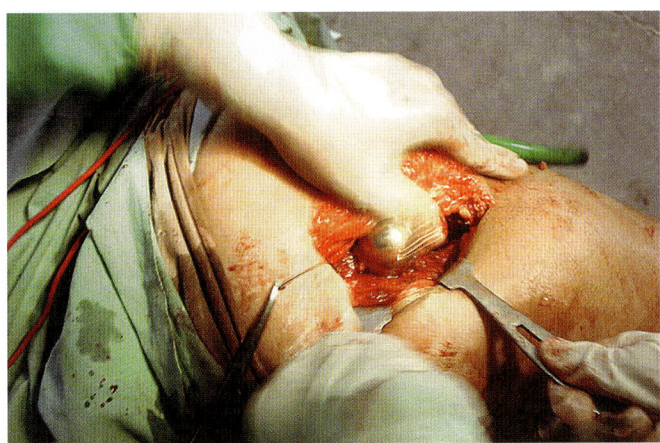

Fig. 52.22: AMP being reduced

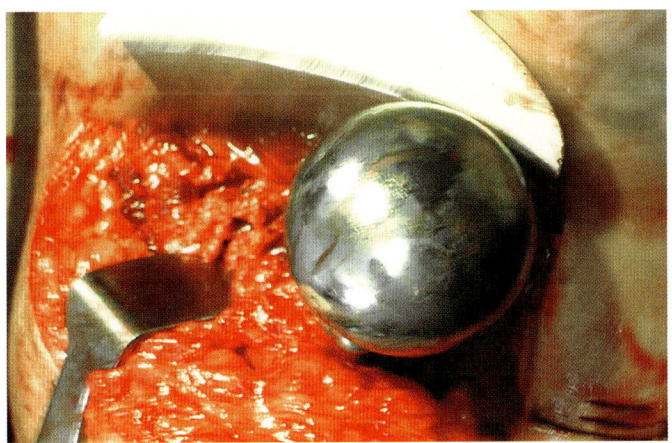

Fig. 52.20: Seating of the prosthesis

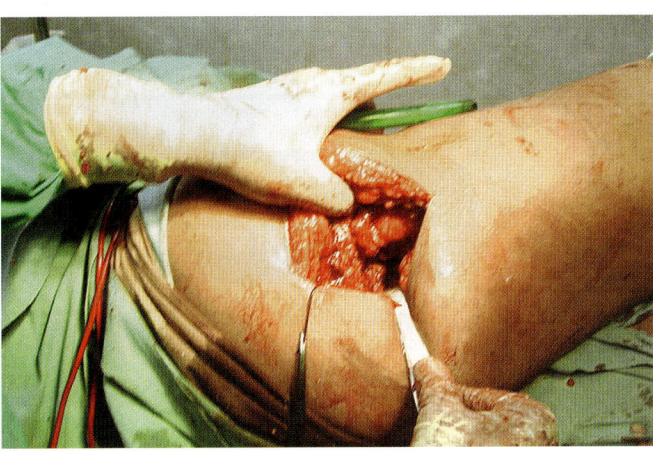

Fig. 52.23: AMP reduced into the acetabulum

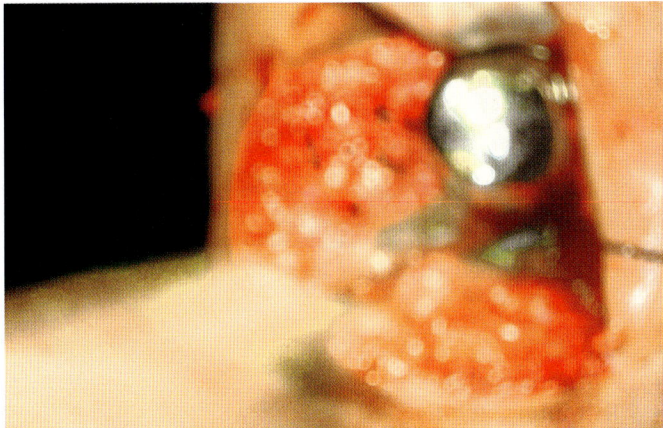

Fig. 52.21: Reducing the AMP

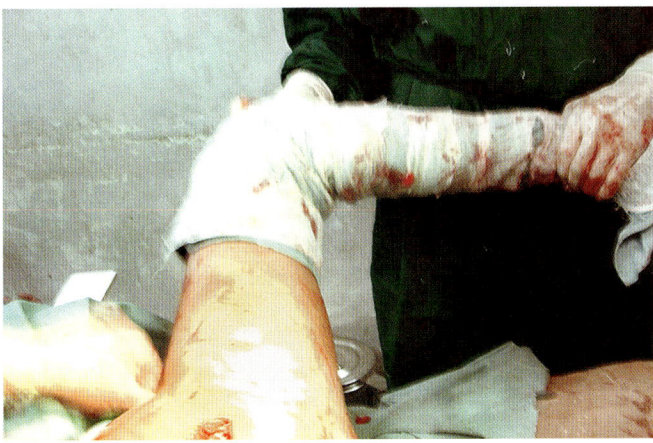

Fig. 52.24: Checking the stability of the reduction

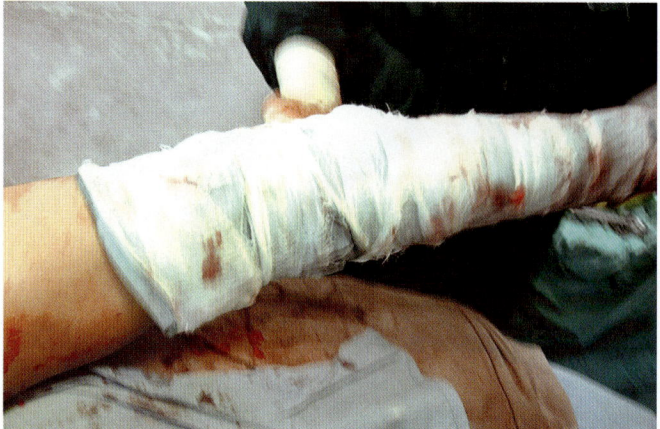

Fig. 52.25: Checking continued

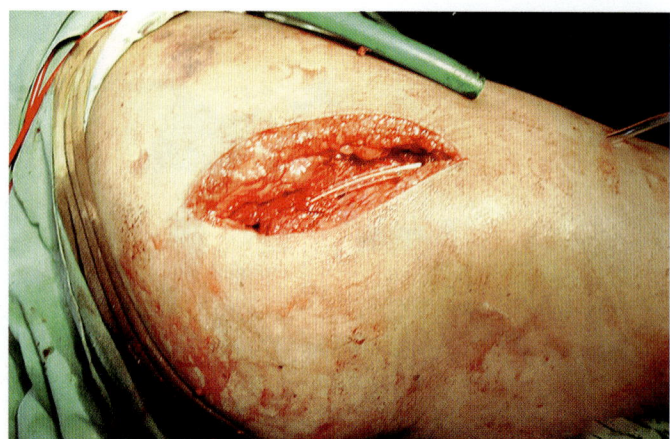

Fig. 52.28: Romovac drain being applied

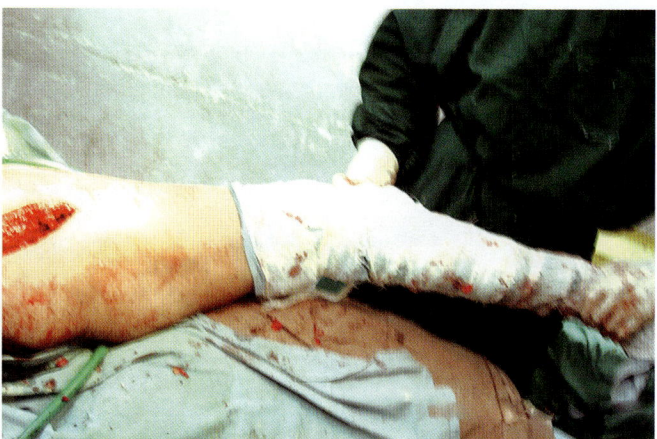

Fig. 52.26: Stability of the reduction confirmed

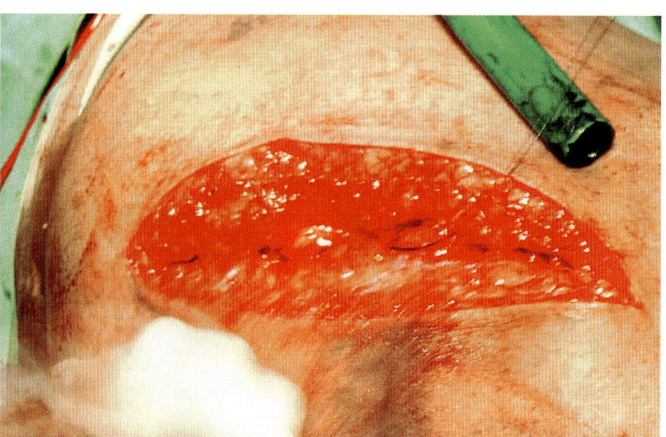

Fig. 52.29: Fascia closure

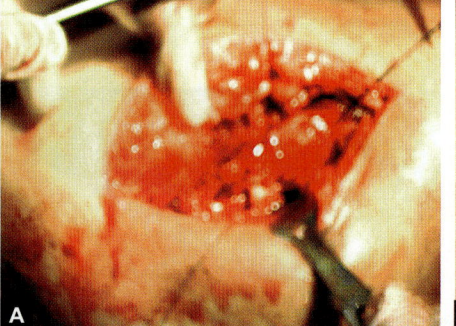 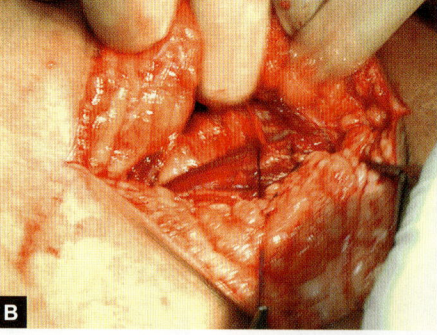 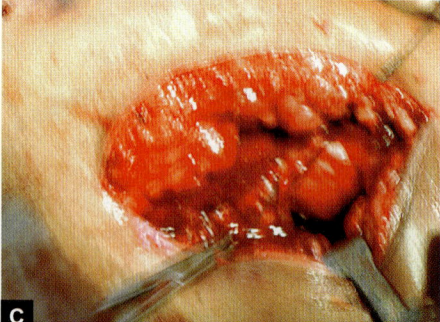

Figs 52.27A to C: (A) The external rotator being repaired; (B) The repair continued; (C) The repair of the external rotators

- Breakage of prosthesis
- Technical errors.

Rare

- DVT
- Shock
- Pulmonary embolism
- Thrombophlebitis
- Fat embolism
- Death.

CHAPTER 52: Common Hip Surgeries **713**

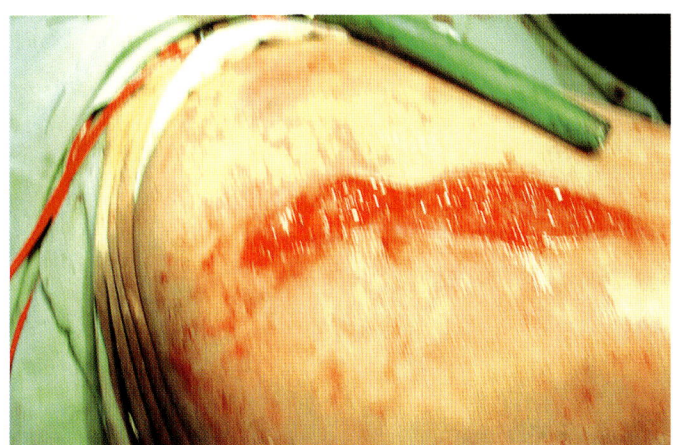

Fig. 52.30: Subcutaneous tissue closure

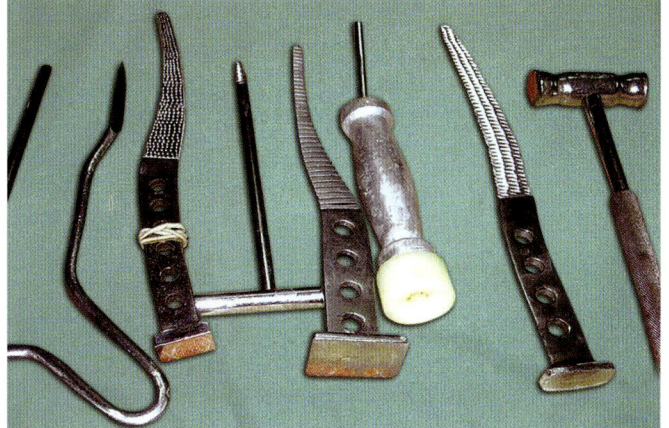

Fig. 52.33: Instruments used for AMP

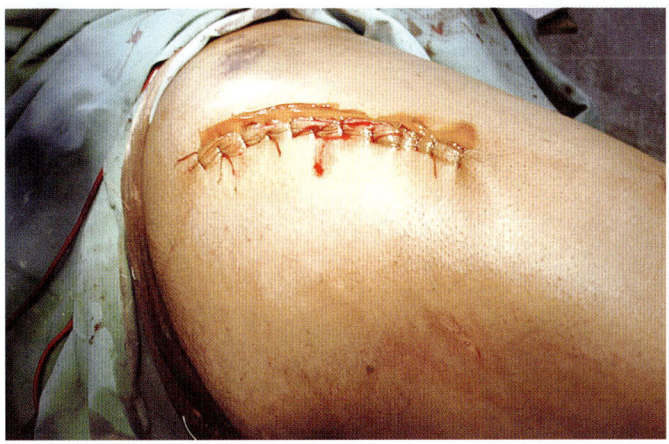

Fig. 52.31: Skin closure

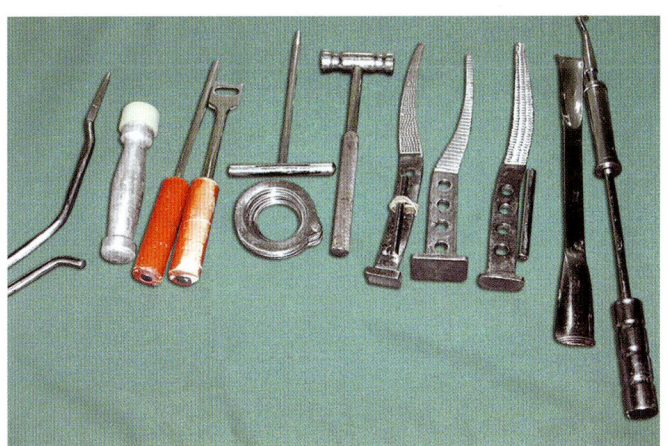

Fig. 52.34: Instruments

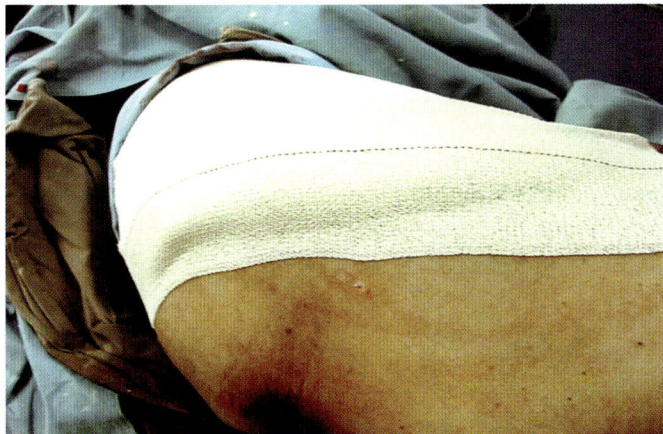

Fig. 52.32: Dynaplast pressure bandage

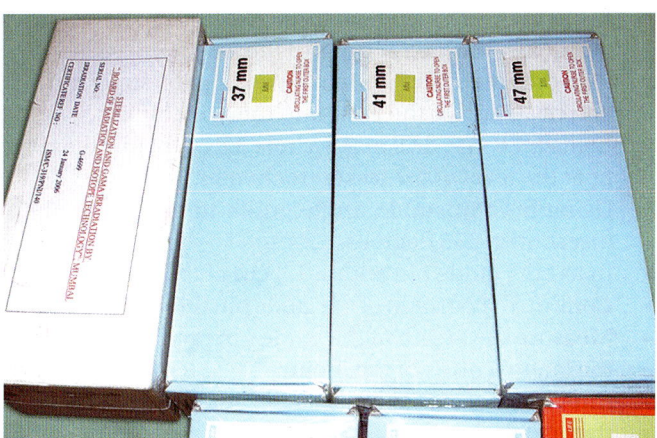

Fig. 52.35: Sterile AMP prosthesis ready for use

714 SECTION 7: Common Surgical Techniques

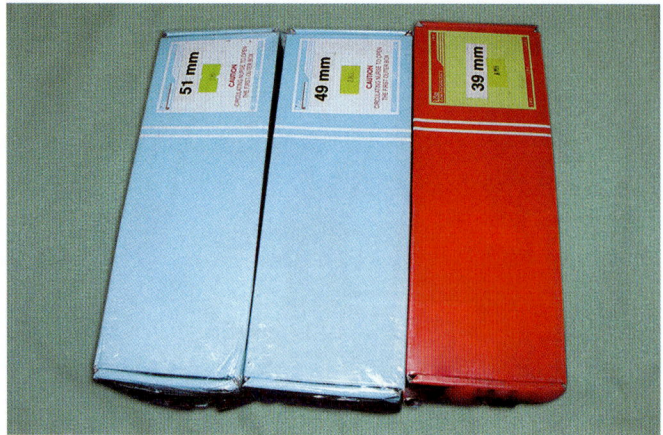

Fig. 52.36: Closer view of the AMP sizes

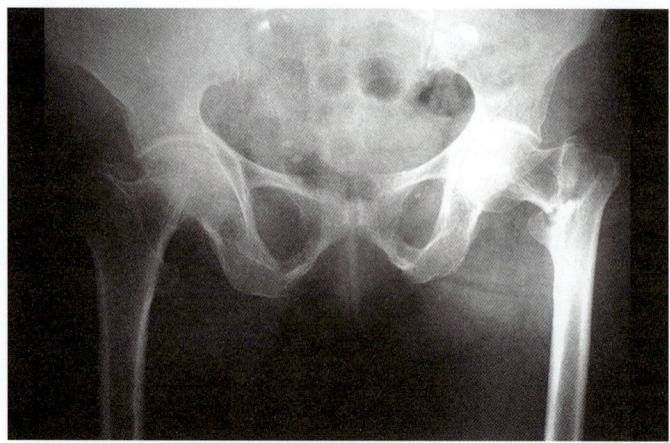

Fig. 52.37: Radiograph of hip—AP view showing pertrochanteric fracture

SURGICAL TECHNIQUE OF AMP PROSTHESIS*

DYNAMIC HIP SCREW (DHS) TECHNIQUE

Indications

To fix trochanteric fractures of femur.

Approach

Lateral approach.

Surgical Steps (Figs 52.37 to 53.52)

- Put the patient on the fracture table, manipulate and reduce the fracture under C-arm control.
- Through the lateral approach, expose the trochanteric area and upper femoral shaft.
- Insert a 2.4 mm guide pin through the mid-lateral cortex just below the lateral ridge of the vastus lateralis.
- Drill the guide pin through the trochanter, superior neck and head across the joint into the acetabulum.
- Using a 4.8 mm drill make a hole 3.8 cm below the ridge or at the level of the lesser trochanter.
- Using an adjustable angle guide to set the angle of insertion at 135 degrees.
- Insert the guide pin within 1.3 cm of the joint margin.
- Confirm the position of the guide pin through the C-arm.
- Measure the length of the guide pin protruding beyond the lateral cortex of the femur.
- After the measurement, drill the guide pin, further into the acetabulum.

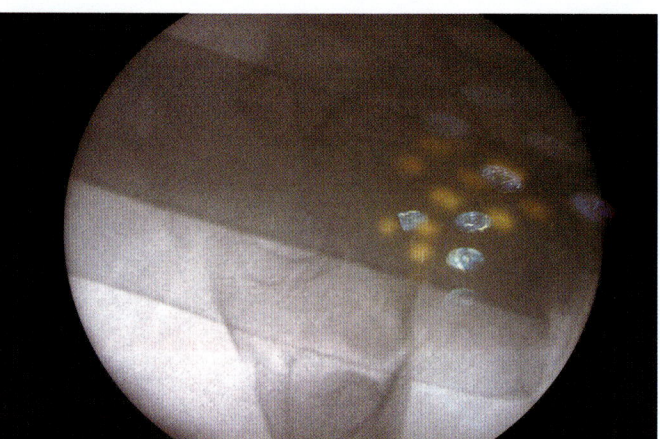

Fig. 52.38: Lateral view of fracture

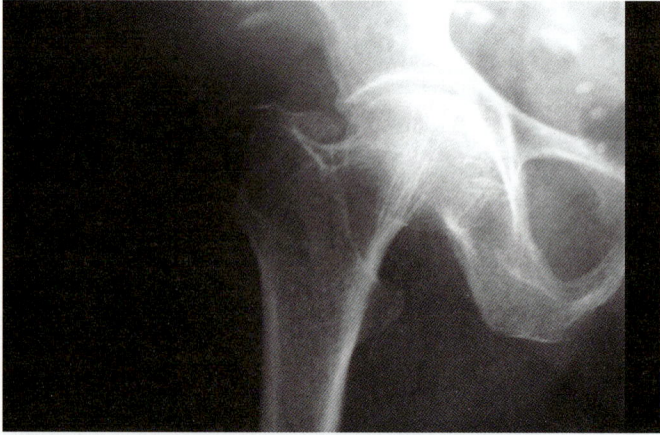

Fig. 52.39: Closure view—normal hip

---

* From "Step by Step Fracture Treatment" by *Dr John Ebnezar*.

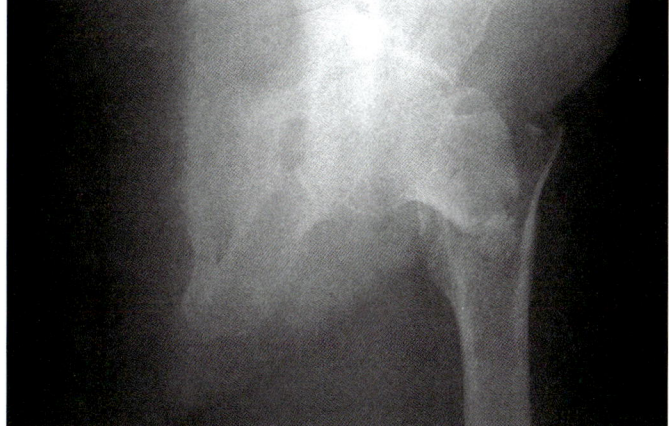

Fig. 52.40: Closer view of fracture

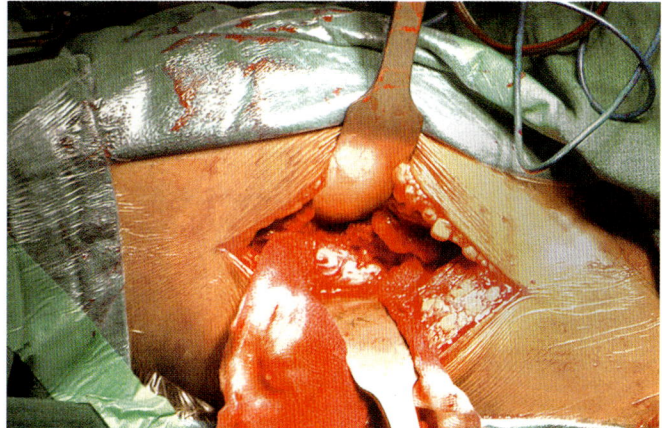

Fig. 52.43: Exposure of the fracture

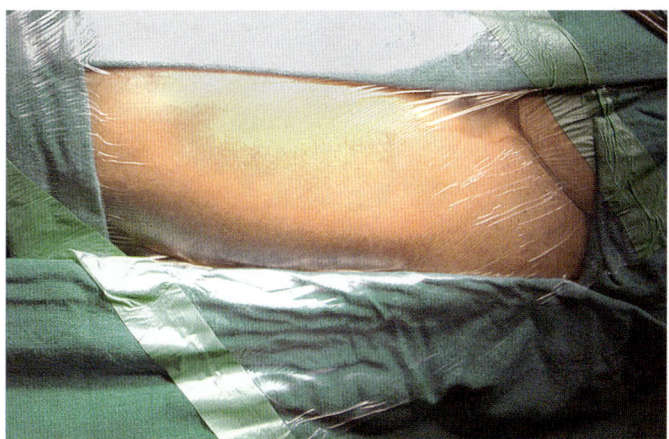

Fig. 52.41: Preparation and draping of the patient

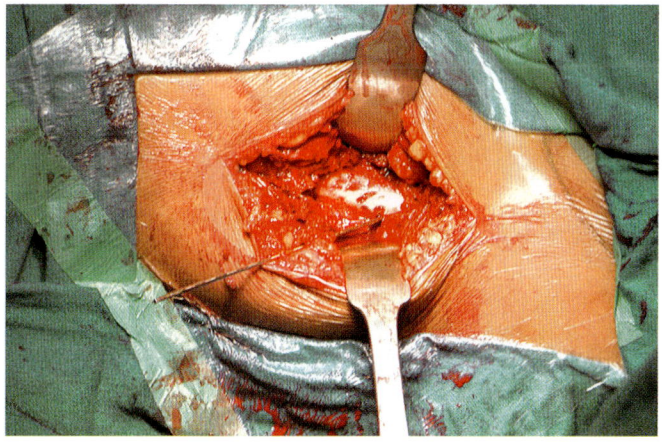

Fig. 52.44: Fracture site exposed

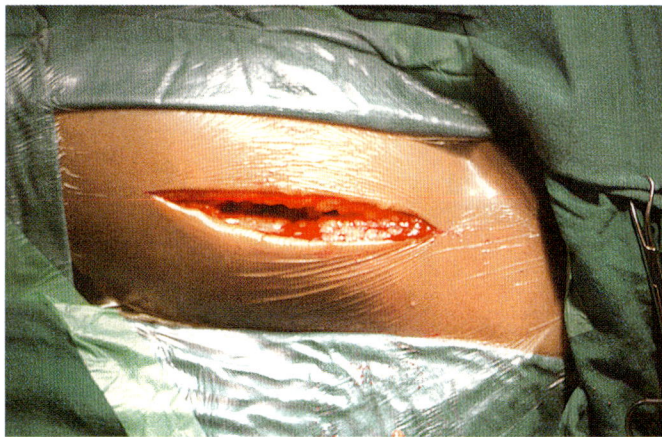

Fig. 52.42: Lateral approach

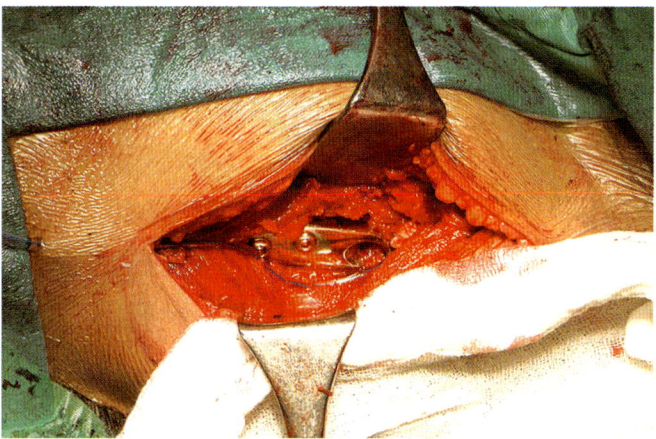

Fig. 52.45: DHS plate and screws fixed

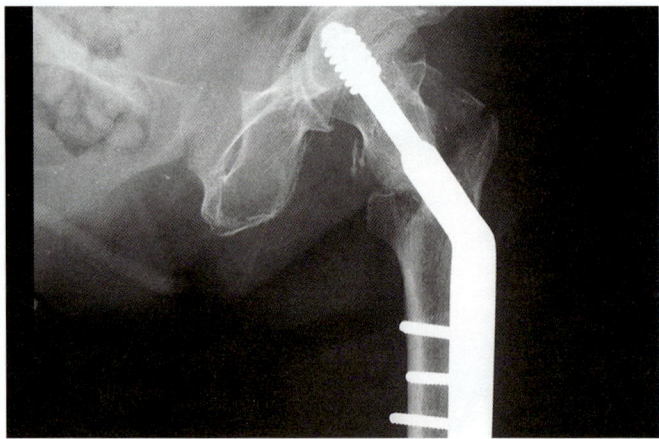

Fig. 52.46: Postoperative film

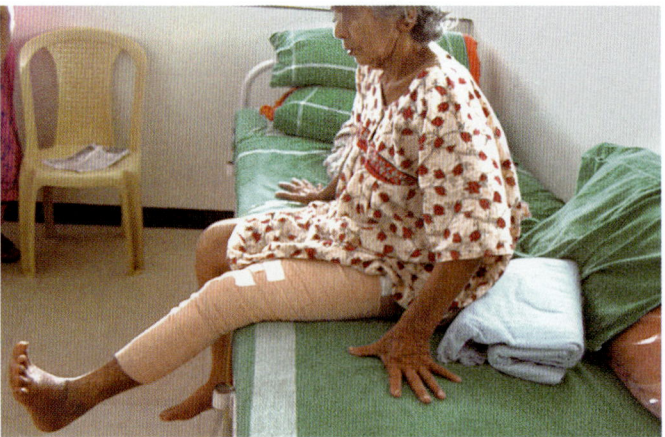

Fig. 52.49: Quadriceps exercises

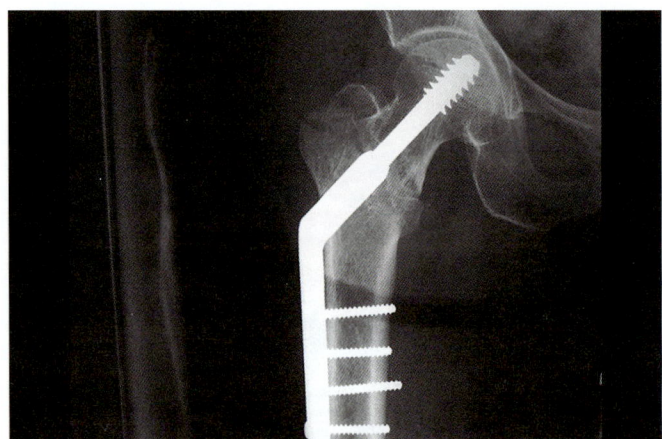

Fig. 52.47: Closer view

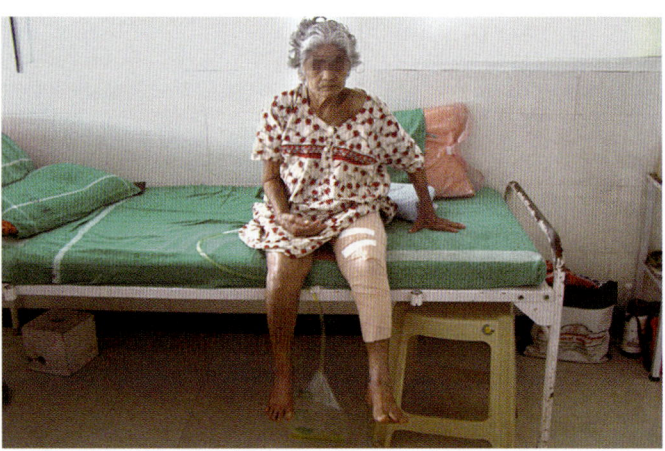

Fig. 52.50: Quadriceps drill

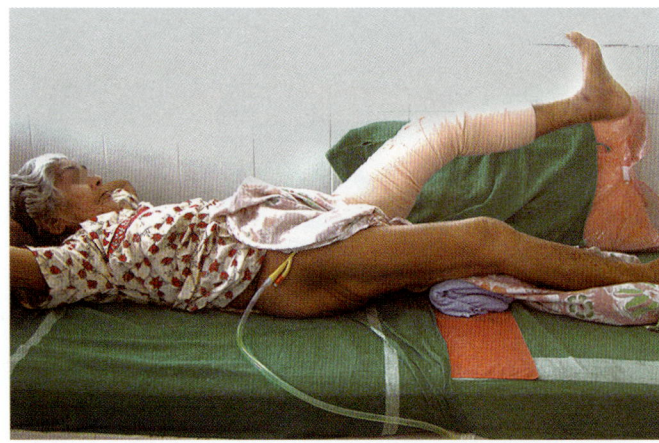

Fig. 52.48: Postoperative rehabilitation

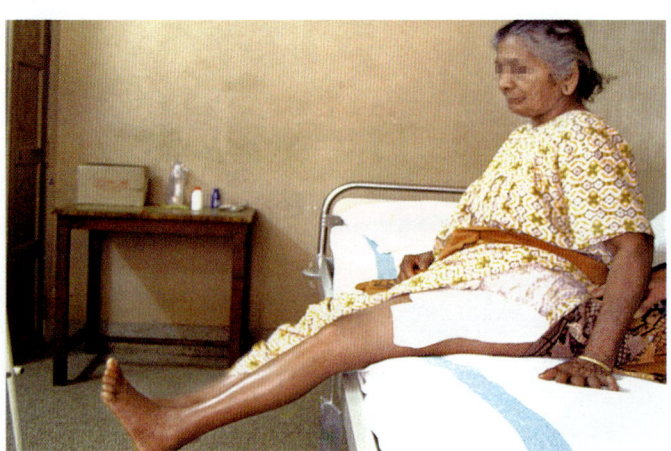

Fig. 52.51: Closer view

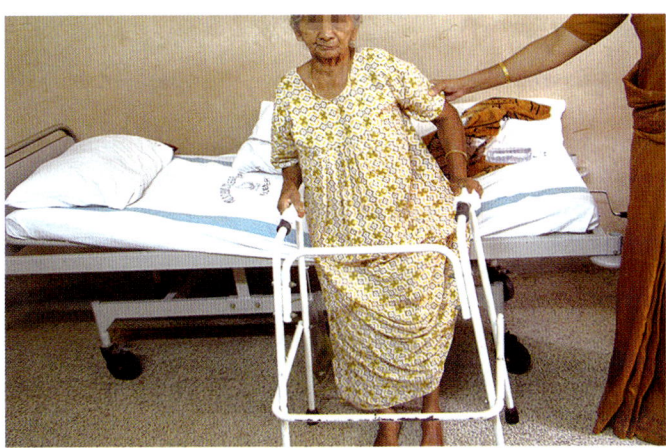

Fig. 52.52: Walking with a walker

- Now for the same length of the protruding guide pin, lock the adjustable depth stop on the reamer.
- Now ream over the guide pin until the depth stops touches the lateral cortex. This will prevent reaming through the head and check this with C-arm.
- During the reaming use the cortical guide sleeve.
- Slowly withdraw the reamer to prevent pulling the guide pin out.
- Now, ream the lateral cortex and trochanter for the plate barrel with a 1.3 cm reamer.
- By using commercial reamers, reaming for the compression screws and the barrel of the side plate can be done at the same reaming.
- Select the lag screw of the correct length by subtracting 1.3 cm from the guide pin measurement.
- Now place the screws such that all of the lag screws threads are within the head fragment.
- Tapping may be required if the bone is hard as in young adults.
- Tapping of the lag screw must be done with a special screw insertion wrench.
- Check for the stability of the fixation.
- Remove the guide pin from the hip and thread the barrel guide into the end of the lag screw shaft.
- Slip the plate barrel over the barrel guide and onto the lag screw shaft.
- Remove the barrel guide, clamp the side plate closely to the femur and screws it securely in place with 3 or 4 screws.
- Thread the compression screw into the distal end of the lag screw shaft and tighten it to compress the fracture
- Before completion of the tightening, release the traction on the leg and check the position with a C-arm.
- Close the wound in layers over a suction drain.

Aftercare

- Patient can be permitted to move the operated limb on the next day.
- Active and active assisted exercises for the hip and knee are done next.
- Bedside standing with a walker can be permitted after the removal of sutures.
- Walker support to be used for walking for at least 3–4 months.
- Weight-bearing can be permitted at the end of 6 weeks.

INTERNAL FIXATION OF FRACTURE NECK OF FEMUR

Indication

Intracapsular fracture neck of femur in young adults.

Choice of Implants

- SP Pin and plate (Not in vogue now).
- Asnis screw.
- Cannulated screws.
- Moore's pins (In children).
- Dynamic screws.

Though there are many choices of implants for internal fixation in fracture neck of femur, the principles of preoperative preparation, reduction technique of the fracture, C-arm or radiographic control, surgical approaches and technique of insertion are the same.

Approach: Lateral approach.

Surgical Steps

- After spinal anesthesia the patient is positioned on a fracture table.
- Closed reduction of the fracture is done under C-arm or radiographic control.
- If the reduction is satisfactory the greater trochanter and the upper end of femur are exposed through a lateral approach after painting and draping.
- Midway between the anterior and posterior cortices of the lateral femur and about 2 cm distal to the inferior edge of the greater trochanter a hole is drilled.
- Guide pin is then passed through this hole at an angle of 45 degrees to the shaft and parallel to the ground.
- Check the position of the guided wire by the C-arm both in the anteroposterior and lateral views. The pins should be in the center of the neck.

- If the position is satisfactory, insert the cannulated screws or Moore's pins parallel to the guidewire and if Richard's screw is used through the guidewire.
- Confirm the position of all the pins as mentioned above.
- In case of pin and plates, fix the plate to the screw and fasten it to the bone with cortical screws.
- Check for the stability of the fracture reduction and fixation.
- Close the wound in layers over a drain.

Aftercare

- Patient can be permitted to move the operated limb on the next day.
- Active and active-assisted exercises for the hip and knee are done next.
- Bedside standing with a walker can be permitted after the removal of sutures.
- Walker support to be used for walking for at least 3–4 months.
- Weight-bearing can be permitted at the end of 6 weeks.

Common Surgery of the Femur

INTRAMEDULLARY NAILING

Indications
Fracture at the level of the isthmus of the femur in adults.

Approach
Midlateral approach.

Surgical Steps
- After spinal anesthesia, the patient is either put in lateral or semilateral position and firmly fastened to the operating table with appropriate fastening materials.
- The patient is painted and draped.
- Closed reduction of the fracture shaft femur is done by traction and counter traction methods.
- The accuracy of the reduction is checked by C-arm.
- If the reduction is satisfactory, the limb is fastened firmly to the table.
- The fracture is exposed through careful dissection and arresting of the bleeders through a lateral or posterolateral approach.
- Care is taken to see that the perforators are identified and ligated firmly.
- Fracture hematoma is drained.
- Trial fracture reduction is carried out under direct vision.
- Now using appropriate sized reamers first the proximal and then the distal fragments are reamed using reamers with progressively increasing sizes.
- The reaming is done in a retrograde manner and the reaming is stopped once it emerges out through the greater trochanter.
- The distal fragment is reamed next.
- After reaming both the fragments, the fracture is now reduced and held firmly.
- Select the appropriate sized Kuntscher's nail.
- Select the nail diameter equal or 1 size more than the reamer to provide a snug fit.
- The open slot of the K-nail is held anterolaterally on the convex (tension) side of the femur.
- The eye of the nail should face posteromedially, so that the extraction of the nail can easily be done at a later stage.
- Now pass the nail through the proximal fragment in a retrograde manner till it emerges out of the greater trochanter.
- Now reduce and hold both the fracture fragments.
- Drive the nail down into the distal fragment leaving the upper end of the nail about 1 inch above the greater trochanter.
- The distal end of the nail should extend upto the level of the proximal pole of the patella.
- Close the wound in layers over a drain after giving a thorough antiseptic wash.
- Apply a pressure bandage.

Aftercare
- Patient can be permitted to move the operated limb on the next day.
- Active and active assisted exercises for the hip and knee are done next.
- Bedside standing with a walker can be permitted after the removal of sutures.
- Walker support to be used for walking for at least 3–4 months.
- Weight-bearing can be permitted at the end of 6 weeks.

INTERLOCKING NAILING

Indications

Fracture of the femur in adults at different levels. Unlike Intramedullary nailing it has a wide indication and is indicated in comminuted fractures, segmental fractures, proximal and distal third fractures, etc.

Approach

Lateral approach at the level of the greater trochanter.

Surgical technique of femoral interlocking are shown in Figures 53.1 to 53.25.

Surgical Steps

- After spinal anesthesia, the patient is firmly fastened to the fracture table.
- The part is painted and draped.
- Closed reduction of the fracture shaft femur is done by traction and manipulation.
- The accuracy of the reduction is checked by C-arm.
- If the reduction is satisfactory, the limb is fastened firmly to the table.
- A short incision is made over the lateral aspect of the greater trochanter.

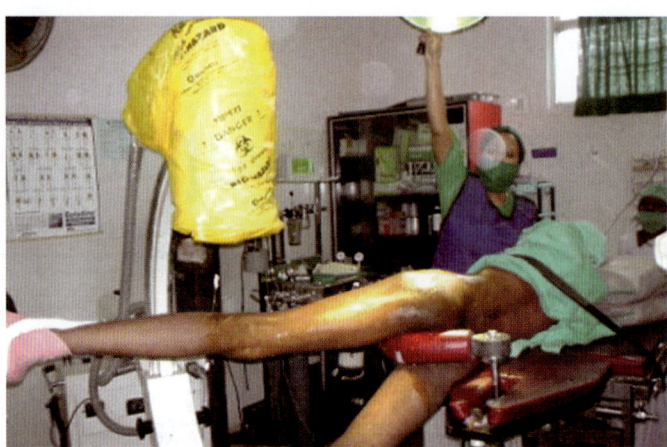

Fig. 53.3: Patient positioning: Probably the best position C-arm accessible all around. Entry into trochanter very easy. Not always possible

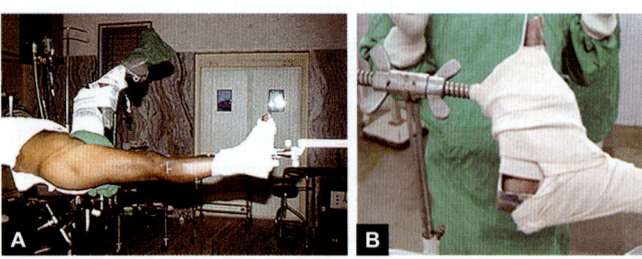

Figs 53.1A and B: (A) Right foot tied under traction. The left leg to be adjusted that it does not come in the way of C-arm visualization of RT femur; (B) While tying the foot to the foot plate the heel should be visible

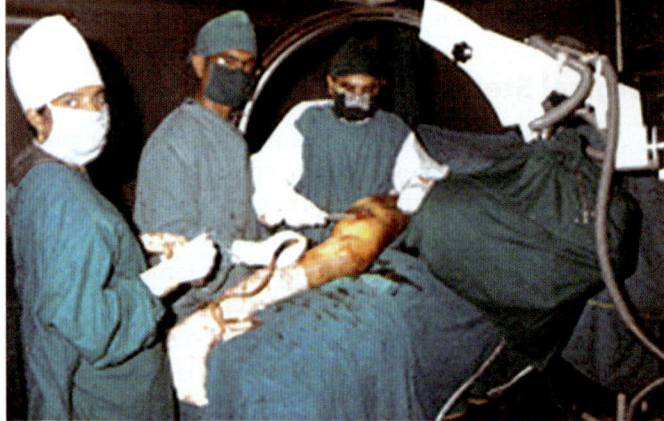

Fig. 53.4: Patient positioning: Lateral position on radiolucent table. Initial time to fix on a traction table saved. But a good extra-assistance needed

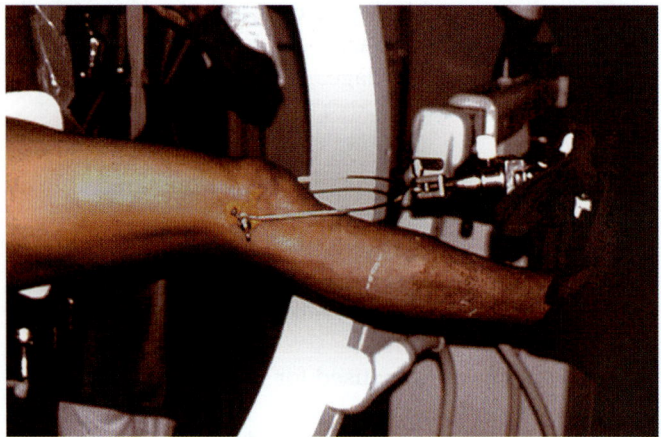

Fig. 53.2: Supracondylar pin traction

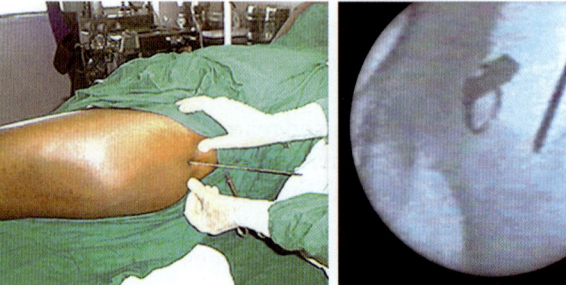

Fig. 53.5: Trochanteric entry: Step number 1

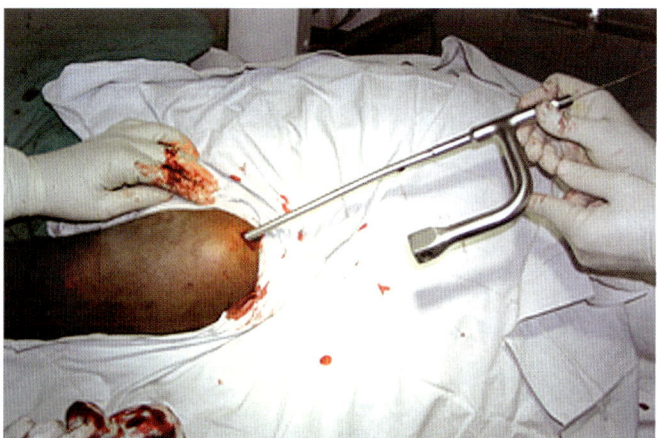

Fig. 50.26: Introduction of the nail

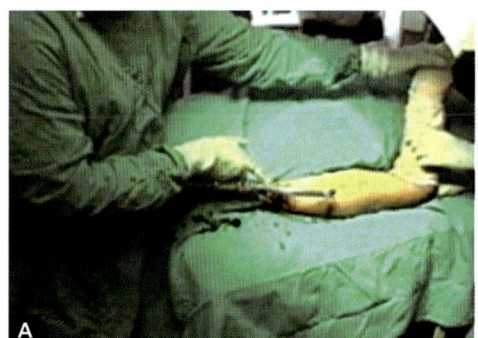
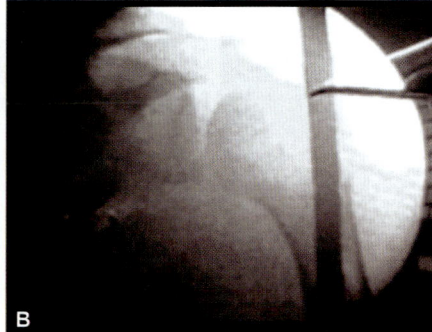
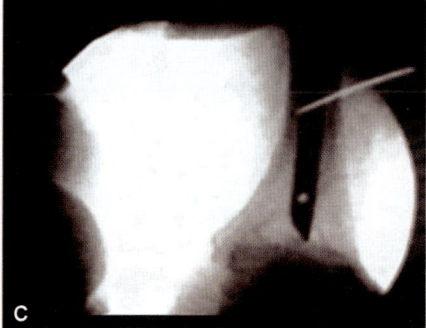

Figs 50.27A to C: Checking nail length

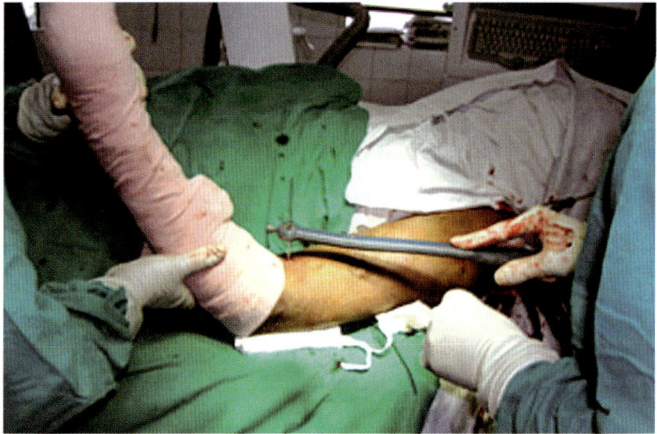

Fig. 50.28: Locating the distal locking hole by a K-wire on a radiolucent handle

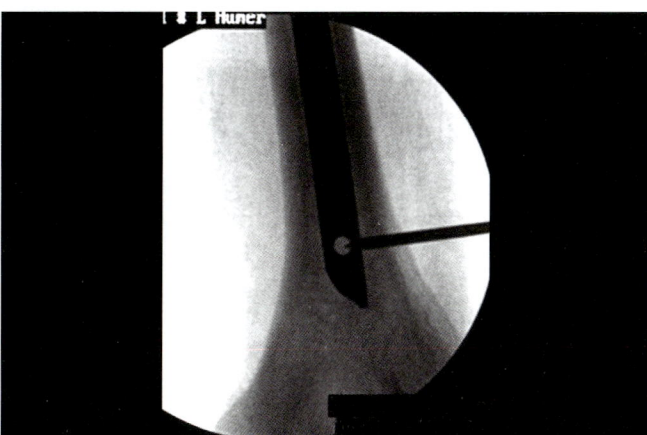

Fig. 50.29: C-arm view

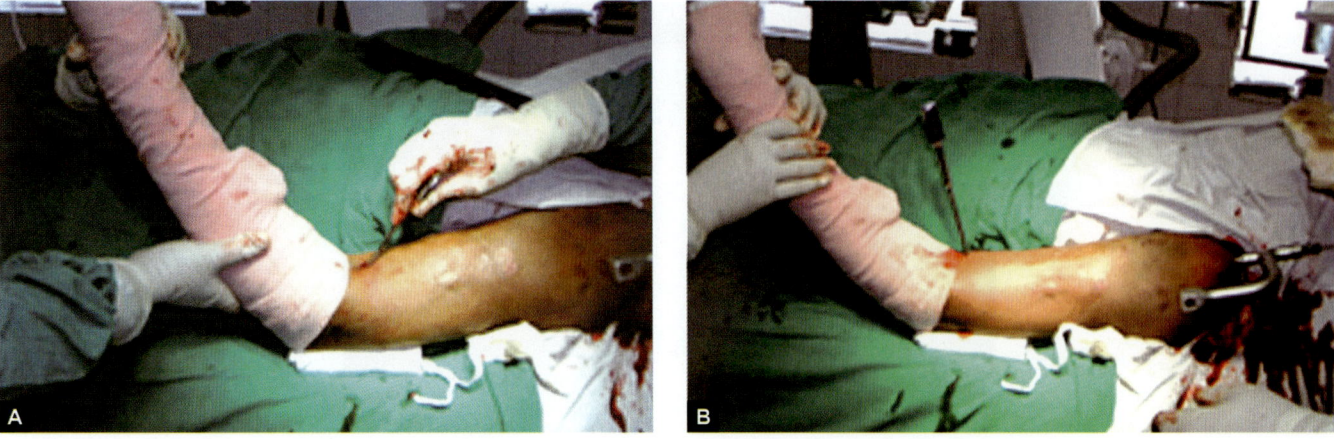

Figs 50.30A and B: (A) Soft tissue clearance; (B) Anterior cortex penetrated

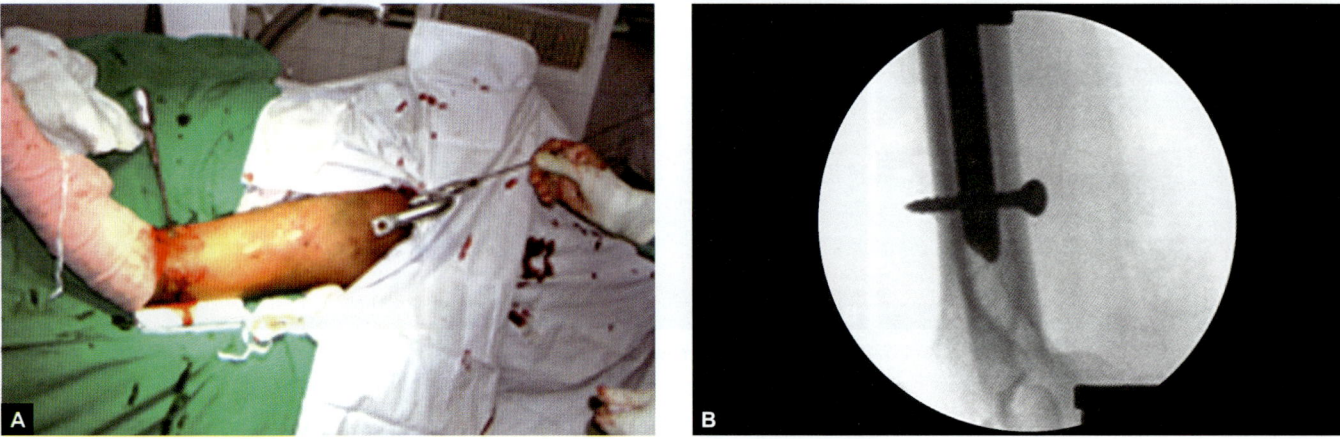

Figs 50.31A and B: (A) Guidewire sounding to confirm; (B) Distal screw introduced

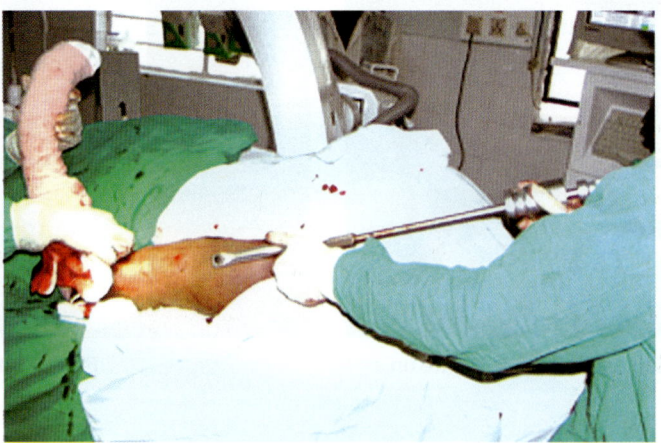

Fig. 50.32: Back slapping to close fracture gap

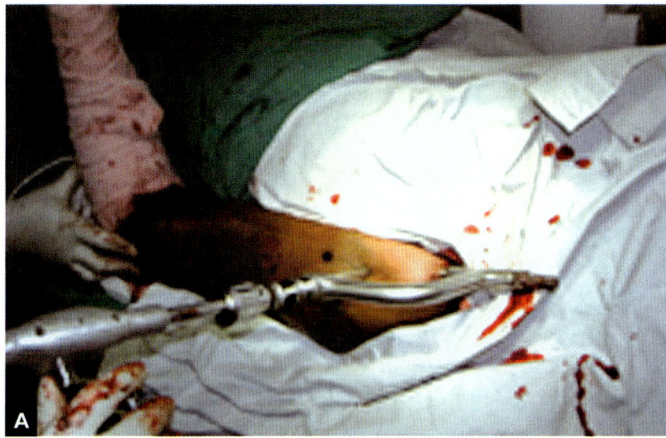
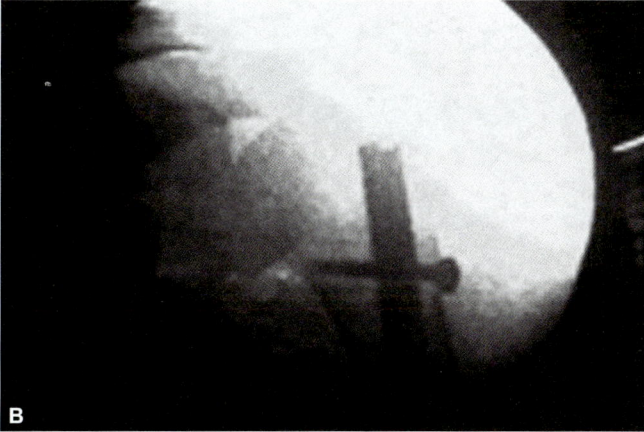

Figs 50.33A and B: (A) Proximal jig; (B) Nail tip is under the surface

SUPRACONDYLAR FRACTURE HUMERUS—PERCUTANEOUS FIXATION**

Technique

Closed reduction and percutaneous pinning.

Indications

Type III Gartland supracondylar fractures of humerus.

Surgical Steps (Figs 50.34 to 50.62)

Method of Closed Reduction of the Supracondylar Fracture

- Under general anesthesia, put the patient prone on the fracture table.
- Identify the landmarks of the posterior triangle of the elbow namely, the medial and lateral epicondyles and the olecranon, and mark them after preparation and draping.
- Reduce the fracture by applying longitudinal traction. Extension and manipulation to correct the lateral tilt, medial impaction and posterior displacement.

Method of Percutaneous Fixation

- Through the condyles, pass 2 K-wires in a criss cross manner, one to exit above the medial epicondyle and the other through the lateral epicondyle.

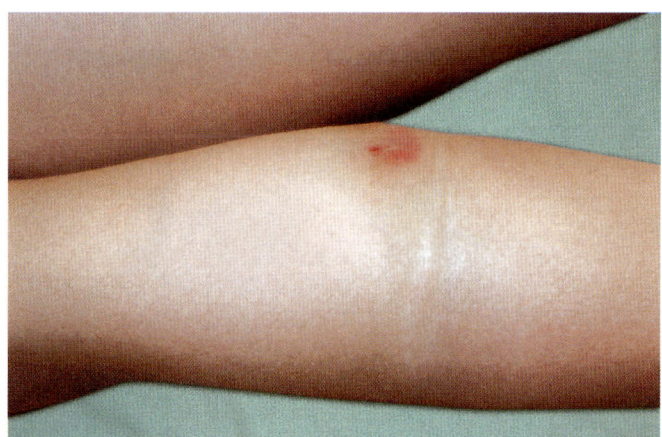

Fig. 50.34: Deformity front view (Clinical photo)

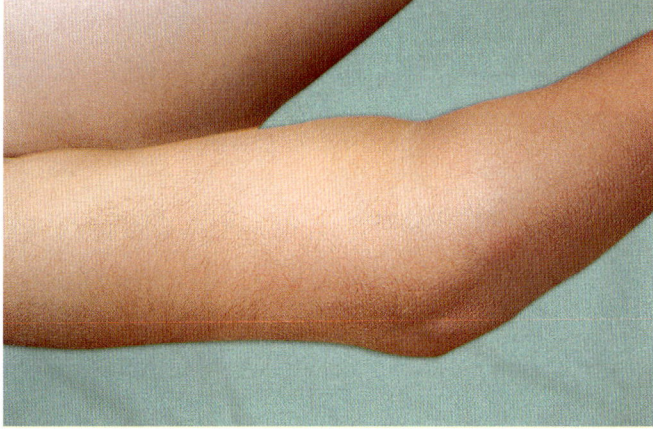

Fig. 50.35: S-shaped deformity side view

**"Step by Step Fracture Treatment" by Dr *John Ebnezar.*

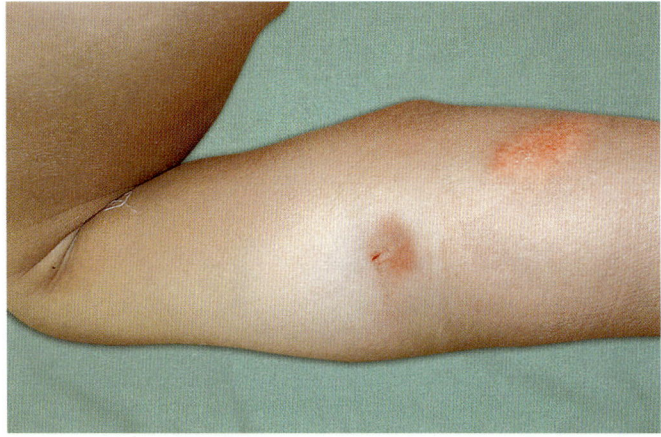

Fig. 50.36: Deformity closer view

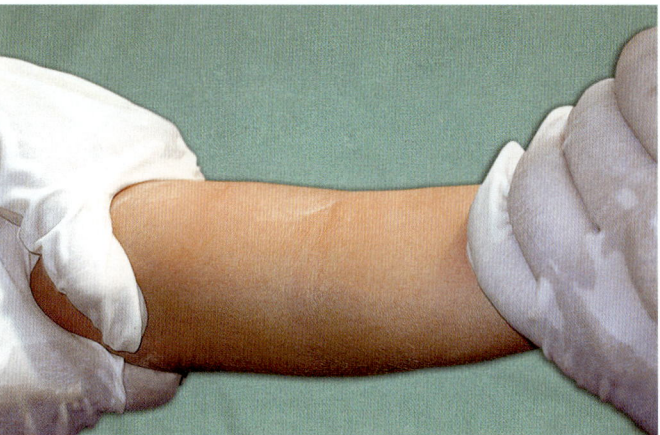

Fig. 50.39: Manipulation of AP displacement

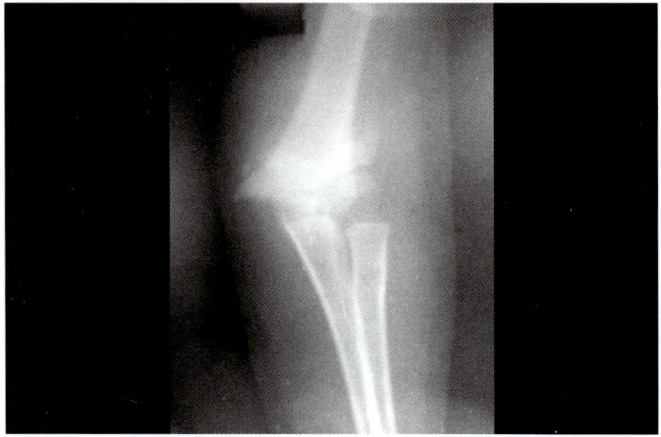

Fig. 50.37: Radiograph—AP view

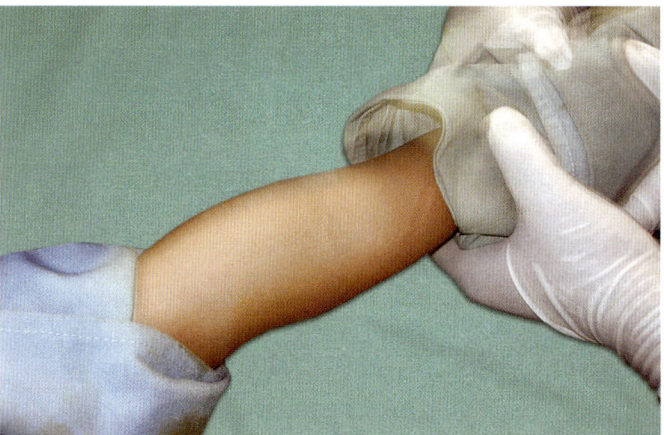

Fig. 50.40: Closed reduction-traction

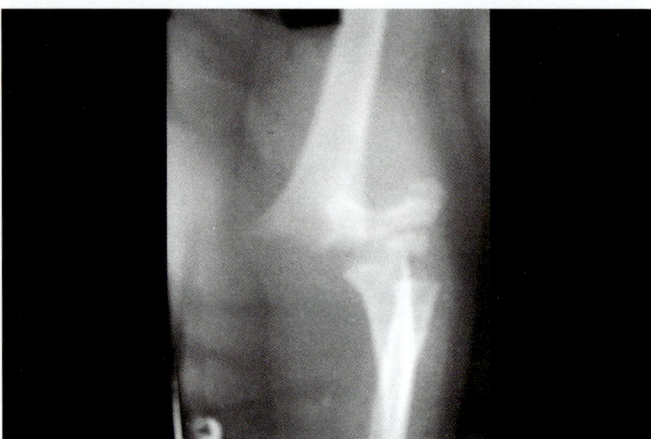

Fig. 50.38: Radiograph—lateral view

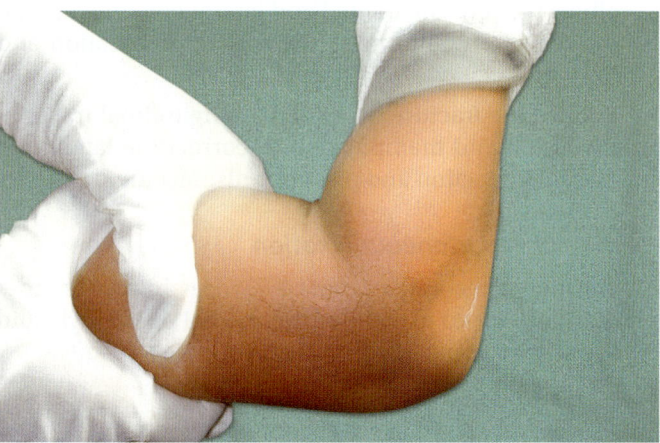

Fig. 50.41: Reduction obtained flexion restored

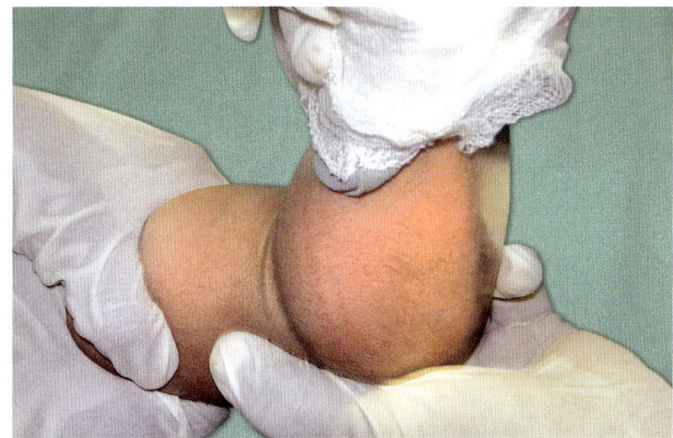

Fig. 50.42: Closed reduction manipulation of sideward displacement

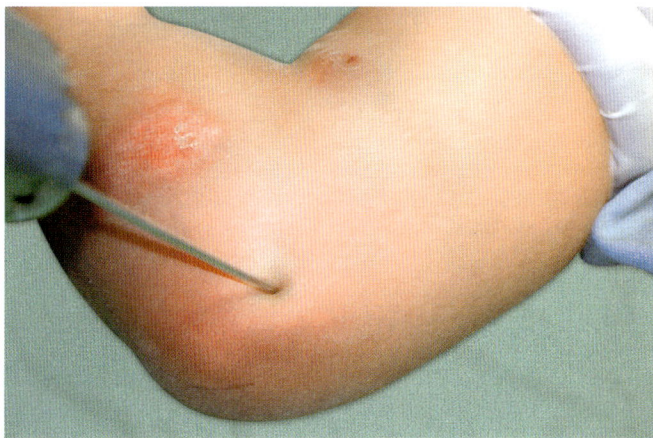

Fig. 50.45: Identifying and marking the point of placement of the medial pin

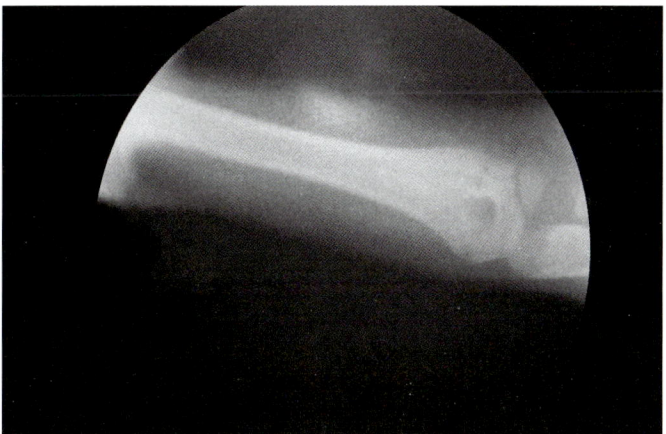

Fig. 50.43: C-arm confirmation—AP view

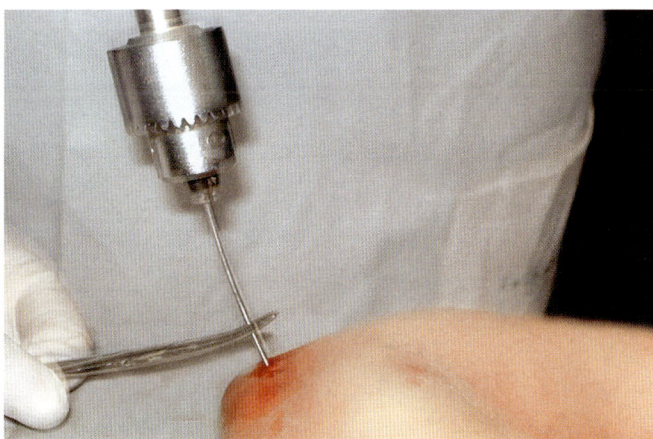

Fig. 50.46: Pin being driven inside

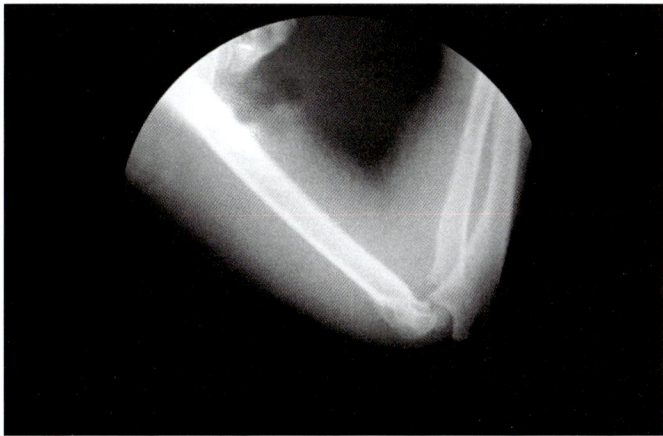

Fig. 50.44: C-arm confirmation—lateral view

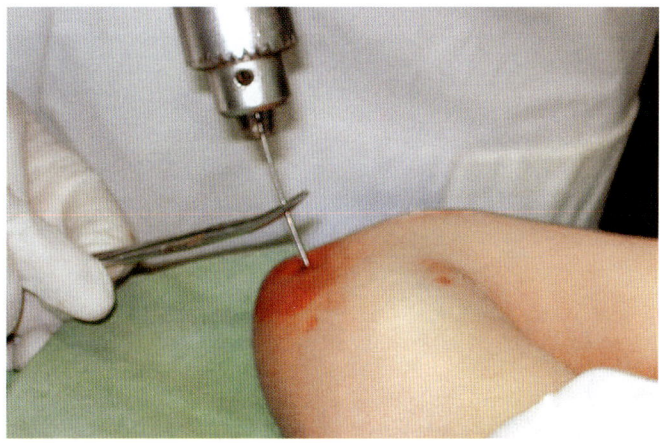

Fig. 50.47: Stabilizing the placement of the pin

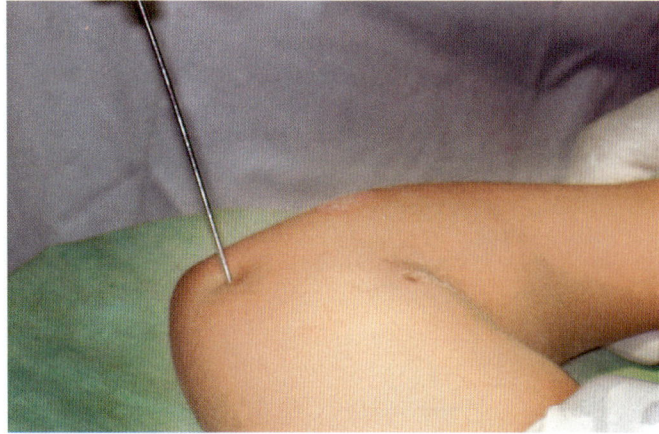

Fig. 50.48: Beginning to penetrate

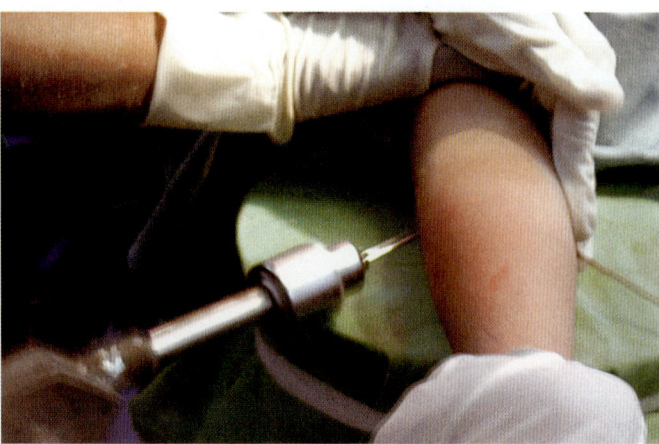

Fig. 50.51: Placement of the lateral pin

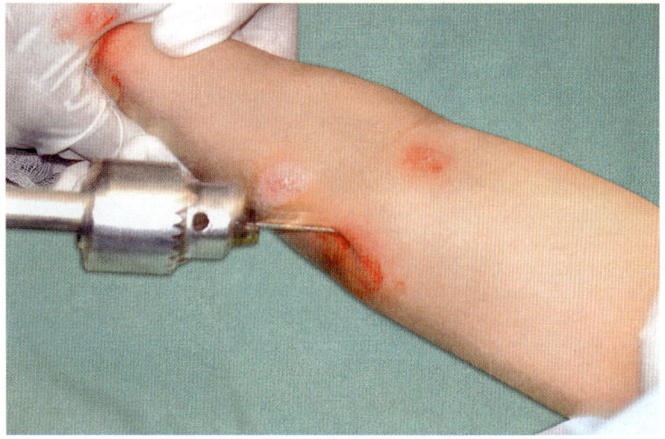

Fig. 50.49: Pin being driven further

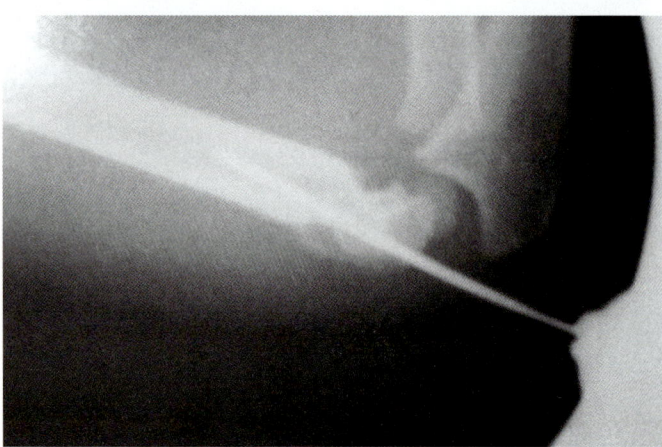

Fig. 50.52: C-arm check of medial pin (Lateral view)

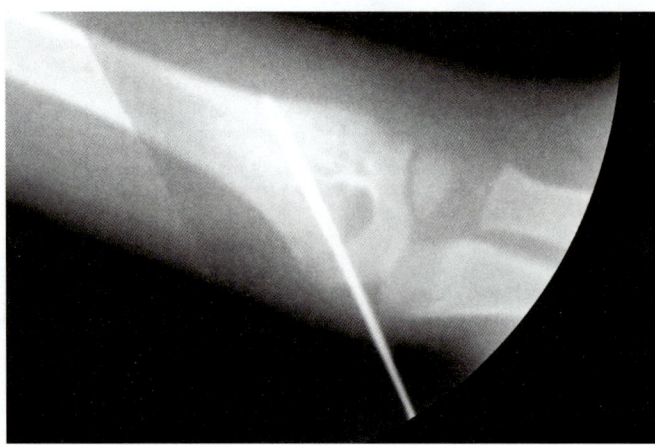

Fig. 50.50: C-arm check medial pin (AP view)

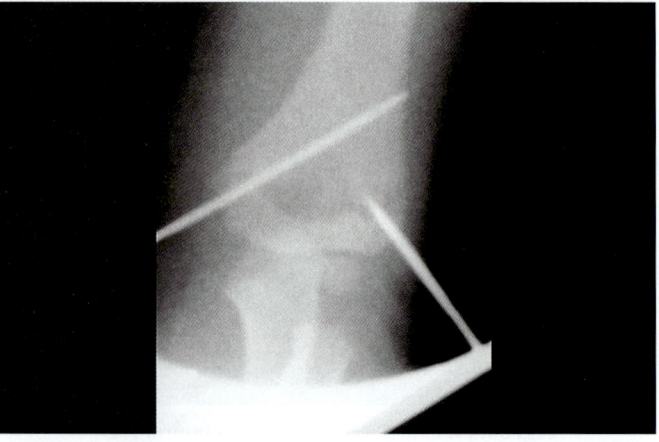

Fig. 50.53: C-arm picture of the lateral pin

CHAPTER 50: Common Surgeries of the Humerus

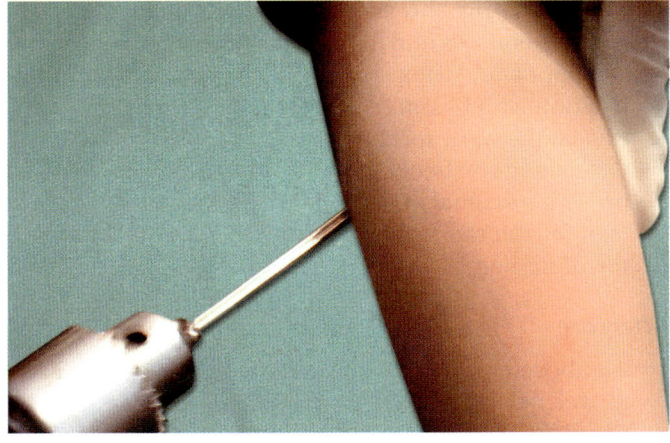

Fig. 50.54: Marking the lateral entry point

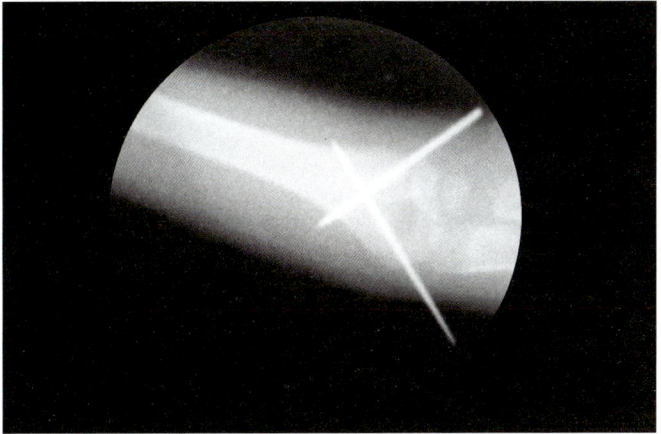

Fig. 50.57: C-arm check of both the pins (AP view)

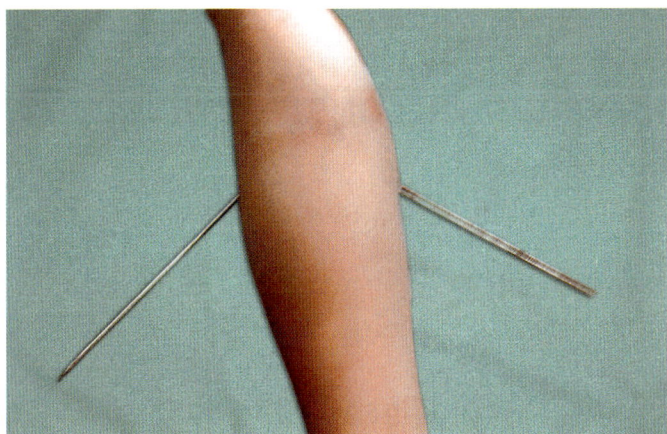

Fig. 50.55: Placement of both the pins

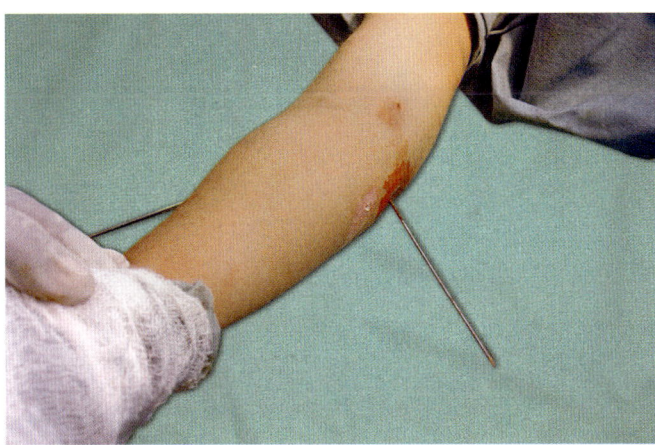

Fig. 50.58: Checking stability in extension

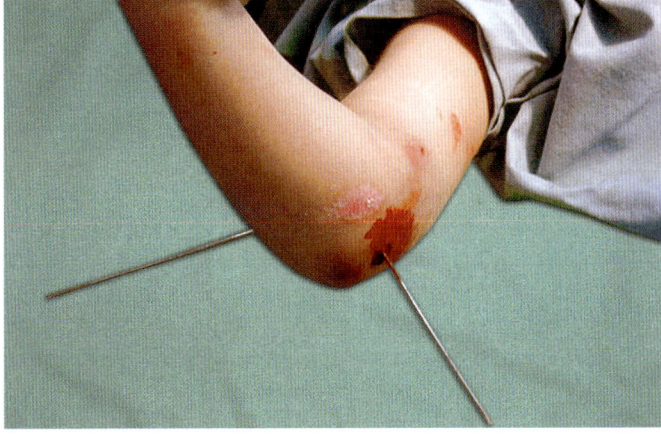

Fig. 50.56: Checking the stability after fixation-flexion

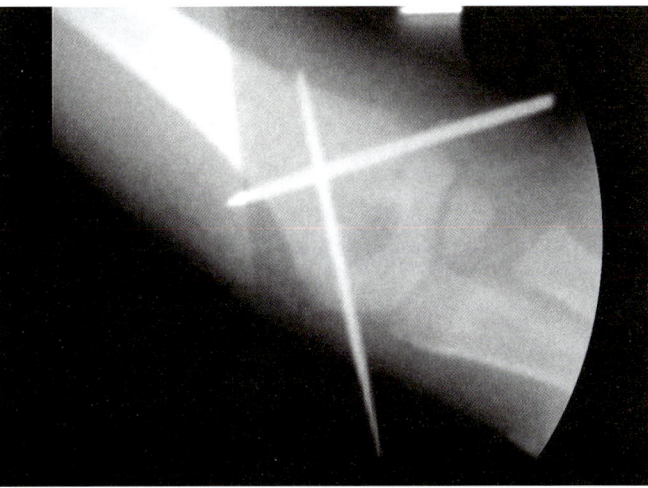

Fig. 50.59: C-arm check—another view

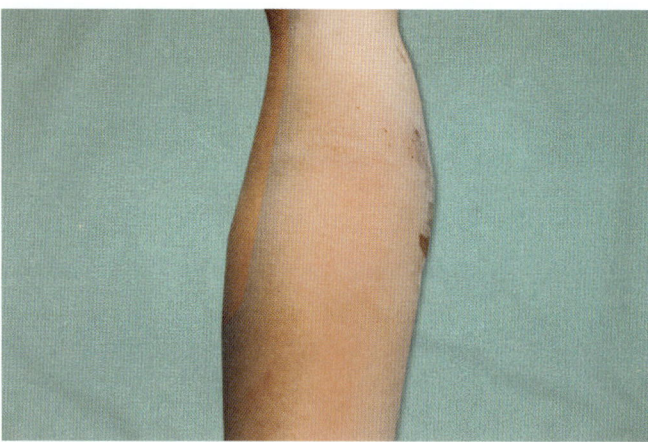

Fig. 50.60: Pins cut at the level of the skin

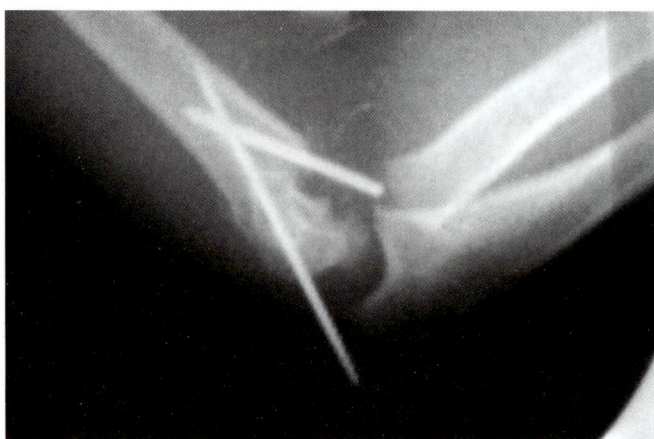

Fig. 50.61: C-arm check—lateral view

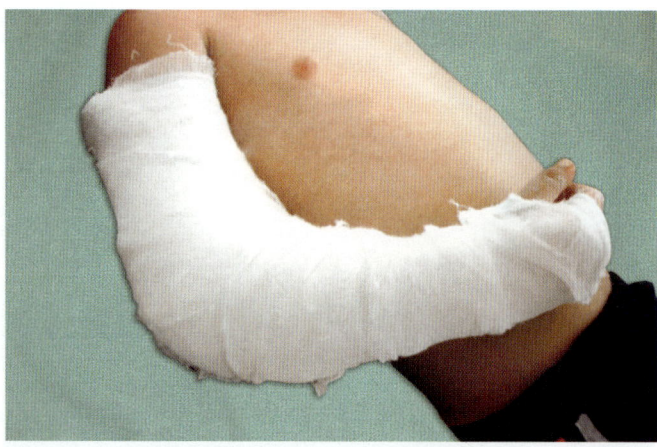

Fig. 50.62: Above elbow plaster slab

- The medial pin should be at an angle of 40 degrees to the humeral axis and directed 10 degrees posterior and the opposite cortex should be engaged. Confirm the position with C-arm.
- Repeat the same for the lateral pins.
- Cut the pins off beneath the skin and bend their ends to prevent proximal migration.
- Feel for the radial pulse and take care not to damage the ulnar nerve.

Aftercare

- An above elbow long slab is applied with elbow in 90 degree flexion.
- Check for the radial, ulnar and median nerve functions.
- Remove the pins after 3 weeks.
- Reapply the plaster slab again.
- Intermittent range of movements exercises are begun after 4 weeks.

INTERCONDYLAR FRACTURE HUMERUS—RECONSTRUCTIONS

Indications

Communized T or Y condylar fractures of the humerus.

Approach

Posterior Campbell approach.

Surgical Steps (Figs 50.63 to 50.86)

- Patient is in prone position after GA and the arm is supported on a short arm board with elbow at right angle.
- Expose the elbow posterior through an incision 5 cm distal to the Olecranon and about 12 cm above the Olecranon tip.
- By careful dissection expose the Olecranon and the triceps tendon.
- Isolate the ulnar nerve.
- Raise a tongue of the triceps aponeurosis and split the triceps in the middle.
- Expose and dissect the fracture fragments carefully without damaging the soft tissue attachments.
- Reorganize and reassemble the fracture fragments of the distal humerus including the epicondyle and condyles.
- Hold the assembled bone fragments firmly with bone holding clamps.
- Using a power drill, fix the assembled fragments with K-wires.

- Fix the major fragments with malleolor or cancellous AO screws. Remove the stabilizing K-wires.
- Now fix the reorganized reassembled and fixed condyles to the humeral shaft by T or Y plates.
- Contour the plates for proper fit.
- Thoroughly irrigate the joint.
- Repair the triceps tongue with multiple interrupted sutures.
- Close the wound in layers over a suction drain.

Aftercare

- A long above elbow posterior slab is applied from the posterior axillary fold to the palm.

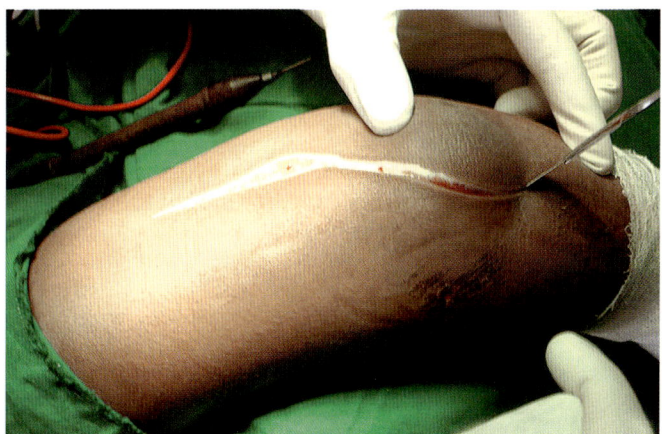

Fig. 50.65: Posterior approach

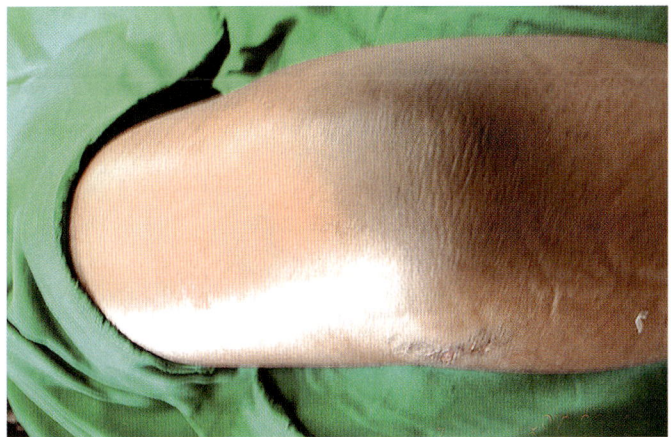

Fig. 50.63: Deformity

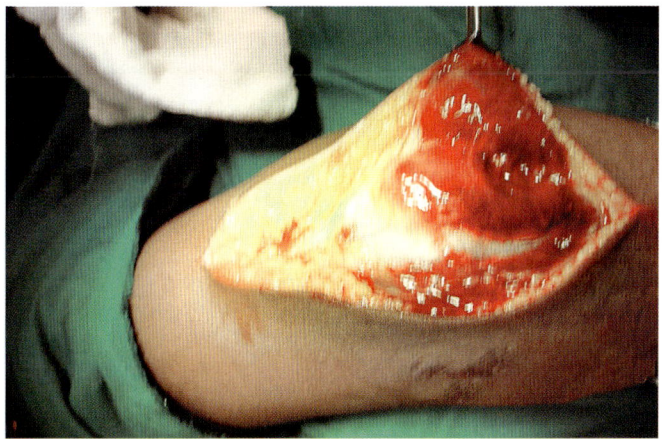

Fig. 50.66: Deep dissection

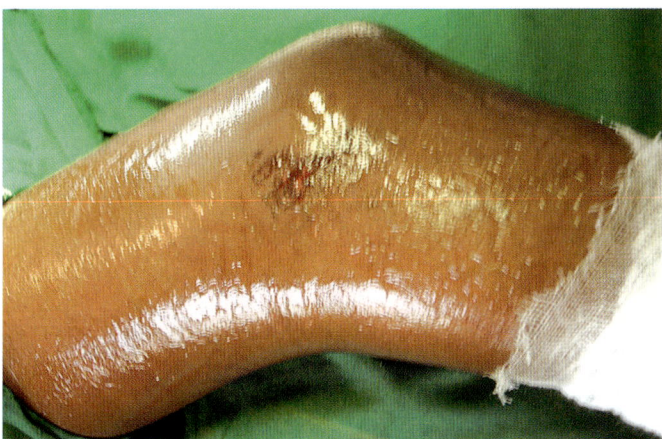

Fig. 50.64: Paint and draping

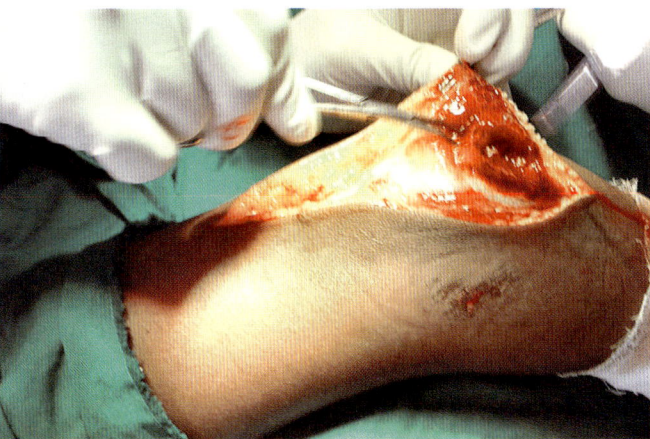

Fig. 50.67: Soft tissue dissection

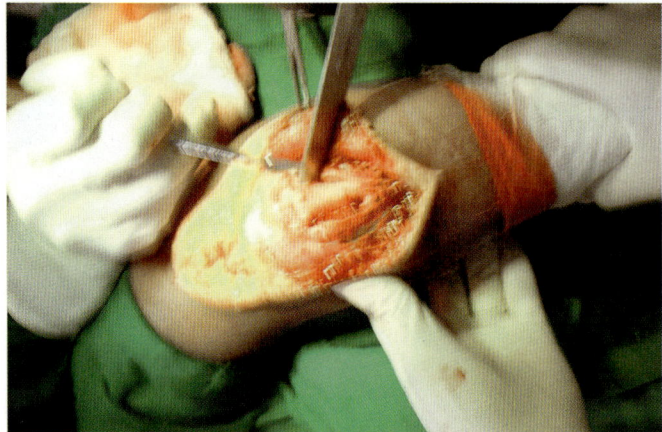

Fig. 50.68: Osteotomizing the olecranon

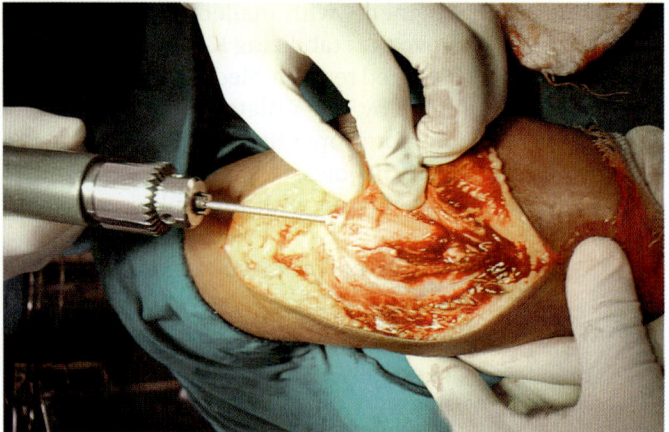

Fig. 50.71: Passing AK wire through the olecranon

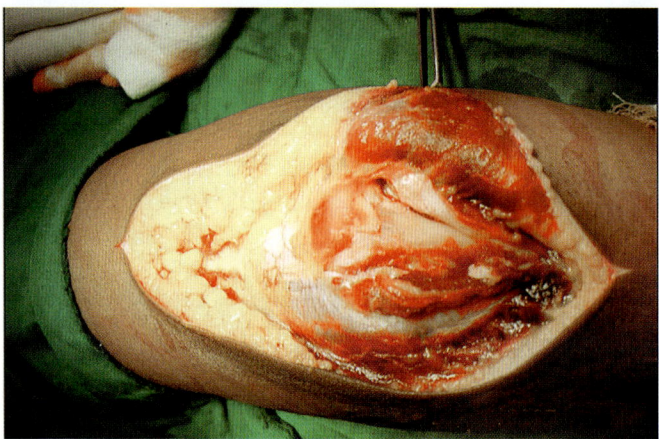

Fig. 50.69: Exposing the olecraon

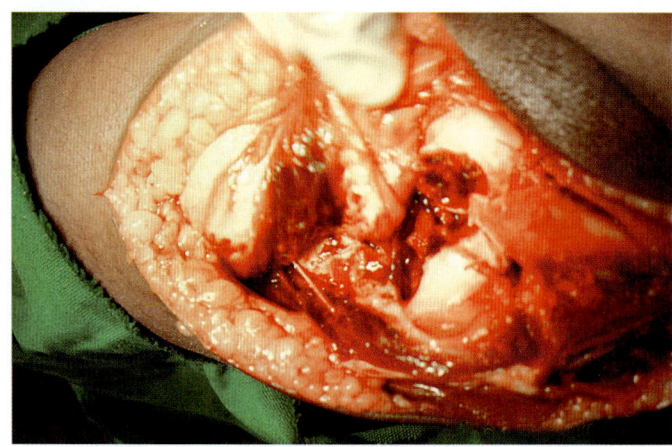

Fig. 50.72: Exposure of the intercondylar fracture

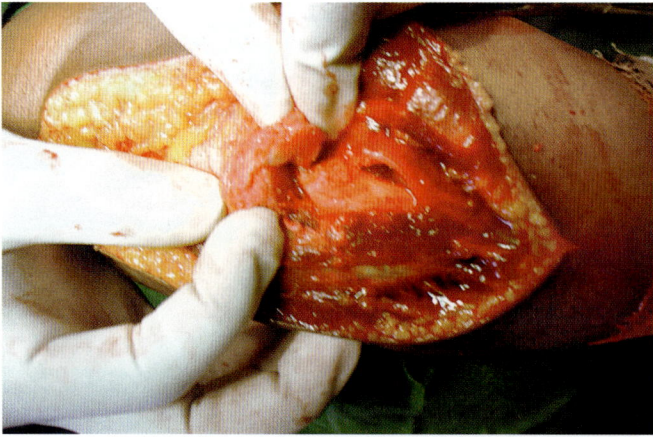

Fig. 50.70: V-shaped olecranon osteotomizing

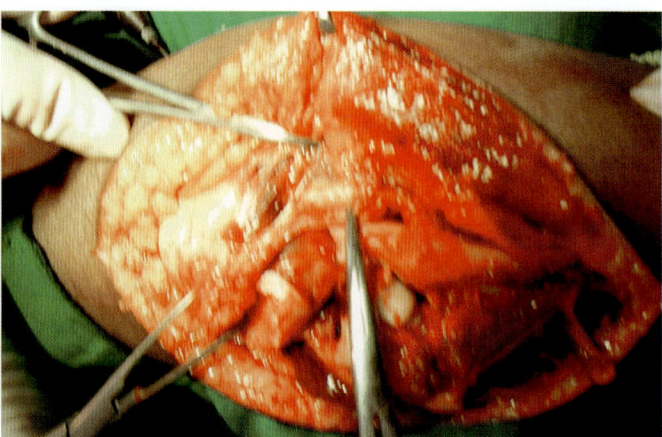

Fig. 50.73: Reflecting the triceps aponeurosis

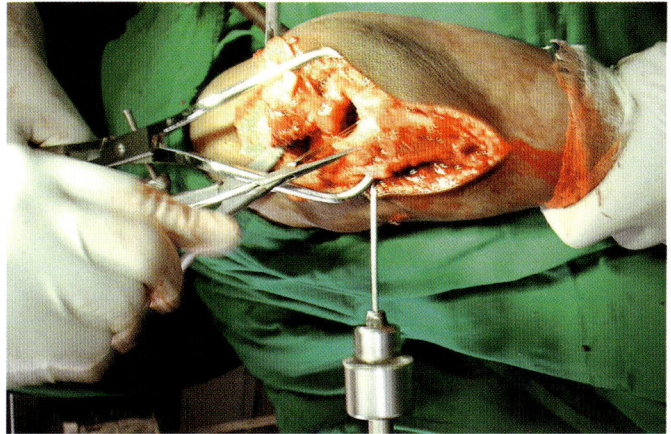

Fig. 50.74: Passing K-wire through the IC area

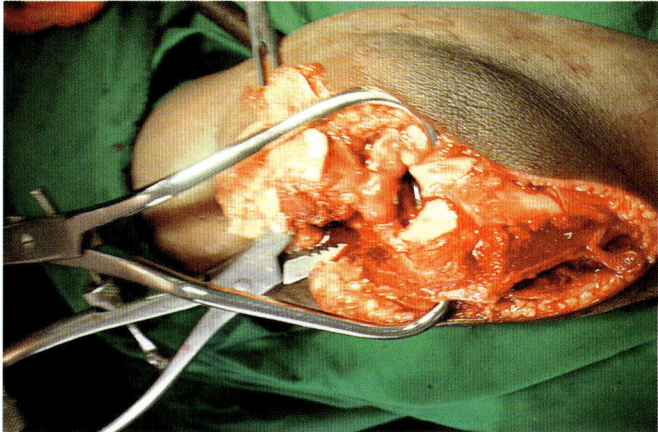

Fig. 50.77: Reduction of the fracture

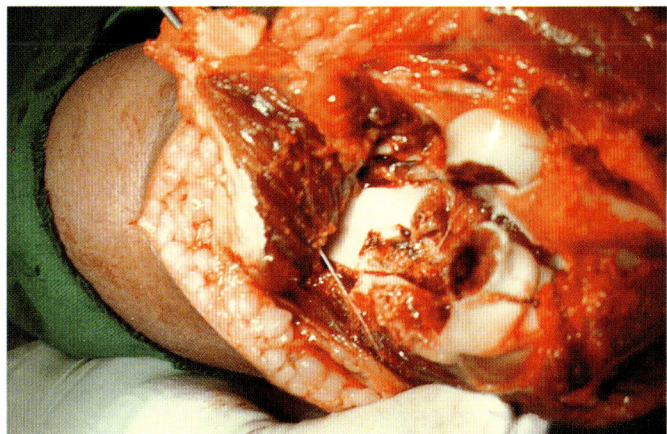

Fig. 50.75: Assembling the fracture fragments

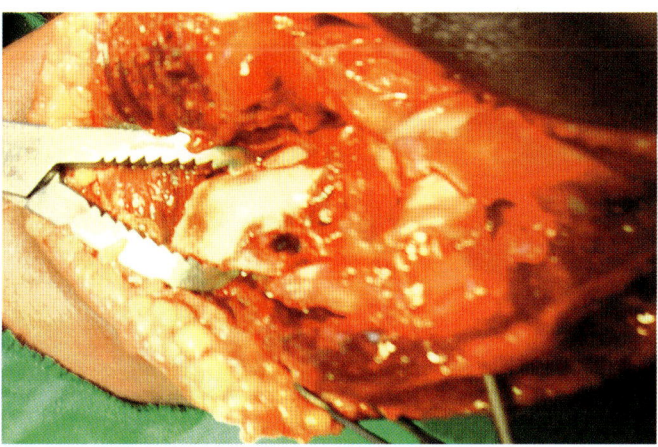

Fig. 50.78: Reconstruction of the fracture

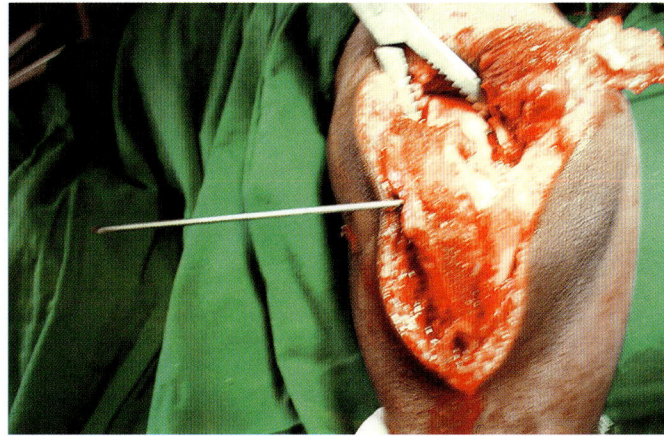

Fig. 50.76: Temporary stabilization with K-wires

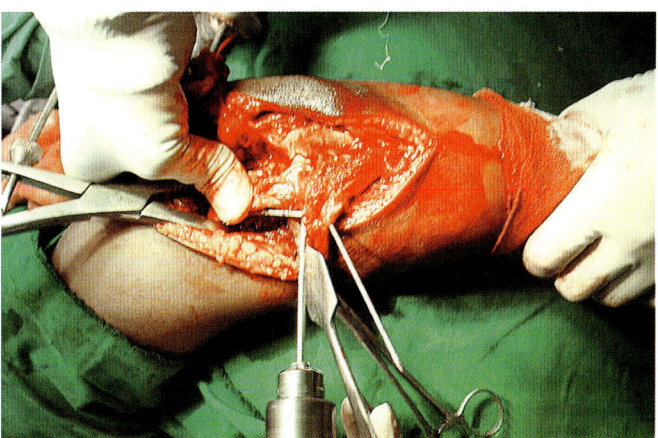

Fig. 50.79: Drilling for the screws

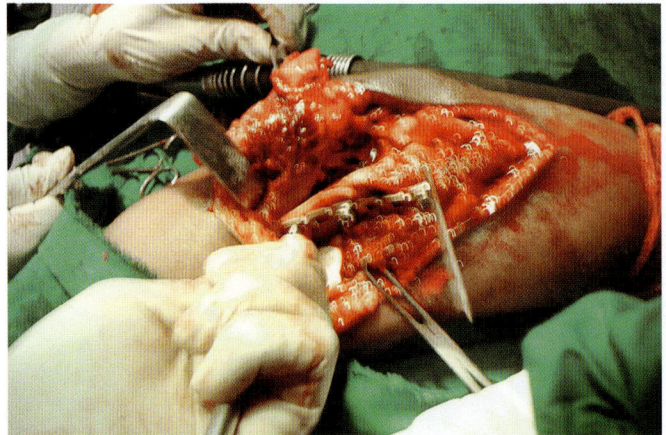

Fig. 50.80: Placement of plate on the other side

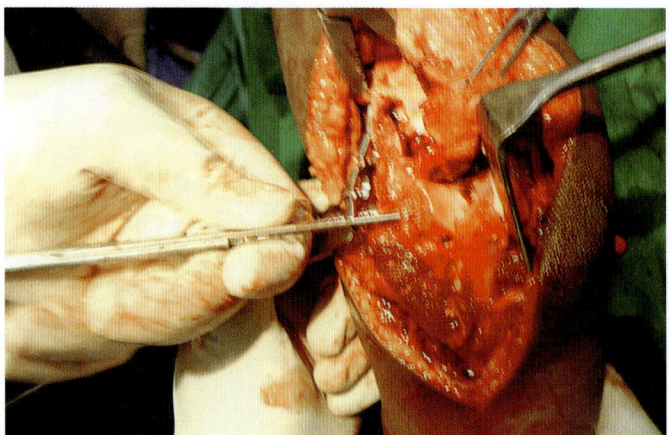

Fig. 50.83: Placement of the plate and screws

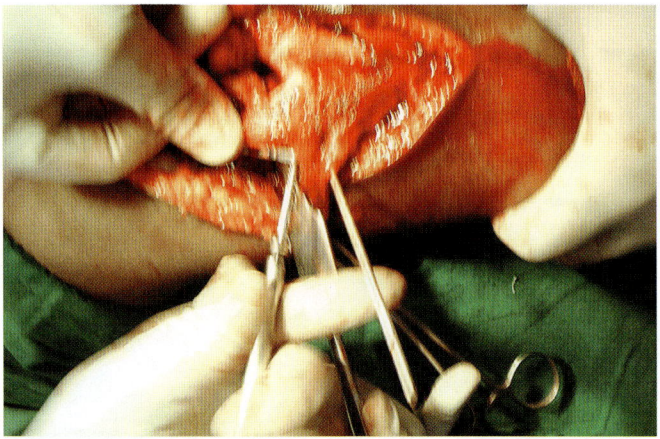

Fig. 50.81: Passing the interfragmentary screws

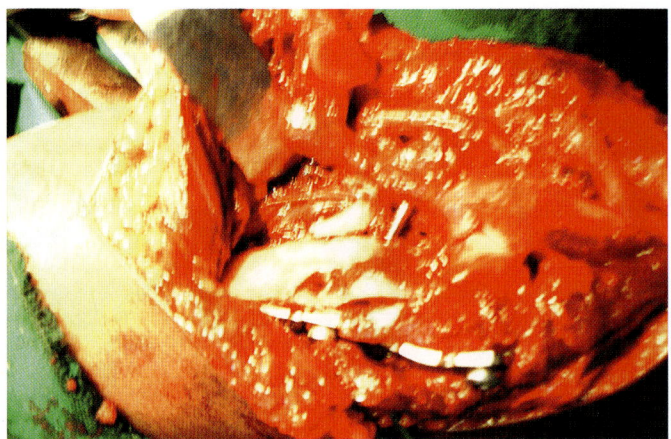

Fig. 50.84: Checking for the stability

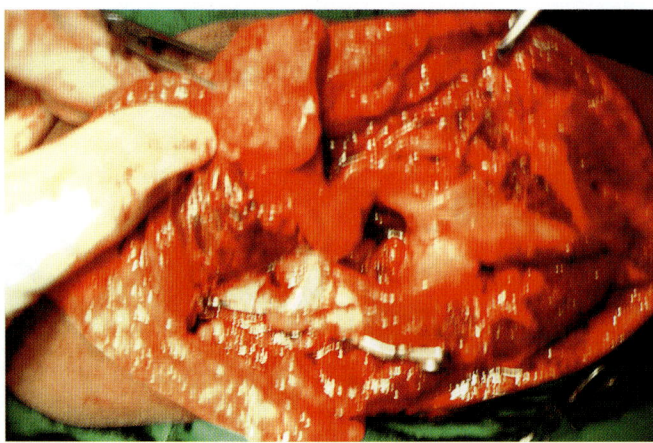

Fig. 50.82: Final construct

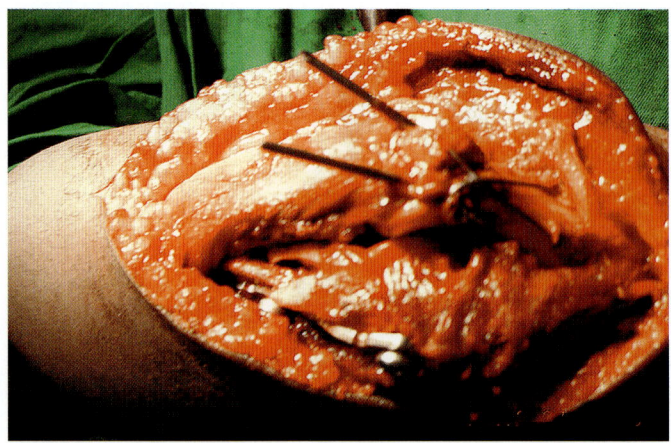

Fig. 50.85: Tension band wiring for olecranon osteotomy

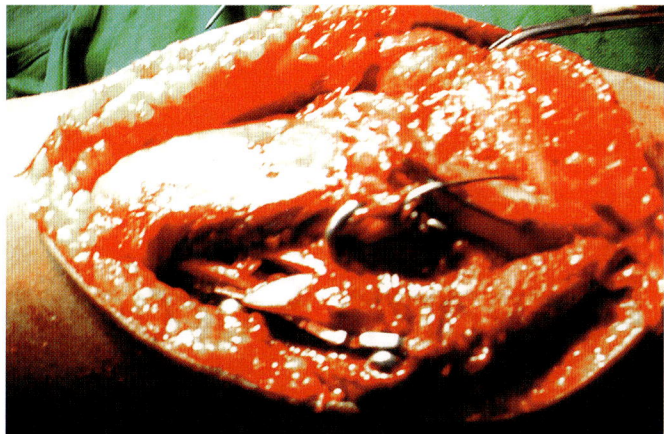

Fig. 50.86: Final reconstruction of the fracture

- By the end of 7th day, gentle active and active-assisted exercises are commenced by removing the splint. It may be reapplied after the exercises.
- By 3 weeks the posterior splint is removed and the exercises are carried out.
- Avoid forceful passive manipulation of the elbow.

51 CHAPTER

Common Forearm Surgeries

EXCISION OF THE RADIAL HEAD

Indications
Comminuted fracture of the head of the radius.

Approach
Posterolateral approach.

Steps
- Make a posterolateral incision from 5 cm distal to the head extending over the radial head and lateral humeral condyle.
- Through the interval between the anconeus and extensor carpi ulnaris muscles expose the fracture.
- Thoroughly irrigate the joint to remove all the debris, blood clots and bone pieces.
- Reflect the periosteum and slowly extricate the head out by carefully leverage.
- Resect the remains of the annular ligament.
- Ensure every piece of the fracture head is removed and check it under C-arm.
- Suture the adjacent soft tissues over the raw end of the bone.
- Close the wound in layers over a drain.

Aftercare
- An above elbow slab is applied with elbow at 90 degrees.
- After 1 week, the splint is removed and the arm is supported in a sling.
- Active and active assisted exercises are now begun.
- Sling is discarded after 3 weeks.
- Step up the exercises to the upper arm gradually.

FOREARM DCP PLATING

Indications
Fracture both bones in adults or fracture radius shaft or ulna.

Approaches
- *Dorsal approach:* This is for fracture ulna.
- *Thompson's approach:* This is fracture of proximal radius.
- *Anterior approach:* This is for distal radius fractures.

Surgical Steps (Figs 51.1 to 51.11)
- Patient is under general anesthesia.
- A pneumatic tourniquet is applied to the upper arm.

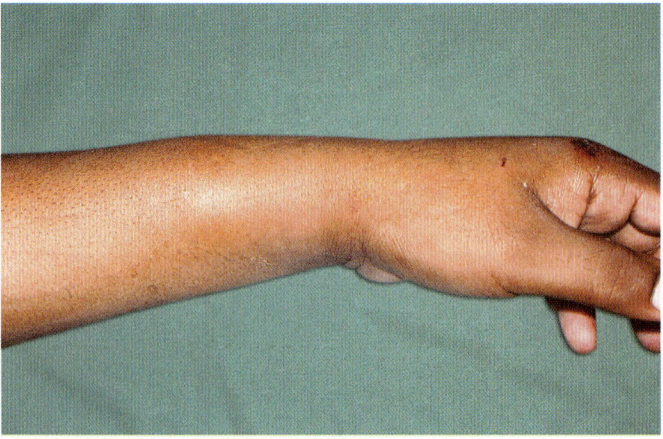

Fig. 51.1: Deformity from the sides (Clinical photo)

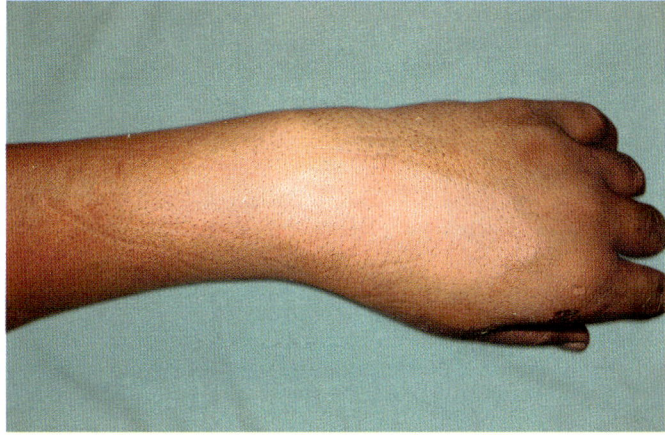

Fig. 51.2: Deformity from above (Clinical photo)

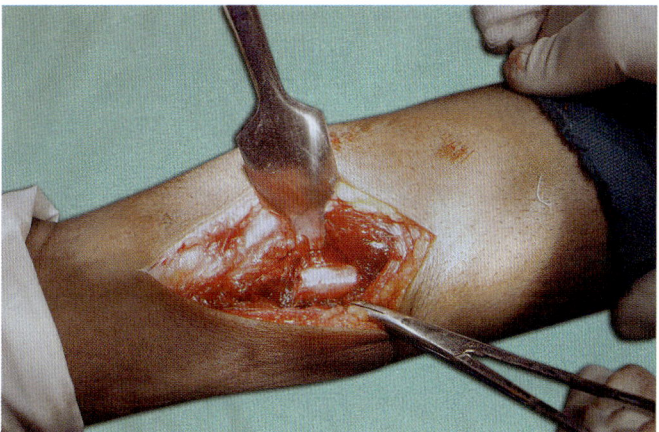

Fig. 51.5: Exposure of the radius

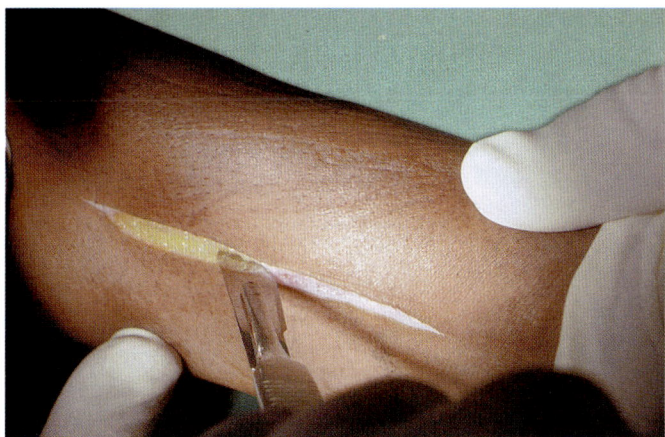

Fig. 51.3: Anterolateral approach

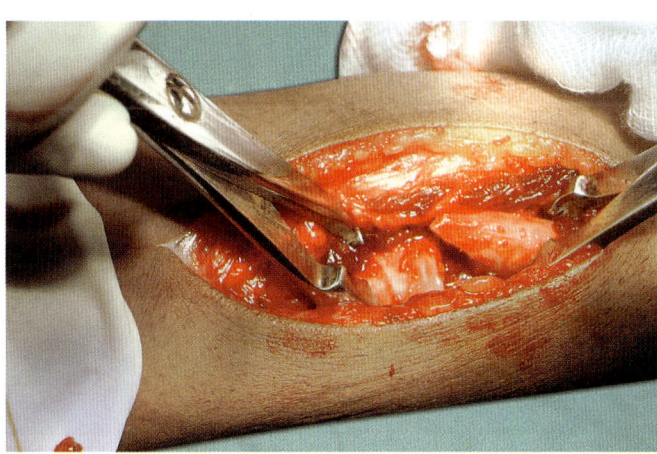

Fig. 51.6: Exposure of the fracture

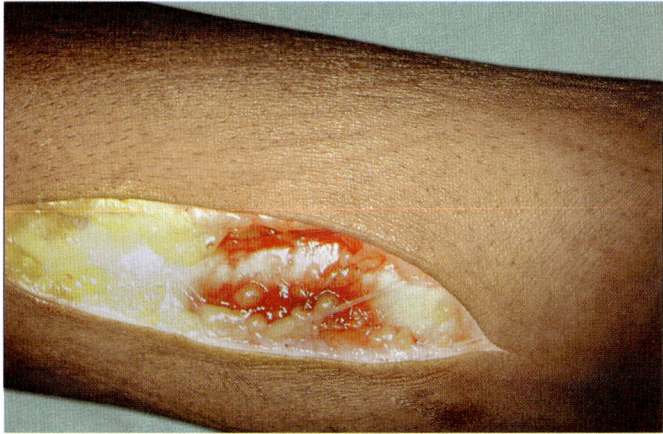

Fig. 51.4: Deep dissection

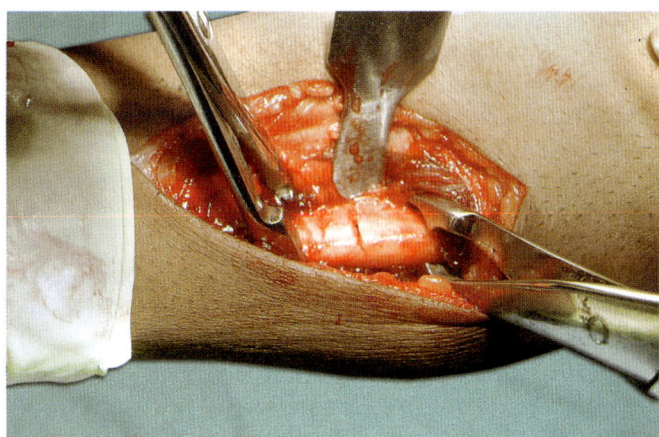

Fig. 51.7: Reduction of the fracture

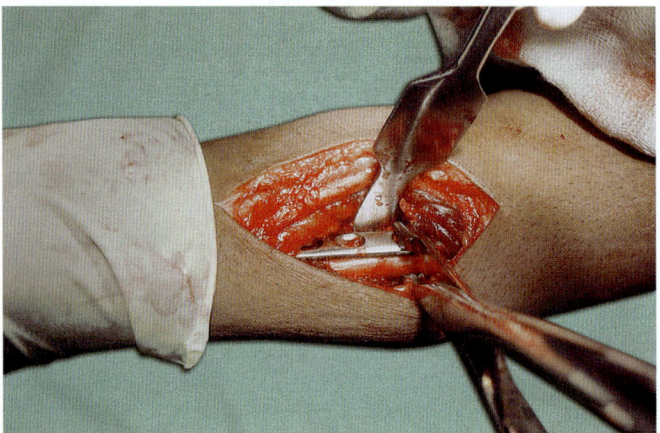

Fig. 51.8: Placement of the plate

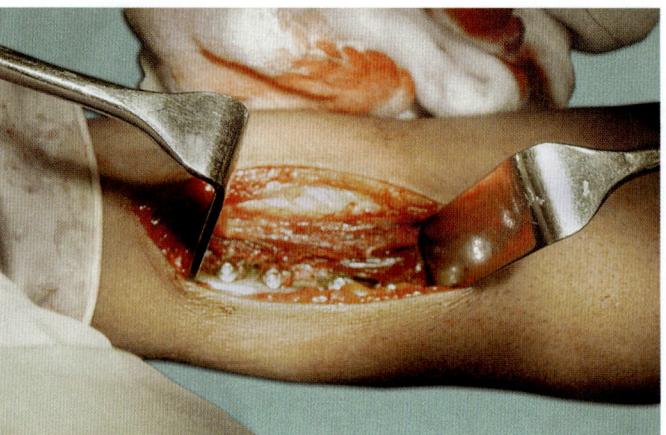

Fig. 51.10: Final placement of plate and screws

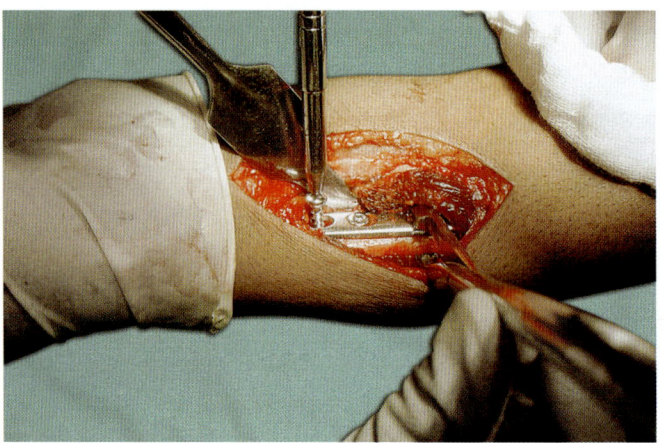

Fig. 51.9: Placement of the cortical screw

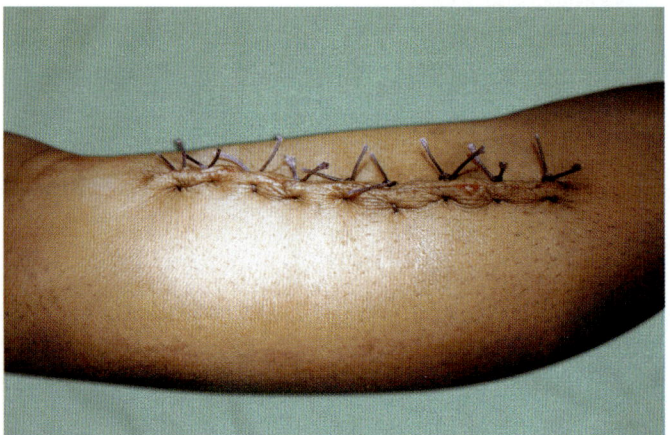

Fig. 51.11: Skin closure

- The part is prepared and draped.
- Expose the ulna first through a 10 cm dorsal incision directly over the subcutaneous border of the ulna centered over the fracture.
- Develop an interval between the flexor carpi ulnaris and extensor carpi ulnaris muscles and incise the periosteum.
- Curette the medullary canal and the fracture serrations to freshen it.
- Attempt to reduce the fracture ulna now.
- Now expose the radius either through a Thompson's approach or Dorsal approach depending on the level of the fractures.
- Expose the fracture radius and deliver it outside the wound.
- Curette the fracture ends and medullary canal with a curette.
- Reduce the fracture radius and hold it with bone holding forceps.
- Decide to fix that fracture first that has less communition and more stable configuration.
- For radius fracture select a 5-holed plate. If the fracture is more comminuted select a longer plate.
- If the fracture is in the proximal half, the plate has to be placed on the dorsal side. If the plate is in the distal half place it on the velar side.
- Using a bone holding forceps, hold the plate in position.
- Place the neutral drill guide in the hole nearest to the fracture site. The neutral guide directs the drill into the exact center of the plate hole.
- The eccentric drill guide locates the drill hole 1 mm off center in the slot of the plate hole always from the fracture. Note that the arrow on the eccentric guide should always point towards the fracture.

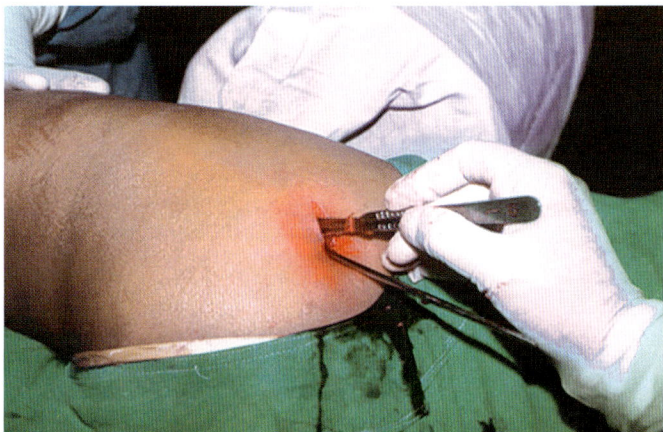

Fig. 53.6: Trochanteric entry: Step number 2

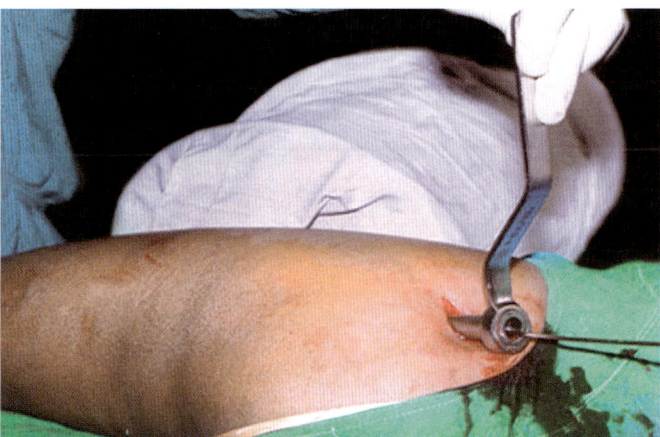

Fig. 53.7: Trochanteric entry: Step number 3

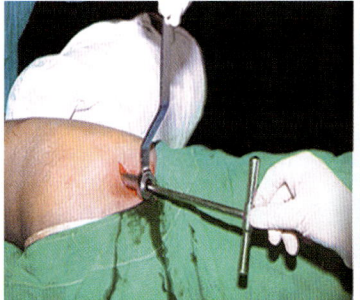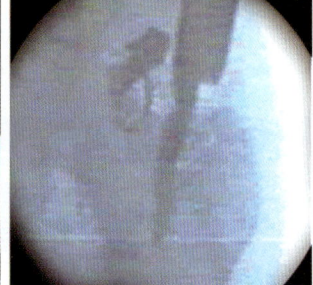

Fig. 53.8: Trochanteric entry: Step number 4

- The piriformis fossa is identified.
- After making a opening in the bone through a bone awl, a guidewire is passed and its position checked in the C-arm.
- If the guidewire is in proper position, it is advanced gently into the distal fragment.
- Manipulation of the fracture is done if there is difficulty in negotiating the guidewire through the fracture.

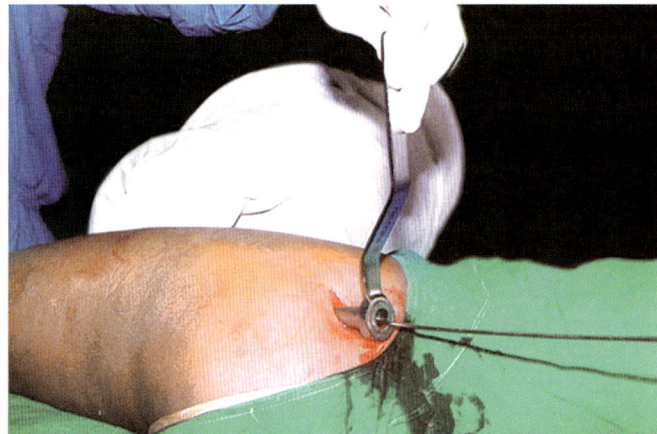

Fig. 53.9: With the sleeve held in place remove the reamer and insert the ball-tipped guidewire. The sleeve helps in locating the entry hole in all the initial steps. The skin incision in small

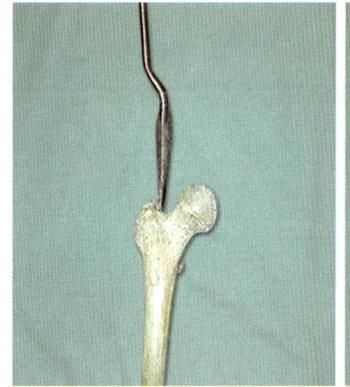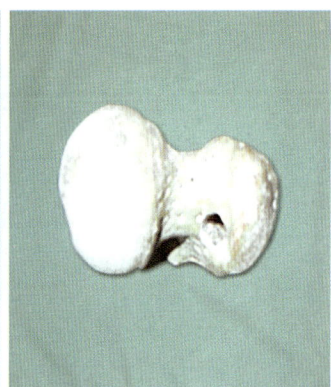

Fig. 53.10: Entry into pyriform fossa shown on bone model

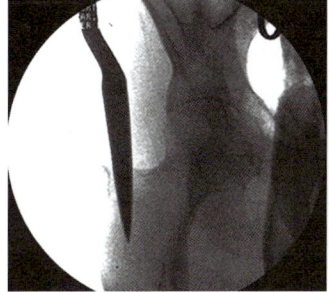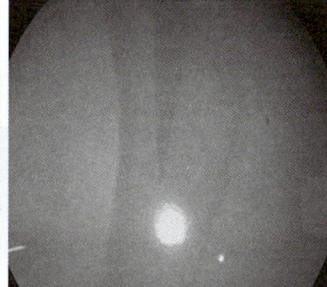

Fig. 53.11: Sharp bone awl inserted under C-arm control, confirmed on both views: Beaded guidewire inserted into the hole created

- Appropriate sized flexible reamers are passed through the guidewire and the femoral canal is reamed.
- Select the appropriate sized interlocking nail.
- Select the nail diameter equal or 1 size more than or equal to the reamer to provide a snug fit.

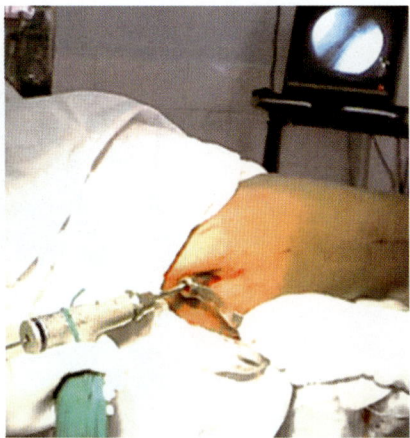

Fig. 53.12: Powered reamer introduced on the guidewire: Reaming is done at least 1 mm more than the chosen nail diameter

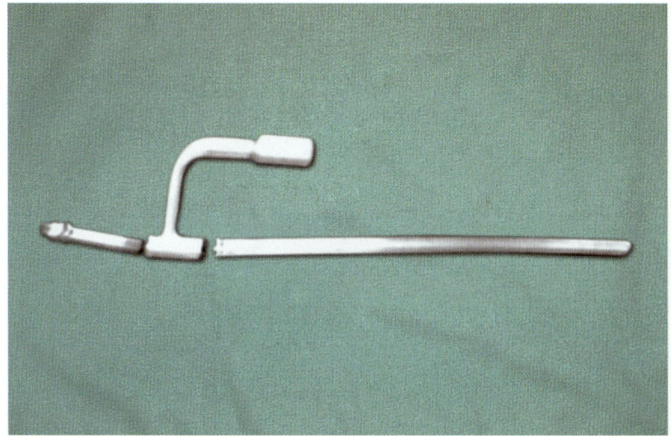

Fig. 53.15: Nail proximal jig assembly

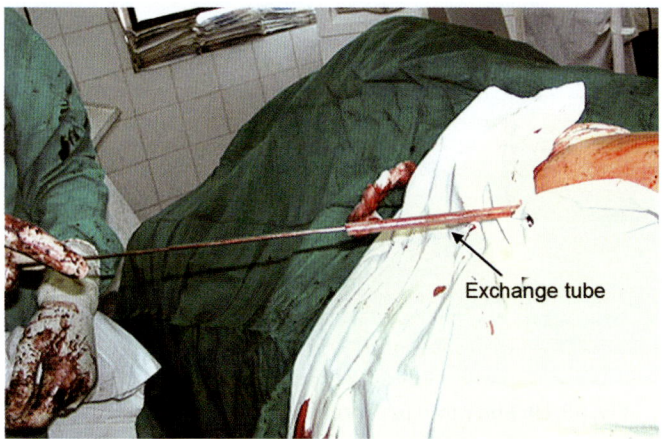

Fig. 53.13: Replace the ball-tipped guidewire with a smooth guidewire using an exchange tube

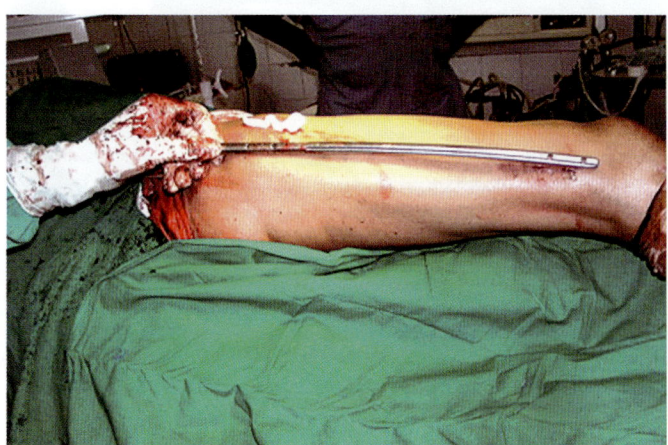

Fig. 53.16: Orientation of the nail

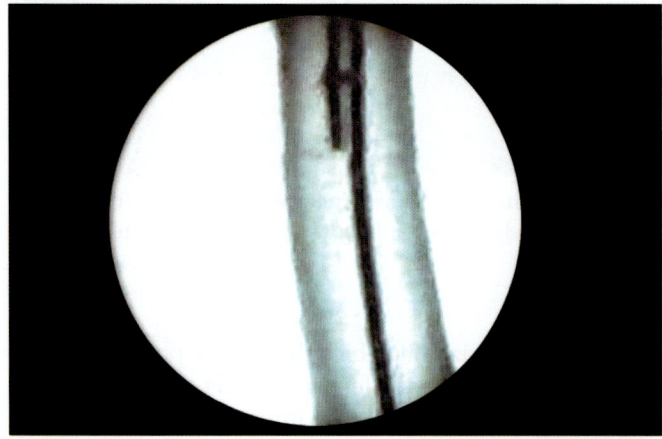

Fig. 53.14: If exchange tube is not available: A smooth guidewire can be inserted by the side and the beaded one removed

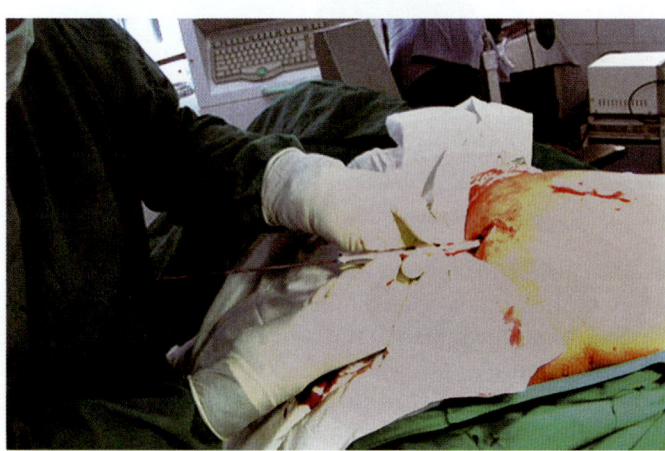

Fig. 53.17: Introduce nail only first and then fit the proximal jig

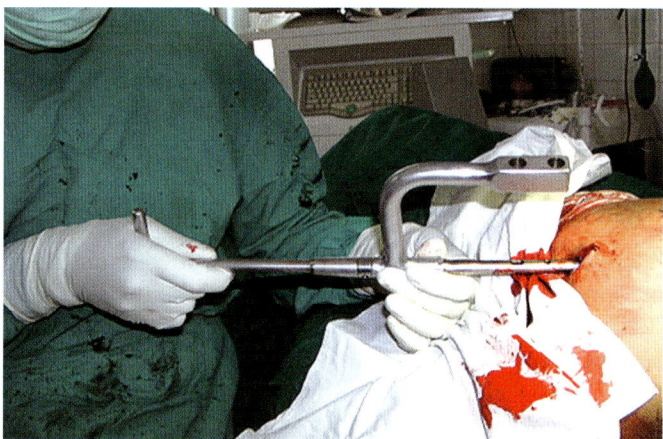

Fig. 53.18: Nail jig assembly to be pushed with hand or gentle hamering: No hard blows

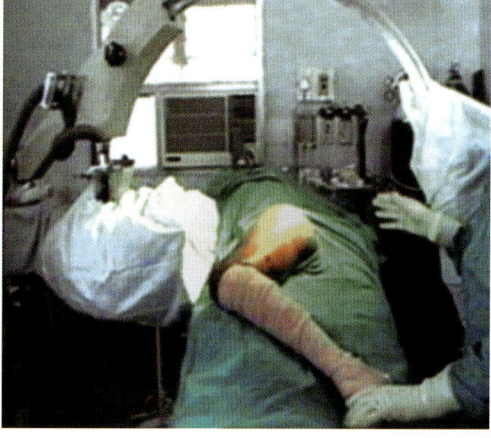

Fig. 53.21: C-arm to be adjusted that the tube is near, camera away from the patient for a magnified image

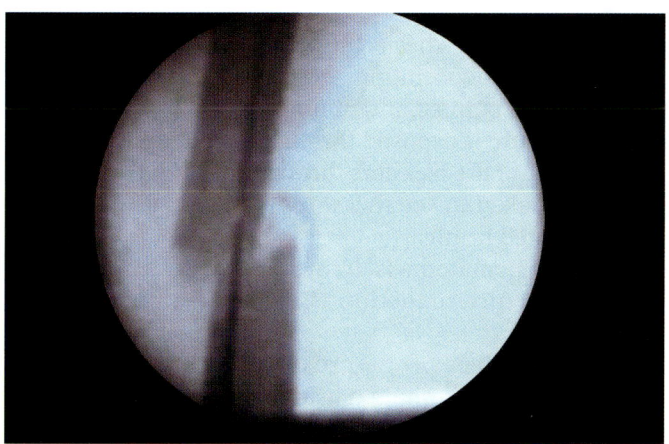

Fig. 53.19: At the fracture site, negotiate the nail into the distal fragment, not to be hammered: One can imagine what will happen when a nail is hammered into the distal fragment, when the guidewire is as shown in the figure; the cortex will be shattered

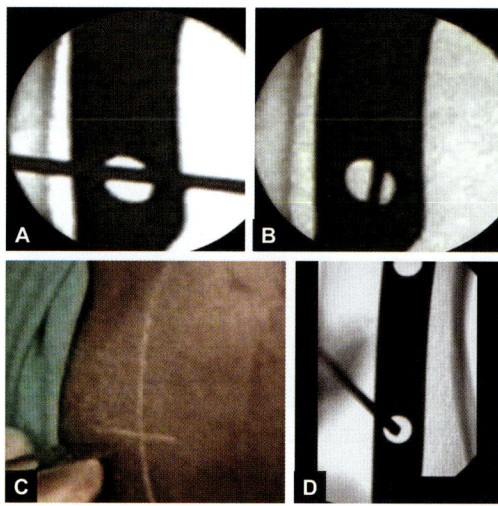

Figs 53.22A to D: Locating the distal hole. Incision made at the junction of the 2 axes: (A) K-wire X-axis; (B) K-wire Y-axis; (C) Skin markings made; (D) Distal hole

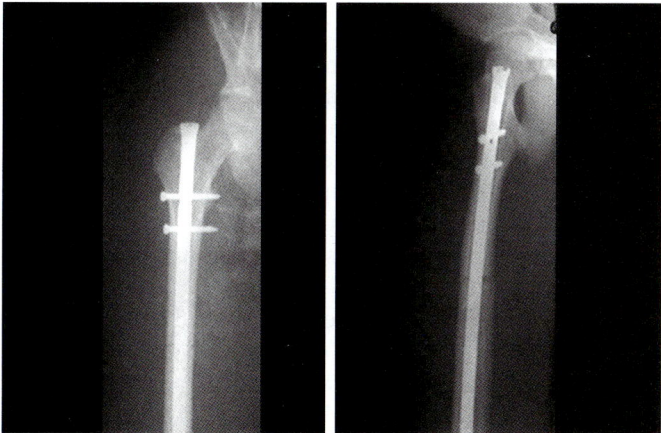

Fig. 53.20: Push the nail till the proximal tip is flush with the trochanter tip

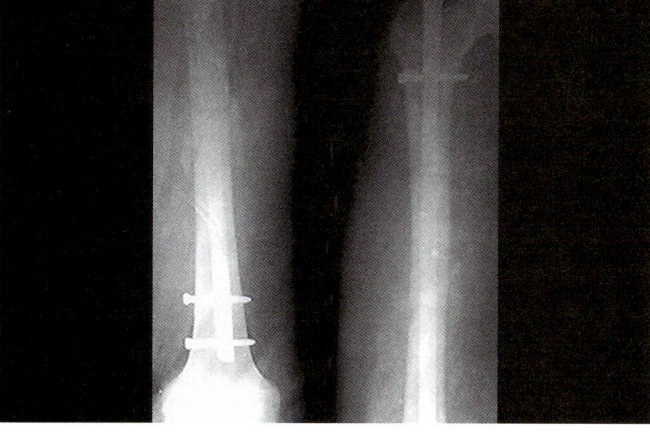

Fig. 53.23: Distal locking done: In the cortical bone preferred proximal dynamic locking: Note screw in upper part of the oval hole

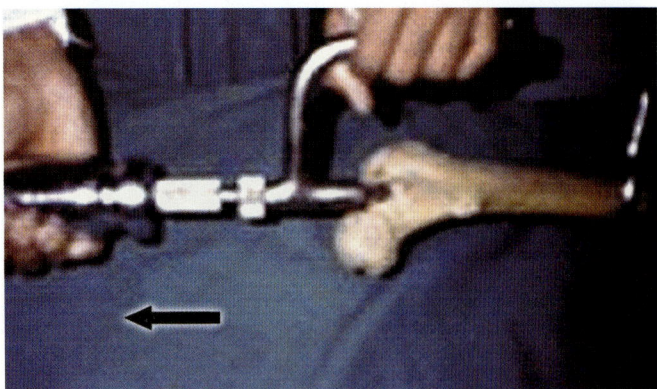

Fig. 53.24: Showing a few back slipping strokes to compress the fracture to avoid any gap at fracture site

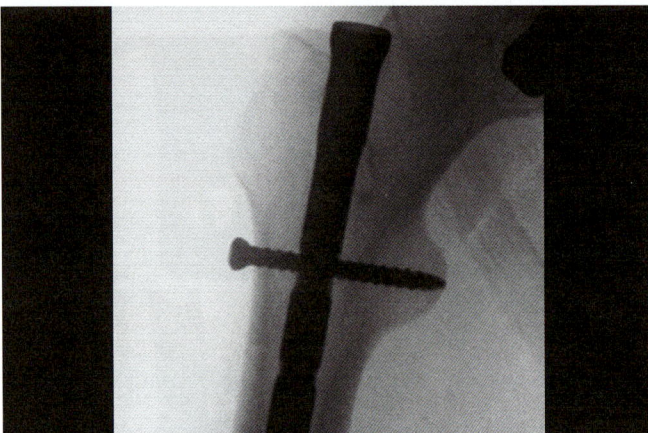

Fig. 53.25: Proximal locking

- Now pass the nail through the proximal fragment in a antegrade manner.
- Now reduce and hold both the fracture fragments and drive the nail down into the distal fragment.
- Two proximal interlocking screws are passed under the guidance of C-arm.
- Then the distal interlocking screws are passed and confirmed with C-arm.
- Close the wound in layers.

Aftercare

- Patient can be permitted to move the operated limb on the next day.
- Active and active assisted exercises for the hip and knee are done next.
- Bedside standing with a walker can be permitted after the removal of sutures.
- Walker support to be used for walking for at least 3–4 weeks.
- Weight-bearing can be permitted at the end of 6 weeks.

DCP PLATING

Indications

Fracture shaft of the femur at various levels including proximal and distal third. Not preferred as the first line. Replaced widely by interlocking nailing and has limited applications.

Approach

Mid-lateral approach.

Surgical Steps

- After spinal anesthesia, the patient is either put in lateral or semilateral position.
- The part is painted and draped.
- The fracture is exposed through careful dissection and arresting of the bleeders through the lateral approach.
- Care is taken to see that the perforators are identified and ligated firmly.
- Fracture hematoma is drained
- Trial fracture reduction is carried out under direct vision.
- Now the edges of the proximal and then the distal fragments are freshened using curettes.
- The fracture is now reduced and held firmly by bone clamps.
- Use a special drill guide for placement of screws. The neutral guide centers the screw at the bottom of the obliquely inclined hole. The load drill guide locates the screw 1 mm eccentrically in the oblique portion of the screw hole.
- Using a 3.2 mm drill bit, drill a hole in the neutral drill hole nearest to the fracture line.
- Tap the hole with a T-tap and insert the first screw. This screw will assume a neutral position with the screw hole.
- Using a local guide, drill a hole next to the fracture in the opposite fragment. Tap it, insert a screw and as it is being tightened, the fracture is compressed.
- Now insert the remaining screws one after another using the neutral guide.
- The outermost distal screws at each end of the plate may be inserted through only one cortex to distribute the forces evenly at the plate ends.
- Check for the stability of the fracture fixation.

- Close the wound in layers over a drain after giving a thorough antiseptic wash.
- Apply a pressure bandage.

Aftercare

- Patient can be permitted to move the operated limb on the next day.
- Active and active assisted exercises for the hip and knee are done next.
- Bedside standing with a walker can be permitted after the removal of sutures.
- Walker support to be used for walking for at least 3–4 months.
- Weight-bearing can be permitted at the end of 8–12 weeks.

54 CHAPTER

Common Surgery of the Patella

PATELLECTOMY

Indications

Comminuted fracture of the Patella.

Approach

Transverse approach.

Surgical Steps

- Put a transverse curved incision about 12.5 cm approximately with the apex of the curve on the distal fragment.
- Expose the anterior surface of the patella and the quadriceps and patellar tendon.
- Give a thorough wash and clear the joint of all loose fragments of bone, cartilage and blood clots.
- Trim away the edges of the capsule and tendon and inspect the trochlear groove of the femur for damages.
- Excise the communized fragments of patella in severe communition.
- *Partial patellectomy:* If only proximal or distal pole is fractured or if less than half of the patella is intact, try to preserve the patella by excising only the badly communized fragments. Using an 18 mm stainless steel wire a purse string suture is applied through the margins of the patellar and quadriceps tendons through the medial and lateral capsular expansions. Tighten the wire with a wire tightened and evaginate the tendon ends completely outside the joint till it makes a circle of about 2 cm in diameter. Twist it firmly and cut it off at the twist, embedding its ends in the quadriceps tendon. This will give the appearance of a small patella.
- Repair the capsular ends with an interrupted suture and appose the quadriceps and patellar tendons.
- Close the wound in layers over a suction drain.

Aftercare

- Apply a long posterior slab from groin to ankle.
- After 3–4 days, quadriceps strengthening exercises can be commenced.
- After 2 weeks, sutures are removed and a cylindrical cast is applied.
- Ambulation can be permitted over a crutch.
- After 3 weeks, commence gentle active and active assisted exercises.
- Discard the crutches after 6–8 weeks.
- Wires can be removed after the fractures have united.

TENSION BAND WIRING (MODIFIED)

Indications

For transverse fractures of patella.

Approach

Anterior approach through a transverse incision as described above.

Surgical Steps (Figs 54.1 to 54.10)

- The first four steps are as described for patellectomy previously.
- Reduce the major proximal and distal fragments accurately and attempt to restore smooth particular surface.

- With the reduced fracture firmly held with clamps, drill two 2.4 mm K-wires from inferior to superior. Through each fragment as parallel as possible.
- Leave the ends of the wires long protruding beyond the patella.
- Now pass a strand of 18 gauze wire transversely through the quadriceps tendon attachment, as closer to the bone as possible, deep to the protruding K-wires, over the anterior surface of the patella, then transversely through the patellar tendon attachment on the inferior fragment and deep to the K-wires, then back over the anterior patellar surface, tighten it at the upper end.
- Pass a second 18 gauze wire loop deep for the protruding wires over the anterior surface of there patella and tighten it firmly.
- Now bend the upper ends of the second K-wire acutely interiorly and cut them short. After cutting, rotate the K-wires 180 degrees, using an impactor; bury the bent ends into the superior margin of the patella posterior to the wire loops.
- Cuts the protruding ends of the K-wires short at the inferior side.
- Repair the retinacular tears with interrupted sutures.
- Close the wound in layers over a suction drain.

Aftercare

- A plaster splint is applied from groin to ankle.
- Walking over crutches is permitted after 2–3 days.
- Gentle range of motion exercises are begun after 5–7 days.
- Isometric quadriceps exercises are started immediately after surgery.

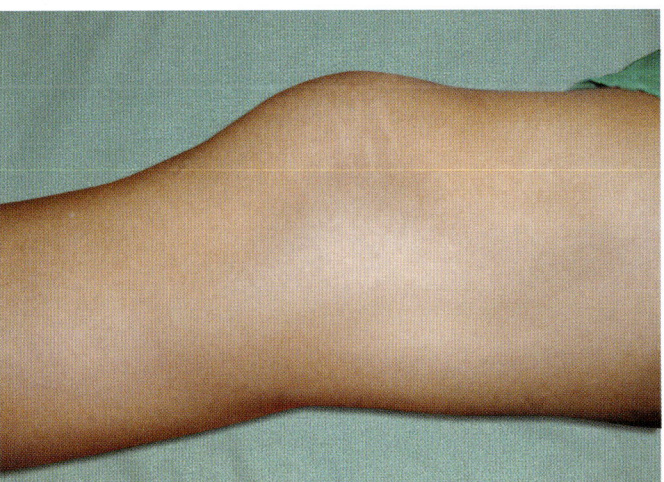

Fig. 54.1: Clinical photo

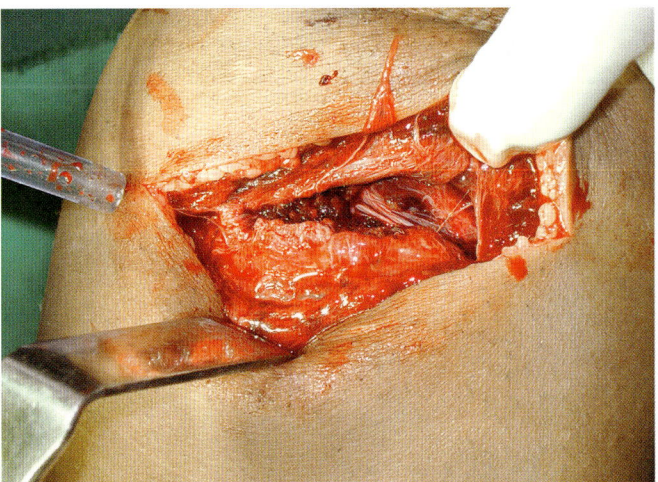

Fig. 54.3: Exposing the fracture

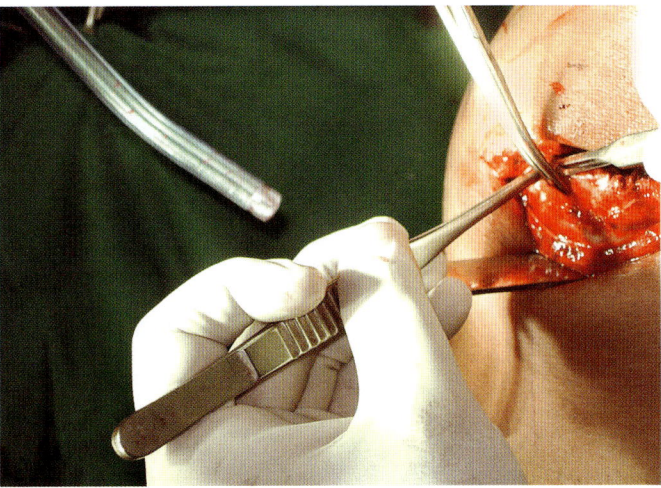

Fig. 54.2: Skin exposure

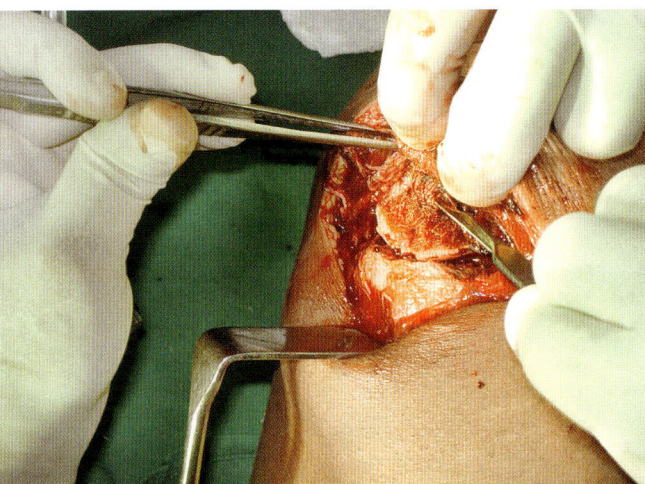

Fig. 54.4: Everting the fracture fragments

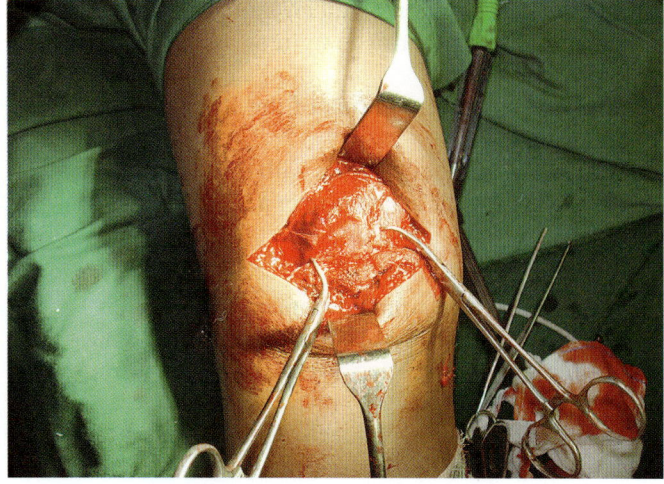

Fig. 54.5: Reduction of the fragments

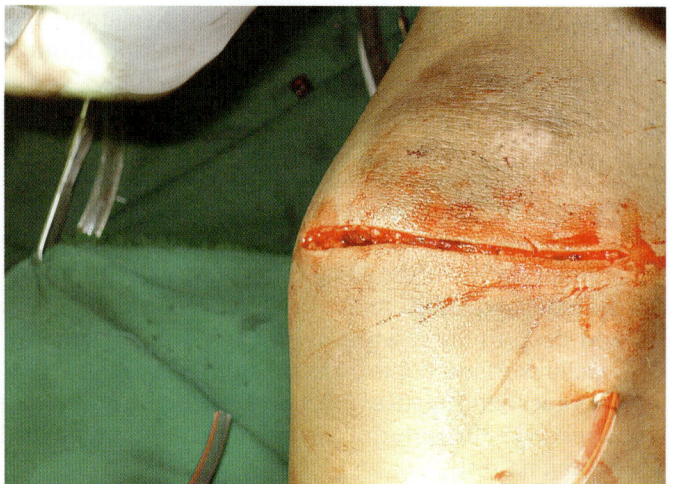

Fig. 54.8: Skin closure

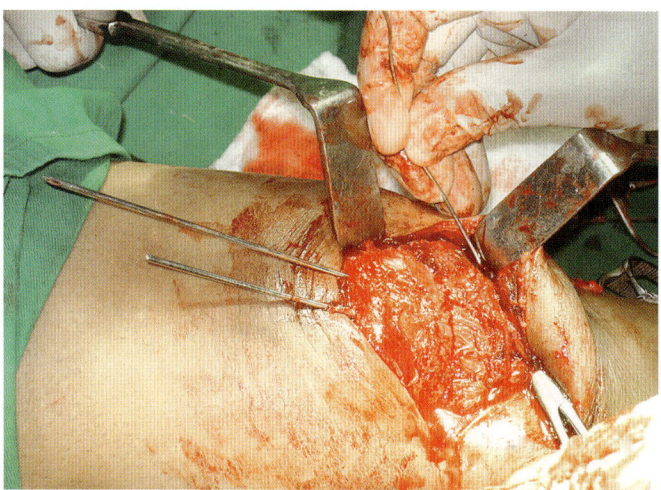

Fig. 54.6: Passing of K-wires

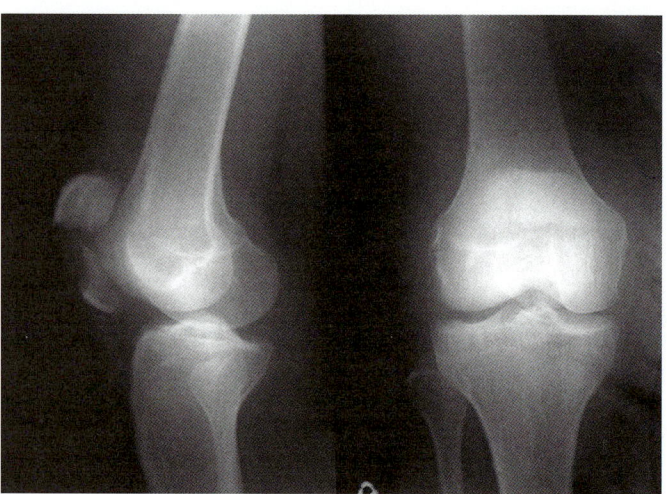

Fig. 54.9: Preoperative X-ray

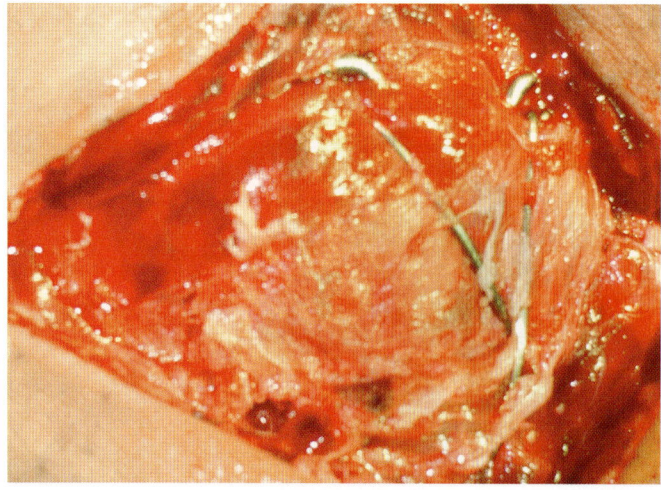

Fig. 54.7: Tension band wiring

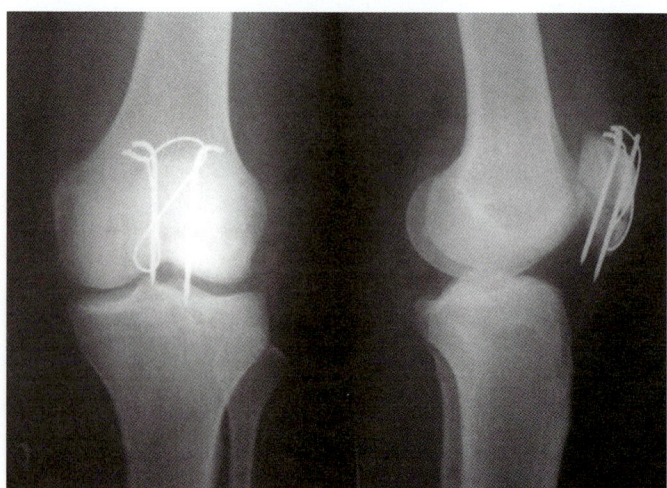

Fig. 54.10: Postoperative X-ray

55

CHAPTER

Common Surgery of the Tibia

DCP PLATING FOR TIBIA

Indications

For short oblique or transverse fractures of the tibia.

Approaches

Anterolateral approach.

Surgical Steps (Figs 55.1 to 55.20)

- Make a longitudinal incision just lateral to the tibial crest.
- Expose the fracture fragments by retracting the muscles laterally.
- Avoid excessive stripping of the periosteum but strip enough to insert a plate.
- Now reduce the fracture by traction and angulations.
- Place the DCP plate on the lateral surface of the tibia, so that it will be covered by the anterior tibial muscles.
- Hold the plate in position over the reduced fracture by two self-retaining bone holding forceps.
- Apply third forceps directly over the fracture at 90 degrees to the other two forceps. Reduce the fracture as anatomically as possible.
- If necessary contour the plate, with a special device to fit the flare of the proximal or distal metaphysis.
- A 6 holed plate is sufficient for transverse fracture but for oblique or comminuted fractures an 8 holed and above plates may be required.
- Use a special drill guide for placement of screws. The neutral guide centers the screw at the bottom of the obliquely inclined hole. The load drill guide locates the screw 1 mm eccentrically in the oblique portion of the screw hole.
- Using a 3.2 mm drill bit, drill a hole in the neutral drill hole nearest to the fracture line.
- Tap the hole with a T-taper and insert the first screw. This screw will assume a neutral position with the screw hole.
- Using a local guide, drill a hole next to the fracture in the opposite fragment. Tap it, insert a screw and as it is being tightened, the fracture is compressed.
- Now insert the remaining screws one after another using the neutral guide.
- The outermost distal screws at each end of the plate may be inserted through only one cortex to distribute the forces evenly at the plate ends.
- Close the wound in layers over a suction drain.

Surgical techniques for DCP plating for tibia as shown in Figures 55.1 to 55.20.

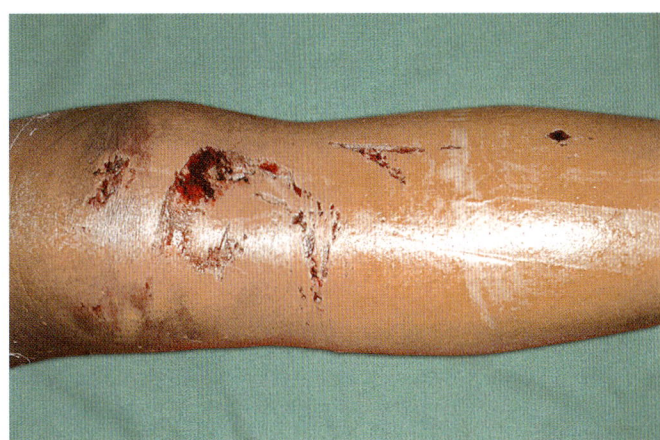

Fig. 55.1: Deformity upper leg

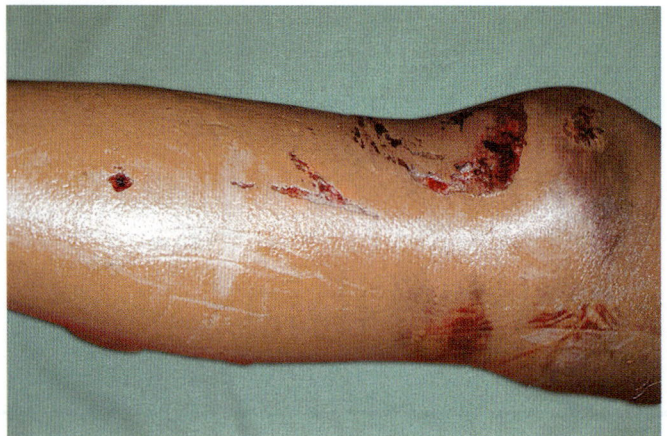

Fig. 55.2: Deformity upper leg from the sides

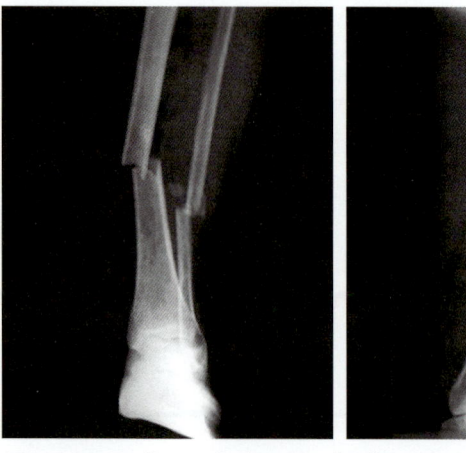

Fig. 55.5: Radiograph showing the fracture in both bones of leg

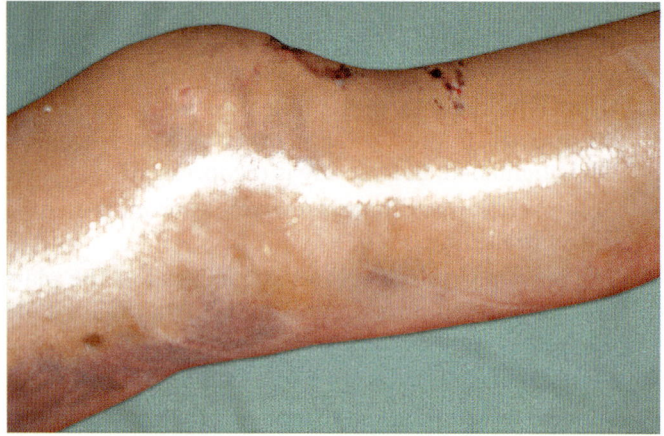

Fig. 55.3: Gross swelling of the knee

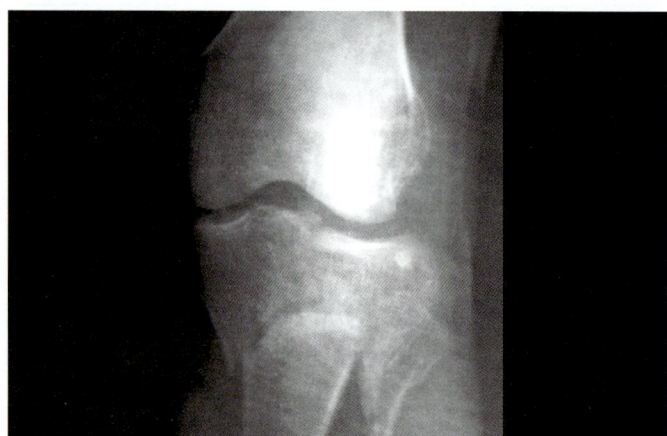

Fig. 55.6: Condylar fractures—AP view

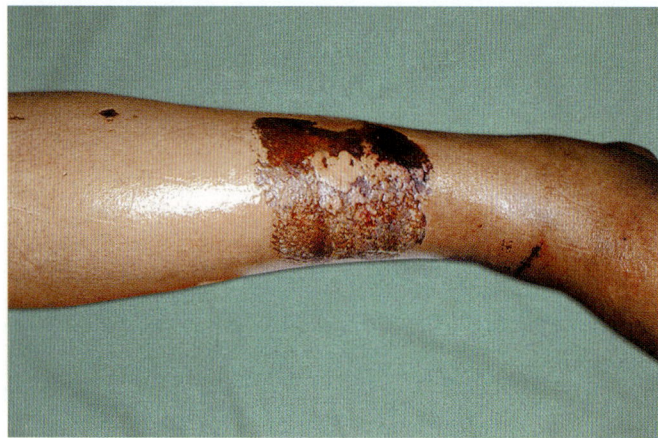

Fig. 55.4: Deformity in lower leg

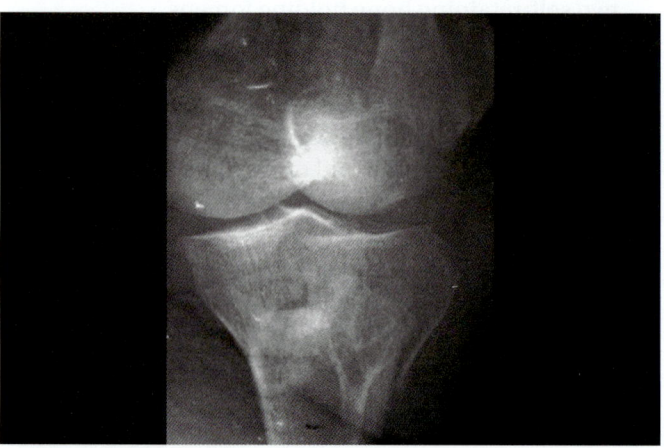

Fig. 55.7: Condylar fractures—Lateral view

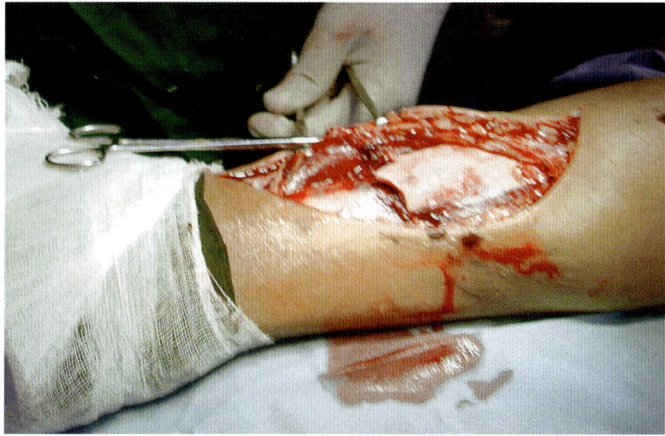

Fig. 55.8: Exposing the leg fractures through anteromedial approach

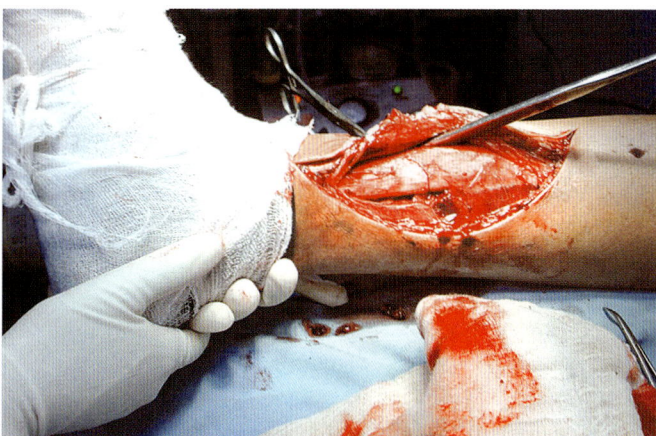

Fig. 55.11: Hairline reduction obtained

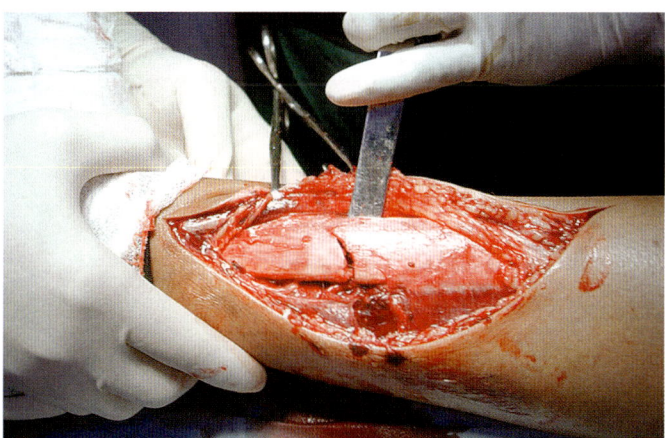

Fig. 55.9: Reduction of the fractures

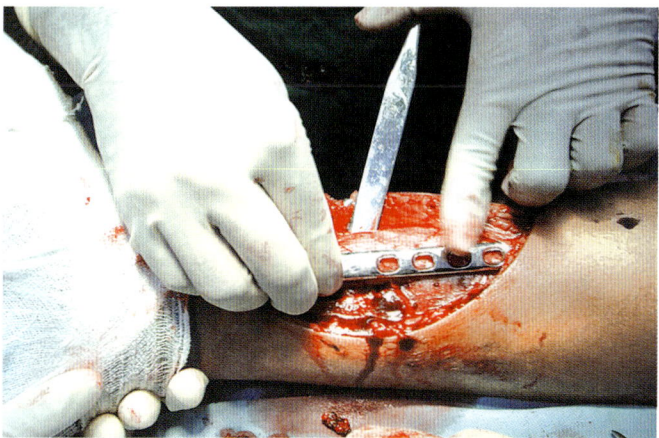

Fig. 55.12: Placement of the 8 holed DCP plate

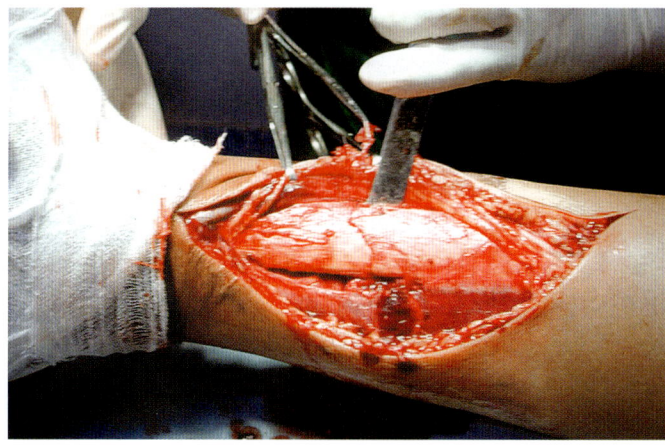

Fig. 55.10: Closer view

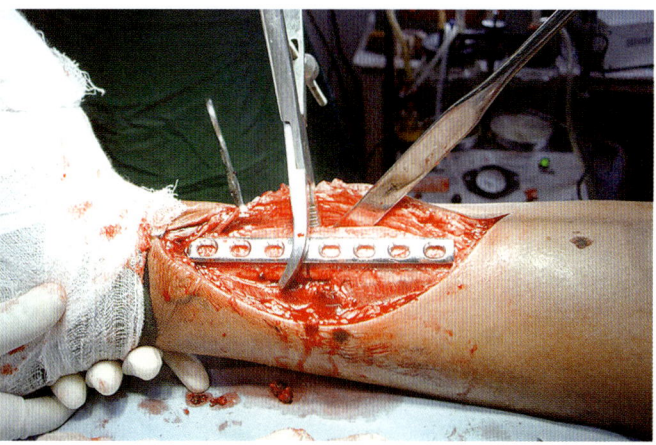

Fig. 55.13: Holding the plate on to the bone through bone clamps

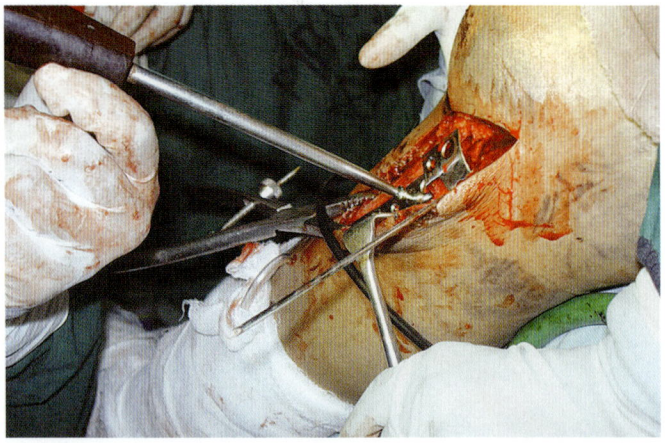

Fig. 55.14: Fixing the plate with screws after drilling and tapping

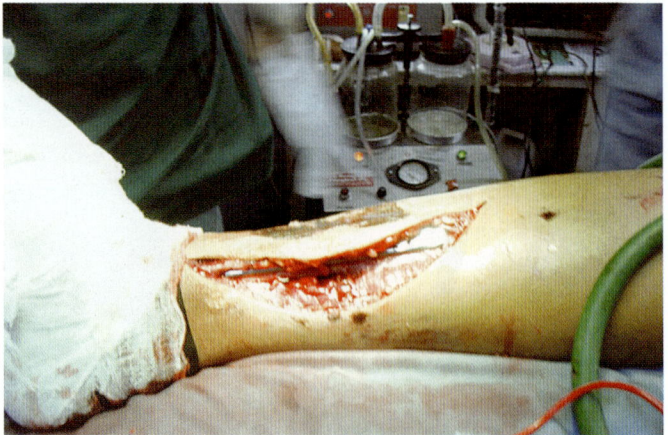

Fig. 55.17A: Closure of the wound

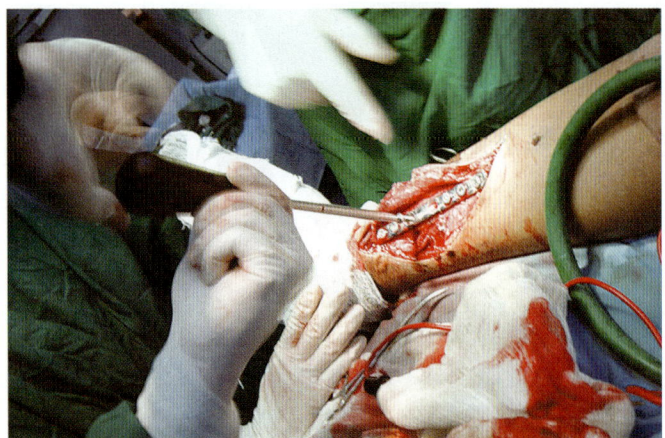

Fig. 55.15: Placing the screws one-by-one

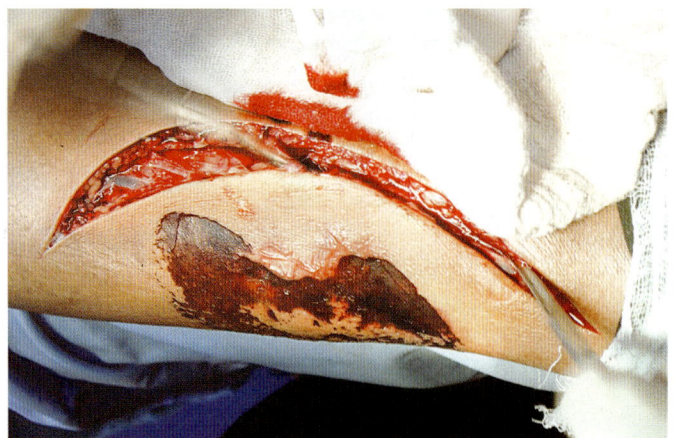

Fig. 55.17B: Placement of a Romovac drain

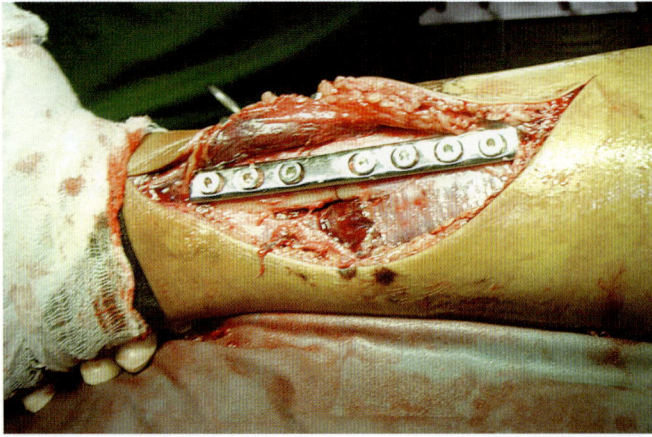

Fig. 55.16: Secure fixation with 8 screws

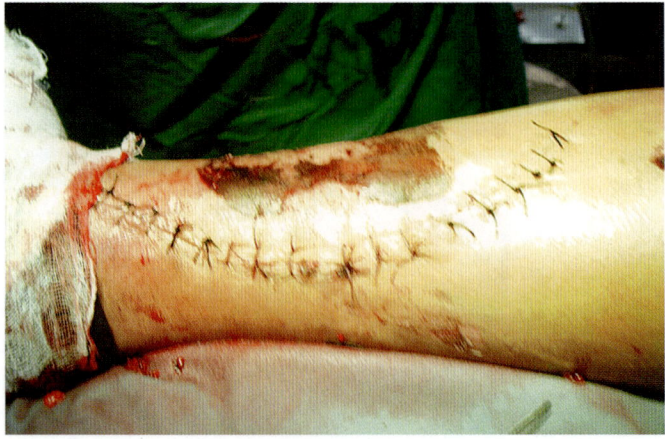

Fig. 55.18: Final skin closure

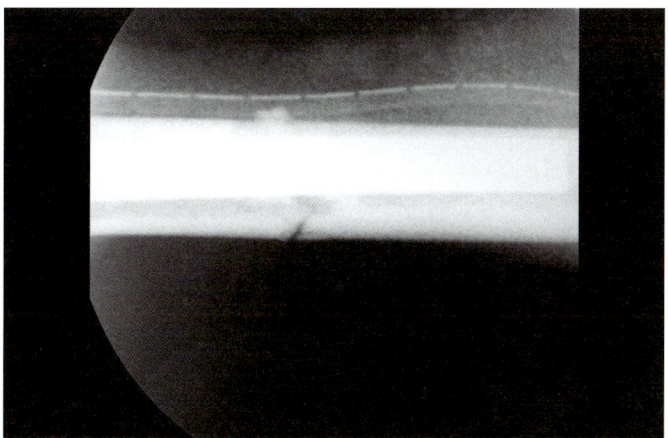

Fig. 55.19: C-arm check—lateral view

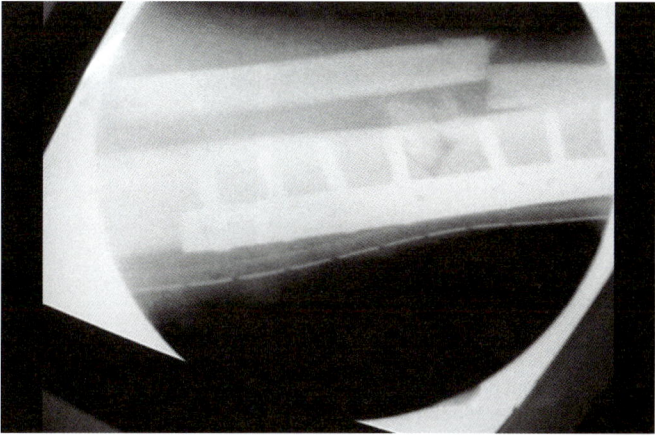

Fig. 55.20: C-arm check of plate fixation

Aftercare

- An above knee cast is applied with knee in slight flexion and the ankle in neutral position.
- This case is used for 3–4 weeks and no weight-bearing is permitted.
- Progressive weight-bearing with crutches is allowed over the next 8–10 weeks.
- Active range of movement exercises is commenced.
- Weight-bearing may be permitted after 12–14 weeks.

INTERLOCKING NAILING OF TIBIA

Indications

Fracture of the tibia in adults at different levels. It is indicated in comminuted fractures, segmental fractures, proximal and distal third fractures, etc.

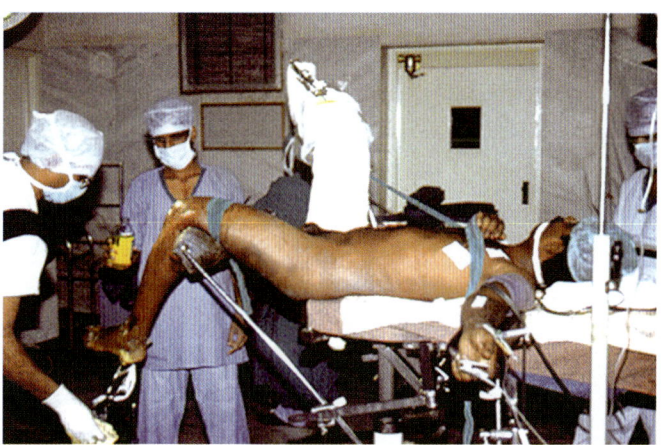

Fig. 55.21: Position of the patient: On a traction table with calcaneal traction

Surgical Steps (Figs 55.21 to 55.36)

- After spinal anesthesia the part is painted and draped.
- Closed reduction of the fracture is done by traction and manipulation.
- The accuracy of the reduction is checked by C-arm.
- A short incision is made over the upper aspect of the tibia through the mid-substance of the ligamentum patellae.
- After making a opening in the bone through a bone awl, a guidewire is passed and its position checked in the C-arm.
- If the guidewire is in proper position, it is advanced gently into the distal fragment.
- Manipulation of the fracture is done if there is difficulty in negotiating the guidewire through the fracture.

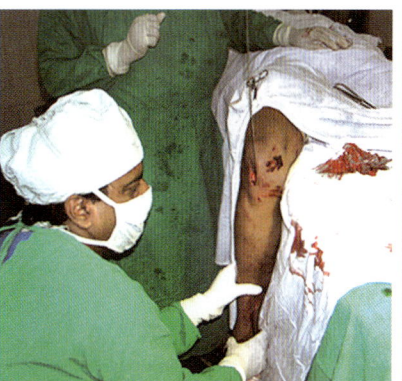 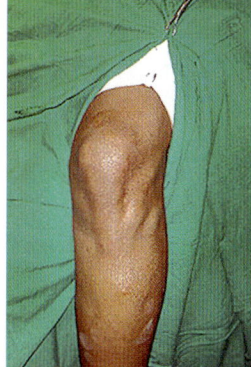

Leg hanging by the side   Or at the end

Fig. 55.22: Patient position on ordinary table

734 SECTION 7: Common Surgical Techniques

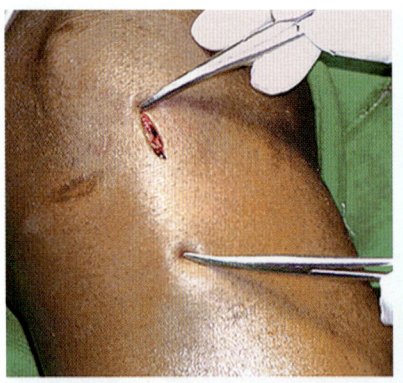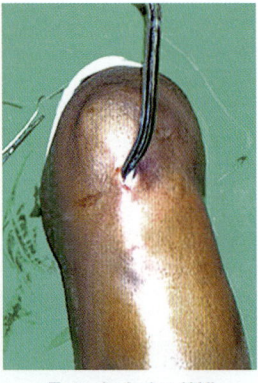

Fig. 55.23: Nail entry

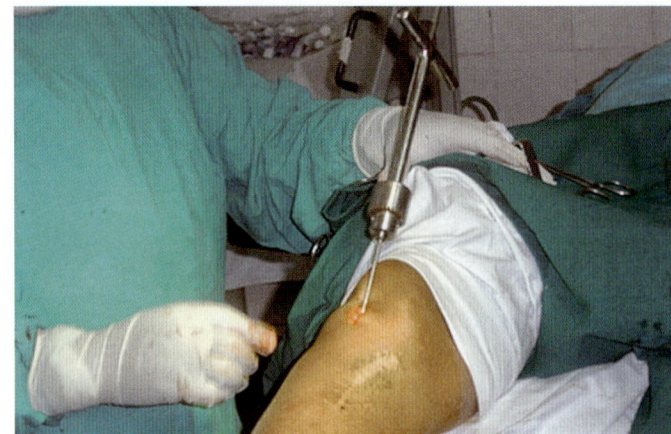

Fig. 55.26: Negotiation of guidewire

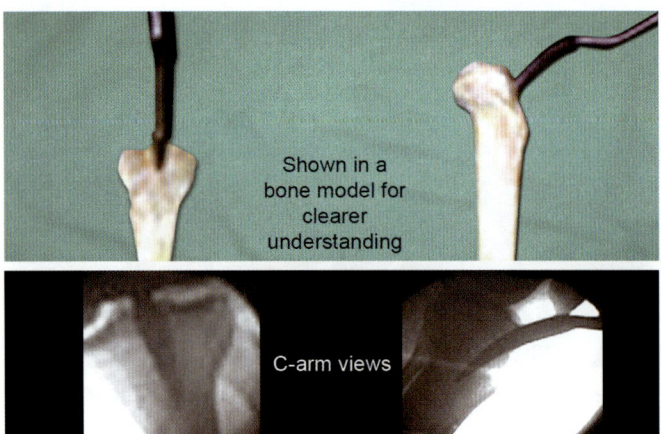

Fig. 55.24: Nail entry (Bone model)

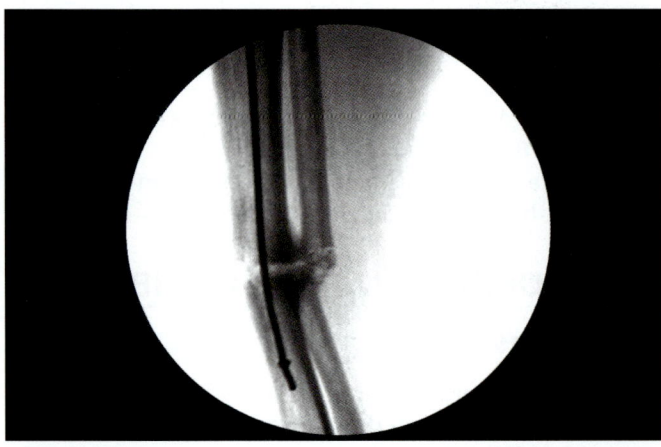

Fig. 55.27: Bend at the tip helps in negotiation of the fracture

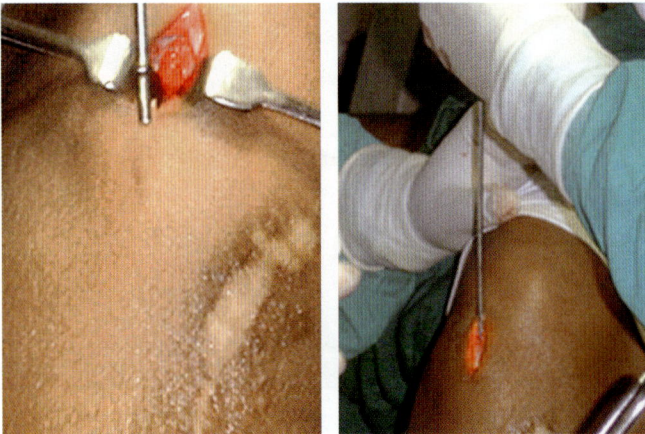

Fig. 55.25: Beaded guidewire entry: Guidewire insertion through the entry hole

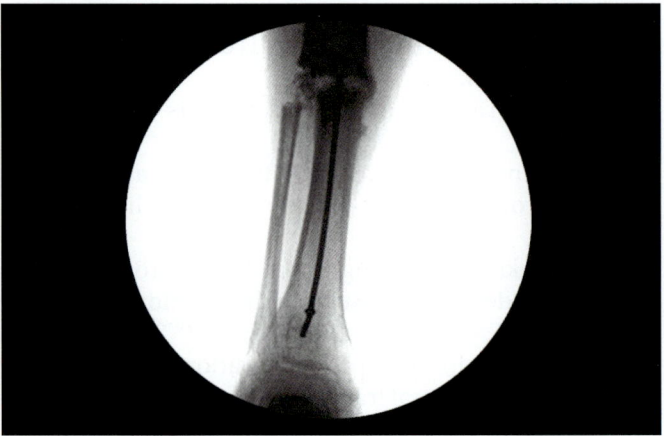

Fig. 55.28: Guidewire up to the ankle

CHAPTER 55: Common Surgery of the Tibia 735

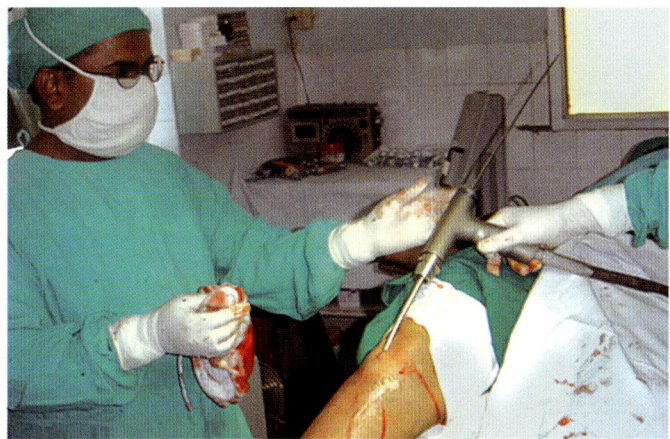

Fig. 55.29: Reaming: Clinical view

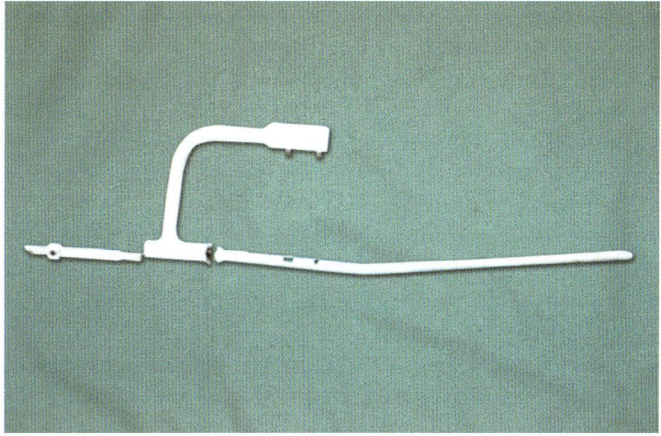

Fig. 55.32: Nail jig assembly: The Herzog bend should be posterior. The jig should be medial (in this case). The holes in the jig should overlie the proximal holes of the nail

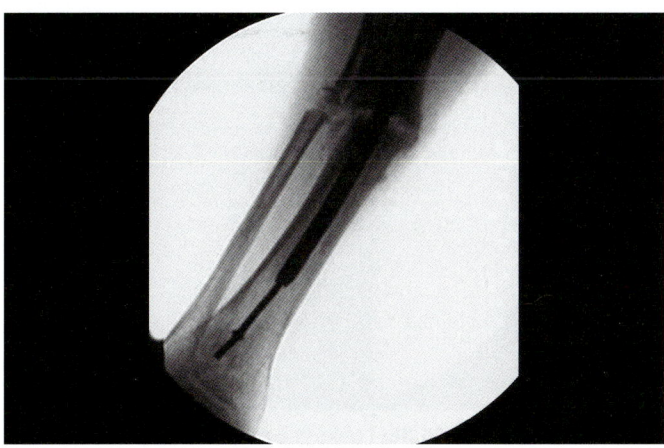

Fig. 55.30: Reaming: Radiographic representation

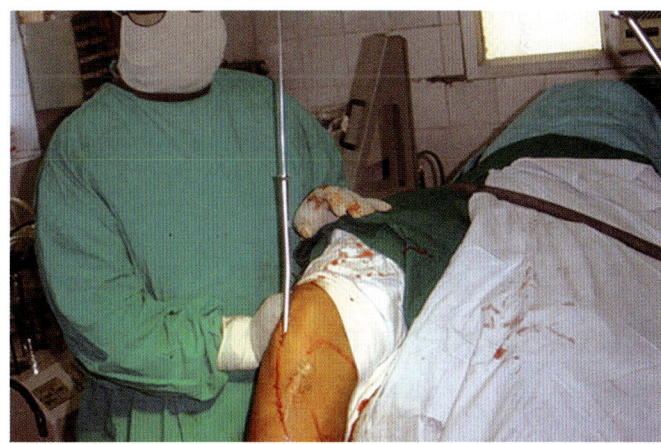

Fig. 55.33: Introduction of the nail: Nail alone inserted on the guidewire first the proximal jig fitted later

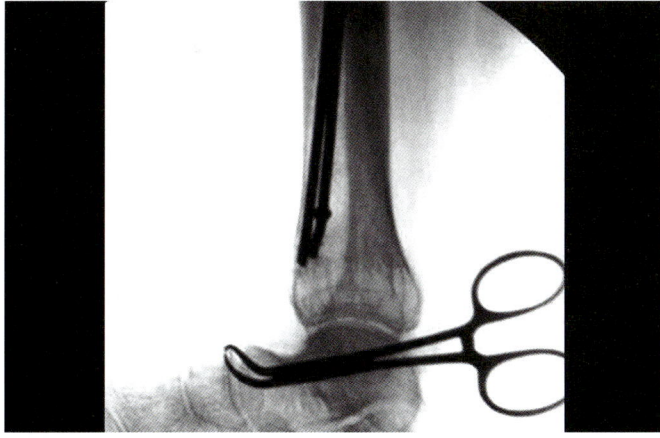

Fig. 55.31: Reaming: Smooth GW inserted by the side of the first one. Now the first will be removed

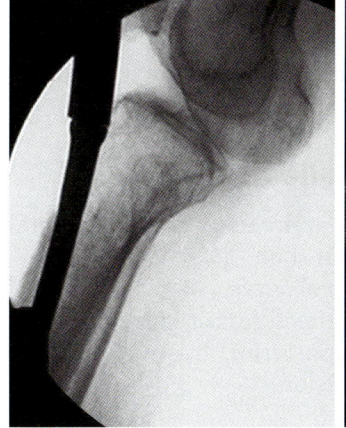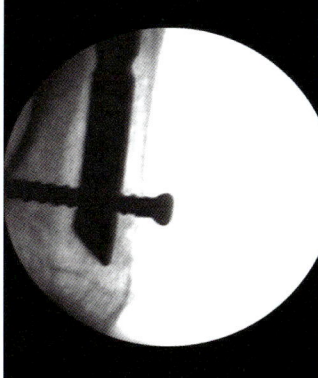

Fig. 55.34: Extent of the nail

- Appropriate sized flexible reamers are passed through the guidewire and the tibial canal is reamed.
- Select the appropriate sized interlocking nail.
- Select the nail diameter equal or 1 size more than or equal to the reamer to provide a snug fit.
- Now pass the nail through the proximal fragment in a antegrade manner.
- Now reduce and hold both the fracture fragments and drive the nail down into the distal fragment.
- Two proximal interlocking screws are passed under the guidance of C-arm.
- Then the distal interlocking screws are passed and confirmed with C-arm.
- Close the wound in layers.

Surgical technique of tibial interlocking nail are shown in Figures 54.21 to 54.36.

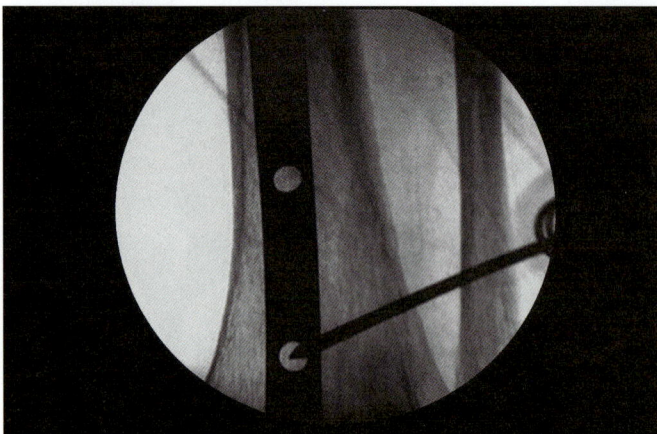

Fig. 55.35: Locking-distal freehand: Images of the holes should be round and big. Note the K-wire in center

Aftercare

- Patient can be permitted to move the operated limb on the next day.
- Active and active assisted exercises for the knee are done next.
- Bedside standing with a walker can be permitted after 2–3 days.
- Walker support to be used for walking for at least 2–3 weeks.
- Weight-bearing can be permitted at the end of 6 weeks.

MALLEOLAR FIXATIONS

Indications

Displaced bimalleolar fractures.

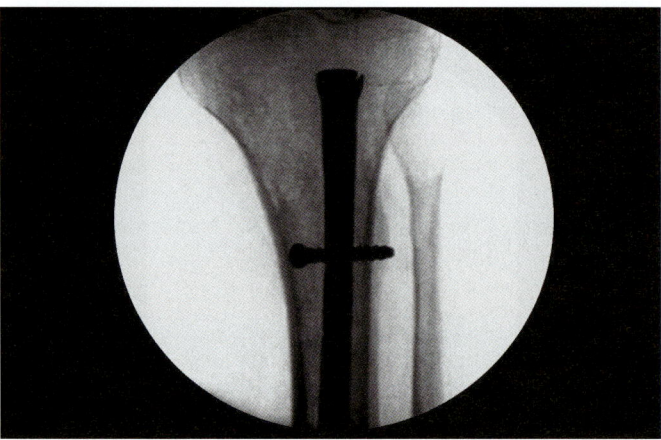

Fig. 55.36: Locking—proximal

Approach

Anterolateral for lateral malleolar fractures, and anteromedial for medial malleolar fractrures. In case of bimalleolar fractures, fix lateral malleolus first.

Surgical technique of medial malleolar fixations is shown in Figures 55.37 to 55.57.

Steps to Fix Lateral Malleolus

- Through the anterolateral approach, expose the lateral malleolus and distal fibular shaft.
- Take care to protect the sural nerve.
- In uncomminuted oblique fracture fix it with 2 malleolar screws from anterior to posterior. This will produce interfragmentary compression.

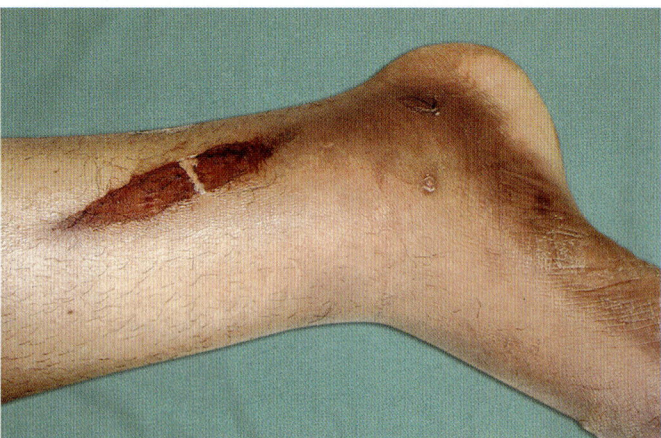

Fig. 55.37: Deformity as viewed from the inner side

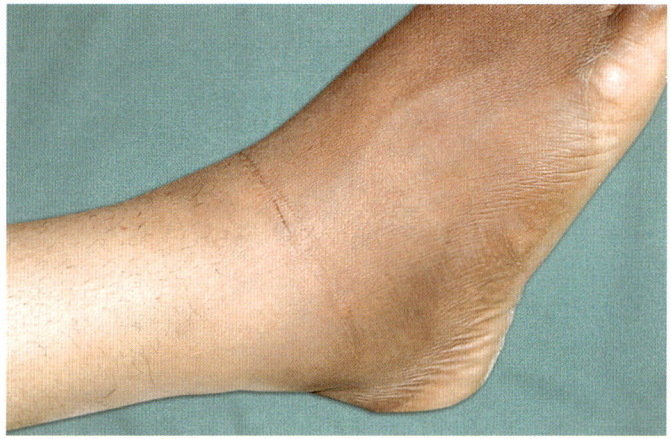

Fig. 55.38: Deformity as viewed from the lateral side

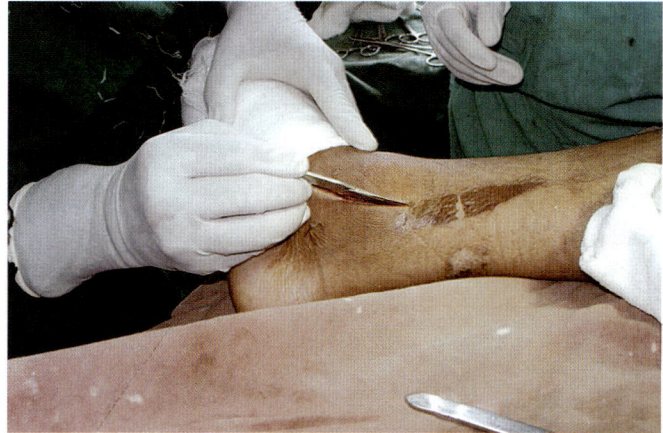

Fig. 55.41: Approach to medial malleolus

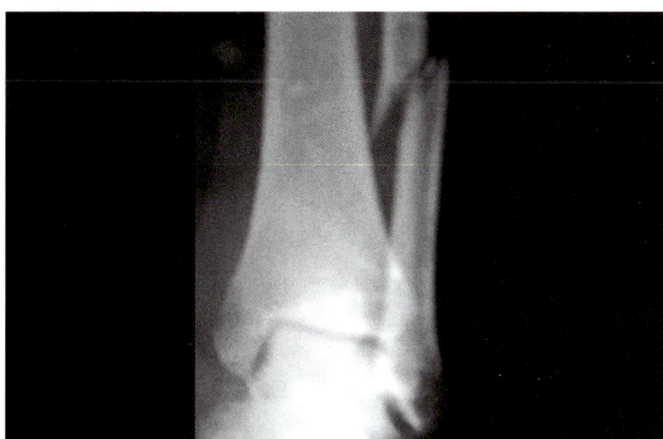

Fig. 55.39: Radiograph—AP view

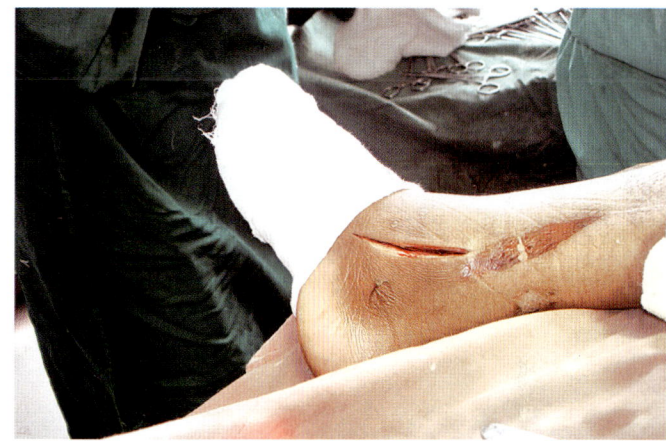

Fig. 55.42: Approach deepened

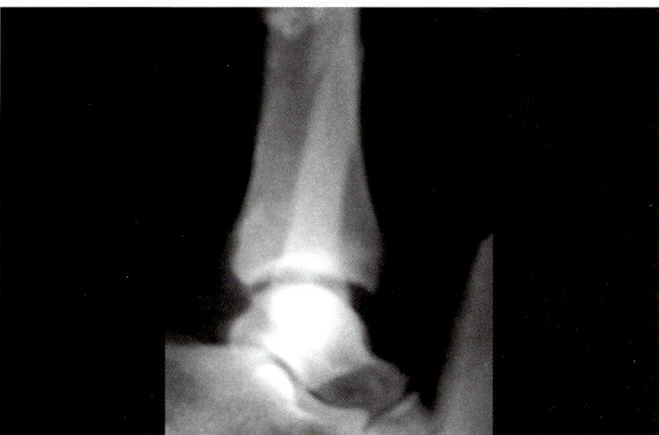

Fig. 55.40: Radiograph—lateral view

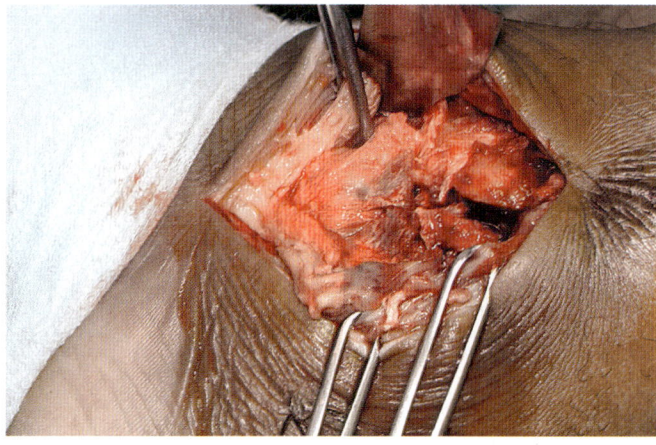

Fig. 55.43: Exposure of the medial malleolus fracture

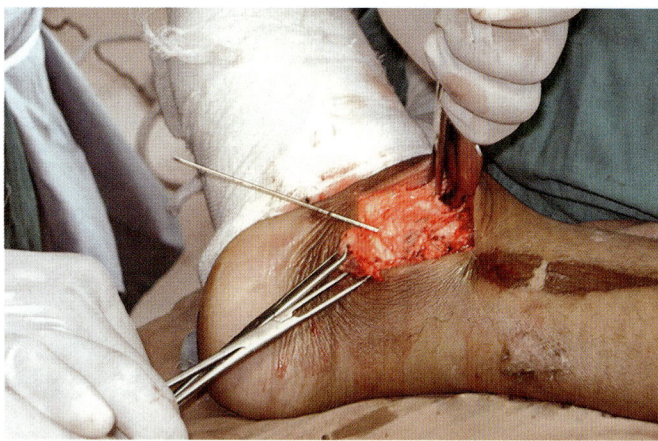

Fig. 55.44: Stabilization of the medial malleolar fracture with K-wire

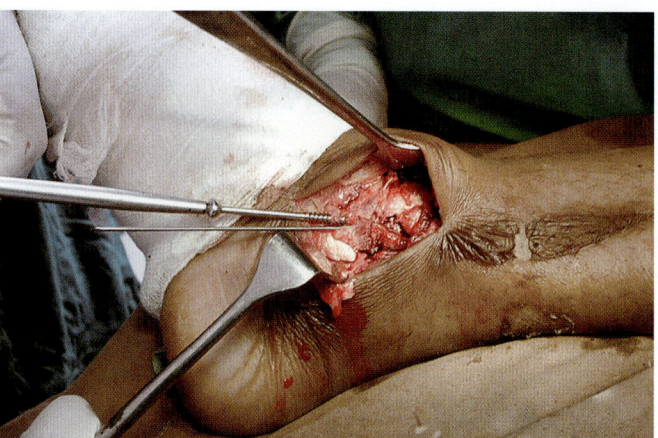

Fig. 55.47: Placement of the malleolar screw

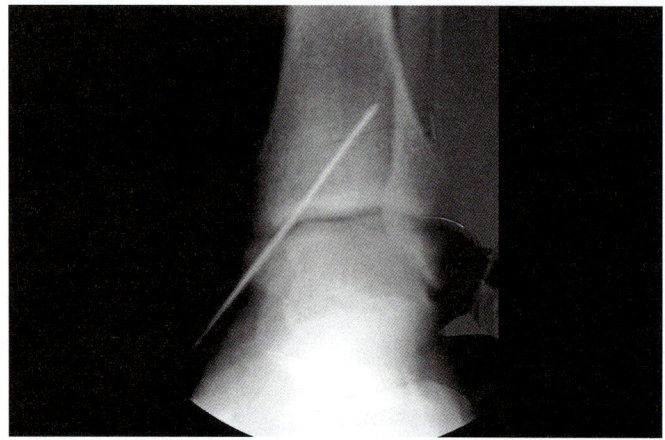

Fig. 55.45: C-arm confirmation—AP view

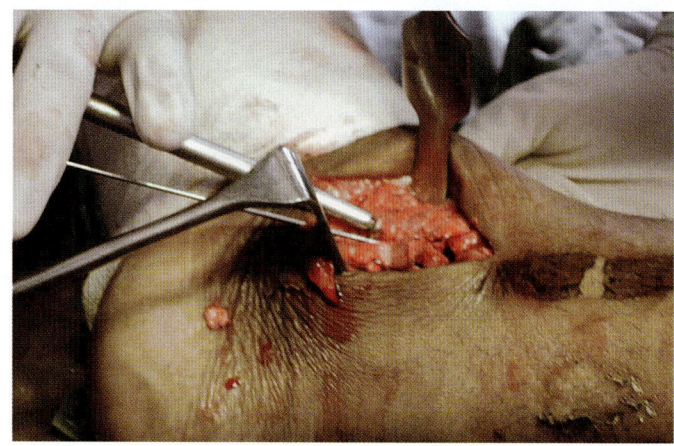

Fig. 55.48: Screw placed deep

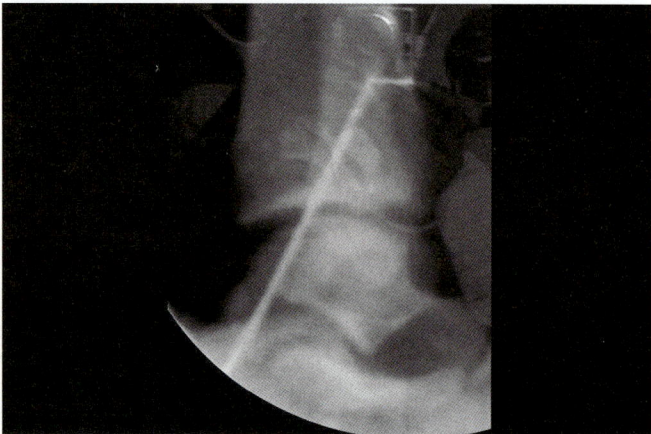

Fig. 55.46: C-arm confirmation—lateral view

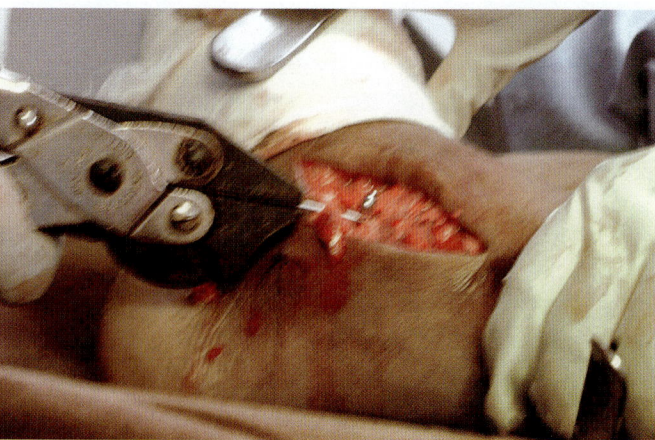

Fig. 55.49: Removal of the K-wire

CHAPTER 55: Common Surgery of the Tibia **739**

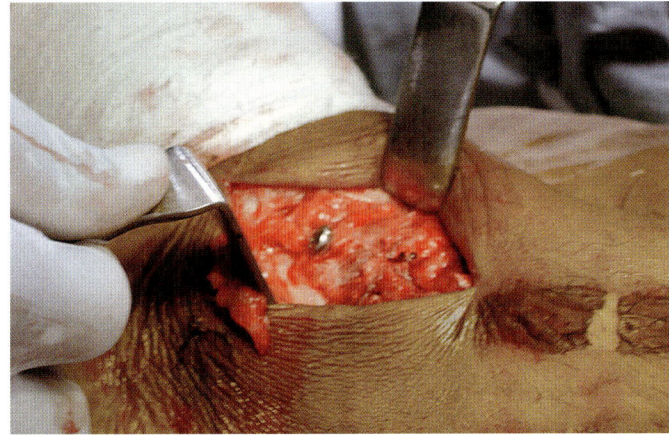

Fig. 55.50: Final placement of the malleolar screw

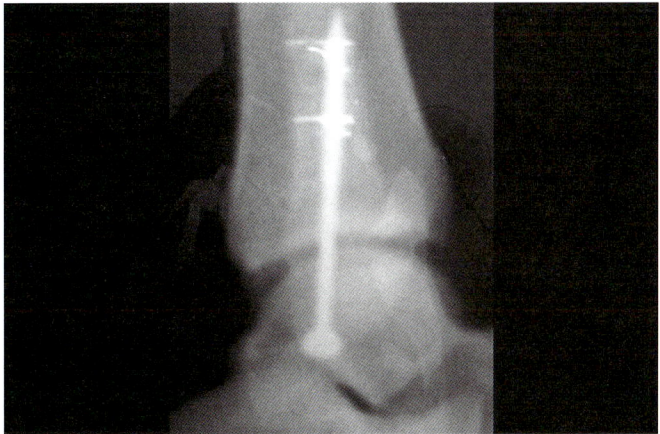

Fig. 55.53: C-arm confirmation of the screw—lateral view

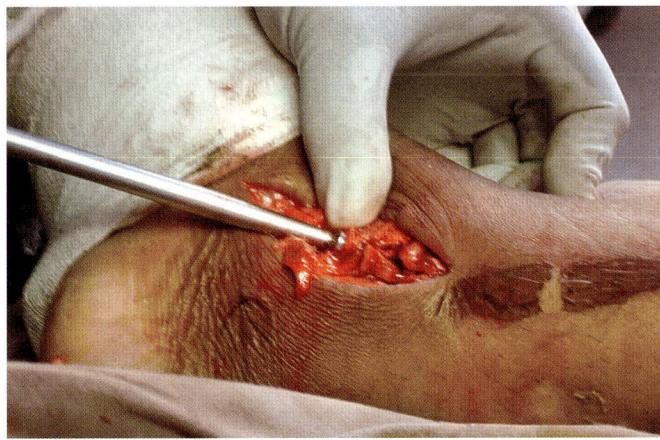

Fig. 55.51: Final tightening

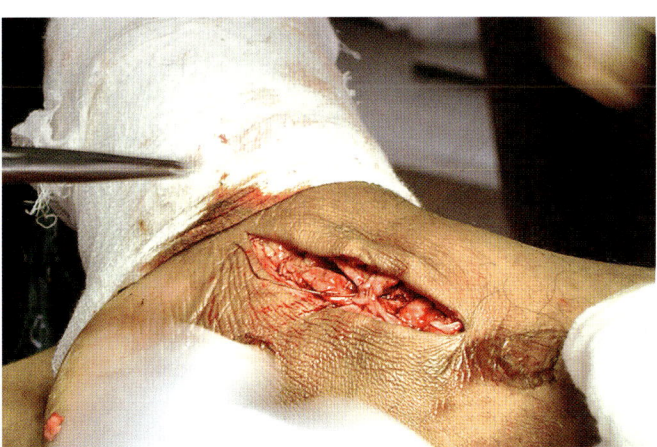

Fig. 55.54: Closure of the periosteum

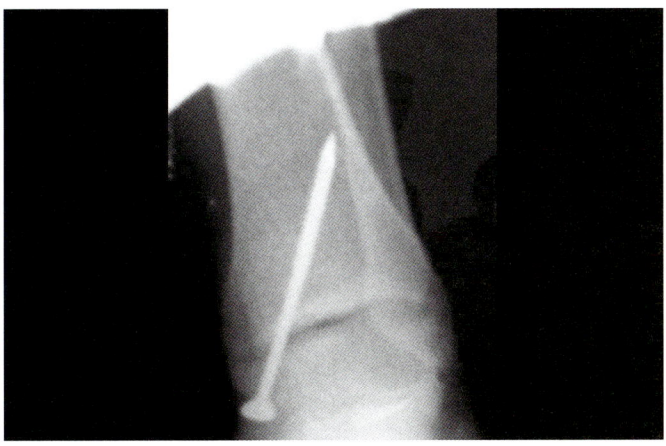

Fig. 55.52: C-arm confirmation of the screw—AP view

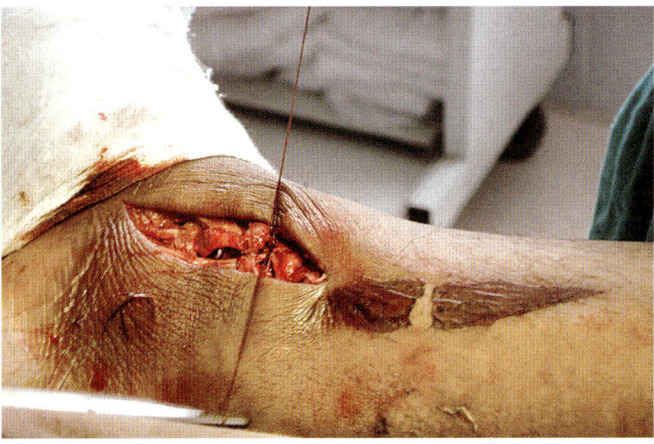

Fig. 55.55: Closure of the muscles

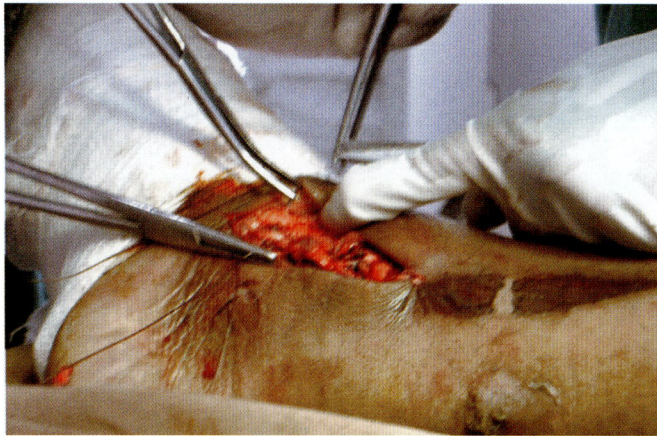

Fig. 55.56: Closure of the deep fascia

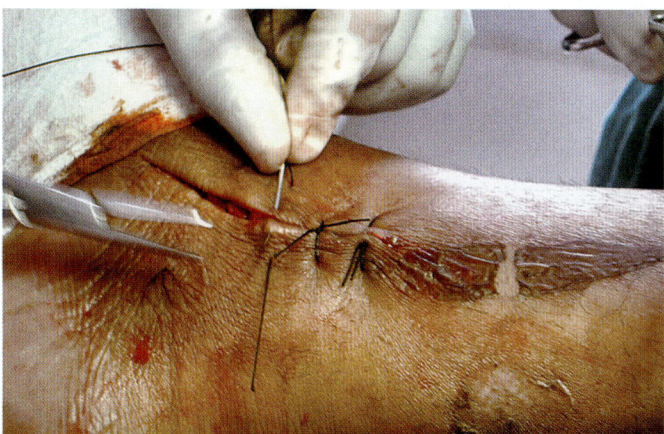

Fig. 55.57: Skin being closed

- Screw length should not be too short so as not to engage the posterior cortex nor too long that it damages the peroneal tendon sheath.
- If the fracture is transverse or if the distal fragment is small, expose the tip of the lateral malleolus by dissecting the calcaneofibular ligament; insert a long screw across the fracture line into the medullary canal of the proximal fragment.
- Fix the fibular fracture with a semi tubular plate if the fracture is above the level of the tibial syndesmosis.

Steps for Medial Malleolus Fixation (Figs 55.37 to 55.57)

- Expose the medial malleolus through a 10 cm long anteromedial curved incision by beginning 5 cm proximal to medial malleolus and ending 2.5 cm distal to the tip of the medial malleolus.
- Usually a fold of periosteum will be interposed between the fracture fragments, release it gently.
- Reduce the fracture and hold it with a towel clip or bone holding clamp.
- Fix it temporarily with 2 small K-wires.
- Next drill a hole through the medial malleolus in a proximal and lateral direction into the tibial metaphysis.
- Now fix the fracture with 1–2 malleolar screws of appropriate size and length determined on the table by suitable measurements.
- Inspect the superomedial corner of the ankle joint to ascertain that the screw has not transgressed that area.
- Confirm the position of the screws under C-arm.
- If the fixation is acceptable, remove the K-wires.
- Close the wound in layers.

Aftercare

- Immobilize the ankle in a below knee cast.
- Remove and reapply the cast after removal of sutures.
- A short leg cast is used for 4–6 weeks.
- Active range of movement exercises can be begun on the 3rd postoperative day and continued for 6 weeks.
- Protected weight-bearing may be permitted and continued till the fracture is united.

Chapter 56

Turco's One Stage Posteromedial Release for Congenital Talipes Equinovarus

Indications

Correction of congenital talipes equinovarus (CTEV) in 6–12 months age group children who have not responded to conservative treatment.

Approach

Turco's one stage posteromedial release (PMR) through Cincinnati incision.

Surgical Steps

- Put a medial incision for about 8–10 cm from the base of the first metatarsal to the tendo-Achilles.
- Curve the incision slightly just below the medial malleolus.
- By careful dissection free the tendons of the tibialis posterior, flexor digitorum longus, flexor hallucis longus and posterior tibial neurovascular structures.
- Free the posterior tibial neurovascular structures and retract it posteriorly.
- Divide the sheaths of the flexor digitorum longus, flexor hallucis longus and the Master Knot of Henry below the navicular bone.
- Divide the calcaneonavicular (spring) ligament and the abnormal origin of abductor hallucis.
- Lengthen the tendo-calcaneus by Z-plasty.
- Expose the posterior capsule of the ankle joint and subtalar joints and incise the capsule.
- Now divide the tibiocalcaneal part of the deltoid ligament.
- Release the deep medial structures and lengthen the tibialis posterior tendon by Z-plasty.
- Open the talonavicular joint mobilize the navicular bone excise that part of the deltoid ligament that inserts on the navicle.
- Release the tibialis posterior from the sustentaculum tali and the spring ligament.
- Detach the spring ligament from the sustentaculum tali.
- On the posterior side, release the superficial layer of the deltoid ligament form the calcaneus.
- Evert the foot and cut the talcalcaneal interosseous ligament.
- Release the bifurcated Y-ligament. Now the navicular bone is completely mobilized.
- Reduce the navicular bone onto the head of the talus and fix this with a K-wire from the dorsum of the first metatarsophalangeal joint transfixing the talonavicular joint.
- Repair the tendo-Achilles with few interrupted sutures
- Suture the tibialis posterior tendon next.
- Close the wound in layers.
- Bend the K-wire, and apply a well-padded long leg case with the ankle in slight dorsiflexion and the knee in slight flexion.

Aftercare

- By 3 weeks, the cast is changed but the sutures are left behind. This is done under general anesthesia (GA).
- By 6 weeks, remove the suture wire and the cast. Apply a new long leg cast with foot held in full correction.
- The second cast must be removed after 4 months.
- Pronator shoes are worn during day and Dennis Browne Splint during night.

Chapter 57

Common Surgery of the Spine

LAMINECTOMY

Indications: Prolapsed intervertebral disk prolapse (IVDP) causing neurological impairment.
Approach: Dorsal approach.

Surgical Steps (Described for L5 Disk Prolapse) (Figs 57.1 to 57.16)

- Identify the spinous process from L3 to S1.
- Make a midline incision extending from the spinous process of L4 vertebra to S1.
- Incise the supraspinous ligament from the 4th lumbar vertebra to the 1st sacral spinous process.
- By subperiosteal dissection strip the muscles from the sides of the lesion.
- Using a self-retaining retractors retract the muscles on other side and expose the required disk space.
- Verify the position of the sacrum by direct vision and deep palpation. This will prevent the mistakes in identifying the disk spaces.
- Obtain hemostasis with electrocautery, bone wax and packs. Take care to leave each pack outside completely.
- Using a curette denude the lamina and ligamentum flavum.
- If exposure is inadequate, remove a small portion of the inferior lamina.
- Hold the ligamentum flavum with an Allis or Kochers make a nick and excise a flap of ligamentum flavum by sharp dissection. Take care not to damage the dura.
- Identify the nerve root retract it medially to visualize the bulging posterior longitudinal ligament.
- Now use Cottonoid patties to tamponade the epidural veins both caudal and cephalic. Cauterize the bleeders carefully.
- The underlying disk should be clearly visible now.
- To expose the herniated disk retract the nerve root using a nerve root retractor.
- If the extruded fragment is not seen, incise the PLL and inspect again.
- If still no herniation is detected then make a search far laterally.
- Now gently remove the disk fragments till the bulge has been decompressed to allow the gentle retraction of the root over the defect.
- Remove all the cottonoids and control the residual bleeding.
- Close the wound in layers with appropriate suture material for different tissues.

Aftercare

- Patient can be allowed to turn in bed the same day.

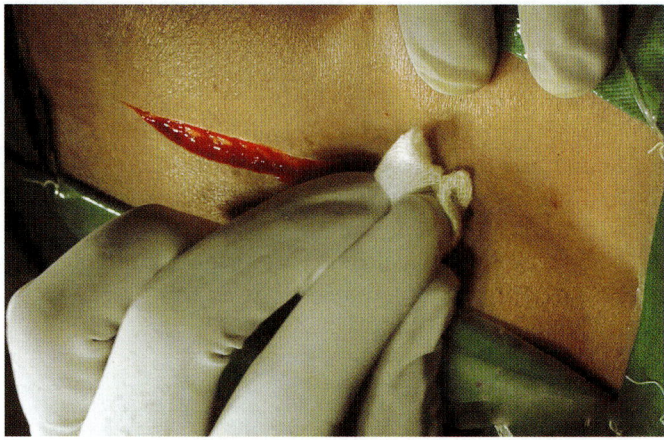

Fig. 57.1: Skin incision

CHAPTER 57: Common Surgery of the Spine **743**

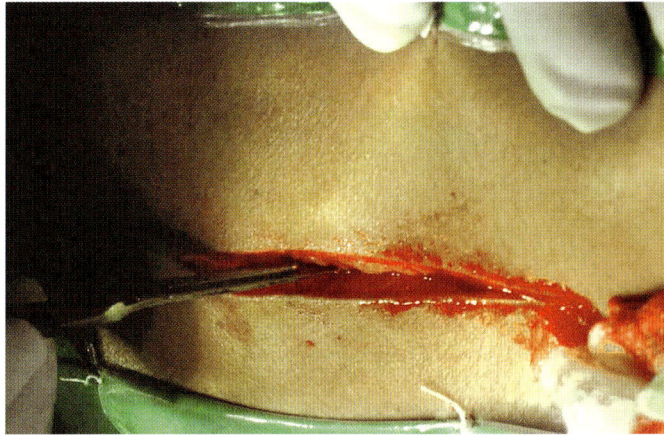

Fig. 57.2: Extending skin incision

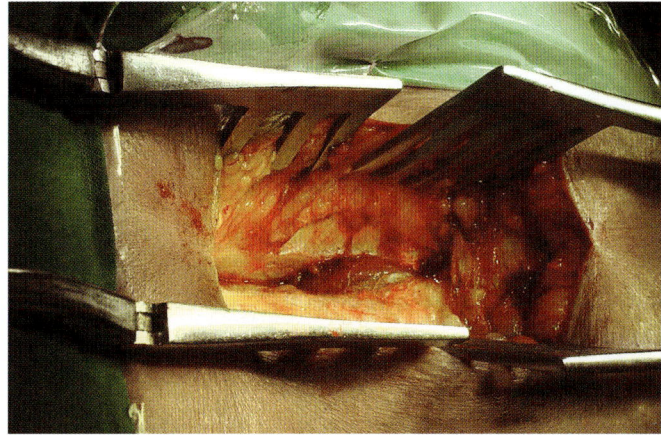

Fig. 57.5: Excision of the supraspinous ligament

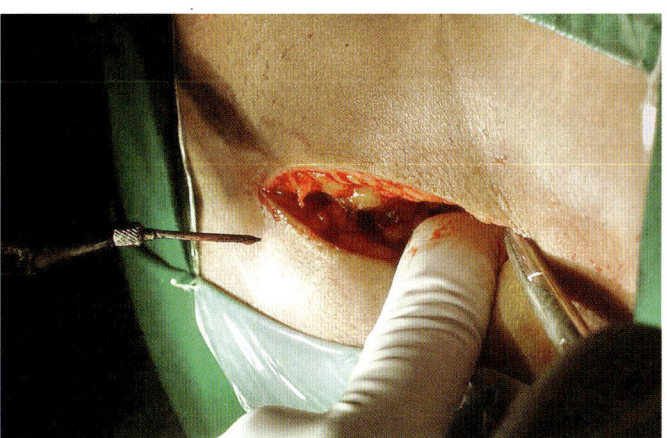

Fig. 57.3: Deepening the incision

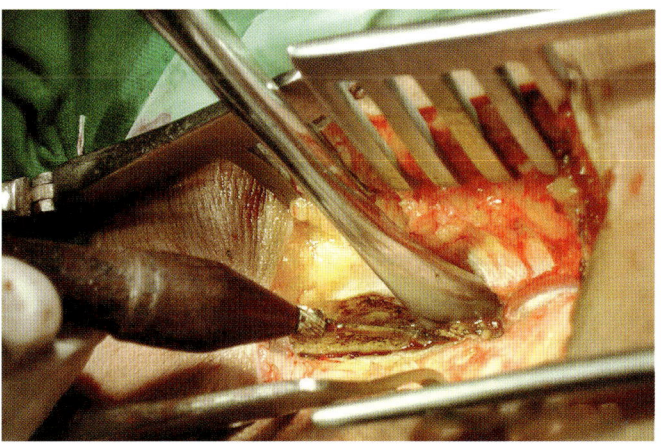

Fig. 57.6: Separating the lumbar muscles

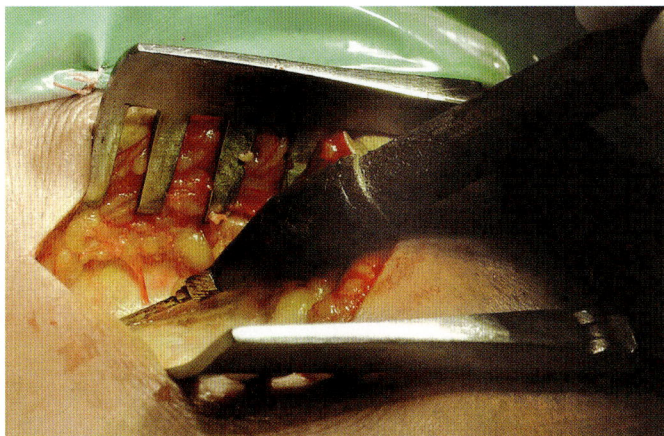

Fig. 57.4: Deep dissection

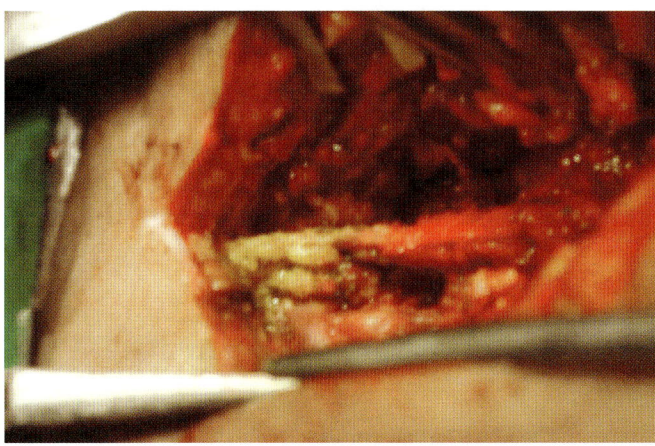

Fig. 57.7: Exposure of the spinous process

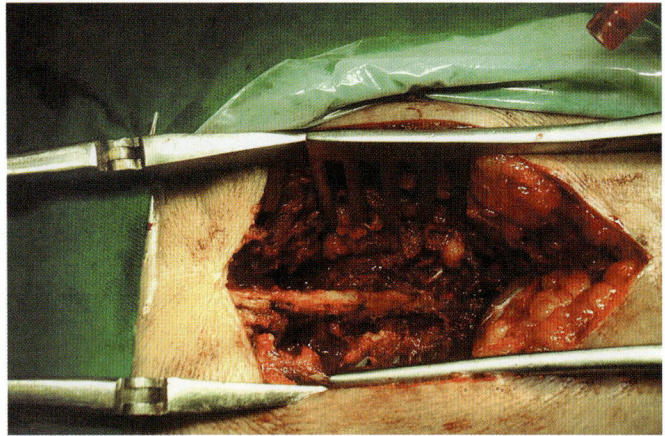

Fig. 57.8: Lamina exposed

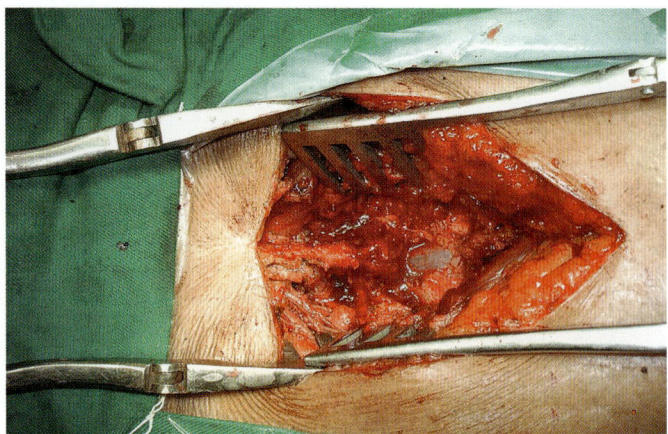

Fig. 57.11: Exposure of the dura

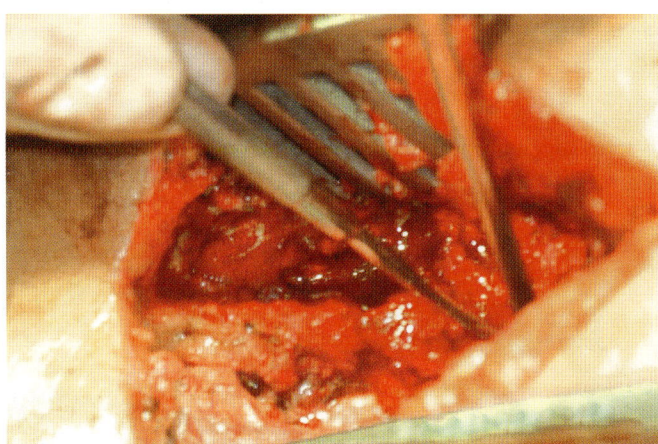

Fig. 57.9: Spinous process excised

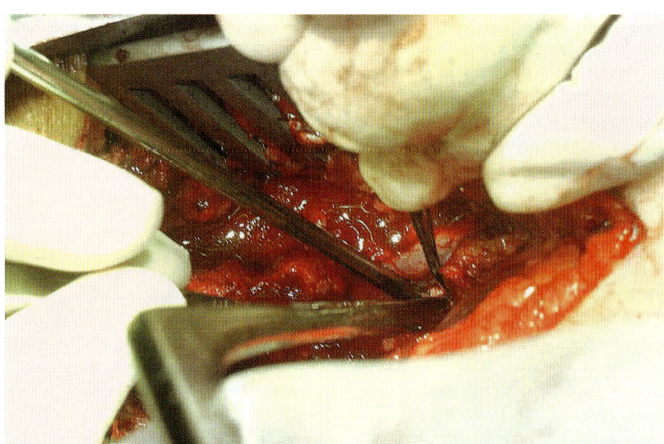

Fig. 57.12: Diskectomy being done

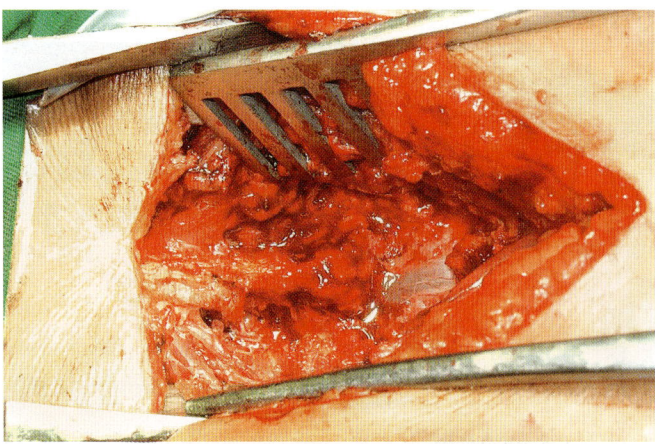

Fig. 57.10: Laminectomy being done

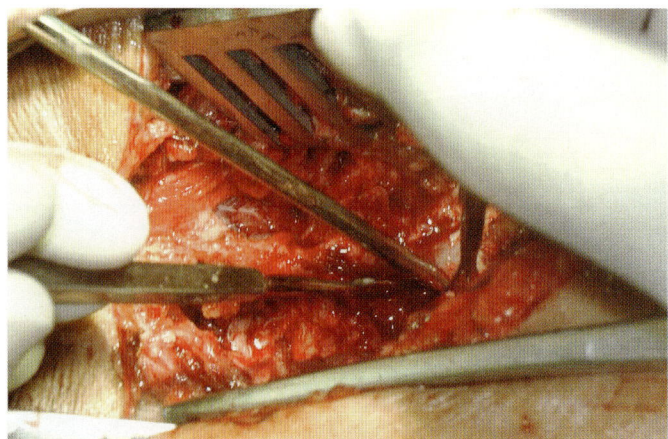

Fig. 57.13: Disk removal continued

- He may be allowed to stand with walker on the same evening and may be allowed to go to the bathroom.
- Walking is permitted after the first postoperative day.
- Isometric abdominal and lower limb exercises are begun.
- Sitting is minimized but walking is encouraged.
- After 4–6 weeks back exercises are commenced.
- After 6th week, lifting, bending, stooping can be allowed.
- Increased sitting may be allowed after 4th week and long trips after 3 months.
- After 8–10th week, lower limb exercises are begun.
- After 12 weeks, patient may be allowed to return to work.

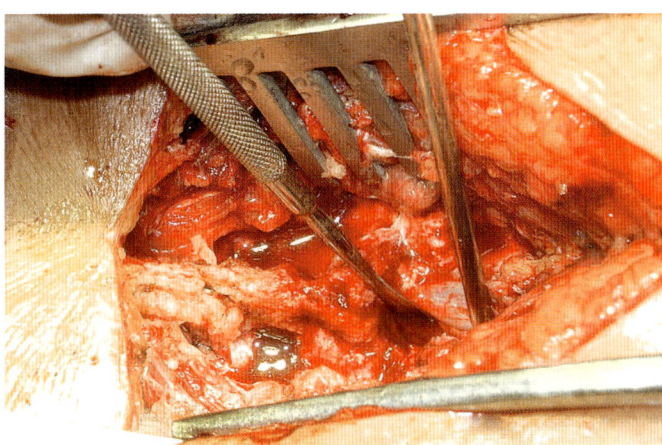

Fig. 57.14: Checking the freed nerve roots

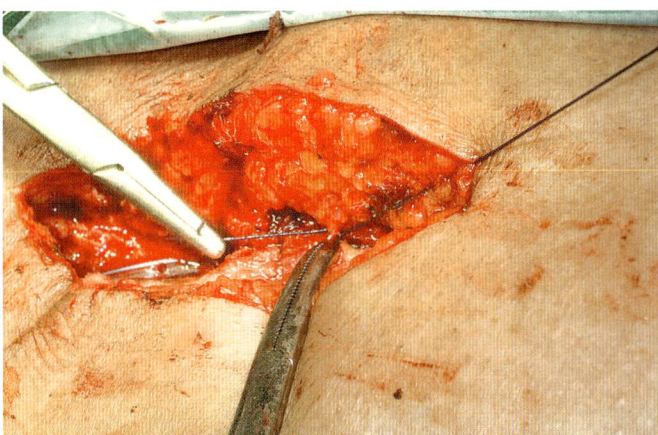

Fig. 57.15: Closure of the wound

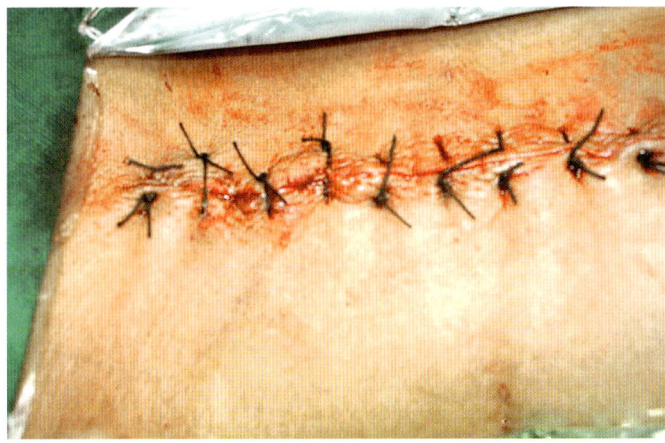

Fig. 57.16: Final skin closure

POSTERIOR INSTRUMENTATION FOR VERTEBRAL COMPRESSION FRACTURES

Indications: Compression fracture of D12 vertebra without neurological deficit.

Approach: Dorsal approach.

Instrumentation: CD rod system.

Surgical Steps (Figs 57.17 to 57.38)

- Identify the spinous process from D8 to L4.
- Make a midline incision extending from the spinous process over the above vertebrae.
- Incise the supraspinous ligament from the above spinous processes.
- By subperiosteal dissection strip the muscles from the sides of the lesion.
- Using a self-retaining retractors retract the muscles on other side and expose the required area.
- Verify the position of the L5 by direct vision and deep palpation.
- Obtain hemostasis with electrocautery, bone wax and packs. Take care to leave each pack outside completely.
- Now identify the point of entry of the pedicle screws.
- Using an awl make a small opening at the pedicle entry point.
- Gently using moderate force proceed through the pedicle with a sharp probe.
- Confirm the position over the C-arm.
- Now tap the pedicle under C-arm control.
- Insert mono- or polyaxial screws and confirm with C-arm.
- Confirm the stability of the screws by trying to pull on it and checking the hold.
- Now similarly pass the other screws above and below.
- Now select the CD rod and size it appropriately.

746 SECTION 7: Common Surgical Techniques

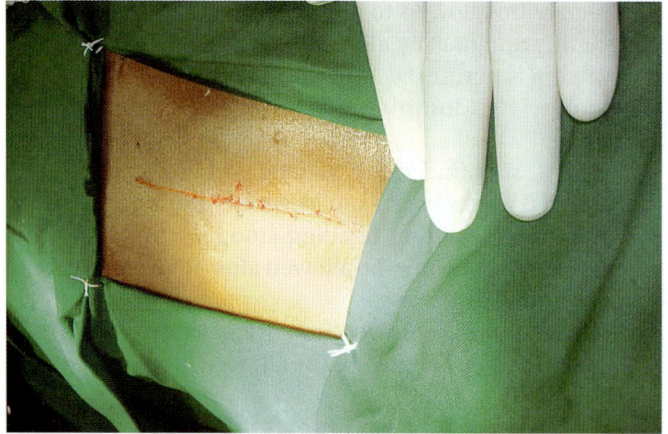

Fig. 57.17: Drape, paint and incision markings

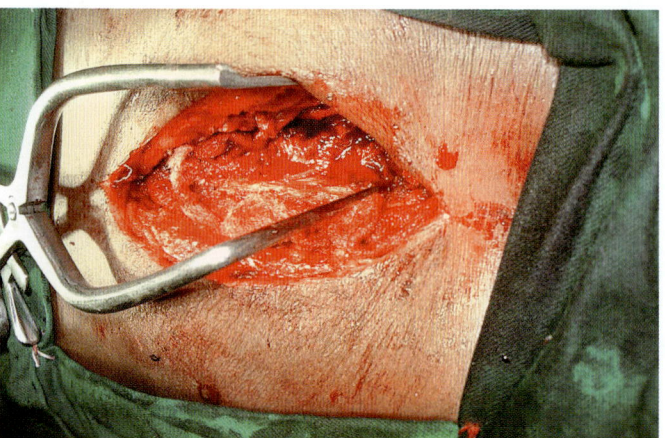

Fig. 57.20: Exposure of the spinous process

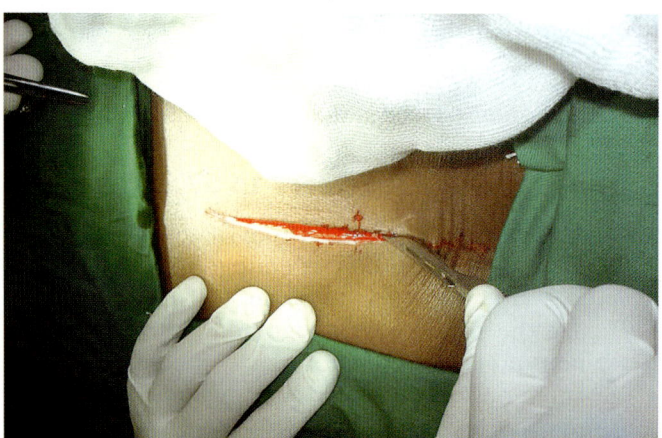

Fig. 57.18: Dorsal incision

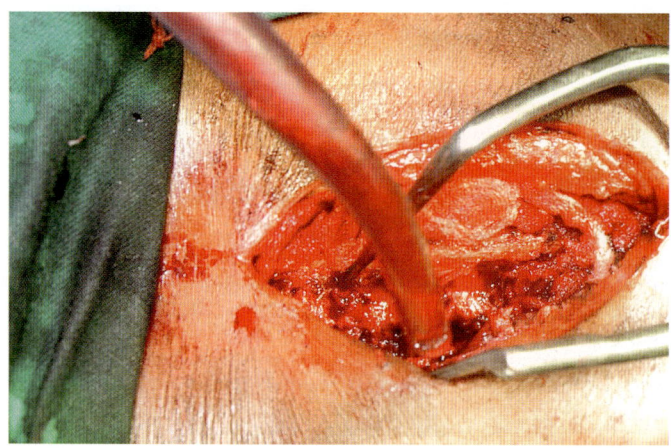

Fig. 57.21: Suction an inescapable routine

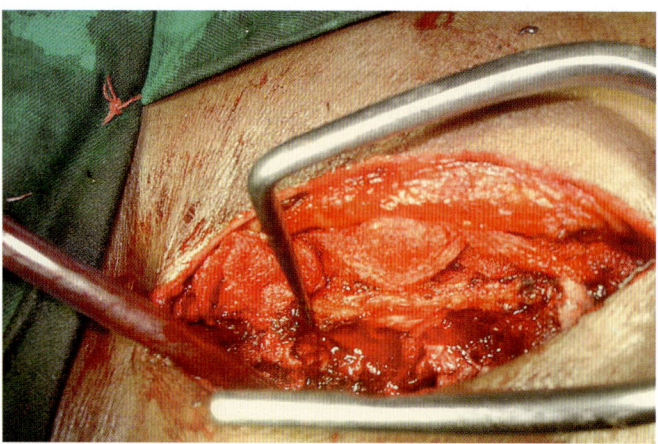

Fig. 57.19: Retraction of spinal muscles

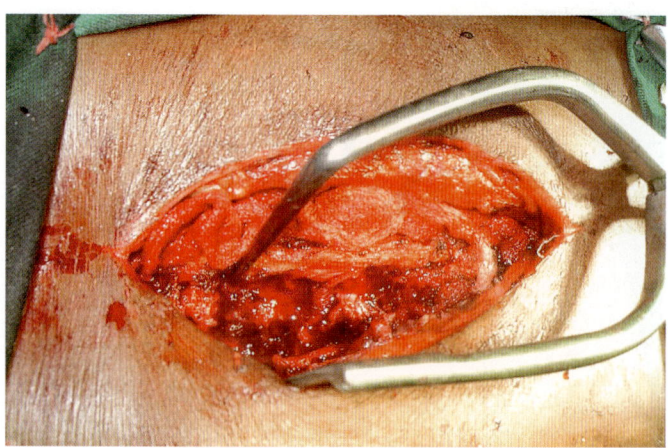

Fig. 57.22: Deep exposure

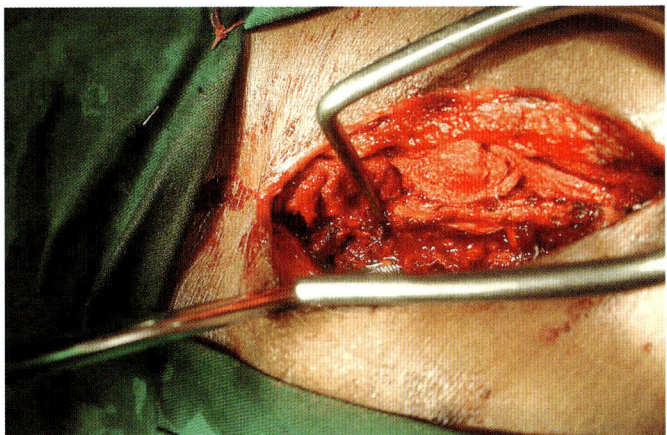

Fig. 57.23: Sideward packing

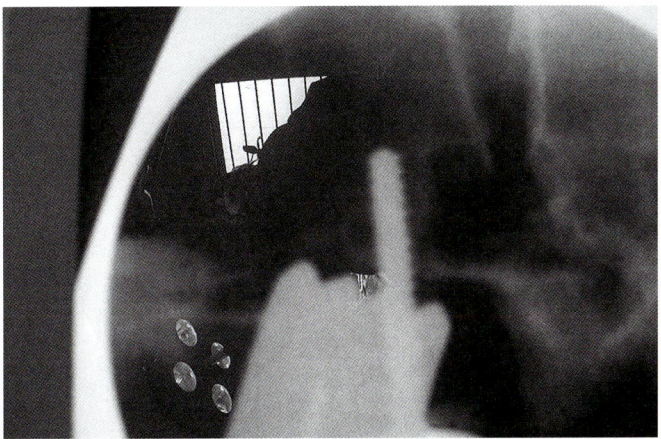

Fig. 57.26: Checking the screw track through C-arm

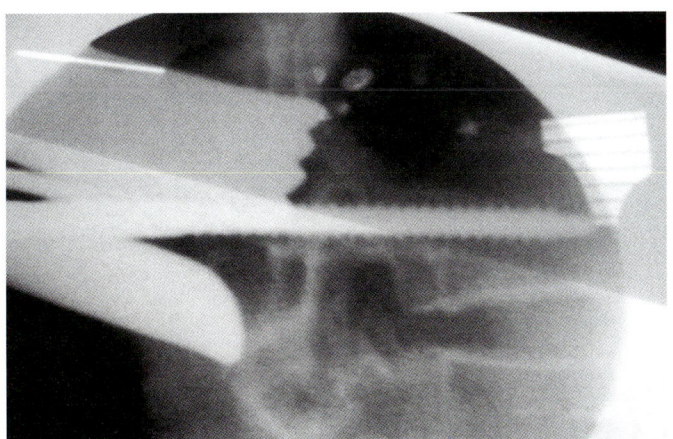

Fig. 57.24: Entry and tapping through pedicle

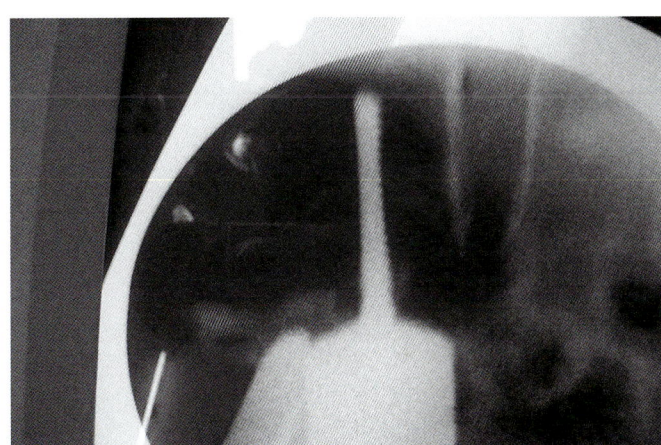

Fig. 57.27: Confirmation of the final screw placement

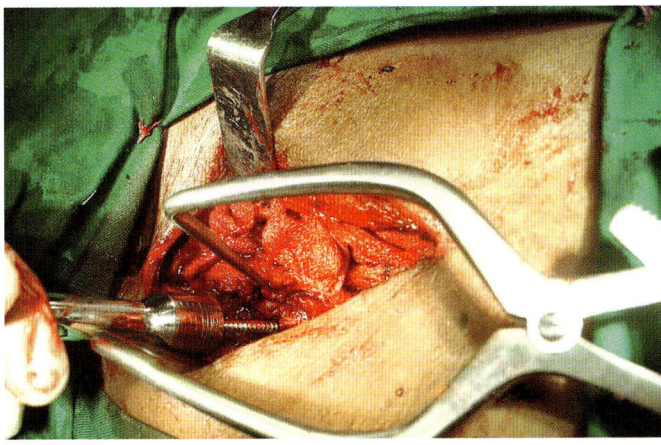

Fig. 57.25: Passing the monoaxial screw

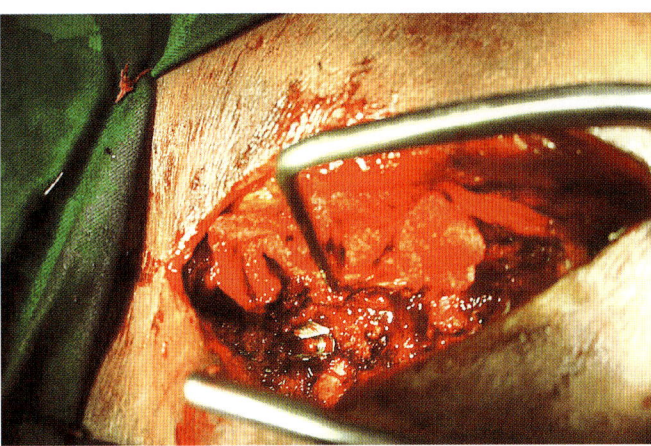

Fig. 57.28: Final seating of the screw

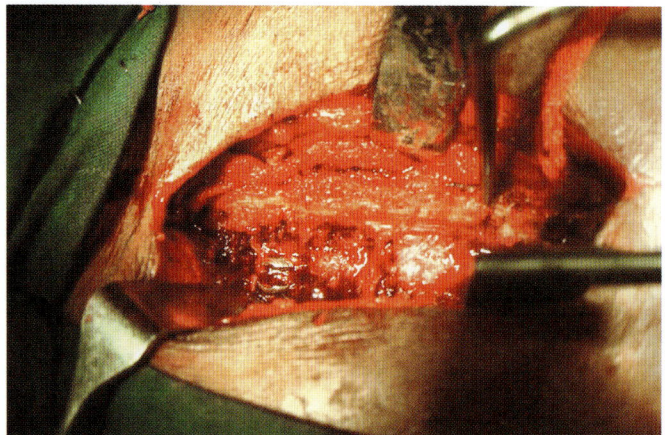

Fig. 57.29: Position of the inserted screws

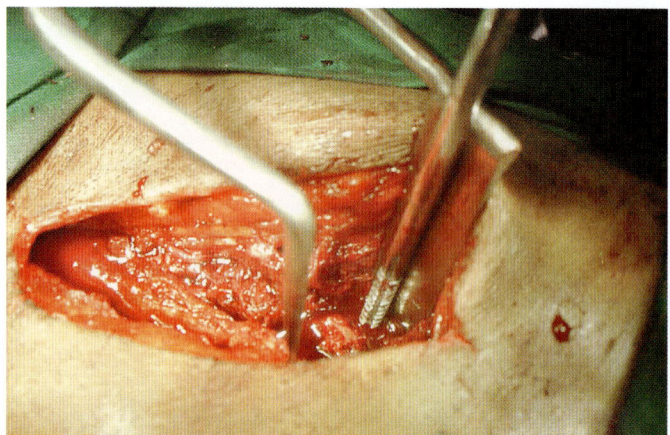

Fig. 57.32: Tapping continued

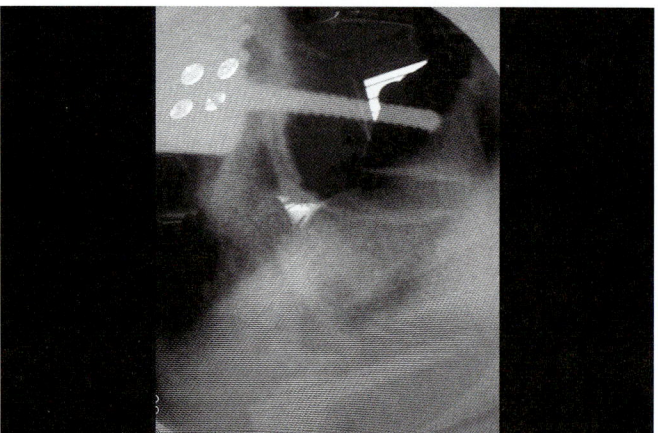

Fig. 57.30: Placement of screws one above and one below

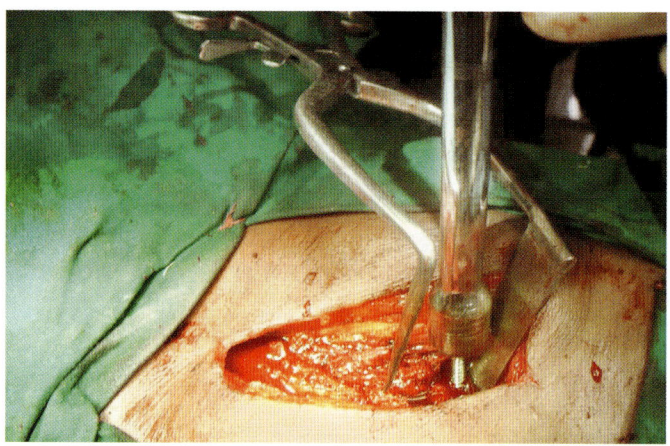

Fig. 57.33: Placement of screwing continued

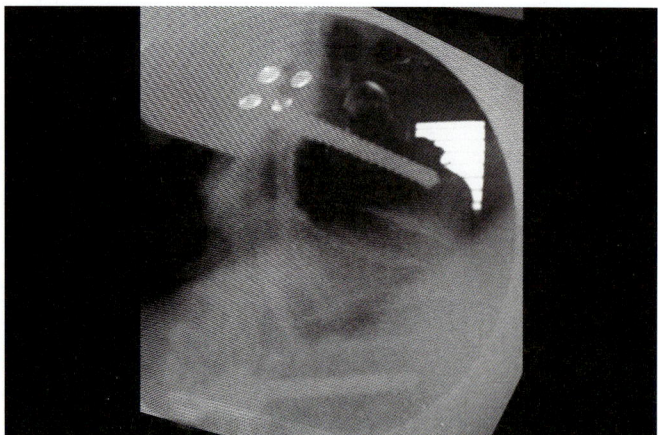

Fig. 57.31: Closer view

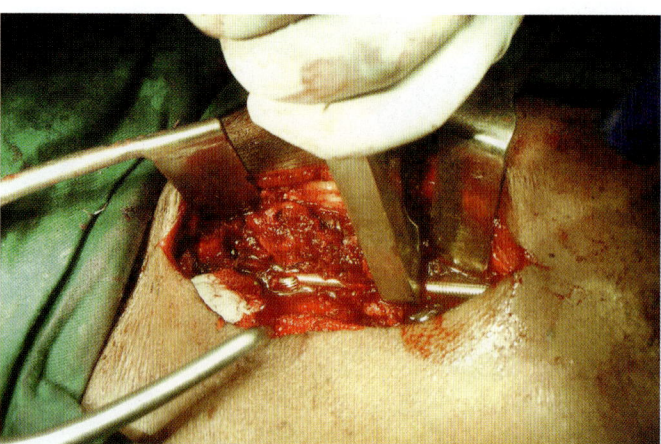

Fig. 57.34: Placement of the rods

CHAPTER 57: Common Surgery of the Spine

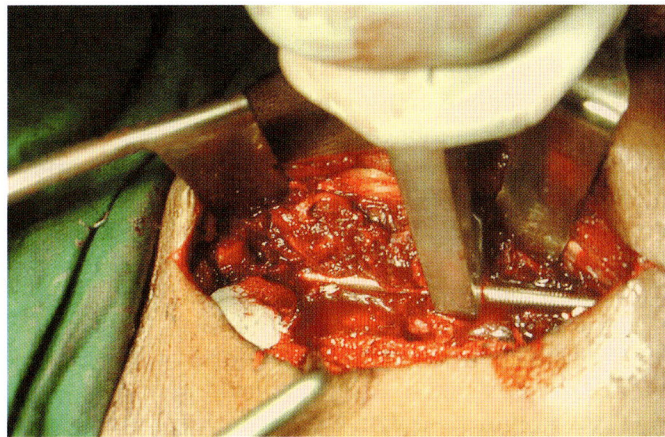

Fig. 57.35: Rod placement on other side

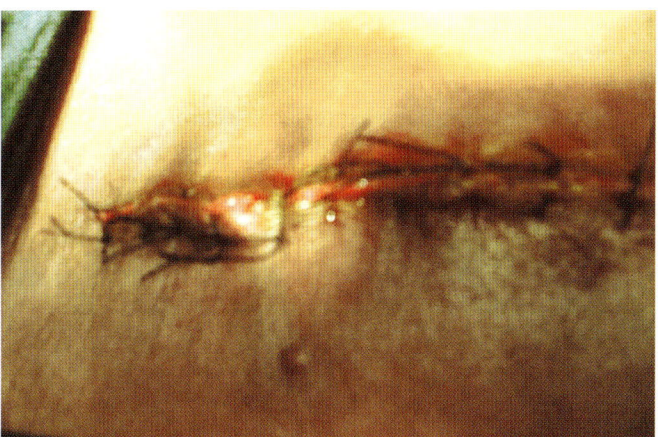

Fig. 57.38: Final skin closure

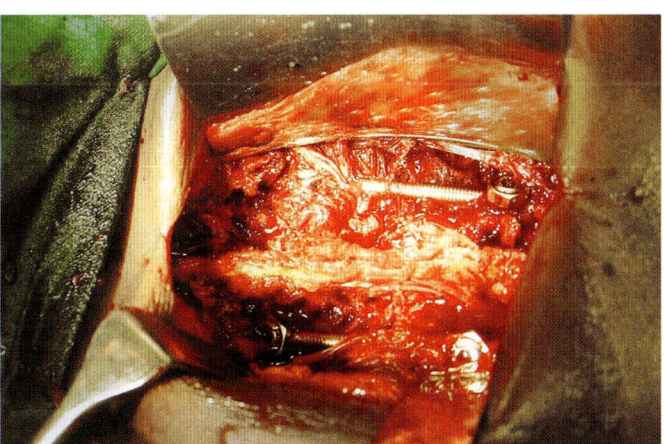

Fig. 57.36: Both rods placement

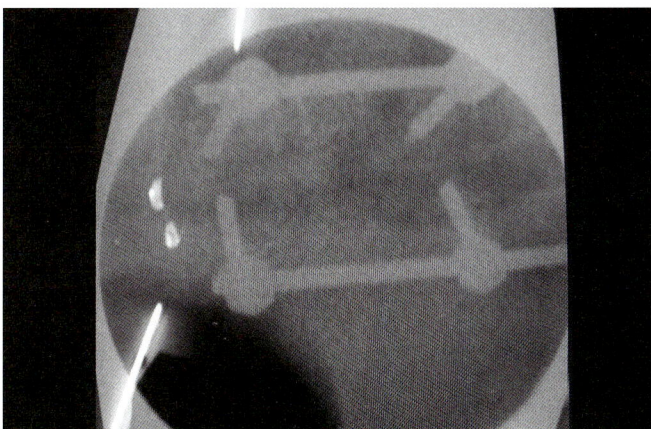

Fig. 57.37: C-arm confirmation

- Bend the rod and configure it the spine curvature.
- Place the rods through the screws above and below.
- Hold the rod firmly through a rod pusher.
- Place the inny and just tighten do not tighten too much as it will be difficult to pass the outy.
- Next insert outy screw cap and tighten both the inny and outy.
- Now check the stability of the construct by gently lifting the CD rod system.
- If the construct is stable, check the position of the rod and screws again on the C-arm.
- If laminectomy is required to decompress carry out these steps.
- Using appropriate rougeurs remove a small portion of the superior and inferior laminae.
- Hold the ligamentum flavum with an Allis or Kochers make a nick and excise a flap of ligamentum flavum by sharp dissection. Take care not to damage the dura.
- Inspect and release the compressed dura.
- Look for the nerve roots on either side for any compressions.
- Remove all the cottonoids and control the residual bleeding.
- Close the wound in layers with appropriate suture material for different tissues.
- Apply a pressure bandage.

Aftercare

- Patient can be allowed to turn in bed the same day.
- He may be allowed to stand with walker on the same evening and may be allowed to go to the bathroom.
- Walking is permitted after the first postoperative day.

- Isometric abdominal and lower limb exercises are begun.
- Sitting is minimized but walking is encouraged.
- After 4–6 weeks back exercises are commenced.
- After 6th week, lifting, bending, stooping can be allowed.
- Increased sitting may be allowed after 4th week and long trips after 3 months.
- After 8–10th week, lower limb exercises are begun.
- After 12 weeks, patient may be allowed to return to work.

POSTERIOR DECOMPRESSION AND SURGICAL STABILIZATION

Indications: Spondylolisthesis of L5 over S1 vertebra without neurological deficit.

Approach: Dorsal approach.

Instrumentation: Moss Miami system.

Surgical Steps (Figs 57.39 to 57.60)

- Identify the spinous process from L1 to S2.
- Make a midline incision extending from the spinous process over the above vertebrae.
- Incise the supraspinous ligament from the above spinous processes.
- By subperiosteal dissection strip the muscles from the sides of the lesion.
- Using a self-retaining retractors retract the muscles on other side and expose the required area.
- Verify the position of the L4, 5 and S1 by direct vision and deep palpation.
- Obtain hemostasis with electrocautery, bone wax and packs. Take care to leave each pack outside completely.
- Now identify the point of entry of the pedicle screws.
- Using an awl make a small opening at the pedicle entry point.

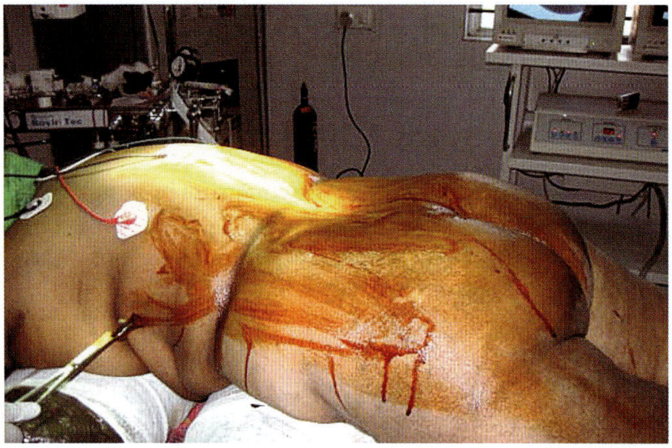

Fig. 57.39: Position and painting

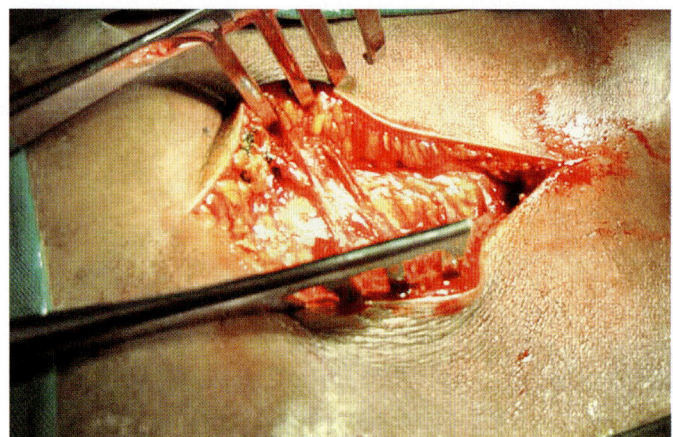

Fig. 57.41: Dissection

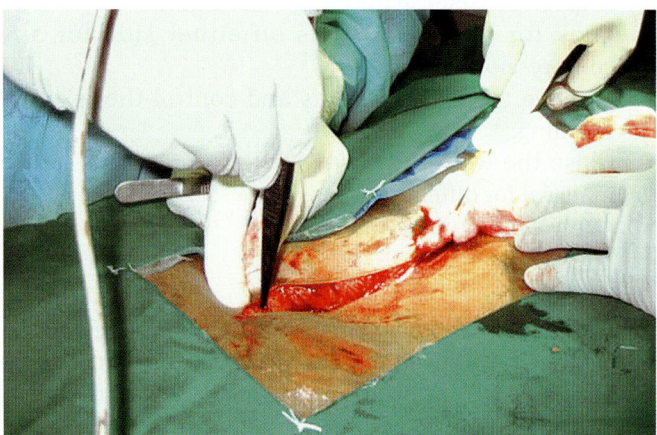

Fig. 57.40: Mid dorsal approach

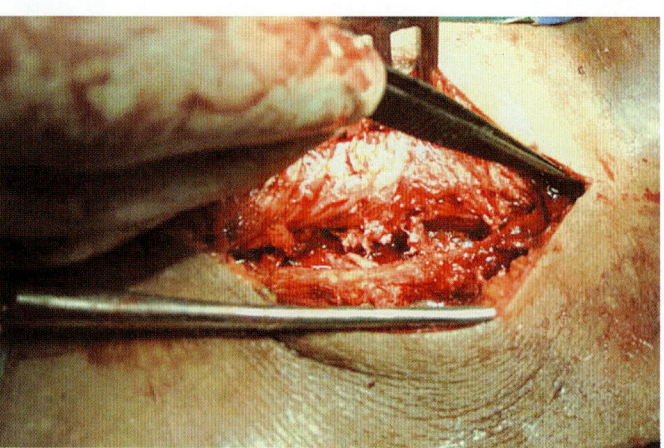

Fig. 57.42: Exposure of the spinous process

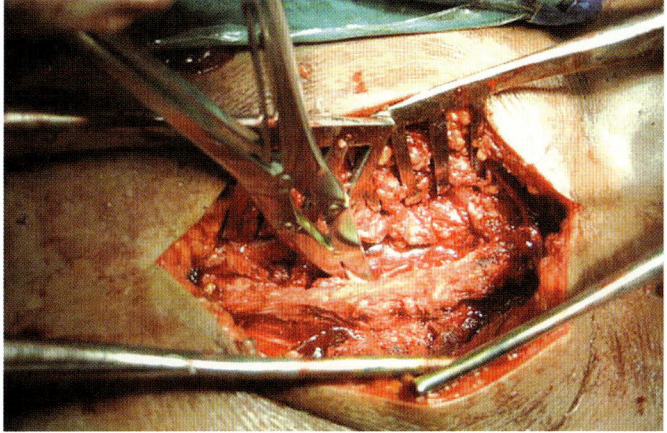

Fig. 57.43: Laminectomy

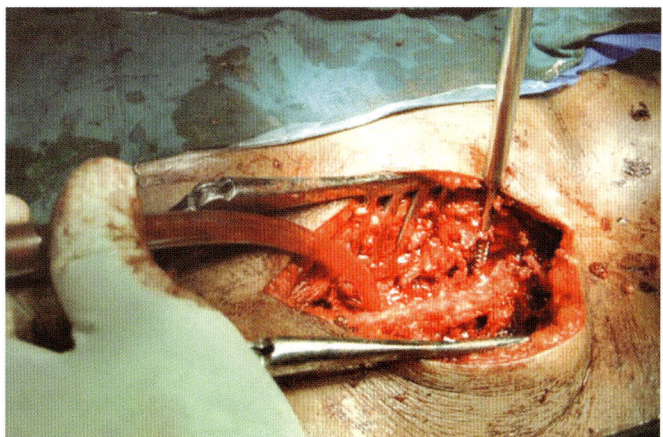

Fig. 57.46: Insertion of the pedicular screws

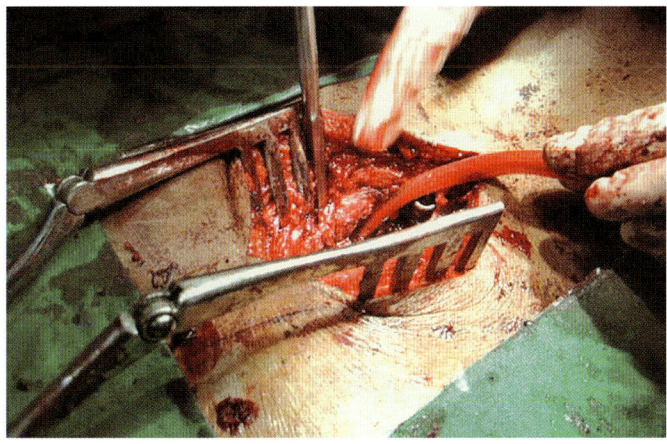

Fig. 57.44: Identifying and penetrating the pedicle

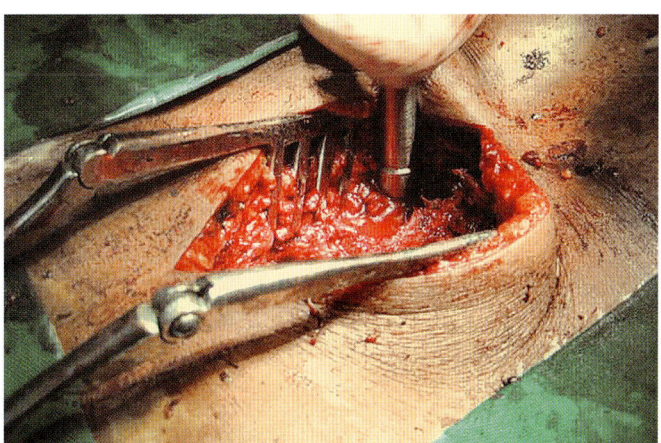

Fig. 57.47: Tightening of the screws

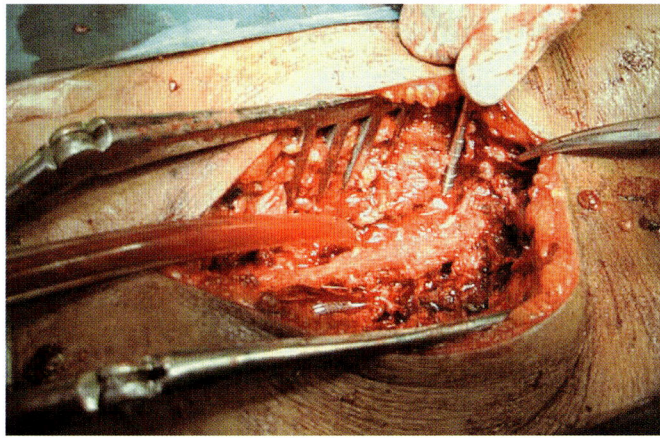

Fig. 57.45: Tapping the pedicle

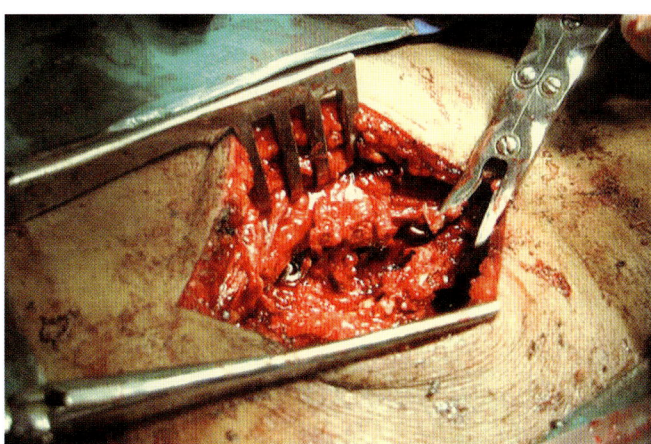

Fig. 57.48: Pedicular screws

752 SECTION 7: Common Surgical Techniques

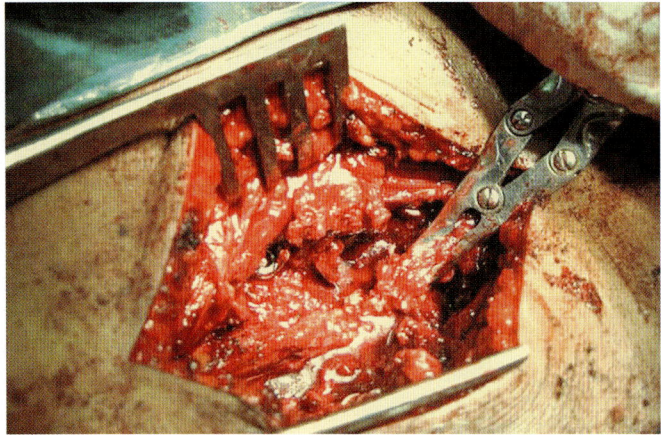

Fig. 57.49: Excision of the spinous process

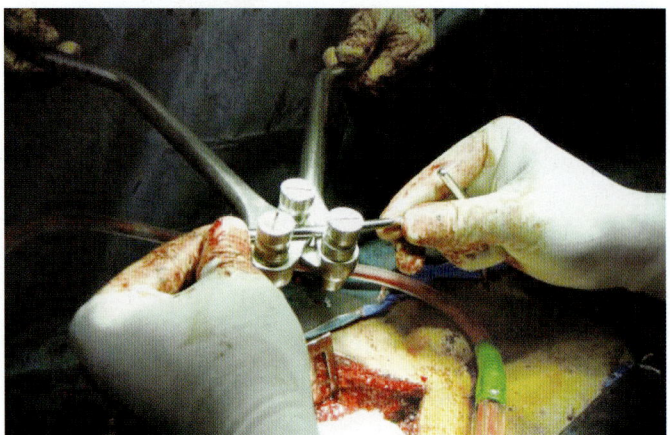

Fig. 57.52: Contouring the CD rods

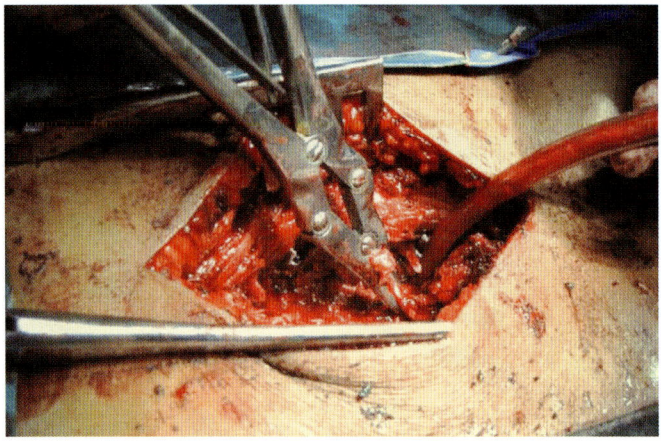

Fig. 57.50: Laminectomy

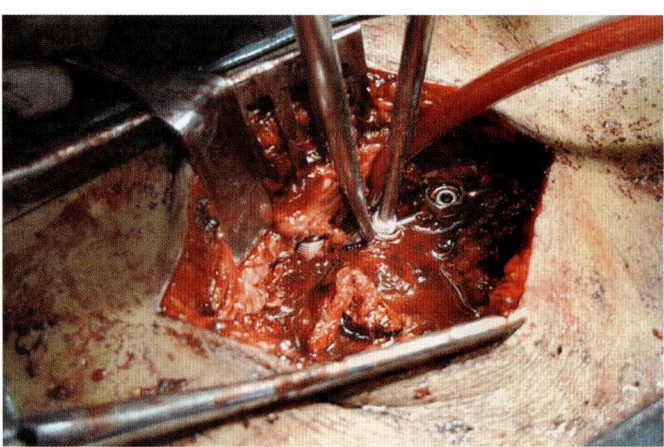

Fig. 57.53: Fixing the rods

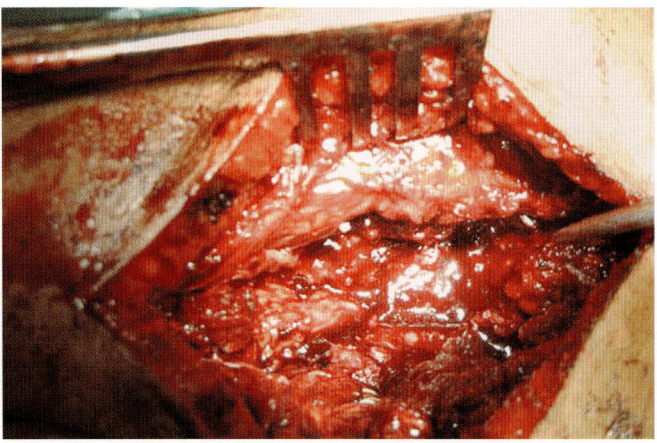

Fig. 57.51: Laminectomy completed

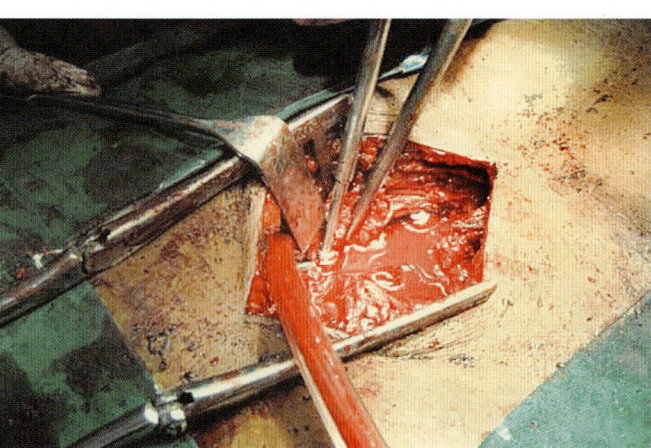

Fig. 57.54: Placement of the inny

CHAPTER 57: Common Surgery of the Spine

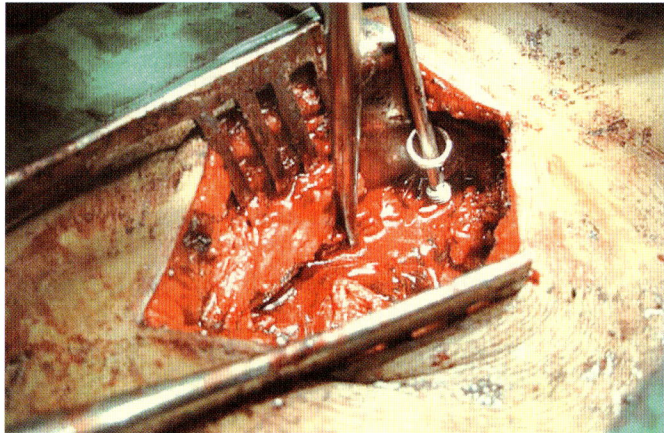

Fig. 57.55: Placing the outy

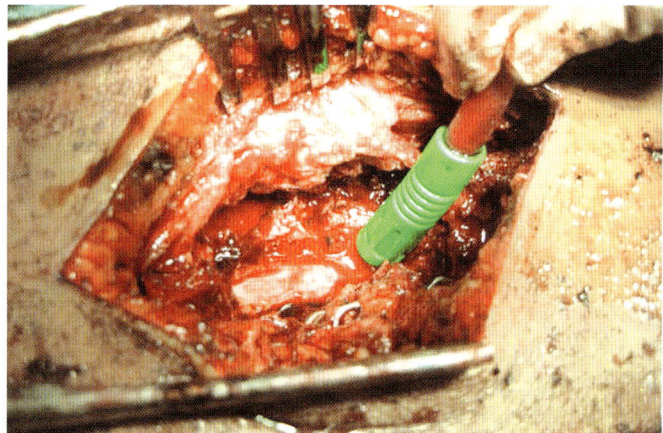

Fig. 57.58: Cleaning the dura of the compression

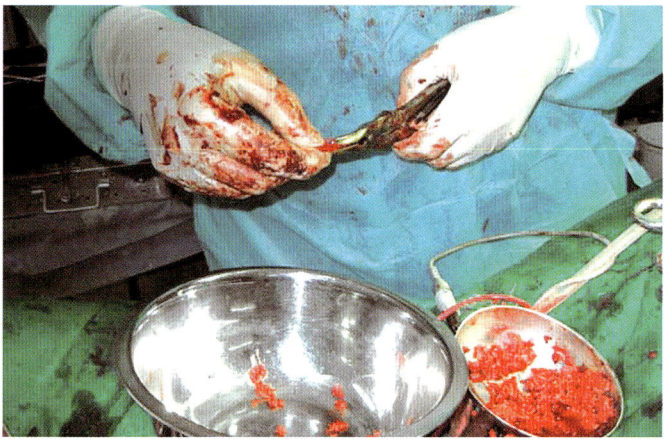

Fig. 57.56: Preparation of the cancellous graft

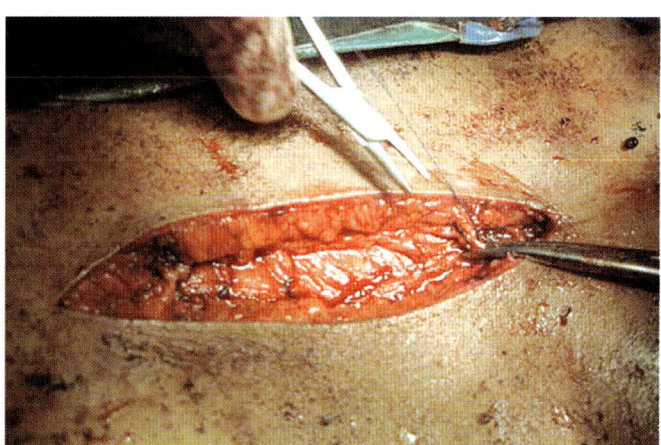

Fig. 57.59: Closure of the layers of muscles

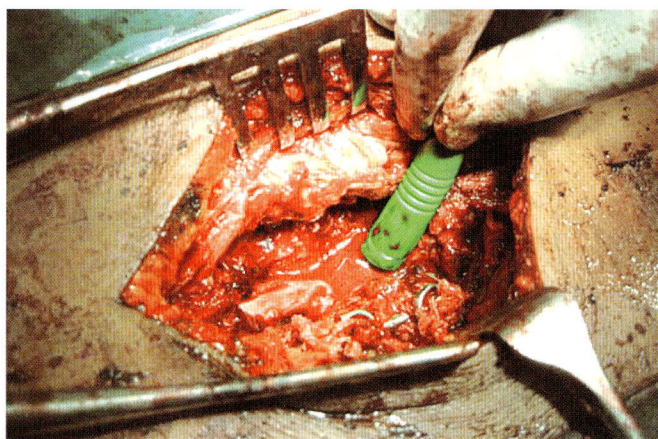

Fig. 57.57: Placement of the grafts

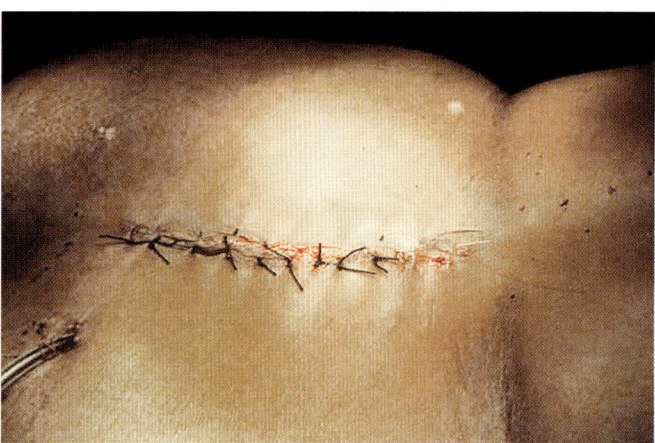

Fig. 57.60: Final skin closure over a drain

- Gently using moderate force proceed through the pedicle with a sharp probe.
- Confirm the position over the C-arm.
- Now tap the pedicle under C-arm control.
- Insert mono- or polyaxial screws and confirm with C-arm.
- Confirm the stability of the screws by trying to pull on it and checking the hold.
- Now similarly pass the other screws above and below.
- Now select the CD rod and size it appropriately.
- Bend the rod and configure it the spine curvature.
- Place the rods through the screws above and below.
- Hold the rod firmly through a rod pusher.
- Place the inny and just tighten do not tighten too much as it will be difficult to pass the outy.
- Next insert outy screw cap and tighten both the inny and outy.
- As the screws are being tightened reduction of the slip happens.
- Now check the stability of the construct by gently lifting the CD rod system.
- If the construct is stable, check the position of the rod and screws again on the C-arm.
- If laminectomy is required to decompress carry out these steps.
- Using appropriate rougeurs remove a small portion of the superior and inferior laminae.
- Hold the ligamentum flavum with an Allis or Kochers make a nick and excise a flap of ligamentum flavum by sharp dissection. Take care not to damage the dura.
- Inspect and release the compressed dura.
- Look for the nerve roots on either side for any compressions.
- Remove all the cottonoids and control the residual bleeding.
- Close the wound in layers with appropriate suture material for different tissues.
- Apply a pressure bandage.

Aftercare

- Patient can be allowed to turn in bed the same day.
- He may be allowed to stand with walker on the same evening and may be allowed to go to the bathroom.
- Walking is permitted after the first postoperative day.
- Isometric abdominal and lower limb exercises are begun.
- Sitting is minimized but walking is encouraged.
- After 4–6 weeks back exercises are commenced.
- After 6th week, lifting, bending, stooping can be allowed.
- Increased sitting may be allowed after 4th week and long trips after 3 months.
- After 8–10th week, lower limb exercises are begun.
- After 12 weeks, patient may be allowed to return to work.

58 CHAPTER

Common Finger and Toe Surgery (Percutaneous Fixations)

Complex and compound finger and toe injuries are managed by closed or open reductions with internal fixations by K-wires through percutaneous techniques as shown in the illustrations below.

FINGER FRACTURE

Technique of K-wire Stabilization of Compound Proximal Phalanx Fractures (Figs 58.1 to 58.10)

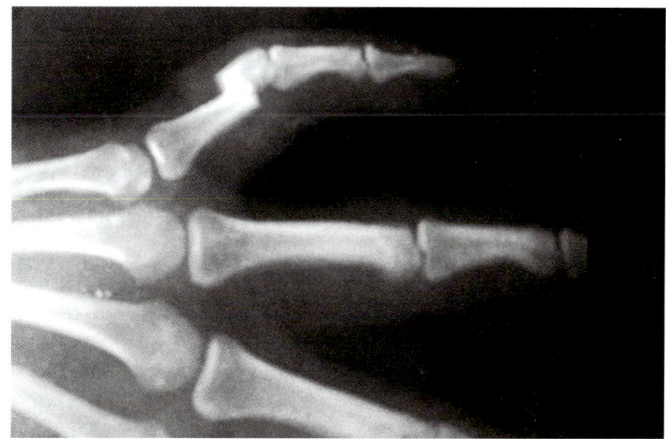

Fig. 58.2: Radiograph showing the fracture of the neck of the proximal phalanx

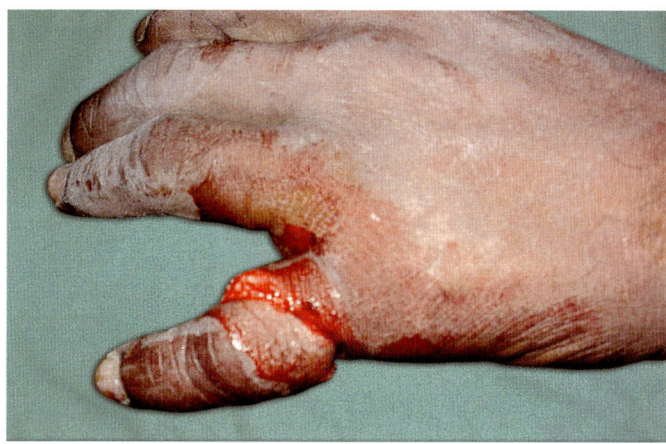

Fig. 58.1: Compound fracture of the proximal phalanx of the little finger

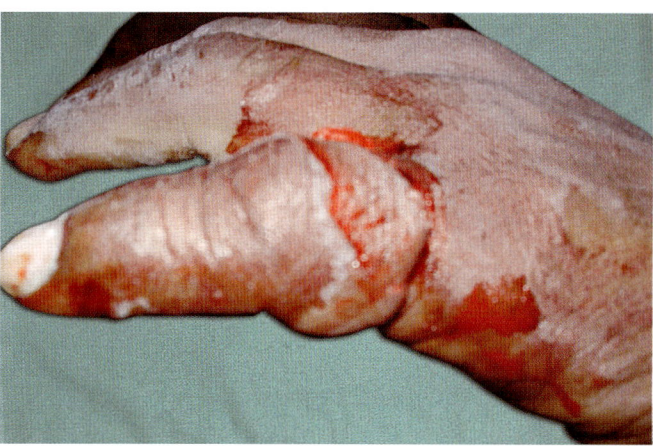

Fig. 58.3: View from the sides

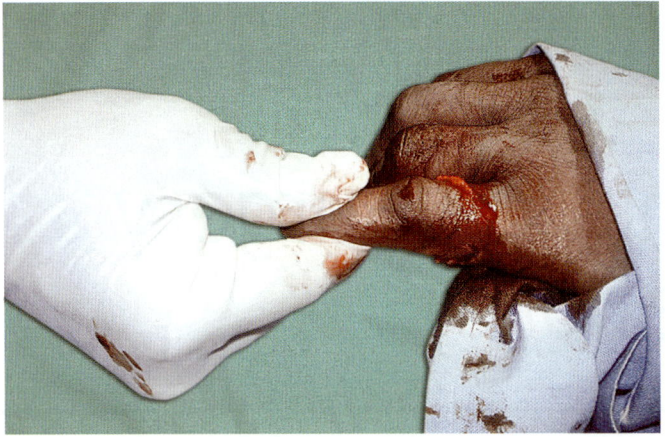

Fig. 58.4: Debridement and reduction

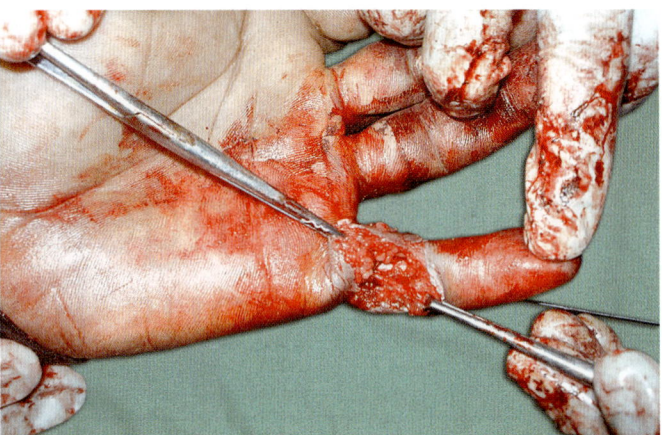

Fig. 58.7: Suturing of the volar side over the K-wire

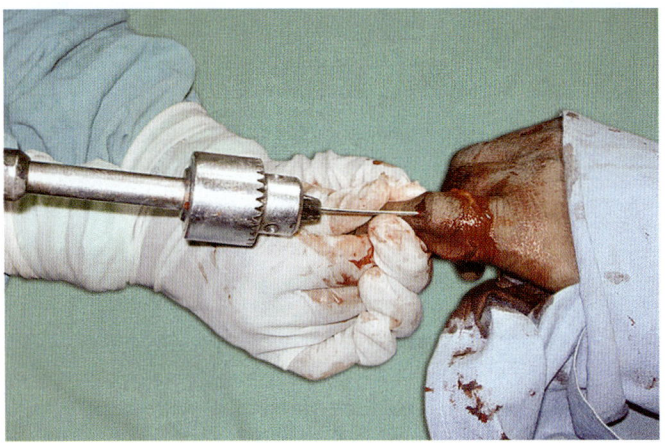

Fig. 58.5: Beginning to fix it with K-wire

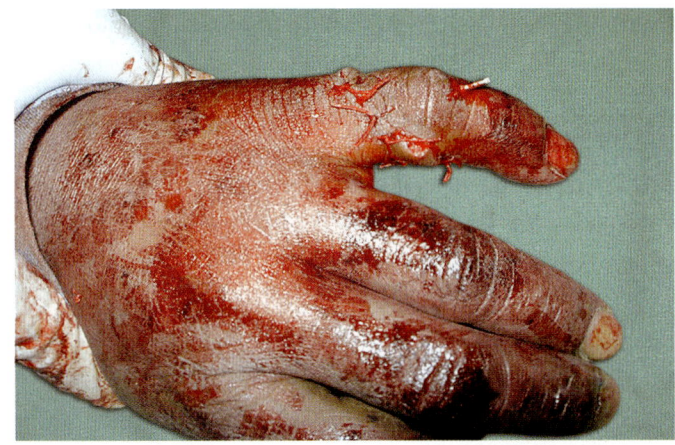

Fig. 58.8: Suturing of the dorsal side

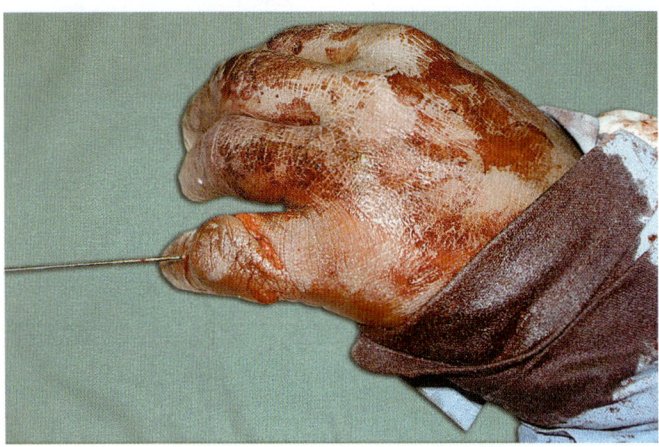

Fig. 58.6: Fixation with K-wire

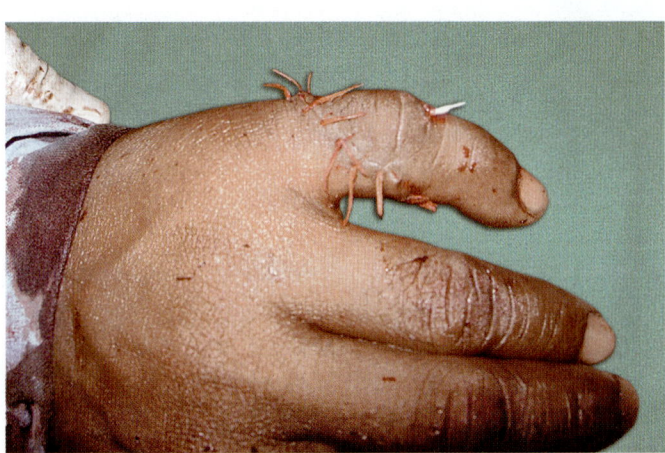

Fig. 58.9: Suturing completed

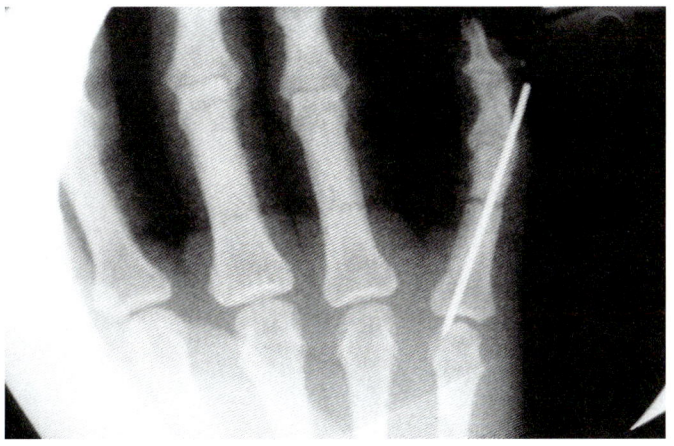

Fig. 58.10: Postreduction and postfixation C-arm view

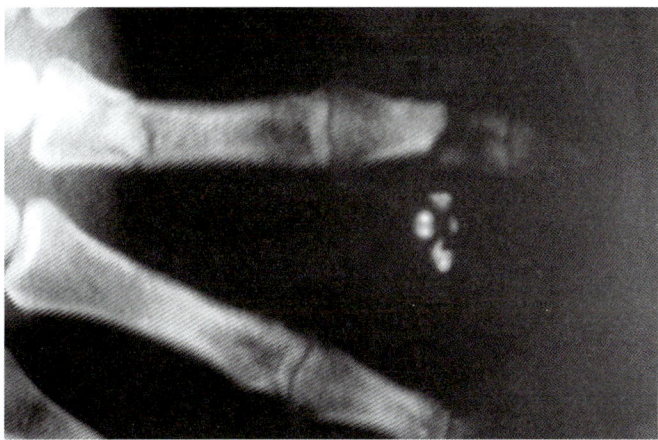

Fig. 58.13: AP view

Technique of Fixation of Ipsilateral Phalangeal Fractures (Figs 58.11 to 58.27)

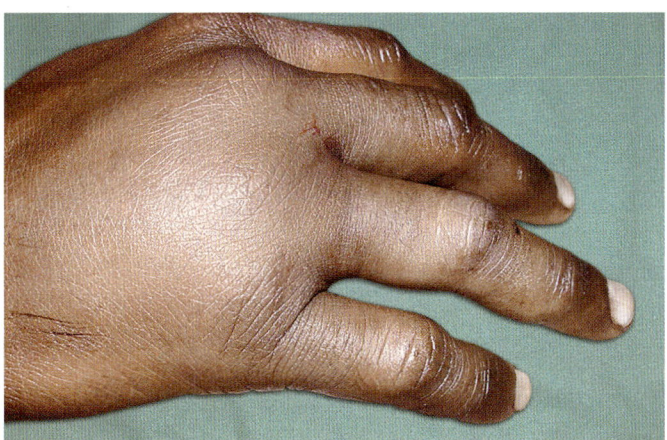

Fig. 58.11: Deformity

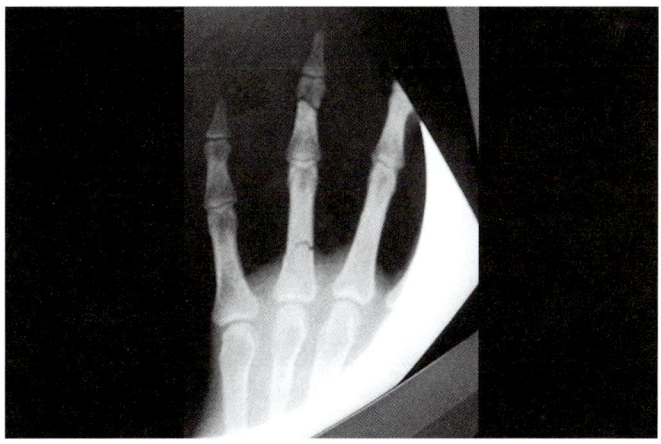

Fig. 58.14: C-arm view after closed reduction of the fractures

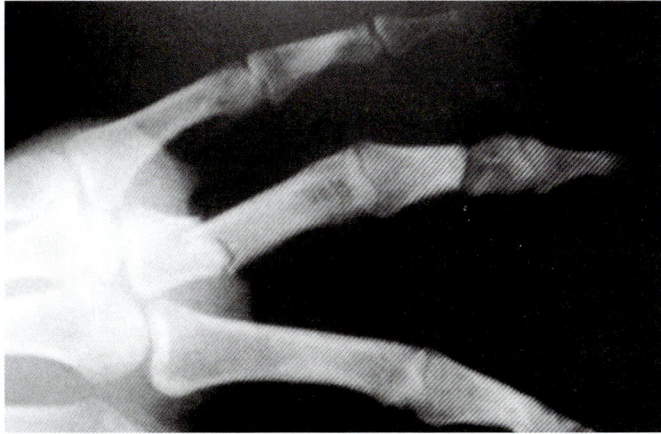

Fig. 58.12: Radiograph showing ipsilateral fractures of the ring finger involving proximal and middle phalanges

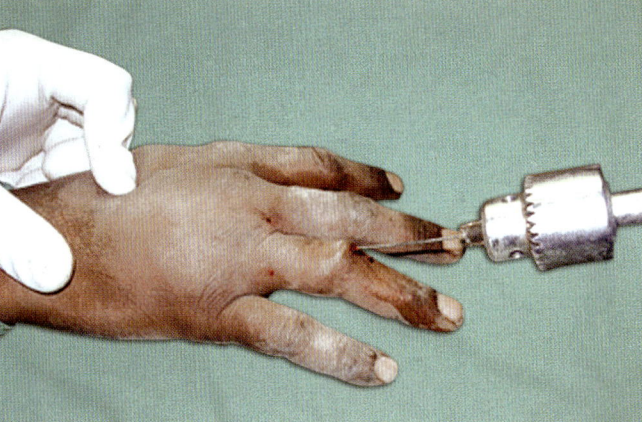

Fig. 58.15: Passing K-wire for the proximal phalanx fracture

758 SECTION 7: Common Surgical Techniques

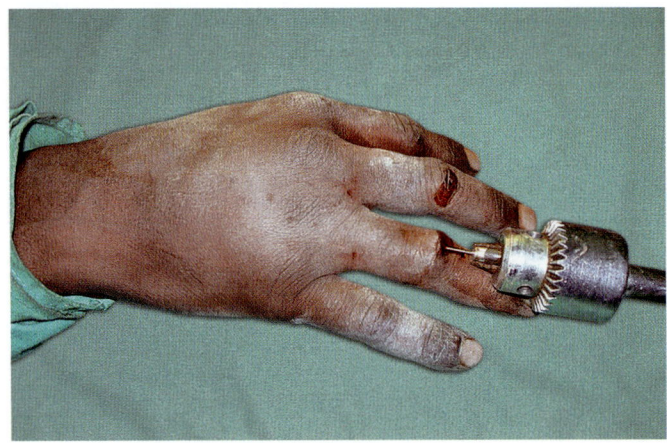

Fig. 58.16: K-wire passed further

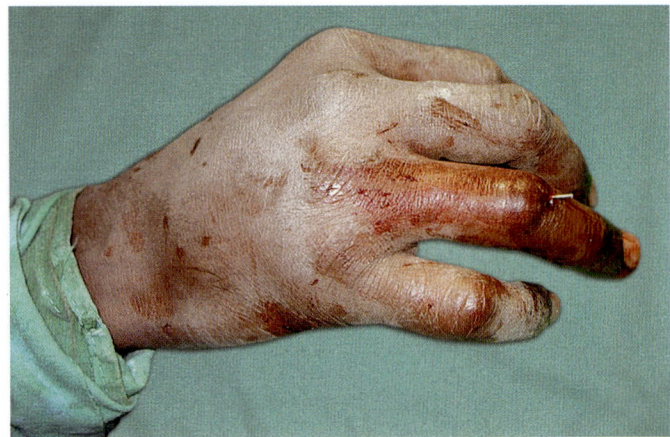

Fig. 58.19: K-wire cut

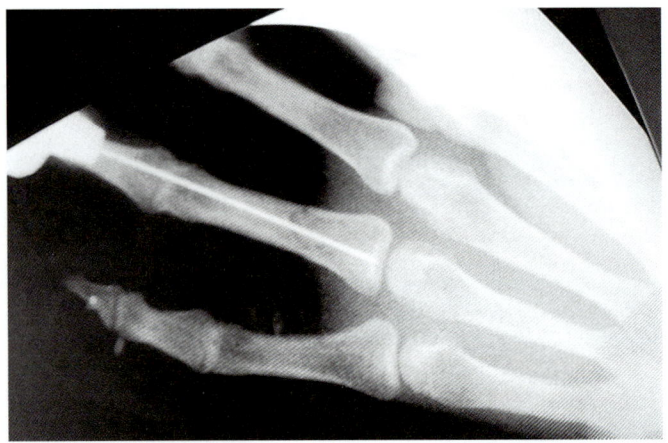

Fig. 58.17: C-arm view of the position of the K-wire

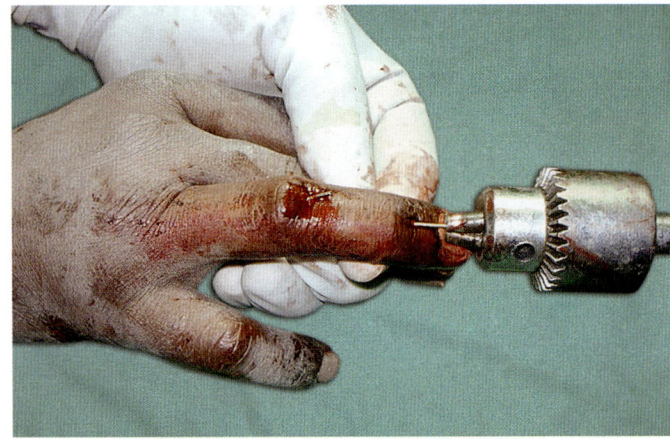

Fig. 58.20: K-wire being passed into the middle phalanx

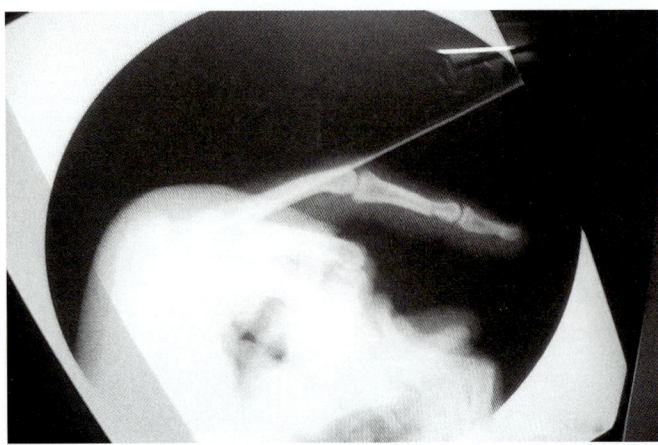

Fig. 58.18: C-arm—lateral view

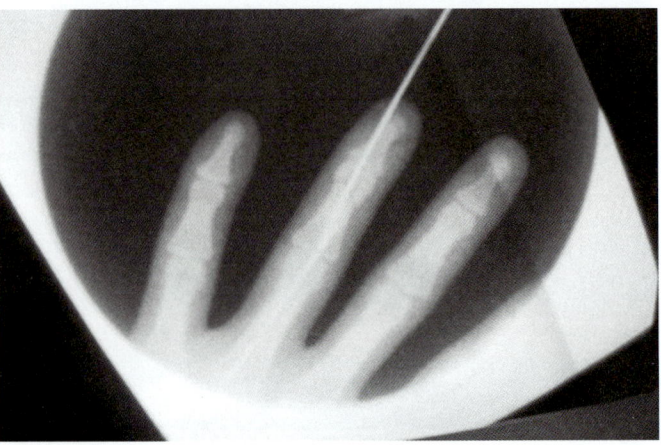

Fig. 58.21: C-arm check—AP view

CHAPTER 58: Common Finger and Toe Surgery (Percutaneous Fixations) **759**

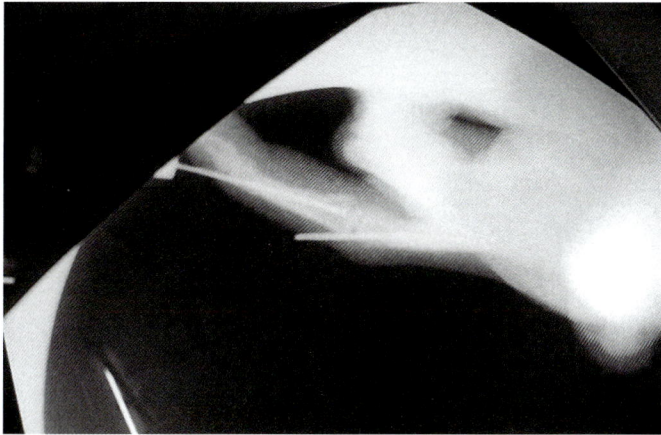

Fig. 58.22: C-arm check—lateral view

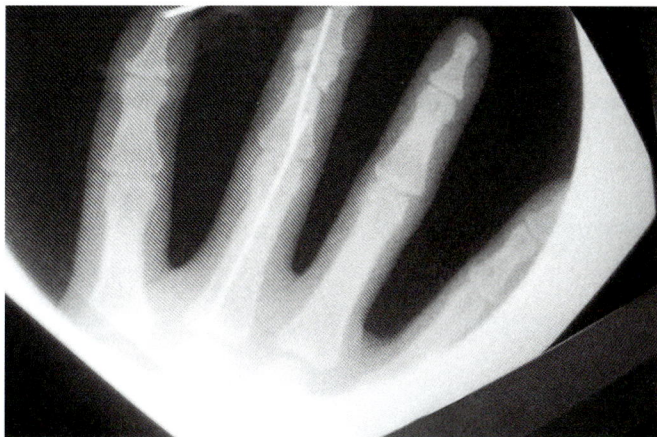

Fig. 58.25: C-arm view of both the pins—AP view

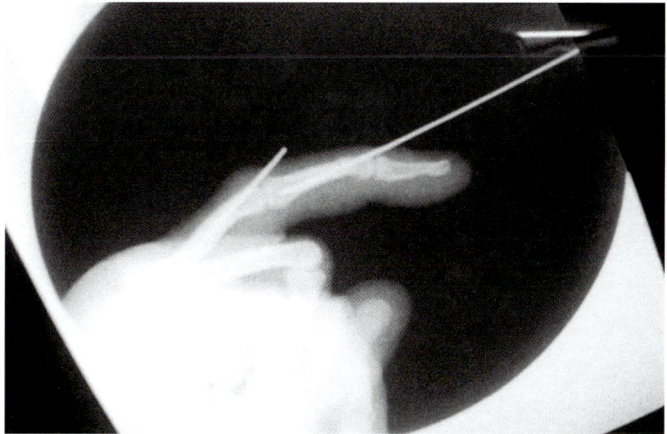

Fig. 58.23: Another view confirming both the pins position

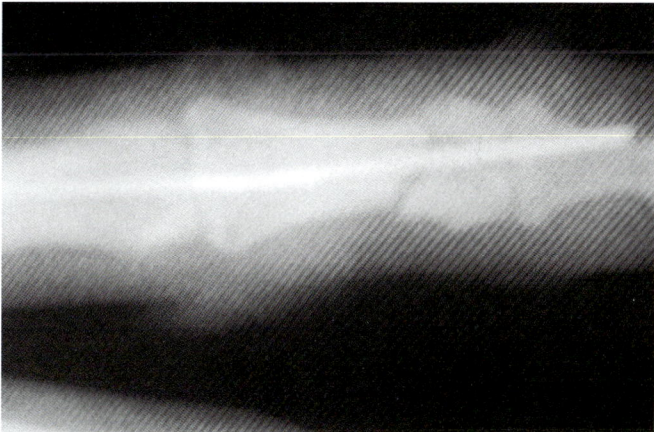

Fig. 58.26: C-arm view of both the pins—lateral view

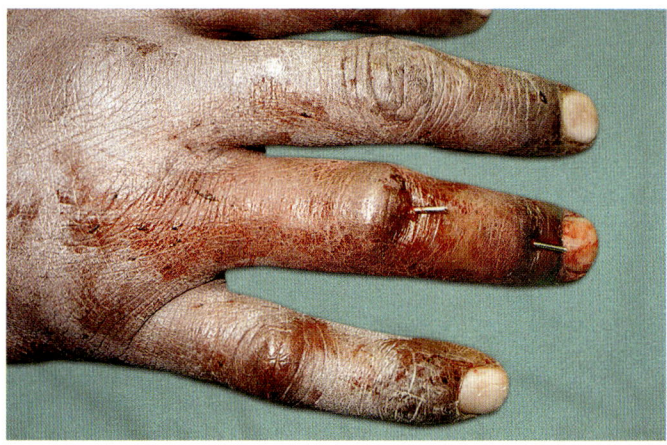

Fig. 58.24: Both the pins cut at the level of the skin

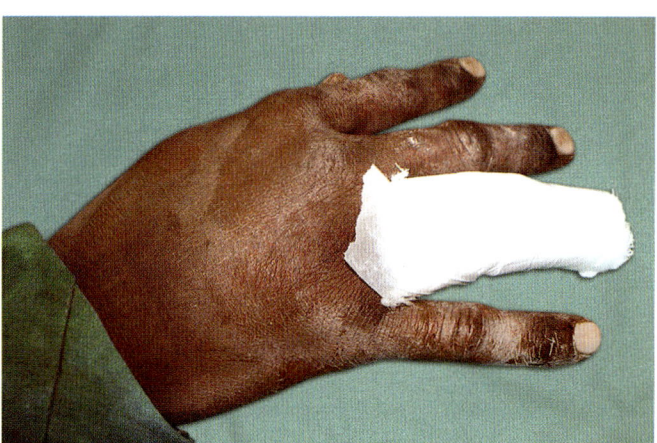

Fig. 58.27: Final dressing

Surgical Technique of K-wire Fixation of a Metacarpal Fracture (Figs 58.28 to 58.44)

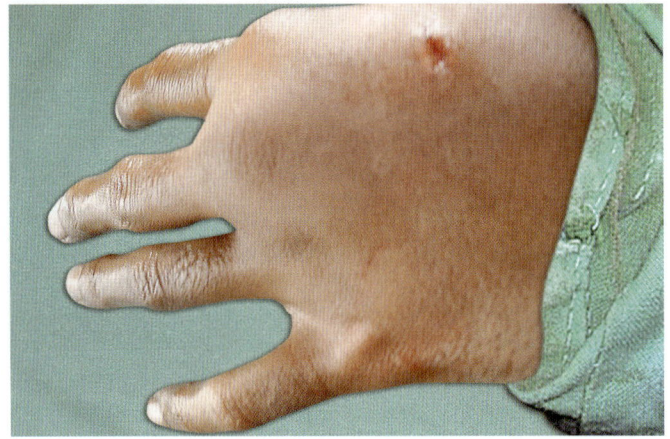

Fig. 58.28: Deformity and pin compound

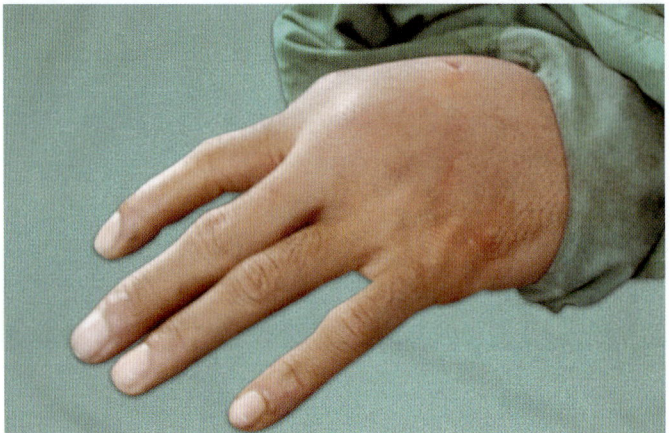

Fig. 58.31: Preparation and draping

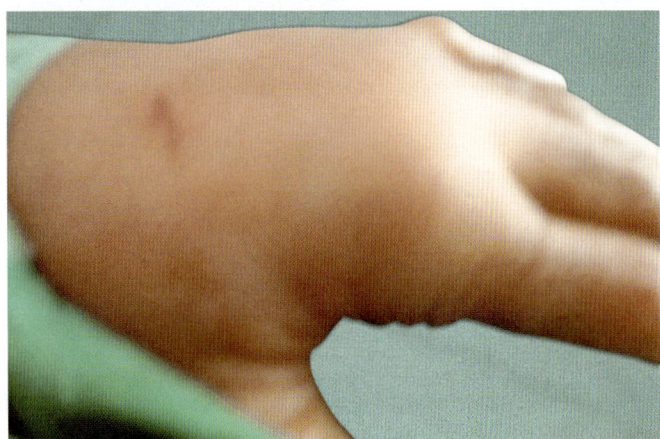

Fig. 58.29: Deformity closer view

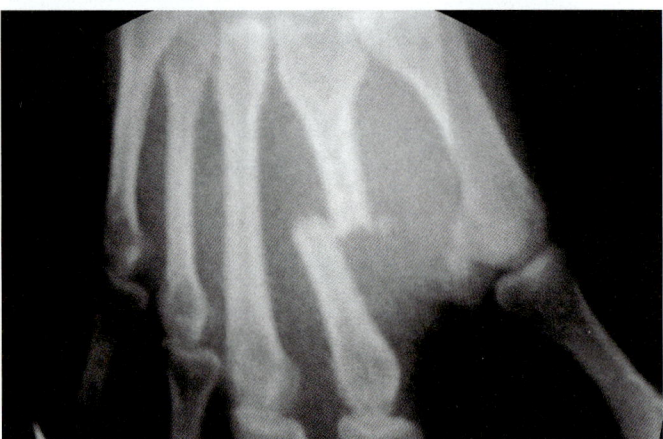

Fig. 58.32: C-arm view

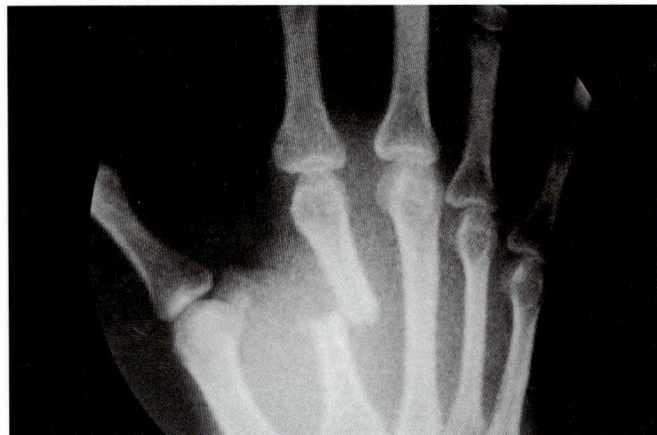

Fig. 58.30: Radiograph showing displaced fracture

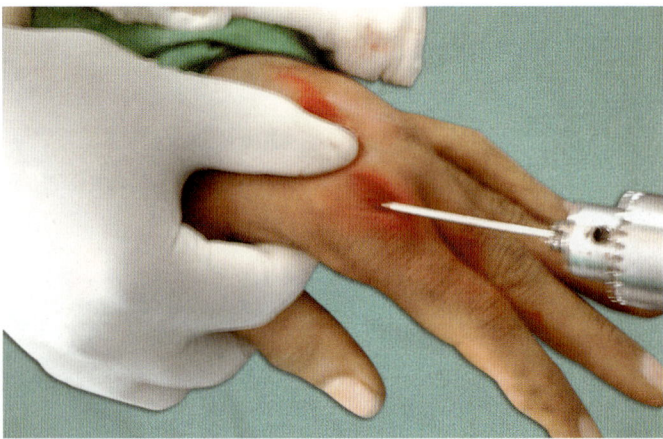

Fig. 58.33: Manipulation and stabilization of fracture and K-wire positioning

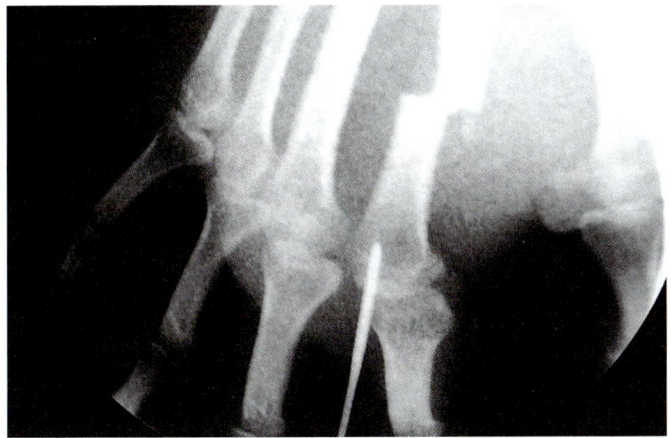

Fig. 58.34: C-arm check pin within the medullary canal

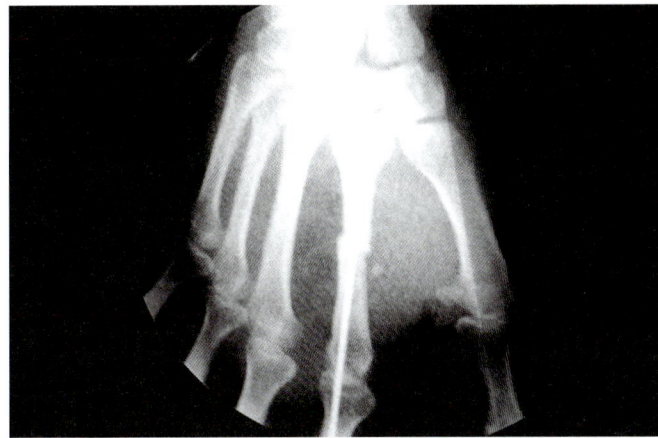

Fig. 58.37: Fracture reduced and pin at the proximal end

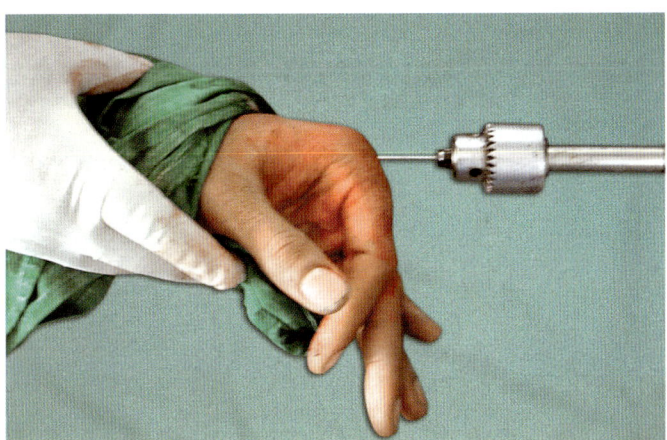

Fig. 58.35: Pin being driven in

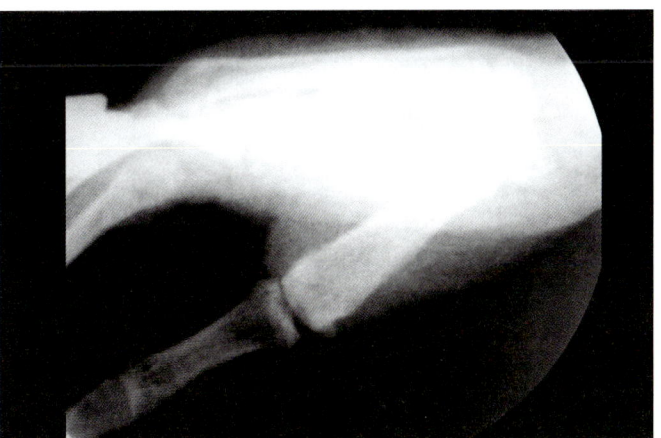

Fig. 58.38: Confirmation in the lateral view

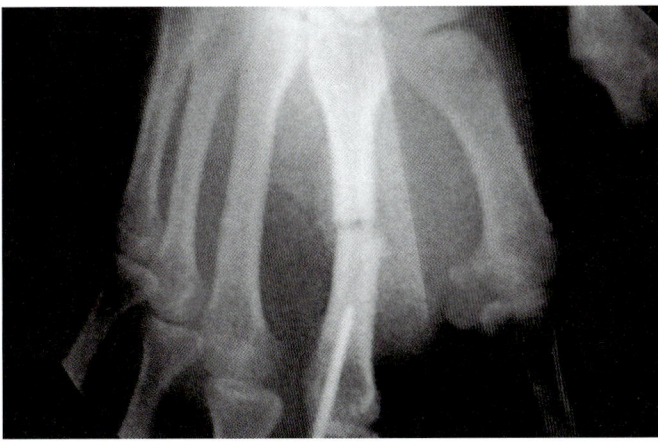

Fig. 58.36: Pin in the center of the medullary canal

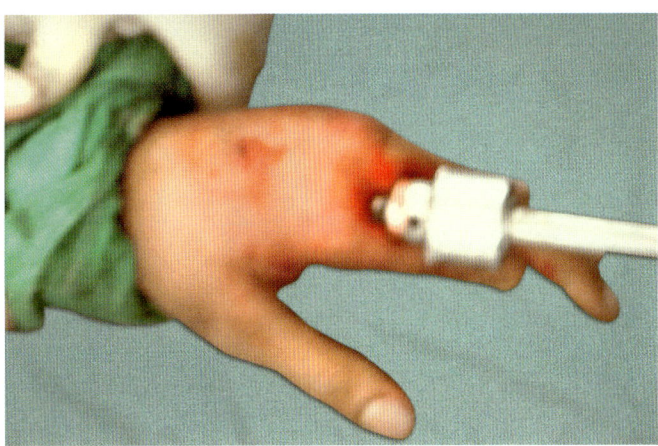

Fig. 58.39: Pin passed completely

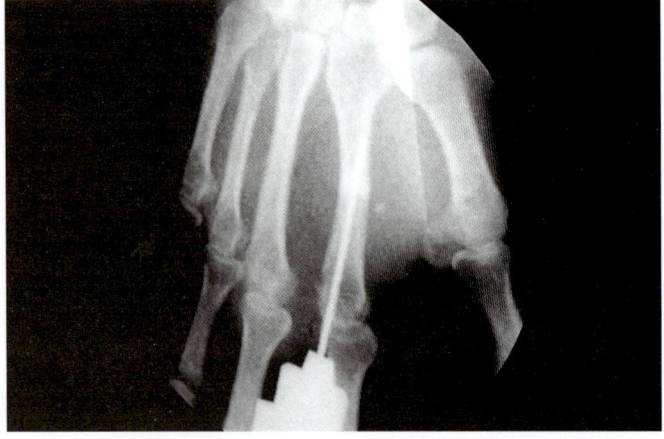

Fig. 58.40: Pin placed within the proximal fragment

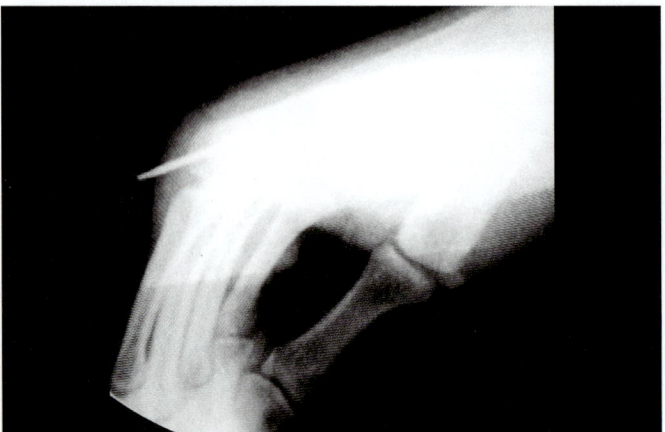

Fig. 58.42: Lateral view

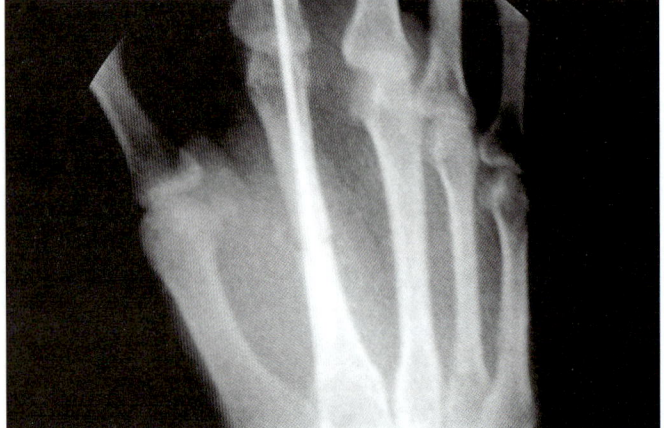

Fig. 58.41: Good fixation

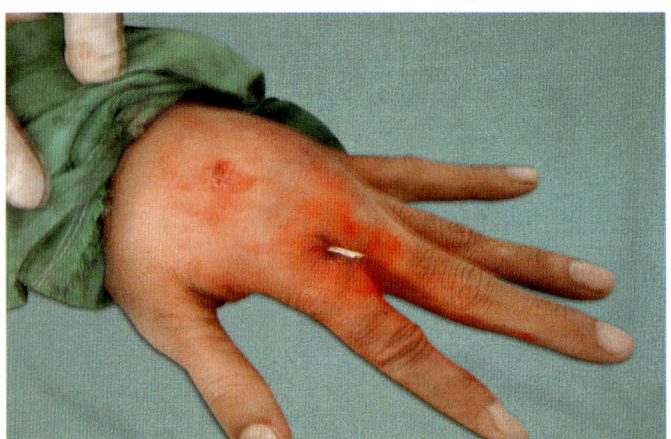

Fig. 58.43: Pin being cut

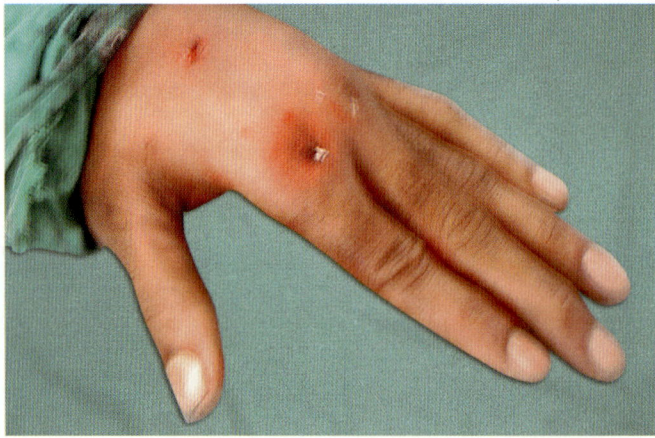

Fig. 58.44: Final pin placement

TOE INJURIES

These are less common than finger injuries. They are usually due to direct injuries from fall of heavy objects on the toes.

SURGICAL TECHNIQUE OF PERCUTANEOUS FIXATION OF TOE FRACTURES (FIGS 58.45 TO 58.59)

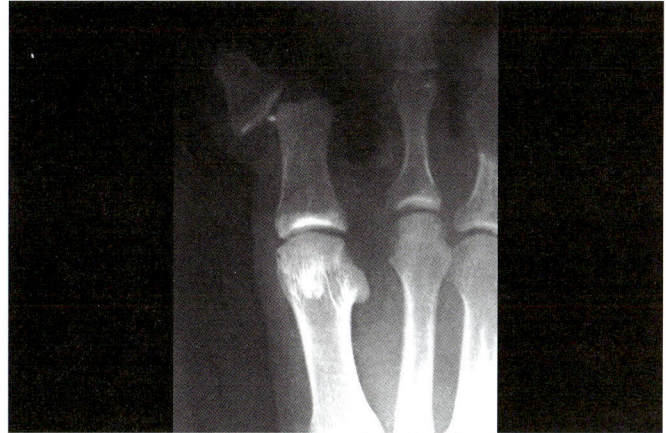

Fig. 58.47: Radiograph of AP view showing dislocation of I MTP joint

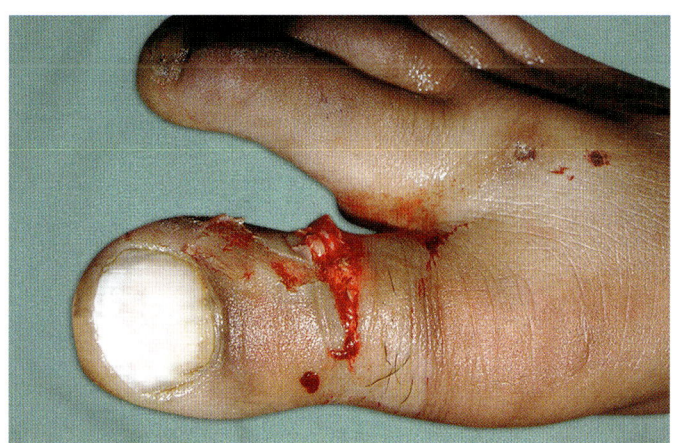

Fig. 58.45: Wound as viewed from the top

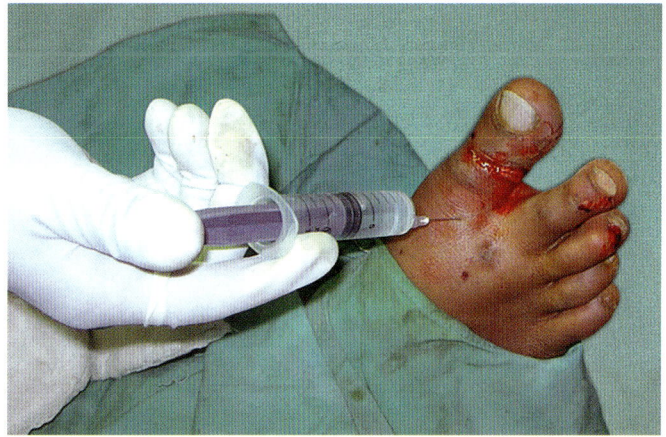

Fig. 58.48: Digital block

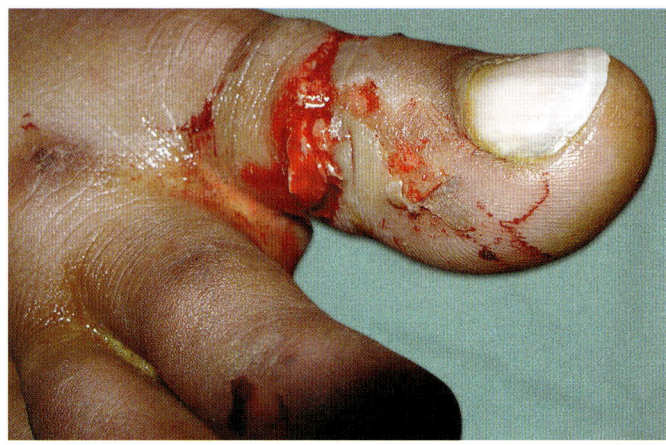

Fig. 58.46: Wound as viewed from the sides

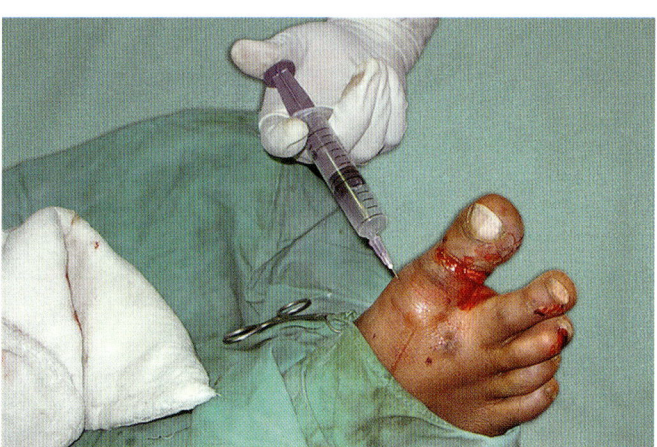

Fig. 58.49: Digital block continued

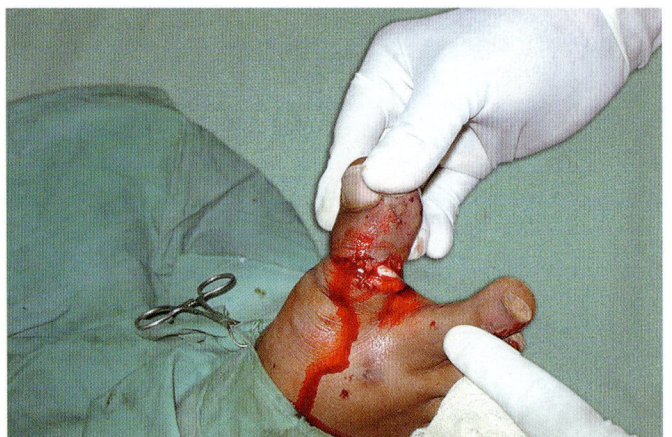

Fig. 58.50: Exposure of the wound

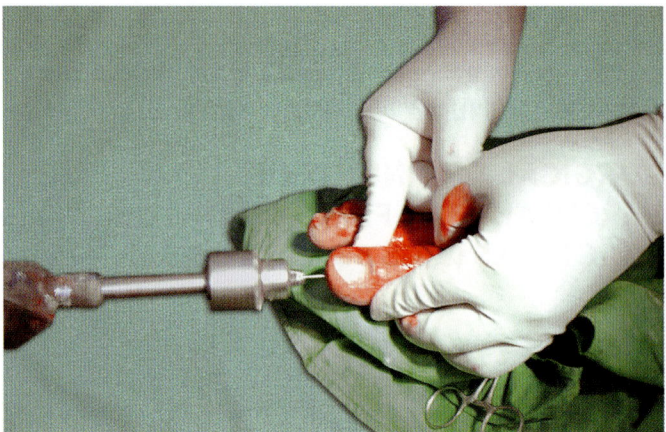

Fig. 58.53: K-wire being driven further

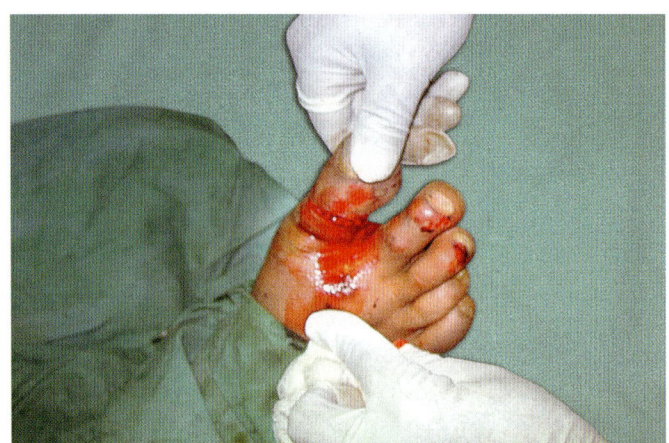

Fig. 58.51: Reduction of the fracture dislocation

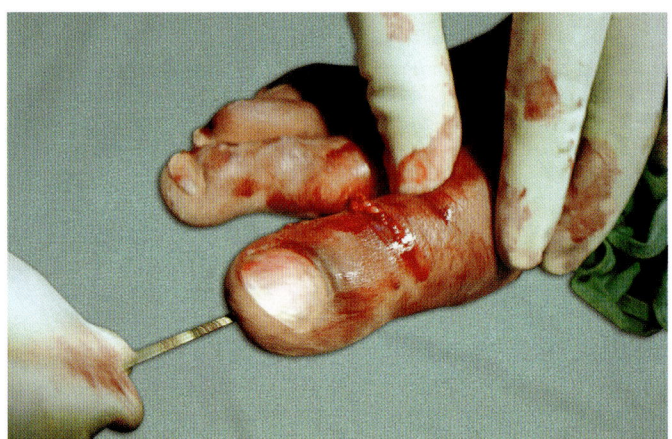

Fig. 58.54: K-wire fixation

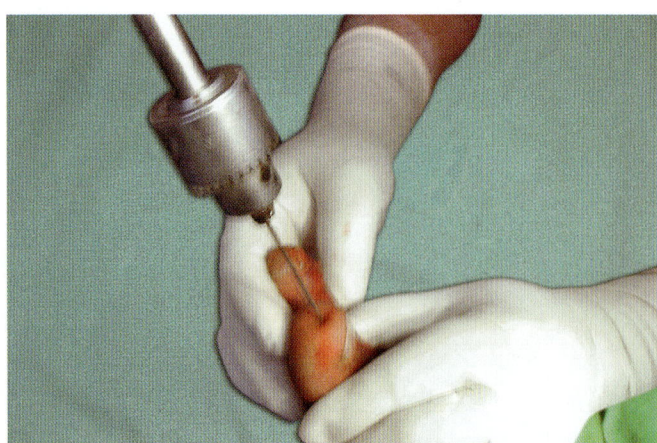

Fig. 58.52: K-wire being passed

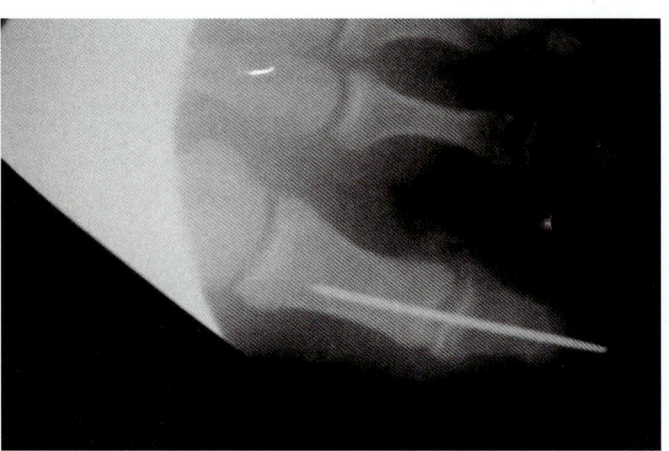

Fig. 58.55: K-wire C-arm view

CHAPTER 58: Common Finger and Toe Surgery (Percutaneous Fixations) **765**

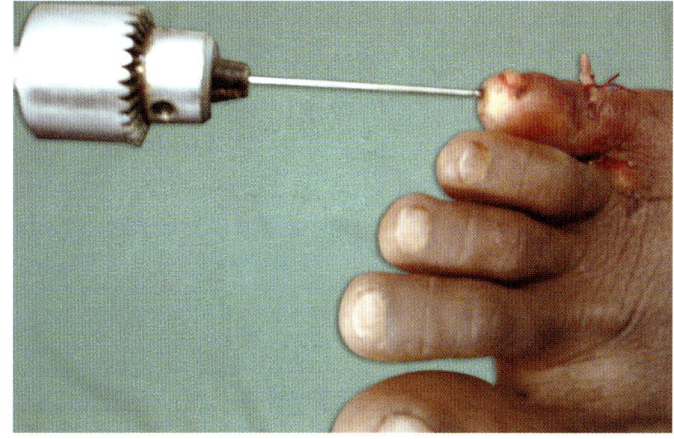

Fig. 58.56: Deformity corrected and being fixed with K-wire

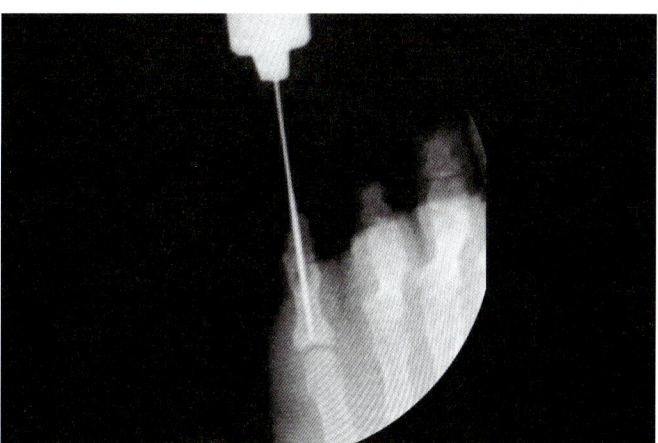

Fig. 58.58: Checking through C-arm

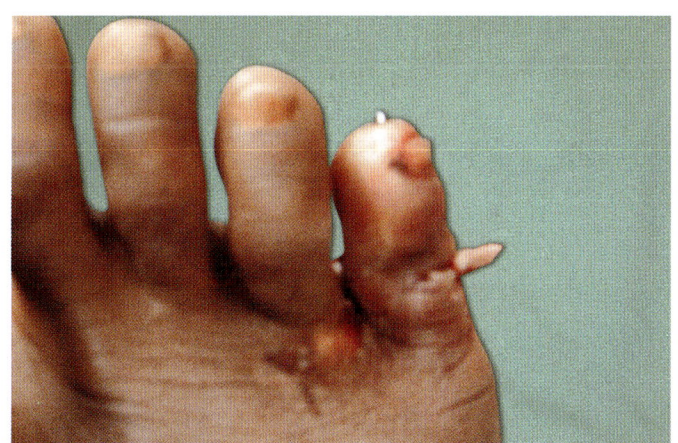

Fig. 58.57: K-wire introduced and positioned

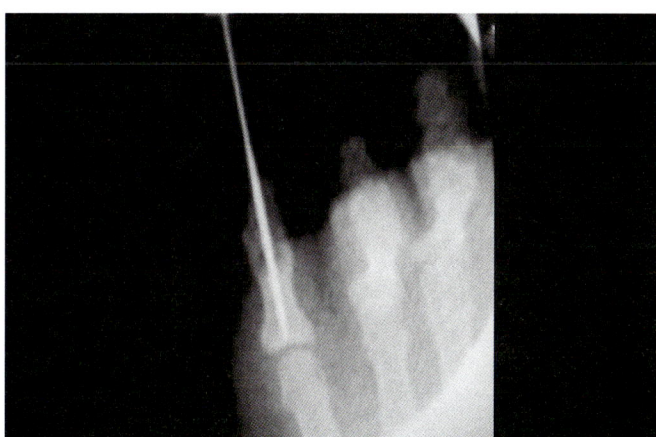

Fig. 58.59: Wire placement final

59
CHAPTER

External Fixation

External fixation of fractures is a great boon in compound injuries. It helps to stabilize the fracture fragments that cannot be fixed internally due to fear of infection. External fixators help to stabilize the fractures while at the same time helps to attend and manage the associated soft tissue injuries.

Surgical Technique of Application of External Fixators (Figs 59.1 to 59.22)

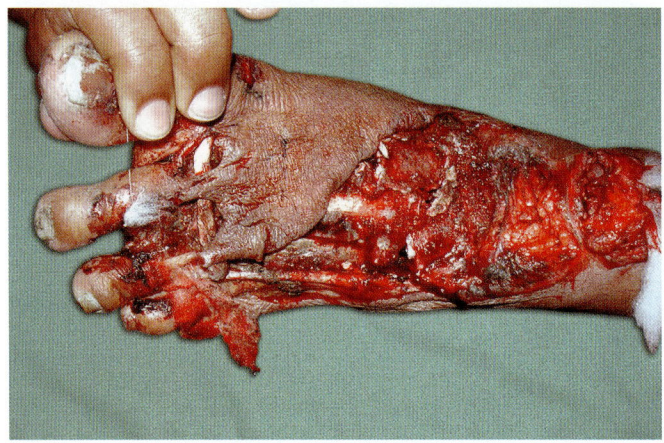

Fig. 59.1: Degloving injury foot

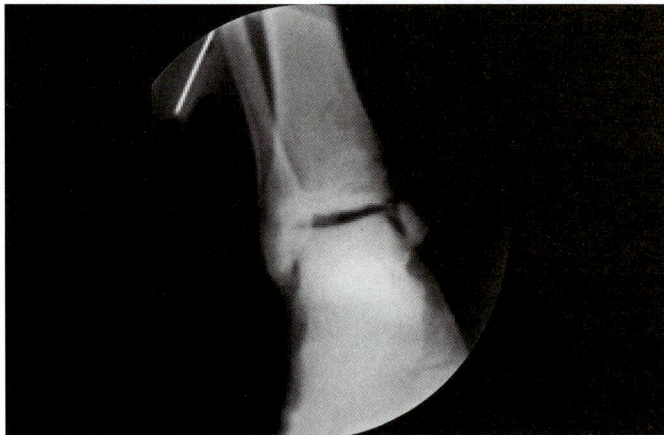

Fig. 59.3: Radiograph shows fracture of medial malleolus

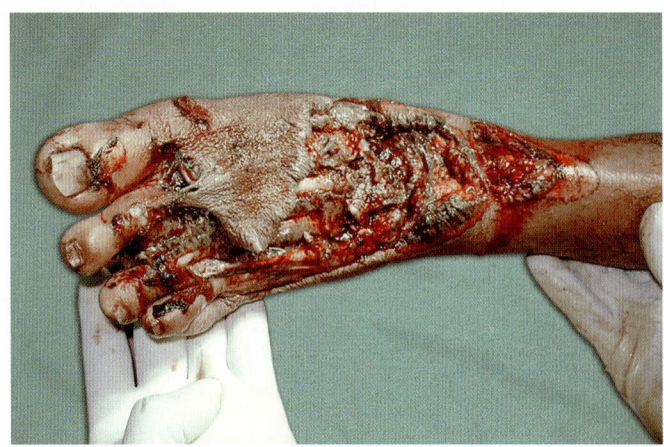

Fig. 59.2: After debridement

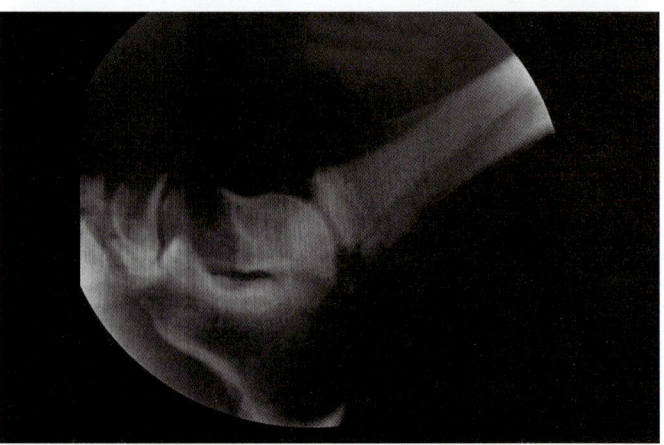

Fig. 59.4: Radiograph shows fracture of lower end fibula

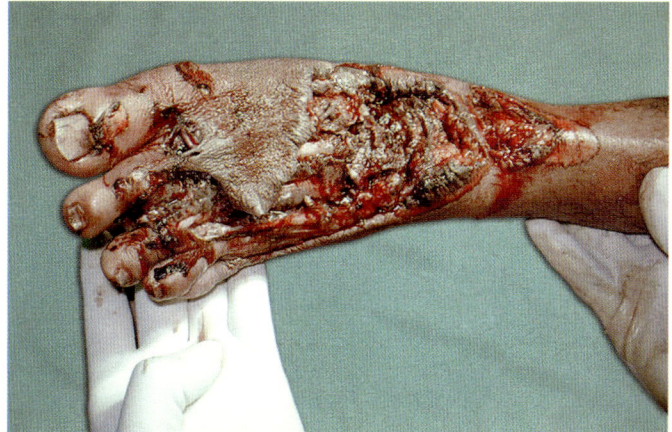

Fig. 59.5: After wound irrigation

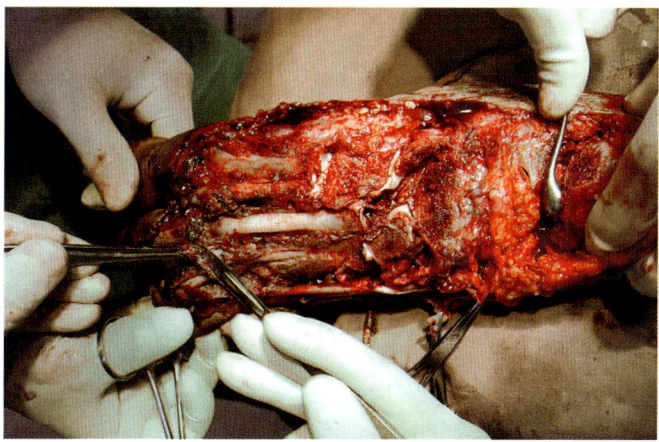

Fig. 59.8: Curetting the exposed bones

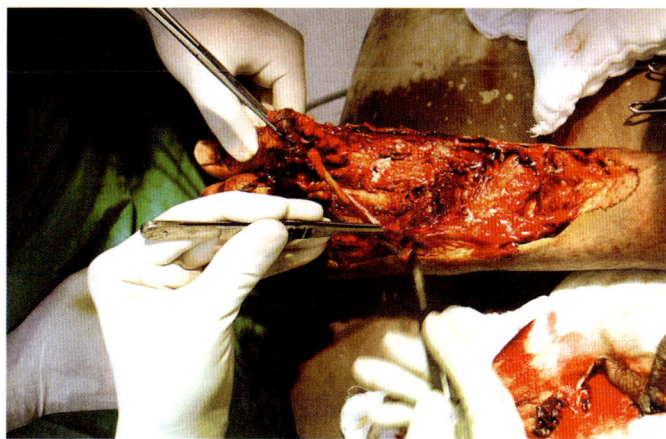

Fig. 59.6: Excision of the dead tissues

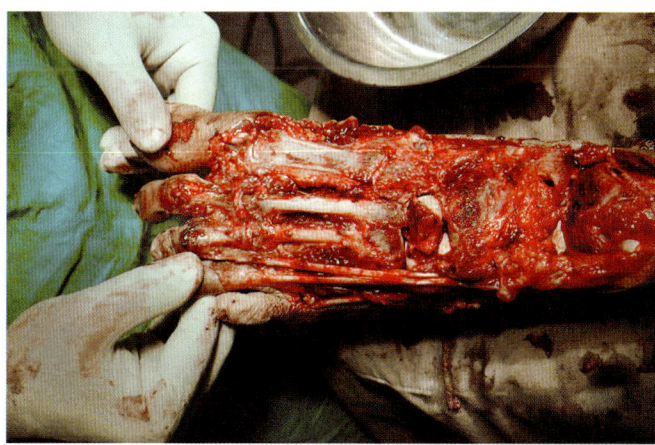

Fig. 59.9: Resurfacing the metatarsals

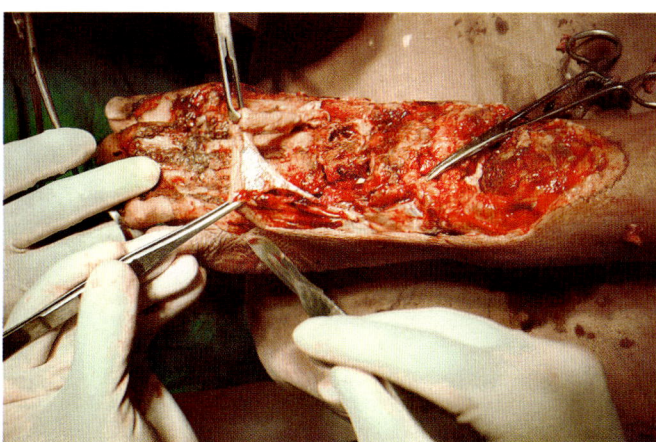

Fig. 59.7: Debridement continued

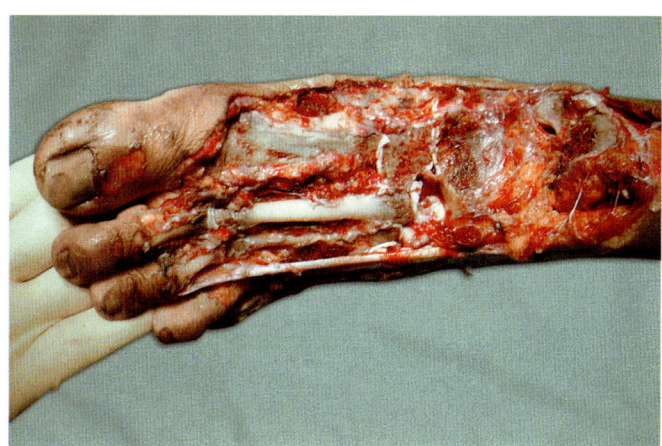

Fig. 59.10: Wound thoroughly washed

768 SECTION 7: Common Surgical Techniques

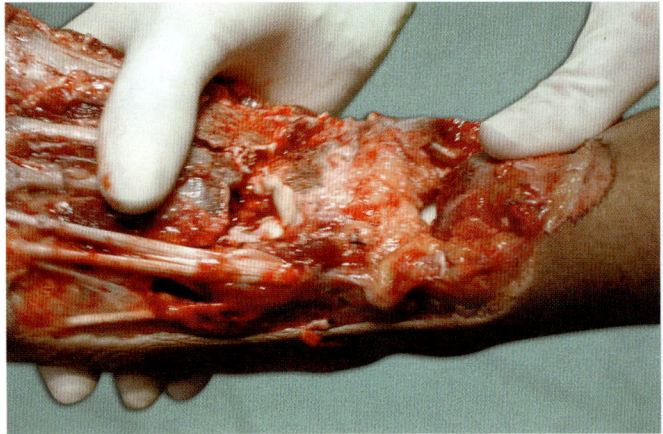

Fig. 59.11: Ankle being stabilized

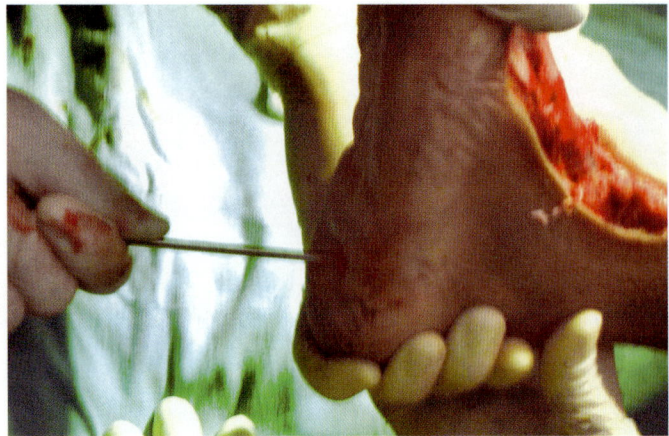

Fig. 59.14: Steinmann pin being driven

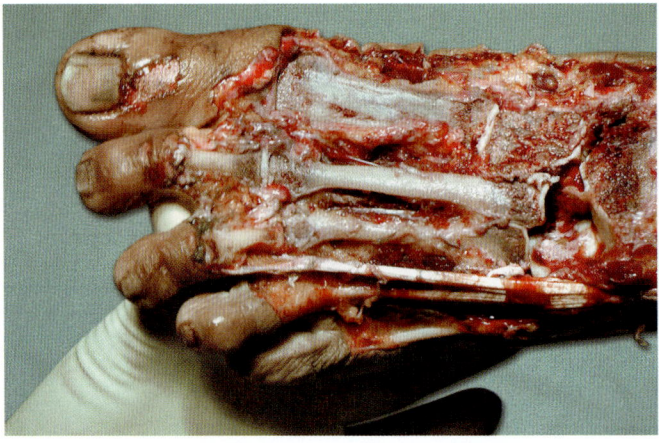

Fig. 59.12: Debridement complete

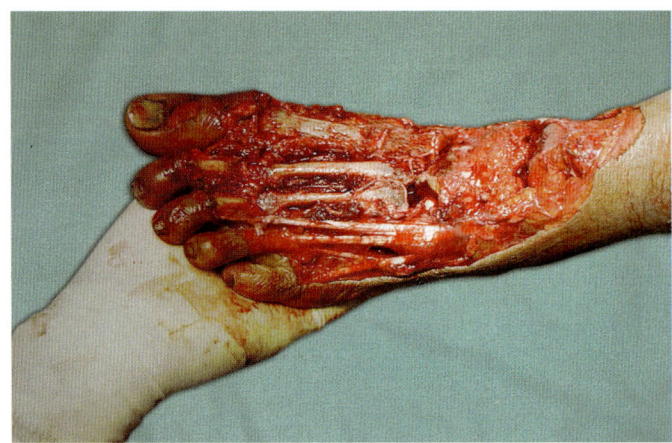

Fig. 59.15: Wound debrided and ankle stabilized

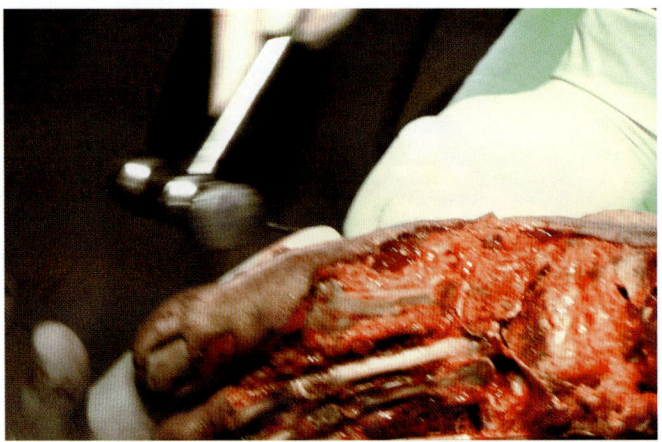

Fig. 59.13: Steinmann pin being driven through the heel

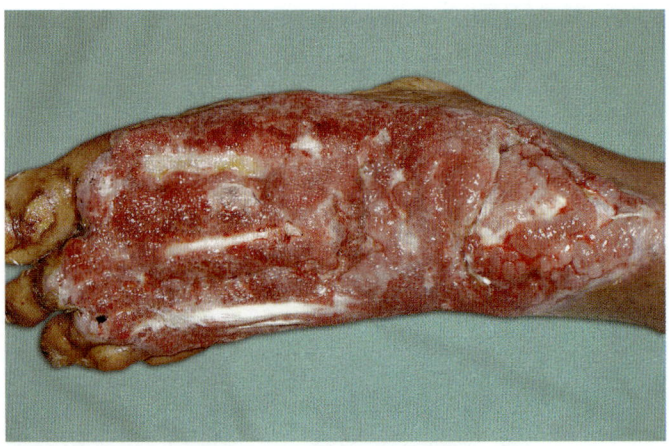

Fig. 59.16: Granulated surfaces of the degloved wound

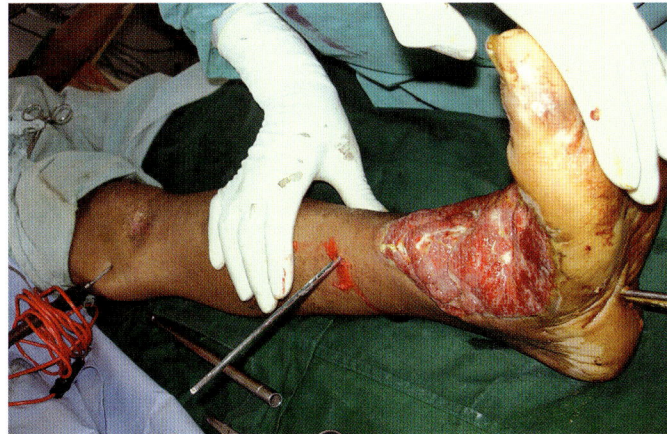

Fig. 59.17: Applying the external fixator—proximal tibial pin

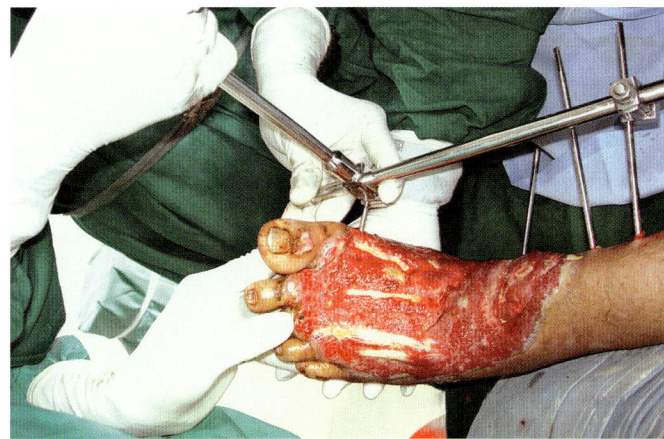

Fig. 59.20: Fixing the frame between tibia and metatarsal

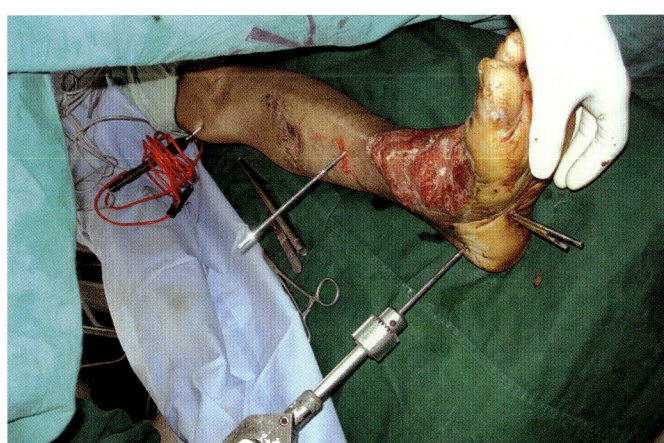

Fig. 59.18: Passing the calcaneal pin

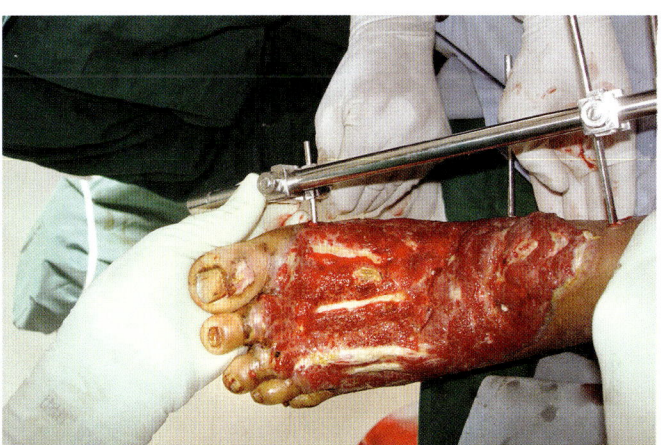

Fig. 59.21: Frame in position

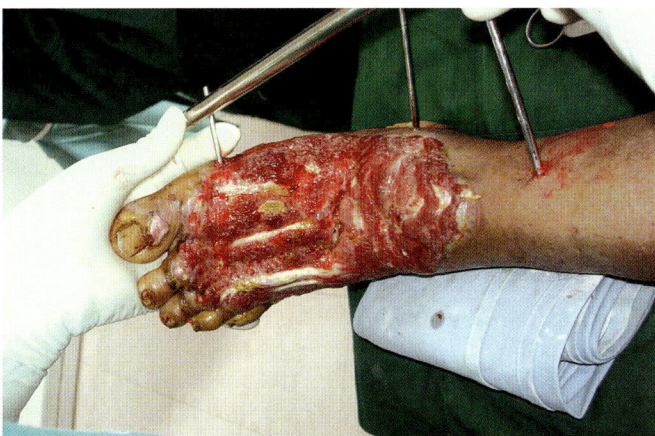

Fig. 59.19: Passing a pin through the metatarsals

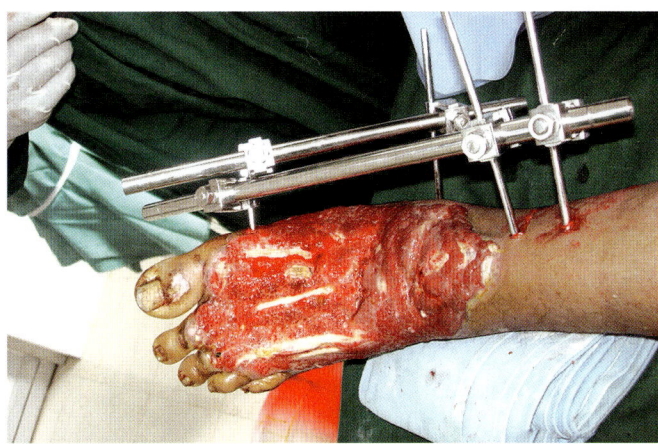

Fig. 59.22: Fixing the frame between metatarsal and heel

SECTION 8

Miscellaneous

- Amputations
- Prosthetics and Orthotics
- Sports Injuries
- Arthroscopy
- Standard Arthroscopy Portals
- 9-Point Diagnostic Knee Arthroscopy
- Arthroplasty
- Evidence-based Orthopedics

Section 8

Miscellaneous

60 CHAPTER

Amputations

INTRODUCTION

Definition

Amputation is defined as removal of the limb through a part of the bone.

Disarticulation is the removal of the limb through the joint.

Incidences

Age: Common in 50–75 years age group.

Sex: 7% men, 25% women.

Limbs: 85% is through the lower limbs, 15% is through the upper limbs.

Indications

Mercifully, due to recent advances in medicine and technology, the incidences of amputations are showing a downhill trend.

However, there are certain specific indications that require amputations (Flowchart 60.1). However, indications are not constant and keep changing according to the age of the patient.

> **Remember**
> The only real absolute indication for amputation is irreparable loss of blood supply of a diseased or injured limb.

> **Quick Facts**
> *Age vs indications in amputations*
> - Children—congenital anomalies
> - Young adults—injuries
> - Elderly—peripheral vascular diseases like TAO.

TYPES

Closed Amputation

This is done most of the times as an elective procedure and may be above knee or below knee, above elbow and below elbow, etc.

Open Amputation

In open amputation, the wound is left open over the amputation stump and is not closed. This is done as an emergency procedure in the face of life-threatening infections. There are two types in this depending upon the skin flaps:
- Open amputations with inverted skin flap
- Circular open amputation in which skin is closed later.

Amputation Levels (Figs 60.1A and B)

Upper Limbs (Fig. 60.2)
- Shoulder disarticulation
- Short above elbow (Fig. 60.1A)
- Standard above elbow (Fig. 60.1B)
- Elbow disarticulation

Flowchart 60.1: Indications for amputations

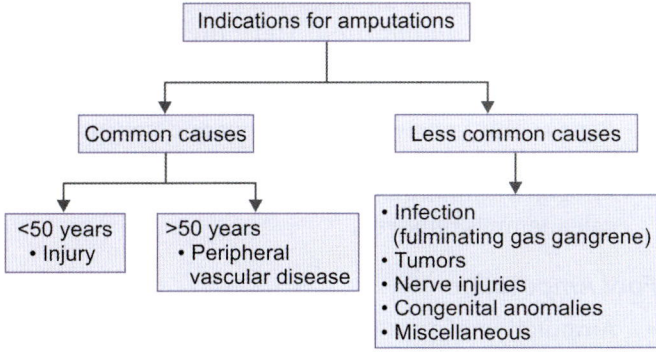

Note: Injury is the most common cause for amputations.

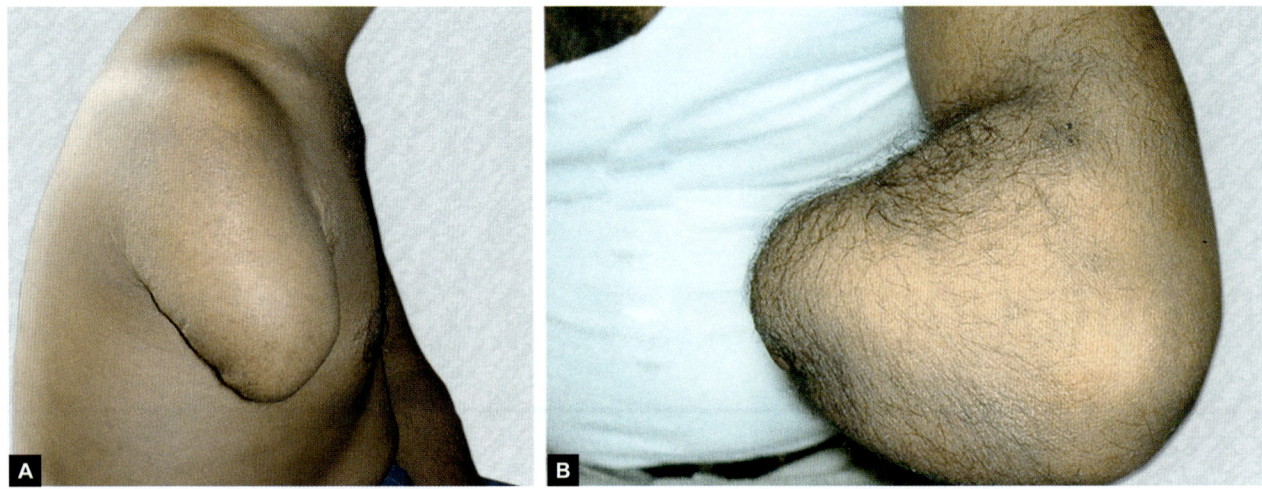

Figs 60.1A and B: Different amputation levels in upper and lower hand: (A) Above elbow; (B) Below elbow

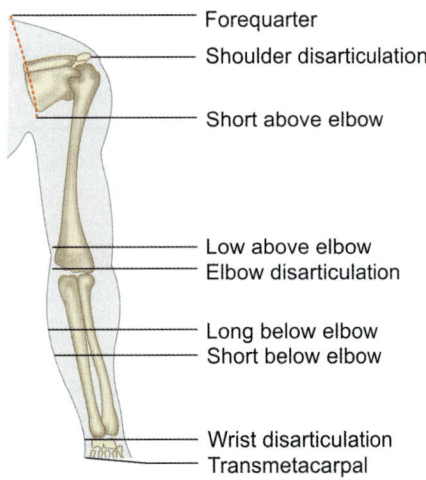

Fig. 60.2: Different levels of amputations in the upper limb

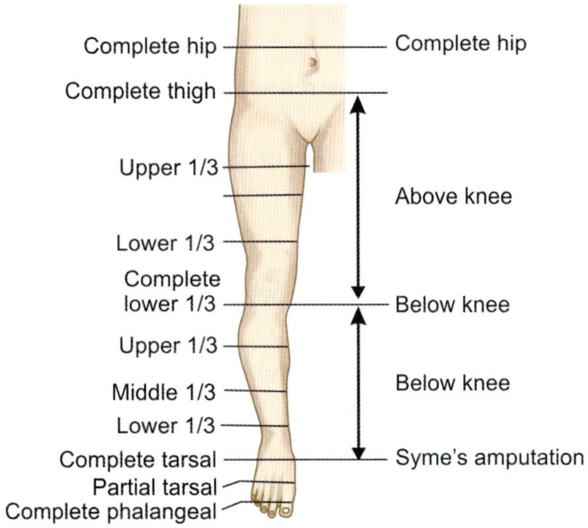

Fig. 60.3: Different levels of amputations in the lower limb

- Very short below elbow
- Medium below elbow
- Long below elbow.

Lower Limbs (Fig. 60.3)

- Hip disarticulation
- Very short above knee
- Short above knee
- Medium above knee
- Long above knee
- Very long above knee
- Knee disarticulation
- Very short below knee
- Short and below knee.

Ankle Amputation

- *Syme's amputation:* Here the level of bone section is 0.6 cm proximal to the ankle joint
- *Sarmiento's amputation:* Here the level is 1.3 cm proximal to the joint
- *Wagner's* is two-stage Syme's amputation
- *Boyd's:* This consists of talectomy and calcaneotibial arthrodesis
- *Pirogoff's amputation:* In this only anterior part of the calcaneum is removed.

Foot Amputation

- Amputation of great toes and other toes
- Amputation through the metatarsal bones

- *Lisfranc's operation:* Amputation is at the level of the tarsometatarsal joints
- *Chopart's operation:* Amputation is through the midtarsal joints.

PRINCIPLES

CLOSED AMPUTATIONS

In this, the skin is closed primarily after amputation.

Tourniquets: These are desirable except in ischemic limbs.

Level of amputation as in the past, the level of amputation is no longer important, thanks to the modern and sophisticated present-day prosthesis.

> **Remember**
> *The cardinal rule*
> Amputate through the tissues that will heal satisfactorily and preserve all possible lengths consistent with good surgical judgment.

- *Skin flaps:* Good skin coverage for the amputation site is of vital importance. The skin should be mobile and sensitive. Location of the scar is not important.
- *Muscles:* The muscle is divided at least 5 cm distal to the level of intended bone section and sutured.

> **Remember**
> *Two methods of muscle suture*
> - *Myodesis:* Here muscle is sutured to the bone.
> - *Myoplasty:* Here muscle is sutured to the opposite muscle group under appropriate tension.

These two techniques of *myodesis* and *myoplasty* help improve the function of the muscles and circulation in the stump and thereby help to prevent phantom pain.
- *Nerves:* The nerves are cut proximally and allowed to retract.
- *Blood vessels* are doubly ligated and cut.
- *Bone:* The bone is sectioned above the level of muscle section.
- *Drains* is removed after 48–72 hours.

OPEN AMPUTATIONS (Guillotine Operation)

In this type of amputation, the skin is not closed primarily and later, any one of the closure methods like secondary closure, reamputation, revision amputation or plastic repair follows it.

Indications

- Severe infections.
- Severe crush injuries.

Types

Open amputations with inverted skin flaps is the method of choice.

Circular open amputation: Here, the wound is kept open and closed secondarily either by secondary suture after a few days, split thickness skin graft, revision of the stump or by reamputation.

AFTER TREATMENT

Two concepts are widely accepted.

Rigid dressing concept: Here, plaster of Paris cast is applied to the stump over the dressing after surgery. This presents the following advantages:
- Prevents edema.
- Enhances wound healing.
- Decreases postoperative pain.
- Encourages early upright posture, which has both physiologic and psychological benefits.
- Reduces hospital stay.
- Helps in early temporary prosthetic fitting.

Soft dressing concept: This is the conventional method wherein the stump is dressed with a sterile dressing and elastocrepe bandages are applied over it (Fig. 60.4). The bed is elevated to facilitate venous drainage and prevent stump edema (Figs 60.4 and 60.5). The sutures are removed after 10–14 days and the muscle exercises are commenced. Prosthetic fitting is taken up as the last step.

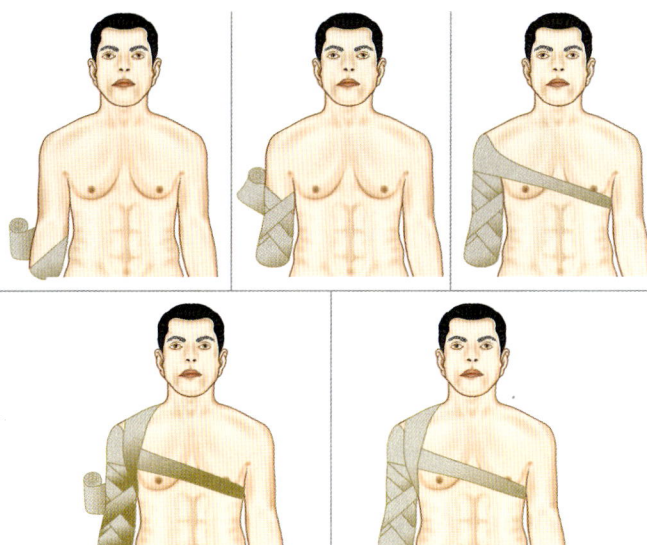

Fig. 60.4: Different steps in the stump bandaging of the above elbow amputation

SECTION 8: Miscellaneous

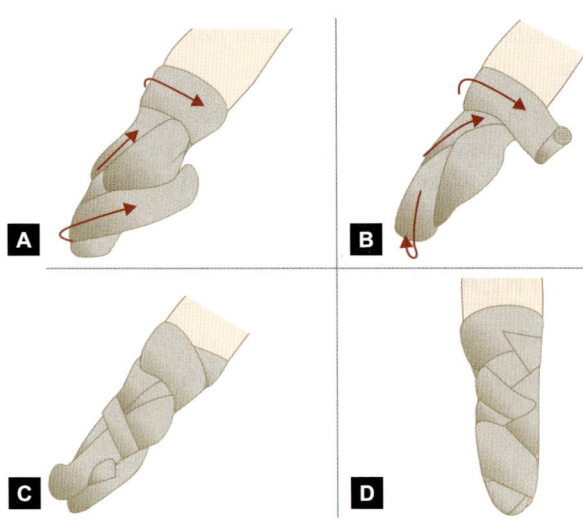

Figs 60.5A to D: Bandaging techniques of the below knee stump: (A and B) Anterior views; (C and D) Posterior views

IMPORTANT AMPUTATIONS OF LOWER EXTREMITY

Amputations of lower extremity accounts for nearly 85% of all amputations. *To successfully use prosthesis, it is desirable to perform amputation of the lower limb at the distal most possible level.*

Above Knee Amputation (Fig. 60.6)

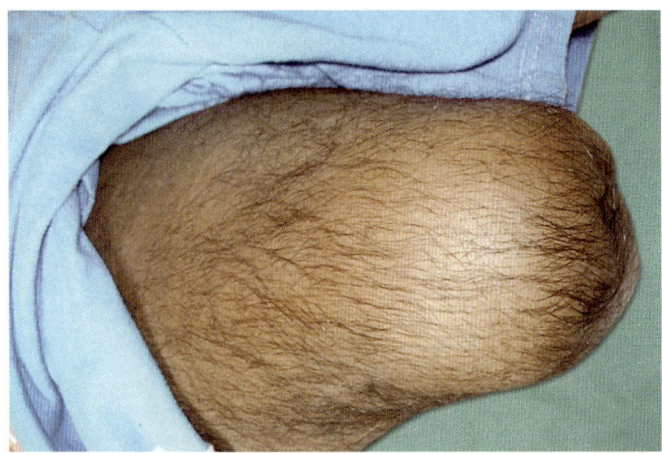

Fig. 60.6: Above knee amputation

Below Knee Amputation

This is the most common amputation performed (Fig. 60.7). Techniques vary in nonischemic and ischemic limbs.

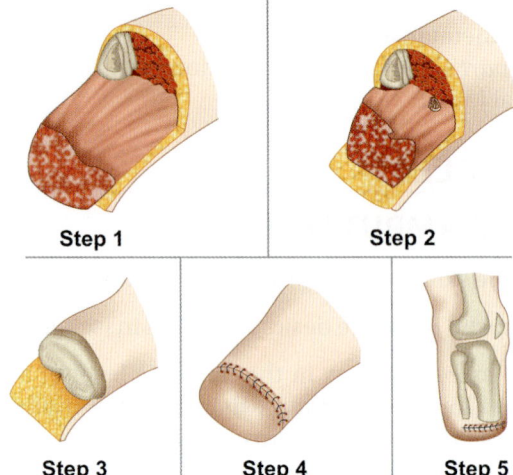

Fig. 60.7: Steps of below knee amputation: Step 1, a long posterior flap is created; Step 2, the edges of the tibia is beveled; Step 3, myoplasty is done; Step 4, the final closure; Step 5, in the final stump, fibula is higher than the tibial stump

Nonischemic limbs: Here, the ideal level of amputation is at the *musculotendinous junction of the gastrocnemius* because distal to this level, the tissues are relatively avascular and soft tissue padding is scanty. Though, soft tissue may heal early, it usually breaks down later due to the prosthetic use and advancing physiologic age.

Ischemic limb: Here, the skin's blood supply is better to the posterior than the anterior. *Hence, a long posterior flap is preferred in ischemic limbs.* To preserve vascular connections, unnecessary dissections are avoided. Unlike in nonischemic limbs, amputation is performed at a higher level. Tension myodesis and myoplasty are contraindicated for fear of damaging the already precarious blood supply.

Knee Disarticulation

This gives an excellent end-bearing stump. Large end-bearing surfaces of the distal femur are naturally suited for weight-bearing and the prosthesis will be stable.

Amputation Through the Thigh

This is second in frequency to the knee. Because knee joint is lost, it is extremely important that the stumps be as long as possible to provide a strong lever arm for the control of prosthesis.

[1]Syme's Amputation

It is indicated in severe crush injuries of the forefoot (Fig. 60.8). A healthy heel pad is required for the successful outcome of this surgery.

---

[1]**James Syme** (1799-1870). Edinburgh British Surgeon described it in 1843.

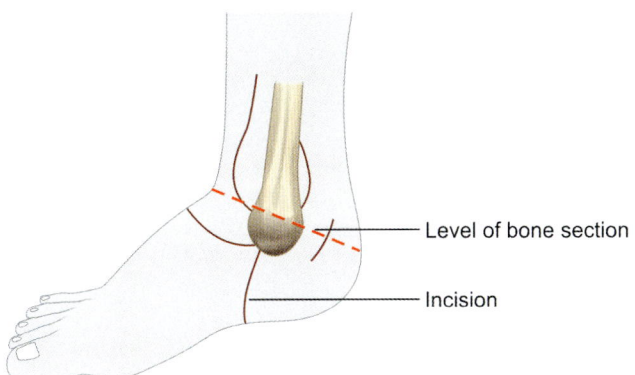

Fig. 60.8: Syme's amputation

COMPLICATIONS

Hematomas: This delays the wound healing and acts as a culture media for the growth of the organisms.

Infections: This is more common in peripheral vascular disease and diabetics.

Necrosis of the skin flaps are usually due to insufficient circulation and require revision amputations.

Contractures: This is largely preventable by positioning the stump properly.

Neuromas form always on the end of a cutaneous nerve and any pain from a neuroma is usually caused by traction on a nerve when it is embedded within the scar tissue.

Phantom sensation: This is a pseudofeeling of the presence of the amputated limb. It could be of a painless or a painful variety.

Causalgia: It is due to division of the peripheral nerves. Even local stimulus stimulates pain.

> **Remember in Amputations**
> - 5% amputations are through the lower limbs.
> - Severe injury forms the most common indication.
> - Level of amputation is no longer important as in the past due to efficient prosthesis.
> - The latest concept is to preserve as much stump length as possible.
> - Guillotine amputations are salvage procedures for life-threatening infections.
> - Stump care is very vital to prevent post-amputation problems.

Prosthetics and Orthotics

PROSTHETICS

Prosthesis in Greek means "in addition". Thus, prosthesis is defined as a replacement or substitution of a missing or a diseased part.

Prosthetics is the theory and practice of the prescription, fitting, design, assessment and production of prosthesis.

Classification

Endoprostheses: These are implants used in orthopedic surgery to replace joints, e.g. Austin Moore prosthesis.

Exoprostheses: These are for replacement externally for a lost part of the limb. They are more extensively used in the lower limbs (Fig. 61.1).

Types

Temporary prosthesis (e.g. pylon): These are used following an amputation until the patient is fitted with permanent prosthesis (Fig. 61.2).

Permanent prosthesis. The following are some of the important ones:

PROSTHESIS FOR THE ABOVE KNEE AMPUTATIONS

Prosthesis for the above knee amputations is required in the following situations:
- For disarticulation of hip and hemipelvectomy (Fig. 61.3).

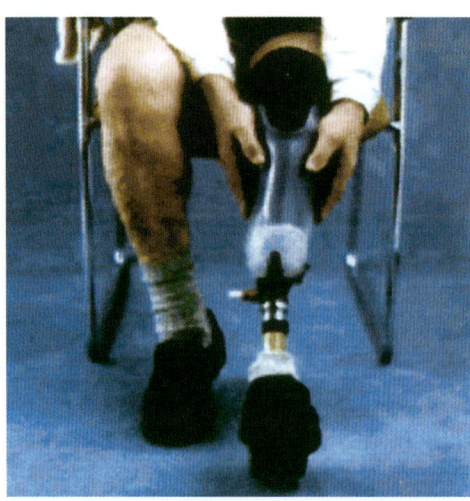

Fig. 61.1: Patient wearing an artificial leg

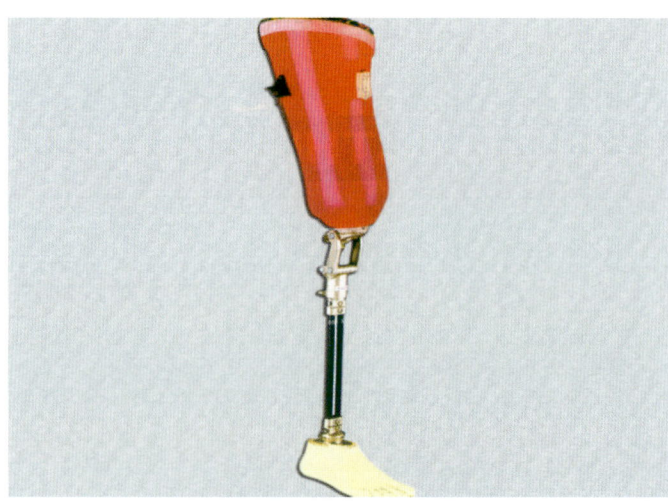

Fig. 61.2: A temporary prosthesis

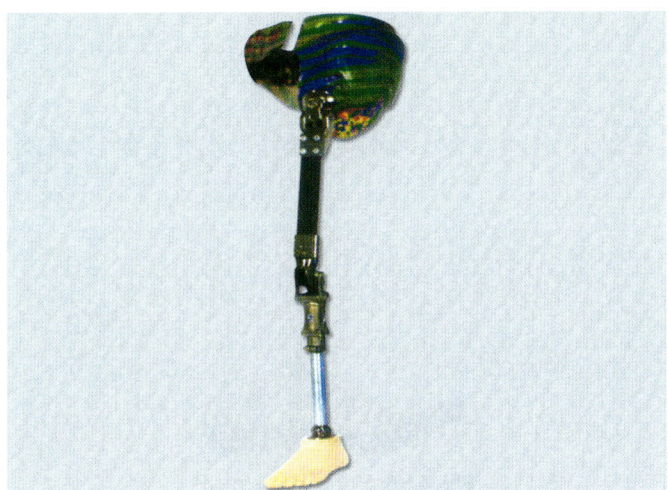

Fig. 61.3: Prosthesis for hemipelvectomy and hip disarticulation

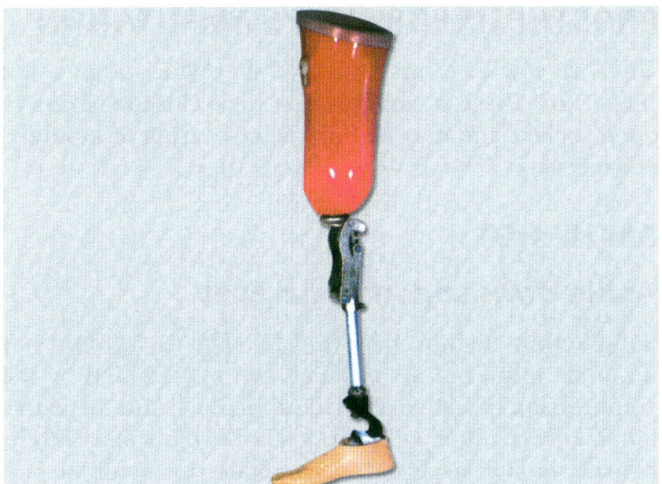

Fig. 61.4: Prosthesis for below knee amputation

- *Transfemoral amputations:* Two types of prostheses are recommended.
  - *Suction-socketed limb:* This is useful in young adults and is best suited for cylindrical stumps. It snuggly fits and has a two-way valve mechanism to maintain negative pressure.
  - *Nonsuction-socketed limb:* Here, no negative pressure is employed to hold the prosthesis, but pelvic bands or harness is made use of for holding.

The advantages of suction-socketed limb are that skin infection is less common, there is freedom from harness of any kind, greater feel of close contact of the prosthesis and the patient feels that it belongs to him or her. Stump socks are not necessary in this variety. On the contrary, the advantages of nonsuction-socketed limb are:
- It is easy to wear,
- There is no perspiration,
- It provides a comfortable fit, and
- There is no difficulty in changing the stump circumference.

Prosthesis for through knee amputation: As already mentioned, knee disarticulation gives a good, stable, long weight-bearing stump, which enables to operate the prosthesis with comfort.

PROSTHESIS FOR BELOW KNEE AMPUTATIONS

Two varieties are described (Fig. 61.4):

Patellar tendon bearing (PTB) prosthesis: In this, the socket is made in such a way that it fits exactly over the patellar tendon and the sides of the tibial condyles such that when in full extension the weight is transferred to some extent through this to the prosthesis (Fig. 61.5). This has the advantage over the conventional prosthesis, which requires the knee supports.

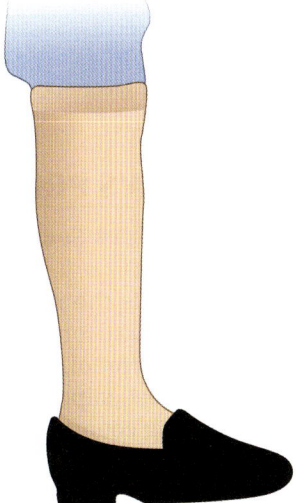

Fig. 61.5: PTB prosthesis

> **Quick Facts**
> *About lower limb prosthesis*
> - Quadrilateral socket prosthesis for above knee amputation.
> - PTB prosthesis for below knee amputation.
> - Syme's prosthesis for Syme's amputation.
> - Shoe fillers for partial foot amputation.

Conventional type prosthesis: This consists of the thigh corset, the side steels, the knee joint, shin piece, ankle joint unit and the footpiece. It definitely has the disadvantage in that it is more cumbersome to put on and use it when compared to the PTB prosthesis.

PROSTHESIS FOR SYME'S AMPUTATION

This is a below knee prosthesis used after Syme's amputation (Fig. 61.6). These prostheses may have closed sockets or open sockets and may be full weight-bearing or modified end-bearing.

SACH FOOT

Ankle Units and Artificial Feet

Solid action cushion heel (SACH) (Fig. 61.7A) foot has no ankle joint, but a simulated action is gained by the compression of wedge-shaped rubber heel and the whole foot is incorporated with various layers of rubber with its density varying, all placed over a wooden insert for the heel and wooden side keel. This allows smooth movements of the foot.

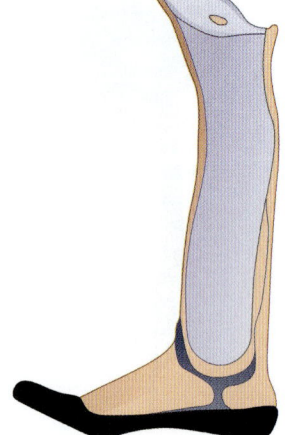

Fig. 61.6: Syme's prosthesis

> **Remember**
> *Aims of prosthetic fitting*
> - To substitute for a lost part.
> - To restore a lost function.
> - In lower limbs, it must provide a comfortable ambulation with minimal expenditure of energy.

JAIPUR FOOT (INDIA'S PRIDE)

- This is the brainchild of Dr PK Sethi and Masterji Ram Chander Sharma of Jaipur.
- Rubber and aluminum is the mainstay. Rubber is waterproof; aluminum is used for the leg piece, because it is cheap, strong and rust proof.
- Unlike the Western model, Jaipur foot is best for foot conditions in developing countries as it allows sitting on the floor, squatting and does not require a shoe (Fig. 61.7B).

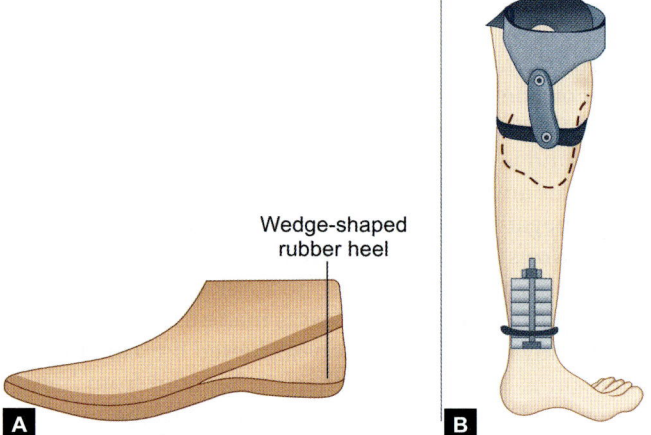

Figs 61.7A and B: (A) SACH foot; (B) Jaipur foot

> **Remember**
> *Prosthesis for lower extremities:*
> Long stump is prosthetically superior to a shorter one because it provides:
> - Longer lever arm.
> - More sensory feedback.
> - Greater area for distribution of pressure forces.

Prosthesis for Upper Limb Amputations

Forequarter amputations: Here, the prosthesis merely serves a cosmetic purpose. A sleeve fitter prosthesis with a plastozoate cap-padded inside with foam and retaining straps is used.

Shoulder Disarticulation (Fig. 61.8)

- *Shoulder piece* extended cap to hold the prosthesis.
- *Elbow piece:* It can be flexed by pulling on the flexion cord with the protractors of the shoulder.
- *Hand piece:* Either cosmetic or splint hook type.

Above elbow amputation: Same as above except that the elbow flexion is stronger due to the action of the arm muscles along with the protractors of the shoulder (Fig. 61.9).

Below elbow amputation: Here there is a cup socket attached to the terminal device through an operational cord. The terminal device can be activated through a loop harness (Fig. 61.10).

For wrist disarticulation: In this, a split socket forearm and a wrist rotation device is provided. A device can be provided to lock for supination and pronation.

ORTHOTICS

Orthosis is an appliance, which is added to the patient to enable better use of that part of the body to which it is fitted.

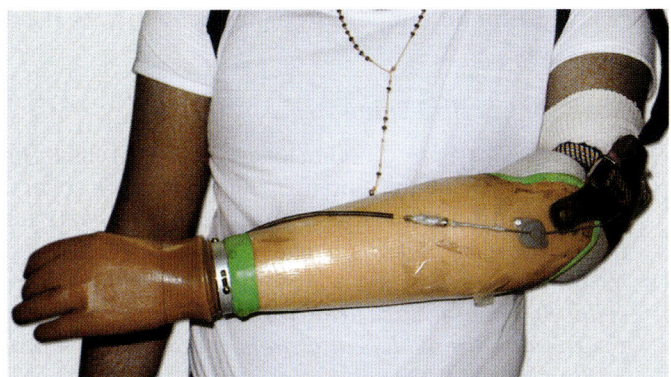

Fig. 61.8: Typical below elbow prosthesis

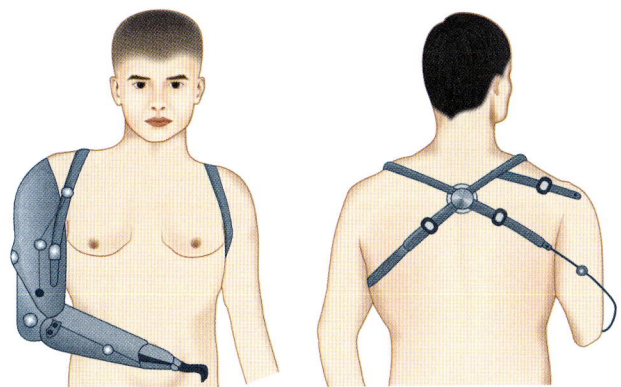

Fig. 61.9: Above elbow prosthesis

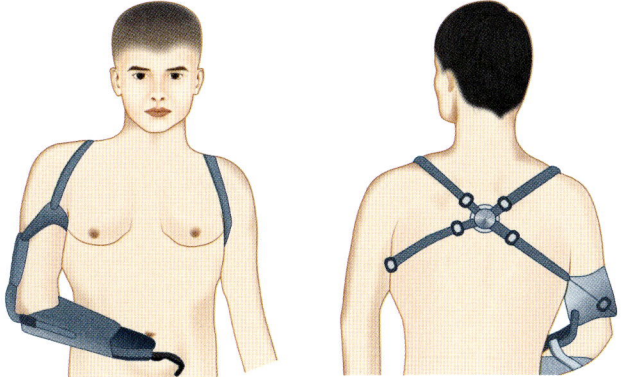

Fig. 61.10: Below elbow prosthesis

Prosthesis replaces a missing part of the body, while an orthosis provides support to a weak part of the body.

An orthotist is a person qualified to measure and fit all types of orthoses.

Classification

One single classification is very difficult. Hence, GK Rose has grouped them as follows:

TABLE 61.1: Major anatomical regions of the body

Upper limb		Lower limbs	Spine
S—Shoulder		H—Hip	C—Cervical
E—Elbow		K—Knee	T—Thoracic
W—Wrist		A—Ankle	L—Lumbar
H—Hand		F—Foot	S—Sacroiliac
F—Fingers	MP	Subtalar	
(2–5)	DIP	Midtarsal	
	PIP	Metatarsal	
Thumb	CM		
	MP		
	IP		

Abbreviations: MP, metacorpo, metatarsophalangeal; DIP, distal interphalangeal; PIP, proximal interphalangeal; CM, carpometacarpal; IP, interphalangeal

- Functional biomechanical
- Functional descriptive
- Nosological (according to disease)
- Regional.

Terminology for orthosis: The three major anatomical regions of the body are divided as follows and the initials are given as in Table 61.1.

Orthotic Facts

Now nomenclature for orthosis has used the first letter of the name of each joint which the orthosis crosses in power sequence, and the letter 'O' for orthosis is attached at the end. Accordingly, we have the following types of orthoses:
a. Cervical orthosis (CO)
b. Cervico-thoraco-lumbo-sacral orthosis (CTLSO)
c. Wrist hand orthoses (WHO)
d. Hip-knee-ankle-foot orthoses (HKAFO)
e. Knee-ankle-foot orthoses (KAFO)
f. Knee orthoses (KO)
g. Ankle foot orthoses (AFO)

Action of orthosis: The action of an orthosis on a joint is indicated by initials, which are as follows:
 F—Free
 A—Assist
 R—Resist
 S—Stop
 H—Hold
 V—Variable
 L—Lock

Varieties

- Spinal orthosis
- Cervical orthosis
- Lower limb orthosis
- Upper limb orthosis

Spinal orthoses: These fall into two categories:
- Supportive
- Corrective.

Functions of spinal orthosis:
- To relieve pain
- To support weakened paralyzed muscles
- To support unstable joints
- To immobilize joints in functional position
- To prevent deformity
- To correct deformity.

Types

Supportive Spinal Orthosis

Belts and corsets: These are most commonly used for the treatment of low backache. *Belts are prescribed for men and corsets for women.* These orthoses encircle the sacral region and extend a variable distance upwards, the term applied to them depends upon their depth posteriorly (sacroiliac, lumbosacral (Fig. 61.11), thoracolumbar). Anteriorly they have buckles.

> **Remember**
> *Role of belts*
> - They do not immobilize the spine but only restrict extremes of forward, lateral flexion and extension.
> - They provide subjective support.
> - They remind the patients to avoid movements.

Rigid spinal brace: All rigid spinal orthoses are constructed based on a metal frame, which takes firm support from the pelvis. To this is added the metal uprights, which are joined by, crossbars and straps, e.g. tailor brace, night tailor brace, etc.

Moulded spinal orthosis of leather, plastic, etc.

Indications for supportive spinal orthosis
- Sacroiliac strain
- Low backache
- Prolapsed intervertebral disk
- Spondylolisthesis, etc.

> **Remember**
> *The mechanisms of pain relief by spinal orthoses*
> - Psychological.
> - Increases intra-abdominal pressure.
> - Decreases lumbar lordosis.
> - Causes local inactivity of associated muscle groups and ligaments.

Corrective Spinal Orthosis

Milwaukee brace: This is an active corrective spinal orthosis used almost exclusively in the ambulant treatment of structural scoliosis (Fig. 61.12). The main aim of Milwaukee brace is to postpone, temporarily or permanently, the need for operation.

Orthosis for Cervical Spine

- *Cervical collar* many different forms of cervical collars or supports are available and are called Thomas's collars. Metal was used earlier, but now thick plastic sheets are preferred. These collars are readymade and are supplied in different sizes or are adjustable. *For a good fit, the collar should be secured firmly around the neck, rest upon the chest and shoulders and support the chin, jaw and occiput* (Fig. 61.13A).
- Sterno-occipital mandibular immobilization (SOMI) brace.
- Four postcervical brace (Fig. 61.13B)
- Halo body orthosis (Fig. 61.13C)
- *Minerva jacket* in lesions of uppermost part of the cervical spine, the forehead must be included in the external support. In such situations, Minerva jacket made from plaster of Paris is used (Fig. 61.14).

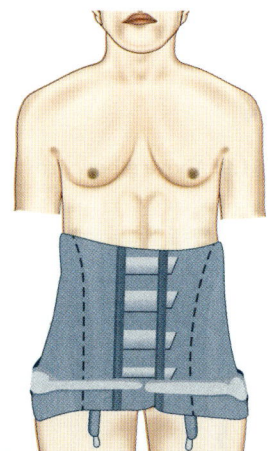

Fig. 61.11: Lumbosacral belt

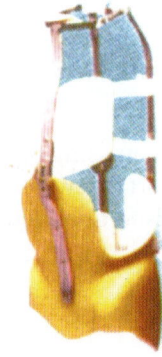

Fig. 61.12: Milwaukee brace

> **Remember**
> *The functions of calipers*
> - It provides stability
> - It relieves weight-bearing
> - It relieves pain
> - It controls deformity
> - It restricts movements
> - It assists movements
> - A combination of the above functions.

LOWER LIMB ORTHOSIS

Caliper is an orthosis for the lower limb, which may be used permanently, or for a very short-time only.

Knee-Ankle-Foot Orthosis (KAFO)

These are either weight relieving or nonweight-relieving calipers (Fig. 61.15A). It consists of the following parts, an upper end that may be made up of ring, cuff or bucket top. It has two sidebars or upright, the knee joint, the ankle joint, a shoe, thigh, knee and calf bands.

Hip-Knee-Ankle-Foot Orthosis (HKAFO) and Lumbosacral Hip-Knee-Ankle-Foot Orthosis (LSHKAFO)

A pelvic band may be attached to the KAFO with or without a hip joint to convert to an HKAFO (Fig. 61.15B). In addition, if this is extended upwards, a lumbosacral support is obtained converting it to an LSHKAFO.

The purpose of the pelvic band at the hip joint is to:
- Prevent development of a flexion deformity in polio, cerebral palsy, etc.
- To increase the stability of spine.

Ankle-Foot Orthosis (AFO)

The ankle joint can be controlled by mechanical ankle joints or by heelstraps (Fig. 61.16) in this below knee orthosis.

All the above lower limb orthoses so far mentioned are useful either to prevent or correct deformities due to polio, cerebral palsy, spina bifida, etc. They can be used either temporarily or permanently.

Footwear and its Modifications

The following are some of the modifications of footwear useful in the clinical situations mentioned as follows:
- *Rocker bar* for hallux rigidus.
- *Outside heel float* for lateral ligament injuries of the ankle.

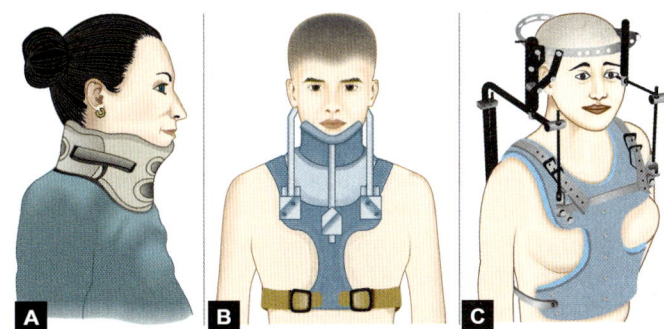

Figs 61.13A to C: Different cervical orthosis: (A) Cervical collar; (B) Four postcervical brace; (C) Halo body orthosis

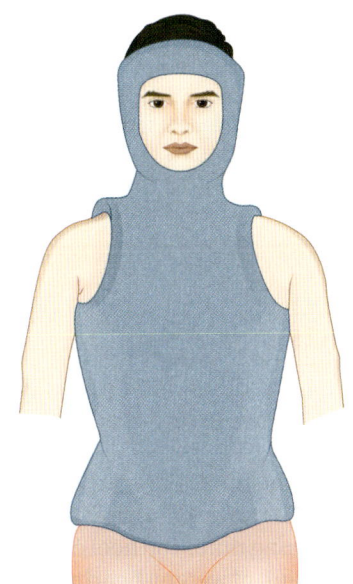

Fig. 61.14: Minerva jacket

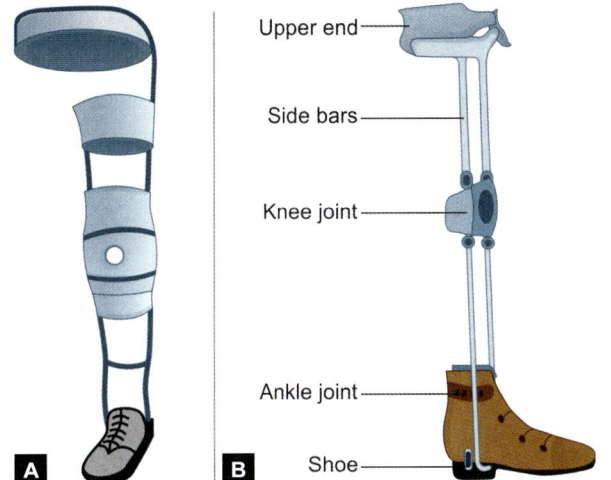

Figs 61.15A and B: (A) Hip knee-ankle-foot orthosis (HKAFO); (B) Knee-ankle-foot orthosis (KAFO)

- *Heel pad* for heel pain (Fig. 61.17A).
- *Medial longitudinal arch support* to relieve pain, the following supports is used:
  - Valgus insole.
  - Thomas heel (extension of medial aspect of the heel).
  - Filling of the medial half of the shank of the shoes (medial shank filler).
- *Metatarsal arch* is supported by the doom-shaped metatarsals bars (Fig. 61.17B).
- *More roomy footwear* to accommodate deformed toes.

Quick Facts
Surgical Footwear

Footwear with	Indications
a. Thomas heel	Flatfoot
b. Arch support	Flatfoot
c. CTEV shoes	For CTEV (Fig. 61.17C)
d. Heel pad	Calcaneal spur and plantar fasciitis
e. Metatarsal pad	For corns
f. Metatarsal bar	Metatarsalgia
g. Medial raise	Genu valgum
h. Lateral raise	Genu varum
i. Universal	For short leg

Foot Supports

The following are the different varieties of heel and foot supports currently in use in orthopedic practice (Figs 61.18 and 61.19).

- **Podotech heel cushion:** For severe pain in heel, ankle, back and anterior knee pain due to injury, overweight or standing for long time. The heel cushion relieves pain by altering the line of weight-bearing. Available in three sizes (Fig. 61.18A).
- **Astro-sorb heel seat:** The cushion protects against stress and relieves pain on the ball of foot from over activity (Fig. 61.18B).
- **Ball of the foot cushion:** Reduces pressure and relieves pain on the ball of foot from over activity (Fig. 61.18C).
- **Stompers gel heel pad:** For knee and back pain, tibial shin pain, athletes and joggers. Place this under the heel and wear shoes. Do not use adhesives (Fig. 61.18D).
- **Duosoft insoles:** For diabetic patients to reduce pain and burning sensation for uncontrolled diabetic neuropathy. Absorbs shock, reduces friction, and disperses weight and protects the foot from harmful forces. Available in two sizes (Fig. 61.18E).
- **Stompers work and sports insoles universal:** To relieve tired, achy legs, try one of the shock absorbing insoles which have a wide variety of uses such as for work on hard surfaces and all sports or simply to relieve the day-to-day stress on feet, knees and back, pain relief for a number of conditions and enhanced cushioning with mild anatomical support (Fig. 61.18F).
- **Star flex:** For use in children above two years who have flatfoot. The Star flex™ orthotic blank is a polyester resin,

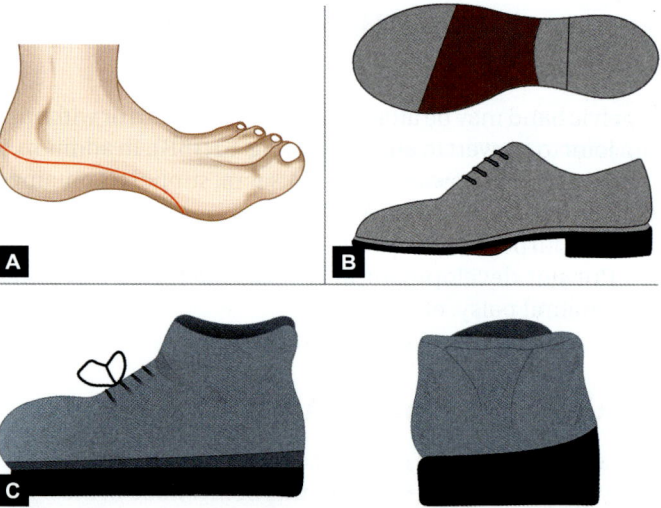

Figs 61.17A to C: (A) UC-BL shoe inserts to relieve heel stress in plantar fasciitis and calcaneal spur; (B) Incorporation of metatarsal bars, under the sole of the footwear; (C) CTEV shoes

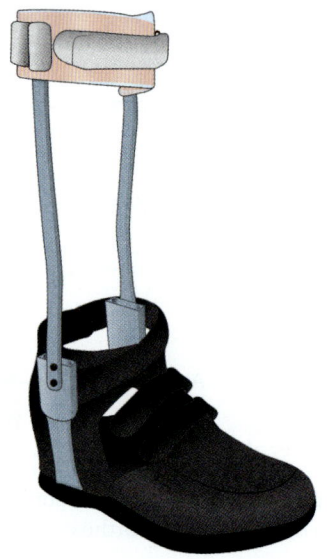

Fig. 61.16: Ankle-foot orthosis (AFO)

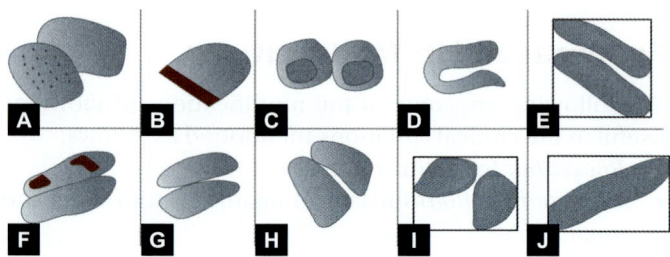

Figs 61.18A to J: Various foot supports

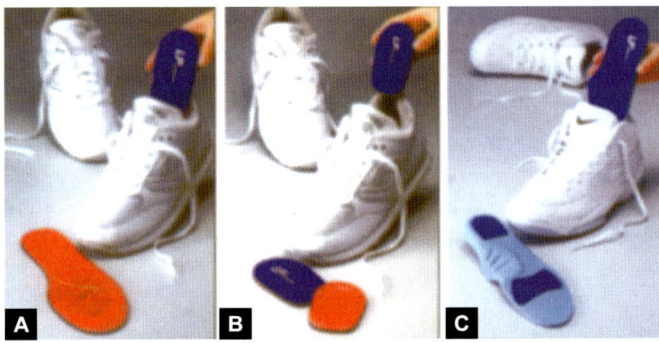

Figs 61.19A to C: Foot inserts

reinforced with glass fiber threads available in three sizes (Fig. 61.18G).
- **Globus heel cup:** For use in children above 18 months who have flatfoot with calcaneo valgus. Available in three sizes (Fig. 61.18H).
- **Valgus pads:** For flatfoot and weak medial arch in adults. To be pasted using rubber adhesive on the inside of the shoes. Available in two sizes (Fig. 61.18I).
- **Trilam insoles:** For adults with plantar fascitis, flatfoot and transverse arch pain. Available in five sizes (Fig. 61.18J).

UPPER LIMB ORTHOSIS

Upper limb orthoses ranges from a simple splint to the very complex varieties, which are manufactured to the following basic requirements:
- Limitation of movements could be either total or partial.
- Exercise of muscles and joint range against energy storing devices such as springs or elastics.
- Replacement of paralyzed muscles using similar devices.
- Preventive deformity control.

BIBLIOGRAPHY

1. Brittain HA. Hindquarter amputation. J Bone and Joint Surg. 1949;31-B:104.
2. Brown PW. The rational selection of treatment for upper extremity amputations. Orthop Clin North Am. 1981;12:843.
3. Burges EM, Romano RL, Traub JE. Immediate post-surgical prosthetic fitting. Prosthetic Study Report Bull Prosthet Res. 1965;10-4:42.
4. Little Wood H. Amputations of the shoulder and at the hip. Br Med J. 1922;381.
5. Malone JW, Moore WS, Goldstone J. Therapeutic and economic impact of a modern amputation program. Am Surg. 1979;189:798.
6. Marquardt E, Correll J. Amputations and prosthesis for the lower limb. Int Orthop. 1984;8:139.
7. McCullough NC. The bilateral lower extremity amputee. Orthop Clin North America. 1972;3:303.
8. Peizer E, Pirrello T. Principles and practice in upper extremity prosthesis. Orthop Clin North Am. 1972;3:197.
9. Phelan JT, Nodular SH. A technique of hemipelvectomy. Surg Gynaecol Obstet. 1964;119:311.
10. Pillet J. The aesthetic hand prosthesis. Orthop Clin North Am. 1981;12:961.
11. Room AJ, Moore WS, Goldstone J. Below knee amputation: a modern approach. Am J Surg. 1977;134:153.
12. Sarmiento A. A modified surgical-prosthetic approach to the Syme's amputation: a follow-up report. Clin Orthop. 1972;85:11.
13. Tooms RE. Amputation surgery in the upper extremity. Orthop Clin North Am. 1972;3:383.
14. Wagner FW (Jr). Amputations of the foot and ankle: status. Clin Orthop. 1977;122:62.
15. Weiss. The prosthesis on the operating room from the neurological point at view. Report of Workshop panel on lower extremity prosthetics fitting, 1966. Committee on prosthetics. Research and Development, National Academy of Sciences.

62 CHAPTER

Sports Injuries

INTRODUCTION

Our cricketing icons; master blaster Sachin Tendulkar, ace spinner Anil Kumble, Nawab of Najafgarh Virender Sehwag, the effervescent VVS Laxman and the rock of Gibraltar Rahul Dravid, S Sree Shanth all were in the news for sports injuries. For once, these injuries outfamed and outshone these cricketing demigods and were discussed and talked by everyone than the cricketers themselves. Therefore, these injuries fall within the gambit of sports medicine, which is in fact a developing science with tremendous potential. With more and more people taking up sports as a career, the sports-related injuries are on the rise.

Sports medicine, like all other branches of medicine, aims at the complete physical, mental and spiritual well-being of a sportsperson. A healthy mind in a healthy body is a concept, which is more true to a sportsperson than anybody else is. Positive thinking, fair play and sportsmanship should be the hallmark of a true sportsman. We, the doctors and the therapists, aim to keep a sportsperson physically fit, so that the rest of the objectives mentioned above are attained automatically.

Like in other branches of medicine so in sports medicine, prevention is better than cure. To prevent sports injuries, the first step is to ascertain whether a person choosing sports is fit to take it. An unfit person taking up sports is a sure prescription for future sports injuries. A fitness testing for those who wish to take up sports, as their career should include various relevant parameters (see Box).

Quick Facts
Sports vs fitness testing
- Muscle power should be adequate.
- Active joint movements.
- Range of passive movements.
- Body balance.
- Coordination skills.
- Symmetrical and coordinated movements between the limbs and the body.
- Elasticity and extensibility of muscles and ligaments.
- Presence of any unwanted or accessory movements.

These and many other factors determine whether a person is fit enough to take to sports.

However, one has to remember that fitness testing is not done only at the initial stages but needs to be done repeatedly at every stage of an athlete or a sportsperson's life. The second stage of prevention of sports-related injuries is assessing whether a sportsman is fit enough to resume the sporting activity after the initial layoff. There is nothing more dangerous than an unfit or a partially fit person resuming the sporting activity. It may spell a doom to his otherwise flourishing career in sports. A sportsperson has to satisfy certain norms before he can finally be sent back to the field (see Box).

Quick Facts
A sportsperson has to satisfy the following norms before he resumes sports:
- Should be able to jump from a height of 1 meter.
- Full range of painless active movements.
- Slight pain at extreme movements against resistance.
- No running limp.
- Can fully squat with one or both legs.
- Can do full press up.
- Can extend the knee with 20 lb × 10 in 45 seconds
- Persons engaged in contact sports should be able to lift 45 lb × 10 in less than 45 seconds
- The sportsperson should be independent of any strapping or support.

If a person satisfies all the above criteria, he can be safely returned back to his passion, i.e. sports.

CLASSIFICATION OF SPORTS INJURIES

Among the various classifications proposed for sports injuries, the one proposed by Williams (1971) is widely used and recommended.

Williams' Classification (Flowchart 62.1)

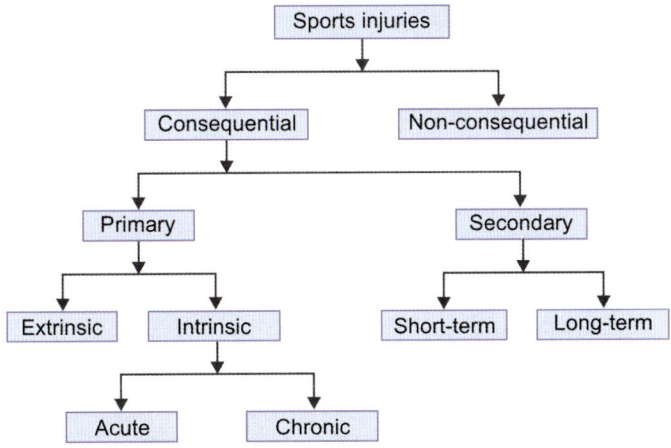

Flowchart 62.1: Williams' classification

Among the Consequential Injuries

Primary Extrinsic

This is further subdivided into:
- *Human:* Black eye due to direct blow.
- *Implemental:* May be incidental (as in blow from a hard ball) or due to overuse (blisters from oars).
- *Vehicular:* Clavicle fracture due to fall from cycle, etc.
- *Environmental:* Injuries in divers.
- *Occupational:* Jumper's knee in athletes, chondromalacia in cyclists, etc.

Primary Intrinsic

This could be acute or chronic.
- *Incidental:* Strains, sprains, etc.
- *Overuse:*
  - Acute, e.g. acute tenosynovitis of wrist extensors in canoeists.
  - Chronic, march fracture in soldiers, etc.

Secondary

Short-term: For example, quadriceps weakness.
Long-term: Degenerative arthritis of the hip, knee, ankle, etc.

No Consequential Injuries

These are not related to sports but are due to injuries either at home or elsewhere and are very not connected to any sports (e.g. slip and fall at home).

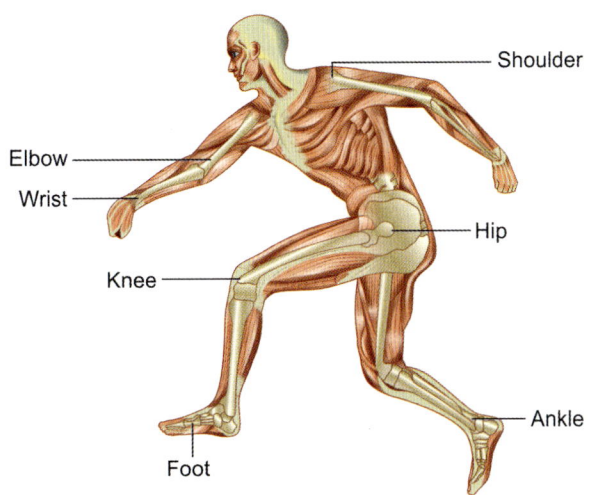

Fig. 62.1: Common sites of soft tissue injuries in sports

COMMON SPORTS INJURIES

Sports medicine usually deals with minor orthopedic problems like soft tissue trauma (Fig. 62.1). Very rarely, there may be serious fractures, head injuries or on the field deaths. There is nothing unusual about these injuries except that a sportsperson demands a 100 percent cure and recovery while an ordinary person is satisfied and happy with a 60–80 percent recovery. The difference is because of the desire of the sportsperson to get back to the sport again, which requires total fitness.

Note: The incidence of sports injuries among all orthopedic injuries is 5–10 percent.

The following are some of the most common sports-related injuries one encounters in clinical practice.

Upper Limbs

- *Shoulder complex*
  - Rotator cuff injuries
  - Shoulder dislocations
  - Fracture clavicle
  - Acromioclavicular injuries
  - Bicipital tendinitis or rupture.
- *Elbow*
  - Tennis elbow (Fig. 62.2)
  - Golfer's elbow
  - Dislocation of elbow.
- *Wrist*
  - Wrist pain
  - Carpal tunnel syndrome.
- *Hand*
  - Mallet injury (Fig. 62.3)
  - Baseball finger
  - Jersey thumb
  - Injuries to the finger joints.

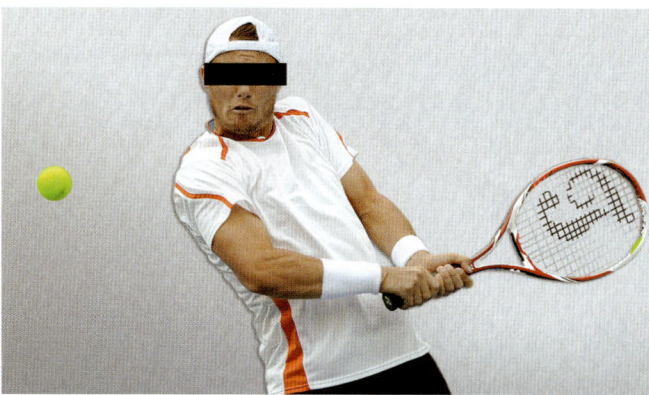

Fig. 62.2: Professional tennis players most commonly suffer from a famous sports disorder tennis elbow

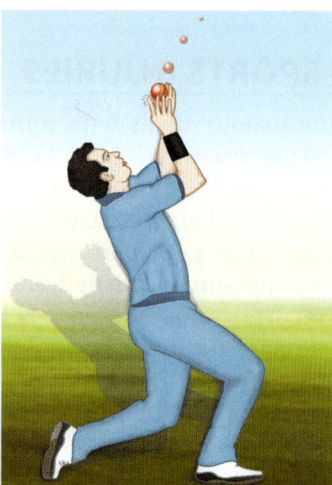

Fig. 62.3: Mechanism of mallet finger injuries in cricketers while trying to catch a ball

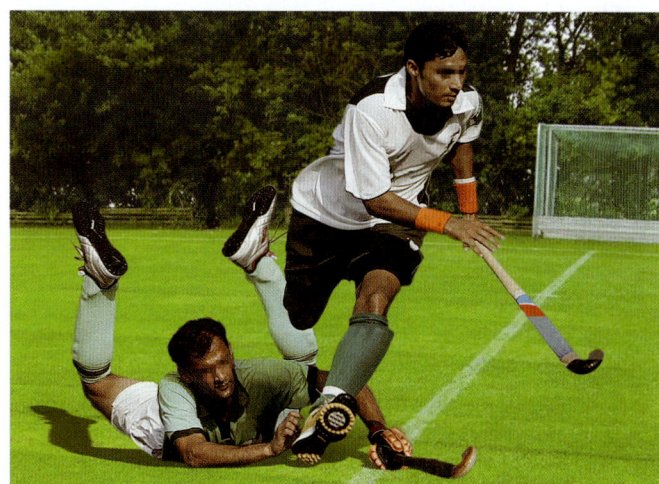

Fig. 62.4: Frequent falls, contact injuries and high-speed activities are the common causes of sports injuries

Lower Limbs

- *Hip*
    - Iliotibial or tract syndrome
    - Quadriceps strain
    - Hip pain
    - Groin pain due to adductor strain.
- *Knee Joint*
    - Jumpers knee
    - Chondromalacia
    - Fracture patella
    - Knee ligament injuries
    - Meniscal injuries.
- *Legs*
    - Calf muscle strain
    - Hamstrings sprain
    - Stress fracture tibia
    - Compartmental syndrome of the leg.
- *Ankle Injuries*
    - Ankle sprain
    - Injuries to tendo-Achilles
    - Tenosynovitis.
- *Foot*
    - March fracture
    - Jones fracture
    - Forefoot injuries
    - Injuries of sesamoid bone of the great toe.

Head, Neck, Trunk and Spine

- Head injuries
- Whiplash injuries
- Rib fractures
- Trunk muscle strains
- Abdomen muscle strain
- Low backache.

All these injuries have been discussed in relevant sections.

Investigations

These are the same as for any orthopedic-related disorders and consists of plain X-ray, CT scan, bone scan, MRI, arthroscopy, arthrography, stress X-rays, etc.

TREATMENT OF SPORTS INJURY

This is discussed under three headings prevention, treatment proper and training.

Preventive Measures

The best way to treat a sports injury is to prevent it from happening. Nothing is better than preventing the injury.

> **Quick Facts**
> *Preventive measures*
> - Proper clinical examination to identify any bodily defects.
> - Fitness training.
> - Correcting the wrong body mechanics and posture.
> - Conditioning exercises to overcome particular deficiencies.
> - Cardiopulmonary conditioning exercises to develop endurance.
> - Proper warm up exercises and relaxation techniques before and after the sports.
> - Wearing proper foot wears and other protective devices like helmet, gloves, etc.
> - To prevent overuse syndrome, taking adequate breaks in between the vigorous sports is advised.
> - Avoiding sports in very high or low temperature climates.
> - Not allowing aggravating minor problems like contusion, sprain, etc. by taking adequate rest and treatment.

Treatment

Treatment of individual sports-related disorders is discussed under suitable sections. However, a mention is made here of the general principles of treatment which is applicable to all sports injuries.

General Principles

- *Concept of RICEMM:* This sums up the early treatment methodology of sports injuries and consists of:
  R—Rest to the injured limb
  I—Ice therapy
  C—Compression bandaging
  E—Elevation of the injured part
  M—Medicines like painkillers, etc.
  M—Modalities like heat, straps, supports, etc.
- After immobilization and rest, early vigorous exercises should be commenced at the earliest to prevent muscle weakness and atrophy.
- To prevent joint stiffness, early mobilization has to be done first by passive movements and later by active movements. To improve the strength, resistive exercises are added.
- Unlike the conventional once a day treatment, a sportsperson needs to be seen at least 2–3 times a day.
- As mentioned earlier, allow resumption of sporting activity only after the sportsperson assumes 100 percent fitness.
- Mind training is as important as physical training. By repeated counseling, improve the psychological status of the patient to avoid depression, anxiety and negative attitudes, which may develop during the injury.
- Orthopedic and surgical treatment to be undertaken at appropriate situations.

Training

The physiotherapist has to train a sportsperson in various exercises to enable him to keep his fitness level very high. After conducting a fitness testing, (mentioned earlier), the therapist has to subject an athlete to various forms of exercises to increase the endurance, strength, running, weightbearing, etc. The following are the various forms of exercises.

Exercises to Increase the Cardiopulmonary Capacity

These exercises are done to increase the endurance level of an athlete or sportsperson.

Exercises to Increase the Muscle Strength

By carefully planned, graded, progressive resistive exercises (PRE), the therapist aims at improving the strength of the muscles of the upper limbs, lower limbs, trunk and spine.

> **Quick Facts**
> *PRE (Progressive Resistive Exercises)*
> - For upper limb muscles—bench press.
> - For lower limb muscles—squatting exercises.
> - For trunk and muscles of the limbs—power clean.

Exercises for Free Weight Training

Strength training with machines has a disadvantage in training only the prime movers. This anomaly is converted by free weight training, which helps to strengthen not only the prime movers but also the synergistic and stabilizing groups of muscles (e.g. exercises with dumb bells). They are also known to increase the tensile strength of the muscles, ligaments and tendons.

Measures to Improve the Agility

The measures to improve the agility levels of sportsperson are two-leg hops, one-leg hop, cross over-run turning, bending and backward running. These exercises help to improve balance, coordination and movements at a faster rate.

Measures to Improve the Speed-Plyometrics

In this, the neuromuscular system is trained to such an extent that it can react very quickly to sudden increase of speed and power, which is so often required in sporting activities.

Measures of Relaxation

After the vigorous workout mentioned above, the sportspersons are taught methods of relaxation and body stretches.

> **Quick Facts**
> *About plyometrics*
> - Hops
> - Speed jumps.
> - Running drills.
> - These above exercises must be done very fast with sudden burst of energy.
> - The speed strength of a sportsperson depends on how fast the muscle action changes from eccentric to concentric ones.
> - This is then followed with graded resistance exercises.

Before an athlete or a sportsperson resumes his sporting activities, a fitness testing is carried out and only then, he is allowed to take to the sports provided he is 100 percent fit.

BIBLIOGRAPHY

1. Bass AL. Rehabilitation after soft tissue injury. Proceedings of the Royal Society of Medicine, 653-56.
2. Fowler JA. Fitness and its components. Physiotherapy, 63.
3. Hornor Z, Werpravnik C. Mechanisms, types and treatment of injuries. British Journal of Sports Medicine, 1:45-6.
4. Williams JGP. Classification of Sports Injuries; 1971.
5. Wright D. Fitness testing after injury. In: Reilly T (Ed). Sports Fitness and Sports Injuries. London: Faber and Faber.

63 CHAPTER

Arthroscopy*

INTRODUCTION

Thousands of years ago, star gazing to unravel the secrets of the skies was a favorite time pass of the yesteryear Greek scientists. The human eye could not match this enthusiasm and belied all their interests. Then came Galileo with his phenomenal invention of a telescope which opened up the secrets of astronomy and behold the beautiful galaxy was now suddenly seen in all its splendor and glory.

Something similar happened in the field of surgery. The morbidity and mortality associated with long incision wide surgical approaches was getting increasingly alienated. The patients and the surgeons yearned for something small and less morbid. The realized that had to open less see more and do more. How could that be possible they wondered. Again that wonder tool called the telescope made this a reality. Peeping inside a joint through a telescope suddenly exposed the joint in all its grandeur. That joint which had a myriad of fascinating structures within it could be accessed for diagnosis and thereafter treatment by a telescopic like instrument that was christened as arthroscopy. Like telescope, arthroscpe revolutinized the way we look and treat joint conditions. Great deeds could now be performed through small nicks courtesy arthroscopy. Joints now heaved a sigh of relief that no longer they need to be subjected to mutilating knives of a marauding surgeon.

WHAT IS ARTHROSCOPY?

It is a 4 mm telescope-like optical instrument (range 1.7–7 mm) used to visualized the inside of a joint, detect pathology if any and then treat it. The angle of inclination of the scope at the tip varies from 25º–90º. The former is commonly used and the latter helps to see corners of the joints. Thus, the equipment of arthroscopy consists of the following:

- An arthroscopies
- A fiber optic light source to adequately and effectively light up the interior of the joints.
- A video camera to catch the glimpses and visualize the joint interiors.
- A TV monitor to see the interiors of the joints in all its grandeur on the screen.

If after introduction and inspection of the joint, a pathology is seen and needs to be tackled by an operation following instruments are required:

- *A Probe:* This is the most vital instrument which is known to extend the surgeons fingers inside the joint to palpate its structures. This also helps in the all important triangulation techniques.
- *Scissors:* Obviously have to be small (3-4 mm) to cut, trim and remove the damaged and frayed joint structures. The jaws of the scissors could be straight or hooked.
- *Punch or Basket Forceps:* This enables to remove or punch the damaged structures and flush it out with saline later. It makes pulling out the forceps out to deliver the debris out unnecessary.
- *Grasping forceps:* Obviously are used to grasp the loose bodies, meniscus, synovial folds, ligaments, etc. while operating.
- *Blade knives:* Inserted through a cannula to prevent damage to surrounding structures and minimize the chances of breakage, blades could be straight, curved, hooked, retrograde, undercutting, etc.
- *Motorized shavers:* These are used to shave the damaged joint structures. To do this there is a hollow rotating cannula with compounding windows within a sheath.
- *Electrocautery:* This is an underwater cutting cautery and is used for cutting and hemostasis purposes.

---
* From "Step by Step Operative Orthopedics" by *Dr John Ebnezar.*

792   SECTION 8: Miscellaneous

- *Laser:* It can be used for cutting purposes that is precise and causes minimal thermal damage. But it has its own disadvantages like bone and joint damage, and is yet to be used widely.
- *Implants* include suture anchors, materials for cartilage repair, tendon and ligament fixation, etc. and can be both metallic or biodegradable with the latter being slightly better.
- *Sheaths and trocars:* To pass and hold arthroscopic instruments.
- *Irrigations systems:* This consists of a 6–6.2 mm sheath to allow ringer lactate or normal saline to flow inside a joint for continuous joint irrigation.
- *Tourniquet* to obtain a bloodless field for surgery.
- *Leg holder* to position the legs properly for the procedure.

INDICATIONS FOR ARTHROSCOPY (FIG. 63.1)

Cartilage Conditions
- Excision of damaged cartilage
- Mosaicplasty.

Synovium Conditions
- Excision of the plicas
- Trimming of the plicas
- Synovial biopsy
- Synvectromy.

Meniscal Pathology
- Repair
- Resect.

Ligament Structures
- Repair
- Reinforce
- Reconstruct.

Loose Bodies
- Crushing
- Removal.

Patellar Problems
- Lateral release
- To correct malt racking.

Joints Pathology
- Arthrolysis
- Debridement
- Shaving
- Stabilization as in recurrent dislocation of shoulder
- Excision of the joints (e.g. ACM joint)
- Fusion of the joints
- To detect and reconstruct tibial plateau fractures.

Operative Procedure (Figs 63.2 and 63.3)
- Under spinal or general anesthesia
- Tourniquet is applied
- Legs are positioned properly
- Painting of the limb is done
- Draping is done next
- Through a anterolateral portal the scope is introduced
- The joint is distended with running RL or saline
- Through a anteromedial portal the instruments are introduced

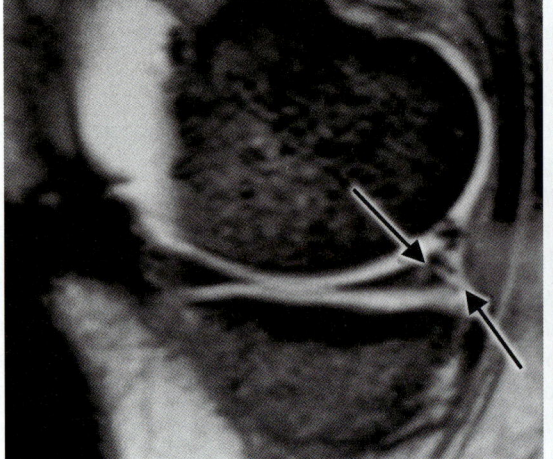
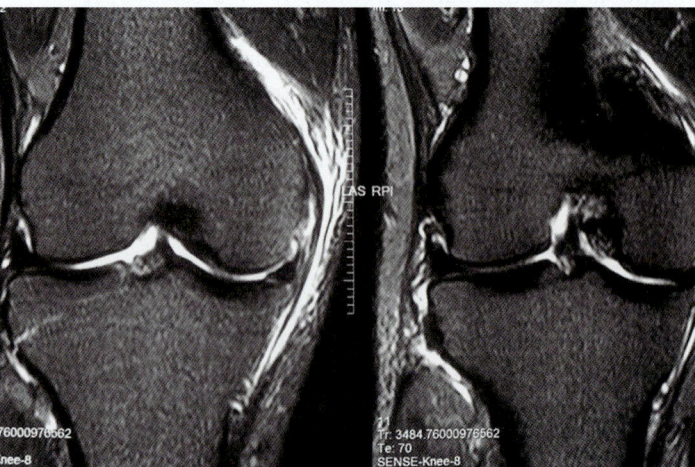

Fig. 63.1: Knee arthroscopy is usually done for meniscal and ACL tears

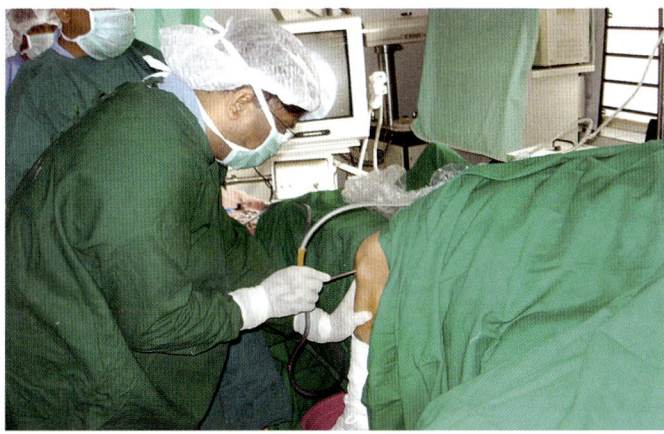

Fig. 63.2: Clinical picture showing knee arthroscopy

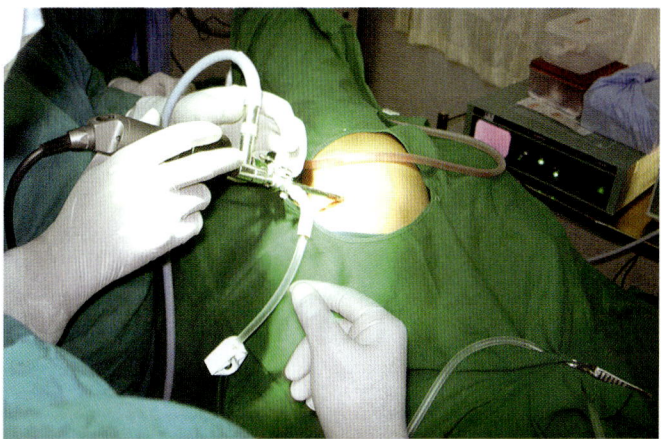

Fig. 63.3: Clinical picture showing shoulder arthroscopy

- The joint structures are now visualized on a TV monitor
- Thorough inspection of the joint structures is done
- Achieve triangulation by bringing the scope and the instruments in front of the telescope
- Joint is continuously irrigated
- The required procedure is carried out
- Thorough joint lavage is done
- Compression bandage applied
- Mobilize the patient the same day or the next day.

Advantages

- Less morbid
- Faster return to activity
- Less bleeding
- Less damage to structures
- Smaller incision and hence smaller scar
- Live joint assessment
- Dynamic joint assessment possible
- Better diagnostic potential
- Faster rehabilitation.

Limitations

- Steep learning curve
- Sophisticated instrumentation
- Good infrastructure needed
- Instruments are costly and expensive
- Not useful in conditions like infection, bleeding diathesis, neuropathic conditions, etc.
- Not useful in recurrent dislocations as in shoulder and patella.

Chapter 64

Standard Arthroscopy Portals*

PATIENT POSITIONING

I do all my knee arthroscopies while sitting on a stool. I do not use a tourniquet. Position a lateral support on the table so that the knee can be stressed to inspect the medial compartment of the knee. Mark the patella, joint line and the portals with a sterile marker. I inject the arthroscopy portals with 20 mL of xylocaine with 1% adrenaline (Figs 64.1 to 64.3).

LATERAL PORT (VISUALIZATION PORT)

I do my visualization port 0.5 cm inferior and 0.5 cm lateral to the inferior pole of the patella. This port is slightly higher than the most commonly described one in the center of the soft spot. The visualization port placed as described helps the arthroscope insertion into the joint without scoring and scuffing the cartilage.

It also helps navigate the arthroscope in the lateral gutter, intercondylar notch and suprapatellar pouch better with relative ease (Figs 64.4 and 64.5).

SUPEROLATERAL PORT (DRAINAGE PORT)

This is placed 2.5 cm lateral and 2.5 cm superior to the superior pole of the patella. This portal can be made using the outside-in technique. This portal can be used to visualize the patellar tracking and hence correct positioning is vital (Fig. 64.6).

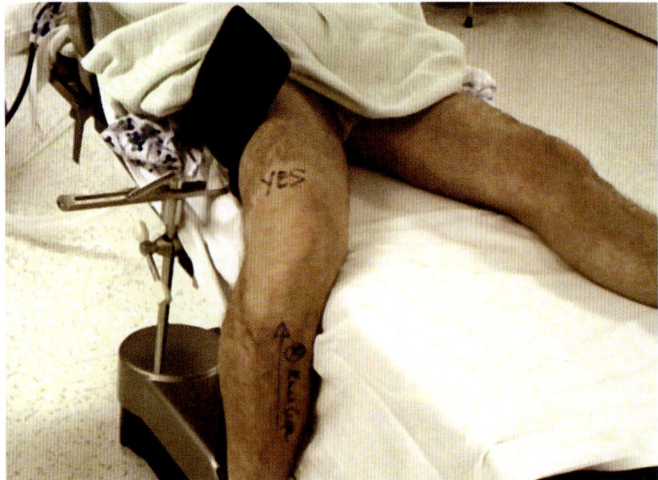

Fig. 64.1: Positioning

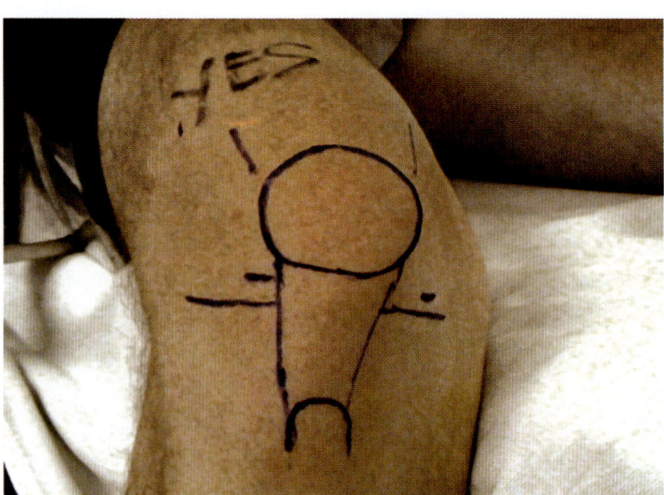

Fig. 64.2: Surface anatomy

---

* From "Step by Step Operative Orthopedics" by *Dr John Ebnezar.*

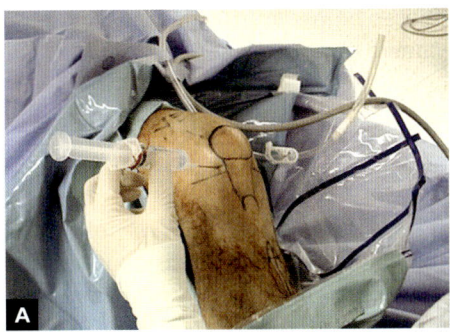 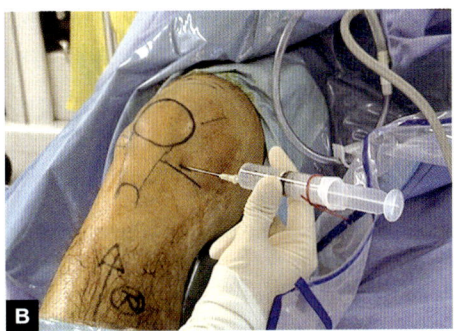 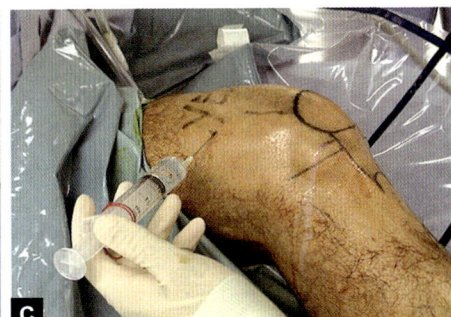

Figs 64.3A to C: Giving local anesthesia

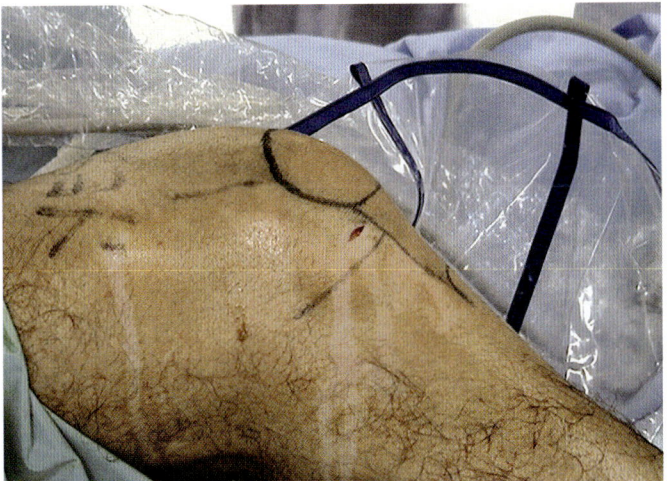

Fig. 64.4: Incision

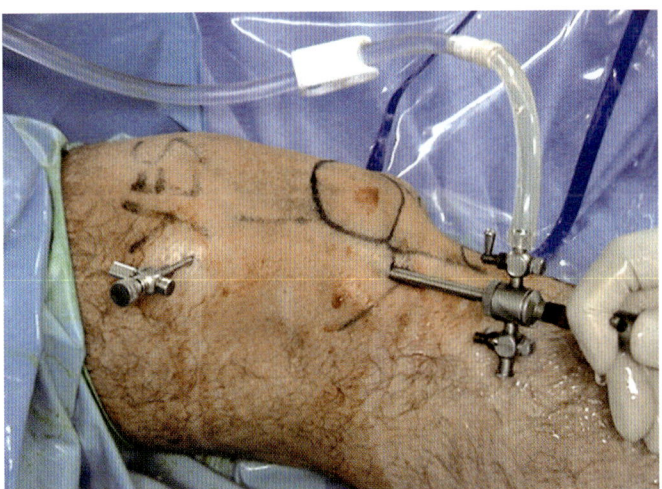

Fig. 64.6: Insertion of the superolateral port under vision

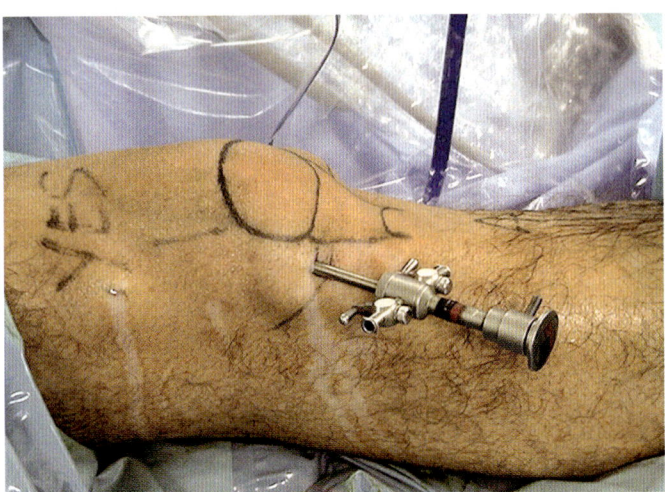

Fig. 64.5: Introduction of anthroscope

MEDIAL PORT (OPERATING PORT)

Mark the exact place of the medial port from outside with a needle. This technique avoids incorrect operating port placement and avoids the struggle to do operative maneuvers.

SUPEROLATERAL PORT (PATELLAR TRACKING PORT)

Enlarging the drainage port can serve as a patellar tracking port. In my opinion, patellar tracking should be assessed using the superolateral port without the tourniquet. The quadriceps muscle is bound by the inflated tourniquet making the patellar tracking assessment imprecise. Make this portal using a switching stick and introduce the sheath of the arthroscope over the stick. Take the switching stick out and introduce the arthroscope to visualize the patella and the tracking (Fig. 64.7).

MY INFEROLATERAL PORT "LATERAL RELEASE PORT"

This port is placed 2.5 cm inferior to the inferior pole of the patella and 2 cm lateral to the patellar tendon. This port is used to introduce the cutting diathermy to do the lateral retinacular release. This port allows the surgeon to complete the lateral release in one step. Not using the tourniquet is very helpful during lateral release as all the bleeders can be visualized and coagulated before cutting them particularly the superolateral geniculate group (Figs 64.8 to 64.10).

OTHER PORTS

Midpatellar Port

This portal is made 1 cm inferior to the inferior pole of the patella through the patellar tendon. Skin incision is marked at the point vertically. A blunt trocar is then introduced through the patellar tendon and the fat pad to gain entry to the joint. This portal is very useful in grasping the dislocated bucket handle portion of the medial meniscus.

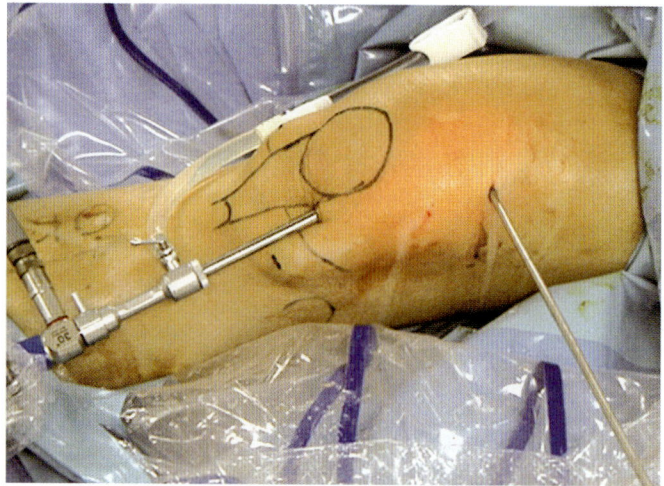

Fig. 64.7: Switching stick in the superolateral port

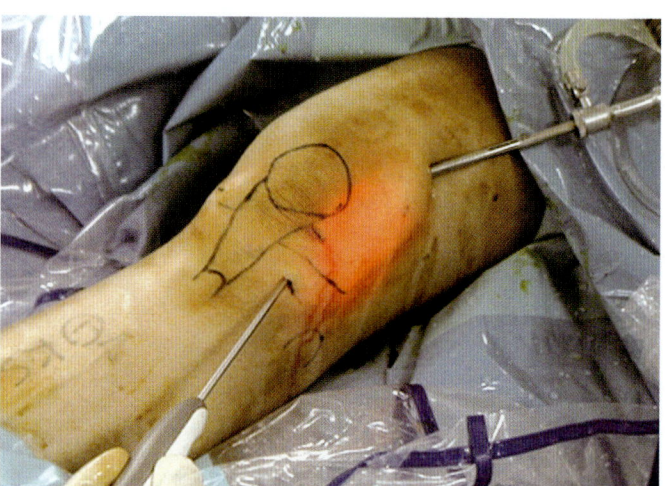

Fig. 64.9: My lateral release portal

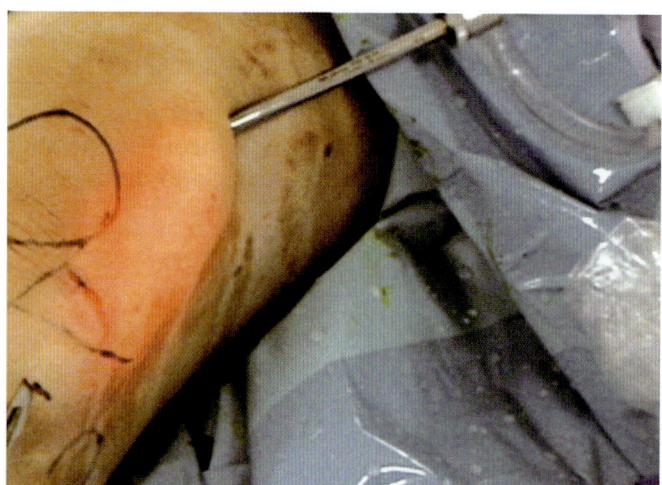

Fig. 64.8: Arthroscope inserted over the switching stick

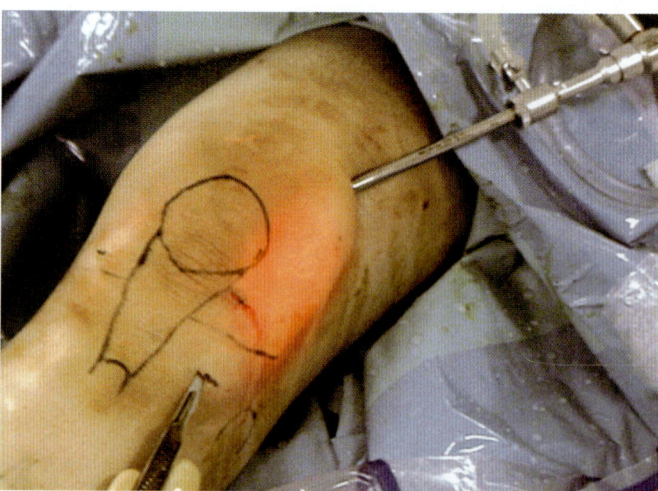

Fig. 64.10: Cutting diathermy through the lateral release portal

CHAPTER 65

9-Point Diagnostic Knee Arthroscopy*

A systematic approach to knee arthroscopy is important to avoid missing pathological lesions. My 9-point arthroscopic technique would help you to inspect the joint and diagnose abnormalities in the knee with ease (Table 65.1). Each point has been further subdivided for the comprehensive evaluation of the joint.

FIRST POINT: SUPRAPATELLAR POUCH

After the arthroscope has been inserted into the joint from the lateral port, the lateral aspect of the suprapatellar pouch is inspected with the knee extended. Drainage portal is made under vision (Figs 65.1 and 65.2). Loose bodies can be found in the suprapatellar pouch. In case of synovitis, biopsy can be taken from here. The light lead is gently turned to inspect the medial aspect of the suprapatellar pouch. Loose bodies can be found here.

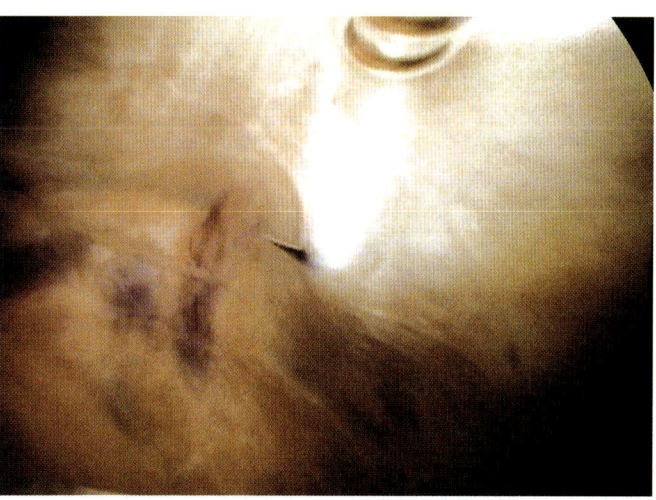

Fig. 65.1: Needle from outside in, marking the superolateral port

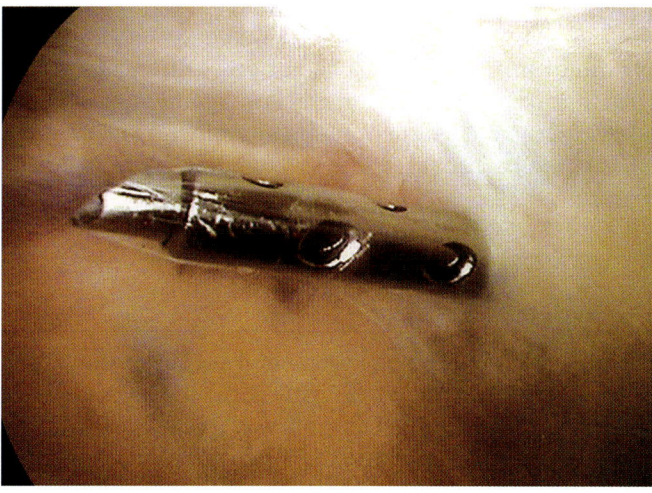

Fig. 65.2: Trocar inserted superolaterally

TABLE 65.1: 9-point arthroscopy

Suprapatellar bursa	Central, medial and lateral parts of the bursa
Patella	All facets from superior to inferior pole
Trochlea	Central, medial, lateral and anterior aspect of the trochlea
Medial gutter	Gutter and plica
Medial compartment	Femur, tibia and meniscus
Anterior cruciate ligament	Integrity and laxity
Lateral compartment	Femur, tibia and meniscus
Lateral gutter	Full length
Patellar tracking	Tracking and patellar cartilage lesions

* From "Step by Step Operative Orthopedics" by *Dr John Ebnezar*.

SECOND POINT: PATELLA

With the light cable pointing towards the ceiling, the patella is visualized (Fig. 65.3). Patella can be visualized from the upper to the lower pole and from medial to lateral to complete the examination. Chondromalacia, chondral wear and osteoarthritis of the patella can be diagnosed.

THIRD POINT: TROCHLEA

With the cable pointing to the floor, the trochlea is inspected from medial to lateral and from the superior to inferior. Trochlear dysplasia, wear and osteoarthritis can be diagnosed.

Sweep the scope past the lower end of the trochlea and visualize it by gently flexing the knee. The fat pad can be inspected during this step.

FOURTH POINT: MEDIAL GUTTER

Gently move the scope into the medial gutter and check for loose bodies and pathological synovial plicae.

FIFTH POINT: MEDIAL COMPARTMENT

The medial condylar cartilage and the medial meniscus is examined (Fig. 65.4). The operating portal can be made by initially marking the site with a needle (Fig. 65.5). Remember the meniscal inspection is not complete until the meniscus is thoroughly probed (superior and inferior surface) (Fig. 65.6). Meniscal tear can be assessed by probing (Fig. 65.7).

SIXTH POINT: INTERCONDYLAR NOTCH AND ANTERIOR CRUCIATE LIGAMENT

Ligamentum mucosum is seen here. Differentiate this structure from the anterior cruciate ligament. Probe the anterior cruciate ligament for its integrity (Figs 65.8A and B). In complete rupture, the empty notch sign is a diagnostic feature.

SEVENTH POINT: LATERAL COMPARTMENT

Park the probe in the posteromedial corner of the lateral joint. Bring the knee in a Figure 4 position. Inspecting the lateral joint is quite easy this way. Inspect the hyaline cartilage of the condyles and the lateral meniscus (Fig. 65.9). Probe the meniscus and assess the popliteus tendon, its hiatus and instability of the lateral meniscus around the popliteus. Anterior cruciate ligament can be inspected again

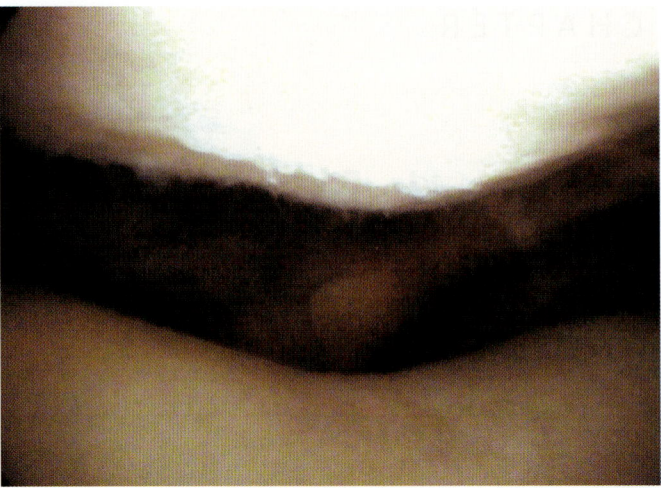

Fig. 65.3: Patellofemoral joint

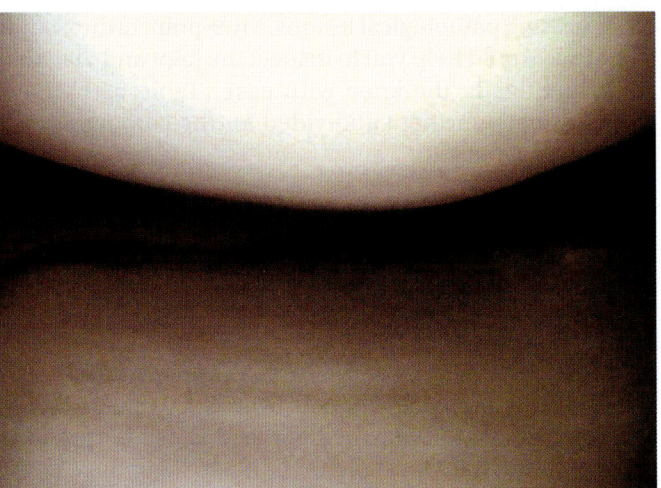

Fig. 65.4: Medial compartment

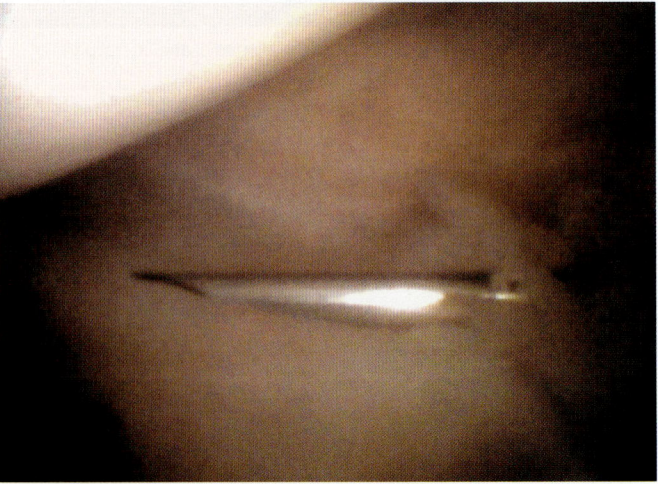

Fig. 65.5: Needle to mark the medial operative port

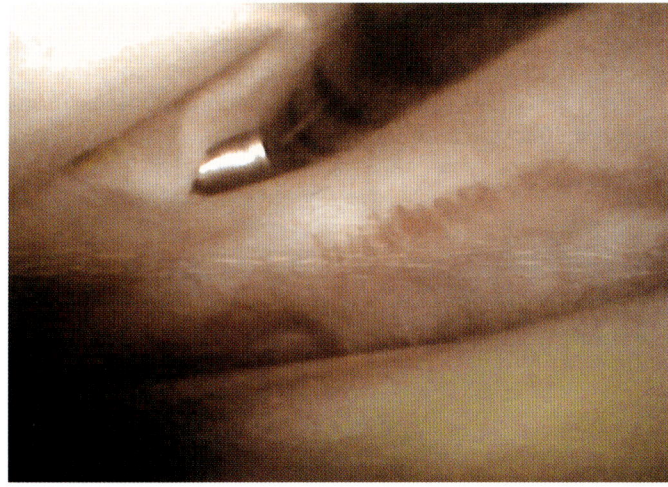

Fig. 65.6: Undersurface of the medial meniscus

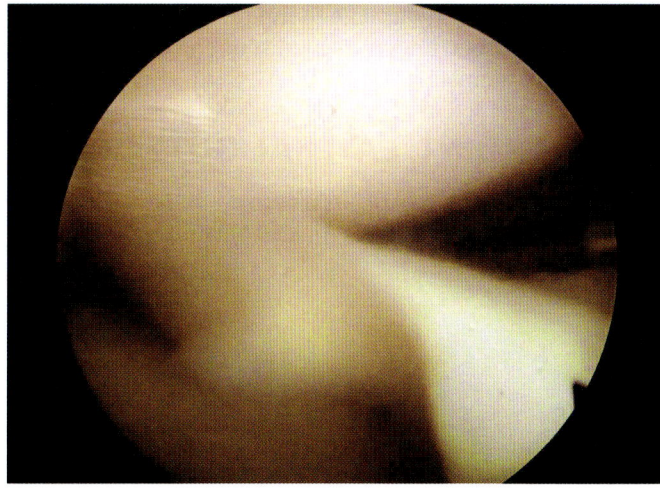

Fig. 65.7: Medial meniscal tear

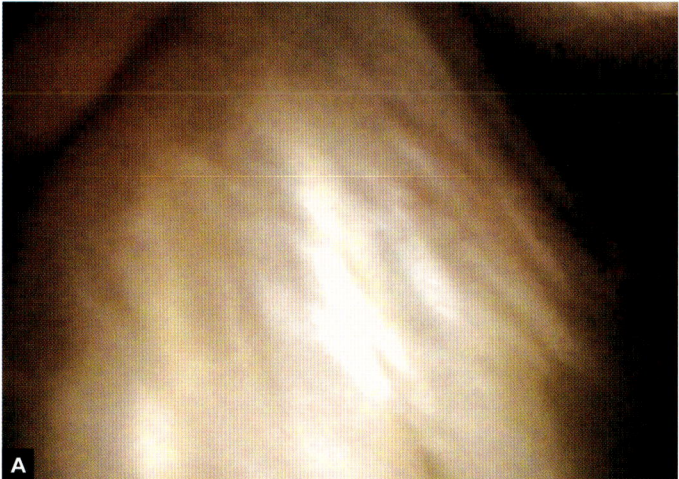
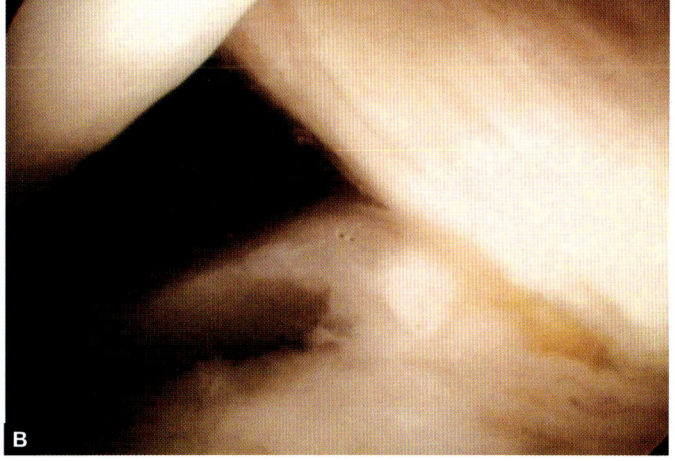

Figs 65.8A and B: Anterior cruciate ligament

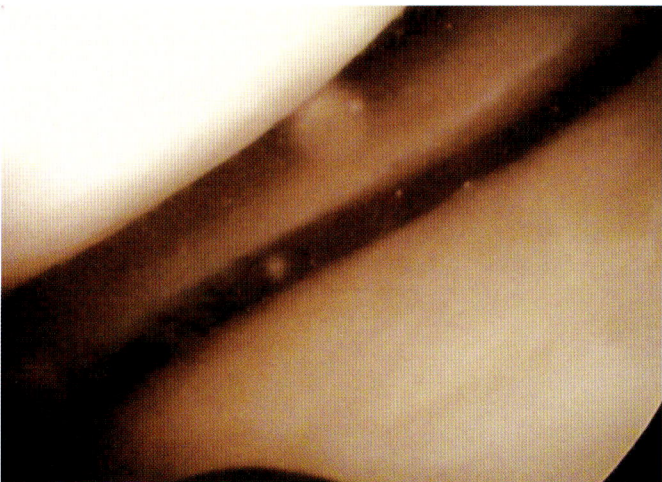

Fig. 65.9: Lateral meniscus

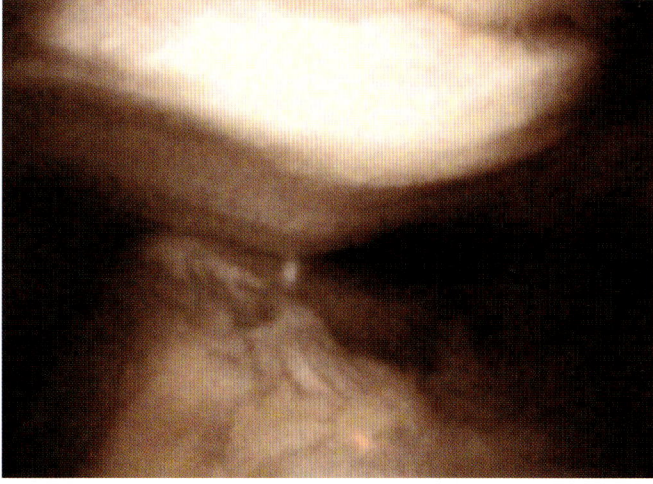

Fig. 65.10: The essential step: Patellofemoral joint from the superolateral portal

in this position. With damage to the posterolateral corner, scarring can be seen under the meniscus and over the lateral aspect of the meniscus.

EIGHTH POINT: LATERAL GUTTER

To complete the diagnostic arthroscopy, inspect the lateral gutter again for loose bodies, pieces of trimmed meniscus and debris.

NINTH POINT: PATELLAR TRACKING

Patellar tracking can be assessed from the superolateral portal (Fig. 65.10). Detailed patellar tracking assessment can be seen in the lateral release section.

CHAPTER 66

Arthroplasty*

INTRODUCTION

Our folklore says that God out of sheer boredom created a man for his company and placed 206 bones and 65 joints within him. Then to give company to man he plucked out a rib from the man and created a woman. He eventually regretted his creation when faced with rebellious Adam and Eve and banished them to earth. They were now made to use their bones and joints for locomotion on earth and this holds good even to this day. Exposed to constant friction due to weight-bearing and locomotion joints wear out. The once free joints now succumb to crippling arthritis.

Till early 1930's, man tried various methods that were essentially nonoperative to alleviate pain. Then came the idea of replacing the worn out joints instead of restoring the ailing joints. Thus, arthroplasty was born. From membrane replacement, glass, metal, alloys, plastics, etc. were used to substitute the joints. After various experimentation, research, we now have a very high quality of implants, technology, infrastructure and expertise to give a near perfect joint.

ARTHROPLASTY

This essentially means replacement of joints and this could be partial or total. When only one part of the joint is removed, it is called partial and is known as hemi replacement arthroplasty. When complete joint is replaced it is called total joint replacement and when one-half of the joint is replaced, it is called unicondylar replacement of the joint. When only diseased surface is resected and resurfaced, it is called resurfacing procedure.

Types of Prosthesis

- Metallic prosthesis on one or both sides of the joints.
- High density polyethylene.
- Ceramic.

Choice of Prosthesis

- Both metals.
- Both ceramics.
- One metallic (Femoral) and one poly (Acetabular).
  Fixation could be cemented or uncemented. The former is used in older people and the latter in younger individuals.

HIP AND KNEE ARTHROPLASTY

Total knee and hip athroplasty have become the definitive treatment for end stage osteoarthritis. They have proved to be reliable and successful allowing patients to resume normal activities. Both knee and hip arthroplasty can be performed using cement or biologic fixation.

In cement fixation, there is mechanical interlock of methyl methacrylate to the interstices of bone. Biological fixation can be either a porous-coated metallic surface that provides bone in-growths fixation or by a grit-blasted metallic surface that provides bone on growth fixation.

The choice of method of fixation remains controversial. In hip arthroplasty, the tendency is towards the use of uncemented prosthesis in younger active patients because cemented prosthesis have reported a higher loosening rate in long-term follow-up. In total knee arthroplasty, the cemented prosthesis have reported good results in long-

---

* From "Step by Step Operative Orthopedics" by *Dr John Ebnezar.*

term follow-up and is more widely used than the cementless ones.

Aseptic loosening is the most common indication for revision surgery. In cemented hip, the most common reason for revision is failure of the cemented acetabular component, while in the uncemented ones the most common cause for failure first the femoral component. In knee arthroplasty aseptic failure can be caused by many factors as component loosening, polyethylene wear, and ligament instability and patellofemoral maltracking.

Articular bearing in hip arthroplasty is mainly on "hard on soft couple", which include metallic heads coupled with polyethylene cup. The other hard on soft couple is ceramic head with polyethylene cup. Titanium alloy heads should be avoided because it is liable to scratching which will cause rapid wear of the polyethylene surface. In knee arthroplasty the majority of articular bearing components are metallic femoral surface (cobalt, chromium) coupled with polyethylene tibial surface.

In 1997, Birmingham hip resurfacing was introduced using metal on metal prosthesis. It is a bone conserving operation with minimal or virtually no dislocation which makes it ideal for young active people.

Indications

- Osteoarthritis.
- Rheumatoid arthritis.
- Secondary osteoarthritis.
- Avascular necrosis of the head of femur.
- Failed hemi replacement arthroplasty.
- Ankylosed hip.
- Tuberculosis hip.

Contraindications

- Infection is an absolute contraindication.
- Poor medical risk.
- Poor anesthetic risk.
- Obesity.
- Neuropathic joints.

Complications

- DVT.
- Fat embolism.
- Infection.
- Breakages of implants.
- Loosening of implants.
- Osteolysis.
- Periprosthetic fractures.
- Dislocation.
- Heterotopic ossification.
- Vascular and nerve injuries.

SURGICAL STEPS OF TOTAL HIP REPLACEMENT (FIGS 66.1 TO 66.26)

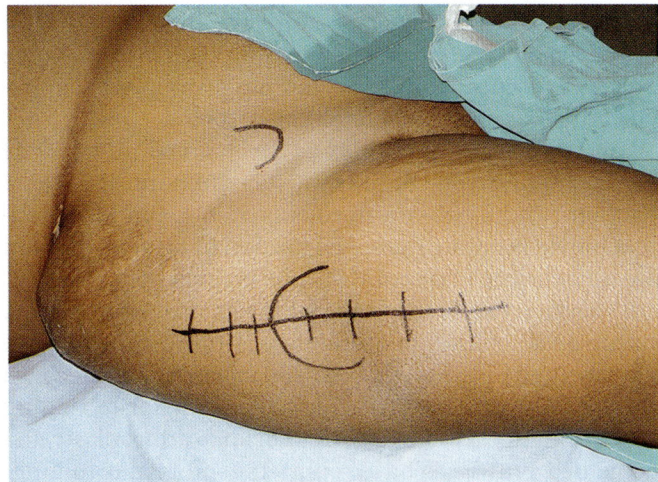

Fig. 66.1: Skin marking

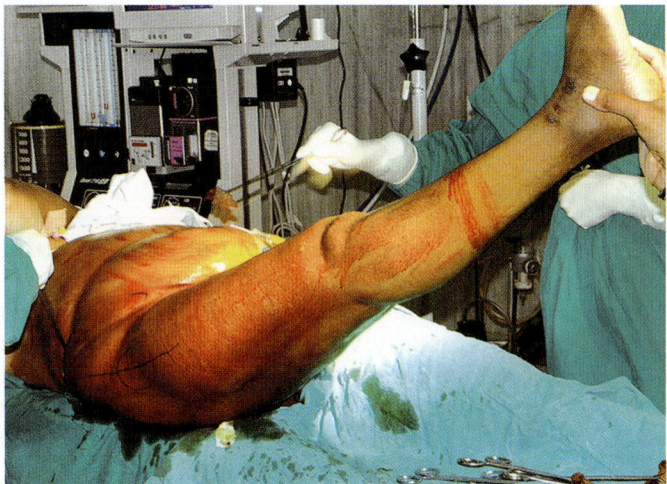

Fig. 66.2: Painting and preparation

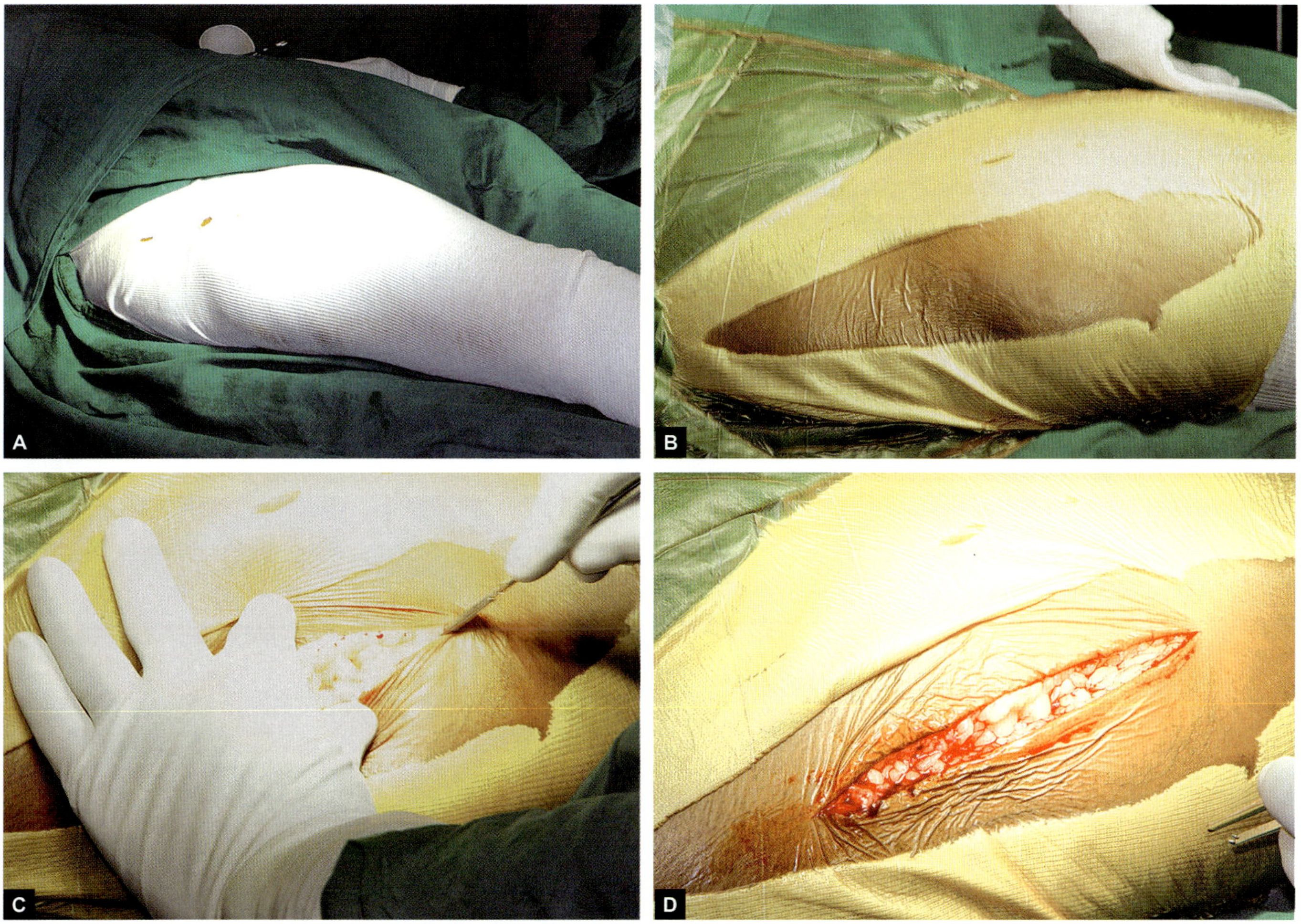

Figs 66.3A to D: Skin incision. Straight lateral incision

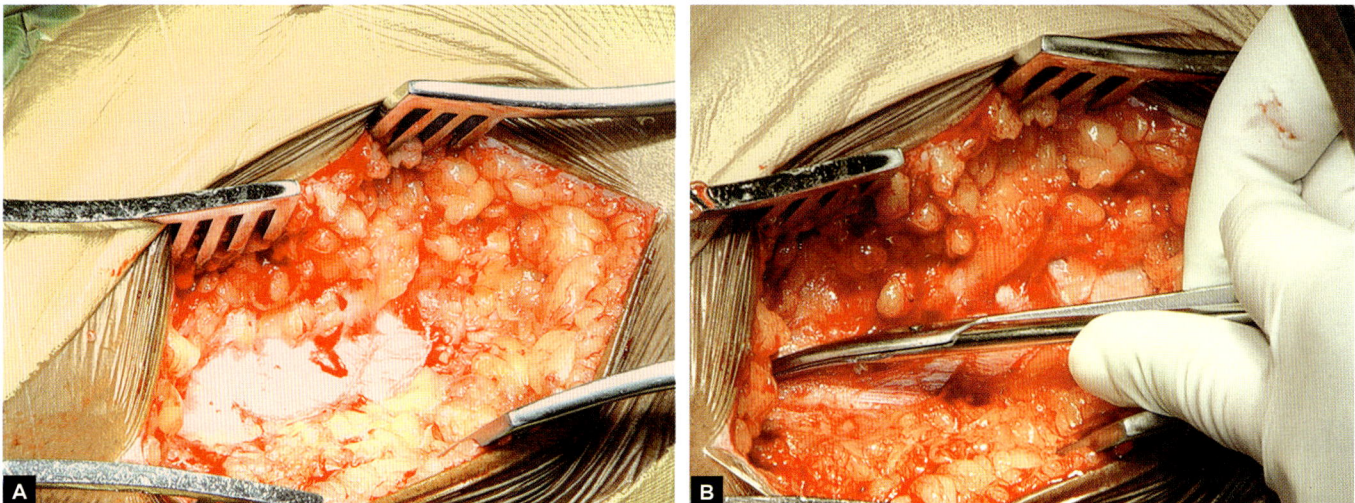

Figs 66.4A and B

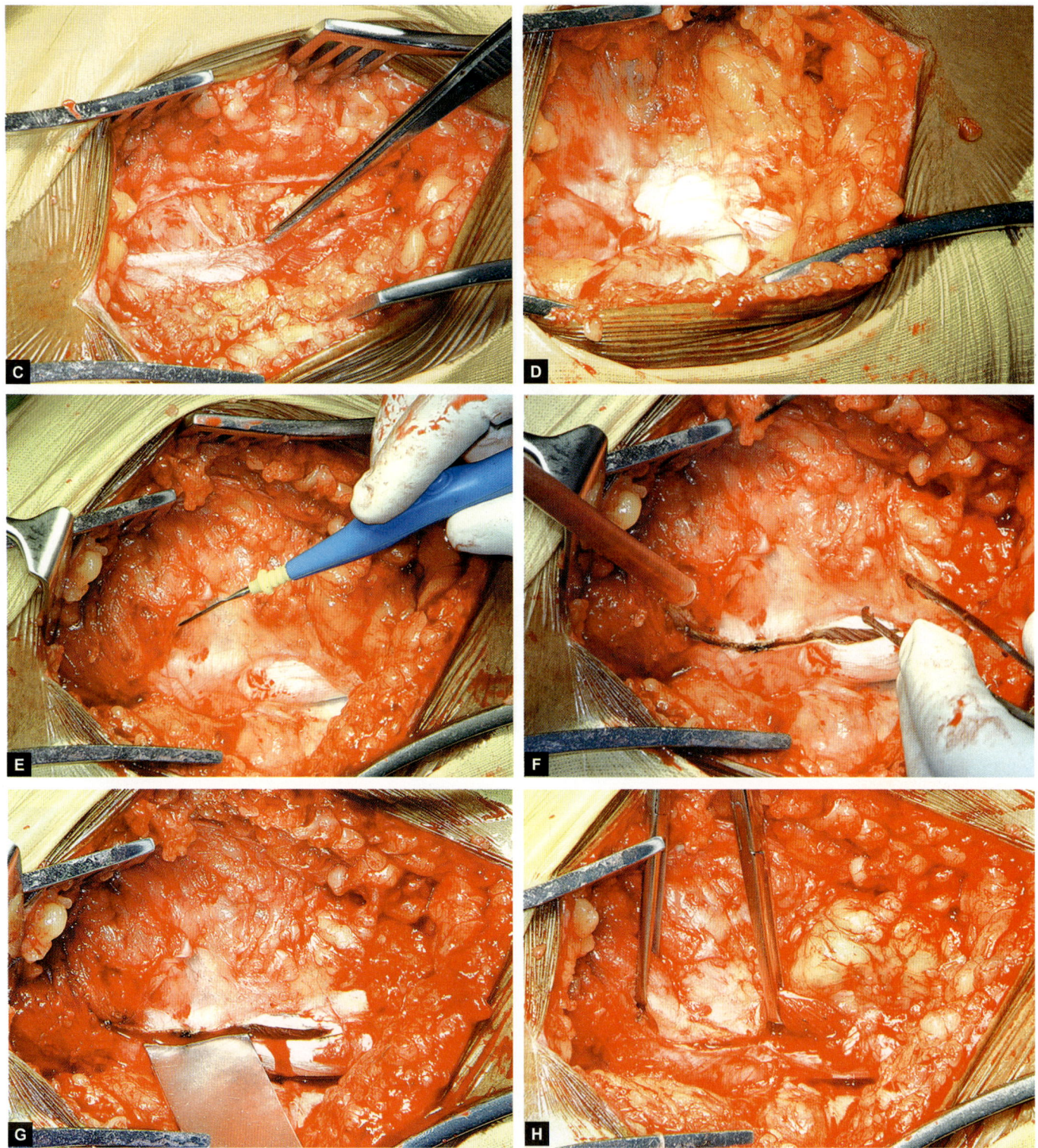

Figs 66.4C to H

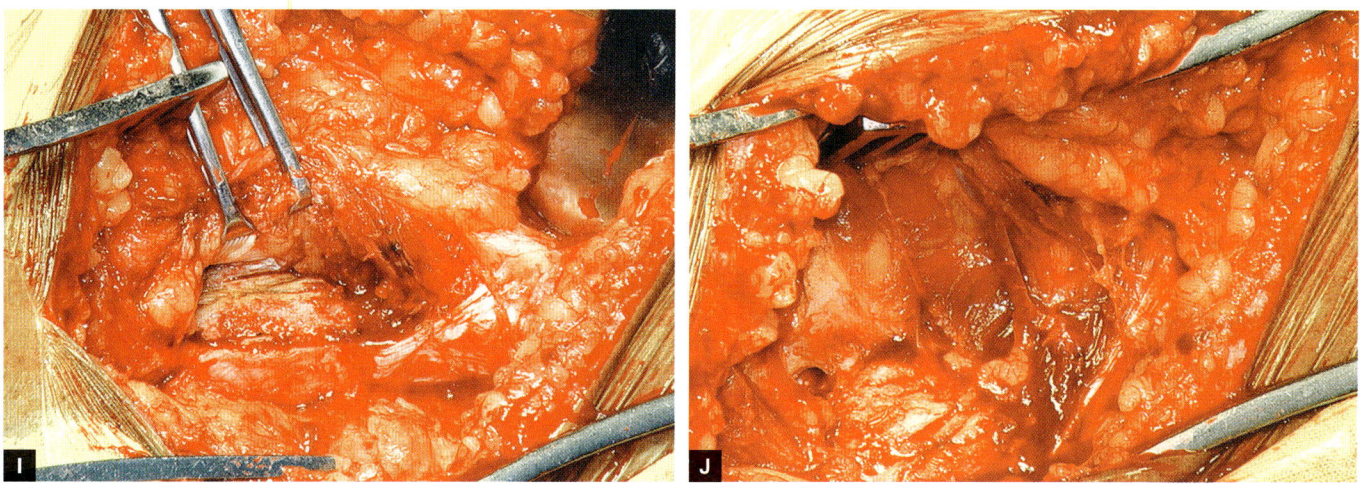

Figs 66.4I and J
Figs 66.4A to J: Modified Hardinge approach

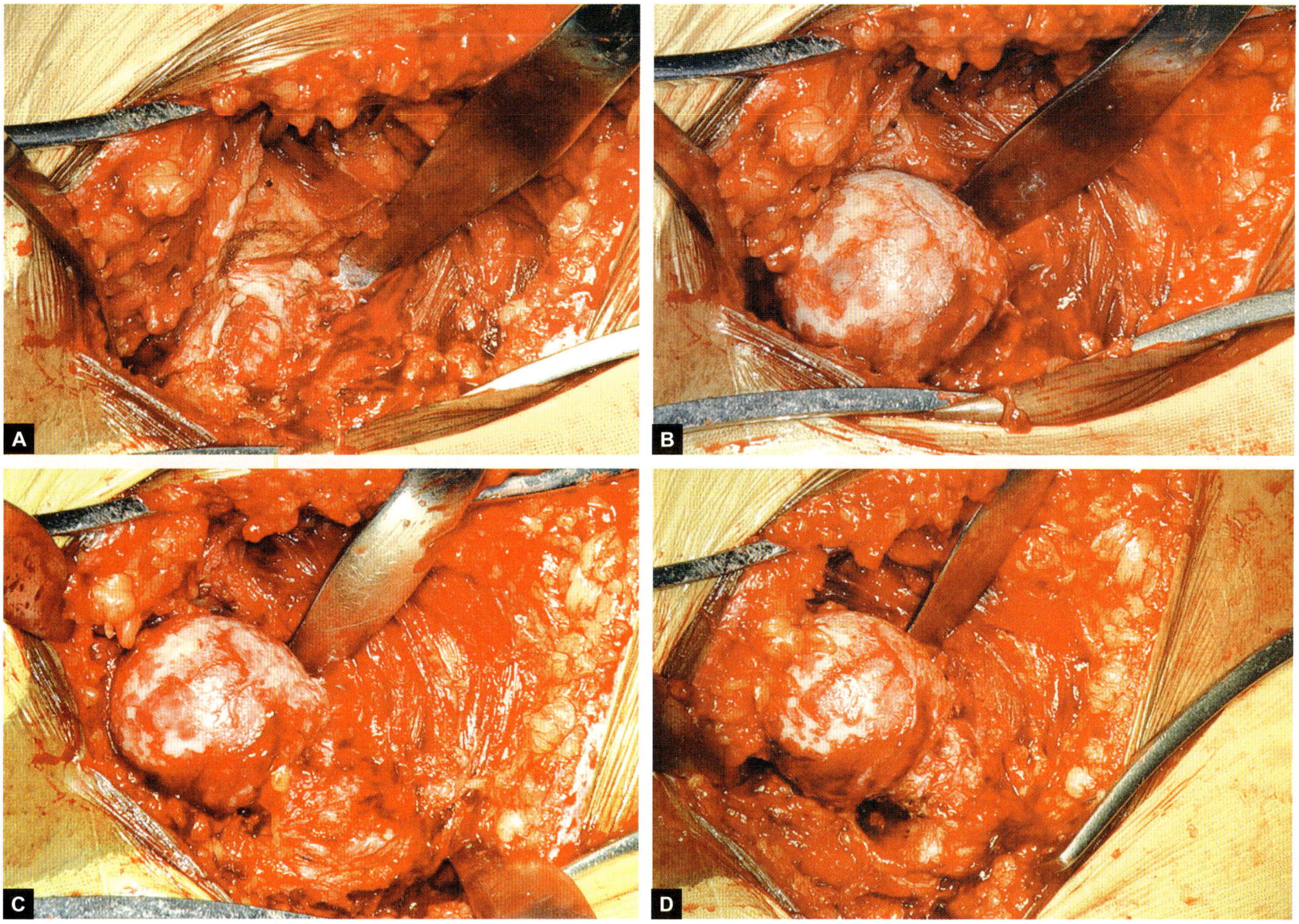

Figs 66.5A to D: Dislocation of femoral head by gentle internal rotation and adduction

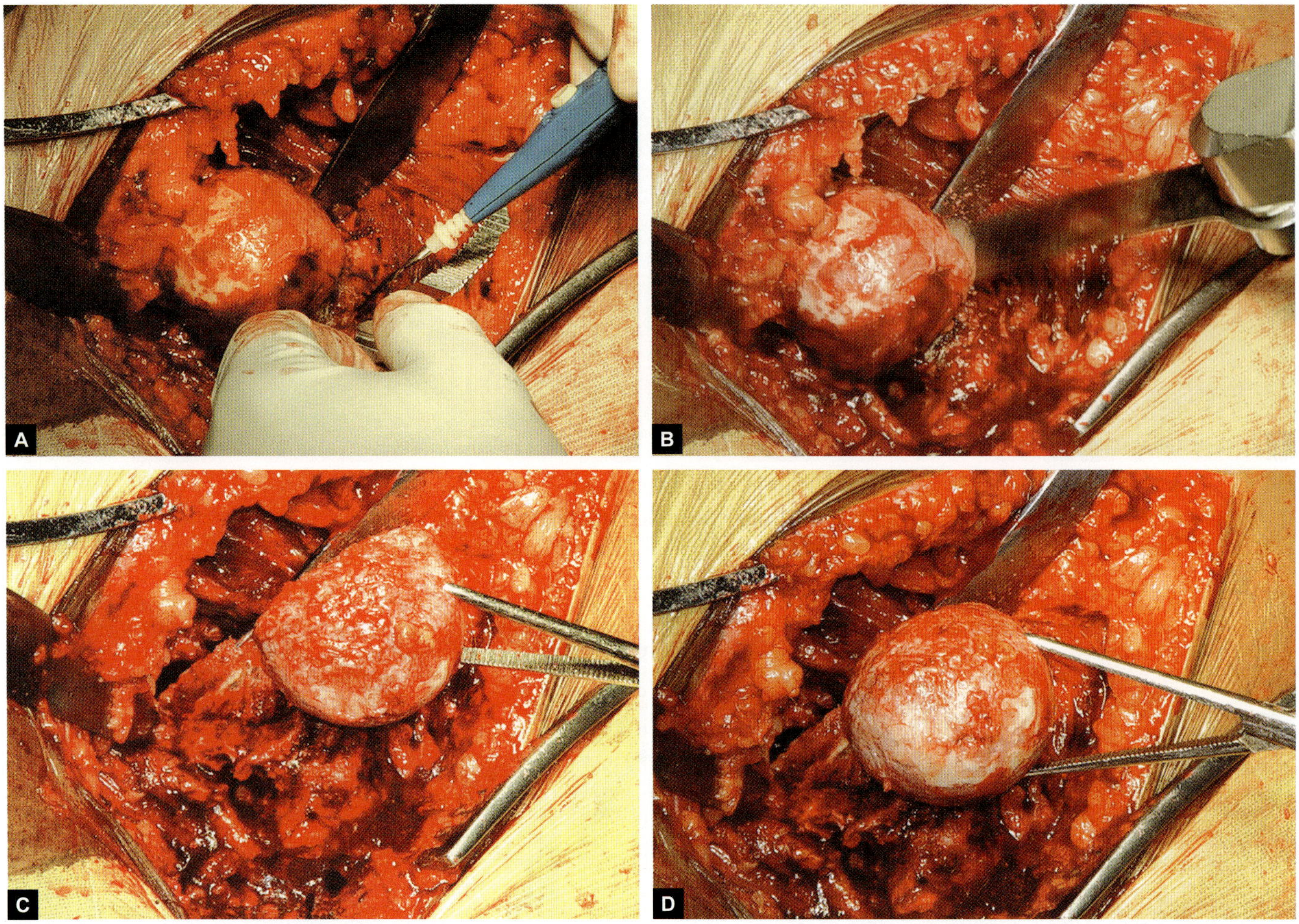

Figs 66.6A to D: Femoral neck osteotomy based on both the intraoperative radiographic measurements and the intraoperative anatomic landmarks

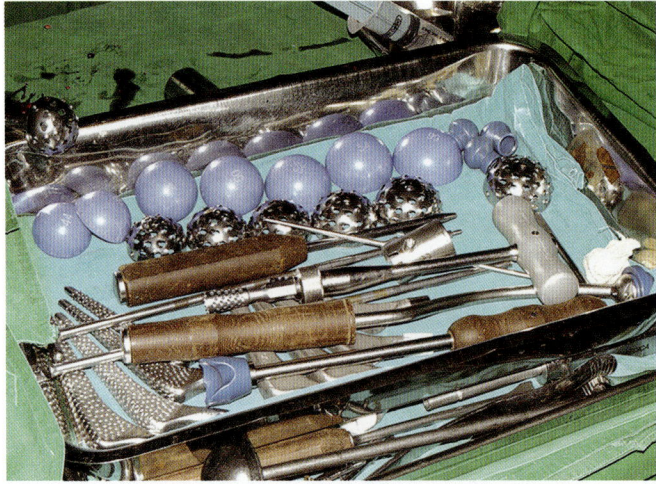

Fig. 66.7: Instruments for acetabular preparation

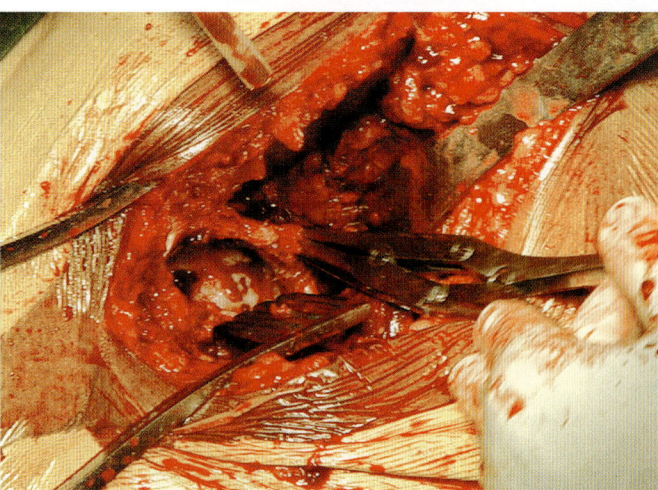

Fig. 66.8: Excision of remnants of acetabular labrum

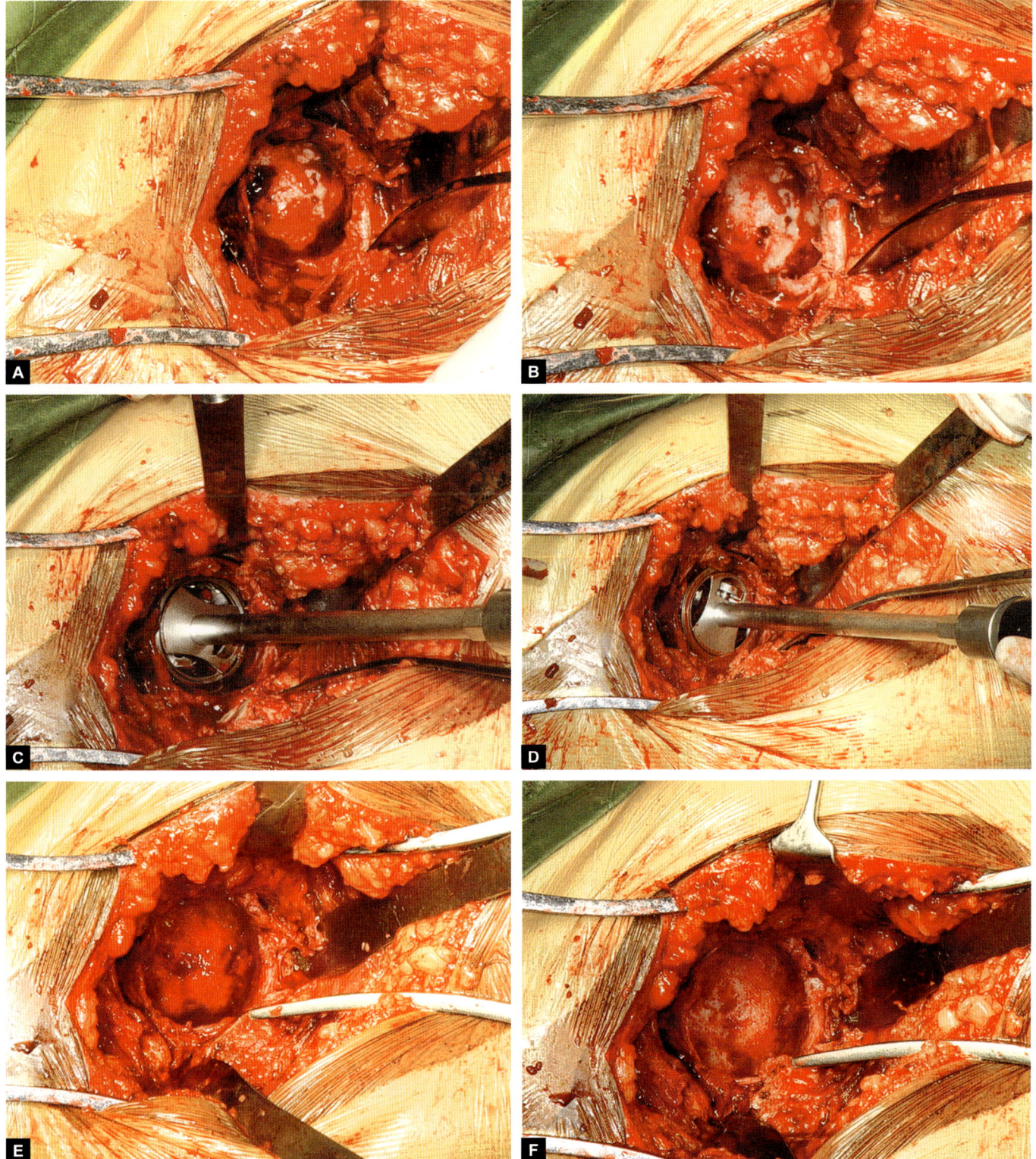

Figs 66.9A to F: Use of acetabular reamers to prepare the acetabulum. Start with a small reamer

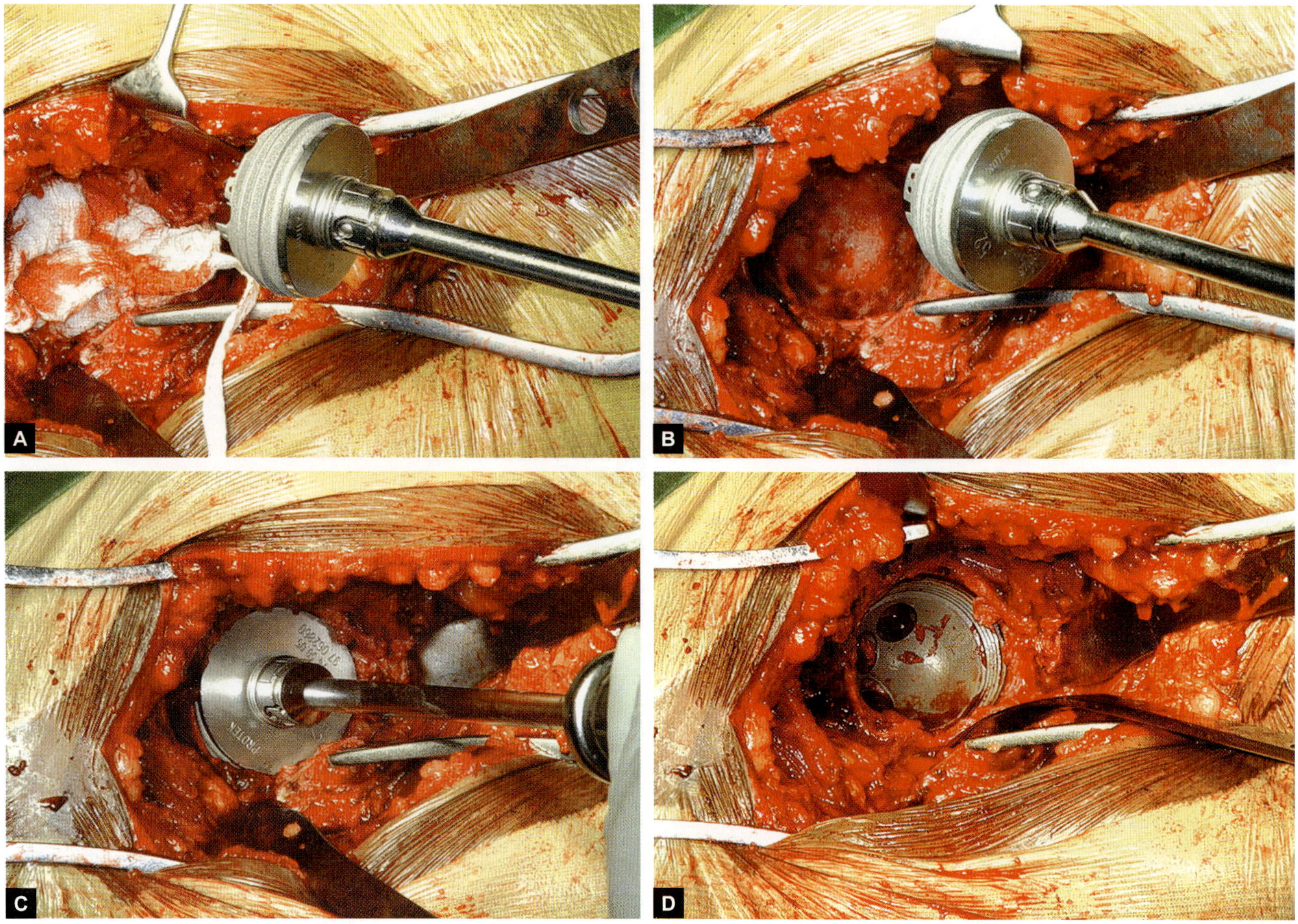

Figs 66.10A to D: Insertion of the acetabular component's shell using the insertion device

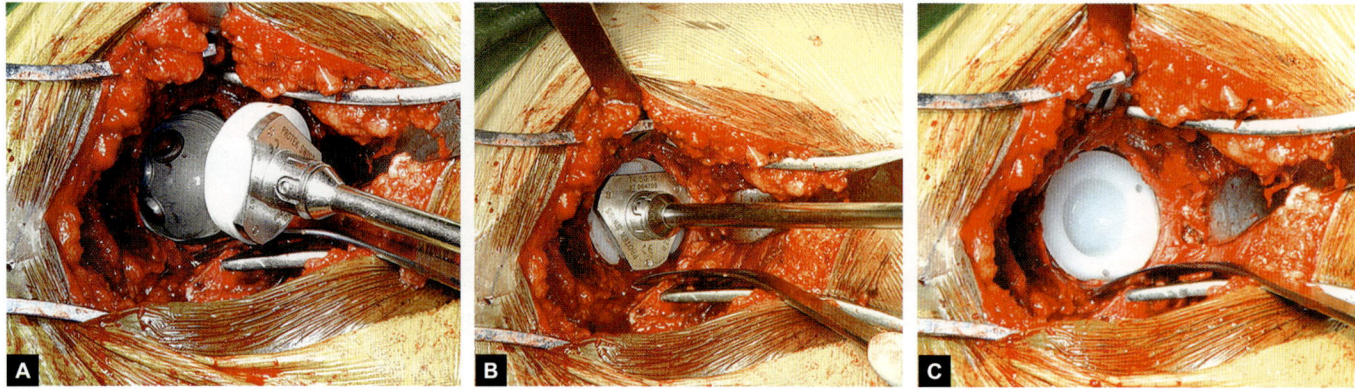

Figs 66.11A to C: Insertion of the polyethylene liner

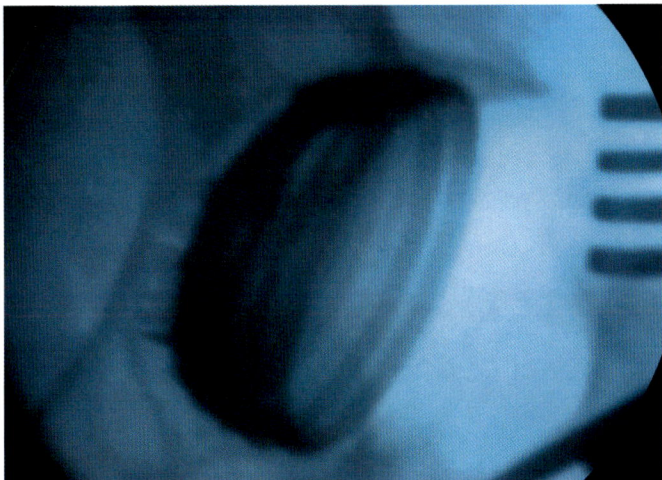

Fig. 66.12: Image intensifier of the acetabular component

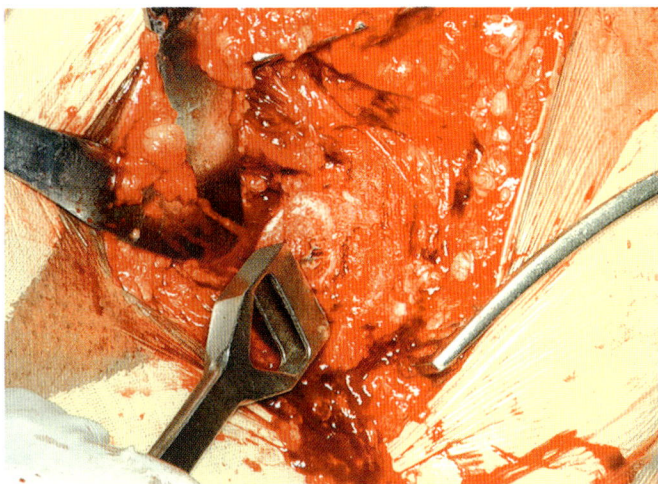

Fig. 66.13: Using box osteotome to remove remnants of bone from the superior femoral neck

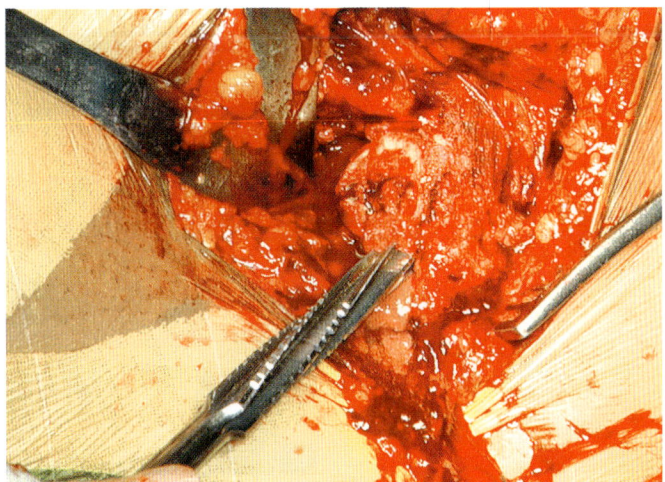

Fig. 66.14: Reaming of the femoral canal

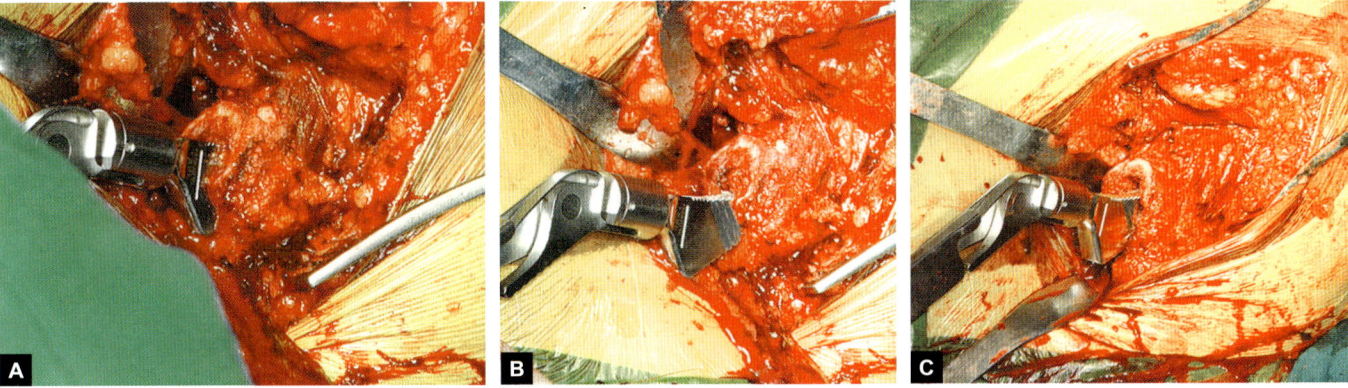

Figs 66.15A to C: Broaching of the proximal femur with sequentially larger broaches until a reasonably snug fit occurs

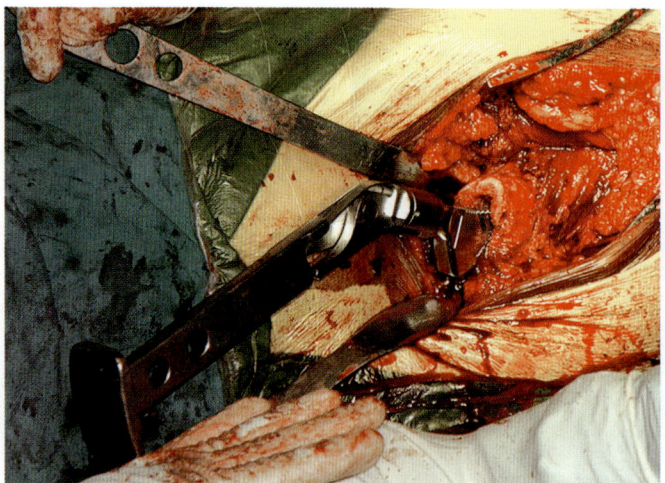

Fig. 66.16: Insertion of the trial implant

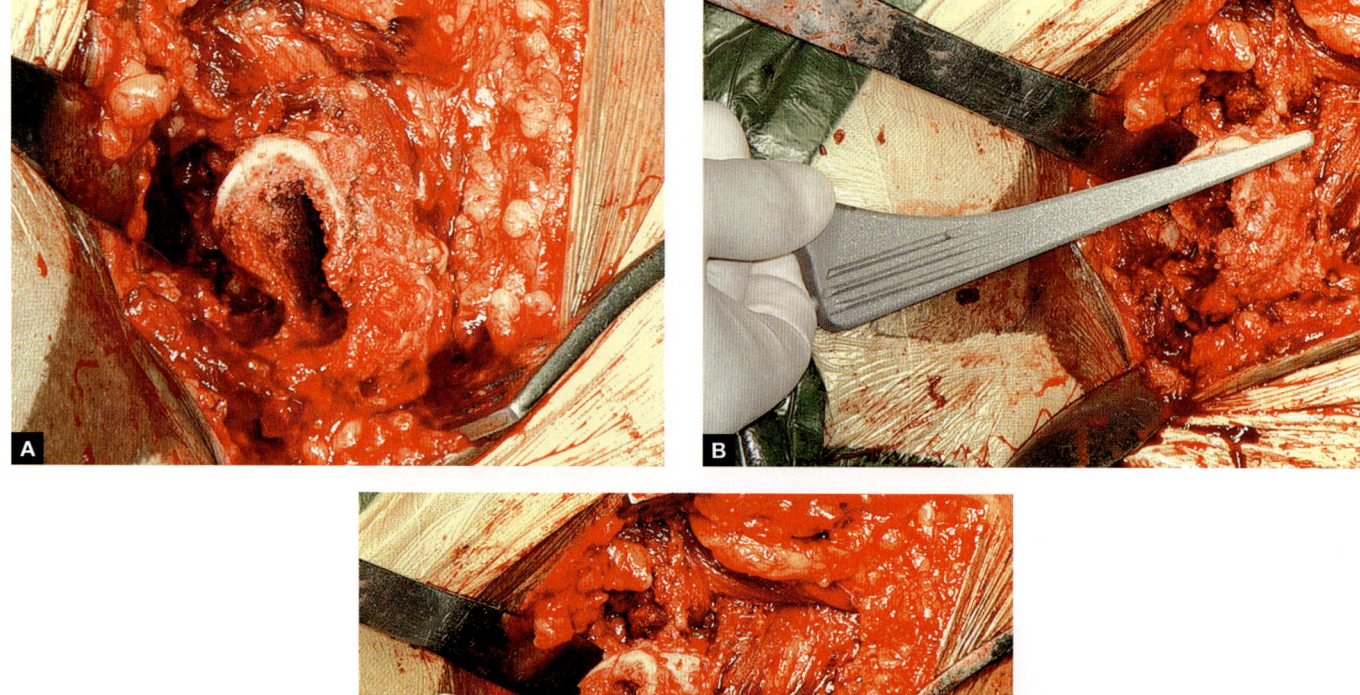

Figs 66.17A to C: Checking of the trial femoral implant

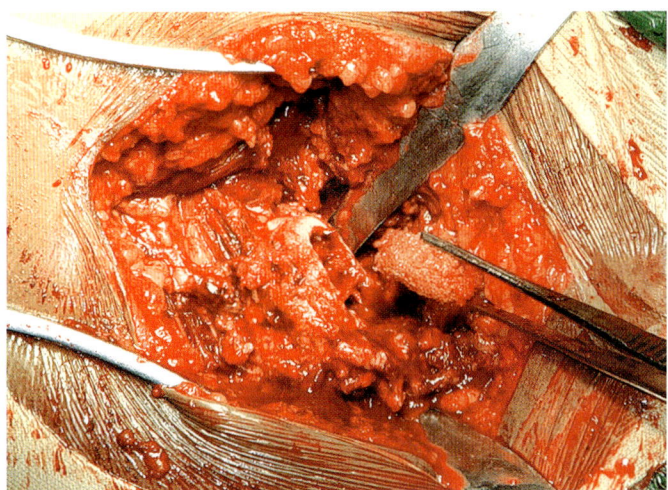

Fig. 66.18: Insertion of the femoral canal plug. It should reside in the femoral canal approximately 2 cm distal to where the end of the stem will sit

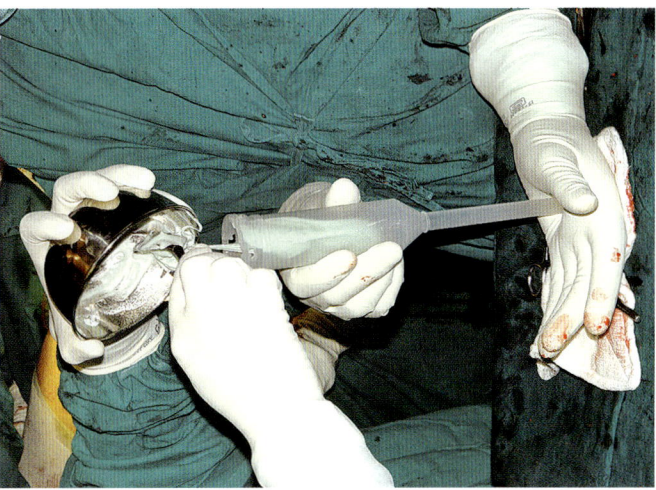

Fig. 66.19: Cement mix. Consider using vacuum mixing technique to enhance cement consistency and reduce overall cement porosity

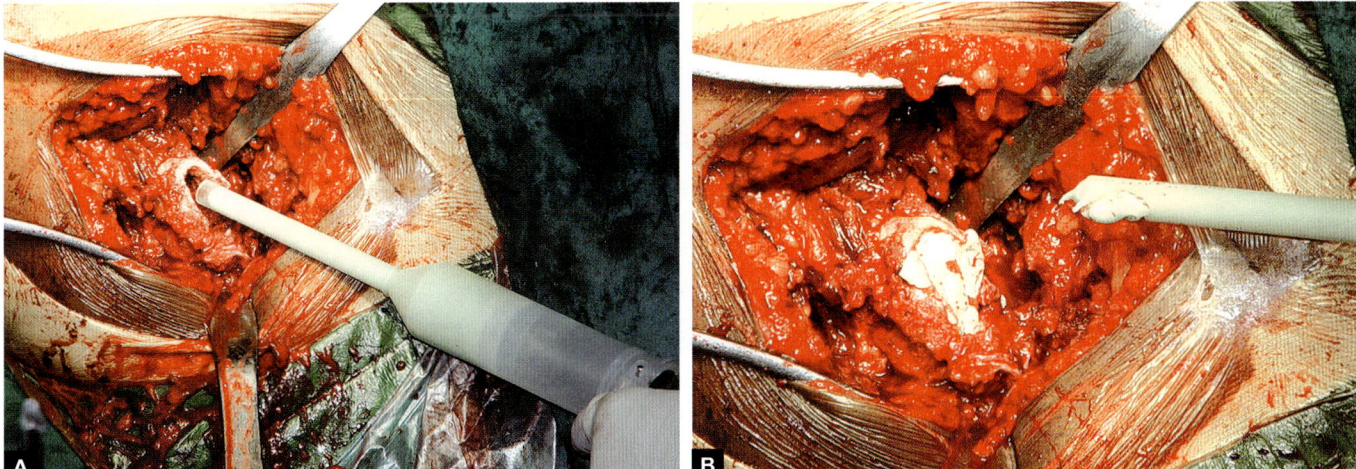

Figs 66.20A and B: Use a cement gun to insert the cement when it reaches a "doughy" state and no longer adheres to the surgical gloves

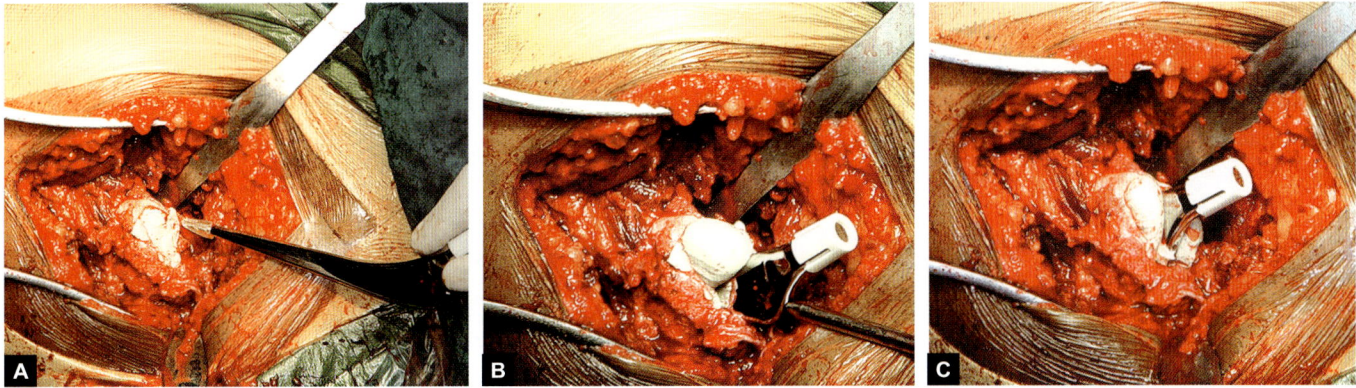

Figs 66.21A to C: Stem insertion using predominately a manual force rather than the mallet

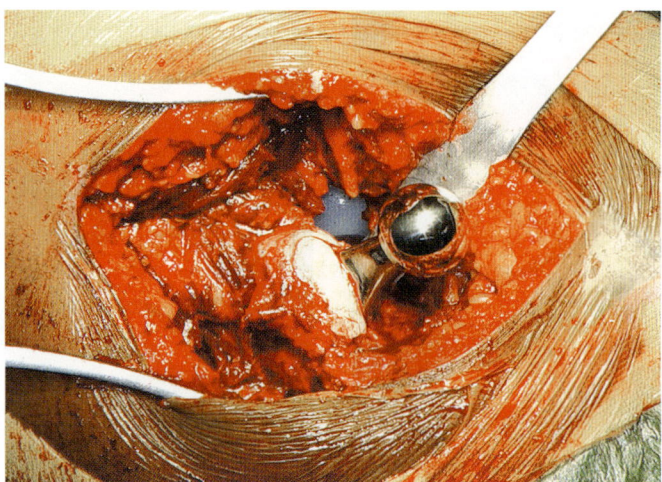

Fig. 66.22: Insertion of the appropriate modular head based on the trial reduction

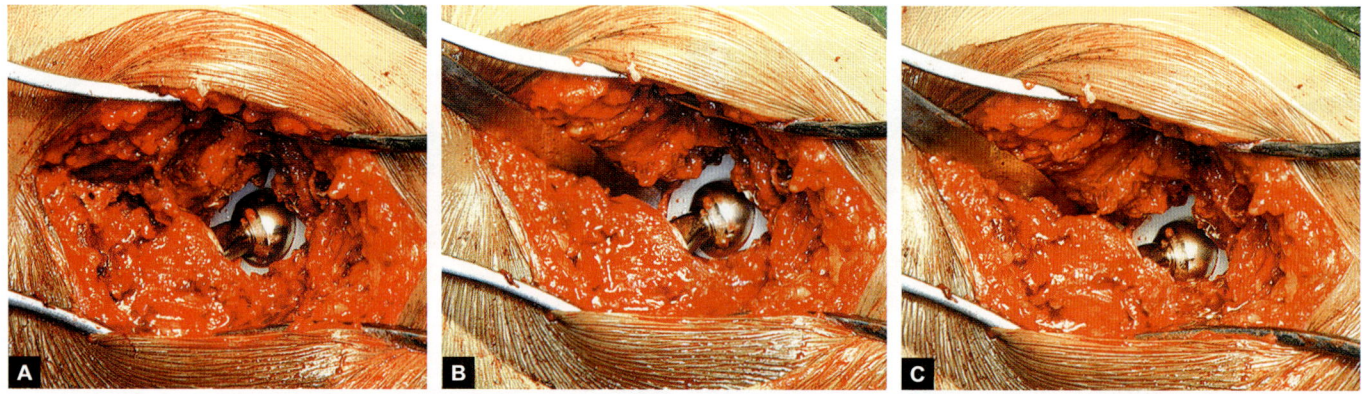

Figs 66.23A to C: Hip reduction and reassessment of stability

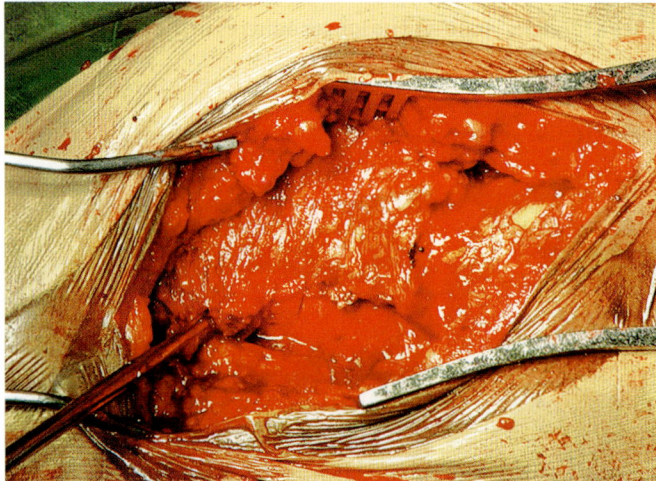

Fig. 66.24: Closure of the abductors using absorbable sutures

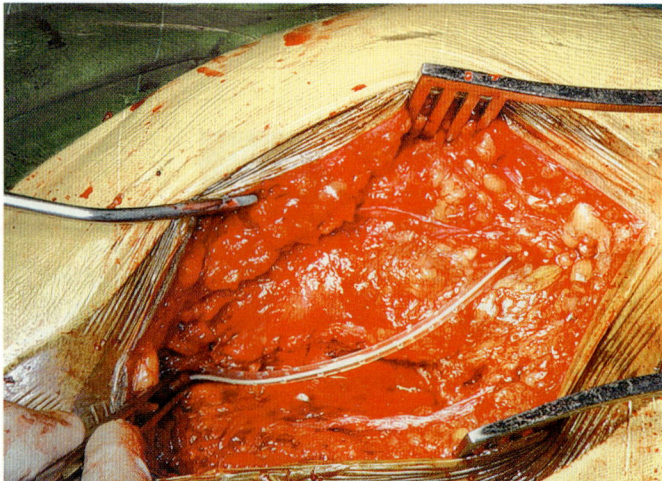

Fig. 66.25: Use of superficial suction drain and closure of the subcutaneous layer

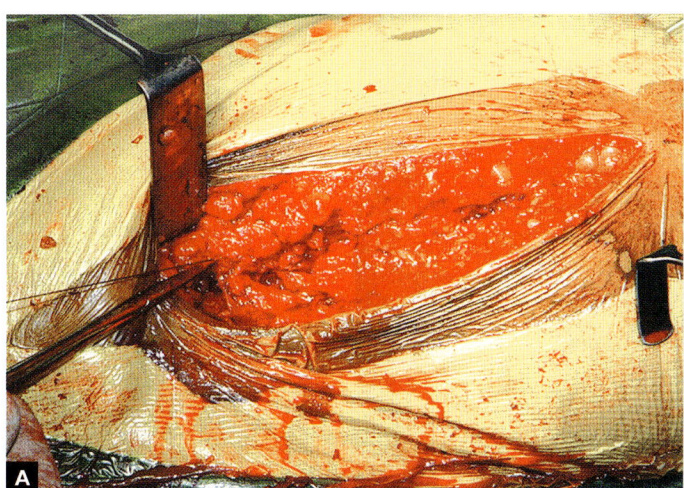
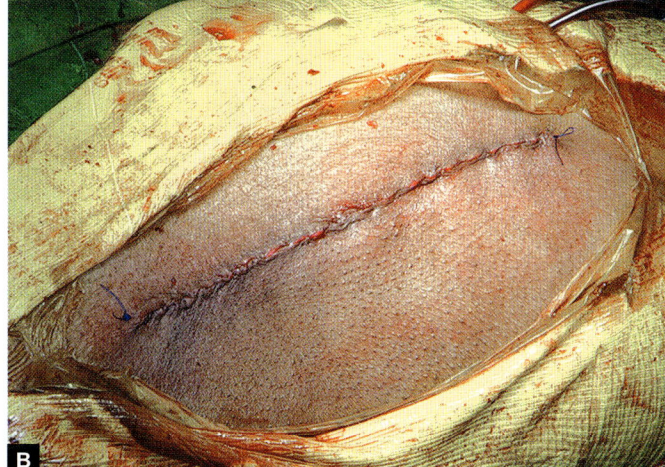

Figs 66.26A and B: Skin closure

SURGICAL STEPS OF TOTAL KNEE REPLACMENT (FIGS 66.27 TO 66.51)

This is increasingly gaining popularity thanks to the high incidences of osteoarthritis of the knee joints world wide. Though not as popular or as successful as total hip replacement, TKR nevertheless is catching the attention of both orthopedic surgeons and patients alike and is being commonly performed across the country.

Types

- Unicondylar replacement.
- Total knee replacement: This could be cemented or uncemented, PCL sacrificing or sparing or rotating platform.

Components

- A metallic femoral component.
- Tibial base plate.
- A plastic component.
- A patellar component.

Indications, contraindications and complications more or less remain the same as for THR.

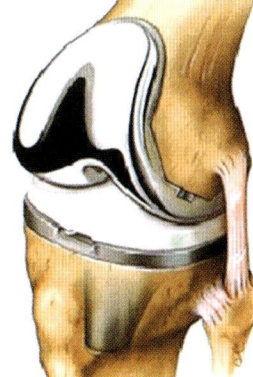
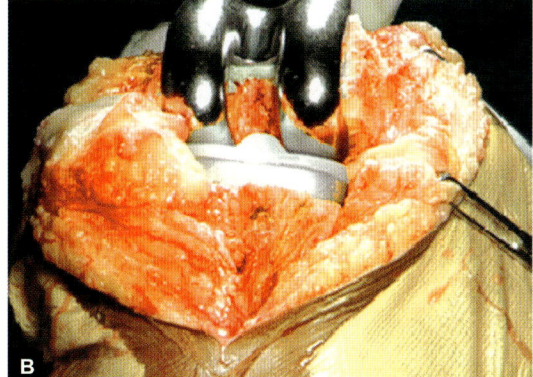
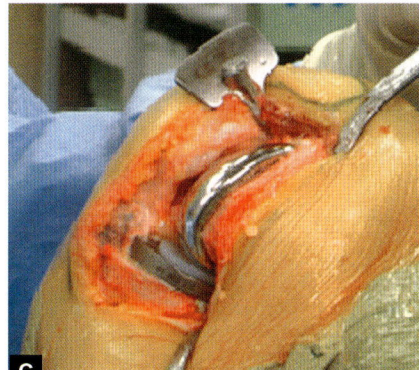

Figs 66.27A to C: Total knee replacement

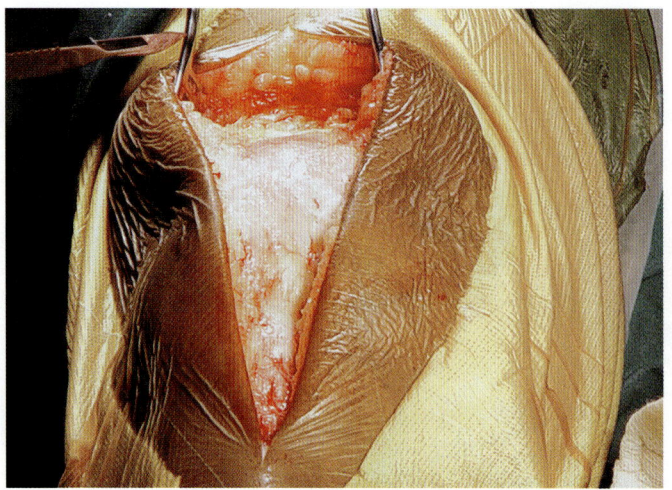

Fig. 66.28: Skin incision. A straight anterior incision

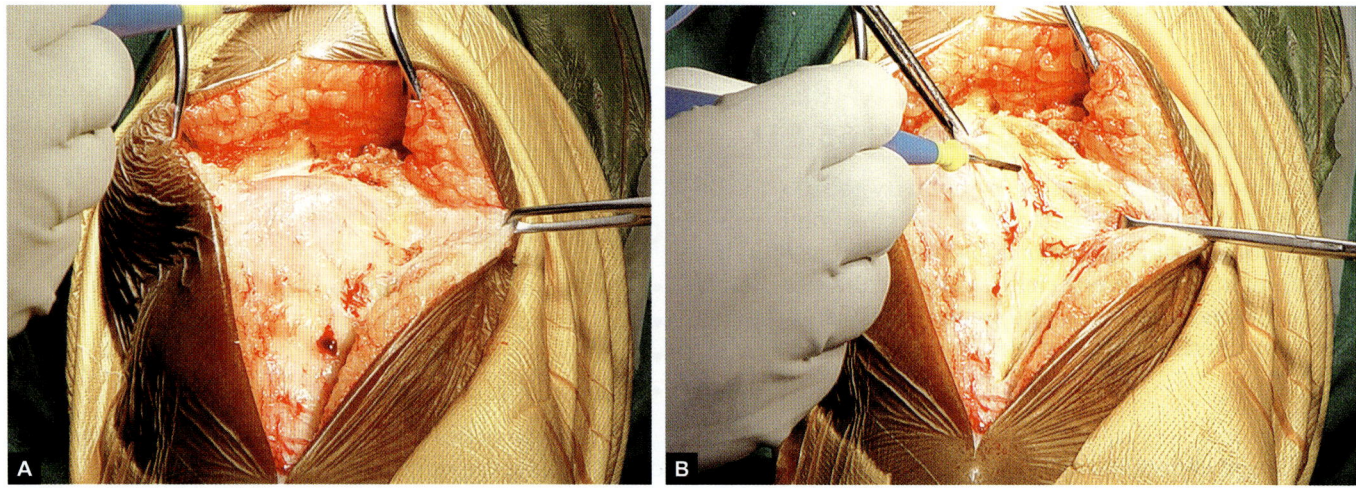

Figs 66.29A and B: Medial parapatellar arthrotomy

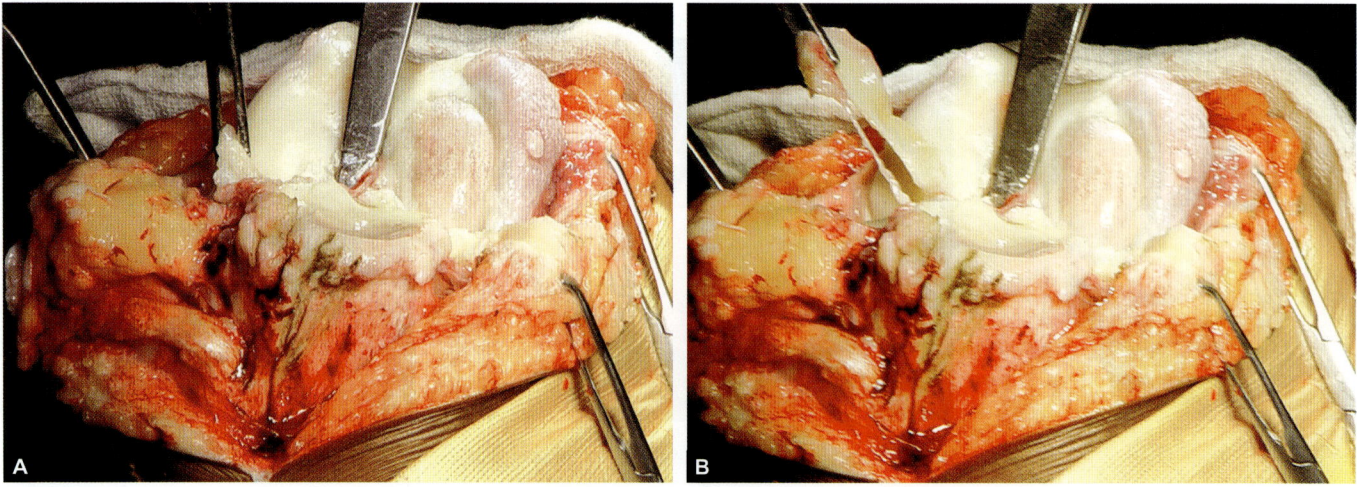

Figs 66.30A and B: Meniscal excision

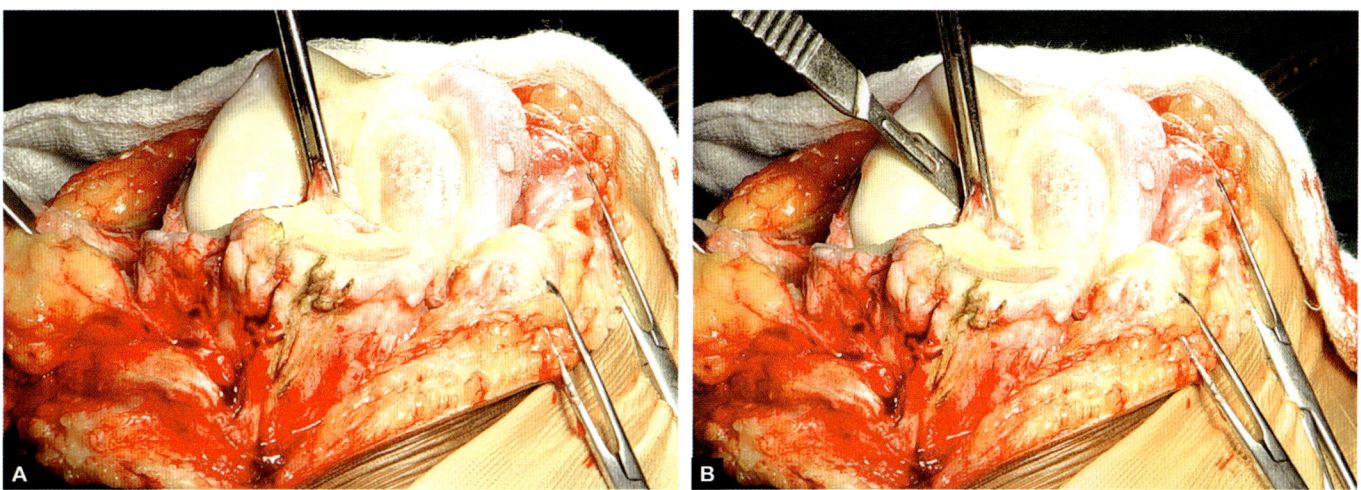

Figs 66.31A and B: Excision of ACL

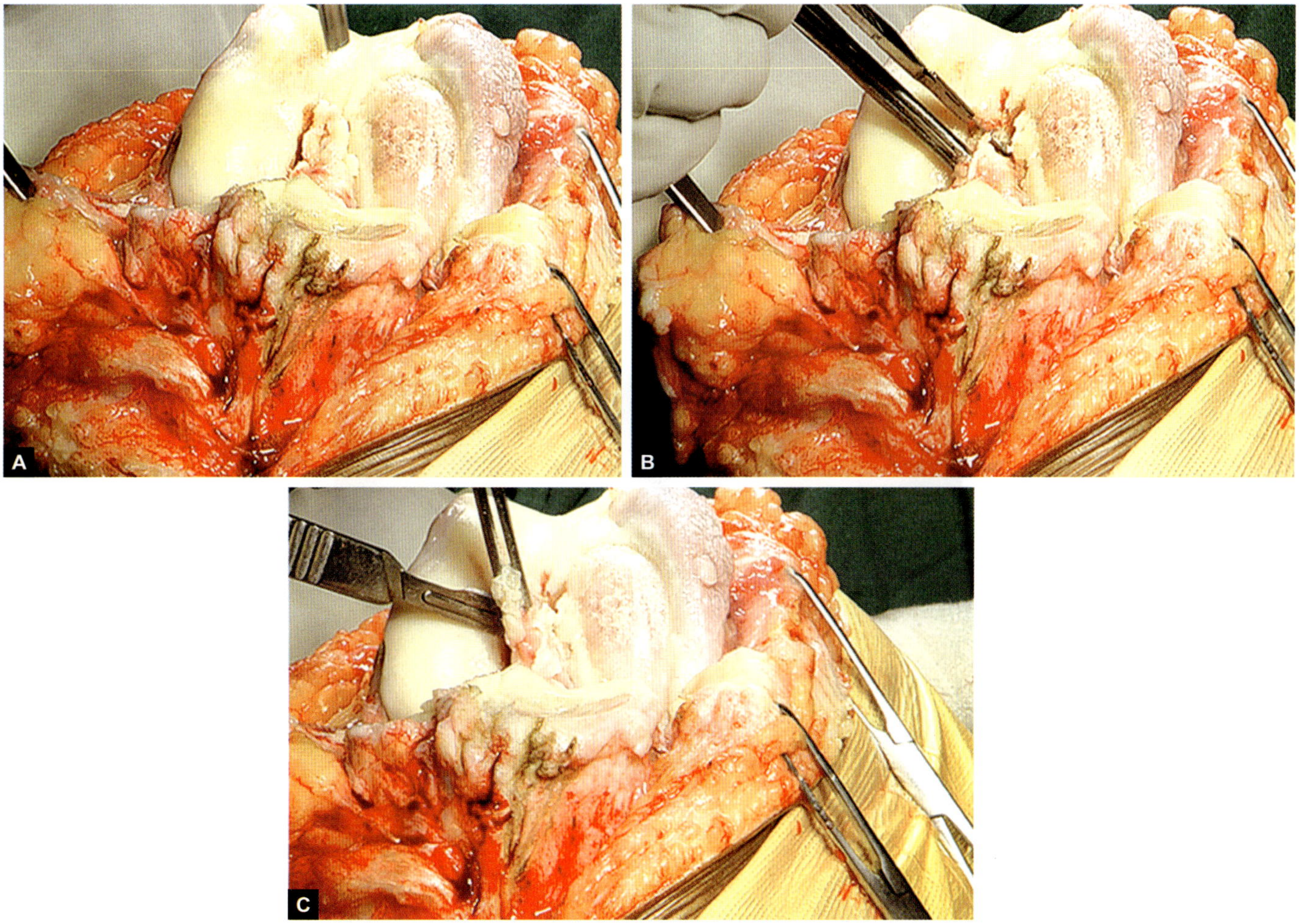

Figs 66.32A to C: Excision of soft tissues from the intercondylar notch

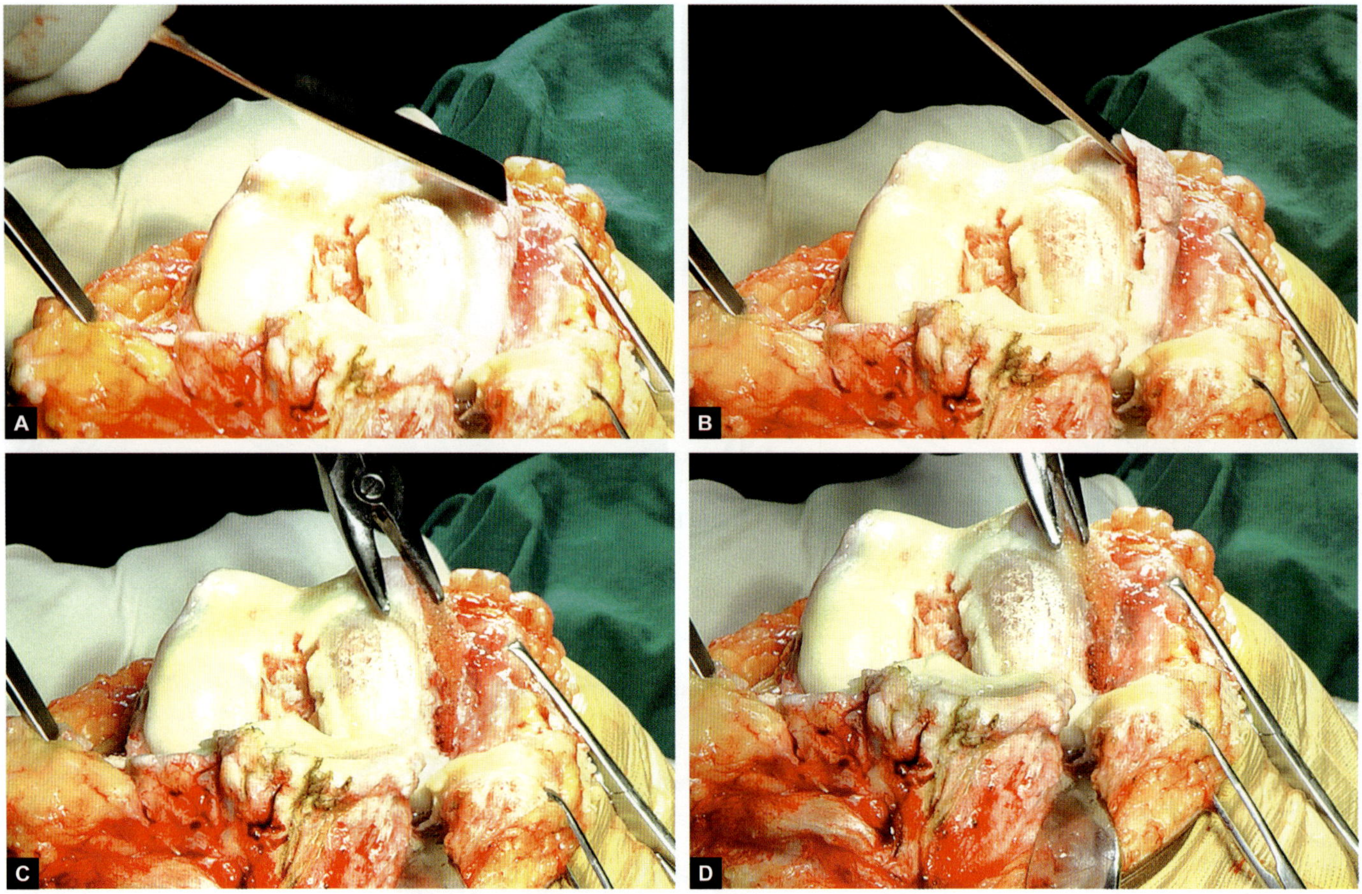

Figs 66.33A to D: Excision of osteophytes using the osteotome

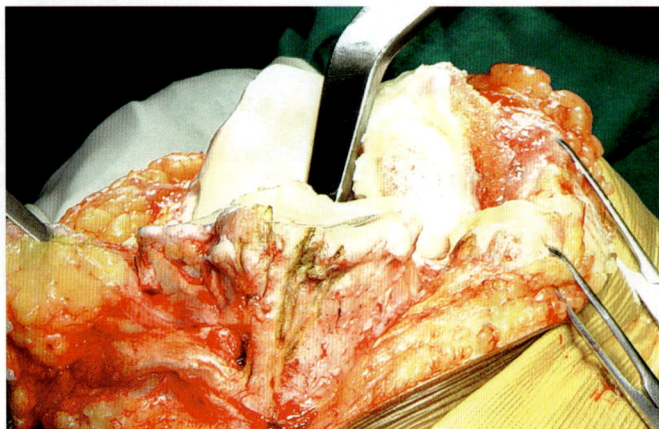

Fig. 66.34: Exposure of the tibial plateau

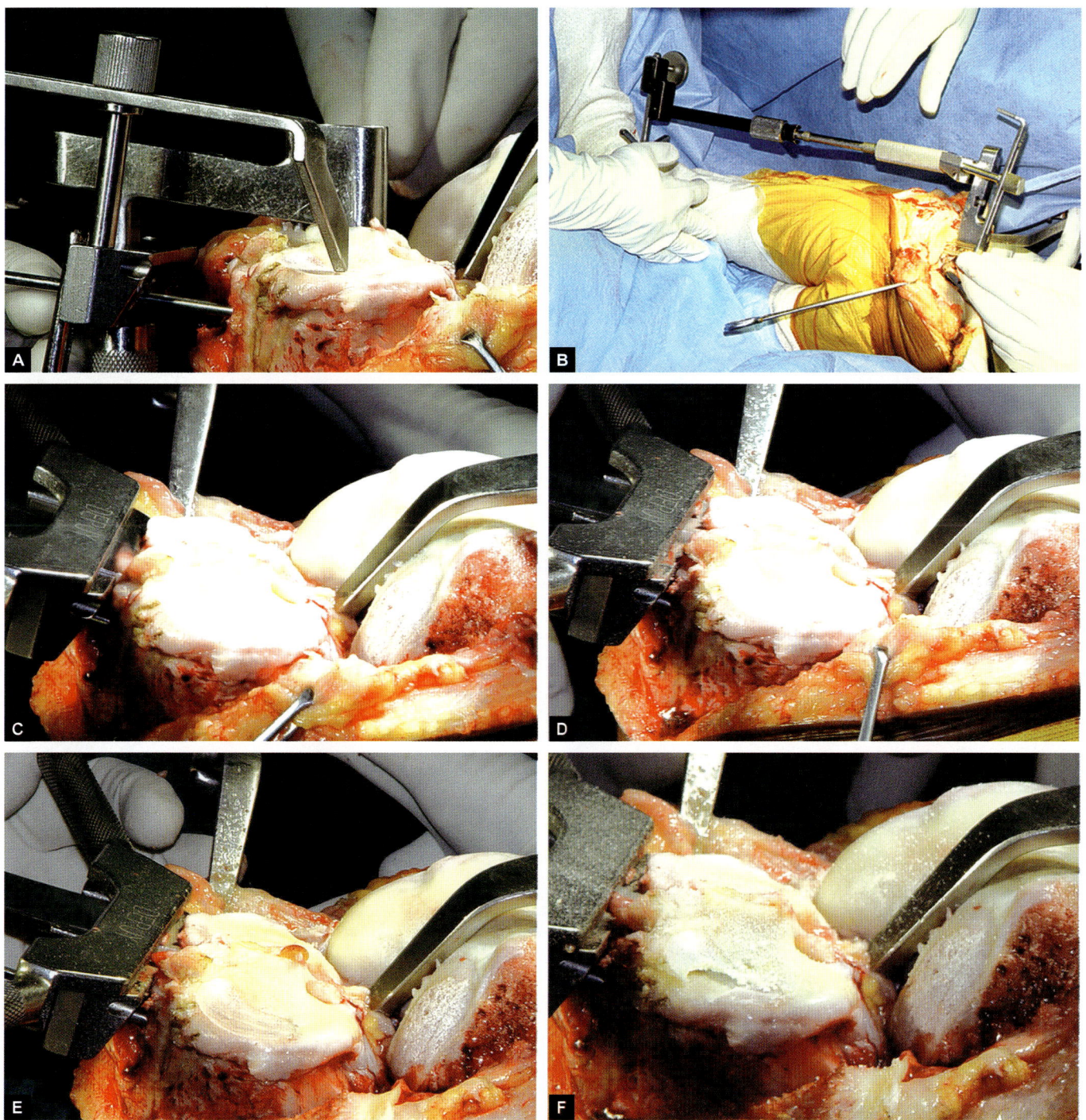

Figs 66.35A to F: Extramedullary tibial alignment guide

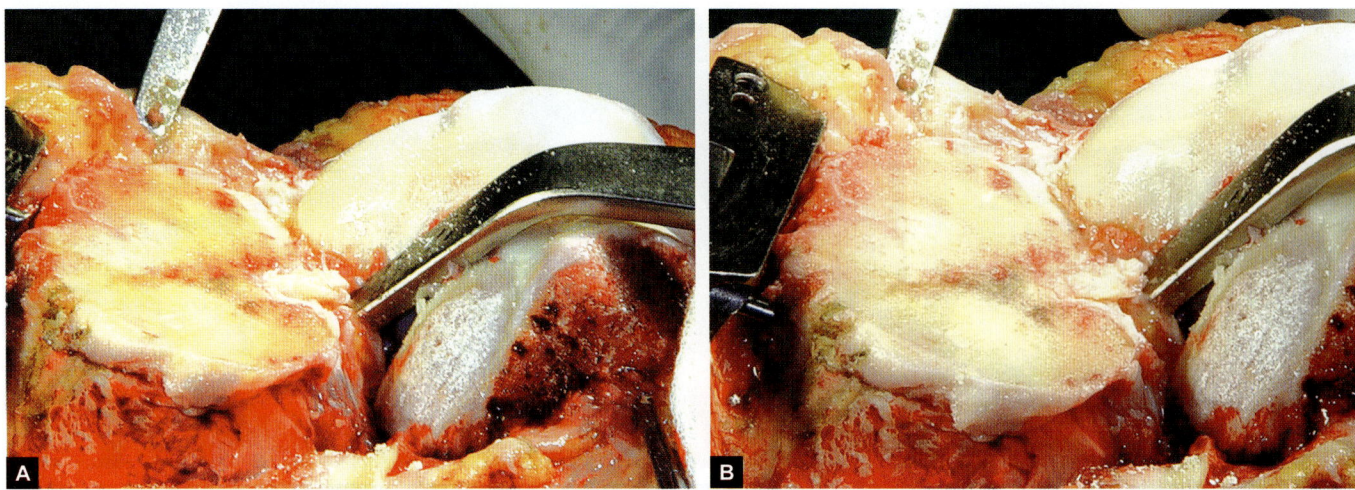

Figs 66.36A and B: Tibia is cut perpendicular to the long axis of the tibia in the frontal plane. Depending on the implant system, the cut should have either a neutral or a slight posterior slope from front to back. Avoid anterior tilt of the proximal tibia cut

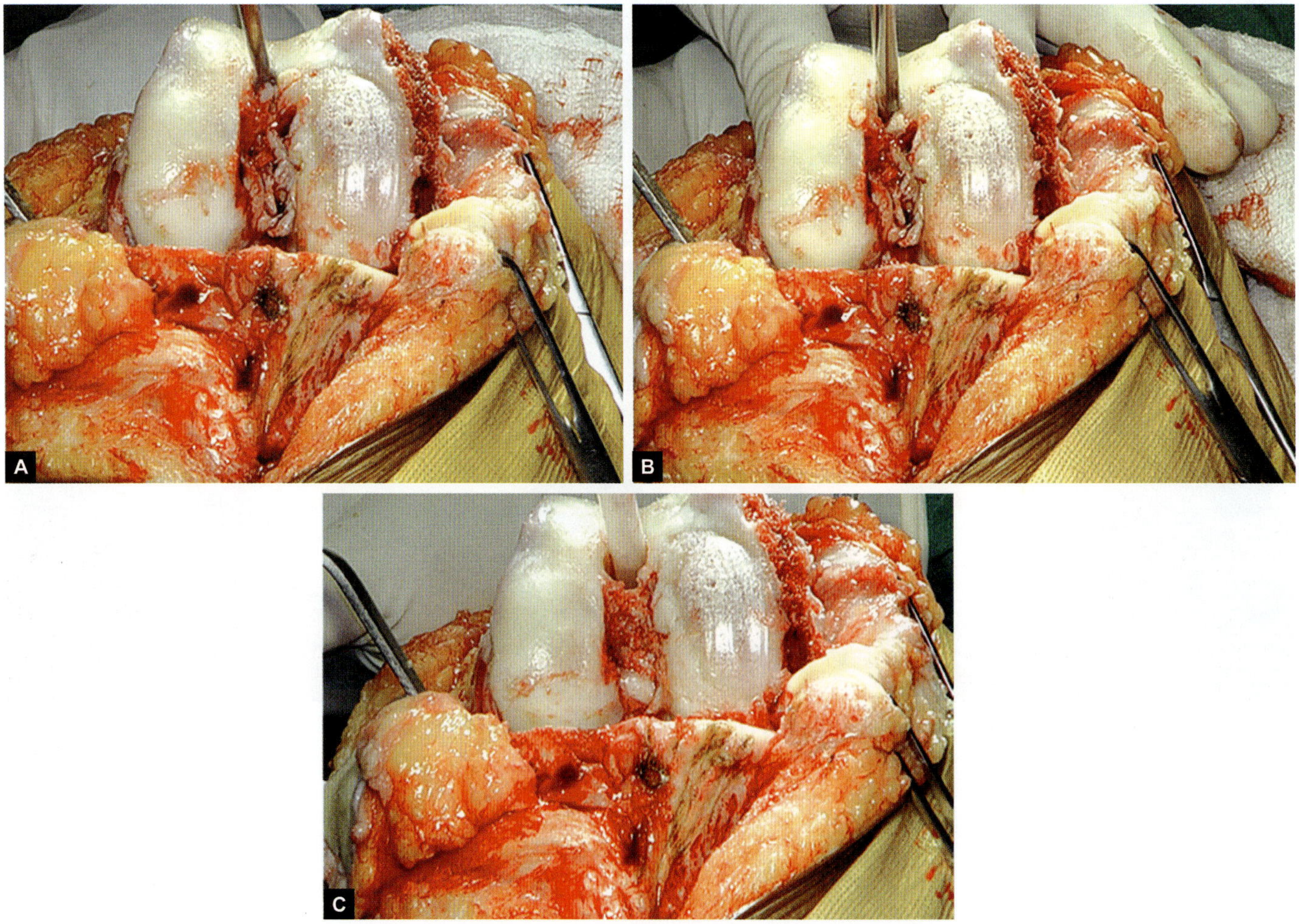

Figs 66.37A to C: Femoral intramedullary starting hole. The hole is place in the intercondylar notch just above the PCL's femoral origin

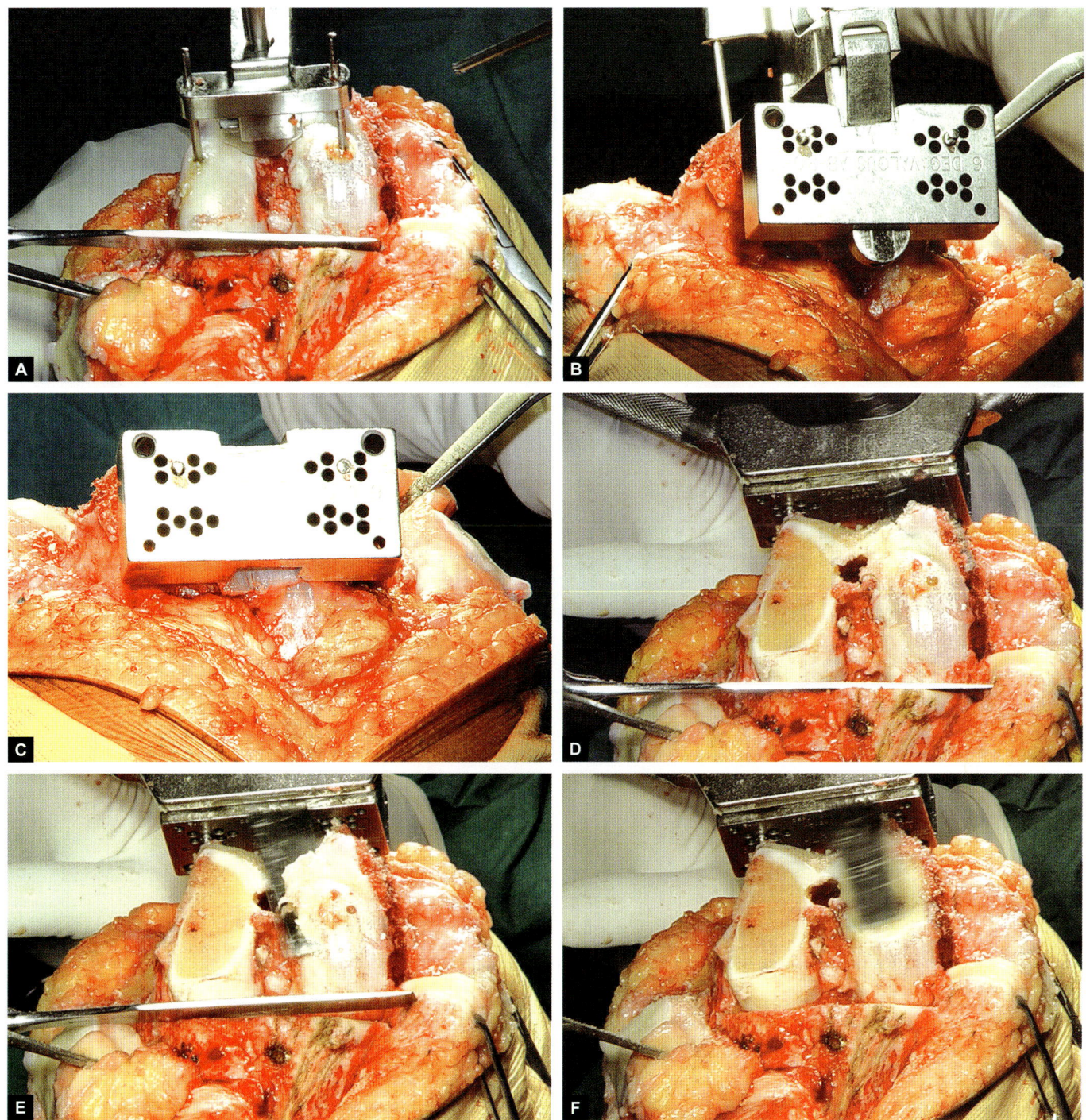

Figs 66.38A to F: Femur cut. The femur is cut in about 5–7 degrees of anatomic valgus

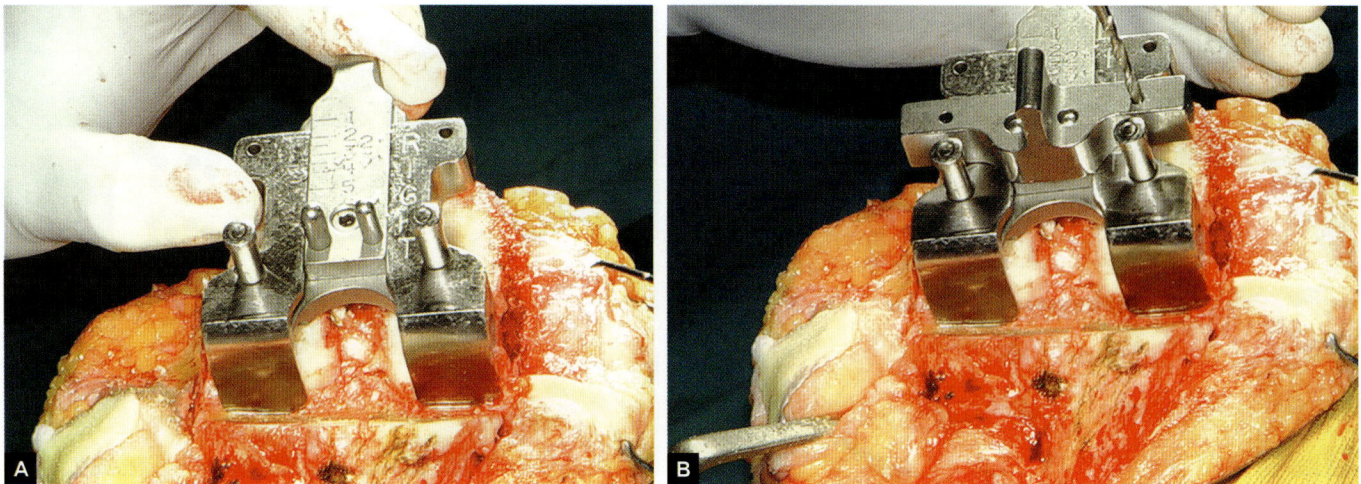

Figs 66.39A and B: Sizing of the femur: Most surgeons tend to downsize the prosthesis if the femur is between sizes

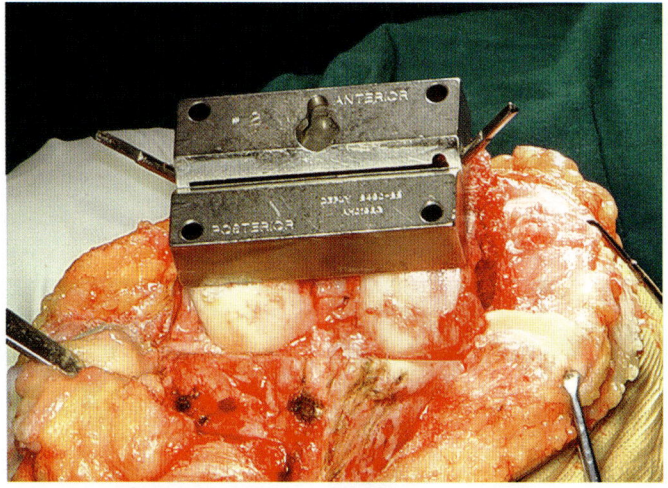

Fig. 66.40: Femoral instrument rotation. Aim to achieve slight external rotation (3°) of the femoral component. Avoid internal rotation

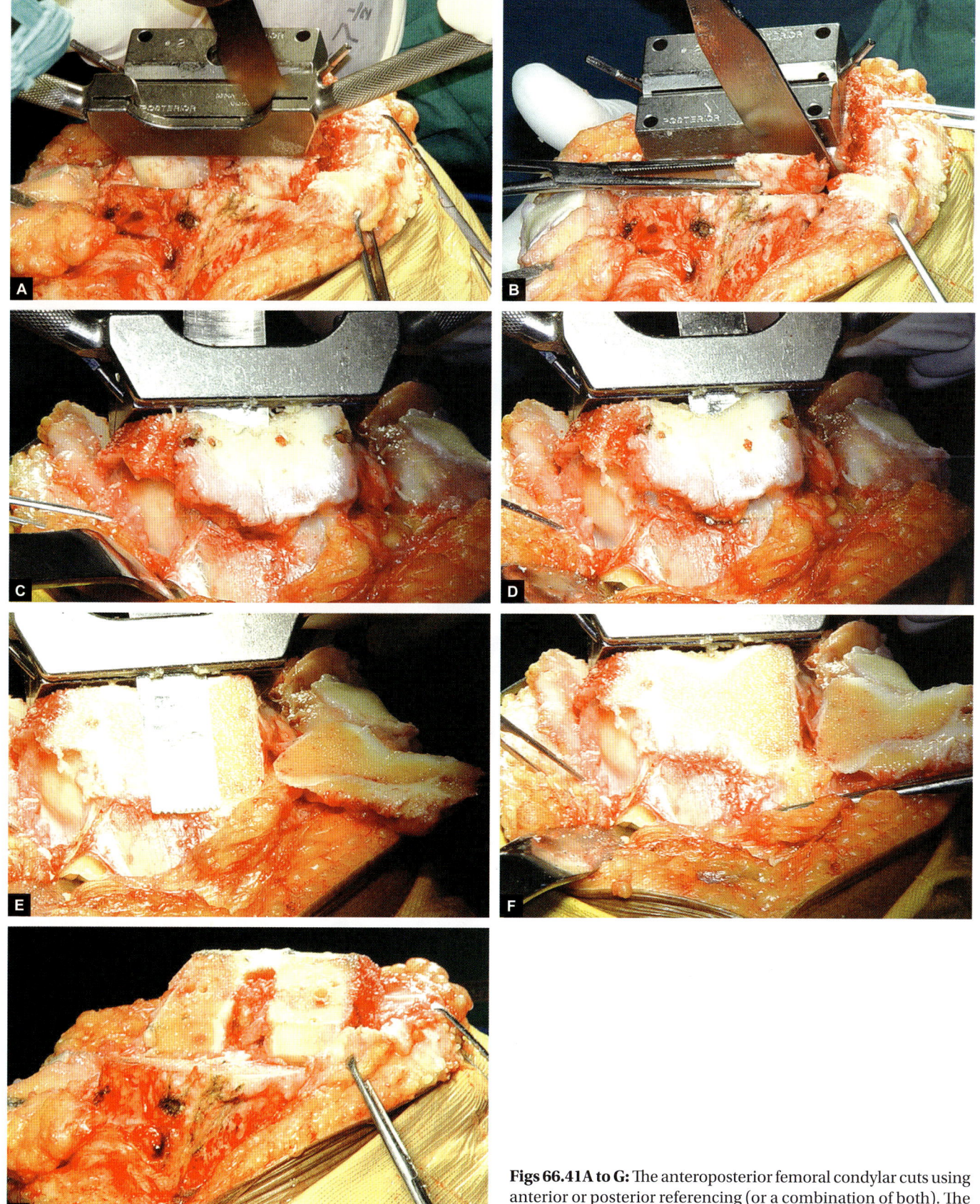

Figs 66.41A to G: The anteroposterior femoral condylar cuts using anterior or posterior referencing (or a combination of both). The anterior and posterior chamber cuts

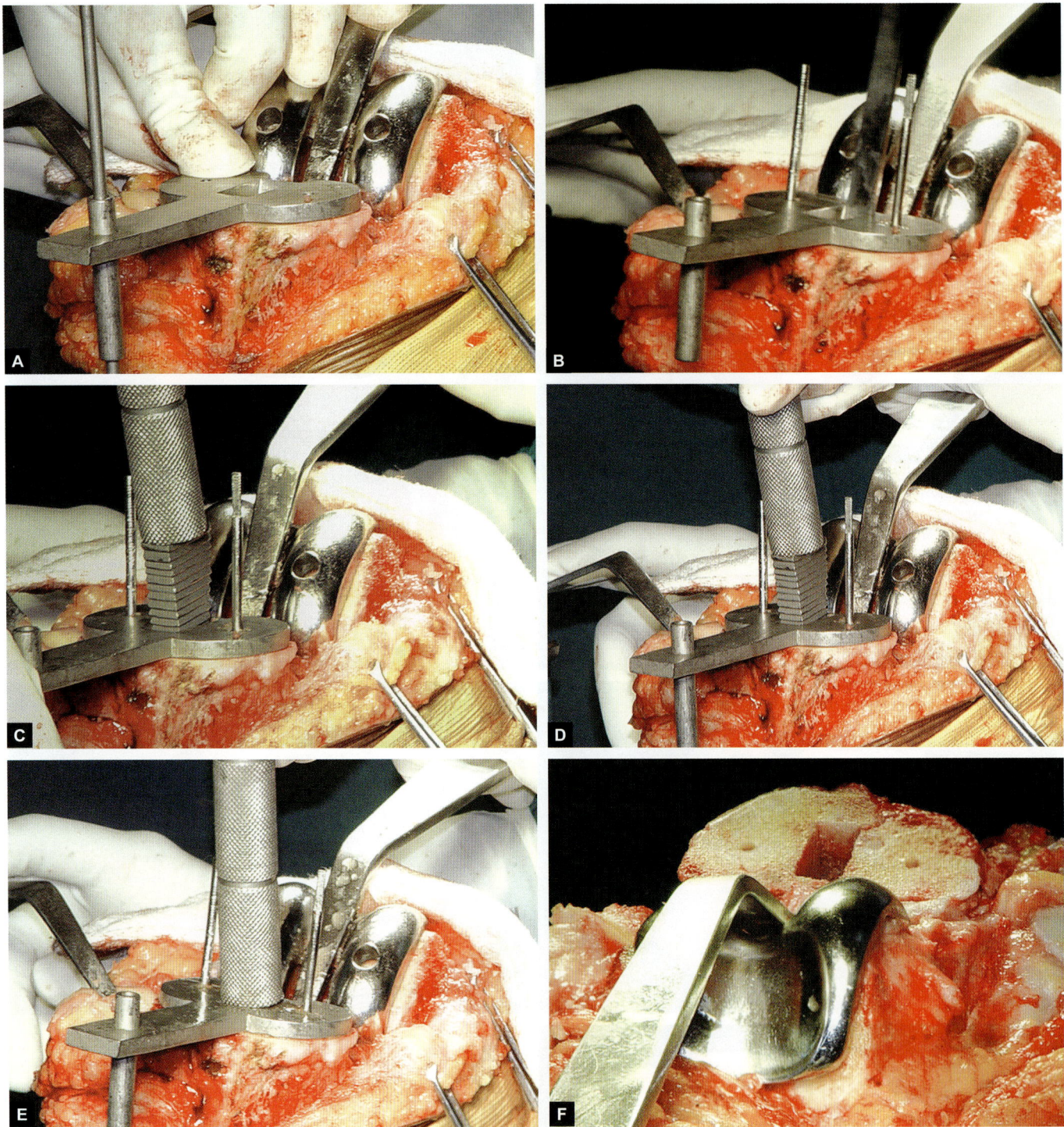

Figs 66.42A to F: Preparation of the proximal tibial base plate utilizing the appropriate instruments. Avoid internal rotation of the tibial component

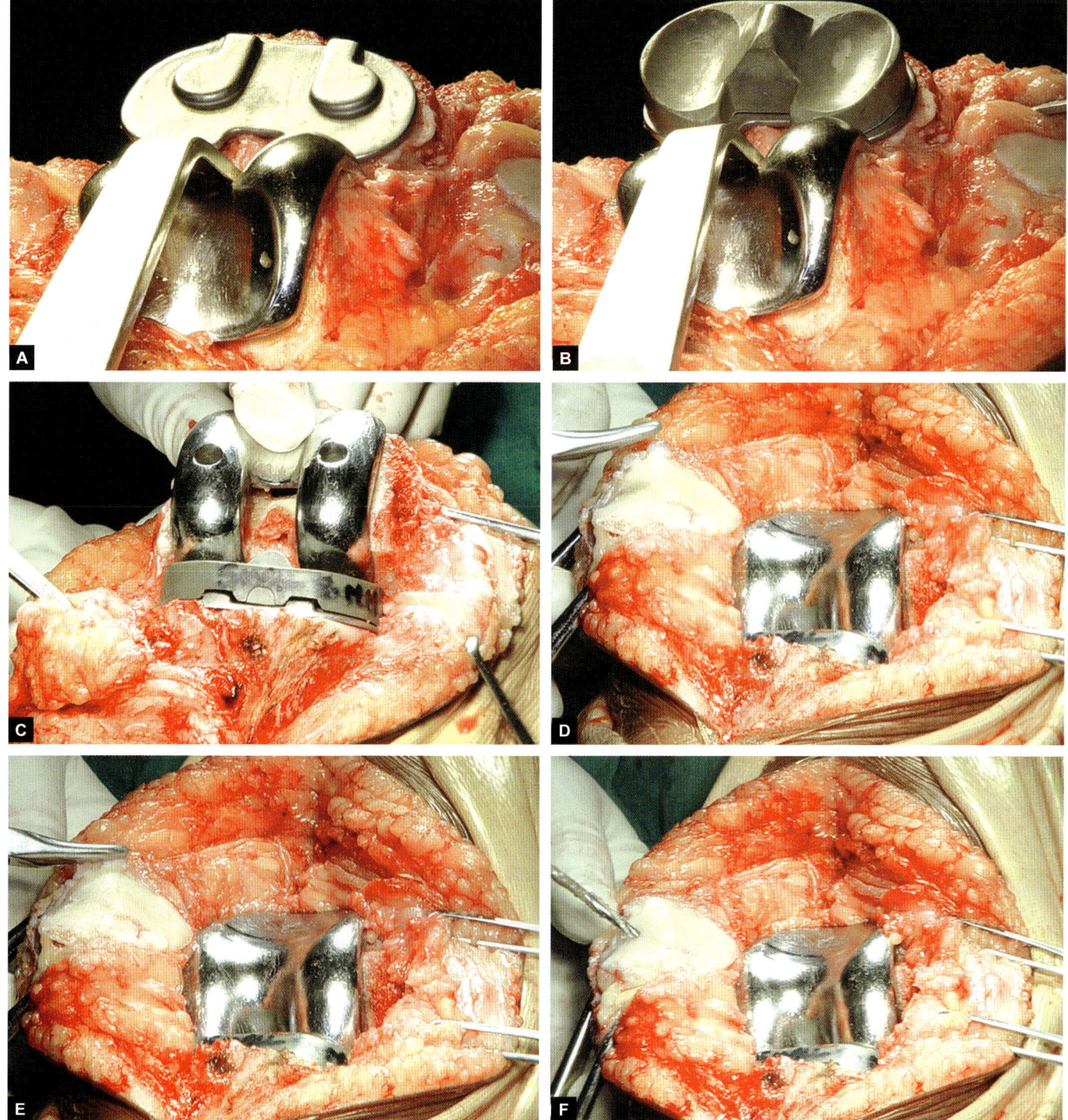

Figs 66.43A to F: Trial reduction

824 SECTION 8: Miscellaneous

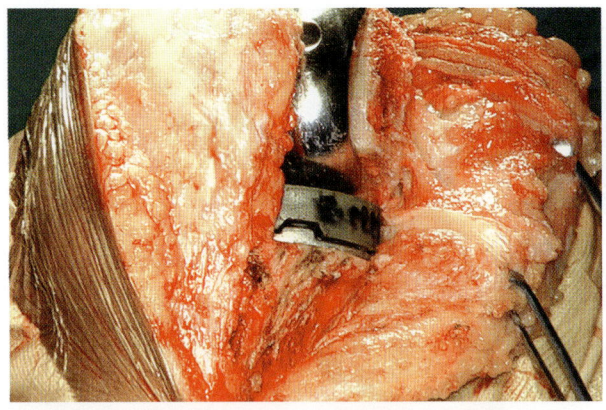

Fig. 66.44: Assessing patellar tracking. The patella should easily track within the femoral components trochlea groove without requiring significant pressure to hold it in place

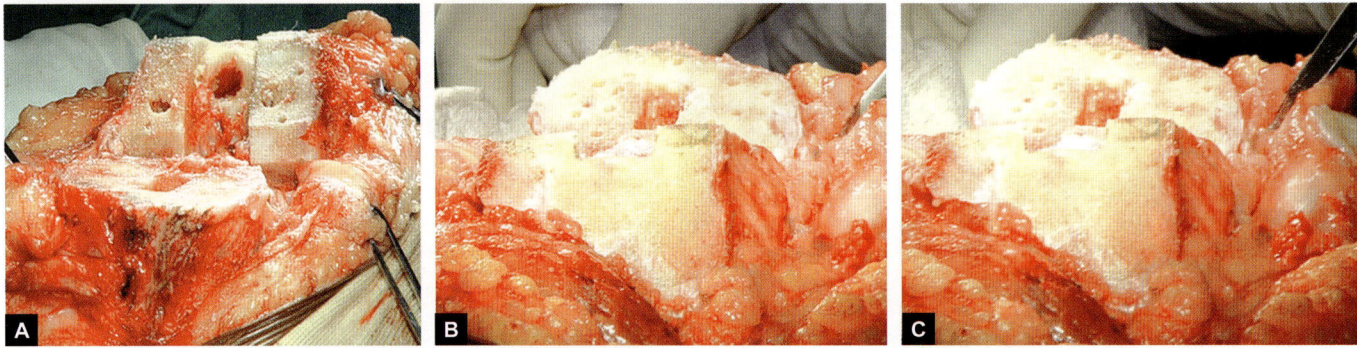

Figs 66.45A to C: Removal of trial component and cleansing of the bony surfaces with a pulsatile lavage

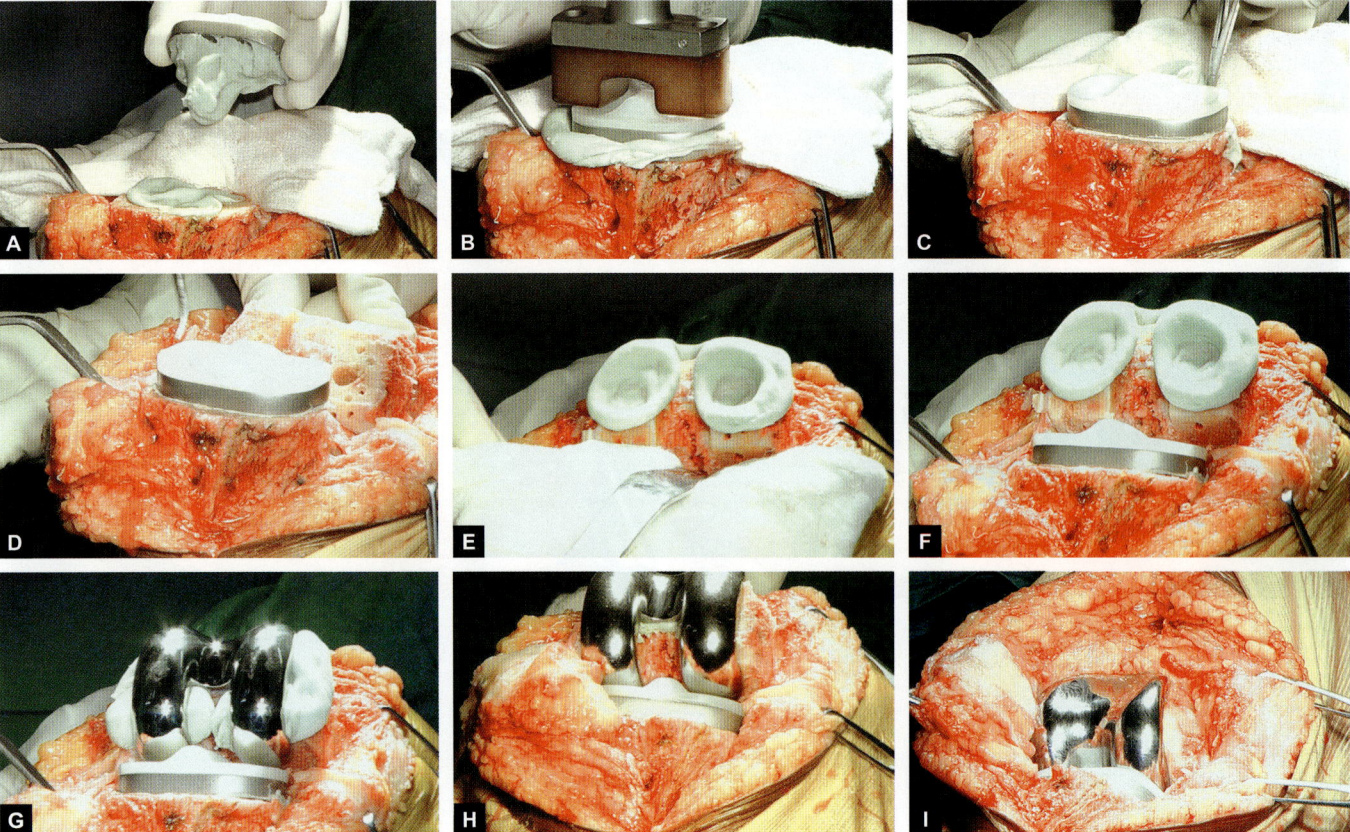

Figs 66.46A to I: Cementing of the tibial and femoral components

CHAPTER 66: Arthroplasty **825**

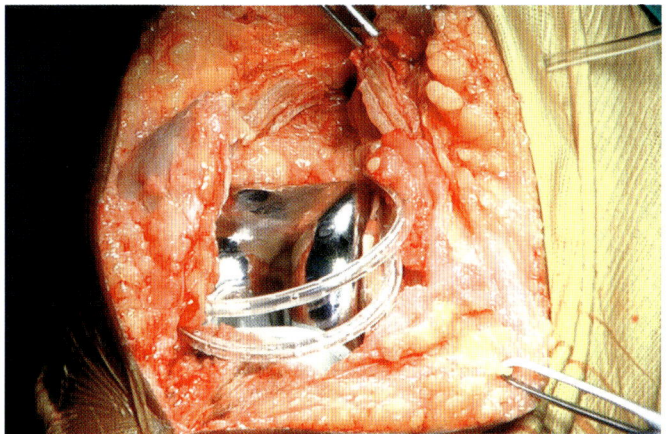

Fig. 66.47: Placing a suction drain through a separate stab incision

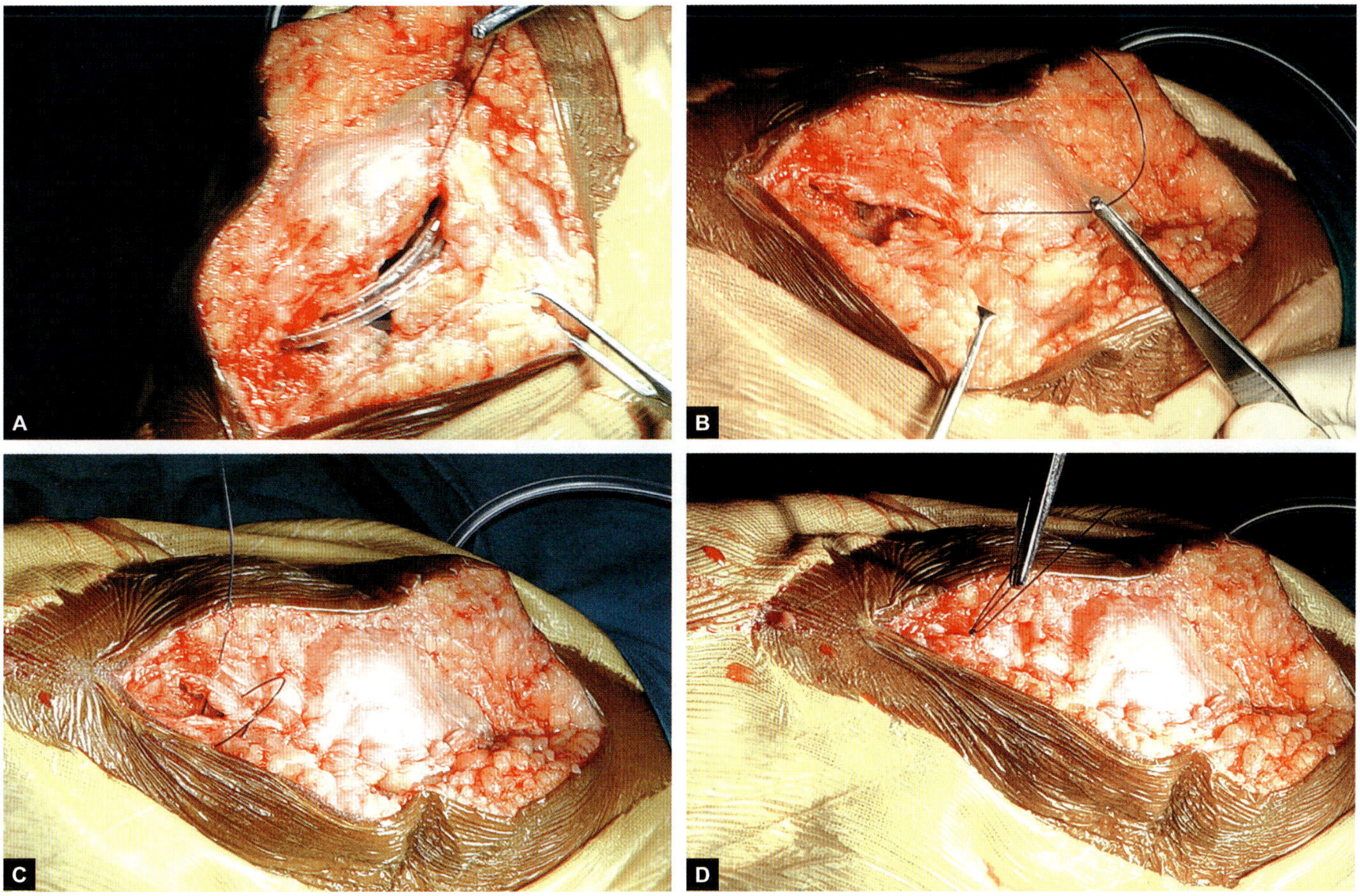

Figs 66.48A to D: Closure of the arthrotomy in meticulous fashion with multiple absorbable sutures

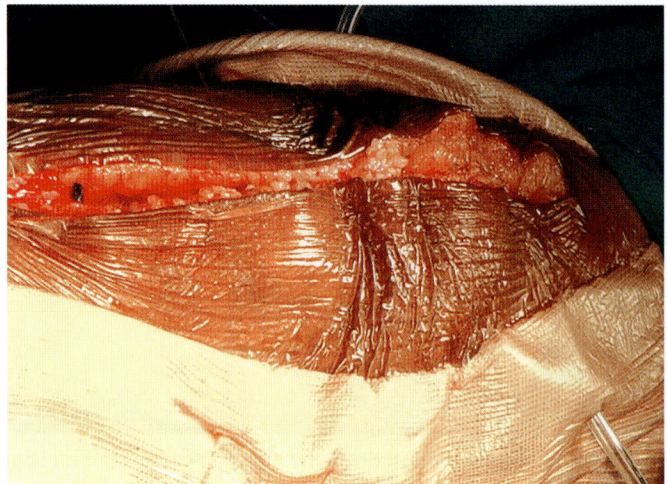

Fig. 66.49: Closure of subcutaneous layer

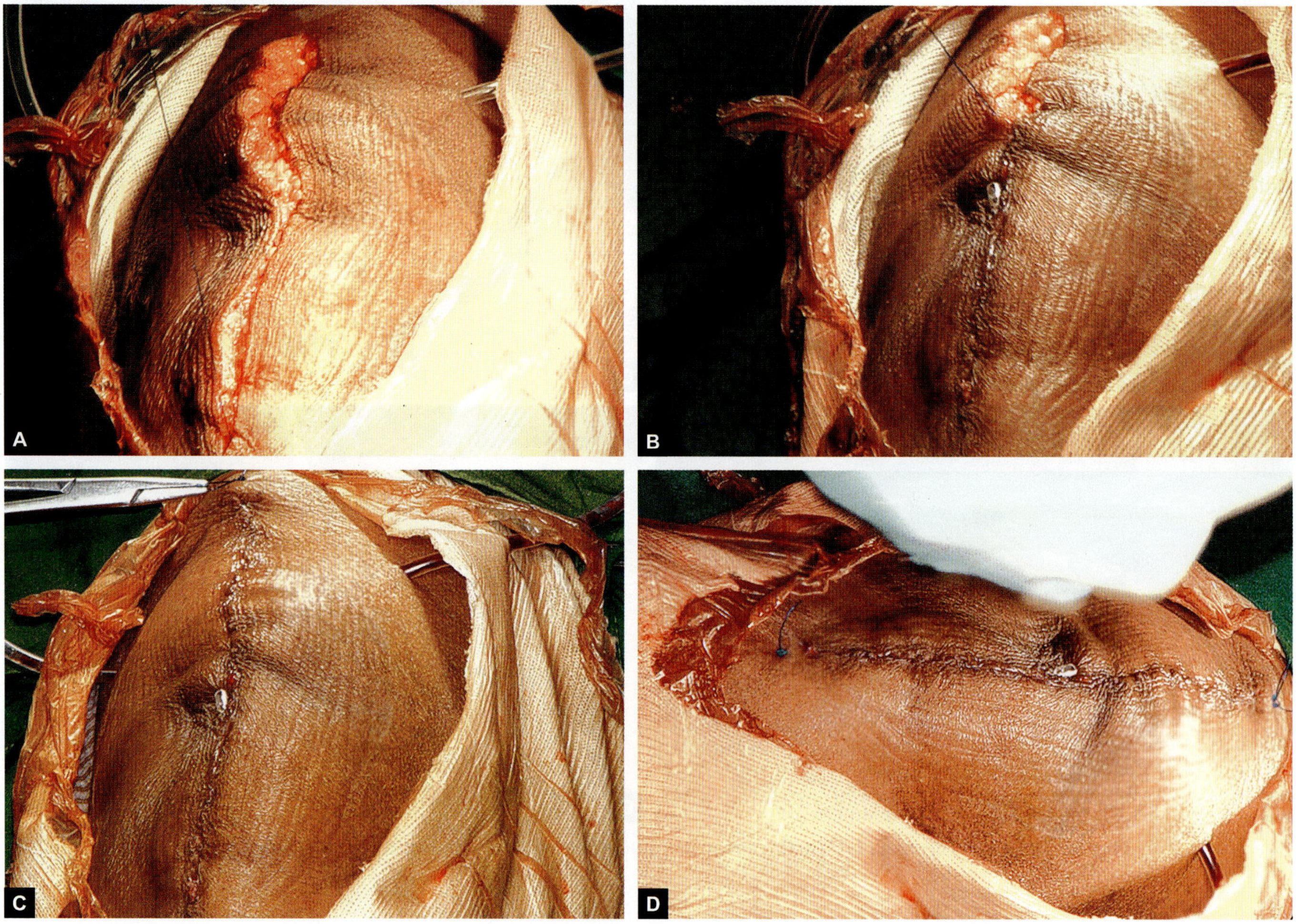

Figs 66.50A to D: Skin closure

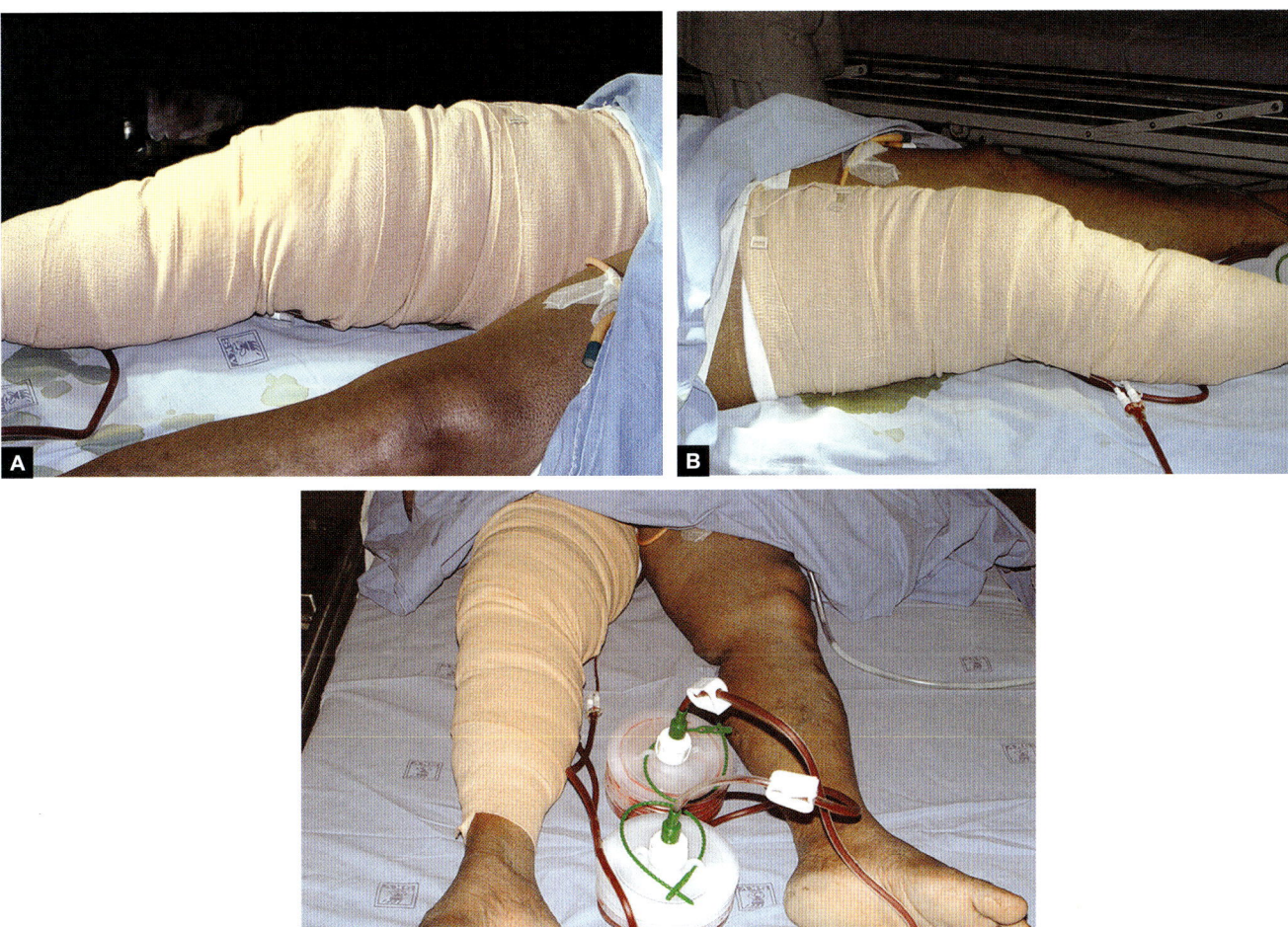

Figs 66.51A to C: Dressing the skin in a sterile fashion with a bulky dressing, wool and crepe

CHAPTER 67

Evidence-based Orthopedics

INTRODUCTION

Evidence and judiciary are two inseparable units. They are inconsequential without each other. Pronouncing a person guilty or not guilty is based on foolproof evidence and not mere evidence. In front of a judge, in an open court, two gentlemen in black coats, one for and against dissect the available evidences against an accused threadbare and each one wants to find out a loophole in the evidence to either support or discard an argument. Listening dispassionately with an analytical mind is the judge who is going to pronounce the judgment based on the veracity of the evidences placed before him. Law is blind but does not buy any argument without proper evidences even though convinced that the accused is guilty.

Real Life Incidences

To quote a popular and recent example in the sensational Aarushi's murder case everyone including the CBI, Court and the public knows that the heinous crime was conducted by her servants. Ironically everyone is a mute spectator as the criminals roam free in the society, reasons lack of evidences. This is travesty of justice that the perpetuators of crime make a mockery of justice. But it is a hard fact. Or on the positive side, take the example of Cine Star Shiney Ahuja's case. That he raped his servant is backed by foolproof DNA evidence that has resulted him remaining confined within the jail. So this is how the judicial systems function and evidence-based judiciary (EBJ) is a well-accepted fact.

If judiciary keeps the society healthy, medicine keeps the people healthy. Principles, practice, drugs used on humans being to keep them healthy also needs to be evidence based as human life is a treasure. Jeopardizing the human life by unproven, unscientific and unfit treatment methods is a crime for one may be deprived of the best treatment options that could make a difference in the morbidity, mortality or recovery. Hitherto the patient was at the mercy of the treating doctor's opinion but now patients are seeking evidences of the diagnostic and treatment methodologies practiced on them. So evidence-based medicine (EBM) is fast gaining ground and is here to stay in the near future. The God like status enjoyed by doctors is a thing of the past for they need to back their actions and deeds with evidences. When all the branches of medicine are brought under the gambit of EBM, orthopedics cannot be far behind and thus evidence-based orthopedics (EBO) has emerged. It is a new paradigm that places less emphasis on expert opinion (authoritarian) but more emphasis to evidences from well conducted and published clinical research (authoritative).

What is EBM?

All these days in our practice two things were involved, patient and the treating doctor. Insinuating between the two now is the clinical research evidence. Thus EBM is a healthy integration of all the three namely patient with his illness, doctor with his clinical expertise and credible evidences based on sound clinical research.[1] Now the expert opinion is backed by expert research evidences for expert medical care. This is EBM for you.

History

Unlike many medical events and practice that has rich history, EBM is a new discovery credited to the recent times. The term was coined by Gordon Guyatt in 1991 and was described by the evidence-based medicine group by

McMaster University. However EBM has still a colorful history starting from an era before Christ.
- 2600 years ago Prophet Daniel conducted a trial on King Nebuchadnezzar's order to the Israelite children to eat a diet of the King's meats and wines.[2]
- Sir James Lind's work on the prevention of Scurvy in 1747.[3]
- May have origins in China BC.
- May have been coined by Dr David Eddy of Kauser Permanente.
- Xavier Bichet, Pierre Louis, Francoid Magendie of post-revolutionary France are credited for the philosophical base.
- Discovery of cowpox vaccine for immunization against smallpox by William Jenner.[4]
- First Cohort trial by Cotton Mather in 1720 about the use of cowpox vaccine against smallpox.[5]
- First RCT was reported in 1931 by J Burns Amberson regarding the treatment of TB.[6]
- In the 1950's, another RCT was carried out on the effect of Streptomycin in TB trials.[7]
- In 1954, a clinical trial on Salk Polio Vaccine was conducted. This is the largest single clinical trial of the 20th century.[7]
- Practiced at McMaster University in the late 1970's.[8]
- In 1980, David Sackett coined the term Critical Appraisal.[9]
- Advances in meta-analysis and systematic reviews started taking place in mid 1980's.[10]
- Prof Gordon Guyatt coined the term EBM in 1991.[1]
- In 1992, first Cochrane center was established by Ian Chambers at Oxford University.[11]
- Second Cochrane center was established in McMaster University in 1994.
- Cochrane collaboration and library was born in 1996.
- JBJS in 2000 introduced a new section evidence-based orthopedics.[12]
- Earliest article to be published about EBO in JBJS was a series of four user's guides to the orthopedic literature by Bhandari, Guyatt et al.[13]
- To classify the quality of study, JBJS introduced 5 levels of evidence rating for all articles submitted for publication.[14]
- In 2002, a study recommending discontinuation of hormone replacement therapy (HRT) in the prevention and treatment of osteoporosis.[15]
- Osteoarthritis Research International (OARSI) group for the first time published an article in 2008, combining expert opinion, with clinical trials and systematic overviews as the highest level of evidence.[16]

Why is EBM Necessary?

Change is the way of life. Right from our evolution nothing has remained static. Due to continuing evolutional changes over centuries we are what we are today. Then how can the treatment and diagnosis of our patients remain the same. It also has to follow the path of change. Earlier medical treatment and decisions were taken on the following grounds:
- Guess work
- Unsystematic observation
- Common sense
- Expert opinion
- Standard and accepted practice.

During this era doctors enjoyed the status of Gods. Everyone followed the advices of doctors as divine and did not question their judgment. If something went wrong they blamed their luck but not the doctor. Such was the implicit faith on doctors in those days. But slowly as people started getting more educated and aware they realized that this method was fraught with lots of dangers and pitfalls.

Pitfalls of this method:
- Improper
- Inadequate
- Faulty treatment
- Legal complications.

Evidence-based medicine is necessary to overcome all the above pitfalls of the earlier medical treatment methods and give quality treatment to the patients.[17] This can be done by systematic reviews of medical literature that include:
- ***Randomized controlled trials***: Here patients are allocated randomly to either a treatment or control group and followed over a period of time for an outcome of interest. They help avoid selection or confounding biases and provide an objective basis for quantifying study outcomes.
- ***Observational studies***: These include large prospective studies followed up over a period of time. Based on the exposure to certain variables, they draw the inferences from groups of patients. Implementation of therapies are not involved in these studies but rather follow groups of patients that have been exposed or analyze patients retrospectively for an exposure that have experienced the outcome of interest. These studies can have bias because the preferences of the patients or the physicians can determine whether patients receive a treatment or control therapy. While the insight and expertise of experienced clinicians cannot be questioned regarding the diagnosis or treatment but they are affected by

a small sample size and human errors of making inferences.[18]

All this will be discussed in greater detail is sections to follow.

When to Practice EBM?

The need to practice EBM is now. In complex clinical situations when decision taking is difficult it is best to practice EBM. If you are reluctant to practice EBM your patients will not shy away from quoting you the EBM and embarrass you. Patients are well informed of late due to the internet boom and easy availability of knowledge over the net, TV, media and other sources. They will not hesitate to question or demand EBM and put you in the dock if you fail to exercise your options well. Let me illustrate with an incident that happened not so recently to my friend who is a very senior and well-known Obstetrician in a corporate hospital in Bengaluru.

Real Life Incidents

It was a case of multipara who was short and had a big baby. She had undergone LSCS for the first child few years back. The obstetrician in question decided to give her vaginal assisted normal delivery though the patient demanded that she be given an option of repeat LSCS to prevent the hazards of scar rupture which according to her is quite high as the literature suggested. But our friend convinced her that incidence of scar rupture is rare and EBM says that this is a better option. Nothing wrong so far only that our friend was unaware that she was dealing with a very well-informed patient who had browsed everything about the pros and cons of various treatment options for previous LSCS births. She was an analytical writer for a software company and had done an extensive analysis about her pregnancy and the outcome perhaps more than her doctor itself.

When the patient set into labor proper monitoring was not done by her junior colleagues. The course of the normal labor was unusually long and there was very slow progress. She kept insisting that she be taken to the OT and LSCS be performed but our doctor friend refused. Patient complained of severe pain abdomen, radiating to both the shoulders and she was very uneasy. The doctor in question should have been alert for a possibility of a scar rupture and palpated the abdomen. But she chose to overlook thinking that as per the evidence available scar rupture is rare and failed to do a simple clinical examination. There was no proper monitoring of the patient and also the child keeping the complications in mind. Everything was taken casually as they thought that scar rupture will not happen as per their EBM analysis. When the general condition of the patient started sinking our senior friend rushed to the labor room and then examined and scanned the patient. To her horror it was detected that the patient had indeed a scar rupture and was serious! Immediate laparotomy was done and an almost still born baby delivered. They could save the mother but were unable to save the baby despite putting it on the ventilator for 2 weeks. The patient was inconsolable.

She accused the doctor of gross negligence. Panicking the doctor said that such incidence are quite common during VAB for repeat LSCS. This was a volte-face where in earlier consultations she had convinced the patient to participate in this trial as the scar rupture was rare! The patient had told her unwillingness to participate in the so called trial of normal labor. She quoted various EBM studies and proved her point to the doctor that she erred in taking the proper decision that cost her the baby and put her through lots of emotional, mental and physical trauma. She widely circulated this error in judgment of her doctor over the internet and there was widespread condemnation of the doctor worldwide. She has threatened to sue the doctor and in all likelihood will win the case too. This is what will happen if we fail to practice a proper EBM. The patient was better informed than the doctor and she had done an extensive research analysis and taken as many as 5 alternate opinions! The doctor was complacent. Patients will fix us for all our decision in days to come. It is high time each and every doctor in all specialties embrace EBM before it is too late.

How to Practice EBM?

The standard medical teaching is when encountered with a patient take proper history, do a clinical examination, order relevant investigations and based on your previous experience institute the treatment what you think is warranted. We were heavily inclined to rely on our past experiences and expert opinions of our teachers and professors under whom we had received our previous medical training. This was OK few decades ago. Now the expectations of the patients are rising and there is very little room for error as patients demand and expect the latest available treatment methods. So the earlier method no longer works. Now the approach should be to assess the patient, formulate your clinical questions by asking the patient, then do a extensive literature survey while the patient is being investigated or planning to be treated, critically examine the studies, now integrate the evidence gathered to the patient in question and later evaluate the outcome and the prognosis.[19] The knowledge gained by all this experience will help you to take decision in future when encountered with a similar case.[20] All these steps are summarized in the Box 67.1.

> **Box 67.1: Quick Facts: Remember the 7 A's**
> - **A**ssess the patient – By clinical examination
> - **A**sk the patient – Formulate a clinical question
> - **A**ccess the information – Literature survey
> - **A**ppraise the evidence – Critically appraise the various indices
> - **A**pply the findings – Integrate the validated evidence with clinical expertise and patient preference before applying
> - **A**ssess the outcome – Evaluate the performance
> - **A**dd the knowledge – For future reference

Who should Practice EBM?

In recent times all practicing clinicians and investigators need to practice EBM. It is beneficial for both the clinicians and the patients to adopt to EBM methods. It gives the best option to the patient and for the clinicians. It gives the satisfaction of executing the best available options supported by strong and good evidence and also provides him immunity from litigation and other problems that may arise due to poor judgments and complications.

Quality of Research: Is it Good or Bad?

Evidence is all right, research analysis is alright but you need to keep in mind that not all evidences and not all research analysis are good and are of standard quality. It is ok if you do not practice EBM but it is not ok if you practice improper EBM based on poor literature and evidences.

> **Note:**
> Only a small proportion of the available research is relevant and is good, interesting and important.

For example: 60,000 articles are published every year in 120 journals. Only 3,500 articles every year meet critical appraisal. 25 articles per year available for clinicians. Only 5–10 articles for authors of evidence-based clinical topic reviews.

What is the Hierarchy of Evidence?

To rate the quality of research evidences available the concept of rating the quality of evidences has been introduced.[1] This alerts the clinician and the patient about the quality of literature they are referring to. Evidences based on good quality randomized controlled trials occupy the top position in the hierarchy while the expert opinion is at the bottom. The following are the hierarchy of evidences currently followed (Box 67.2):
1. Systematic reviews.
2. Critically appraised topics (Evidence syntheses).
3. Critically appraised individual articles (Article synopsis).
4. Randomized controlled trials.
5. Cohort studies.
6. Case Control Studies (Case series/Case reports).
7. Background information/Expert opinion.

> **Box 67.2: Quick Facts: What is the Level of Evidence of the Research?**
> Level 1: Systematic review of RCT
> Level 2: Single RCT
> Level 3: Systematic review of observational studies addressing the patient important outcomes
> Level 4: Single observational studies addressing patient important outcomes
> Level 5: Unsystematic clinical observations

> **Note:**
> RCT's have the highest value as it eliminates bias so common with observational studies.

What is the Type of Study?

You have now understood what a good study is and a bad study, what is the level of literature evidences. Now you need to know what the various types of literature studies available are. There are three types described:
1. *Therapeutic study:* Aims to determine efficacy or adversity of a treatment method. This is the commonest study encountered in orthopedic practice.
2. *Diagnostic study:* This helps to detect the presence or absence of specific condition by an intervention.
3. *Prognostic study*: This predicts the outcome of the patient's condition.

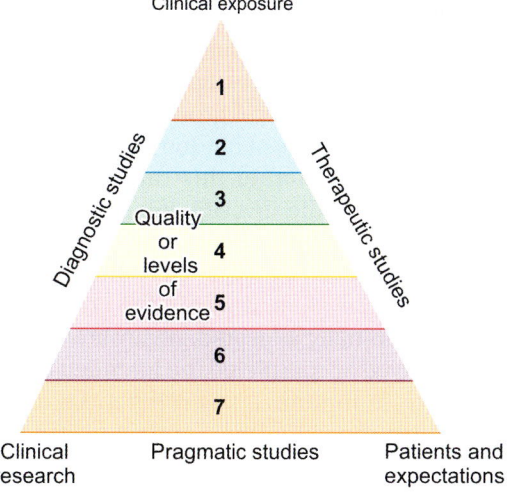

Fig. 67.1: The EBM triad puts its entire spectrum in a nutshell

Levels of evidence
1. Systematic reviews
2. Critically appraised topics (Evidence syntheses)
3. Critically appraised individual articles (Article synopsis)
4. Randomized controlled trials (RCT's)
5. Cohort studies
6. Case controlled studies/Case series/Reports
7. Background information/Expert opinions

EBM Triad

This triad puts the entire EBM in a nutshell (Fig. 67.1).

User's Guide

How to Critically Appraise a Level 1 (RCT) Research Article and What is the Role of the User's Guide?

You have come across a literature pertaining to the diagnosis or treatment of your patient. You have also ascertained that the said literature is good and is rated high. Is that enough? No, not all literature is good and trustworthy. You now need to critically assess the research and not just assess it. It is advised to observe the following guidelines in critically judging an article based on RCT study. To give an effective care to our patients, EBM helps to amalgamate experience and education with relevant literature. According to the *User's guide*[21] to the medical literature a therapeutic study should answer three important questions:

1. Are the results valid or is the study believable?
2. What are the results? Is the result big and precise?
3. How can the results apply to patient care? Is it applicable to my patient?

   Now let us evaluate each one in greater details.
1. **Are the results valid?** This can be done by analyzing whether the study results support a cause effect relationship between the treatment and the observed outcome. This is called the internal validity and the results are said to be valid if the following conditions or criteria's are fulfilled:
   - *Randomization:* Here some method of chance (e.g. flip of a coin) is used to assign patients to treatment groups, study or control groups to eliminate bias. Box 67.3 shows types of randomization.
   - *Concealment:* Whether this randomization was concealed from the investigator, patient, observer and analyst (Box 67.4).
   - *Intention to treat analysis*: Here the patients are followed and evaluated within the group to which they were initially allocated, regardless of whether they received or completed the intended treatment.
   - *Blinding:* To minimize any differences in patient care other than the intervention under investigation it is necessary to keep the patient, clnicians, outcome assessors and statisticians unaware of the group to which the patient was allocated. In double blind study, both the patient, the clinician or the researcher are blind to the treatment allocation (Box 67.5). Unlike in drug trials where in the physicians can be blinded, it is difficult to blind a surgeon during surgical trials.

   Note:
   Blinding a patient helps eliminate psychological or placebo effect.

   - *Follow up:* Adequate follow up is a must, to consider the study as valid. Remember the 5 and 20 rule. If less than 5 percent of the patients are lost to follow up then the effect on the outcome is considered minimal and if 20 percent or more of the patients are lost to follow up, the validity of the study is poor (Box 67.6).

   Box 67.3: Quick Facts: Methods of Randomization
   - Use of computerized random number generator or random number table (Most common and reliable)
   - Use date of birth
   - Use alternate days
   - Use patient's hospital chart number
   - Use toss of a coin
   - Use patient's preference
   - Use surgeon's preference

   Box 67.4: Concealment Facts: Types of Concealment of the Randomization
   - Remote call center telephone randomization
   - Opaque envelopes of equal weight

   Box 67.5: Blinding Facts: Concerning Surgical Trials
   - It is *always* possible to blind a data analyst
   - *Almost always* blind the outcome assessors
   - It is possible to *occasionally* blind the patient
   - Surgeon can *never* be blinded

   Box 67.6: Quick Recap: Is the Study Believable? The Criteria's of Internal Validity
   - Were the patients randomized?
   - Was the randomization concealed?
   - Was the intention to treat (IT) analysis?
   - Were the prognostic factors balanced?
   - Was blinding followed?
   - Was the follow-up complete?

   User guides mentions all these criteria's in greater detail. If all these question are answered satisfactorily then the study is said to be valid (Table 67.1).
2. **What are the results?** To know what are the results two values need to be looked into, namely its magnitude and precision.

   Magnitude: It is important to find out the magnitude of the treatment effect to know what impact the intervention has had on the subjects under study. It is easy to interpret the outcome if the patient's response is either a definite yes or no eliminating the gray are in between. To know the magnitude of the treatment effect two measures need to be followed:
   a. *Summary measures:* This measures central tendency along with the dispersions (Standard deviation, standard error, variance, range).
   b. *Outcome measures:* This includes incidence, prevalence and various risk parameters like:
      - Absolute risk (AR).

TABLE 67.1: User's guide to randomized trials in orthopedics

Validity
- Did experimental and control groups begin the study with a similar prognosis?
- Were patients randomized?
- Was randomization concealed?
- Were all patients in the treatment and control groups similar with respect to known prognostic factors?
- Did experimental and control groups retain a similar prognosis after the study started?

Blinding:
- Did investigators avoid effects of patient awareness of allocation
- Were patients blinded?
- Were aspects of care that affect prognosis similar in the two groups: were clinicians blinded?
- Was outcome assessed in a uniform way in experimental and control groups:
  - Were those assessing outcome blinded?
  - Was follow up complete?

Results
- How large was the treatment effect?
- How precise was the estimate of the treatment effect?

Applicability
- Can the results be applied to my patient?
- Were all clinically important outcomes considered?
- Are the likely treatment benefits worth the potential harm and costs?

- Absolute risk reduction (ARR).
- Number needed to treat (NNT).
- Relative risk (RR).
- Relative risk reduction (RRR).
- Hazard ratio (HR).

Precision: After ascertaining the *magnitude* of the treatment effect, it is imperative to find out the *precision* of the study. The estimate of the magnitude of a treatment effect is called a point estimate. But it is extremely unlikely that this estimate will be precise but may lie between ranges of values called the confidence interval.[22] Two methods are employed to achieve this namely the p-value and the confidence interval.

a. *P-value:* It is the *probability* that the treatment effect has happened by chance alone in a long trial is depicted by the p-value. It tells us whether the results obtained by the study are due to chance or by choice of the intervention. In other words is the study statistically significant. This is answered by observing the p-values which is normally set at 5 percent ($p<0.05$). If the p value is less than this level then the study results are actual and not due to chance. If it is above this value then the results are not statistically significant and could be due to chance.

Limitations:
- The p-value does not tell how important this actual difference is. Even a small difference that is clinically insignificant can be shown as statistically significant. This is revealed by the minimally important difference (MID).
- It does not tell us the range over which the effect can possibly happen. This is taken care by the confidence interval.

Minimally important difference (MID): It represents the smallest difference in this actual difference. Even a small difference that is clinically insignificant can be shown as statistically significant.

b. *Confidence interval (CI):* This depicts the range of values within which we can be confidant that the true value for the whole population lies. Normally a confidence interval of 95 percent is accepted as a standard by statisticians who mean that if a study is repeated 100 times the point estimate will remain within this interval 95 times. CI is related to the sample size. Bigger the sample size narrower will be the CI and greater will be the precision of the study.

Note:
More the sample size more will be the CI.

Outcome of the studies: This could be positive, indeterminate or negative.

Positive study: Here the CI is above and not overlapping the MID in statistically significant studies ($p<0.05$).

Indeterminate study: Here the CI crosses the MID in statistically significant studies ($p<0.05$) and in statistically significant results ($p>0.05$) the upper limit of CI overlaps the MID.

Negative study: Here the results are statistically insignificant ($p>0.05$) and the CI lies below MID.

Note:
Statistically significance, MID and CI is necessary to identify whether a study is positive, indeterminate or negative.

Sample size: A bigger sample size makes a study more authentic than a study with a smaller sample size. To either support or refute the use of intervention it is important to know whether the sample size was large enough or the CI was narrow enough. To achieve these following steps needs to be fulfilled:
- State the upper and lower limits of the stated range.
- Introduce the concept of *minimally important treatment effect* which means the smallest amount of benefit that would justify the initiation of the therapy under investigation. If the study is statistically significant but fails to surpass the MITF then it would be deemed as inappropriate as no benefit is conferred.

How to assess the adequacy of the sample size based on the results?

Positive study: If the CI is positive, the adequacy of the sample size is determined by looking at the lower limit of the interval and ascertaining if it lies above the MITF. If true then the adequacy of the sample size is sufficient.

Negative study: Here the treatment group is no better than the control group and the CI is negative. Now inspect the upper limit of the range, if found below zero, then the sample is adequate and the treatment can be ruled out. On the other hand if the upper limit is above zero, the trial does not have an adequate sample size to dismiss the treatment.[23]

3. **Is the study applicable to my patient?** Every clinician is interested to know how effective and relevant is the study to this patient? To do this the following things needs to be done:
   a. *Compare* the characteristics of study participants in your clinical patients? This can be done by determining the research question which involves the following criteria's (PICOT):
      P – Patient
      I – Intervention
      C – Control
      O – Outcome of interest
      T – Time frame
   b. *Know the types of trial:* Was it explanatory or pragmatic?
      In explanatory trial, the trial is conducted in an ideal situation and by expert clinicians and in highly compliant patients.
      In pragmatic trial: Here the trial is completed under usual situations in usual circumstances. Most of the studies les in between the two.
   c. *Applicability:* Can be further determined by looking at the inclusion and exclusion criteria's and other criteria's of a study.
   d. *Cost effectiveness (CE):* Any treatment to be effective has to be cost effective and affordable to your patients and answer the question is it really worth the increased cost, apart from knowing the benefits and risks of the treatment in question. Now let us deal with the CE analysis.

COST EFFECTIVENESS ANALYSIS

It is alright to have procedures and treatment methods that are far superior to the available treatment options. But it is not alright if the same comes with a prohibitive higher treatment costs that will pinch the pockets of your patients. Hence it is imperative that a full economic analysis must consider both the costs and outcomes of the alternative treatment methods. Thus it is imperative that CEA be carried out along with the RCT's where both the efficacy and cost data are collected prospectively.[24] The ideal scenario that is desirable from a new treatment option that it should be both less costly and more effective (Box 67.7).

> **Box 67.7: Quick Facts: Look at the Permutations in Cost Effectiveness Analysis**
> 1. Less costly/more effective – Accept and adopt
> 2. More costly/less effective – Discard
> 3. Less costly/less effective – Weak dominance[3]
> 4. More costly/more effective – A challenge in decision making. Hence the ideal scenario would be to look at the first option.
>
> *Note:* It is important to know that costs may vary among population's treatment providers and geographical locations like the patient outcomes that may vary between populations.

STUDIES OTHER THAN RCT

EBM is not only about RCT's. In fact RCT's unfortunately form a very small percentage of all scientific studies (Only 3%). This implies that there are other studies which are being advocated with greater frequencies though they are not in the same pedestal as RCT's. Let us now know about these other studies.

Cohort Study

A group of individuals that share similar characteristics is called a Cohort. Cohort studies identify equal sized groups with or without an exposure of interest and follow them forward in time to determine outcomes.[25]

Types

1. *Prospective cohort study:* Here before the onset of the study, the exposures are identified and then followed forward.
2. *Retrospective cohort study:* Here the outcomes have already happened even before the study was initiated.

Advantages: Where randomization is not feasible these studies help to identify infrequent and harmful outcomes of intervention.

Disadvantages: It is affected by confounding variables and surveillance bias.

Case control study: These are entirely retrospective studies. Identify a group of people with a specific outcome and label them as the case group. Then a control group is selected based on a similar group of individuals with the same demographics but without the outcome of interests. Now analyze these groups for previous exposures to suspected harmful agents and determine if they influence the target outcome.

Advantages: It helps to investigate outcomes that are rare or slow to develop since the outcome here has already occurred.

Disadvantages: They are affected by confounding variables and recall bias.

Case Series

This could be multiple patients (Case series) or single patient (Case report). These simply report on variables thought to be causally linked with the outcome of interest. They do not provide a comparison with the control group.

Though placed on the lower level of the hierarchy of evidence it serves the following beneficial purposes:
- It helps the clinicians to generate clinical questions and hypothesis for future or further studies.
- It helps to identify substantial adverse events that have changed the standard of treatment.

Diagnostic Study

Using a reference standard or gold standard as comparison, the efficacy of the diagnostic tests under question must be studied. A test that is well accepted and accurate diagnostic tool in the medical community is called the gold standard. To describe the performance of a diagnostic test, two indices are used:
1. *Sensitivity:* This is the proportion of diseased individuals with a positive test result or the true positives.
2. *Specificity:* This is the proportion of non-diseased persons with a negative test result or the true negatives.

DECISION ANALYSIS STUDY

Is it not true that our whole life is based on the choices we make? Right choices or decisions make our life successful and the wrong ones make our life miserable. It is said that when we pick up a stick we pick up the other end too. God has given us the great capacity to make our own choices in all spheres of life and it is fully under our control but once we make a choice the consequences is not under our control.

Now apply the same logic to the clinical trials. Faced with a clinical situation you have done a painstaking research analysis of the various treatment options and now you are faced with taking decision as to which treatment options is the best for your patient. This decision making is extremely vital in achieving the best possible outcome. This can be achieved by rigorous and objective analysis of the outcomes and probabilities and is known as the decision analysis.

Decision analysis is an objective, explicit method to represent specific decision problems using models and allows the user to apply EBM to a particular clinical scenario. This requires the construction of a decision tree that illustrates all plausible relationships, alternatives and outcomes involved with a given decision. By incorporating both probabilities and outcome values, a decision analysis model expresses its conclusion in terms of average expected results.[26]

Components of Decision Analysis

1. *Probabilities:* This is a quantities estimate of the chance or likelihood that a given outcome will occur and is derived from a systematic and rigorous analysis of available literature particularly the RCT's. To help in the decision making processes these estimated probabilities are then incorporated into the decision tree.
2. *Outcome variables:* These are summary measurements of a particular outcome and are expressed in the form of:
   - Life years
   - Quality adjusted life years (QALY's)
   - Costs
   - Utilities.

These are derived from the literature or from expert opinion or patient's choice. The next step is to multiply outcome values by their respective probabilities and obtain the calculation. The model then expresses its conclusion in terms of an average expected results interpreted as life years, days of treatment, cost or other variables depending on the clinical context. These final values represent the baseline values that can undergo further analysis in a decision tree and is called the sensitivity analysis.

Sensitivity Analysis

Due to biologic variations, differing techniques and expertise, discrepancies in literature baseline probabilities and outcome values are often associated with some uncertainties. Moreover the difference between the options may be quite small though they may show one method is preferred over the other. In such situations a sensitivity analysis is performed by varying probabilities and outcome values. This helps to explore the uncertainty of data and to examine what are the effects of variability or probabilities and outcome values in an expected outcome.

This allows a clinician to choose a preferred method of treatment and explores the various variables that may influence the final decision. Thus decision analysis has developed into a powerful and effective technique for variety of clinical application. It thus helps in determining the best course of action.

QUALITY OF REPORTING

Evidence-based decision hinges not just on available literature but on good literature. How to ascertain that the available literature is good and reliable. Well this can be done by subjecting each level of evidence through their own quality control check lists (Table 67.2). Let us first begin with the mother all evidences, the RCT. Therapeutic studies

TABLE 67.2: Checklists for various studies

Checklist	Number of items	Study type evaluated
1. CONSORT	22	RCT'S
2. CLEART NPT	15	RCT'S
3. QUOROM	18	Meta-analysis of RCT's
4. STROBE	22	Observational studies (Cohort, case control and cross sectional)
5. MOOSE	35	Meta-analysis of observational studies

are the most common class of study found in orthopedic literature.

1. **RCT's:** These occupy the top level of hierarchy of evidence simply because these studies eliminates bias by ensuring that both the treatment and control groups are balanced for both the known and unknown prognostic factors. Here the subjects have an equal chance of being either in the study or control group by chance and not by choice. However, the quality of reporting in orthopedic RCT is of poor quality and needs effort to improve it.[27,28] RCT's to be of top standard it should meet other criteria's apart from mere randomization namely:
   - Concealment of randomization
   - Blinding
   - Loss to follow up
   - Sample size calculation
   - Following the intention to treat principle.

   To improve the quality of orthopedic RCT's reporting the following quality checklists needs to be applied:
   a. *Detsky quality index:* This includes 14 items and a score of >75% is deemed a high quality RCT's. Only 68% of the reported RCT's meet these criterias.
   b. *CONSORT criteria:* It is a 22 item checklist and a flow diagram first published in journal of American Medical Association (JAMA) in 1996. This criterion focuses on reporting of trial design, analysis, interpretation and participant progress. So poor is the quality of reporting, that more than 70% of the RCT studies did not meet even half of the CONSORT criteria.[29]

   It is appalling to note that only 11.3% of published articles are considered to be of level 1 evidence and even among these the reporting quality is considered to be poor causing concern and hence the value of these checklists. RCT'S in particular constitute only 3% of these orthopedic literatures.

2. **Systematic reviews:** Unlike unsystematic literature reviews, systematic reviews are more likely to be quoted as evidences[30] and they follow the eight step process:
   a. Formulating a hypothesis.
   b. Identifying the inclusion and exclusion criterias.
   c. Searching for the studies.
   d. Selecting the studies.
   e. Checking the study quality.
   f. Extracting data.
   g. Result of the analysis.
   h. Interpretation of the results.

   But like RCT's, the quality of rigorous methodological reporting of the systematic reviews is found to be only 15% and is a cause of concern.[31]

Meta-analysis: One of the most beneficial aspects of following a systematic review is meta-analysis. This is a quantitative analysis of results across many studies to arrive at the single best estimate of treatment effect. This helps eliminate bias and is an important tool for practitioners while making treatment decisions.

For methodological consideration of systematic reviews the quality of reporting of meta-analysis (QUOROM) was developed.[32] This helps the readers to critically appraise the meta-analysis. Based on these criteria it is observed that only 15% of the systematic reviews is correct while a whopping 85% gives biased results.

By improving the quality of RCT's and overcoming its shortcomings will help overcome the shortcomings of systematic reviews. But on the flip side it is observed that the majority of published orthopedic systematic reviews are non-randomized trials due to apparent lack of RCT studies.

Publication Bias

Another factor that affects systematic reviews is the *publication bias* where positive trials are published more frequently than negative trials.[33] This tilts the balance heavily towards positive affects and creates bias even in the most rigorously followed systematic analysis. This is known as positive outcome bias. In a trial, it has been noted that nearly 70% of the positive studies were published against the 10% of the neutral studies. This is a serious problem and can result in severe bias.

These checklists provide invaluable source guidance to authors, journals, editorial and readers to critically appraise the published reports.

DEVELOPING AN EVIDENCE-BASED BALANCE SHEET

After all this painstaking procedures of research analysis it is now time to prepare a balance sheet of the evidence-based procedure by adopting the following four procedures:

1. Identification of alternative treatments available to the patients.

TABLE 67.3: Showing the problems and their solutions in EBM

Problems	Solutions
Resources and commitments in terms of time and money that needs to be delivered away from actual patient care	Evaluate against opportunity cost, follow-on and abandonment option costs. Evidence based practice wins hands down as a strategic investment
Finding and evaluating the evidence is costly in terms of time	Use EPR
Lack of skills in computer use and locating evidence	Train personnel. This is not an issue with the generation next
Resources needed to acquire and maintain databases	Availability in electronic form and increased usage will bring the prices down
Searching may only result in discovering gaps in medical knowledge	One must seriously doubt our capabilities and question our insecurities
Poor indexing may lead to frustration of futile literature searches	Use online searches and make all literature available searchable online
The quality and quantity of research mostly unknown	Use refined studies performed real-time using EPR
Demands a high degree of statistics knowledge	Use EPR that have the calculations as well as their interpretations built-in
Viewed as a form of rationing	Evidence-based medicine is about improving the quality of patient care. It is just as likely to show that effective interventions are underused as to show that ineffective procedures are over-used

2. Identification of the health outcomes that are affected by treatment.
3. Estimation of the probabilities or magnitudes of each of the health outcomes for each of the treatment methods.
4. Displaying the information in a table.

COMMUNICATION TO A PATIENT

Once you have zeroed on the best possible treatment options after careful analysis, communicating the same to the patients effectively and convincingly poses a bigger challenge to the clinicians. As in life so in EBM lack of proper communication skills can give rise to lots of confusion and sometimes may be reason for litigations. Hence due care need to be exercised while communicating facts and figures to the patients.[34] Some of the better ways of doing this are:

1. *Paternalistic method:* Here the clinician makes the decisions.
2. *Patient independent model:* Here the patient makes the decision based on the facts presented by the clinician.
3. *Relationship centered model:* This is the best model. Here the physicians establish a relationship with the patient and their families and both participate in the decision making process with mutual trust. This two way process seems to be ideal.[35]

Tools for Communication

You have decided to communicate and you have chosen your method of doing so. But you need to know the different tools available for effective communications. One cannot follow a set pattern as each patient is different and hence different tools and strategies need to be used to communicate[36] namely:

- Verbal, written or video information presented in a structured format.
- To use aids like illustrations and graphs, bar charts and pictographs, etc.

Appliances for Communication

The following five approaches may be used to communicate to your patients the results of an orthopedic study:
- Relative risk
- Relative risk reduction
- Odds ratio
- Absolute risk reduction
- Number needed to treat.

Detailed descriptions about these approaches are outside the scope of this book and the students are advised to refer bigger books on this subject.

Note:
It is important to note that the same rules do not apply to each patient and different yardstick needs to be used to convince the patients better.

Problems in EBM

EBM is not without problems. But however the benefits far outweigh the problems and should not come in the way of putting EBM into use. The problems and their solutions are depicted in Table 67.3.

REFERENCES

1. Sackett DL, Rosenberg WM, Gray JA, Haynes RB, Richardson WS. Evidence-based medicine: What it is and what is not. Br Med J. 1996;312:71-2.

2. Neuhauser D, Daniel DM. Using the Bible to teach quality improvement methods. Qual Saf Health Care. 2004;13:153-5.
3. Lind J. A treatise of the Scurvy in Three parts: Containing an inquiry into the Nature, Causes and Cure of that Disease, Together with a Critical and Chronological View of What Has been published on the subject. London; 1753.
4. Gross CP, Sepkowitz KA. The myth of the medical breakthrough: Smallpox, Vaccination and Jenner reconsidered. Int J Infect Dis. 1998;3:53-60.
5. Best M, Neuhauser D, Slavin L, Cotton Mather, you dog, damn you! I will inoculate you with this: with a pox to you: Small pox inoculation, Boston, 1721. Qual Saf Health Care. 2004;13:82-3.
6. Amberson J, McMohan B, Pinner M. A clinical trial of sanocrysin in pulmonary tuberculosis. Am Rev Tuber. 1931;24:401-35.
7. Medical Research Council. Streptomycin treatment of pulmonary tuberculosis. Br Med J. 1948;2:769-82.
8. Evidence-Based Medicine Working Group. Evidence-based medicine: A new approach to teaching the practice of medicine. JAMA. 1992;268:2420-5.
9. Sackett DL, Haynes RB, Tugwell P. Clinical epidemiology: A basic science for clinical medicine. Boston; Little, Brown and Co; 1985.
10. Montori VM, Swiontkowski MF, Cook DJ. Methodologic issues in systematic reviews and meta-analyses. Clin Orthop Relat Res. 2003;413:43-54.
11. Jadad AR, Cook DJ, Jones A, Klassen TP, Tuuwell P, Moher M, et al. Methodology and reports of systematic reviews and meta-analyses: A comparison of Cochrane reviews with articles published in paper-based journals, JAMA. 2003;280:278-80.
12. Swiontkowski MF, Wright JG. Introducing a new journal section: Evidence-based orthopedics. Bone Joint Surg. 2000;82:759.
13. Bhandari M, Guyatt GH, Swiontkowski MF. User's guide to the orthopedic literature: How to use an article about a surgical therapy? J Bone Joint Surg Am. 2001:83:916-26.
14. Wright JG, Swiontkowski MF, Heckman JD. Introducing levels of evidence to the journal. J Bone-Joint Surg Am. 2003;85:1-3.
15. Writing Group for the Women's Health Initiative Investigators. Risks and benefits of estrogen plus progestin in healthy postmenopausal women: Principal results from the Women's Health Initiative randomized controlled trial. JAMA. 2002;288:323-33.
16. Zhang W, Moskowitz RW, Nuki G, Abramson S, Altman RD, Arden N, et al. OARSI recommendations for the management of hip and knee osteoarthritis, part I: Critical appraisal of existing treatment guidelines and systematic review of current research evidence. Osteoarthritis Cartilage. 2008; 15:981-1000.
17. Haynes RB, Strauss SE. Evidence-based medicine: How to practice and teach EBM. Edingurgh, New York: Elsevier/Churchill Livingstone; 2005.
18. User's guides to the medical literature; Essentials of evidence-based clinical practice. Chicago.H: American Medical Association; 2002.
19. Haynes RB, Strauss SE. Evidence-based medicine; How to practice and teach EBM. Edingurgh, New York: Elsevier/Churchill Livingstone; 2005.
20. Hanson B, Bhandari M, Audige L, Helfet D. The need for education in evidence-based orthopedics. Acta Orthop Scand. 2004;75:328-32.
21. Guyatt GH, Rennie D. User's guides to the medical literature: Essentials of evidence-based clinical practice. Chicago, IL: American Medical Association; 2002.
22. Altman DG, Gore SM, Gardner MJ, Pocock SJ. Statistical guidelines for contributors to medical journals. In: Gardner MJ, Altman DG, (Eds). Statistics with confidence. Confidence intervals and statistical guidelines, London: British Medical Journal; 1989.p.83100.
23. Detsky AS, Sackett DL. When was a "negative" trial big enough? How many patients you needed depends on what you found. Arch Intern Med. 1985;145:709-15.
24. Busse JW, Heetveld MJ. Critical appraisal of the orthopedic literature: Therapeutic and economic analysis. Injury. 2006;37:312-20.
25. Grimes DA, Schuyltz KF. An overview of clinical research: The lay of the land. Lancet. 2002;359:57-61.
26. Graham B, Detsky AS. The application of decision analysis to the surgical treatment of early osteoarthritis of the wrist. J Bone Joint Surg Br. 2001;83:650-4.
27. Agha R, Cooper D, Muir G. The reporting quality of randomized controlled trials in surgery: A systematic reviewing J Surg. 2007;5:413-22.
28. Jacquier I, Boutron I, Moher D, Roy C, Ravaud P. The reporting of randomized clinical trials using a surgical intervention is in need of immediate improvement: A systematic review. Ann Surg. 2006;244:677-83.
29. Mills E, Wu P, Gagnier J, Heels-Ansdell D, Montori B. An analysis of general medical and specialist journals that endorse CONSORT found that reporting was not enforced consistently. J Clin Epidemiology. 2005;58:662-7.
30. Moher D, Tetzlaff J, Tricco AC, Sampson M, Altman DG. Epidemiology and reporting characteristics of systematic reviews. PLos Med. 2007;4:447-55.
31. Bhandari M, Morrow F, Kulkarni AV, Tornetta P 3rd. Meta-analysis in orthopedic surgery: A systematic review of their methodologies. J Bone Joint Surg Am. 2001;83:15-24.
32. Moher D, Cook DJ, Eastwood S, Olkin I, Rennie D, Stroup DF. Improving the quality of reports of meta-analyses of randomized controlled trials: the QUOROM statement. Lancet. 1999;354:1896-900.
33. Hasenboehler EA, Choudhary IK, Newman JT, Smith WR, Ziran BH, Stahel PF. Bias towards publishing positive results in orthopedic and general surgery: A patient safety issue? Patient Safe Surg. 2007;1:4-9.
34. Hoff rage U, Lindsey S, Hertwig R, Gigerenzer G. Medicine: Communicating statistical information. Science. 2000;290:2261-2.
35. Quill TE, Brody H. Physician recommendations and patient autonomy: Finding a balance between physician power and patient choice. Ann Intern Med. 1996;125:763-9.
36. Trevena LJ, Davey HM, Baratt A, Butow P, Caldwell P. A systematic review on communicating with patients about evidence. J eval Clin Pract. 2006;12:13-23.

Appendices

Appendix I: Instruments and Implants in Orthopedics

For convenience and easy understanding, instruments used in orthopedic surgery can be categorized into three groups:
1. General surgical instruments
2. Regular orthopedic instruments
3. Instruments used in special orthopedic situations.
   Now let us try to analyze each one in detail.

GENERAL SURGICAL INSTRUMENTS

- Surgical knife and blade is used to incise the skin and soft tissues.
- Artery forceps is used to catch the bleeding vessels.
- Allis forceps is used to catch the soft tissues.
- Retractors are used to retract the soft tissues.
- Scissors are used to cut the soft tissues.
- Tissue holding forceps, needles, etc.

The general surgical instruments help in the initial stage of surgery, for exposure, to deal with the soft tissue structures, to expose the bones, etc.

REGULAR ORTHOPEDIC INSTRUMENTS

After reaching the bone, general orthopedic instruments help to deal with the bone to place implants, etc. The following are the general orthopedic instruments mentioned in order of priority:

BONE HOLDING, PLATE HOLDING AND ROD HOLDING INSTRUMENTS

Instruments

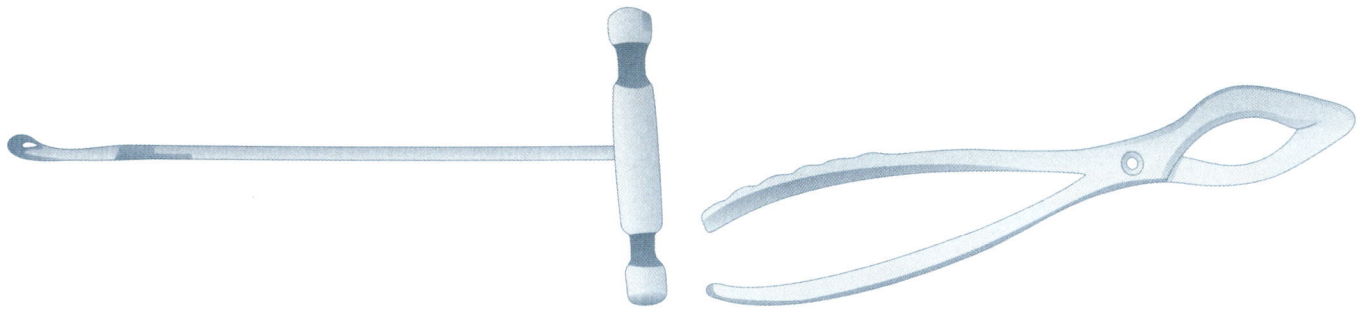

1. Bone hook
2. Fergusson's lion-toothed bone holding forceps

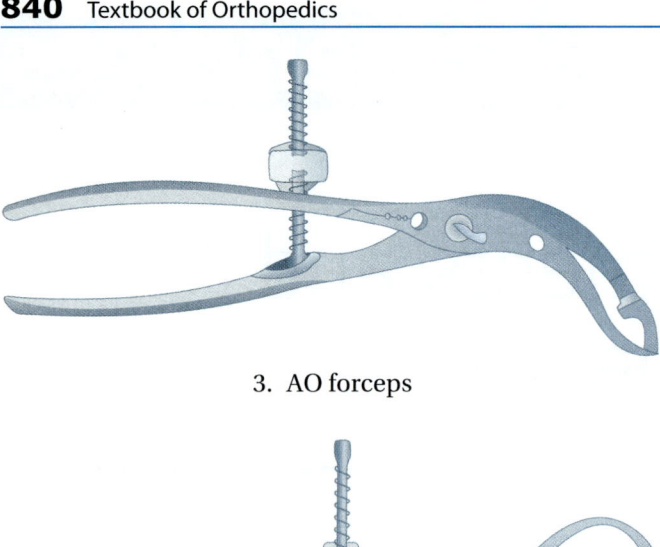

3. AO forceps

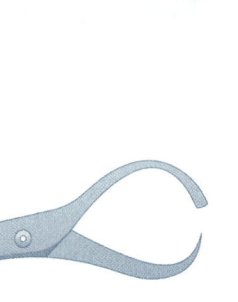

4. Patella forceps

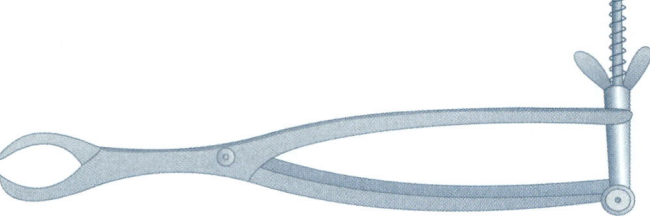

5. Heygroves bone holding forceps (sizes 8"/10"/12")

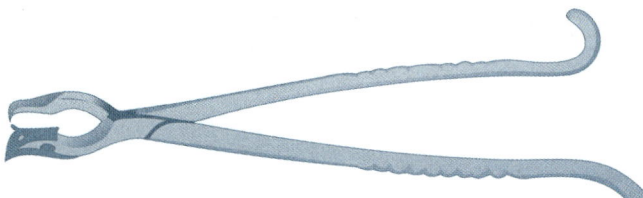

6. Lane's Fagg's bone holding (sizes 12 ½")

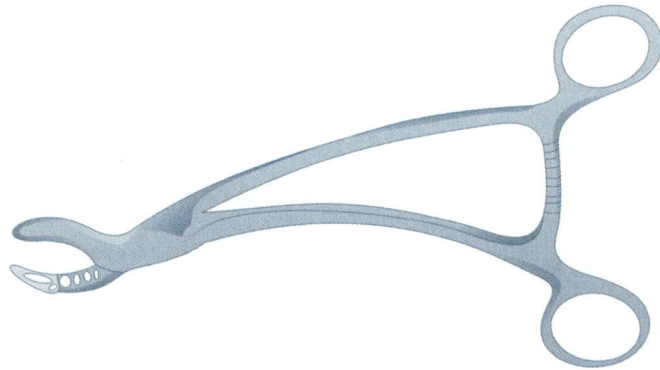

7. Burn's bone holding forceps

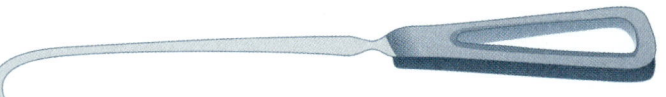

8. Kocher's bone hook (sizes: small/medium/large)

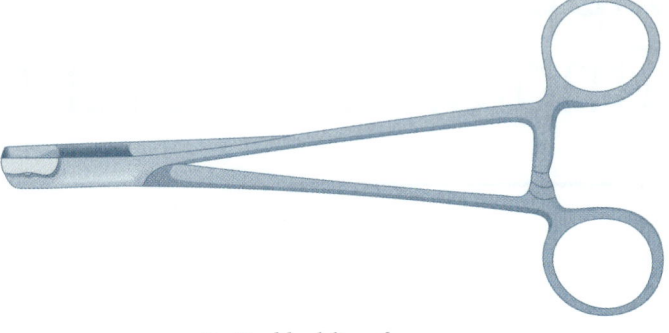

9. Rod holding forceps

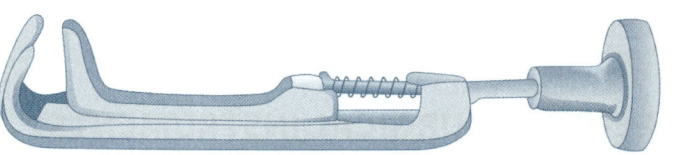

10. Lowman's bone holding clamp (sizes 4", 5", 8")

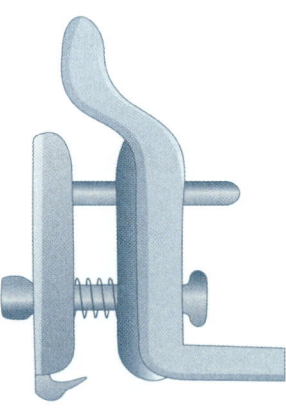

11. Müller's compression device with handle

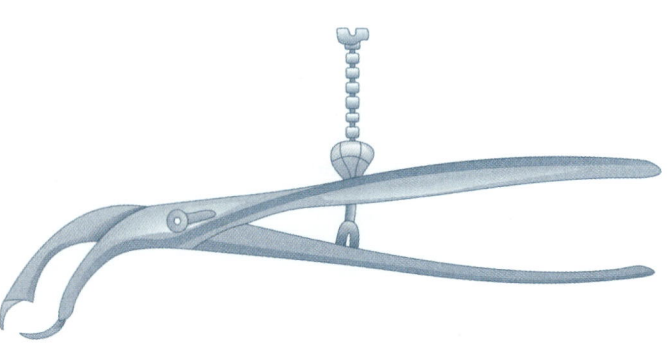

12. Self-centering bone holding forceps

Appendix I: Instruments and Implants in Orthopedics **841**

Instruments from 1-8 are used to pick-up and hold the bone firmly during surgery, instrument number 9 is used to hold and steady the intramedullary nails. Number 10 is to hold the plate to the bone for fixation.

INSTRUMENTS USED TO CUT, NIBBLE, CURETTE AND MAKE HOLES IN THE BONES

Instruments

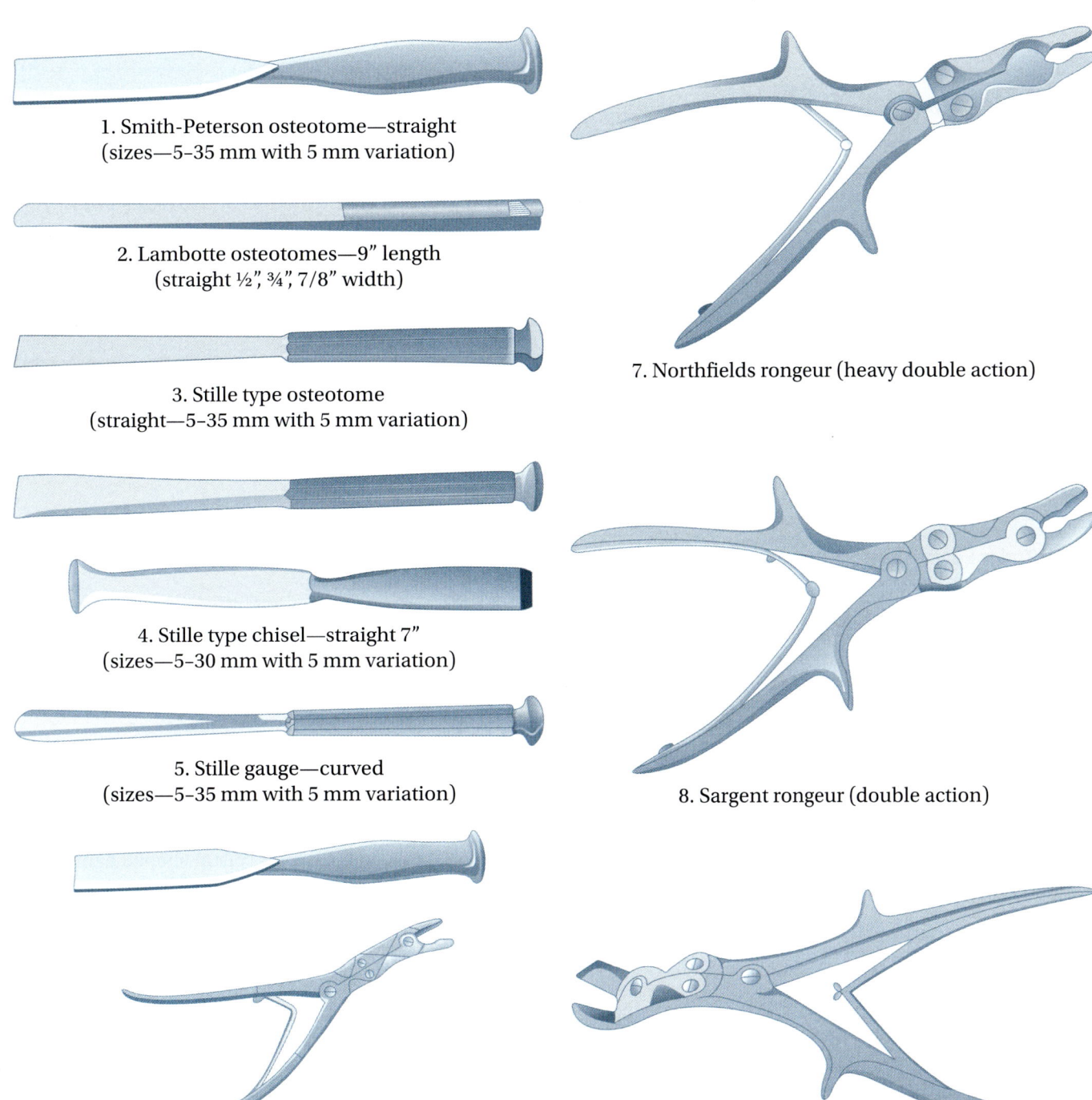

1. Smith-Peterson osteotome—straight (sizes—5-35 mm with 5 mm variation)
2. Lambotte osteotomes—9" length (straight ½", ¾", 7/8" width)
3. Stille type osteotome (straight—5-35 mm with 5 mm variation)
4. Stille type chisel—straight 7" (sizes—5-30 mm with 5 mm variation)
5. Stille gauge—curved (sizes—5-35 mm with 5 mm variation)
6. Leksell's rongeur (double action)
7. Northfields rongeur (heavy double action)
8. Sargent rongeur (double action)
9. Stille-Horsley bone cutting forceps (10" length)

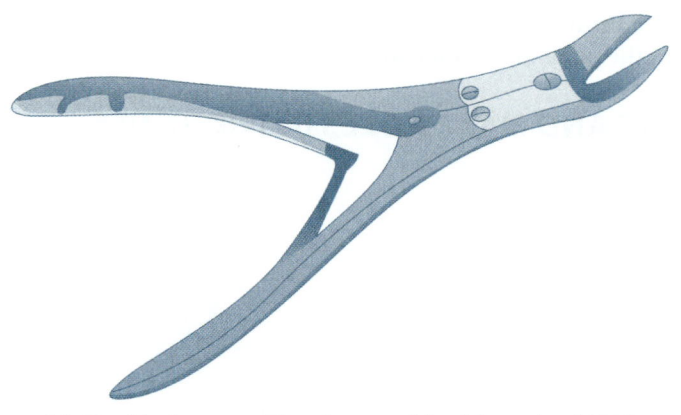

10. Ruskin bone cutting forceps (double action) 7½"

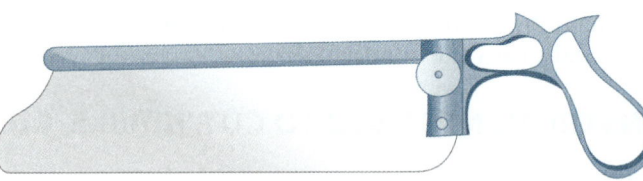

12. Amputation saw

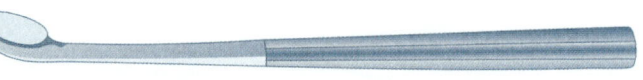

13. Cup curette (sizes 3–10 mm)

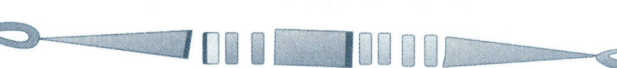

14. Volkman curette double ended (sizes 4 mm)

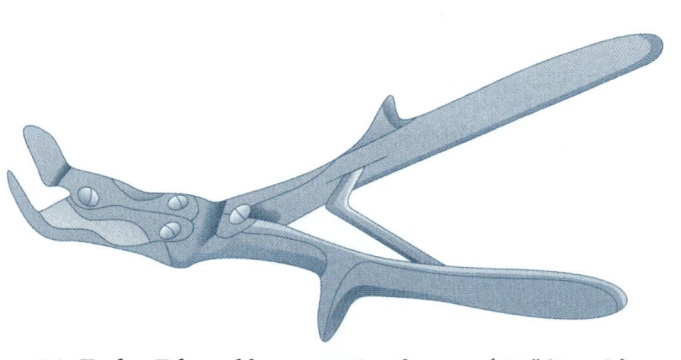

11. Tudor Edward bone cutting forceps (9½" length)

15. Kuntscher's diamond pointed AWL

MISCELLANEOUS ORTHOPEDIC INSTRUMENTS

Instruments

Periosteal Elevators

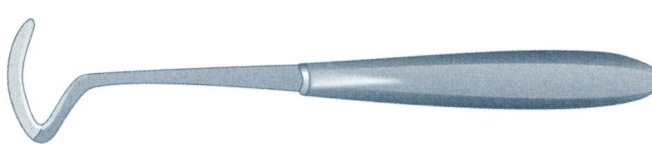

1. Doyan's periosteal elevator adult—right/left

2. Farabeuf Rugine Straight/Curved

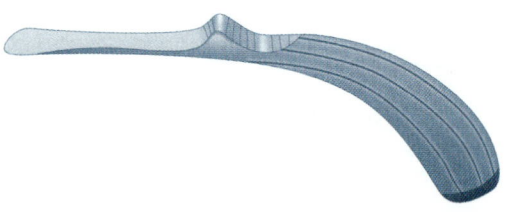

3. Jone's periosteal elevator (pistol-shaped handle)

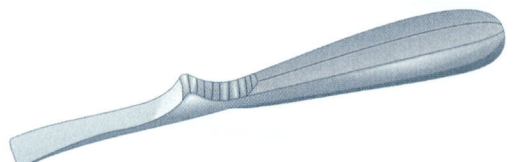

4. Mitchell elevator—straight 8¼"

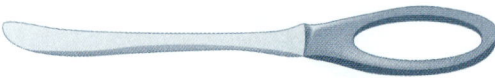

5. Bristows periosteal elevator

Bone Levers

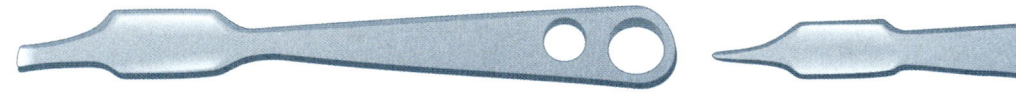

1. Retractor wide tip—width 22 mm
2. Retractor long narrow tip (for hip surgery)—width 18 mm

Fracture Reduction Forceps

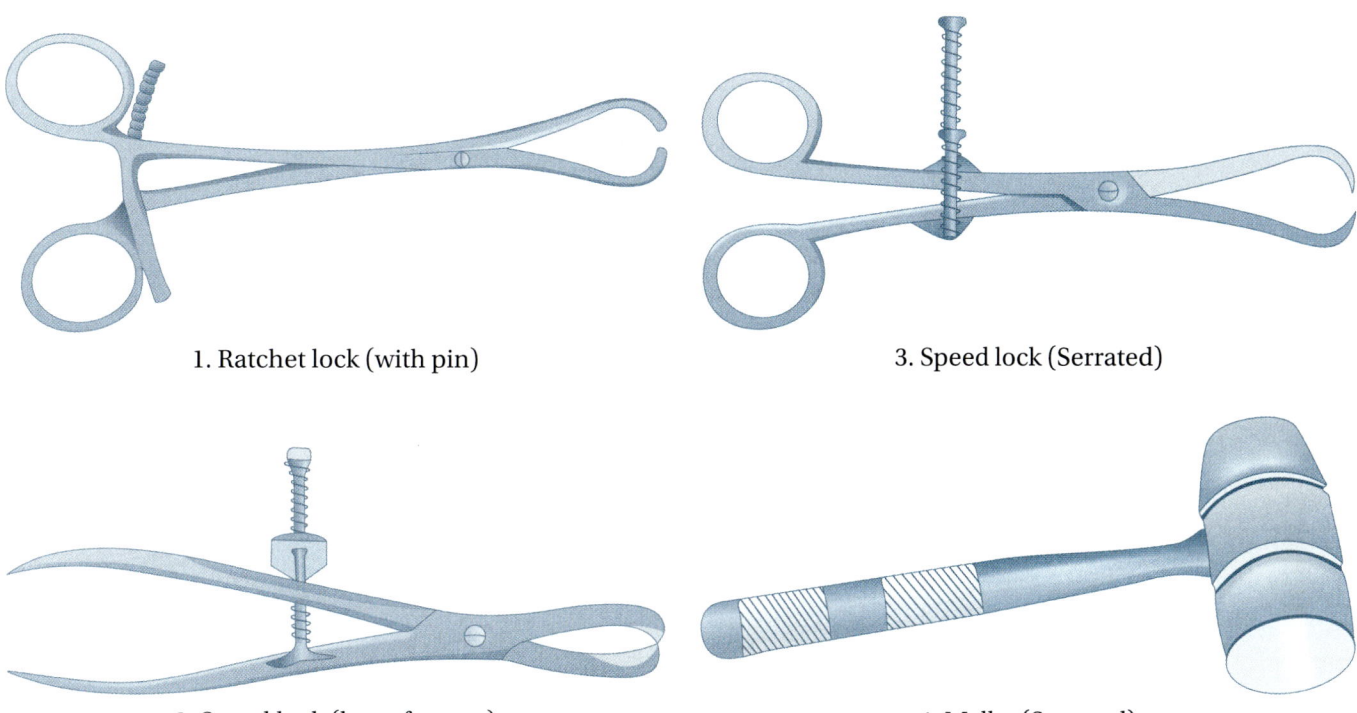

1. Ratchet lock (with pin)
3. Speed lock (Serrated)
2. Speed lock (large forceps)
4. Mallet (Serrated)

INSTRUMENTS USED FOR INSERTION OF PLATE AND SCREWS

Instruments

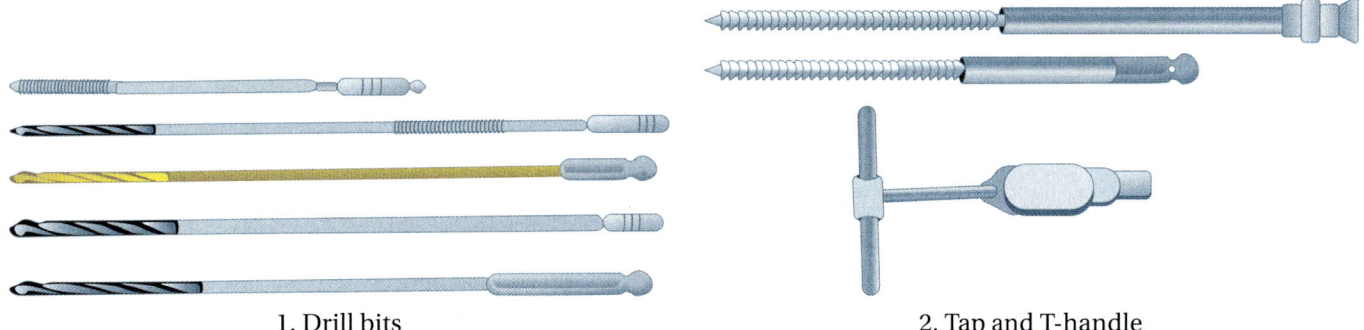

1. Drill bits
2. Tap and T-handle

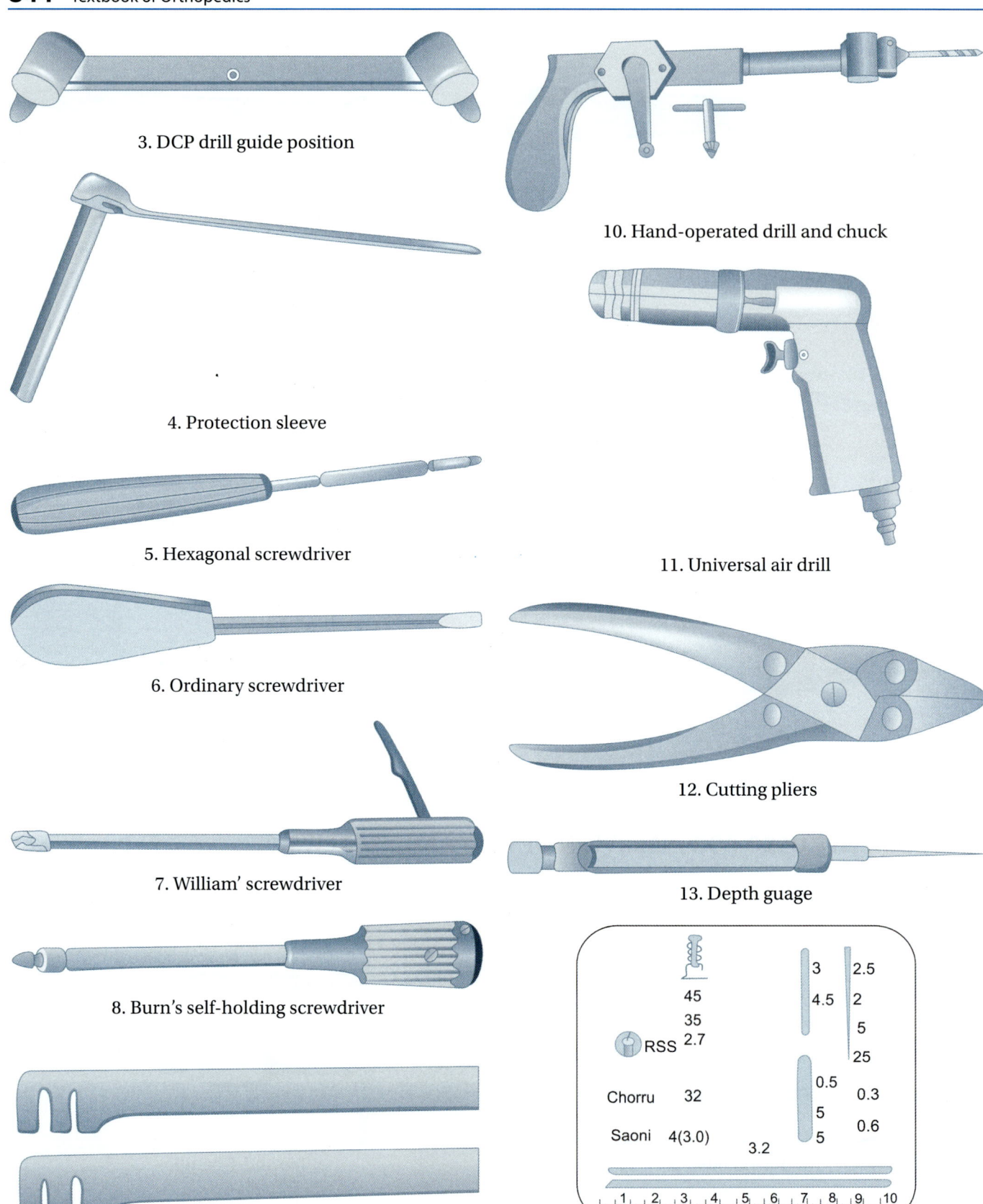

INSTRUMENTS USED FOR CUTTING PLASTER CASTS

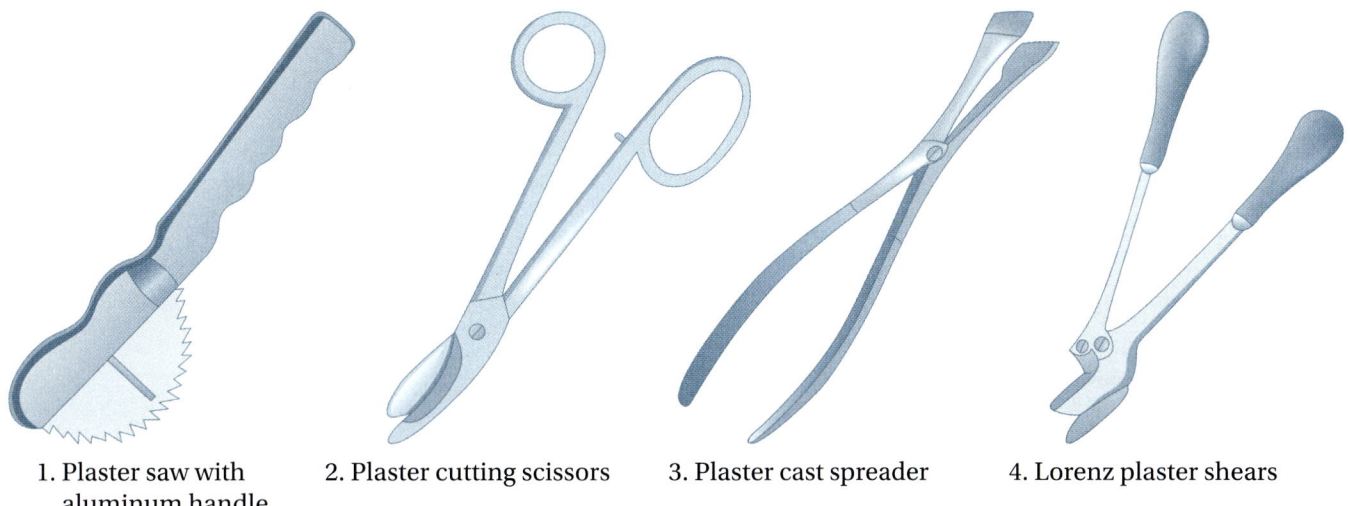

1. Plaster saw with aluminum handle
2. Plaster cutting scissors
3. Plaster cast spreader
4. Lorenz plaster shears

INSTRUMENTS USED FOR WIRE INSERTION

Instruments

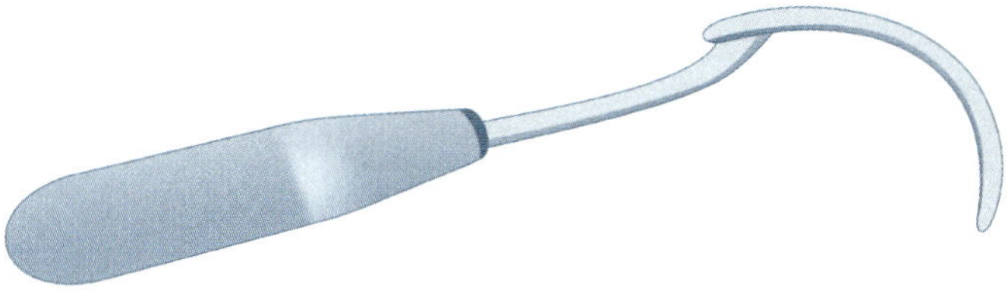

1. Wire sleeve
2. Wire tightener 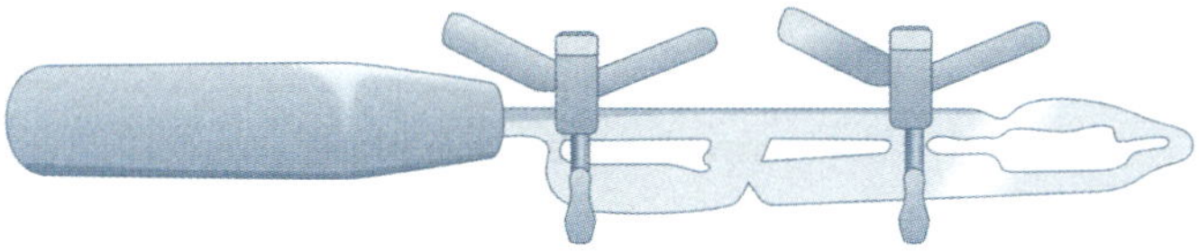
3. Wire bender 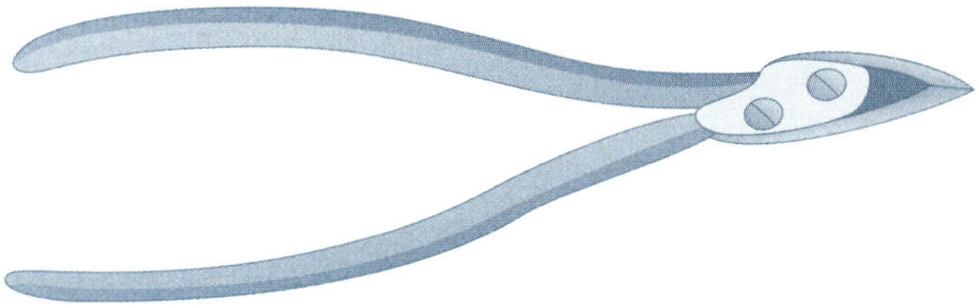
4. Wire cutter 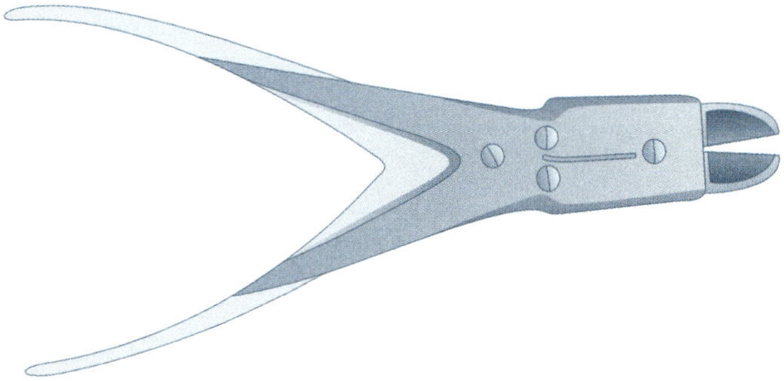
5. Cerclage wire 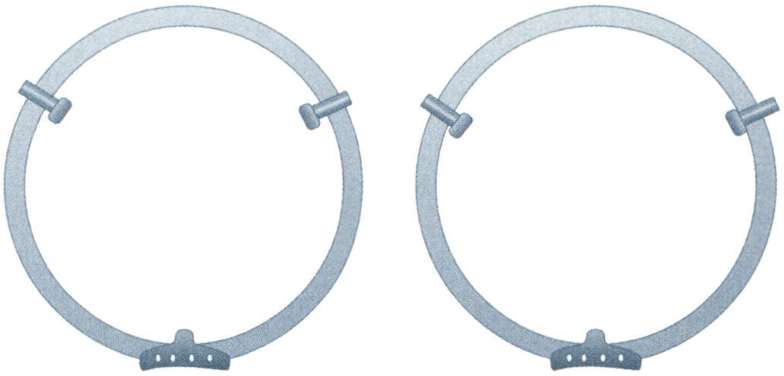
6. Kirschner wire

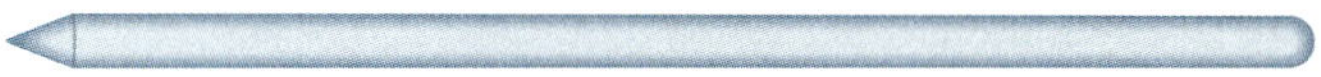

846 Textbook of Orthopedics

IMPLANTS IN ORTHOPEDICS

Different Types of Plates Used in Orthopedics

Instruments

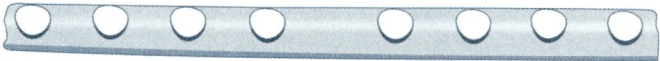
1. Semitubular plate

2. Narrow DCP 4.5

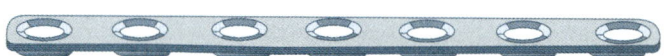
3. Narrow LC-DCP 4.5

4. Broad DCP 4.5

5. Broad LC-DCP 4.5

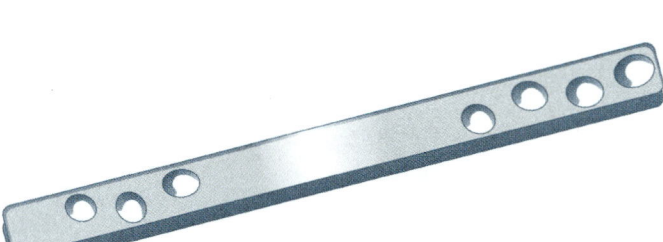
6. Form plates

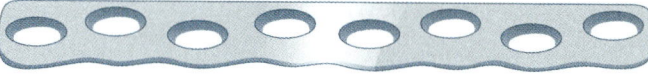
7. Broad lengthening plate

8. Narrow lengthening plate

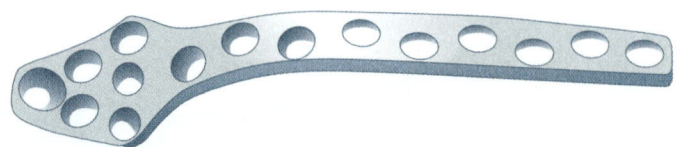
9. Cobra head plate

> **Semitubular Plate is Used for Fracture of Subcutaneous Bones like Ulna**
> *Note:*
> - Narrow DCP—is used for tibia and is not intended for femur
> - Broad DCP—is used for femur and humerus and is not intended for tibia
> - LC-DCP—is a limited contact dynamic compression plate.

Different Sets of Screws

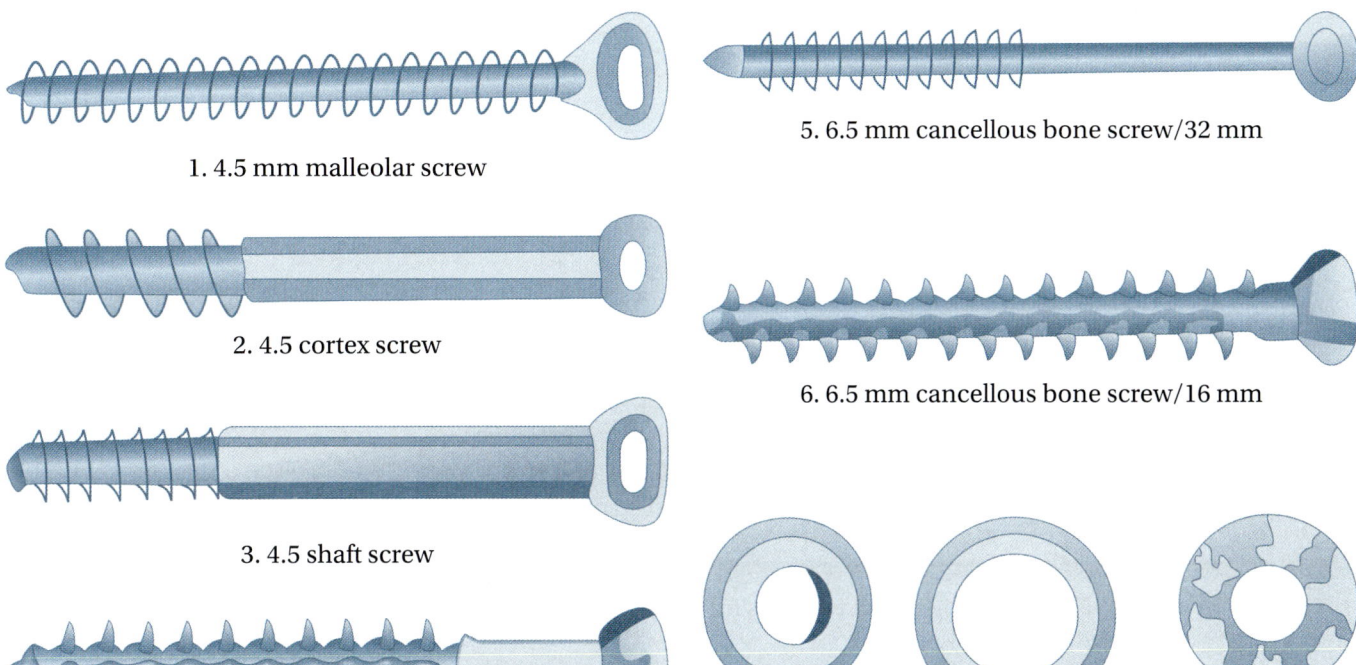

1. 4.5 mm malleolar screw
2. 4.5 cortex screw
3. 4.5 shaft screw
4. 6.5 mm cancellous bone screw/fully threaded
5. 6.5 mm cancellous bone screw/32 mm
6. 6.5 mm cancellous bone screw/16 mm
7. Nuts and washers

DYNAMIC HIP AND ANKLE IMPLANTS

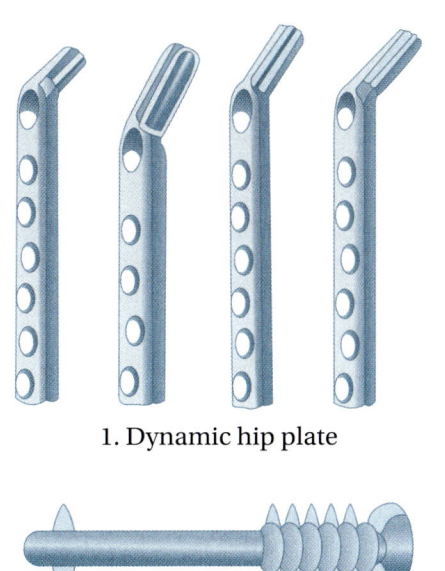

1. Dynamic hip plate
2. DHS locking device

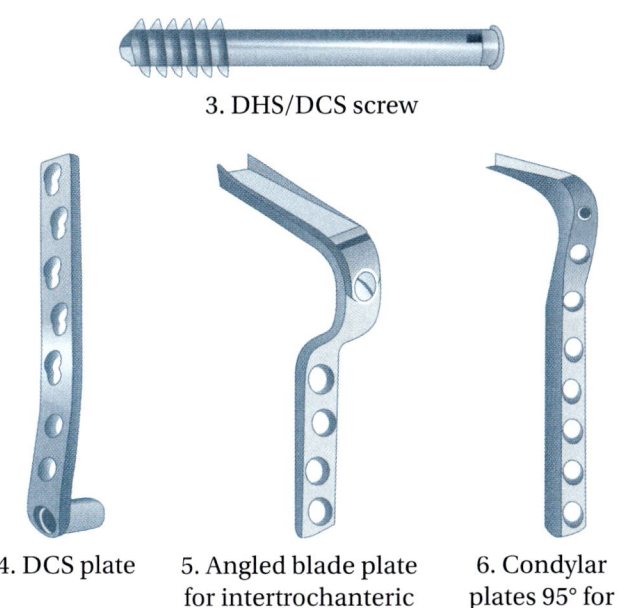

3. DHS/DCS screw
4. DCS plate
5. Angled blade plate for intertrochanteric femoral osteotomies in adults
6. Condylar plates 95° for small adults and adolescents

SOME OF THE SPECIAL PLATES USED IN ORTHOPEDICS

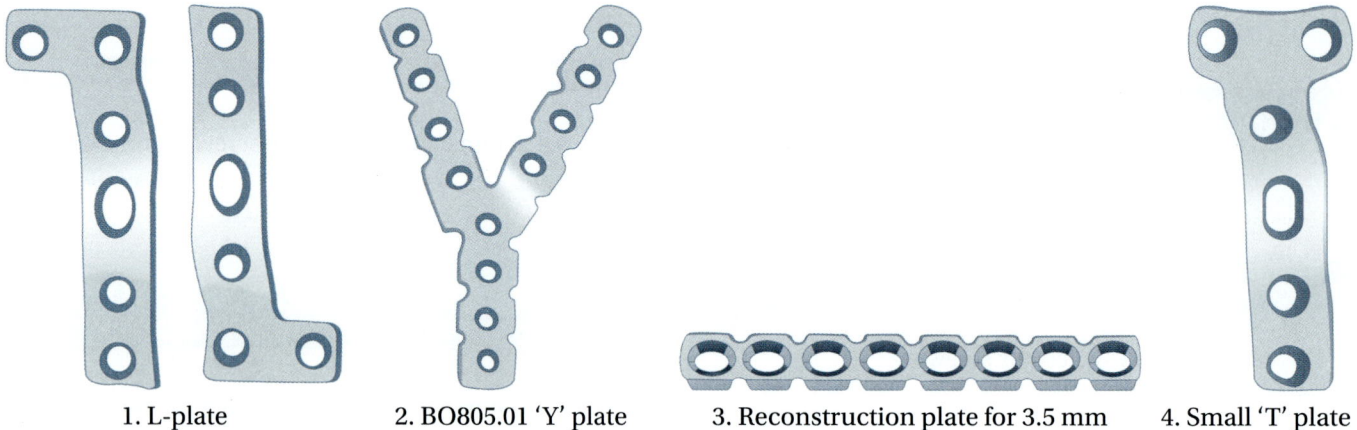

1. L-plate
2. BO805.01 'Y' plate
3. Reconstruction plate for 3.5 mm
4. Small 'T' plate

DIFFERENT CONVENTIONAL INTRAMEDULLARY NAILS

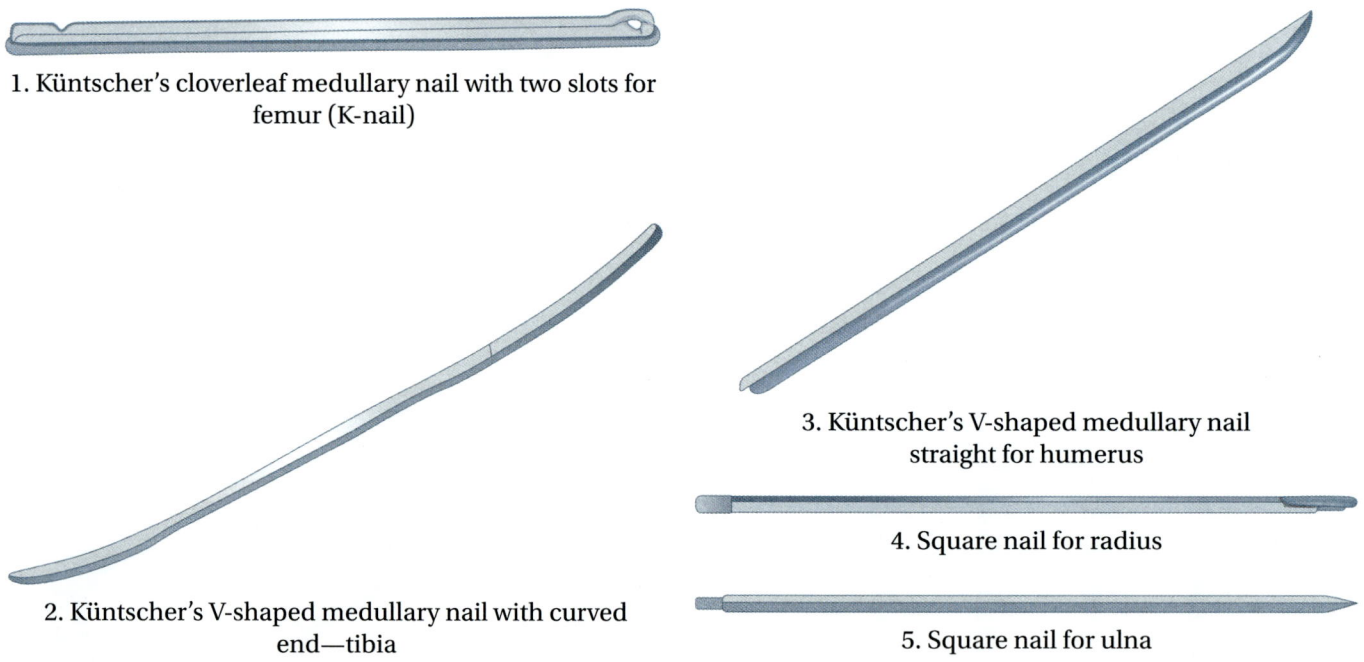

1. Küntscher's cloverleaf medullary nail with two slots for femur (K-nail)
2. Küntscher's V-shaped medullary nail with curved end—tibia
3. Küntscher's V-shaped medullary nail straight for humerus
4. Square nail for radius
5. Square nail for ulna

INSTRUMENTS USED FOR K-NAIL INSERTION FOR FEMUR

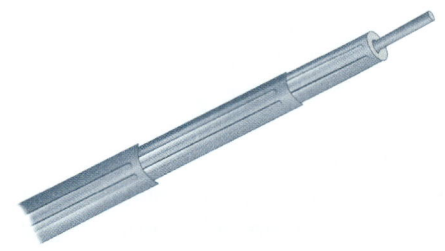 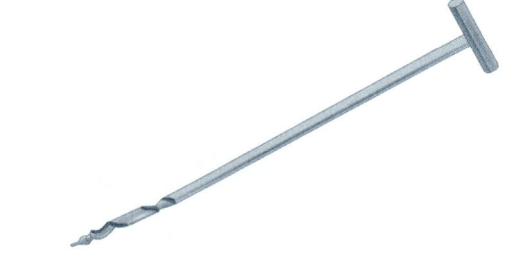

1. Nail set
2. Intramedullary reamer (sizes 6–15 mm with 1 mm variation)

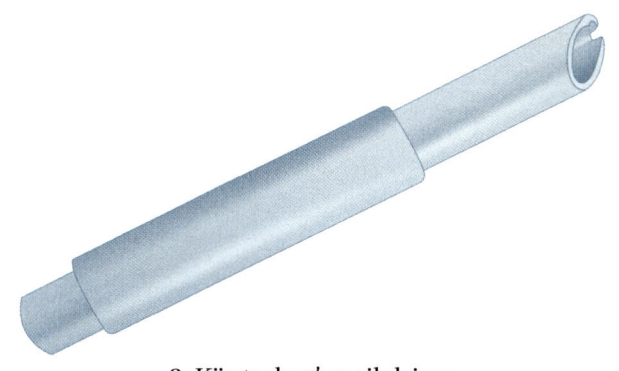

3. Küntscher's nail driver

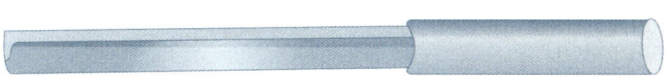

4. Küntscher's nail punch for final tapping

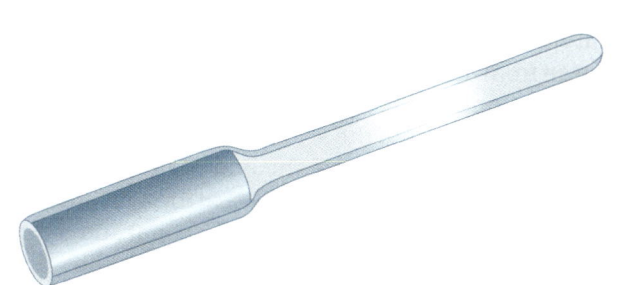

5. K-nail impactor

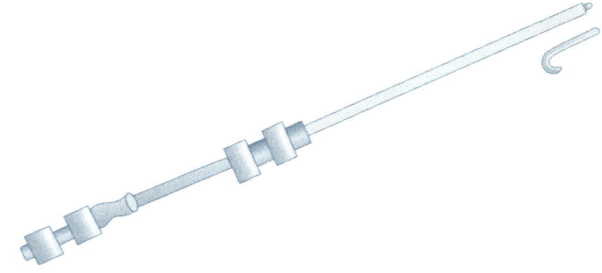

6. K-nail extractor with two hooks

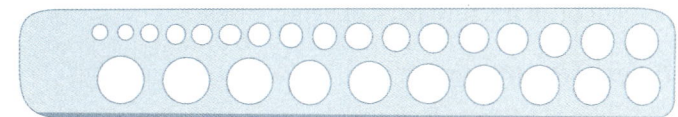

7. Diameter measuring gauge

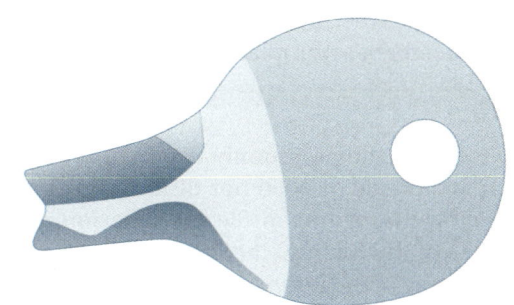

8. Tissue protector

KÜNTSCHER'S CLOVERLEAF* INTRAMEDULLARY NAIL

For information about intramedullary nail, its requirements, mode of action, and its varieties please refer to page 70. The technique of nail insertion is described on page 218.

Methods of Insertion

It could be either open or closed. A comparative study is presented here.

Open technique	Closed technique
Advantages	*Advantages*
Good anatomic reduction can be obtained	All the disadvantages of open technique are absent
Disadvantages	*Disadvantages*
• Infection is more common	• Technically difficult.
• Exposure time is more	• Require sophisticated equipment
• Fat embolism may occur	• Expensive

- Blood loss is more
- Fracture hematoma is lost
- Tissue trauma is more expensive.

PROSTHESIS OF THE HIP

Prostheses are used for replacement of head of femur following nonunion and avascular necrosis due to fracture neck of femur.

Advantages

- It helps to mobilize the patients early.
- It eliminates the complications like avascular necrosis, nonunion, fixation failure, etc.

Disadvantages

- Function after hemireplacement arthroplasty and prosthesis is not equal to patient's own femoral head.
- The surgery is extensive and time consuming.

---

*So called because on cross-section the nail has colorleaf shape and this gives good rotational stability.

Indications (9 Ps)

- **P**oor general health.
- **P**athological fracture.
- **P**orosis.
- **P**auwels type III fracture.
- **P**hysiological age 60 years and above.
- **P**araplegia and paresis.
- **P**aget's disease.
- **P**rimary internal fixation failed.
- **P**oor union (nonunion and delayed union).

Primary prosthesis replacement is required only in 10 percent of all fracture neck of femur cases.

Types of Prosthesis

There are two types of hemireplacement prostheses used in orthopedic practice, the Austin Moore prosthesis and the Thompson prosthesis (Figs AI.1A and B). Table AI.1 shows the differences between the two varieties of prostheses used in hemireplacement arthroplasty.

Approaches

Posterior: This is the commonly used approach. In this approach, incidence of posterior dislocation is common due to poor healing of the capsule due to flexion, adduction contractures of the hip and increased incidence of sepsis due to proximity of the perineum.

Anterior: This is less commonly employed and is known to cause increased incidence of fracture shaft femur.

Technique of Prosthesis Insertion (Moore's)

The hip can be approached either by the anterior (Watson Jones), lateral (Gibson's) or posterior (Moore's or Southern)

TABLE AI.1: Differences in prostheses

Features prosthesis	Austin Moore's prosthesis	Thompson's
Indications	Fracture neck femur with at least 1/4" calcar femoral left intact	For fracture neck femur with no calcar
Neck	Present	Absent
Collar	Present	Absent
Bone cement	Not required	Always required
Holes	Present	Absent
Locking mechanism	Self-locking	Not self-locking

approaches. The one commonly preferred is the Moore's approach.

The hip is exposed through the posterior approach and the hip is dislocated posteriorly and the head is removed. The medullary canal of the neck and upper shaft is opened and reshaped with a rasp. A notch is cut in the proximal end of the greater trochanter. Now measure the size of the head removed from the acetabulum and select a prosthesis of the same size. Confirm the size of the prosthesis so chosen by inserting it directly into the acetabulum. Now using a hand saw or a motor saw, prepare the end of the femoral neck leaving about 1.3 cm of the calcar to seat the A-M prosthesis. The prosthesis is now inserted into the canal and reduced back into the acetabulum. A check is made for the stability of the prosthesis. Close the wound needed in layers. No external immobilization is required. After two weeks, active and passive movements are begun and the patient can begin to walk between parallel bars after 2-3 weeks.

Complications

- *Infection*: This is due to poor aseptic measures and due to close proximity to the perineum. Incidence is 2–20 percent.
- *Dislocation of prosthesis:* This is rare in posterior approach. Incidence is 1–10 percent.
- *Fracture of femoral shaft:* This can occur if the stem of the prosthesis is forced into an improperly reamed medullary canal and while trying to reduce the head into the acetabulum. The incidence is 4–5 percent.
- *Breakage of prosthesis:* This is a rare complication and can be due to undue stress and strains or faulty material.
- *Pain:* This can be due to tightness into the acetabulum due to the large size of the prosthesis. If the size is too small, the joint will be painful and unstable.
- *Heterotropic calcification*: This is seen in some patients in the dissected gluteal muscles and the capsule.
- *Damage to the acetabular articular cartilage*: This is due to excessive and constant pressure of the prosthesis over the acetabular cartilage.

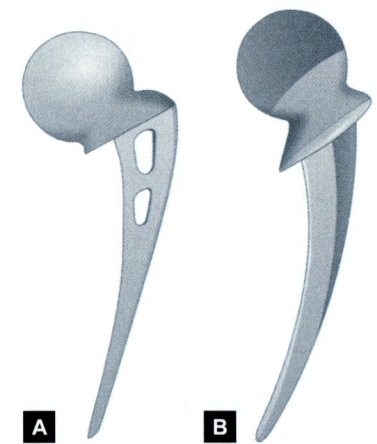

Figs AI.1A and B: (A) Austin Moore and (B) Thompson's prosthesis

DIFFERENT HIP IMPLANTS

1. Fixed angles nails and plates (sizes 2.5"–7" with 0.25")

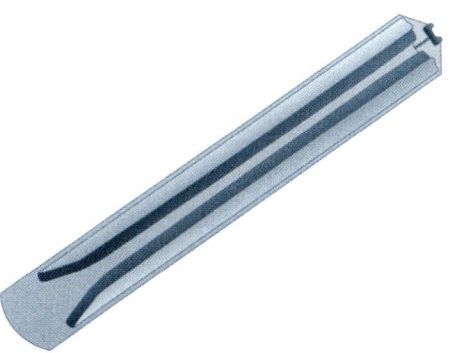 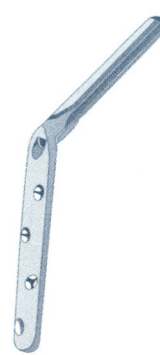

a. Smith-Peterson nail

b. Jewett nail 120 DEG, pin length 2.5"–4" with 0.25" variation (Plate sizes 3–6 holes)

2. Hip fixation pins

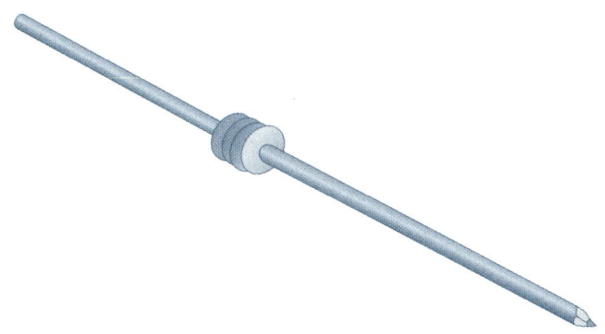 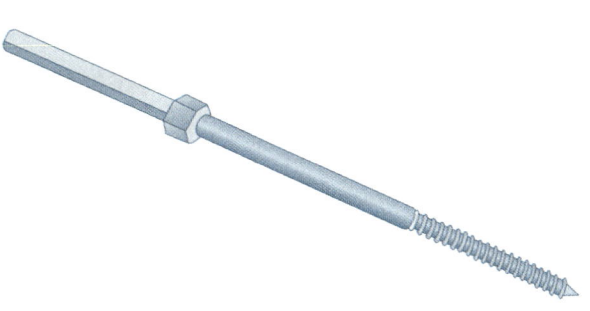

a. Moore pin with two nuts
Sizes 2.5"–5" with 0.25" variation

b. Knowles pin 4 mm diameter
Sizes 2.5"–5" with 0.25" variation

3. Hemi-hip replacement prosthesis

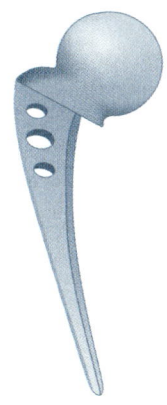 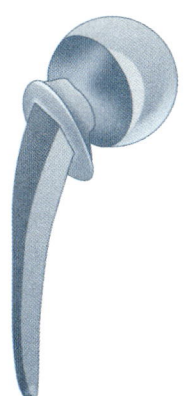

a. Austin Moore prosthesis
Sizes 35–55 mm with 2 mm variation

b. Thompson prosthesis
Sizes 35–55 mm with 2 mm variation

4. Hip screws

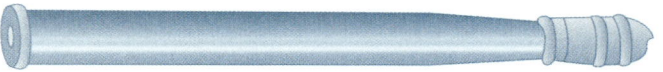

a. Garden screw—short tapping
Sizes 2.25"–5" with 0.25" variation

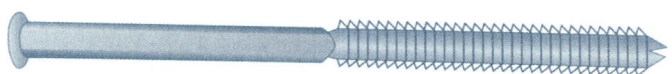

b. Garden screw—extended tapping
Sizes 2.25"–5" with 0.25" variation

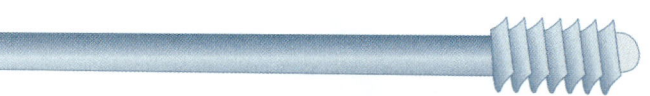

c. Cannulated hip screws (CHS).
Length: 50–115 mm with 5 mm variation

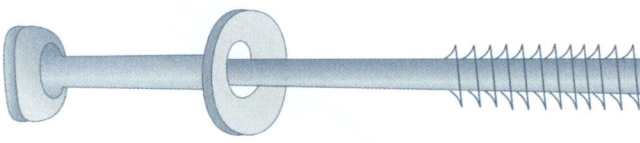

d. Cannulated bolts
Sizes 2.5"–4.5" with 4.25" variation

5. Osteotomy fixation plates

a. Kessel plate 3 or 4.7 mm thick. Sizes 5 or 6 holes

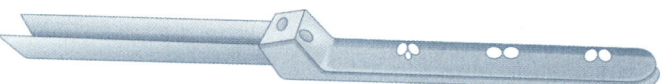

b. Wainwright plate, Blade sizes 2"–2.5" plate sizes 3 and 4 holes

INSTRUMENTS USED FOR HIP HEMIREPLACEMENT SURGERY

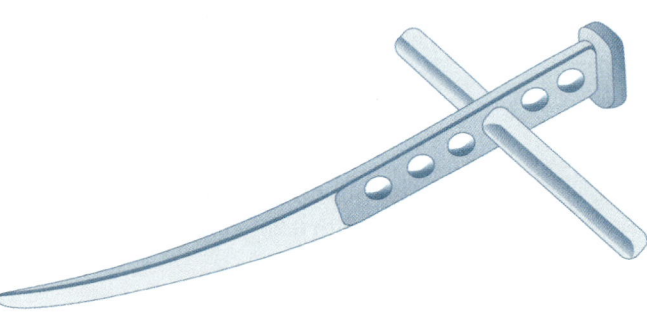

1. Rasp for intramedullary canal reaming for AM prosthesis

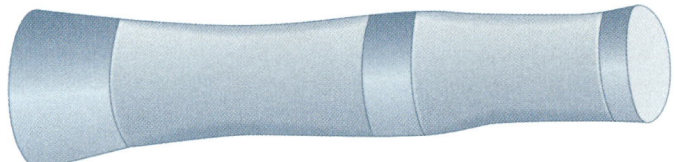

3. Alluminum impactor for AM prosthesis

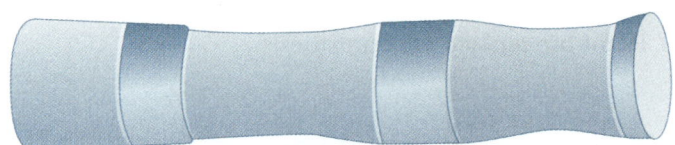

4. Alluminum impactor with tufnol head for AM prosthesis

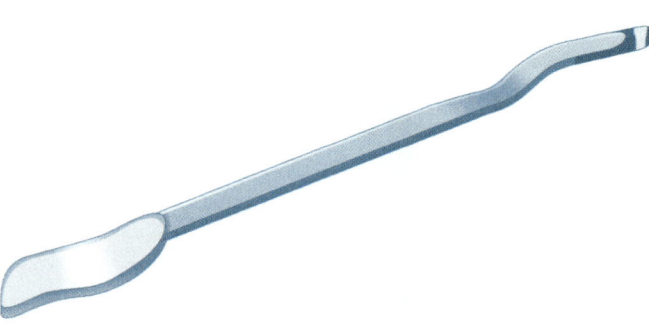

2. Murphy skid

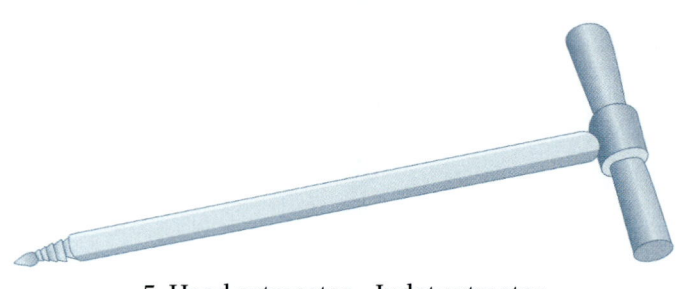

5. Head extracator—Judet extractor

INSTRUMENTS USED FOR SMITH-PETERSON NAILING

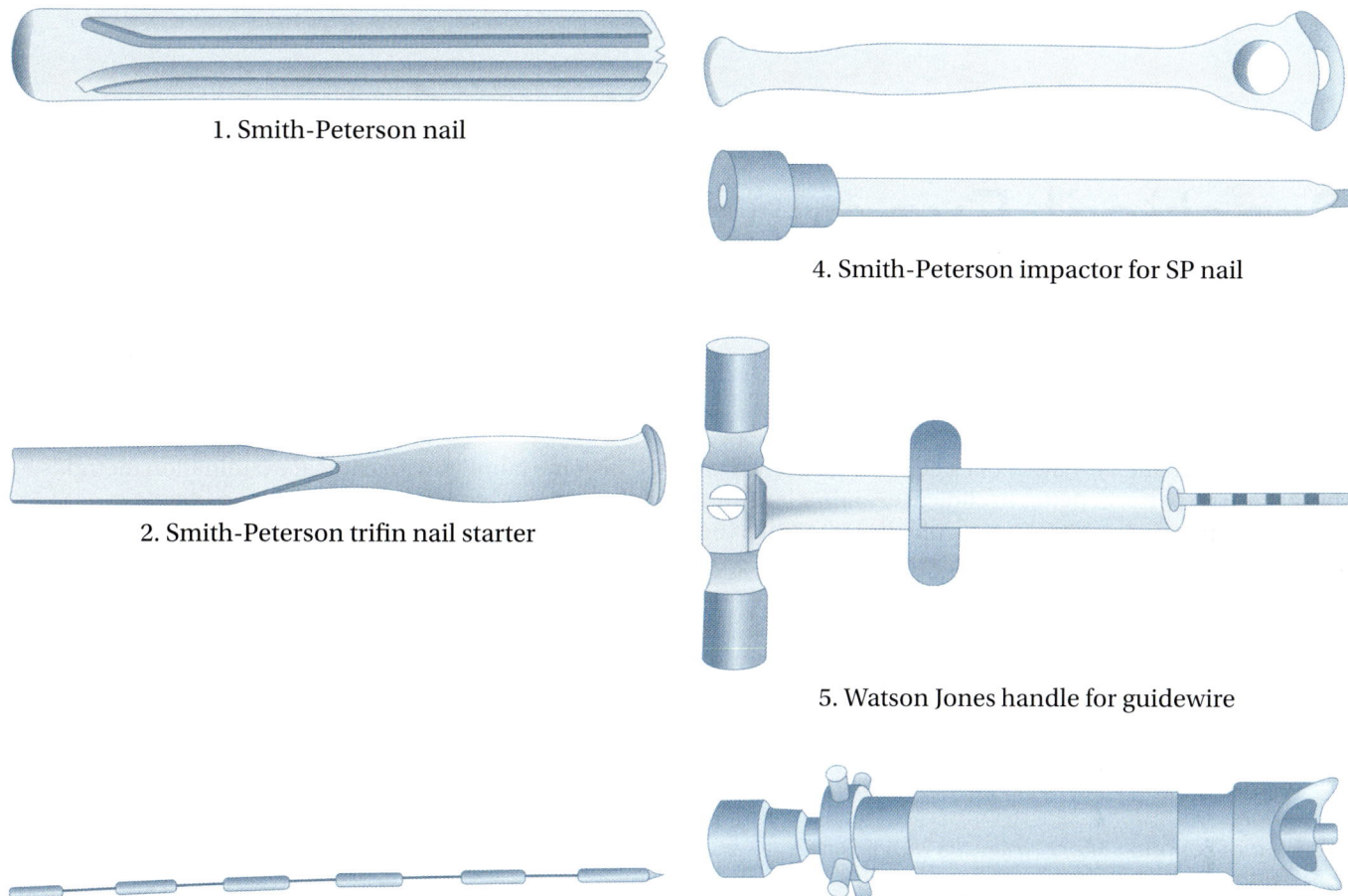

1. Smith-Peterson nail
2. Smith-Peterson trifin nail starter
3. Guidewire—calibrated 9° for SP nail
4. Smith-Peterson impactor for SP nail
5. Watson Jones handle for guidewire
6. Extractor/impactor for SP nail

Appendix II: Guidelines for Practical Examinations

Time and again students have requested me to give practical suggestions to perform better in clinical examination. This section is intended to give some guidelines to help the students to fare better in the practical examinations. *I would like to remind the students that this is only a guideline and not a passport to success.* I can only give clues, but it is the student who has to perform. One has to develop his own method built upon the information given here.

This section is presented under the following headings:
- *Guidelines to perform well in the clinical examination.*
- *Common pitfalls which can be avoided during the examination.*
- *A list of common short cases, the diagnostic clues and pitfalls in each case.*

(Remember only the common cases are mentioned here. There could be a few others also).

Apart from clinical presentation of short cases, a practical examination consists of viva voce which is mainly oral question and answers identifying radiographs of classical cases, instruments and specimens. The important radiographs have been given at the end of each chapter and the instruments have been clearly displayed on the chapter on implants. One need to read them prior to the examinations.

GUIDELINES TO FARE BETTER IN CLINICAL EXAMINATION IN ORTHOPEDICS

- Attend the clinical postings regularly.
- See all the examination cases at least once during the postings or later.
- Read standard books on orthopedics right from the beginning and not at the time of examination.
- Become familiar with clinical examination methods by reading and practicing the correct methods.
- Present as many cases as possible during the clinical postings. This will make you fluent and boost your confidence.
- Inculcate the habit of discussion with the staff, professor and fellow students.
- Try to understand the principles behind treatment, etc.

Do not read for the examination sake. Read to acquire knowledge, since you are going to practice in future. *Examination should just be a part of the exercise and not your goal.*

- In cases of ambiguity, do not give a very accurate diagnosis even though you are very sure. This creates suspicion and hence always give a differential diagnosis.
- Do not argue even though you feel that the examiner is wrong. Mildly, but firmly, express your opinion.
- Do not depend on luck. Try to do things correctly and minimize the errors. Always put up a brave front, look straight into the examiner's eye. Remember luck always favors the brave.
- Do not cry and try to gain examiner's sympathy. Snatch the result with both your hands rather than spread your hands pleading for results.
- Keep cool, use plenty of common sense and be opportunistic. Remember hardwork always pays.
- Certain amount of tension is unavoidable, but do not be overcome by it.
- Keep all the instruments needed for examination in proper shape.
- Remember the examiners were students once and they know all the trials, tribulations and mischiefs. So do not bluff and try to outsmart them.

- Usually clear-cut and straight forward spotters are given in the examination. Diagnosis is not a problem, but discussion is.

AVOID THE FOLLOWING PITFALLS IN THE EXAMINATION HALL

- Make your own diagnosis.
- Do not heed to prompts by examination experts.
- Be cautious with the patients. Fed-up with repeated examination by many students and you, they may mislead you.
- Do not look into the case papers, as things may be erroneous in it.
- Follow a methodical and analytical approach.
- Do not stop after making a diagnosis, look beyond for complications and other changes.
- Make a common diagnosis and be skeptical about rare diagnosis.
- Be on your guard if you are the first student or the last student in the examination. *A fresh examiner and a tired examiner both are dangerous.*
- When things are going tough, keep yourself cool, have presence of mind and look for clues. *Never panic even in extremely difficult situations.*
- By making smart, intelligent moves always lead the examiners into areas of your strength and do not get led into areas of your weakness.

INSTRUMENTS REQUIRED FOR CLINICAL EXAMINATION

- Measuring tape
- Skin marker
- Knee hammer
- Goniometer
- Common pin
- Cotton
- Stethoscope.

COMMON EXAMINATION CASES

Case	Relevant clues	Pitfalls	Ref. page
I. Upper limb • Cubitus varus	• History of old trauma • Gunstock deformity • Loss of carrying angle (compare with opposite elbow) • Movements of elbow full • Arms short	• 95% of cases are due to old supracondylar fracture • 5% other causes • Measurements to be interpreted cautiously The bony measurements are not very useful but are useful in acute cases	138
• Unreduced posterior dislocation of elbow	• History of old trauma • Slightly older child • Fixed flexion deformity of elbow movements are definitely restricted • Wasting of muscles and forearm is short	• Likely to confuse with old supracondylar fracture of humerus • See for points above • Look for other complications of posterior dislocation of elbow	146
• Malunion Colles' fracture	• History of old trauma • Usually patient is an elderly female but not necessarily • Dinner fork deformity if present helps but if absent does not rule out diagnosis • If styloid processes are at the same level, it clinches the diagnosis with certainty • Movements of the wrist decreased	• Dinner fork deformity. If present, helps in the diagnosis; but if absent, does not rule out	629
• Claw hand	• Classical claw hand deformity • Look whether total or ulnar • History of trauma ± • Look for features of leprosy • Carry out tests for all three peripheral nerves • Look for wasting of hypothenar and intermetatarsal space • Trophic changes may be present	• If total, lesion could be higher • Leprosy is a common cause • If ulnar, lesion could be low down • Do not confuse with Dupuytren's contracture. Here, there is flexion of both MP and IP joints. In clawing, there is extension of MP joints and flexion of IP joints of the fingers • VIC is another important differential diagnosis	325

Contd...

Contd...

Case	Relevant clues	Pitfalls	Ref. page
• Dupuytren's contracture	• Long history • Usually affects little and ring finger • See above • Flexion of both MP and IP joints • Examine the other hand also • Cord-like structure felt on the ulnar aspect of palmar fascia • Peripheral nerve tests are usually normal	• Likely to be confused with claw hand	380
• Wrist drop	• Inability of extend wrist, thumbs, and MP joints of the fingers • Extension of IP joints is present. It is brought about by intrinsic muscles of the hand, supplied by ulnar nerve and median nerve	• Tendency to ignore the diagnosis on seeing extension of fingers of IP joints	331
• VIC	• Old history of trauma • Old supracondylar fracture in child • Old both bone fracture in adults • Extensive forearm scarring • Forearm thin, atrophic • Function of elbow and wrist joints are affected • Peripheral nerves affected • Volkmann's sign, if present is characteristic • Claw hand deformity	• Confused with other causes of claw hand • Confused with Dupuytren's contracture	33
• Rheumatoid hand	• Chronic history • Bilateral, symmetrical • Other joints involved • Swan neck. Boutonnière deformity ulnar deviation, etc. • Generalized pain, swelling	• Confused with other hand anomalies described above	566
II. Lower limbs • Genu valgum	• If bilateral, could be idiopathic • If unilateral, look for history of trauma or infection • Deformity is the only complaint if idiopathic • Intermalleolar distance is increased • Late onset genu valgum is a feature of renal rickets (11–14 years) • Movements usually are full range	• In idiopathic variety deformity is the only complaint • Late onset deformity is common with renal rickets • Lock carefully for any general causes, other accompanying deformities, etc.	405
• Genu varum	• Spot diagnosis • Deformity is the only complaint in the idiopathic variety • If unilateral, look for infection and trauma • Common deformity in OA knee • Movements are usually normal	• Not to be confused with genu valgum	407
III. Foot • CTEV	• Present since birth • Classical five deformities • In idiopathic, deformity is the only complaint • Look for other causes • Examine spine and other features of congenital disorders	• If generalized and rigid, suspect AMC • Defect in the spine with a tuft of hair, etc. Suspect spina bifida • Carefully check for muscle imbalance	485
• Foot-drop	• Traumatic history • Leprosy is a common cause • If complete, inability to dorsiflex, evert and invert • Look for trophic ulcers • Follow the course of sciatic nerve to detect the cause	• Always check whether foot-drop is complete or incomplete • Common peroneal nerve affection, either due to trauma or leprosy is the most common cause of foot-drop	334
IV. General • Chronic osteomyelitis *Any bones not joints*	• Chronic history • History of acute osteomyelitis • Characteristic point in history is discharge of bony spicules • Irregular bone thickening • Multiple scars and sinuses adherent to bone • Movements of neighboring joints are decreased • Wasting of the muscles • Sprouting granulation tissue is seen	• Septic arthritis. Here joint movements grossly disturbed unlike chronic osteomyelitis • Ewing's sarcoma	527

Contd...

Contd...

Case	Relevant clues	Pitfalls	Ref. page
• **TB spine** • **TB hip** • **TB knee** • **TB shoulder** • **TB ankle**	• Chronic history • Constitutional symptoms • Monoarticular • Gross wasting of muscles • Movements markedly affected • Lymphadenopathy	• Other joint disorders	536 544 550 552 553

Tumors	Diagnostic clues	Pitfalls	Ref. page
Exostosis Common sites are: • Lower end of radius • Around knee joints • Around shoulder	• Bony hard swelling at the ends of long bones • Immobile • Chronic • Movements of neighboring joints may be decreased • No symptom unless associated with complications	• Look for multiple exostosis which is a developmental disorder	598
Osteoclastoma Common sites: • Lower end of radius • Lower end of femur • Upper end of tibia • Upper end of fibula	• General condition of the patient is normal • Slightly longer history • Young adults • Epiphyseal ends of long bones • No dilated veins • Egg shell crackling may be present or absent • Joint movements are usually affected late • Age: Slightly middle age group is affected	• Confused with osteomyelitis • Malignant bone tumor • Other bone cysts	609
Chondrosarcoma	• Usually a long history • Metaphyseal ends of long bones • Huge size • Patient usually not very moribund	Confused with osteosarcoma which has: • Short history • Patient is more cachectic • Dilated veins are present • Other features of malignancy • Slightly younger patient	601
Ewing's sarcoma	• 5–15 years of age • Very short history • Diaphysis situation • History of fever present • Features of malignancy present	• Confused with acute osteomyelitis • Look for features of osteomyelitis	612

Nonunion of any bone characteristic sites	Diagnostic clues	Confused with	Ref. page
• Lower end of tibia • Patella • Both bones forearm • Neck of femur • Humerus lower 1/3	• History of trauma • Prolonged history of treatment • Painless abnormal mobility • Loss of function • Wasting • In infected nonunion, look for features of chronic osteomyelitis, sinus scars, implants, etc.	• Delayed union • Malunited fracture • Pseudarthrosis tibia	35

Malunion of any bone sites	Diagnostic clues	Confused with	Ref. page
• Humerus shaft • Supracondylar fracture of humerus • Both bones forearm • Femur • Tibia • Clavicle	• History of trauma • History of long treatment • History of treatment by quacks • Cosmetic deformity • Shortening • Altered function • Wasting of muscles	• Nonunion • Delayed union • Deformities due to other causes	44

Glossary

IMPORTANT CLASSIFICATIONS IN ORTHOPEDICS

Spine

- Allen's—for cervical spine injuries.
- Anderson and D'Alonzo—for odontoid process fractures.
- McAffee's—for thoracolumbar fractures.

Upper Limbs

- Neer's—for proximal humeral fractures.
- Gartland's—for supracondylar fracture of the humerus (extension type).
- Bado's—for Monteggia's fractures in adults.
- John Wein's—for Monteggia's fractures in children.
- Stimson's—for posterior dislocation of the elbow joint.
- Shorbe's—for side swipe injuries of the elbow.
- Colton's—for olecranon fractures.
- Frykmann's—for Colles' and Smith's fractures
- Mason's—for radial head fractures.

Pelvis Fractures

- Key and Conwell's
- Tile's.

Lower Limbs

Hip Joint

- Garden's—for fracture neck of femur (intracapsular).
- Pauwell—for intracapsular fracture neck of femur.
- Perlington—for intracapsular fracture neck of femur.
- Delbet's—for fracture neck of femur in children.
- Seinsheimer's—for subtrochanteric fracture of femur.
- Thompson Epstein—for fracture dislocation of the hip.
- Fielding's—for subtrochanteric fracture of the femur.
- Judet—for central dislocation of the hip.
- Neer—for supracondylar fracture of the femur.

Knee and Proximal Tibia

- Smillie's—for menisci injury.
- Hohl and Moore's—for fracture of the proximal tibia.
- Elli's—for fracture of shaft of tibia and fibula.

Ankle

- Lauge Hansen—for ankle injuries.
- Dennis Weber—for ankle injuries.

Foot

- Essex-Lopresti—for calcaneal fractures.

Peripheral Nerve Injuries

- Sunderland.
- Seddon.

Epiphyseal Injuries

- Salter and Harris.

Miscellaneous

- Gustilo and Anderson's—for open or compound fractures.

IMPORTANT RADIOLOGICAL APPEARANCES

Hip Joint

- Trethovan' sign—seen in slipped capital femoral epiphysis.
- Risser's sign—seen in iliac bone epiphysis.
- Shenton's line—for hip dislocations and displaced hip fractures.
- Hilgenreiner's line—for congenital dislocation of hip (CDH).
- Perkin's line—for CDH.
- Sagging rope sign—for Perthes' disease.
- Tear drop sign—for Perthes' disease.
- Garden's criteria—for fracture neck of femur.
- Salter extrusion angle—Perthes' disease.

Knee Joint

Insaal and Blumensaat's lines—for patella alta.

Ankle Joint

- Hawkin's sign—avascular necrosis talus.
- Böhler's angle—for calcaneum.
- Crucial angle of Gissane—for calcaneum.

Shoulder

- Goldie's sign—for periarthritis or frozen shoulder.
- Maloney's line—for shoulder joint, similar to the Shenton's line.

Elbow Joint

- Crescent sign—absence of the normal radiolucent gap of the elbow on the lateral view.
- Tear drop sign—seen in the lateral view of the elbow.
- Anterior humeral line—a line drawn along the anterior border of the distal humeral shaft.
- Fish tail sign—the sharp anterior border of the proximal fragment in supracondylar fracture of the humerus.
- Coronoid line—a line directed proximally along the anterior border of the coronoid process of the ulna.
- Bauman's angle—angle between the horizontal line of the elbow and the line drawn through the lateral epiphysis and the long axis of the forearm.
- Mac Laughlin's line—a straight line drawn along the center of the shaft of the radius cuts the capitulum in the center irrespective of the position of the elbow.

Hand

- Kaplan's lesion—presence of a sesamoid bone within the metacarpophalangeal joint of the finger (commonly index).
- Scapholunate angle—for carpal injuries.

Spine

- Aneurysmal sign—Pott's spine (anterior type).
- Scottish terrier sign—for spondylolysis due to fracture in pars.

Infection

- Sequestrum—seen in chronic osteomyelitis.
- Cloacae and involucrum—chronic osteomyelitis.
- Spina ventosa—tubercular dactylitis.
- Protrusio acetabuli, Mortal Pestle appearance—TB hip.
- Concertina collapse—TB spine.

Metabolic Disorders

- Champagne glass appearance—rickets.
- Moth-eaten appearance—renal rickets.
- Looser's or Milkman's line—osteomalacia.
- Pin head stippling—primary hyperthyroidism.
- Ground glass and biconcave vertebrae—osteoporosis.
- White line of Frankel—scurvy.
- Scurvy line—scurvy.
- Wimberger's line—scurvy.
- Pelkan spur—scurvy.

Developmental Disorders

- Shepherd's crook deformity—fibrous dysplasia.
- Ribbon ribs—von Recklinghausen's disease.
- Marble bone—osteopetrosis.
- Quadrilateral ilium—achondroplasia.

Congenital Disorders

- Von Rosen's line—CDH.
- Kite's index—congenital talipes equinovarus (CTEV).
- Hourglass tibia—congenital pseudarthrosis of tibia.

Bone Tumors

- Soap-bubble appearance—seen in giant cell tumor.
- Onion peel—seen in Ewing's sarcoma.
- Sunrise sign—seen in osteogenic sarcoma.

- Codman's triangle—seen in osteogenic sarcoma.
- Nidus—osteoid osteoma.
- Fluffy, cotton-wool, bread crumb or popcorn—chondrosarcoma.
- Pedicle sign—multiple myeloma.

IMPORTANT FRACTURES WITH EPONYMS

Spine

- Hangman's fracture—fracture pedicle lamina of C_2 vertebra.
- Jefferson's fracture—fracture of C_1 vertebra.
- Whiplash injury—ligament injury of the neck.
- Chance fracture—horizontal avulsion fracture of lumbar spine.

Upper Limbs

- Essex-Lopresti fracture—fracture head of the radius with dislocation of the inferior radioulnar joint.
- Night stick fracture—fracture of the shaft of the ulna.
- Galeazzi fracture—fracture distal radius with subluxation or dislocation of the inferior radioulnar joint.
- Fracture of necessity—other name for Galeazzi.
- Reverse Monteggia's fracture—other name for Galeazzi.
- Colles' fracture—fracture distal end of radius.
- Smith's fracture—fracture distal end of radius with palmar displacement.
- Chauffeur's fracture—fracture of the radial styloid process.
- Bennett's fracture—intra-articular fracture of the base of the first metacarpal bone.
- Rolando's fracture—extra-articular fracture of the base of the first metacarpal bone.
- Jersey finger—avulsion of flexor digitorum profundus from its insertion on distal phalanx.
- Baseball thumb—avulsion of ulnar collateral ligament.
- Mallet's finger or baseball finger—avulsion of the extensor tendon from base of the distal phalanx.
- Barton's fracture—rim fracture of the distal end of the radius.

Pelvis

Malgaigne's fracture—disruption of the pelvic ring with injury to the pubic symphysis and sacroiliac joint on the same side.

Lower Limbs

- Dash board fracture—fracture patella.
- Bumper's fracture—comminuted lateral condyle fracture tibia.
- Pott's fracture—bimalleolar fracture.
- Cotton's fracture—trimalleolar fracture.
- Aviator's fracture—fracture neck of the talus.
- Jone's fracture—fracture base of the fifth metatarsal bone.
- March fracture—stress fracture of the second metatarsal bone.

IMPORTANT CLINICAL TESTS IN ORTHOPEDICS

Neck

Adson's test—for thoracic outlet syndrome.

Shoulder Joint

Tests for anterior dislocation of shoulder:
- Bryant's test.
- Callaway's test.
- Dugas test.
- Hamilton ruler test.
- Regiment badge test—for axillary nerve injury.

Elbow Joint

- Cozen's test—for tennis elbow.
- Gunstock deformity—malunited supracondylar fracture humerus.
- S-shaped deformity—seen in supracondylar fracture humerus.

Forearm

Volkmann's test—for Volkmann's ischemia of the forearm.

Wrist Joint

- Wrist drop—for radial nerve injury.
- Thumb and finger drops—for radial nerve injury.
- Finkelstein's test—for de Quervain's disease.

Hand

- Police tip deformity—for Erb's palsy.
- Claw hand—for ulnar nerve injury.
- Benediction test—for median nerve injury.
- Ape thumb deformity—for median nerve injury.
- Pointing index—for median nerve injury.
- Kanaval sign—for ulnar nerve bursitis.
- Froment's sign—for ulnar nerve injury.
- Tinel's sign—for peripheral nerve injury recovery.

Spine

- Anvil test—percussion by the fist thumping to elicit spine tenderness.
- Straight leg raising test (SLRT)—passive straight leg raising test in disk prolapse.
- Fazerstazan test—SLRT with dorsiflexion of the foot.
- Lasègue test—hip-flexed, knee-flexed and the leg is slowly straightened.
- Buckling sign—after doing SLRT knee is suddenly flexed.
- Sicard's test—after doing SLRT great toe is dorsiflexed.
- Well leg raise test—SLRT of the normal leg.
- Bilateral SLRT—SLRT of both the legs.
- Femoral nerve stretch test—reverse SLRT for high disk prolapse.
- Coin test—for TB spine.

Sacroiliac Joint

- Pump handle test.
- Gaenslon's test.

Hip Joint

- Barlow's test—test for CDH in the newborn.
- Ortolani's test—test for CDH in infant between 3 and 9 months.
- Galeazzi's test—knee flexion test for CDH.
- Thomas test—for fixed flexion deformity of the hip.
- Trendelenburg test—test for abductor mechanism of the hip.
- Ober test—test for iliotibial band contracture as in polio.

Pelvis

- Destot's sign—pelvic fracture.
- Roux's sign—pelvic fracture.
- Earle's sign—pelvic fracture.

Knee Joint

- Lachman's test—anterior drawer test at 30 degrees knee flexion in acute injuries.
- Drawer's test—for anterior cruciate ligament (ACL) tear.
- McMurray's test—test for meniscal injuries.
- Ludloff's test—for avulsion of the lesser trochanter.
- Apley's compression test—for meniscal injuries.
- Apley's distraction test—for knee collateral ligament injuries.
- O'donoghue's triad—injury to the medial meniscus, medial collateral and anterior cruciate ligaments.
- Pivot shift test—for ACL tear.

IMPORTANT ORTHOPEDIC SURGERIES BY NAMES

Upper Limbs

Shoulder Joint

- Putti-Platt's—overlapping and tightening of subscapularis tendon for recurrent dislocation of shoulder.
- Ban Kart's—detached anterior structures attached to glenoid rim by sutures.
- Bristow's—transplantation of coracoid process to anterior rim of the glenoid cavity in recurrent dislocation of shoulder.
- Staple capsulorrhaphy of Destot's and Roux—same as Ban Kart's but staples used instead of sutures.
- Magnusan and Stack—lateral advancement of subscapularis tendon.
- Eden Hybinette—anterior bone graft over glenoid and scapular neck.
- Mac Laughlin—for posterior dislocation of the shoulder.

Elbow Joint

- French osteotomy—lateral closed wedge osteotomy for cubitus varus.
- King's osteotomy—medial open wedge osteotomy for cubitus varus.
- Max page—releasing of structures from medial epicondyle of humerus for VIC.

Wrist Joint

- Fernandez—dorsal wedge osteotomy for Colles.
- Campbell—lateral wedge osteotomy for Colles.

Lower Limbs

Hip Joint

- Souter—release of structures arising from anterior superior iliac spine (ASIS) for polio.
- Yount—sectioning of iliotibial band.
- Meyer—muscle pedicle (quadratus femoris) graft for posterior wall comminution in fracture neck of femur.
- Girdle stone—surgical excision of the hip joint.

Knee Joint

- Wilson—for flexion deformity of the knee.
- Hauser—for recurrent dislocation of the patella.
- Campbell—for recurrent dislocation of patella.

Foot

- Triple arthrodesis—fusion of the subtalar, talonavicular and calcaneocuboid joints.
- Lambrinudi—for severe equinus deformity of the foot.
- Dwyer—lateral closed osteotomy for varus foot deformity.
- Evan—resection of calcaneocuboid joint for CTEV.
- Garceau—transfers of tibialis anterior to middle cuneiform for CTEV.
- Turco—one-stage release of posteromedial structures in mild CTEV.
- MacKay—one-stage release of posteromedial and posterolateral structures in severe CTEV.
- Grice-Green—subtalar fusion.
- Jones'—surgical correction of foot deformity.
- Keller's—surgical correction of halux valgus deformity.
- Steindler's—release of plantar fascia short plantar muscles and long plantar ligament in cavus foot deformity.

TERMINOLOGIES ASSOCIATED WITH FRACTURES

- Fracture—a break in the continuity of the bone.
- Simple fracture—fracture that does not have an open wound in the skin.
- Compound or open—fracture in which there is an open wound at the skin or soft parts that leads into the fracture.
- Comminuted—fracture with multiple fragments.
- Avulsion fracture—small fracture near a joint that usually has a ligament or tendon attached to it.
- Impacted fracture—fracture whose ends are driven into each other.
- Displaced fracture—fracture whose ends are separated.
- Undisplaced fracture—fracture whose ends are not separated.
- Greenstick fracture—incomplete fracture due to break in one cortex of the bone in children.
- Pathologic fracture—fracture that occurs due to bone weakness due to a local or generalized bone disorder.
- Intra-articular fracture—fracture that involves the joint surface of a bone.
- Fatigue or stress fracture—fracture due to repeat minor stresses.
- Taurus or buckle fracture—fracture caused by compression of the cortex most commonly in the distal region.
- Epiphyseal fracture—fracture of the growth plate usually in the long bones.
- Occult or hidden fracture—as clinical condition that suggests a fracture. Radiographs 2-3 weeks later may show the fracture line or a new bone formation.
- Nonunion—complete failure of fracture union.
- Malunion—union of a fractured bones in a position other than anatomical.
- Cross-union—side-to-side union of fracture.

IMPORTANT ORTHOPEDIC TERMINOLOGIES

Joint

- Ankylosis—restriction of joint motion.
- Arthrodesis—surgical fusion of a joint.
- Arthroplasty—surgery to restore motion and function to a joint.
- Arthrotomy—opening of a joint.
- Effusion—escapes of fluid into a joint cavity.
- Dislocation—complete disruption in the continuity of a joint.
- Subluxation—partial disruption in the continuity of the joint.
- Fracture dislocation—dislocation that occurs in conjunction with a fracture of the bone if incomplete it is called fracture subluxation.
- Osteoarthritis—degeneration of a joint.
- Osteophytes—new bone growth due to degeneration of the joint.
- Arthrocentesis—joint aspiration.
- Arthroscopy—inspection of a joint through an arthroscopy.
- Strain—muscle tears.
- Sprain—ligament tears.
- Genu—pertains to knee.
- Cubitus—pertains to the elbow.

Movements

- Flexion—forward bending of the joint.
- Extension—backward bending of a joint.
- Abduction—movement away from the midline.
- Adduction—movement towards the midline.
- Pronation—to rotate the forearm in such a way that the palm looks downwards when the arm is in the anatomical position.
- Supination—to rotate the forearm in such a way that the palm looks forwards when the arm is in the anatomical position.
- Eversion—turning outward of the foot.
- Inversion—turning inward of the foot.

Spine

- Spondylitis—inflammatory condition of the spine.
- Spondylosis—degenerative condition of the spine.

- Spondylolysis—defect in the pars interarticularis of the vertebra.
- Spondylolisthesis—slipping of one vertebra over the other.
- Kyphosis—curvature of the spine with posterior convexity.
- Lordosis—curvature of the spine with anterior convexity.
- Scoliosis—abnormal lateral curvature of the spine.
- Radicular pain—shooting pain due to a spinal nerve involvement.
- Sciatica—shooting pain along the course of the sciatic nerve.
- Laminotomy—opening made in the lamina.
- Hemilaminectomy—partial removal of the lamina.
- Laminectomy—complete removal of the lamina.
- Fenestration—opening made in ligamentum flavum between two laminae.

Foot and Ankle

- Equinus—plantar flexion of the foot.
- Calcaneus—dorsiflexion of the foot.
- Planus—flat foot.
- Cavus—hollow foot.
- Talipes—talus (ankle) + pes (foot).
- Pes—foot.
- Hallux—great toe.

Tendons and Nerves

- Tenotomy—cutting a tendon.
- Tenodesis—attaching a tendon to another tendon or bone.
- Tenolysis—freeing a tendon from adhesions.
- Tendon transfer—transferring a tendon from one site to the other.
- Neurolysis—freeing a nerve from adhesions.
- Neurorrhaphy—repairing a sectioned nerve.
- Neurectomy—sectioning a nerve.

IMPORTANT OSTEOTOMIES IN ORTHOPEDICS

Upper Limbs

- French—for cubitus varus deformity.
- King's—for cubitus varus deformity.

Hip Joint

- McMurray—for nonunion fracture neck femur.
- Shanz—for nonunion fracture neck femur.
- Pauwel—for nonunion fracture neck femur.
- Salter—for CDH.
- Pemberton—for CDH.
- Steel—for CDH.
- Chiari—for CDH.
- Derotation osteotomy—for CDH.
- Innominate osteotomy—for Perthes.

Knee

High tibial osteotomy (HTO) for genu varum deformity in osteoarthritis.

Spine

Spinal osteotomy—for ankylosing spondylitis.

Foot

Dwyer's—for varus deformity of the heel.

Clinical Examination Methods in Orthopedics

- Examination of a Bony Swelling
- Examination of Shoulder Joint
- Examination of Elbow Joint
- Examination of Wrist Joint
- Examination of Hip Joint
- Examination of Knee Joint
- Examination of Sacroiliac Joint
- Examination of Spine

CHAPTER 1

Examination of a Bony Swelling

A lesion in the bone could be congenital, developmental, metabolic, infective, inflammatory, neoplastic or traumatic. To diagnose a bony lesion, a proper history and an accurate examination is necessary.

HISTORY

Age of Onset

Ewing's sarcoma is seen in children less than 10 years. Osteogenic sarcoma in the second decade, multiple myeloma in the fourth decade, etc.

Thus, the age of onset of a bony lesion has a special reference to the diagnosis.

Sex

Osteoid osteoma, osteomyelitis, osteogenic sarcoma are more common in males.

Role of Trauma

Trauma could be a contributory factor (e.g. fracture and its problems like malunion, nonunion, etc.) or could be a precipitating factor or aggravating factor (e.g. osteogenic sarcoma, Perthes' disease, tuberculosis, etc.).

Thus, trauma has a definite role to play in the development of a bony lesion.

Pain

This is the most common complaint given by the patient with a bony lesion. The nature and intensity of the pain varies. It could be acute and severe as in acute osteomyelitis, osteogenic sarcoma, etc. or dull aching as in giant cell tumor, tuberculosis, etc. If the patient complains of night cries, it is suggestive of TB arthritis, if a young male patient complains of pain in the tibia disturbing the normal sleep and relieved by taking aspirin, it could more likely be a case of osteoid osteoma.

Duration

This will be short in acute osteomyelitis, osteogenic sarcoma, etc. but long in cases of chronic osteomyelitis, benign bone tumors, etc.

Deformity

Deformities may develop due to the effects of a bony lesion near the growth plate in children (e.g. genu varum or valgum) (Figs 1.1A and B). Malunion or nonunion of fractures can also cause deformities.

In congenital problems like congenital talipes equinovarus (CTEV) or developmental disorders like osteogenesis imperfecta, the patient can present with deformity as the main complaint.

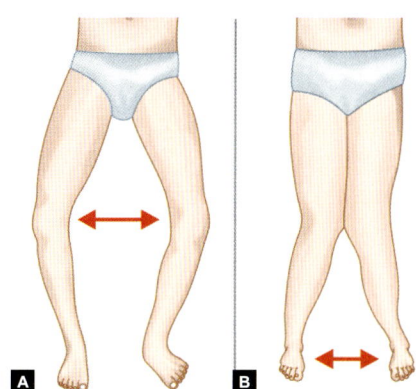

Figs 1.1A and B: Various knee deformities: (A) Genu varum: (B) Genu valgum

Other Complaints

There may be complaints of restriction of movements, discharging sinuses, limp, etc. Constitutional symptoms are present in tuberculosis, malignancy, etc.

PHYSICAL EXAMINATION OF A BONY LESION

Inspection

It is important to make the patient as comfortable as possible and the examining part should be adequately exposed and examined in broad daylight. Look for the following points during inspection:

- *Site of the lesion:* An accurate diagnosis of the bony lesion can be made depending upon the site of involvement (Figs 1.2A to D). Hence, determine first whether the lesion is epiphyseal (e.g. giant cell tumor—GCT), metaphyseal (e.g. osteomyelitis) or diaphyseal (e.g. Ewing's sarcoma).
- *Extent of involvement:* After having established the site of lesion, it is now important to determine the extent of bone involvement. In GCT, one aspect of the bone is involved while in osteogenic sarcoma, the entire circumference of the bone may be involved.
- *Color and texture of the overlying skin:* The skin will be stretched and shiny with dilated veins in osteogenic sarcoma and will appear more red. In GCT, the skin may be just stretched and shiny.
- *Presence of any scars or sinuses:* These indicate the presence of chronic osteomyelitis or old infections.
- *Deformities:* Like cubitus varus or valgus, genu valgus or varus, flexion deformities, etc. should be looked for.

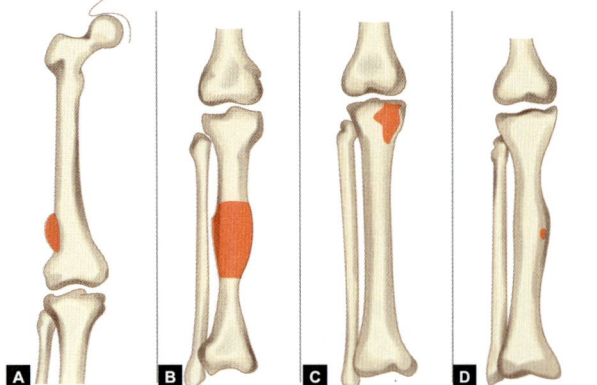

Figs 1.2A to D: The different sites of a bony swelling: (A) Metaphyseal (osteogenic sarcoma); (B) Diaphyseal (Ewing's sarcoma); (C) Epiphyseal (GCT); (D) One aspect of diaphysis (osteoid osteoma)

- *Length of the bone:* Due to the effects of a bony lesion, there could be alteration in the length of the bone like shortening (common) or lengthening (rare).
- *Shape of the lesion:* Find out whether the lesion is globular, oval, etc. by a 3-dimensional examination.
- *Size of the lesion:* Huge swelling is commonly seen in osteogenic sarcoma, chondrosarcoma, etc. Medium-to-small sized swellings are common in bone cysts, GCT, etc.
- *Surface:* In benign bone tumors, the surface is smooth and regular; while in chronic osteomyelitis, malignant bone tumor the surface may be irregular.
- *Edge of the swelling:* Determine whether the edge of the swelling is indistinct or clearly defined.
- *Pressure effects:* Edema of the limb distal to the swelling indicates the pressure effect.
- *Gait:* Find out whether the patient has limp, antalgic gait, short-limbed gait, etc.
- Look for muscle wasting proximal and distal to the swelling.

Palpation

In this step, effort is made to confirm most of the findings observed during inspection.

- *Local rise of temperature:* This is elicited by examining the bony lesion with the dorsum of the hand since it helps detect even minor changes in the temperature, as this is the most sensitive part. Increased warmth indicates increased inflammatory activity of the bony lesion. Compare this with the opposite side.
- *Tenderness* has to be elicited and graded carefully as described previously.
- *Size and shape:* The size and shape of the swelling is measured and expressed in centimeters.
- *Consistency:* The whole swelling is gently palpated and the consistency is graded as follows:
  - Grade I—very soft (like jelly)
  - Grade II—soft (as a relaxed muscle)
  - Grade III—firm (as a contracted muscle)
  - Grade IV—hard (as a contracted biceps)
  - Grade V—stony or bone hard.

  Bony lesions are usually hard, but there can be variable consistency as in osteogenic sarcoma or egg shell crackle like consistency as in GCT.
- Situation of the bony lesion by careful palpation, determine:
  - Whether the swelling is epiphyseal (e.g. GCT).
  - Whether near the epiphyseal line (e.g. exostosis).
  - Whether the swelling envelopes the whole circumference or is eccentric (e.g. GCT).
  - Whether swelling is metaphyseal (e.g. osteomyelitis).

- Whether swelling is diaphyseal (e.g. Ewing's sarcoma).

Diagnostic Facts

Bone site	Lesions
• Epiphysis	• GCT
• Epiphyseal line	• Epiphysitis
• Metaphysis	• Exostosis
	• Osteomyelitis
	• Brodie's abscess
	• Osteogenic sarcoma
	• Bone cysts
• Diaphysis	• Ewing's sarcoma
	• Eosinophilic granuloma

- Palpate the surface and find out whether it is regular or irregular.
- *Edge:* In soft tissue tumors like lipoma, the edge of the swelling slips under the examining finger.
- *Fluctuation:* This can be elicited in a cystic swelling.
- *Translucency:* This can be demonstrated in a cystic swelling.
- *Fixity of the swelling:* A bony lesion is usually fixed to the underlying bone and cannot be moved independent of it.
- *Plane of the swelling:* It is important to determine the anatomical plane of the swelling. By putting the muscle over the swelling into contraction, the plane of the swelling can be determined:
  - If it is situated on the bone beneath the muscle—the swelling reduces in size.
  - If in the muscle—gets fixed and slightly reduces in size.
  - Above the muscle—no change in the size of the swelling.
- *Scars and sinuses:* The presence of scars and sinuses near a bony lesion indicates an old infection and chronic osteomyelitis (Fig. 1.3). Find out whether the sinuses are old and healed or contains sprouting granulation tissue. If present, it indicates a nonhealing sinus and could be due to:
  - Anerobic infection
  - Sequestrum
  - Foreign bodies
  - Epithelialization of the sinus tract
  - Diabetes
  - Steroid treatment
  - Secondary infection
  - Neoplasm
  - Anemia and debility.
- Neurovascular status: It is important to determine the effects of the swelling due to compression of the nerves and vessels.

Due to the compression over the vessels, there could be distal limb edema, discoloration of skin and weak or absent peripheral pulses.

Compression over the nerves causes impairment of the neurological status of the limb distal to the lesion. Examination of the sensory system, motor system and reflexes has to be carried out.

Movements

The movements of the neighboring joints near the bony lesion could be restricted due to:
- The mechanical block created by the swelling near the vicinity of a joint.
- Soft tissue and muscle contractures.
- Intra-articular extension of the swelling (e.g. osteogenic sarcoma).
- Neurovascular compression.

Measurements

The limb is measured for shortening, lengthening and wasting of the muscles. This is compared with the normal side (*see page 349-350).

OTHER EXAMINATIONS

A complete systemic examination is carried out to find out if the bony lesion is a local manifestation of a generalized disorder.
- Find out if similar swellings are present elsewhere. In multiple exostoses, bony hard swellings are found at various sites.
- Examine the thyroid, breast, lungs for evidence of primary.
- Examine the local draining lymph nodes.

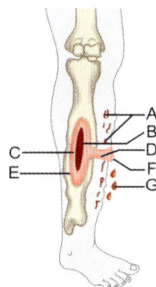

Fig. 1.3: Features in chronic osteomyelitis: (A) Multiple scars and sinuses, (B) Sequestrum, (C) Cavity, (D) Sinus tract, (E) Irregular thickening of bone, (F) Sprouting granulation tissue, (G) Discharge of bony spicules and pus

---

* See *Textbook of Orthopedics*, John Ebnezar, 5th Edition.

After completing the above examination of a bony lesion, an attempt is made to arrive at a proper diagnosis as follows:
- Is the lump congenital? If so, it will be present since birth or appears within a few months or years after birth.
- Is the lump developmental? If so, it will be seen during the developmental phase of the skeletal system and will be most of the times generalized.
- Is it traumatic? If so, there will be definite history of trauma and the patient could have suffered a fracture or dislocation and now could be presenting as a late complication of fractures like malunion, nonunion, contractures, deformity, etc.
- Is it inflammatory? If so, the patient will show features of inflammatory disorders like polyarthritis, systemic involvement, etc.
- Is it infective? If so, the patient will give history of fever, pain, swelling, etc. in acute infections and chronic discharging sinuses in old infections, etc.
- Is it neoplastic? If so in benign, long duration, slow growth, painless, no constitutional symptoms, etc. and if malignant, fast growing, cachexia, constitutional symptoms, etc.
- If it does not fall into any of the above categories, it could be due to:
  – Metabolic origin
  – Degenerative origin
  – Hormonal origin
  – Idiopathic.

Quick Recap
Examination of a bony lesion
- Age of onset
- Trauma
- Sext
- Duration of symptoms
- Where is the swelling—epiphyseal, metaphyseal or diaphyseal?
- How much bone circumference is affected—half/entire?
- Plane of the swelling—bone/muscle/above the muscle
- Scars and sinuses—indicate chronic infections
- Size, shape, surface and edges
- Consistency—hard/variable/egg shell crackles
- Fixity
- Pressure effects
- Movements of the neighboring joints
- Measurements done to know the length of the limb and extent of muscle wasting
- Neurovascular status
- Constitutional symptoms

2 CHAPTER

Examination of Shoulder Joint

Shoulder joint is an extremely mobile ball and socket synovial joint. Because of its high mobility, it is very unstable and more prone to injuries. The shoulder consists of a series of four articulations:
1. The glenohumeral joint (true shoulder joint).
2. The acromioclavicular joint.
3. The sternoclavicular joint.
4. The scapulothoracic joint.

The three primary functions of the shoulder are:
1. Suspension of the upper limb.
2. Fixation for motion.
3. Provision of a fulcrum for the upper extremity.

The following are some of the problems peculiar to the shoulder joint:
- Rotator cuff tears.
- Painful arc or impingement syndrome.
- Frozen shoulder.

The examination of the shoulder consists of history, observations, physical examination and certain special tests.

HISTORY

A patient with shoulder joint problems presents with the following complaints.

Pain

This is the first and the most common complaint. Injuries of the shoulder give rise to acute and severe pain. In chronic disorders, pain is dull aching. In painful arc syndrome, the patient complains of pain only during the midrange of abduction. In arthritis, the patient complains of pain all over the shoulder joint.

The pain in the shoulder joint could be a "true" shoulder pain or it could be a "referred pain" from the cervical spine or thorax.

In the true shoulder pain, the pain is seldom confined to the shoulder joint itself. It usually radiates from a point near the tip of the acromion down the lateral side of the arm to the level of deltoid insertion. *True shoulder pain will never extend below the elbow joint* (Fig. 2.1).

In pain referred from the cervical spine, it starts from the base of the neck, radiates to the top of the shoulder down the lateral side of the arm to the elbow. Unlike the true shoulder pain, the referred pain from the cervical spine frequently extends below the elbow into the forearm and hand and is accompanied by a feeling of pins and needles (paresthesiae) (Fig. 2.2).

Swelling

The swelling could be due to injury or arthritis.

Deformity

In anterior dislocation of the shoulder there will be anterior prominence and the arm will be held in internal rotation.

Loss of Contour

This may be due to shoulder dislocation or due to wasting of deltoid muscle in tuberculosis (TB), rheumatoid arthritis, etc.

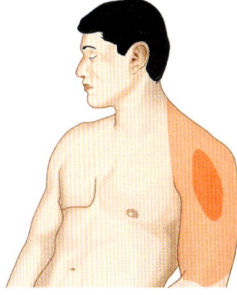

Fig. 2.1: Region of distribution of pain in frozen shoulder

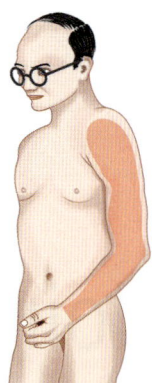

Fig. 2.2: Distribution of radiating pain in cervical spondylosis

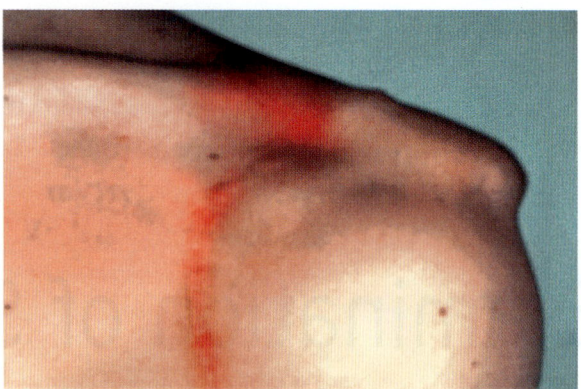

Fig. 2.3: ACM joint injury, the clinical appearance

Restriction and Loss of Movements

This is particularly seen in frozen shoulder, arthritis, etc.

PHYSICAL EXAMINATION OF THE SHOULDER JOINT

Inspection

The patient is stripped down to the waist and is examined in a sitting position. Inspection is carried out from the front, sides, behind and above.

From the Front

First note, whether there is any prominence of the sternoclavicular joint. If present, it indicates sternoclavicular joint subluxation or dislocation. Next, look for any deformity along the clavicle. If seen, it could be due to malunion or nonunion of a fracture clavicle. Any prominence near the area of acromioclavicular joint indicates subluxation or dislocation (Fig. 2.3). Lastly, look for any wasting of the deltoid muscle. If present, it could be due to axillary nerve palsy or a chronic disease like TB, rheumatoid arthritis, etc.

From Behind

Here, the structure to be noted most is the scapula. Look whether the scapula is placed high or low, normal or small in size and if, there is any winging of the scapula (due to paralysis of serratus anterior).

From Above

Look for asymmetry of the supraclavicular fossae on both the sides. Swelling of the shoulder and any deformity of the clavicle are the other points to be looked for.

From the Sides

Note whether there is any swelling of the joint, flattening of the shoulder (anterior dislocation) or rounded fullness of the shoulder (due to effusion).

The following points are also noticed during inspection:
- *Attitude:* In diseases of the shoulder, the position adopted are usually flexion, adduction and medial rotation.
- Wasting of the supraspinatus or infraspinatus muscles.
- Wasting of deltoid or rotator cuff muscles.

> **Note:**
> Rotator cuff muscles comprise those muscles, which fuse with the joint capsule namely the supraspinatus, subscapularis, infraspinatus and teres minor.

> **Quick Facts**
> *Inspection: Shoulder joint*
> - From front look for the prominence of:
>   - Sternoclavicular joint
>   - Deformity of clavicle
>   - Acromioclavicular joint
>   - Wasting of the deltoid muscle
> - From behind—look for the position of the scapula, supra- and infraspinatus wasting
> - From above—look for asymmetry of the supraclavicular fossae
> - From sides—swelling, flattening or rounded fullness of the joint

Palpation

- *Local temperature:* Feel for the local rise of temperature.
- *Tenderness:* Try to elicit the tenderness along the following points:
  - Just below the acromion—supraspinatus tendinitis.
  - Just below the acromion and the arm abducted—subdeltoid bursitis.

- Along the coracoid process—this is the anterior aspect of the joint.
- Posteriorly.
- All round the joint—in arthritis.
- *Swelling:* If this is due to effusion in the joint, it is best palpated in the axilla, as it is difficult to palpate through the deltoid. Swelling and tenderness beneath the acromion process is due to subdeltoid bursitis.
- The sternoclavicular and the acromioclavicular joint are also palpated for swelling, tenderness, etc.

Movements

Movements as already mentioned, shoulder joint is highly mobile and consists of (Fig. 2.4):

Flexion (Normal Range is 180°)

Flexion is best tested with the patient seated. Both active and passive movements are tested.

Extension (Normal Range is 45°)

Best tested in the seated position.

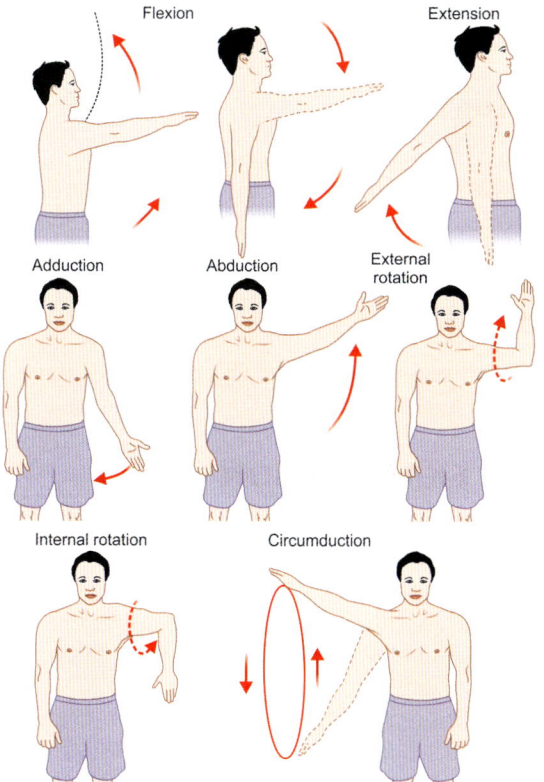

Fig. 2.4: Different shoulder movements

Abduction (Normal Range is 180°)

Best tested in the standing position and both the shoulders are tested simultaneously for comparison.

First 25–30° of abduction of the shoulder joint takes place only at the glenohumeral joint. Later, for every 15° of abduction, glenohumeral joint contributes 10°, and the movement of scapula and clavicle contributes 5°. Thus, totally in 180° of abduction, 100–120° is at the glenohumeral joint and 60–80° is due to forward rotation of scapula and elevation of clavicle. For this reason, in total ankylosis of glenohumeral joint, about 60–80° of abduction is still possible due to the rotation of scapula and elevation of the clavicle.

Thus, to know how much abduction is actually taking place at glenohumeral joint and to know whether the glenohumeral joint is ankylosed, the scapula should be fixed while determining both the active and passive movements of the abduction.

When the patient is actively carrying out the abduction simultaneously on both the sides, observe the following:
- Does the patient shrug his shoulder at the beginning of abduction? If yes, suspect rupture of supraspinatus.
- Is the pain felt in the midrange of abduction and the extremes of movement painless? If yes, suspect subacromial bursitis.
- Is there a sharp pain felt only above 90° of abduction? If yes, it points towards acromioclavicular joint arthritis.
- Is the whole range of abduction painful? If yes, it indicates arthritis of the glenohumeral joint.
- Is the abduction very much restricted? If yes, suspect frozen shoulder (Fig. 2.5).
- Is the abduction nil, when the scapula is fixed? If yes, suspect bony ankylosis.

> **Quick Facts**
> *Abduction shoulder*
> - This is the most important movement of the shoulder
> - Normal range is 180°
> - Both the active and passive movements are tested simultaneously for both shoulders
> - Pain:
>   - Initial—supraspinatus rupture
>   - Midrange—subacromial bursitis
>   - More than 90°—ACM joint arthritis
>   - All through—glenohumeral arthritis
> - Out of 180° abduction—100–120° is by glenohumeral, 60–80° is by scapula and clavicle. Thus, abduction can still take place even if glenohumeral joint is ankylosed

Adduction

This cannot take place beyond the neutral because the arm encounters the body. With the arm held horizontal to

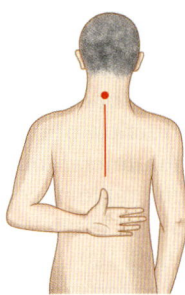

Fig. 2.5: Test to detect frozen shoulder (The distance between the thumb and the base of the neck is increased)

the floor, the elbow in full extension and the hand pointed anteriorly, the patient is asked to adduct the arm across the body.

Rotations

Both internal and external rotations are tested in supine and sitting positions. In supine position, the upper arm is parallel to the long axis of the body and in slight abduction. The elbow is flexed to 90° perpendicular to the examining table and the internal and external rotations are tested. Normal range of internal rotation is 80°.

External Rotation

Sixty degrees in standing position, the upper arm is held in 90° of abduction and the elbow in 90° of flexion and the patient is asked to rotate, the forearm internally and externally from the horizontal. Normal range is 50–90° each.

Other Ways to Test Rotations

- Elbow is fixed to the sides of the trunk, and the forearm is moved laterally. Normal range is 70°.
- With the patient seated, instruct the patient to reach the back. This tests the internal rotation.
- Instruct the patient to place the hand behind the head. This tests the external rotation in abduction.

Useful Facts
About rotations
- Unlike in abduction, scapula has little or no role in shoulder rotations
- Hence, by testing the passive rotation of the shoulder, it is possible to detect the affection of the glenohumeral joint alone

Note:
- Both the active and passive movements of the shoulder should be tested.
- Both the shoulder joints should be examined simultaneously for various movements for purposes of comparison.

---

*See *Textbook of Orthopedics*, John Ebnezar, 5th Edition.

- Abduction and adduction take place in the plane of the scapula, which is rotated 30° anterior and medial. Thus, in abduction, the arm is carried "laterally and forward".
- Flexion and extension take place at right angles to the plane of the scapula. Hence, the arm is carried "forwards and medially".

TESTS FOR SHOULDER JOINT

Apprehension Test

There is a look of apprehension or the patient resists any attempt made to dislocate the shoulder joint.

Bryant's Sign

Lowering of the axillary folds suggests dislocation.

Callaway's Test

Girth of the affected shoulder is increased in dislocation.

Duga's Test

The patient is seated and places the hand of the affected shoulder on the opposite shoulder. The patient is instructed to touch the chest with the elbow.

Inability to do so indicates shoulder subluxation or dislocation.

Hamilton's Test

Normally, it is not possible to touch the acromion and lateral epicondyle by placing a ruler by the side of the arm due to the rounded contour of the shoulder. In dislocation, this becomes possible.

Painful Arc Test

For subacromial bursitis refer Figure 2.6 (*see page 371 for description).

OTHER EXAMINATION

- Examine the cervical spine.
- Examine the acromioclavicular and sternoclavicular joints.
- Neurovascular examination of the upper limbs:
  – Winging of scapula—long thoracic nerve of bell is paralyzed.
  – Regimental badge anesthesia and loss of deltoid power—damage to axillary nerve (Fig. 2.7).
- Systemic examination for tuberculosis, rheumatoid arthritis, etc.

Examination of Shoulder Joint

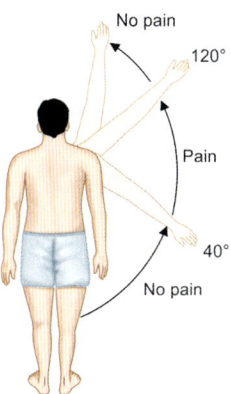

Fig. 2.6: Pain occurs in the impingement syndrome between 40-120° of shoulder abduction as it is in a position that the supraspinatus tendon is impinged against the undersurface of the acromion and head of the humerus. Rest of the movements are painless (painful are syndrome)

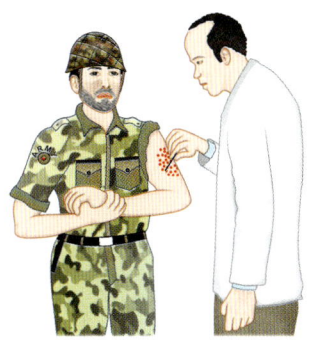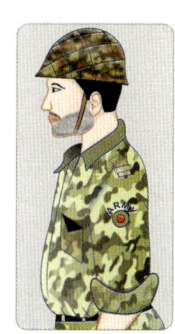

Fig. 2.7: The 'regimental badge' sign

Recap Order of Shoulder Examination
- History
- Inspection
- Palpation
- Movements
- Special tests
- Examination of cervical spine
- Neurovascular examination of the upper limbs
- Systemic examination for TB, RA, etc.

Quick Facts
Important shoulder disorders

Dislocation of shoulder	(*see page 121)
Subacromial bursitis	(*see page 369)
Rotator cuff injury	(*see page 368)
Frozen shoulder	(*see page 366)
TB arthritis (caries sicca)	(*see page 552)
Rheumatoid arthritis	(*see page 567)
Proximal humeral fracture	
Exostosis	
Bone cysts	
Sprengel's shoulder	(*see page 472)

---

*See *Textbook of Orthopedics*, John Ebnezar, 5th Edition.

CHAPTER 3

Examination of Elbow Joint

The elbow is a freely movable joint with three distinct articulations:
- *Humeroulnar joint:* This is a hinge joint. Flexion and extension take place here. Hence, this is the "true" elbow joint.
- *Humeroradial joint:* This is a pivot joint.
- *Superior radioulnar joint:* This is a pivot joint and together with the humeroradial joint provides axial rotation of the forearm.

Elbow joint is commonly injured joint in the childhood. The problems affecting the elbow could be intra-articular or extra-articular. TB arthritis and rheumatoid arthritis are some of the common intra-articular problems while the tennis elbow, golfer's elbow and the student's elbow are some of the famous extra-articular problems of the elbow.

Supracondylar fractures, posterior dislocation of the elbow and fracture head of the radius are some of the common elbow injuries.

The examination of the elbow consists of history, inspection and physical examination.

HISTORY

Patients with elbow disorders usually complain of pain, stiffness and deformity.

Pain

Pain in the elbow could be due to disorders of the elbow joint or could be a referred pain from the neck or shoulder. True elbow pain usually does not extend to the forearm or hand whereas pain from the neck usually radiates below the elbow.

Depending upon whether the problem is intra-articular or extra-articular, the pain pattern in the elbow varies.

In intra-articular problems, the patient complains of pain all over the joint (e.g. arthritis).

In extra-articular problems, pain is usually localized to one area as follows:
- Medial side—medial epicondylitis (e.g. golfer's elbow).
- Lateral side—lateral epicondylitis (e.g. tennis elbow).
- Posterior aspect—olecranon bursitis (e.g. student's elbow).
- Anterior aspect—bicipitoradial bursitis.

Thus, it is important to determine the character and location of pain. Activities that precipitate, aggravate, or relieve the symptoms should be carefully recorded.

> **Vital Facts**
> *Referred pain at elbow*
> - Myocardial infarction
> - Cervical root lesions
> - Thoracic outlet syndrome
> - Subdeltoid bursitis
> - Psychogenic pain
> - Carpal tunnel syndrome
>   – Retrograde pain

Stiffness and Loss of Movements

Elbow joint is notorious to develop stiffness and loss of movements early.

Trauma

Most of the elbow disorders in children and young adults are due to trauma. Fall from height or road traffic accidents (RTA) are the usual causes. Supracondylar fractures of humerus, fracture head of the radius and posterior dislocation of the elbow are some of the well-known problems in these groups. Due to the injury, there could be damage to the neurovascular structures in and around the elbow joint and the patient can complain of vascular or neurological problems.

Deformity

Patients with elbow deformity usually give a history of childhood injury mismanaged or treated by an osteopath (e.g. cubitus varus deformity in supracondylar fracture humerus).

Inspection

The physical examination of the elbow joint begins with a systematic inspection of the joint and extremity. The entire arm including the elbow, forearm and hand should be exposed. The following points should be noted during inspection:

- *Carrying angle:* Like the knee joint a true elbow joint is never straight. The carrying angle is determined by measuring the angle between the longitudinal axis of the arm and forearm when the elbow is fully extended and the forearm supinated. Normally, this angle is about 10° in males and 15-20° in females (due to wider pelvis). Carrying angle is reduced in cubitus varus deformity (*see page 132).

  Note: Why carrying angle?
  This angle helps the upper limb to clear the pelvis while the arm swings during walking.

- *Deformities* of the elbow are very much revealed and consist of the following:
  - *Flexion deformity:* Fixed flexion deformity is the commonest elbow deformity since flexion is the position of ease.
  - *Cubitus varus deformity*—(Fig. 3.1) *(gunstock deformity)* this is usually due to malunited supracondylar fracture in children.
  - *Cubitus valgus deformity:* This is commonly due to malunited lateral condyle fractures of humerus and rarely due to supracondylar fractures (Fig. 3.1).
- *Swelling:* Around the elbow joint could be due to effusion, synovial thickening, periarticular soft tissue inflammation, soft tissue mass, bony enlargement or deformity. The swelling could be generalized or localized. If generalized, it is usually due to effusion in the joint. The features are:
  - Swelling all around the joint.
  - Normal hollows on either side of the olecranon process are obliterated.
  - Fullness in the cubital fossae.

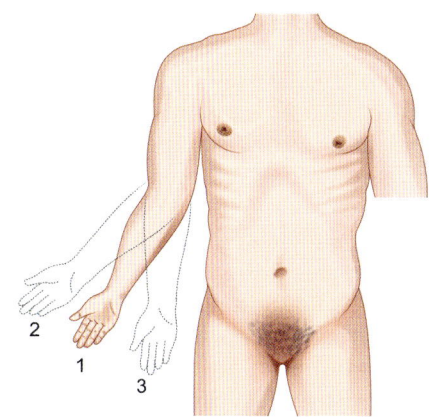

Fig. 3.1: Carrying angle of elbow: (1) Normal, (2) increased (cubitus valgus), and (3) decreased (cubitus varus)

  If localized:
  - Swelling over the olecranon process—olecranon bursitis.
  - Swelling over front of the joint—bicipitoradial bursitis.
- Inspect the soft tissues and skin about the anterior, posterior, medial and lateral surfaces of the joint. The presence and location of scars, sinuses, discoloration, etc. should be noted.
- *Muscle wasting:* Look for wasting of the arm and forearm muscles.

> **Quick Facts**
> *Inspection elbow*
> - Carrying angle
> - Deformities
> - Swelling
> - Soft tissues and skin
> - Muscle wasting.

Palpation

After inspection, a systematic palpation of the elbow joint and adjacent soft tissues should be done. The patient can be examined while sitting or supine, but it is essential that the elbow and extremity be as relaxed as possible. The following points are noted:
- *Local temperature* will be raised in arthritis and bursitis.
- *Tenderness:* The site of tenderness can give clue to the diagnosis.
  - All over the joint—could be arthritis.
  - Over lateral epicondyle—tennis elbow.
  - Over medial epicondyle—golfer's elbow.
  - Over olecranon process—student's elbow.

---

*See *Textbook of Orthopedics*, John Ebnezar, 5th Edition.

- Over cubital fossae—bicipitoradial bursitis.
- Over radial head—fracture head of radius.
- *Bony landmarks:* On the lateral side, the most important bony landmark are the lateral epicondyle. Lateral supracondylar ridge of the humerus is just proximal to it and the lateral surface of the capitellum is just distal. The radial head is palpable approximately 3 cm distal to the lateral epicondyle and is best palpated by holding the elbow in slight flexion and simultaneously rotating the forearm. Feel for the tenderness, crepitus or synovial thickening during this procedure.

The most prominent part on the medial side is the medial epicondyle. Just proximal to it is the medial supracondylar ridge. Just posterior to the medial epicondyle is the ulnar notch of the humerus where ulnar nerve can be palpated.

Posteriorly, the olecranon, the triceps tendon and the olecranon fossae are easily palpable.

Bony relations (Figs 3.2A and B) with the elbow flexed to 90°, the lines connecting the lateral and medial epicondyles and the olecranon process form a near isosceles triangle when viewed from behind. When the elbow is extended, these three structures come to lie in a straight line. The interpretation of these bony points is done as follows:
- Isosceles triangle—normal or supracondylar fracture of the humerus.
- Apex altered (olecranon shifted)—posterior dislocation of elbow.
- Base of the triangle altered—intercondylar or condylar or epicondylar fractures.

Anteriorly, palpate the margins of the cubital fossae and its contents.
- *Swelling* due to effusion can easily be palpated in the region bordered by the lateral epicondyle, radial head and the lateral margin of the olecranon.
- Palpate the lower end of the humerus, upper end of the radius and ulna for any bony thickening.

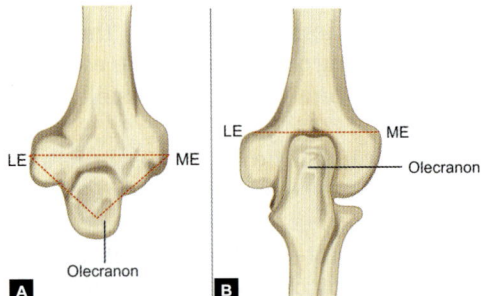

Figs 3.2A and B: Relationship between the three bony points of the elbow in flexion and extension between LE—lateral and olecranon epicondyle, ME—medial epicondyle

- Palpate the supratrochlear and axillary lymph nodes (supratrochlear lymph node is situated on the anterior aspect of the medial intermuscular septum 1 cm above the medial epicondyle. It can be best felt in the flexed position of the elbow. If enlarged on both sides, it indicates syphilis).

Quick Facts
Palpation of elbow
- Feel for the local raise of temperature
- The site of the tenderness gives clue to the diagnosis
- Bony landmarks:
  - Medial side—medial epicondyle
    Medial supracondylar ridge
  - Lateral side—lateral epicondyle
    Lateral supracondylar ridge
  - Posteriorly—the olecranon
    The olecranon fossa
- Posteriorly, the three bony points (lateral and medial epicondyle and olecranon) form an isosceles triangle in 90° flexion and lie in a straight line on extension
- Effusion best palpated on the lateral side
- Palpate for bony thickening
- Palpate for supratrochlear and axillary lymph nodes

Movements

Elbow movements should be recorded and measured after completion of inspection and palpation. Elbow movements are flexion, extension, and rotations (supination and pronation).

Flexion

Range

Elbow flexion is measured from the fully extended position (0°) to about 140–150° and this is recorded as (0–140°). In some patients, the elbow can be extended beyond 0° to say 15–20°. This is called hyperextension (HE) and is recorded as 20° HE-140° flexion. In an individual, where there is a fixed flexion deformity (FFD) of say 40°, the movement is recorded as 40° FFD-140° flexion.

Prime Movers

- Biceps [C_{5-6} musculocutaneous nerve (Figs 3.3A and B)].
- Brachialis (musculocutaneous nerve).
- Brachioradialis (radial nerve).

Extension

- *Normal* is neutral or 0°.
- *Prime movers* are triceps and anconeus (C_{7-8}).

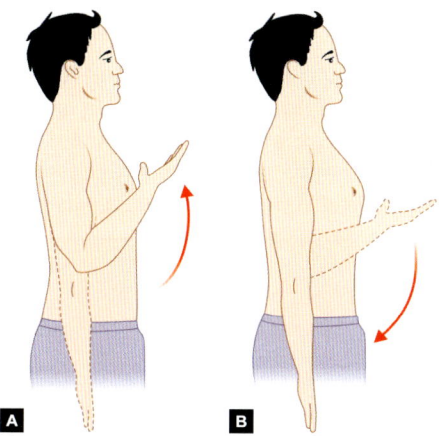

Figs 3.3A and B: Elbow movements: (A) Flexion; (B) Extension

Supination/Pronation Method

The patient is seated, the side places arm firmly, the elbow is held at 90° flexion and the thumb is straight up. Rotation of the forearm with palm facing down is pronation and is normally 45–80° and the opposite movement is supination and is about 85° (Figs 3.4A to C).

Muscles Supination

Prime movers are biceps/supinator. *Accessory muscles* are brachioradialis.

Pronation

Prime movers are pronator quadratus and pronator teres. *Accessory muscles* are flexor carporadialis.

> **Note:**
> Most of the activities of daily living can be completed using approximately 50° of pronation and 50° of supination.

MEASUREMENTS

The following measurements are of importance in elbow joint disorders:

Limb Length Measurements

The length of the entire upper limb should be measured and compared to the normal side (Fig. 3.5).

Method

Arm length has to be measured between the angle of the acromion and the lateral epicondyle, while the forearm length has to be recorded between the lateral epicondyle and the radial styloid process.

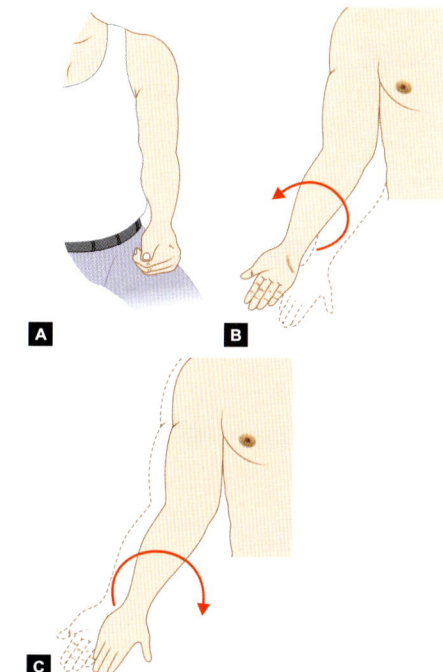

Figs 3.4A to C: Method of examination of supination and pronation: (A) Elbow flexed to 90° and held at the sides; (B) Supination; (C) Pronation

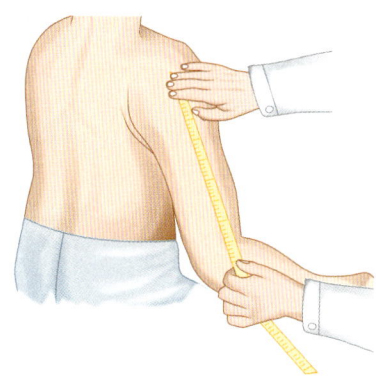

Fig. 3.5: Method of upper arm length measurement

Methods to identify the three bony points:

Angle of Acromion

Palpate laterally along the spine of the scapula. The point at which it meets the acromion process is the 'angle of the acromion'. Mark it.

Like in the hip joint, the true measurement has to be taken from the top of the head of humerus. Nevertheless, since this is not practically possible, the nearest bony landmark, the angle of the acromion is chosen.

Lateral Epicondyle

Palpates the lateral supracondylar ridge and run the finger down along the ridge. The most prominent bony point felt at the end of the ridge is the lateral epicondyle.

Radial Styloid Process

The forearm is pronated and the wrist is slightly flexed. Feel the radial and ulnar styloid processes simultaneously with the index fingers, which are bent to 90° at the PIP joint. Mark the third point.

Wasting of Muscles

Mark the identical points on the upper arms and forearms on both sides and measure the girth of the muscles.

Deformity Estimation

- *Cubitus varus or valgus:* Draw a straight line along the long axis of the arm and forearm, measure the angle and compare it with the normal side.
- *Flexion deformity:* The angle between the long axis of the forearm and the straight line is the angle of fixed flexion deformity.

SPECIAL TESTS

Cozen's Test (for Lateral Epicondylitis)

Affected elbow is slightly flexed and pronated. The patient is instructed to make a fist and actively dorsiflex the hand and wrist against full resistance. If this produces pain at or near the lateral epicondyle, it is suggestive of tennis elbow (Fig. 3.6).

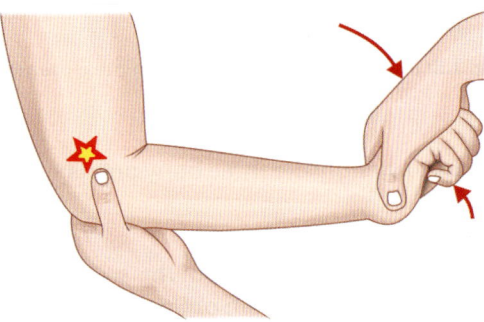

Fig. 3.6: Method of performing the Cozen's test

Golfer's Elbow Test (Reverse Cozen's Test)

The elbow is in slight flexion. The hand and wrist of the patient is in supination. Steady pressure is applied to the supinated hand in an attempt to extend the elbow. The patient resists this movement with active flexion. If pain is elicited at the medial epicondyle, it suggests golfer's elbow.

Quick Facts

Movements/measurements
- Flexion normal 0–140°
  In 20° HE 20–140°
  In 20° FFD 20–140°
- Extension normal is 0°
- Supination normal is 75–80°
- Pronation normal is 85°
- Arm length is taken from the angle of acromion to the lateral epicondyle
- Forearm length is taken from the lateral epicondyle to the radial styloid process
- Estimate the deformity and wasting
- Cozen's test—for tennis elbow
- Golfer's elbow—reverse Cozen's test

Note: HE—hyperextension, FFD—fixed flexion deformity

OTHER EXAMINATIONS

Examine the shoulder joint, the neck and the wrist joints. Systemic examination is required in TB and rheumatoid arthritis.

IMPORTANT ELBOW DISORDERS

- Cubitus varus deformity   (*see page 138)
- Posterior dislocation of elbow (*see page 141)
- Fracture of radial head   (*see page 147)
- Tennis elbow   (*see page 373)
- Golfer's elbow   (*see page 376)
- Olecranon bursitis   (*see page 377)
- TB elbow
- Rheumatoid arthritis   (*see page 566)
- Myositis ossificans   (*see page 39)

Quick Facts

Order of examination
- History
- Inspection
- Palpation
- Measurements
- Special tests
- Examination of neck, shoulder and wrist joints
- Systemic examination in tuberculosis and rheumatoid arthritis

---

*See *Textbook of Orthopedics*, John Ebnezar, 5th Edition.

CHAPTER 4

Examination of Wrist Joint

Wrist joint is not a single joint but consists of multiple articulations, which include the distal radioulnar joint, the radiocarpal joint, the ulnocarpal joint, the midcarpal joint between the proximal and distal carpal rows and the intercarpal joints. The intrinsic ligaments bind all the carpal bones together, while the extrinsic ligaments, the palmar and dorsal radiocarpal ligaments connect the carpal bones to the radius. Stability of the wrist joint depends upon the geometry of adjacent articular surfaces and the ligaments.

HISTORY

Trauma

Trauma has a definite role to play in most of the common wrist disorders. The history could be a slip and fall in the bathroom usually by elderly women (Colles' fracture) (Fig. 4.1), fall from height (scaphoid and other carpal bone injuries), Chauffeur's fracture (e.g. fracture radial styloid process) or sports injuries.

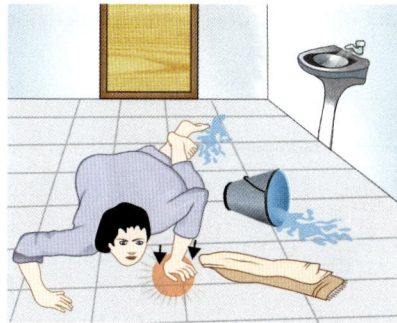

Fig. 4.1: Colles' fracture is usually due to a slip and fall on the outstretched hands in elderly females

Pain

This is the most common complaint in wrist disorders. Pain is severe in acute injuries, while it is dull and chronic in tuberculosis (TB), giant cell tumor (GCT), etc.

Swelling

This could be diffuse as in cellulitis, Sudecks' dystrophy or localized as in case of ganglion, GCT, etc.

Restriction of Movements

Restriction of wrist movements is the other usual complaints.

Deformity

This is the main complaint in cases of malunited Colles' fracture.

PHYSICAL EXAMINATION OF WRIST JOINT

Inspection

For inspection, the entire forearm, wrist and hand should be exposed and any clothing or jewellery should be removed. Inspect the dorsal, radial, ulnar and volar surfaces of the wrist.

Deformity

The following are some of the important deformities of the wrist:
- Radial deviation of hand—marked in Madelung's deformity, radial club hand.

- Ulnar deviation and swan-neck deformity, etc—seen in rheumatoid arthritis (Fig. 4.2A).
- Dinner fork deformity—old Colles' fracture (Fig. 4.3).

Swelling

Swelling caused by intra-articular wrist disorders is typically seen on the dorsal, radial and ulnar surfaces of the joint.

Localized swellings could be due to ganglion, rheumatoid nodule (Fig. 4.2B) or tumors. Eccentric swelling near the lower end of radius could be due to GCT. Compound palmar ganglion is a swelling at both the wrist and palm. Cross-fluctuation is positive. This is commonly seen in TB and rheumatoid arthritis.

Generalized swelling could be due to cellulitis, Sudeck's osteodystrophy, etc.

Scars and Sinuses

If present, indicates old healed infection or chronic osteomyelitis.

Muscle Wasting

Look for wasting of the hypothenar, forearm muscles and dorsum of the hand.

Palpation

Palpation is done with the patient seated or supine. For convenience, the wrist is divided into four zones for palpation (radial, dorsal, ulnar and palmar).

Local Rise of Temperature

Feel for the local rise of temperature over the swelling and the wrist joint.

Tenderness

Palpate and grade the tenderness (*see page 18). Tenderness over the wrist joint line indicates arthritis, tenderness in the anatomical snuffbox (fracture of scaphoid bone); tenderness over the lateral surface of the wrist indicates de Quervain's disease.

Deformity

In dinner fork deformity, due to malunited Colles' fracture, both the radial and ulnar styloid processes will be at the same level; while normally, the ulnar styloid process is 1.3 cm higher than the radial styloid process (Figs 4.4A and B).

Swelling

The swelling is palpated for tenderness, consistency, fluctuation, edge, surface, etc.

RANGE OF MOVEMENTS

The radiocarpal and midcarpal joints provide movements in two planes (Fig. 4.5).
- Flexion (palmar flexion) and extension (dorsiflexion).
- Radial and ulnar deviation.
- Supination and pronation takes place in the inferior radioulnar joint.

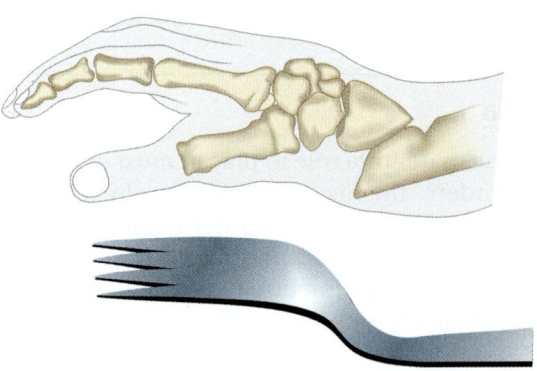

Fig. 4.3: Colles' fracture (A dinner fork deformity)

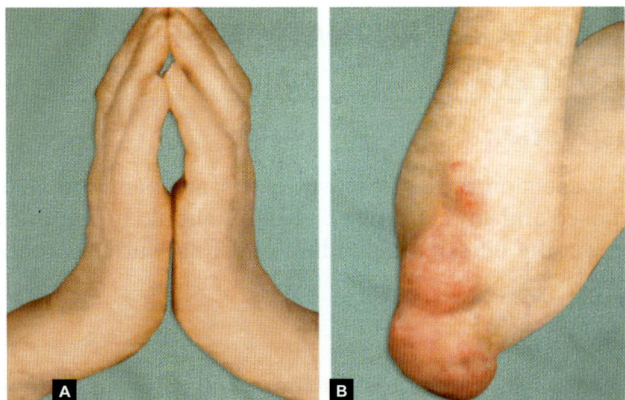

Figs 4.2A and B: Rheumatic features of the hand and the elbow

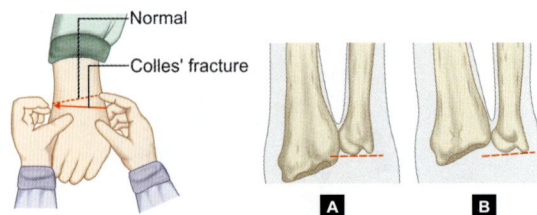

Figs 4.4A and B: Styloid process test: (A) Normal; (B) In Colles' fractures

---

* see *Textbook of Orthopedics*, John Ebnezar, 5th Edition.

Natural Position for Wrist Measurement

Longitudinal axis of the third metacarpal bone is parallel to the longitudinal axis of the forearm. Both active and passive movements are done and compared on both sides.

Normal Range

This is approximately 80° of flexion, 70° of extension, radial deviation 20° and ulnar deviation of 30°.

Procedure

Indian salutation method (for dorsiflexion of wrist): This tests the extension of the wrist. Both the hands are joined, together in a position of doing *Namaskar*. The elbows are slowly lifted keeping the hands in firm apposition (Fig. 4.6A). The angle formed by the dorsum of the hand and forearm is measured and compared with the normal side.

Reverse Indian salutation method (for wrist palmar flexion): Here, exact reverse is done to the method described above. The dorsum of the hand is placed in firm contact with each other and the elbows are lowered as far as possible. The angle formed between the hand and forearm is the range of flexion of the wrist (Fig. 4.6B).

Pronation supination: This method has already been described.

Measurements

The length of the arm and forearm is measured. Girth of the forearm is measured, on both sides from a fixed point.

SPECIAL TESTS FOR IMPORTANT WRIST DISORDERS

Finkelstein's Test

This test is for de Quervain's disease (Fig. 4.7).

Procedure

The elbow is flexed, forearm is pronated. Ask the patient to make a "fist" over the thumb. Now suddenly push the hand into ulnar deviation. The test is positive if the patient complains of pain in the region of abductor pollicis longus and extensor pollicis brevis.

Finsterer's Sign

Percussion at the proximal head of the third metacarpal bone with the arm pronated, if elicits pain, suggests Keinböck's disease of the lunate.

Maisonneuve's Sign

The arm is pronated with the elbow flexed. The hand and wrist are actively dorsiflexed. If marked hyperextension of the wrist is seen, the test is positive and it is seen is old malunited Colles' fracture.

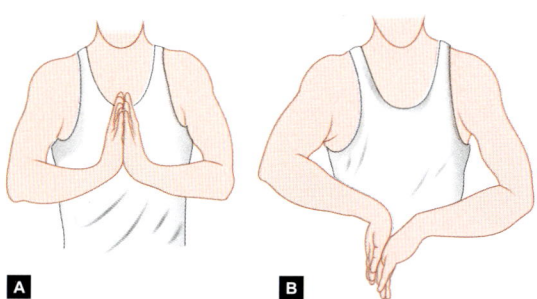

Figs 4.6A and B: Test for wrist: (A) Dorsiflexion; (B) Palmar flexion

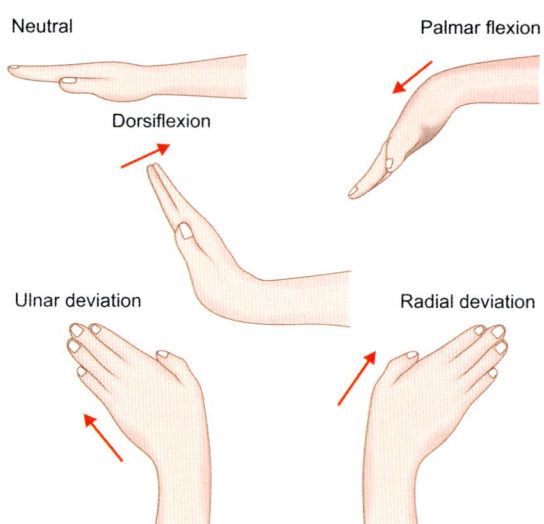

Fig. 4.5: Various movements of the wrist

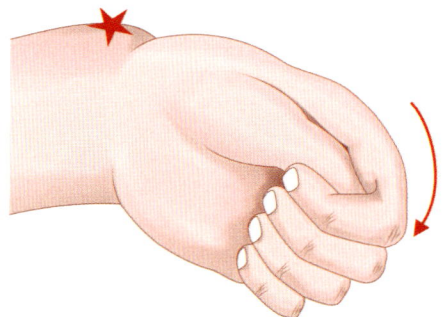

Fig. 4.7: Finkelstein's test

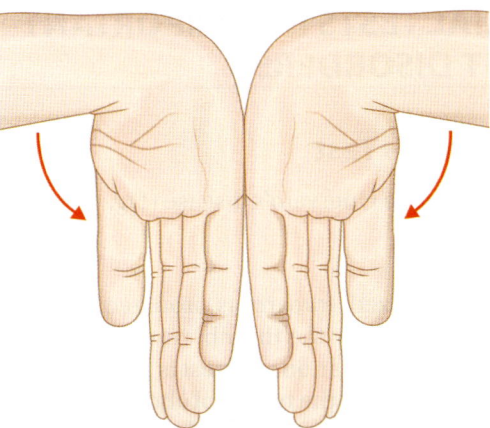

Fig. 4.8: Phalen's test

Phalen's Sign (Dorsal)

In this test, both the hands are approximated at the dorsal surfaces for at least 60 seconds. Median nerve paresthesia indicates a positive test. This test indicates carpal tunnel syndrome (Fig. 4.8).

Carpal Lift Test

Here, the finger to be examined is lifted against resistance, while the other fingers are fixed. If pain is elicited, the test is positive and it is the earliest sign of carpal bone fracture even before X-ray.

> **Quick Recap**
> *Special tests for wrist*
> - Finkelstein's test for de Quervain's disease
> - Finsterer's sign—for Kienböck's disease
> - Maisonneuve's sign—for old malunited Colles' fracture
> - Phalen's sign—for carpal tunnel syndrome (Prayer sign)
> - Carpal lift test—for carpal bone fractures
> - Bracelet test—for rheumatoid arthritis
> - Bunnel Litter—for OA of DCP joint
> - Allen's test—for entrapment of vessels at wrist
>
> *Important disorders of the wrist*
> - *Congenital:* Madelung's deformity
> - *Inflammatory:* Rheumatoid arthritis
> - *Infective:* TB arthritis, etc.
> - *Traumatic*
>   – Colles' fracture   (*see page 621)
>   – Scaphoid fracture   (*see page 171)
>   – Chauffeur's fracture   (*see page 166)
>   – Lunate fracture   (*see page 177)
> - *Neoplastic:* GCT
> - *Bone cysts:* Unicameral/aneurysmal bone cyst
> - *Tenosynovitis:*
>   – Compound palmar ganglion   (*see page 384)
>   – de Quervain's disease   (*see page 378)
>   – Carpal tunnel syndrome   (*see page 381)
>   – Ganglion   (*see page 379)

---

*See *Textbook of Orthopedics*, John Ebnezar, 5th Edition.

5
CHAPTER

Examination of Hip Joint

Hip joint is a remarkable piece of God's creation designed to carry the weight of the body and at the same time help in locomotion. It is extremely sturdy and stable than the shoulder joint though less mobile.

The acetabular component of the pelvic bone and the femoral head, neck, greater and lesser trochanters of the femur constitute the hip joint. The surface palpable bony landmarks of paramount importance while conducting the clinical examinations are the anterosuperior iliac spines, the greater trochanter and the pubis anteriorly; the iliac crests, the posterosuperior iliac spines, the ischial tuberosity and the greater trochanter posteriorly. Next to spine, the hip joint is the most commonly affected part of the skeletal system (Fig. 5.1).

> **Remember**
> *About hip joint*
> - It is a multiaxial ball and socket joint
> - It is the biggest and most stable joint of the body
> - It has maximum stability because of the deep insertion of the head of the femur into the acetabulum
> - It consists of femoral and pelvic components
> - Femoral nerve supplies the hip flexors and the knee extensors and hence the hip pain usually refers to the knee
> - It is the second most commonly affected part of the skeletal system.

HISTORY

How Does the Patient with Hip Disorders Present?

Interestingly, a patient with a hip problem can present with either symptoms (e.g. pain, commonest symptom) or signs (e.g. limp, commonest sign) or both. The following are the common modes of presentations in order of importance.

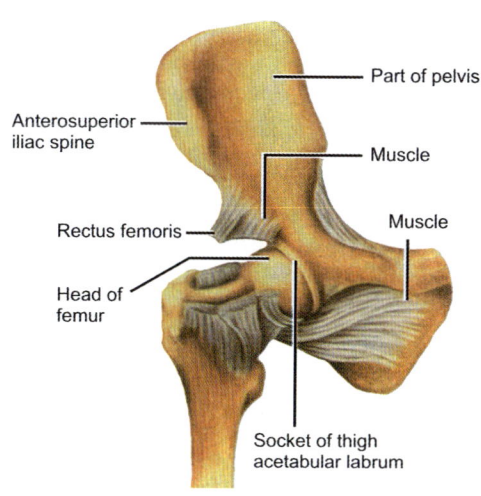

Fig. 5.1: Anatomical structure of the hip joint

Pain

This is the most common complaint of a patient with a hip disorder. Characteristically, if the pain is due to the hip proper, it is experienced in the groin or in front of the thigh or rarely in the knee. Nevertheless, utmost caution is required to interpret the referred pain from the spine or the pelvis felt in the groin. Table 5.1 helps to categories *true hip pain* from the *referred hip pain*.

Limp

This is the second commonest complaint. It could be painful as in acute hip condition (e.g. arthritis) or painless as in congenital dislocation of hip (CDH). *Limp is usually noticed and told by the relatives than by the patient himself.*

TABLE 5.1: Features of true hip pain and referred hip pain

Features	True hip pain	Referred hip pain
Site	Felt mainly in the groin, front or inner side of the thigh or rarely in the knee	If from the spine, pain is felt in the glutei region
Radiation	To the knee and never below the knee	To the back, outer side of the thigh, back of the thigh and leg
Aggravating factors	Decreased by walking	Increased by walking, decreased by stooping, sneezing, lifting, etc.

Important Presenting Signs

Gait Disorders

Since the hip joint is mainly concerned with gait and locomotion, it is but natural that patients with hip disorders have alteration in the normal gait pattern, which varies according to the cause (discussed later).

Problems with Hip Joint Activities

The patient can present with problems like inability or difficulty in sitting, squatting or walking. The reasons could be painful muscle spasms, joint adhesions or arthritis.

Movements

There could be restriction of all movements (e.g. arthritis) or a few movements (e.g. decreased abduction as in CDH).

Deformity

The patient can present with flexion, abduction, adduction or rotational deformities of the hip.

Other Relevant Points

Age

A look at Table 5.2 indicates the importance of age in hip conditions.

TABLE 5.2: Common hip problems according to age

Age in years	Common hip problem
0–2	Congenital dislocation of hip (CDH)
2–5	Tuberculosis hip
8–10	Perthes' disease
10–20	SCFE (slipped capital femoral epiphysis)
20–50	Osteoarthritis (usually secondary)
50–80	Osteoarthritis (usually primary)

Sex

Perthes' disease and tuberculosis are more commonly seen in males, while slipped capital femoral epiphysis, rheumatoid arthritis, etc. are common in females.

Trauma

This could be the cause (e.g. neck femur) or a precipitating or aggravating factor (e.g. Perthes' disease, tuberculosis, etc).

Duration

Longer duration of symptoms and signs are noticeable in chronic disorders like tuberculosis, rheumatoid arthritis, etc.

Constitutional Symptoms

These are commonly seen in problems like tuberculosis, rheumatoid arthritis, etc.

CLINICAL EXAMINATION

Most of the conditions affecting the hip joint can fairly be diagnosed accurately by a good, methodical and proper clinical examination. A student is advised to understand and master the techniques of the art of correct clinical examination of the hip joint, to enable him to arrive at a proper diagnosis.

Ideally, the hip joint should be examined in four positions namely walking, standing, lying and sitting in that order. Nevertheless, sometimes the condition of the patient dictates the choice; for example, if the patient is non-ambulatory, examination of the patient in lying down position is the correct choice. The examination methods include inspection, palpation, measurements and movements.

Preparation for the Examination

The best way to examine the hip joint is that the patients have no clothing on the body. However, this is ideally possible only in children and is impractical in adults especially women, for obvious practical reasons. Hence, a man is allowed to keep his shirts on and cover the genitalia. For females, adequate cover should be provided to cover the private parts and the presence of a *female attendant* or *nurse* cannot be less emphasized in females and it is in them that the hip joint examination provides the greatest difficulty.

Examination in Walking (Gait)

A proper inspection of the gait gives an insight into the hip problem, which the patient might have been affected with.

List of Tools Required for Hip Joint Examination
- *Measuring tape:* Measurement is usually recorded in centimeters and not inches. This is the single most important tool in the examination of hip joint.
- *Skin marking pencil:* It is advisable to use a skin marking pencil to mark the bony points and joint lines and not the routine ink or ball pens.
- *Goniometry:* This is the correct way of measuring the range of movements of the joint.
- *Knee hammer* to examine knee jerk, etc.
- *Tools for per rectal examination:* Per rectal examination are especially recommended in central dislocation of the hip, cold abscess, etc.

Method of examination: The legs of the examining patient should be adequately exposed and the feet should be bare. There should be no constricting clothing like gown, etc. The patient should walk away from the examiner first, then turn around at a given point and come towards him again.

Points to be noted: During the examination of gait, the following points should be noted; Can the patient walk? Does he or she walk in a straight line? Does he fall? Does he or she walk with a limp? If so, does he or she lurch towards the affected side (e.g. coxa vara, CDH) or does he or she lean towards the sound side (e.g. arthritis) or does he or she waddle or lurch on both sides? Is the patient carrying a walking stick and holding it in the same hand or opposite hand?

Hip Gait Disorders

Normal gait and its pattern have been discussed earlier (*see page 346). The following are some of the important gait disorders due to hip diseases.

Short Leg Gait

In cases where the limb has become short due to hip diseases, the patient tries to bring the foot to the ground by tilting the affected half of the body down. In other words, the head of the patient will be lowered towards the involved side when in the stance phase.

Circumduction Gait

In cases of stiff hip, the patient tries to clear the ground by circumducting the whole limb. Here the pelvis will translate during the gait rather than the femur.

Trendelenburg Gait

This is like gait of a duck. Here the body is thrown backwards, there is an increased lumbar lordosis and the feet are held widely apart. The body sways or lurches "side-to-side" instead of the "up and down" movement seen in the short limb gait.

---
*See *Textbook of Orthopedics,* John Ebnezar, 5th Edition.

This type of gait is seen in the disorders where there is a failure of the "abductor mechanism of the hip".

Antalgic Gait

In painful disorders of the hip, the patient naturally tries to avoid weight bearing on the affected side. Therefore, he quickly takes off the weight from the ground and bends towards the normal side. He may also carry a walking stick for the same purpose on the opposite hand.

Gluteus Maximus Gait

This is seen in weakness or paralysis of the gluteus maximus muscle. Here the patient lurches backwards during the stance phase on the involved side.

In Toe Gait

Here the patient walks with both the feet turned inwards. Seen in patients with femoral anteversion.

Quick Facts
About gait
- Gait is the index of hip diseases
- Antalgic gait is the commonest gait disorder. Here the stance phase on the involved side is shortened and the swing phase on the contralateral side is prolonged
- In short limb gait, the patient has an up and down movement and no lurch
- In Trendelenburg gait, the patient lurches to the affected side
- In gluteus maximus gait, the patient lurches backwards

EXAMINATION IN STANDING POSITION

Having examined the gait, examinations are now carried out in the standing position, particularly if the patient is ambulatory. First the clinician examines the patient from the front, sides and then from the back. It is to be noted that examination in standing position is predominantly "inspection" and it is advisable to proceed from above downwards to avoid errors.

Spine

This is best seen from the sides. Increase in the lumbar lordosis of the spine suggests a compensatory mechanism to conceal a fixed flexion deformity (FFD) of the hip.

The Level of Anterosuperior Iliac Spine (ASIS)

Normally, both the ASISs should be in the same horizontal line and should be at 90° to the vertical line or spine (Fig. 5.2). In this position, pelvis is said to be "square."

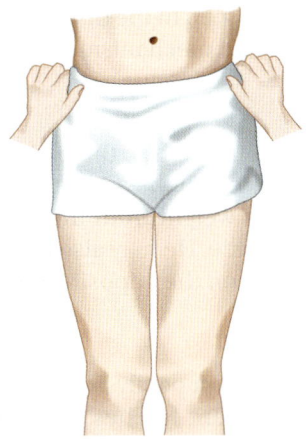

Fig. 5.2: Examination of the level of ASIS on both sides

Flowchart 5.1: ASIS on both sides

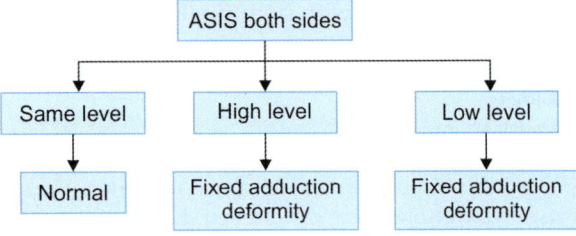

The ASIS will be at a higher level in fixed adduction deformity, and lower in fixed abduction deformity (Flowchart 5.1).

Swelling

Swellings in and around the hip joint indicate the following:
- *Swelling in the glutei regions:*
  - Cold abscess (soft in consistency).
  - Head of femur in posterior dislocation of hip (hard and moves with femur).
- *Swelling in the femoral triangle:*
  - Cold abscess.
  - Enlarged inguinal group of lymph nodes.
  - Head of femur in anterior dislocation of hip.
- *Swelling in the trochanteric region:*
  - Inflamed trochanteric region.
  - Malunited trochanteric fracture.
  - Growth (neoplastic).
- *Swelling in the medial aspect of the thigh:*
  - Cold abscess.
  - Ruptured iliopsoas tendon.

Old Healed Scars and Sinuses

The presence of these indicates chronic hip disorders like tuberculosis, osteomyelitis, etc.

Wasting of Muscles

This is particularly noted in the glutei, thigh and hamstring muscles and indicates chronic disorders of the hip.

Asymmetry of Glutei Folds

Indicates posterior dislocation of hip, CDH, etc.

Stance

A patient with pain in the hip due to arthritis tends to bear most of the weight on the *normal* leg to lessen the weight bearing.

Shortening of the Lower Limb

The limb may be really short (no pelvic tilt) or apparently short (pelvic tilt present). To enable the patient to keep the limb on the ground and thus walk, the following "compensatory" changes take place (Figs 5.3A and B).

Same side	*Opposite side*
• Downward pelvic tilt • Plantar flexion of the foot	• Knee held in slight flexion to shorten the 'normal' limb and thus attempt at length equalization

Level of Patella

The level and position of patella gives valuable clinical "clues" for diagnosis of hip disorders:
- Both patella at the same level and pointing slightly outwards (5–15°)—*normal.*

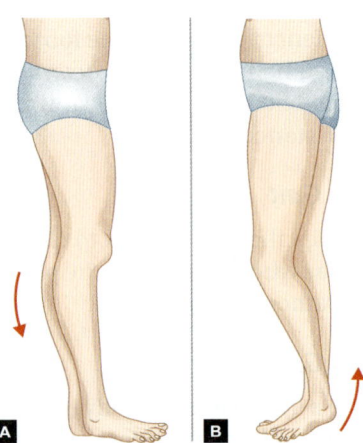

Figs 5.3A and B: Compensation for lower limb shortening by plantar flexion of foot on: (A) Affected side; (B) Knee flexion on opposite side

- Patella rotated outwards more than 15°—*suggests fixed external rotation deformity.*
- Patella looking "straight" or inwards *suggests fixed internal rotation deformity.*
- Patella shifted up—*shortening of the limb or fixed adduction deformity.*
- Patella shifted down—*apparent lengthening or fixed abduction deformity.*

Level of Popliteal Fossa

Alteration of the level of popliteal folds when viewed from the back indicates discrepancies in the length of the legs.

Equinus of the (Ipsilateral) Foot and Flexion of the Contralateral Knee

This has been already explained.

IMPORTANT TESTS IN STANDING POSITION

Trendelenburg Test

This is discussed in detail later.

Block Test

In this test, wooden blocks are used to block the short leg until the pelvis is in level (Fig. 5.4). By measuring the height of the wooden blocks, "true leg shortening" can be obtained.

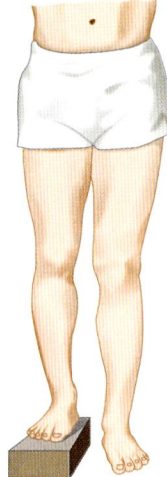

Fig. 5.4: Measurement of true shortening test in the standing position

---

*See *Textbook of Orthopedics,* John Ebnezar, 5th Edition.

> **Quick Facts**
> What to look for in different positions:
> *From front:*
> - Pelvic tilt
> - Shortening
> - Gait
> - Level of patella.
>
> *From sides:* Increased lumbar lordosis
> *From back:* Fullness in the glutei region

> **Quick Facts**
> *Inspection*
> - In ambulatory patients, examination in standing position is the method of choice
> - In standing position, predominant examination method is inspection
> - ASIS at higher level—fixed adduction deformity
> - ASIS at lower level—fixed abduction deformity
> - Lumbar lordosis—indicates concealed fixed flexion deformity
> - Rotational deformities indicated by level of patella
> - Equinus of the ipsilateral foot and flexion of the contralateral knee indicate compensation due to limb shortening
> - Trendelenburg test—for the abductor mechanism of the hip
> - Block test—an accurate method to measure shortening in standing position.

EXAMINATION IN THE LYING DOWN POSITION

Considerable skill is required to carry out a proper clinical examination of the hip in the lying down position and it consists of four steps.

Step I (Routine Examination)

Here, most of the inspectory findings noted during examination of the hip in the standing position are confirmed. The most commonly employed method of examination in this step is *palpation* and is best carried out in the following order:

- Feel for the rise in local temperature of the structures around the hip joint by the dorsum of the hand. It indicates "acute" or "acute-on-chronic" condition.
- Elicit and grade tenderness over the anterior hip, joint lines (e.g. arthritis), over the trochanter (e.g. bursal inflammation, fracture trochanter, etc.) or over a swelling (*see page 18 for grading of tenderness).
- Feel and palpate for a bony hard mass (e.g. head of femur) in the glutei region or in the femoral triangle. A soft mass in these areas indicate soft tissue tumors or cold abscess.
- The greater trochanter: The greater trochanter could be tender (fractured or inflamed bursa), thickened (malunited trochanteric fracture or growth), shifted

up (fracture neck femur or dislocation), or not easily palpable (due to rotation as in femoral anteversion).
- Look for increased lumbar lordosis (called swayback deformity) as indicated by the easy passage of clinician's hand beneath the spine and examination table in the supine position (Fig. 5.5A).
- Palpate both the ASIS on both the sides simultaneously and find out their levels (see Fig. 5.2).
- Feel for the femoral artery pulsation. Normally, it should be just felt. If felt prominently, it could be due to the anteriorly dislocated femoral head. If difficult to feel it could be due to lack of support of the posteriorly dislocated femoral head (called vascular sign of Narath positive).
- Test for the mobility of the scars and sinuses. Fixity of these to underlying structures indicates chronic infection.
- Feel and examine the enlarged group of inguinal lymph nodes.

Quick Facts

Step I
- Palpation is the method of choice
- Feel for local rise of temperature
- Elicit and grade tenderness
- Feel and palpate for bony hard or soft tissue mass in various locations
- Feel for the greater trochanter. It could be tender, thickened, shifted up or not felt prominently
- Look for lumbar lordosis and levels of ASIS
- Feel for femoral artery pulsation. If not felt, vascular sign of Narath is said to be positive
- Test for fixity of the scars and sinuses
- Examine the local lymph nodes

Interesting Facts

About greater trochanter
The greater trochanter is not felt easily in the following conditions:
- Obesity
- External rotation of the thigh as in fracture neck femur
- Internal rotation of the femur in anteversion
- Inflamed or thickened bursal sac

Step II (Deformity Estimation)

In this step, efforts are made to identify and interpret the following deformities of the hip:
- Fixed flexion deformity
- Fixed adduction deformity
- Fixed abduction deformity
- Fixed rotational deformities.

Fixed Flexion Deformity

Fixed flexion deformity is the most common deformity of a hip disease. The reasons for this being:

- In the position of flexion, the joint capacity is "maximum" and hence can accumulate more synovial fluid, which is increased due to synovitis.
- In this position the articular capsule of the hip 'relaxes' the most and thus lessens the effects of pain, spasm and distensions.
- The flexors of the hip are more powerful than the extensors.

Features of Fixed Flexion Deformity (FFD)

Attitude: Normally, in supine position, the back of the patient rests against the examining table and it is difficult to pass the hand underneath the spine. However, if a patient has fixed flexion deformity, there is increased lumbar lordosis and the clinician can easily pass the hand between the back and the table.

Methods to Unveil the Deformity:

Thomas test

Indication: in unilateral fixed flexion deformity of the hip.

Principle: It is to obliterate the increased lumbar lordosis and to reveal the FFD.

Method: This test consists of three steps:
- *Step 1:* The patient lies supine. With the palm of the hand facing upwards, the clinician passes the hand beneath the spine (Fig. 5.5A).
- *Step 2:* Now flex the "Normal" hip until the thigh touches the abdomen. Now the hand can "feel" the spine and this suggests the "obliteration" of the lumbar lordosis (Fig. 5.5B).
- *Step 3:* The affected hip now shows flexion and the concealed deformity stands revealed. *The angle formed between the back of the thigh and the table is the angle of fixed flexion deformity.*

Caution

The thigh should not be overflexed beyond the point of obliteration of lumbar lordosis, especially in children, as this will raise the pelvis and the deformity appears exaggerated.

Limitations of the test: This test is not useful in bilateral fixed flexion deformity.

Problems of the test: The angle measured between the thigh and the bed is significantly inaccurate because:
- The pelvic fixation is actually incomplete.

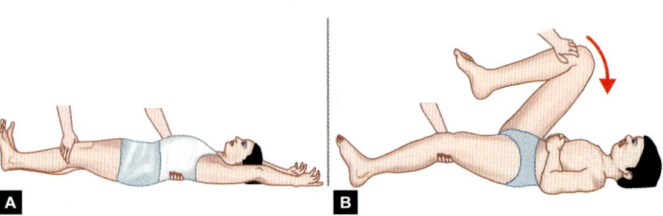

Figs 5.5A and B: Step 1 and step 2 of the Thomas test

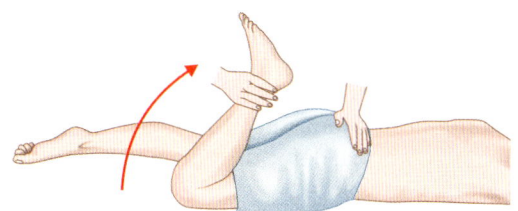

Fig. 5.6: Method of performing the prone test for bilateral FFD of the hip

- The angle formed by the thigh and the table is altered considerably by motion of the thigh with respect to the pelvis and motion of the pelvis with respect to the table.

Prone test:
Indication: In bilateral fixed flexion deformity of the hip where Thomas test cannot be done.

Method: The patient is in the prone position with the body at the edge of the table and the legs hanging out. With the hand of the clinician supporting the lumbar spine, the angle between the body and the thigh is measured and this is the angle of fixed flexion deformity (Fig. 5.6).

> **Important Facts**
> *When to say the patient has FFD*
> - When you can perform the Thomas test
> - The patient lies prone and cannot extend the hip
> - The examiner cannot lift the thigh into extension without simultaneously lifting the patient's pelvis

> **Quick Facts**
> *About fixed flexion deformity (FFD)*
> - Commonest deformity of the hip
> - Compensation is seen mainly in the spine in the form of increased lumbar lordosis. This is also called as "swayback deformity"
> - Thomas test is useful only in unilateral FFD of the hip
> - Prone test helps to measure bilateral FFD
> - FFD signifies loss of hip extension.

Fixed Adduction Deformity

Attitude: The patient lies with the pelvis tilted up on the affected side.
Effects: Due to the fixed adduction deformity:
- The patient cannot keep the feet on the ground.
- The pelvis is tilted up and the ASIS at the affected side is on a higher level.
- The affected limb 'appears' short.
- The angle between the horizontal axis of the pelvis and the long axis of the limb is more than 90°.

Compensatory mechanisms: As mentioned earlier in patients with fixed adduction deformity, the foot is off the ground. To enable the patient to walk again, the following compensatory mechanism develops:

- Spine tilts towards the normal side (convexity on the opposite side).
- ASIS is at a higher level on the affected side due to pelvic tilt.
- Apparent shortening of the affected limb (due to pelvic tilt).

> **Note:**
> The rule of thumb is for every 10° of adduction deformity, 3 cm of "apparent shortening" develops.

Methods to Measure the Deformity (Table 5.3)

Decompensation method: This method aims at revealing the "concealed" deformity. Here the affected limb is adducted till both the ASIS (Figs 5.7A and B) come to lie in the same horizontal line and at right angles to the midline of the body, the angle between the long axis of the limb and the straight line is the angle of fixed "adduction."

Kothari's method: Measure the angle formed between the interspinous line connecting the two ASIS and the horizontal line drawn from the sound ASIS. This angle is formed at the sound side, is above the horizontal line, and is the angle of "fixed adduction deformity".

Significance: Fixed adduction deformity signifies that there can be further adduction in the line of the deformity but there can be no abduction.

Fixed Abduction Deformity

Attitude: The patient lies with the pelvis tilted down.
Effects:
- The patient cannot keep the limb on the ground.
- The limb "appears" lengthened.

TABLE 5.3: Compensatory mechanisms for different deformities

Deformities	Length of the limbs	ASIS	Spine	Compensation	Signifies
Flexion deformity (Commonest)	No change	Same level	↑ Lordosis	↑ Lordosis	No extension further flexion possible
Adduction deformity (Next common)	Apparent shortening	Higher-level	Scoliosis (convexity opposite side)	1. Scoliosis 2. Pelvic tilt	No abduction, further free adduction
Abduction deformity	Apparent lengthening	Lower side	Scoliosis (convexity same side)	1. Scoliosis 2. Pelvic tilt	No adduction further, free abduction
Rotational deformity	No change	Same level	Normal	No compensation	No opposite movements

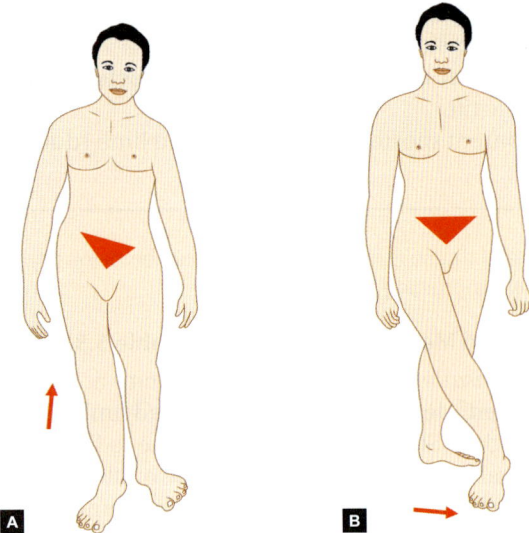

Figs 5.7A and B: Method of squaring of the pelvis by the decompensation method

Compensatory mechanism: To counter the above effects:
- Spine tilts with convexity towards the affected side.
- ASIS is at a lower level due to pelvic tilt.
- Apparent lengthening, again due to pelvic tilt.
- Angle between the transverse axis of the pelvis and the long axis of the limb is more than 90°.

Estimations of the Angle of Fixed Abduction:

Method of decompensation: Here the "concealed" deformity is "revealed." The affected limb is abducted until the interspinous line becomes horizontal and is at right angles to the body. The angle between the long axis of the limb and the straight line is the angle of fixed abduction deformity.

Kothari's method: Measure the angle formed between the interspinous line and the horizontal line drawn from the sound ASIS. Such an angle is formed at the sound side "below" the horizontal line.

> **Significance:** Fixed abduction deformity signifies no free "adduction" movement but only further abduction.

Fixed Medial or Lateral Rotational Deformities

Attitude: The patient lies with the limb in either internal (medial) or external rotation (lateral).

Effects
- The limb is not off the ground.
- There is no apparent shortening or lengthening.

Compensatory mechanism: Nil, as these deformities do not keep the leg off the ground.

Methods of Estimation
- Note the direction of the patella. Normally, the anterior surface of the patella is 5–10° externally rotated. In the lateral rotational deformity, the angle will be more and in medial rotational deformity, the patella looks towards the ceiling or inwards.
- The direction of the toes.
- In fixed lateral rotational deformity, the limb cannot be rotated to "neutral position". The angle by which it falls short of neutral position when rotated medially is the angle of fixed lateral rotation.

> **Quick Facts**
> *About compensatory mechanism*
> - Develops only if the deformity keeps the foot off the ground
> - Develops from structures in and around the hip joint namely the spine and pelvis
> - It conceals the deformity
> - It enables the patient to walk again
> - It has to be undone to estimate the deformity.

Step III (Measurements of the Limb Length)

Measurement of the limb length gives a lot of vital information and clues about the effects of the hip disease. The important measurements are:
- Apparent length of the whole limb.
- Actual or true length of the limb.
- Individual bone lengths.

Apparent Length of the Whole Limb

Due to the bone or joint diseases, the limbs may appear of different lengths. The apparent length of the whole limb is recorded by measuring from any fixed point in the midline of the trunk like the xiphisternum, umbilicus, etc. to the tip of the medial malleolus *without correcting any of the existing fixed deformities.*

The recording of the apparent length gives two vital information:
- The extent to which the skeleton has adopted to keep both the legs parallel and both feet flat on the ground when the patient stands up.
- It also tells about the effect of a joint deformity on the length of the whole limb.

Technique of Measuring (Fig. 5.8) the Apparent Length (in Supine Position)

Step I: Place the limbs parallel to one another and in line with the trunk.

Step II: Measurement is made bilaterally from any fixed point in the midline of the trunk (e.g. umbilicus) to the apex of each medial malleoli.

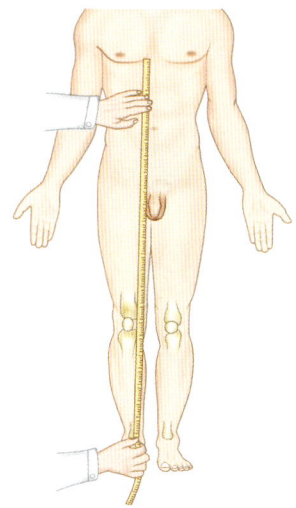

Fig. 5.8: Measurement of apparent shortening

Step III: Determine the true length of the limb (discussed next).

> **Note:**
> Apparent length test is an index of the functional length of the lower limbs.

It is noted that apparent lengthening is seen in abduction deformity of the hip and apparent shortening in adduction deformity. *Pelvis tilts sideways to make the legs parallel.* This test suggests a "leg length discrepancy due to pelvic obliquity". Pelvic tilting with heel discrepancy indicates apparent shortening of the limb. The apparent shortening may be accompanied by some true shortening. The discrepancy at the heels provides a measure of the degree.

> **Note:**
> It is necessary to measure the apparent discrepancy only when there is a correctible pelvic tilt.

Actual, Real, or True Length of a Limb

This is the combined length of the bones and joints not altered by the position of the spine, pelvis or hip joints. In other words, real length of the limb is to be obtained after eliminating the compensatory mechanisms. The real length of the limb has to be measured between the ASIS and the tip of the medial malleolus with the joints being in the "identical" positions (Figs 5.9A to C).

Why should the joints be in identical positions to measure the real length?

Ideally, the real shortening has to be measured from the top of the femoral head to the heel or medial malleolus. Since clinically it is impossible to measure from the top of the femoral head, the nearest convenient bony landmark, the ASIS is chosen. Thus, position of the hip and the ASIS influences the measurement.

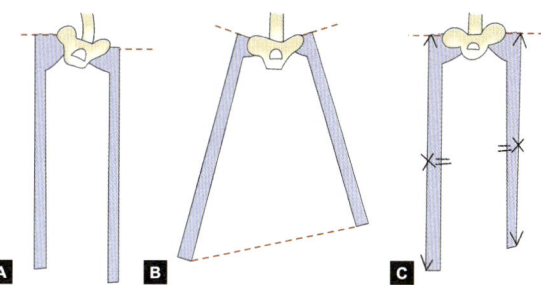

Figs 5.9A to C: Importance of joint positions in measurement of real lengths of lower limbs: (A) Real lengths should not be measured in different joint position; (B) To measure real length bring both the lower limbs to the same position; (C) Measure individual bones to detect site of shortening

The distance between the ASIS and the medial malleolus is "less" in adduction and 'more' in abduction and not the "same". Therefore, both the limbs should be in either "adduction" or "abduction" to get the true length of the lower limbs. This can be done by bringing both the ASIS at the same level by "squaring" before recording the real lengths.

> **What is Squaring of Pelvis?**
> Normally, the horizontal line joining the two ASIS is at a right angle to the midline of the body or the spine. In this position, the pelvis is said to be "level" or square with the spine. In fixed adduction or abduction deformities, this no longer happens. Before recording the real length of the limbs in these deformities, the two ASISs should be brought in the same line by either adducting the limb in adduction deformity or by abducting the limb in abduction deformity. This process of bringing the two ASISs in the same line by either adducting or abducting is called "squaring of the pelvis". For reasons already mentioned, squaring of the pelvis is the prerequisite before measuring the real lengths of the limbs.

Technique to Measure the Actual Leg Length

Step I: **The** patient is supine. First, bring the two limbs to the same identical position by squaring the pelvis.

Step II: **Fix** the tape measure to the ASIS with a flat metal end. The metal end is placed immediately distal to the ASIS and this end is pushed against the ASIS. The thumb is then pressed firmly backwards against the bone and the tape end. This procedure provides rigid fixation of the tape against the bone.

Step III: **At** the medial malleolus, the tip of the index finger is placed immediately distal to the medial malleolus and pushed up against it. The thumbnail is brought down against the tip of the index finger so that the tape measure is pinched between them (Figs 5.10A and B). The point of measurement is indicated by the thumbnail.

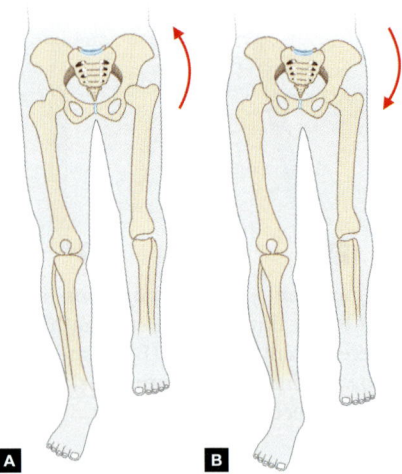

Figs 5.10A and B: Measurement of true limb shortening: (A) Adduction deformity; (B) After squaring of pelvis

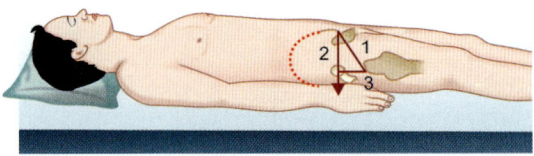

Fig. 5.11: Method of construction of Bryant's triangle

After recording the actual length of the limb, if there is 'real' shortening, it is now imperative to find out the source of the shortening whether it is 'supratrochanteric' or 'infratrochanteric'.

Supratrochanteric Shortening

Here the shortening is above the trochanter.

Causes

- Coxa vara
- CDH
- Fracture neck femur
- Dislocation of hip
- Arthritis of hip—TB or rheumatoid.

Methods of Measurement

- *Bryant's triangle*
  - This triangle is constructed on both sides as follows:
    - *Line 1:* This is drawn between the ASIS and the greater trochanter.
    - *Line 2:* This is an imaginary line dropped perpendicular to the examination table from the ASIS.
    - *Line 3:* This is a vertical line drawn from the greater trochanter to line two above.
  - Bryant's triangle is drawn on both sides and the length of the lines is measured and compared (Fig. 5.11). The difference in the lengths of the third line indicates the upward shift of the trochanter and confirms the supratrochanteric shortening (this is the most important line).
  - The difference in the lengths of the first line indicates anterior or posterior shift of the greater trochanter.

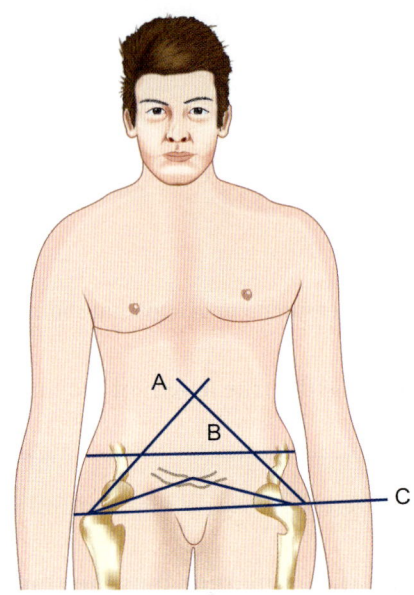

Fig. 5.12: Method of construction of: (A) Schoemaker's line, (B) Chiene's line, (C) Morris bitrochanteric line

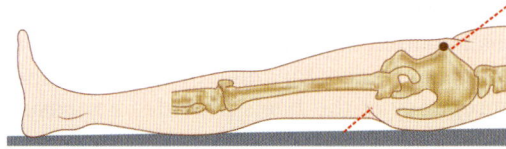

Fig. 5.13: Method of construction of Nelaton's line

Limitations of this test: This test is not useful in bilateral hip disease.

- *Schoemaker's line:* The lines joining the greater trochanter and the ASIS when extended up from both sides (Fig. 5.12A):
  - May cross above the umbilicus in the midline—normal.
  - May cross above the umbilicus away from the midline—supratrochanteric shortening on one side.
  - May cross in the midline below the umbilicus—bilateral supratrochanteric shortening.
- *Nelaton's line:* The patient lies on the side. A line is drawn from the ischial tuberosity to the ASIS. Normally, the greater trochanter just touches this line. If it lies above this line, supratrochanteric shortening is confirmed (Fig. 5.13).

Advantage: In this test, upward displacement of the greater trochanter can be demonstrated without having to compare it with the opposite side unlike in the Bryant's triangle.

If Shortening is Below the Trochanter

If Bryant's triangle, Nelaton's line, etc. are normal, the cause of the real shortening could be below the trochanter.

Causes
- Old malunited fracture femur.
- Old fracture tibia.
- Growth disturbances.

Method of Estimation
- *Galleazi's or Allen's test:* The patient is supine. Slightly flex both the hips and knees, square the heels together by placing a hand behind the heels and record the observations.
    - *In femoral shortening:* Here both the thighs are level but the knee is lower than the normal one. The leg is also slightly "behind" the normal leg.
    - *In tibial shortening:* Here both the legs are level, but the thighs are not level and the knee appears pushed forwards.
- *Direct measurement:* Tibial shortening is now confirmed by taking direct measurement from the medial joint line to the medial malleolus.

True Length of the Individual Bones

After having obtained the "apparent" or "true" lengths of the limb, an attempt is now made to measure the true length of the individual bones. This can be obtained by measuring between two recognizable bony landmarks like ASIS to medial joint line for length of the femur and from the medial joint line to the medial malleolus for *the length of the leg.*

A Quick Recap
About the scheme of hip measurements
- Measurements are best taken with the patient in supine position
- If the patient has 'correctible pelvic tilt', record the apparent length of the limb first
- Then, next eliminate this pelvic tilt by 'squaring' the pelvis. Measure the real or true length of the limb
- Once real shortening is detected, find out whether the shortening is above or below the trochanter
- Lastly, measure the individual lengths of each bone to confirm where the shortening is

Interesting Facts
Do you know the types of shortening?
- *Apparent shortening:* Here the limb is not short, but 'appears' short due to pelvic tilt (about 10° of pelvic tilt creates 3 cm of apparent shortening)
- *True shortening:* Here the limb is actually short due to the pathology above or below the trochanter
- *Relative true shortening:* Here the limb appears short because of the lengthening of the other limb (i.e. pathology is in the other limb). The causes could be:
  a. Coxa valga due to polio
  b. Stimulation of growth epiphysis in children due to trauma, growth or infection

Screening Tests for Quick Diagnosis

Test	Possibility
Lumbar lordosis (Swayback deformity)	Fixed flexion deformity
ASIS shifted up	Fixed adduction deformity
ASIS tilted down	Fixed abduction deformity
Patella externally rotated >10°	Fixed external rotation deformity
Patella facing inwards	Fixed internal rotation deformity
Pelvic tilt with heel discrepancy	Apparent shortening
No pelvic tilt but heel discrepancy	True shortening
Equinus ipsilateral and contralateral knee flexion	True shortening

Tests for Infratrochanteric Shortening
- Galeazzi's or Allis test
- Actual measurement of the limbs

Step IV (Examination of the Movements of the Hip Joint)

Hip joint is a multiaxial ball and socket joint with flexion, extension, adduction, abduction, internal or medial rotation, external or lateral rotation and circumduction.

Flexion
- *Normal range:* With the thigh flexed, it is 0-120°. With the thigh extended, it is 0-75-90° (due to tight hamstrings) (Fig. 5.14).
- *Muscles*
    - *Prime movers* are iliopsoas and iliacus.
    - *Accessory muscles* are rectus femoris, sartorius tensor fascia latae, pectineus, adductor brevis, longus, and oblique fibers of adductor magnus.
- *Methods of examination*
    - *Sitting posture:* The patient sits with the hip and knee flexed. By holding the edge of the table, the pelvis gets fixed. The examiner further stabilizes the pelvis with one hand and provides resistance to hip flexion with his other hand proximal to the knee.
    - *Supine method:* If the patient does not have fixed flexion deformity, flexion of the hip is tested with both the knees flexed and extended. If there is FFD,

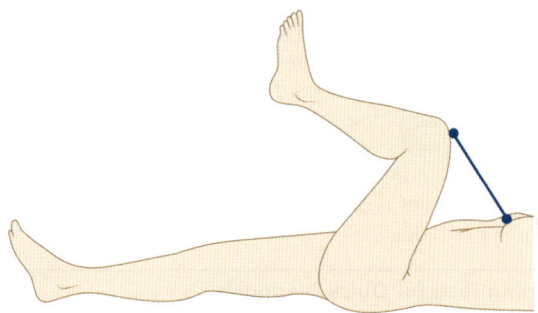

Fig. 5.14: Hip flexion

Thomas test is done first and the angle is recorded. Further, flexion is then done and measured.

Extension

- *Normal range:* 0–15°.
- *Muscles*
  - *Prime movers*—gluteus maximus muscle.
  - *Accessory muscles*—semimembranosus, semitendinosus, and long head of biceps.
- *Method:* The patient is in prone position. The examiner passively lifts the thigh from the bed to record the extension (Fig. 5.15A).

Adduction

- *Normal range:* 30°.
- *Muscles:* Adductor magnus, brevis, longus, pectineus and gracilis.
- *Method:* The patient is supine. The examiner fixes the pelvis by holding the ASIS and the limb is adducted. Note at what level the limb crosses the opposite thigh:
  - In the middle 1/3—normal
  - In the upper 1/3—↑adduction (e.g. CDH⁺)
  - In the lower 1/3 or less—↑adduction.

If there is fixed adduction deformity, square the pelvis and then test for further adduction.

Abduction

- *Normal range:* 45°.
- *Muscles*
  - *Prime movers*—gluteus medius.
  - *Accessory muscles*—gluteus minimus, tensor fasciae latae, upper fibers of gluteus maximus.
- *Method*
  - The patient is in supine position. Steady the pelvis by fixing the ASIS and the limb is slowly abducted and the angle is measured (Fig. 5.15B).
  - In fixed abduction deformity, first square the pelvis and then test for further "free" abduction and compare with the normal limb.

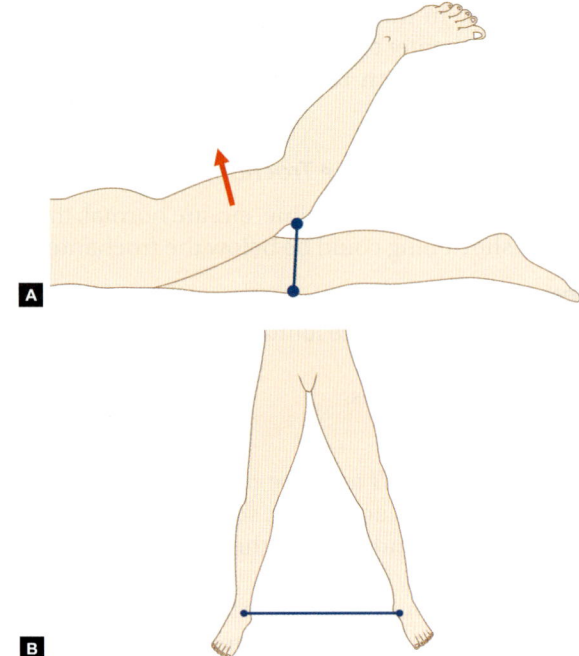

Figs 5.15A and B: (A) Method of recording hip extension; (B) Method of recording hip abduction and adduction

Internal Rotation

- *Normal range:* 35–40°.
- *Muscles*
  - *Prime movers*—gluteus minimus, tensor fasciae latae.
  - *Accessory muscles*—gluteus medius, semitendinosus and semimembranosus.

External Rotation

- *Normal range:* 45°.
- *Muscles:*
  - *Prime movers*—obturator externus and internus, piriformis, superior and inferior gemelli and gluteus maximus.
  - *Accessory muscle*—sartorius.

Methods of Examination

In supine position
- By rolling the limb gently sideways in the supine position, internal and external rotations can be determined by looking at the direction of the toes and patella.
- By flexing the hip and knee to 90°, both the legs are simultaneously rotated internally or externally and the range is recorded (Figs 5.16A and B).

In the prone position: Hip is extended and the knee is flexed to 90°. The patient is asked to internally and externally rotate and the range is recorded (Fig. 5.17).

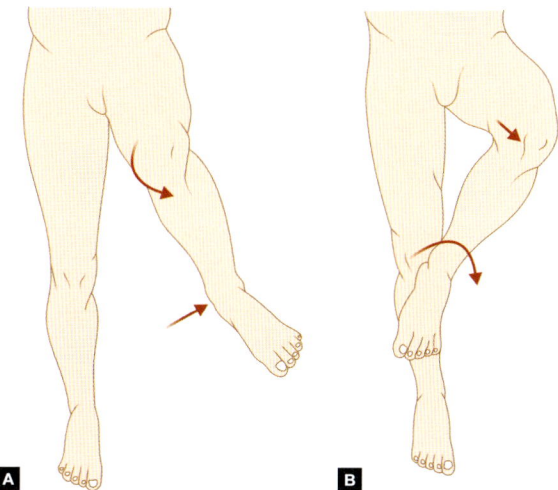

Figs 5.16A and B: Method of recording hip: (A) Internal rotation; (B) External rotation

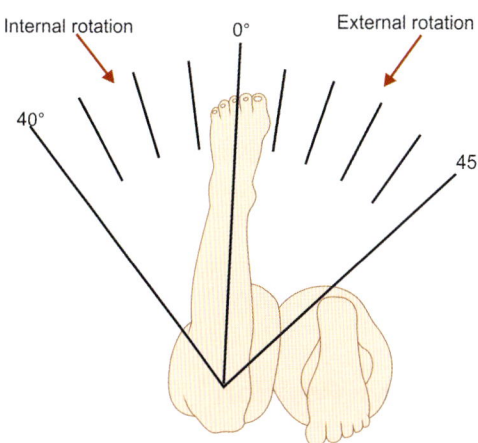

Fig. 5.17: Measurement of hip rotations in prone position

TESTS FOR HIP STABILITY

A normal stable hip is required for locomotion, walking, etc. The stability of the hip is dependent upon a good abductor mechanism of the hip. The following tests enable to determine the stability of the hip.

In Standing Position

Trendelenburg Test

Principle: This is a test for the abductor mechanism of the hip. The abductor mechanism of the hip consists of the head of the femur (fulcrum), the neck of the femur (lever) and the abductor mechanism (power).

In the normal posture, the weight of the body is distributed equally on both the lower limbs and the center of gravity falls between the two limbs. If, for example, left limb is lifted, the weight of the body and the weight of the left lower limb now falls on the right lower limb. Consequently, the center of gravity automatically shifts to the left to maintain balance. This tends to pull the opposite pelvis down. To counter this pelvic tilt, on the left side, the right abductor muscles of the hip contract and pull the (left) side of the pelvis up and prevent it from sinking. If there is a failure of the abductor mechanism, this no longer happens and the pelvis on the opposite side sinks.

Test (Figs 5.18A and B)

The patient is first asked to stand on the normal limb. The pelvis on the opposite side rises (or alternatively the iliac crest will be low on the standing side and high on the side of the elevated leg) due to the intact abductor mechanism of the hip on the normal side. The patient is now made to stand on the affected limb. Due to the faulty abductor mechanism,

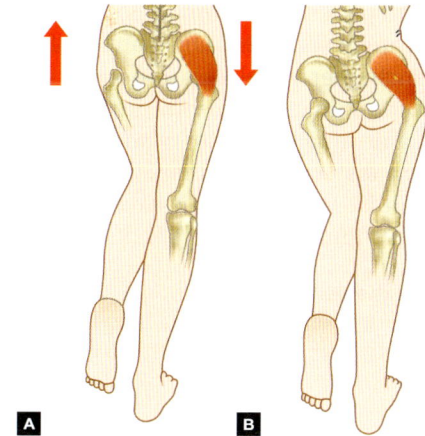

Figs 5.18A and B: Showing Trendelenburg test: (A) Normal; (B) Positive

the opposite side of the pelvis sinks (or alternatively the iliac crest will be high on the standing side and low on the side of the elevated leg). The test is said to be positive.

Causes

- *Failure in power:* Gluteus medius weakness or paralysis due to polio, etc.
- *Failure in lever:* Fracture neck femur, trochanteric fracture, etc.
- *Failure in fulcrum:* Arthritis due to TB and rheumatoid, dislocation of hip, etc.

  Sometimes, two or more factors operate:

  In upward dislocation of the hip, there is a failure in the fulcrum and slack abductor muscles due to upward shift of the greater trochanter.

Note:
False positives are seen in 10% of the patients with hip pain.

Quick Facts
Trendelenburg test
- It is a test for stability of the hip and the ability of the hip abductors to stabilize the pelvis on the femur
- Test the abductor mechanism of the hip
- Important causes:
  - Glutei weakness or paralysis (polio)
  - Glutei inhibition (due to hip pain)
  - Glutei insufficiency (due to coxa vara)
  - CDH
- False-positive results are seen in 10% of the cases
- Positive test suggests the insufficiency of the hip abductor mechanism

In Lying Down Position

Telescopy Test

Principle: This is a test for hip stability.

Procedure: The patient is in supine position, the patient's knee and hip are flexed to 90°. One hand is placed beneath the greater trochanter to feel for it. The femur is now pushed down into the examination table. The femur and leg are then lifted up. In a normal hip, little movement occurs during the action. In a dislocated hip, there will be a lot of relative movement felt by the hand. This excessive movement is called the telescoping of the hip (Fig. 5.19).

Limitations of the Test
- It is not useful in painful conditions of the hip as the patient is unable to flex the hip
- It is difficult to perform in fat or obese people
- This test is mainly useful in neonates and children where it is easy to perform
- Particularly useful in conditions like:
  - CDH
  - Old and neglected posterior dislocation of the hip
  - Nonunion fracture neck femur

Other Tests

Measurement of muscle wasting: The thigh and the leg muscles are measured for muscle wasting as follows.

Marks are made at a convenient distance from the ASIS or from the patella (say about 18 cm up) on both the sides and the measurement is taken. The difference between the circumference of the two thighs or leg is the amount of wasting (Fig. 5.20).

Quick Facts
Order of hip joint examination
- Clinical history
- Preparation and tools for the examination

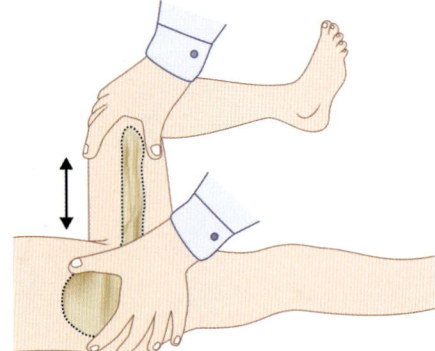

Fig. 5.19: Telescopy test (Examination of hip)

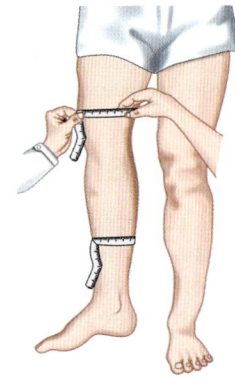

Fig. 5.20: Measurement of the lower limb girth

- Examination in walking—mainly inspection
- Examination in standing—mainly inspection
- Examination in lying positions—mainly palpation

This has four important steps:
Step I: Routine examination
Step II: Deformity assessment
Step III: Measurement of limb length
Step IV: Movements
- Tests for hip stability
  - Standing—Trendelenburg test
  - Lying—telescopy test
- Important special tests:
  - FABERE test
  - Stinchfield test.
- Examination of SI joints, spine, etc.
- Systemic examination
- PR examination

Quick Facts
Important different pathological conditions of the hip:
- Congenital:
  - CDH　　　　　　　　　　(*see page 477)
  - Coxa vara　　　　　　　(*see page 369)

---

*See *Textbook of Orthopedics,* John Ebnezar, 5th Edition.

- *Infective:*
  - Acute septic arthritis (*see page 556)
  - Chronic tuberculosis arthritis. (*see page 547)
- *Traumatic:*
  - Fracture neck femur (*see page 631)
  - Trochanteric fracture (*see page 642)
  - Dislocation of hip joint (*see page 199)
    (Post/ant/central)
- *Inflammatory:*
  - Rheumatoid arthritis (*see page 564)
- *Degenerative disorders:*
  - OA (*see page 666)
- *Neoplastic disorders:*
  - Benign
- *Non-specific:*
  - Perthes' (*see page 397)
  - Slipped capital
    Femoral epiphysis (*see page 403)

---

*See *Textbook of Orthopedics,* John Ebnezar, 5th Edition.

6
CHAPTER

Examination of Knee Joint

The knee joint is at the end of two long lever arms—the tibia and the femur. It is particularly susceptible to traumatic injury.

The knee joint is not a "true" hinge joint as presumed to be. It consists of two components: (i) the patellofemoral joint (this is an example of saddle joint), and (ii) the femorotibial joint (hinge joint) (Flowchart 6.1). Thus, the knee joint in its true form is a "compound synovial joint" (Fig. 6.1).

The knee joint lacks the stability of the hip, because little stability is furnished by the rounded contours of the femoral condyles and the flat tibial plateau. For stability, the knee must depend largely upon the soft tissues, the capsule, the quadriceps muscle and the four ligaments—the tibial collateral, the fibular collateral, and the anterior and posterior cruciate ligaments. The knee joint is an unusual joint, because it contains ligaments deep within the joint (the cruciates). The knee joint represents a challenge for diagnosis and treatment.

PROBLEMS RELATED TO KNEE

The knee joint could be affected due to a generalized disorder like developmental, metabolic, rheumatoid, etc. or it could be just a local manifestation of diseases peculiar to knee. These problems could be traumatic or nontraumatic. If traumatic, it could be a high velocity and vehicular trauma or sports-related injuries. Nontraumatic causes could be either infective or noninfective. Noninfective causes could be developmental disorder, growth arrest, tumors, inflammatory conditions, etc. Problems due to the many bursae and patella also could disable the knee. Overall, a myriad number of diseases and disorders can affect the knee joint (Flowchart 6.2).

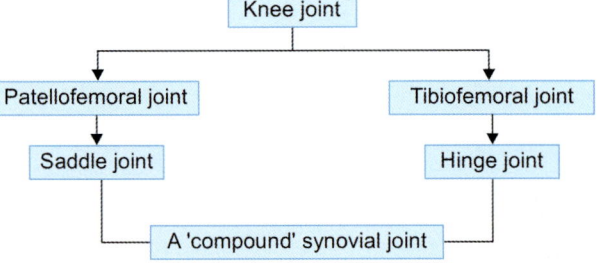

Flowchart 6.1: Components of knee joint

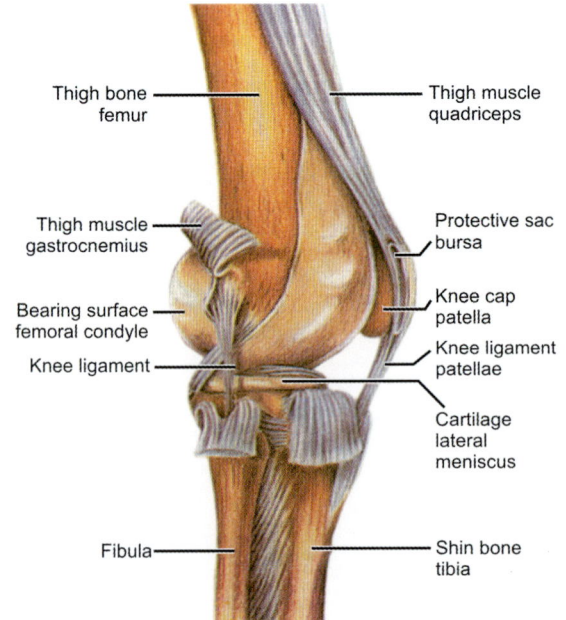

Fig. 6.1: Anatomical structure of knee joint

Flowchart 6.2: Problems associated with knee joint

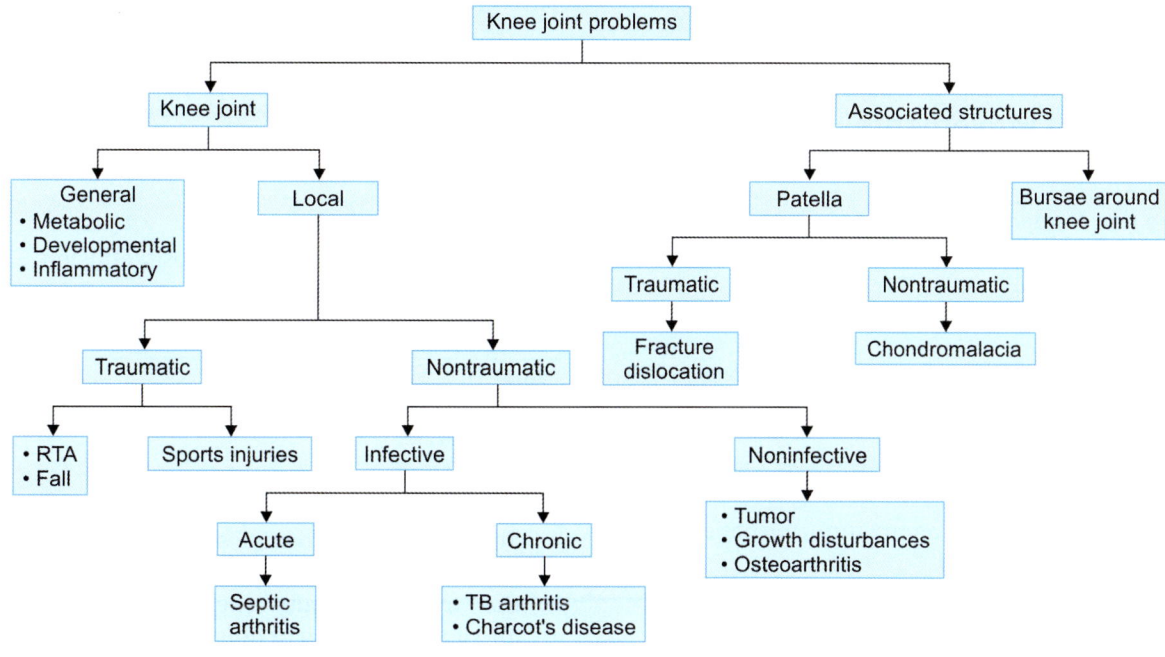

> **Interesting Facts Peculiar to the Knee**
> - A normal knee joint is never straight. It has on an average 7° valgus (men: 3–5°, women: 5–7°)
> - It is a combination of two joints
> - It is a superficial joint and is more prone to injuries
> - The support and stability of the knee joint is mainly due to the capsule, the quadriceps, cruciates and collaterals. These are very vulnerable for injuries, especially due to sports
> - Though a hinge joint, slight rotational and sideward movement is possible in flexion of the knee
> - A stiff knee is a disabled knee
> - There are plenty of bursae around the knee and each could be a site of the disease

CLINICAL EXAMINATIONS

This consists of history, observation and physical examination.

HISTORY

A patient with knee problems usually presents with the following complaints.

Pain

This may be acute or chronic and there may be a history of trauma. History of night cries if present suggests TB arthritis.

Swelling

This could be due to effusion or synovial membrane thickening and could be general or local (Flowchart 6.3). The duration of the swelling following trauma gives a clue to the probable diagnosis—if a swelling develops within 2 hours of the injury, it suggests hemarthrosis; and if it develops after 2 to 24 hours, it suggests traumatic synovitis. Approximately 75% of the cases of hemarthrosis are due to anterior cruciate ligament (ACL) tears.

Localized swellings could be due to bursal enlargement.

Flowchart 6.3: Type of swelling of knee joint

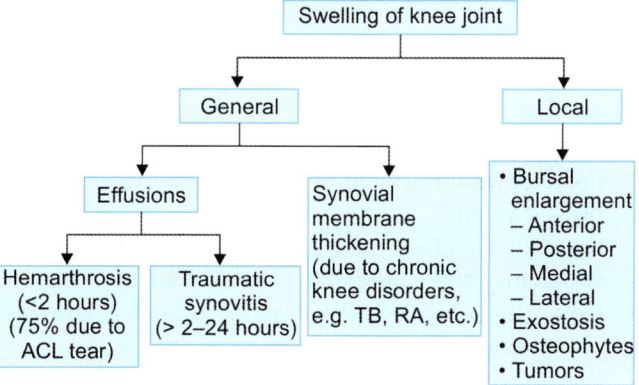

Limp

This may be due to pain, muscle spasm, stiffness or arthritis.

Restriction of Movements

Locking

Could be due to menisci tear or loose bodies. In locking, the patient complains of inability to complete the last few degrees of extension.

> **Note:**
> - Locking is inability to extend the knee for the last few degrees
> - Springy block suggests—menisci tear
> - Rigid block suggests—loose bodies or fixed flexion deformity.

Deformity

In genu valgum, varum and recurvatum, the patient usually presents with the deformity.

> **Quick Facts**
> - Pain is the common presenting complaint
> - History of night cries suggests TB arthritis
> - Duration of swelling after injury
>   – <2 hours—hemarthrosis (75% due to ACL tear)
>   – >2 hours—traumatic synovitis
> - In genu varum and valgum, deformity is the main complaint
> - Locking and giving way are the usual mechanical symptoms

PHYSICAL EXAMINATION OF THE KNEE

As in the other parts of the body, examination of knee joint consists of inspection, palpation, measurements, movements and stability tests peculiar to the knee.

Preparation

The whole limb to be examined is exposed with the patient wearing short trousers. Examination of the knee is carried out from the front, sides and back.

Inspection

Inspection is carried out in the following order:
- First look at the height and weight of the patient.
- Look for standing alignment of the knee, which should be 3–7° valgus.
- Look for the abnormality of the feet like flat feet, etc. which may contribute to the knee problems.
- Gait—the patient could walk with a limp (e.g. arthritis), circumduction (stiff knee), etc.
- Wasting of the thigh and leg muscles are to be noted.

Swelling

This could be due to intra-articular or extra-articular causes. If all the natural depressions above, below and by the sides of the patella are obliterated, the cause could be intra-articular. In extra-articular causes, not all the natural fossae will be obliterated and the swelling usually extends over the patella.

Limits of the Swelling
- Confined to knee—hemarthrosis/effusion.
- Beyond knee—could be infectious, tumors or major injuries.

> **Note:**
> *Localized swellings* around the knee could be due to bursitis, exostosis or osteophytes.

Deformity

- The usual knee deformities are genu valgum, varum and recurvatum. The other deformity peculiar to TB knee is the "triple deformity" (flexion, posterior subluxation and lateral rotation of tibia).
- Look for old scars, sinuses, etc. as evidences of injury, surgery, trauma or infections.
- Look for the position of the patella whether lateral, high or low.

> **Quick Facts**
> *Inspection: look for*
> - Normal alignment of knee
> - Observe the gait
> - Wasting of muscles
> - Swelling of knee—whether confined to knee, beyond knee or localized
> - *Deformities:*
>   – Flexion deformity—commonest
>   – Genu varum—rickets/OA
>   – Genu valgum—rheumatoid
>   – Genu recurvatum—congenital
>   – Triple displacement—tuberculosis knee

Palpation

Temperature

Feel for the local rise of temperature with the dorsum of the hand.

Tenderness

Elicit the tenderness and grade it as described earlier.

Test for the Extensor Mechanism

The extensor mechanism of the knee consists of the quadriceps muscle, patella, patellar ligament and the tibial tubercle. Palpate these for tenderness, wasting, loss of continuity, etc.

Swelling

Swelling of the joint is usually due to effusion within the joint, which indicates damage to the joint and the presence of a major cause must always be ruled out. Synovial membrane thickness is the other common cause.

Contents of Knee Effusion
- Synovial fluid (common)
- Blood
- Pus

Types of Swelling
- *Small:* In these cases, there will be bulging of the sides of the patellar ligament and obliteration of the hollows of the medial and lateral edges of patella.
- *Medium.*
- *Large:* All the findings noted in the small and medium effusions and distension of suprapatellar pouch.
- *Localized:* Due to osteophytes, exostosis, bursa, cysts, etc.

Swelling due to Synovial Membrane Thickness

Swelling due to synovial membrane thickness is usually due to chronic inflammatory disorders. The features of the swelling due to the synovial membrane thickness are:
- Most prominent usually above the patella near the suprapatellar pouch.
- Boggy to feel.
- Local raise of temperature.

Tests

The following tests help to evaluate the swellings of the knee:
- Patellar tap test.
- Fluid displacement test.
- Fluctuation test.

Quick Facts
Is there a huge swelling of the knee? Think of the following possibilities:
- Soft tissue injuries of the knee
- Fracture, infections, tumors, etc. of the distal femur
- Malignant synovioma
- Massive knee effusions due to hemarthrosis, etc.
- Cellulitis
- Synovial membrane thickening

Patellar Tap Test

This test (Fig. 6.2) is carried out as follows:

Step 1: In the horizontal position, a considerable amount of excessive synovial fluid gravitates into the suprapatellar pouch. From 6" above the patella, excess fluid in the

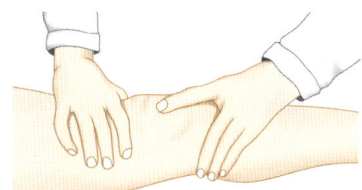

Fig. 6.2: Patellar tap test

suprapatellar pouch is driven back into the joint by sliding down firmly with index finger and the thumb.

Step 2: The tips of the three fingers and the thumb of the free hand is placed over the anterior surface of the patella and a quick "jerk" is given downwards. If the fluid is present, a "click" is heard as the patella can be felt to strike on the femoral condyle and "bounces" back.

Limitations
The patellar tap is not always reliable. It is negative in:
a. Tense swelling due to too much fluid.
b. Small swelling due to too little fluid.
Thus, it is positive only in "moderate" knee effusions.

Fluid Displacement Tests

These tests (Fig. 6.3) help to detect small effusions. Two methods are described below:

Type 1: Evacuate the suprapatellar pouch as mentioned in the previous test and stroke the medial or lateral side of the joint and look for 'distension' of the other side.

Type 2: Pressure is applied over one of the obliterated hollows on either side of the ligamentum patellae. The pressure is slowly released and an observation is made for "refilling" of the hollow by the fluid.

Limitations: These tests are not useful if the effusion is large and tense.

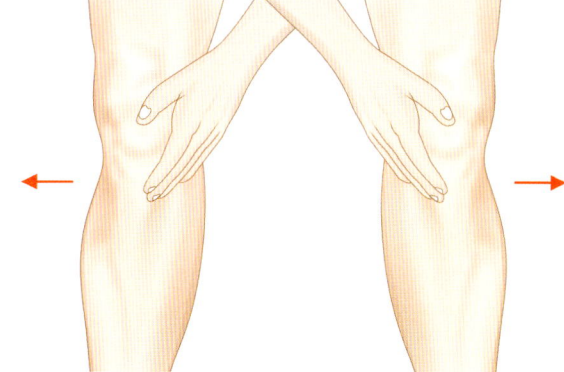

Fig. 6.3: Examination of knee joint—fluid displacement test

Fluctuation Test

This test is particularly useful in large knee joint effusions (Fig. 6.4).

Method

Step 1: The patient is in the supine position. Excessive fluid in the suprapatellar pouch is squeezed with the index finger and thumb of the left hand and held in that position.

Step 2: With the thumb and index finger of the (right) hand on either side of the ligamentum patellae, pressure is applied and the (left) hand feels this transmission of force.

Limitations: This test is negative in small effusions.

Localized Swelling of the Knee

The knee joint swellings could be due to intra-articular or extra-articular causes (Flowchart 6.4). These are due to enlarged bursa and cysts, which are present all round the knee, and has been discussed earlier. The important characteristics about them are their 'reducibility' on compression and their relation to the tendons (*see page 411).

Exostosis and growth arising from the lower end of femur, upper end of tibia and fibula are the other causes of localized bony hard swellings around the knee. All these structures should be carefully palpated and evaluated.

Patella

It is very important to carry out a systematic examination of the patella as described below:

Position: Position of the patella. Is it high, low or laterally placed?

Tenderness: Palpate for the tenderness over the anterior surface, upper, lower, medial and lateral borders. Push the patella laterally and palpate the surface underneath.

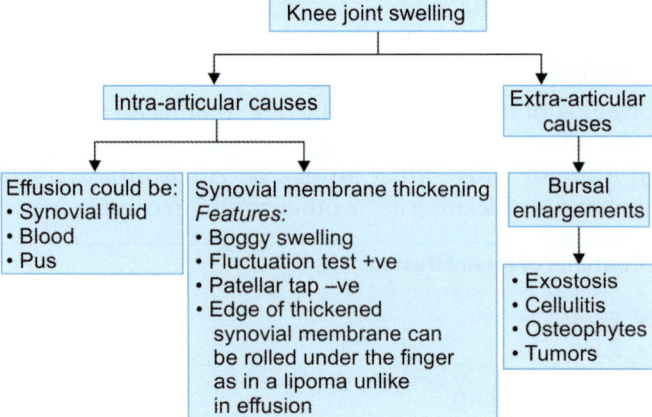

Flowchart 6.4: Causes of knee joint swelling

Tests for effusion
- Displacement test—for mild effusion
- Paellar tap—for moderate effusion
- Fluctuation test—for large effusion

Mobility: The patella can normally be moved up and down and side-to-side up to 25–50% of its width in both the directions. Note whether this normal mobility is maintained or restricted (retropatellar arthritis).

Q-ANGLE (QUADRICEPS ANGLE)

Definition

The Q-angle is defined as the angle between the quadriceps tendon (primarily the rectus femoris) and the patellar tendon (Fig. 6.5).

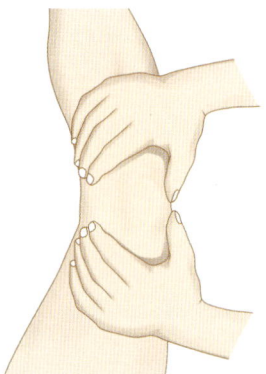

Fig. 6.4: Fluctuation test

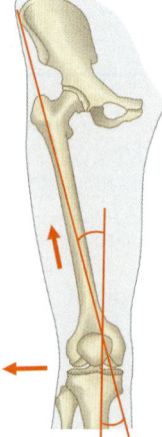

Fig. 6.5: Q-angle

---

*See *Textbook of Orthopedics,* John Ebnezar, 5th Edition.

Step 1: First, ensure that the lower limbs are at a right angle to the line that joins the two anterosuperior iliac spines (ASIS).

Step 2: A line is then drawn from the ASIS to the midpoint of the patella.

Step 3: Another line is drawn from the tibial tubercle to the midpoint of the patella.

The angle formed by the intersection of these two lines is the Q-angle.

Interpretation

When the knee is straight, the normal Q-angle for males is 15° and for females, it is 18°. Any angle less than 13° may be associated with patellofemoral dysfunctions or patella alta. Any angle more than 18° is associated with patellofemoral dysfunction, subluxating patella, genu valgum, increased femoral anteversions and lateral tibial torsions.

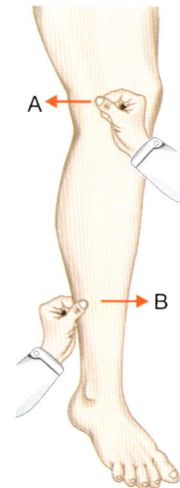

Fig. 6.6: Method of eliciting joint: (A) Line tenderness, (B) Bony tenderness

> **Quick Facts**
> *Q-angle*
> - Also called patellofemoral angle
> - Normal is 13–18°
> - The foot and hip should be placed in neutral position before recording
> - If measured in seated position, Q-angle should be 0°
> - During the test, the quadriceps should be relaxed
> - In children an increased Q-angle presents as genu valgum

Joint Line Tenderness

It is important to elicit joint line tenderness in arthritis, menisci injury or collateral ligament injuries.

Method: The patient is supine. To mark the joint line, flex and extend the knee slowly and feel for the gap between the femoral and tibial condyles. Mark this with a skin pencil on both sides. Now palpate systematically for tenderness from front-to-back and at the points of attachments of the collateral ligaments (Fig. 6.6).

TESTS PECULIAR TO KNEE

As mentioned earlier, the stability of the knee depends on the soft tissues, the capsule, the meniscus, the quadriceps, the cruciates and the collateral ligaments. To detect the integrity of the above structures, stability tests are carried out.

TESTS FOR COLLATERALS

Abduction or Valgus Stress Test

This test is done to detect the medial collateral ligament injury (Fig. 6.7).

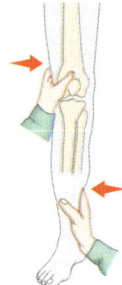

Fig. 6.7: Abduction or valgus stress test

Procedure

The patient is in supine position with the knee extended. Stand on the ipsilateral side of the patient and place one hand against the lateral aspect of the knee at the joint line. Now grasp the ankle with the other hand and attempt to drag the leg laterally to open the medial side of the knee joint. If there is evidence of pain above, below or at the joint line, the test is positive for medial collateral ligament injury.

Adduction Stress or Varus Stress Test

This test is to detect the lateral collateral ligament injury (Fig. 6.8).

Procedure

The patient is supine with knee extended. Standing on the ipsilateral side of the patella, place one hand against the medial aspect of the knee. Grip the ankle with the other hand and draw the leg medially in an attempt to open the lateral side of the knee joint. If the patient complains of pain above, below or at the joint line, the test is positive.

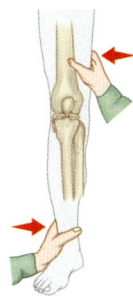

Fig. 6.8: Adduction or varus stress test

Note:
After doing the above tests in extension, it has to be repeated with the knee in 30° flexion.

TESTS FOR CRUCIATES

Anterior Drawer's Test

This is a one-plane test for anterior instability as it tests the anterior cruciate ligament (ACL).

Procedure

The patient is supine. The knee is flexed to 90° and the hip to 45°. The examiner sits on the forefoot of the patient. The hands of the examiner are placed around the tibia to ensure that the hamstring muscles are relaxed. The tibia is then pulled forwards on the femur. The normal amount of movement that should be present is 6 mm. If the tibia moves forward over the femur more than 6 mm, the test is said to be positive (Fig. 6.9).

Note:
If the test is positive, the following structures could be injured: (i) The ACL (the anteromedial bundle), (ii) the posteromedial and posterolateral capsule, (iii) the deep fibers of medial collateral ligament, (iv) the iliotibial band (v) the posterior oblique ligament, and (vi) the arcuate popliteus complex.

Posterior Drawer's Test

Procedure

Following the anterior movement of the tibia on the femur, the posterior movement of the tibia on the femur should be completed and the tibia is pushed back on the femur.

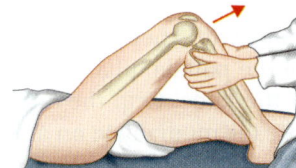

Fig. 6.9: Anterior Drawer's test

The test is said to be positive if there is a large amount of posterior movement.

Note:
If the above test is positive, the following structures could be damaged: (i) The posterior cruciate ligament, (ii) the anterior cruciate ligament, (iii) the arcuate popliteus complex, and (iv) the posterior oblique ligament.

TESTS FOR MENISCI

McMurray's Sign (Figs 6.10A to D)

The presence of this sign indicates injury to the menisci.

Procedure

The patient is supine and the thigh is flexed until the heel touches the buttocks. One hand of the examiner grasps the knee and the other hand the heel. The examiner internally rotates the leg and slowly extends it (test for lateral meniscus). Then the examiner externally rotates and extends the leg (test for medial meniscus). McMurray's sign is said to be present if a painful click or snap is heard at some point in the arc. The higher the leg is raised when the snap is heard, posterior the lesion is.

Reliable Facts
Consistent and reliable signs of a torn meniscus:
- Joint line tenderness
- Springy block to full extension
- Quadriceps atrophy

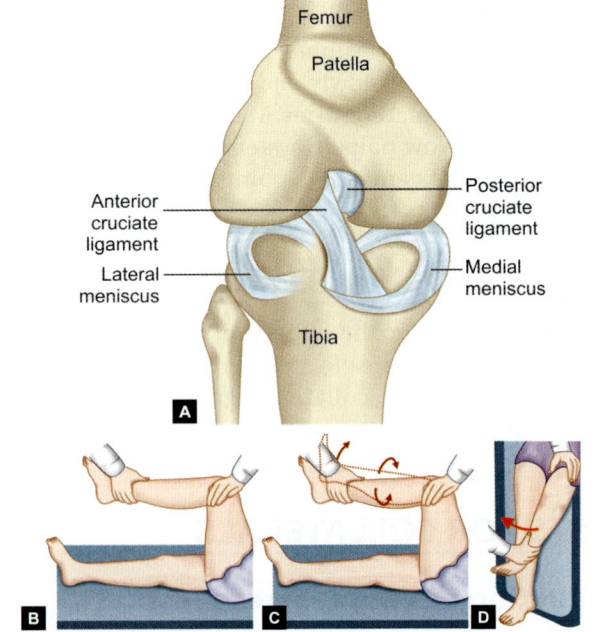

Figs 6.10A to D: (A) Anatomy; (B to D) Steps of performing the McMurray's test

Apleys' Compression and Distraction Tests

Procedure

This test consists of four steps (Figs 6.11A and B):

Steps 1: The patient is lying prone. The examiner grasps the foot of the affected limb, internally rotates and slowly flexes the knee to 90° (test for lateral meniscus).

Step 2: The above test is repeated with the leg externally rotated (test for medial meniscus).

Step 3: The examiner then places his knee in the popliteal fossa of the patient and anchors it to the examination table. By lifting the foot, the examiner strongly distracts the patient's knee joint. This is followed by rapid internal (lateral collateral ligament) and external rotations (for medial collateral ligament).

Step 4: This procedure is repeated with strong downward pressure on the patient's foot.

Lachman Test

This test indicates injury to the anterior cruciate ligament. This is a test especially for the posterolateral band, one plane, and anterior instability (Fig. 6.12).

Procedure

The patient is supine and the knee of the patient is flexed to 30°. The examiner then stabilizes the patient's femur with one hand; while with the other hand, the tibia is moved forward.

The test is said to be positive if there is a soft end feel and if the intrapatellar tendon slope disappears.

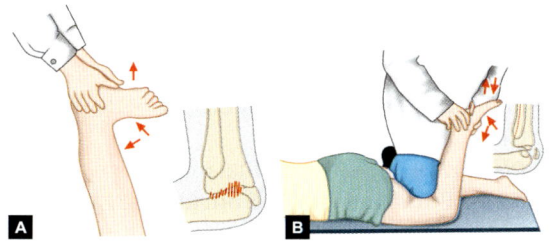

Figs 6.11A and B: Apleys' compression (A) and distraction tests (B)

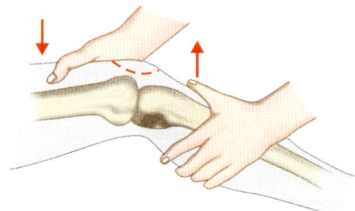

Fig. 6.12: Lachman's test

Note:
The following structures could be injured if the above test is positive:
- The anterior cruciate ligament (especially the posterolateral bundle).
- The posterior oblique ligament.
- The arcuate popliteus complex.

Quick Facts
Stability Tests
- Tests for collaterals
  - Abduction or valgus stress test—for medial collateral ligament injury
  - Adduction or varus stress test—for lateral collateral ligament injury
  - Apley's distraction tests
- Tests for cruciates
  - Anterior Drawer test—for ACL injury (especially anteromedial bundle)
  - Posterior Drawer test—for PCL tears
  - Lachman's test—for ACL injury (especially posterolateral bundle)
- Tests for menisci
  - McMurray's sign
  - Apley's grinding or compression tests

EXAMINATION OF MOVEMENTS

The important movements taking place at the knee joint are flexion and extension. In a semiflexed position, slight side-to-side and rocking movements are possible.

Flexion

The normal range of knee flexion is 130–150°.

Muscles

- *Prime movers*—biceps femoris, semimembranosus, and semitendinosus.
- *Accessory muscles*—popliteus, sartorius, gracilis, and gastrocnemius.

Muscle Testing

The patient is prone. The examiner places one hand over the pelvis to stabilize, it while he offers graded resistance with the other hand at the ankle as the patient attempts to flex the knee. If knee flexion is tested with the ankle externally rotated, biceps femoris is tested and if the ankle is rotated medially, semimembranosus and semitendinosus are tested.

Procedure to Record Flexion

- In the prone position, the patient is asked to flex both the knees simultaneously and the distance between the heels to buttock is noted (Fig. 6.13A).

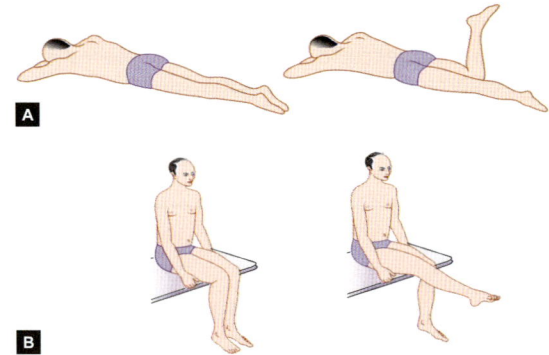

Figs 6.13A and B: Method of recording knee movements: (A) Prone position; (B) Sitting position

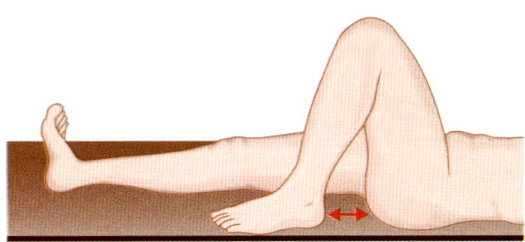

Fig. 6.14: Loss of terminal flexion in osteoarthritis knee

- In supine position, the patient is asked to flex the knee and the heel to buttock distance is measured by a tape (Fig. 6.14).
- In sitting position, the patient is asked to flex and extend the knee holding the edge of the table (Fig. 6.13B).

> **Rule of Thumb**
> For every 1 cm distance restriction, there is 1.5° loss of flexion.
> *Advantages*
> - Gives a very accurate reading even in small alterations of flexions
> - Helps in checking daily or weekly progress

Extension

Normal Range
The knee should normally extend to a straight line (0°) and occasionally can hyperextend to 15° in some women.

Measurement
The degree of extension is determined by measuring the angle between the thigh and the leg.

Prime Movers
Quadriceps femoris.

Muscle Testing
The patient sits with the legs hanging over the edge of the table. The examiner then stabilizes the thigh by placing one hand over the pelvis or proximal thigh. Against the resistance provided by the examiner, the patient slowly extends the knee through its range of motion (Fig. 6.13B).

Look for the following impairments during knee extension:
- Springy block to full extension—suspect bucket handle tear due to menisci injury.
- Rigid block to full extension—loose bodies or fixed flexion deformity (FFD).

Measurements
- *Measurement of the length of the thigh:* Length of the thigh is recorded by taking a measurement between the ASIS and the medial joint line of the knee.
- *Measurement of the length of the leg:* This is done by recording the length between the medial joint line and the medial malleolus.
- Breadth of the lower end of femur and upper end of tibia is recorded by using a caliper.
- Distance between the tibial tubercle and the head of the fibula is recorded.
- To measure the muscle wasting, circumference of the thigh and muscles are recorded from fixed points on both sides (e.g. about 6–7" above the joint line) (Fig. 6.15).
- Measurement of deformities around the knee:
  - *Genu valgum deformity*
    Intermalleolar distance or gap: In children, the examiner rotates the legs until the patella are vertical. The legs are brought together to touch lightly at the knee. A measurement is made between the malleoli. Serial measurements every 6 months are made to check the progress (Fig. 6.16).
    Plumb line: Normally, a line drawn from ASIS to the center of patella strikes the medial malleolus. In genu valgum, the medial malleolus will be lateral to this line. The distance between this line and the medial malleolus is the measure of the deformity.
  - *Genu varum deformity*
    Plumb line: Here the medial malleolus will be medial to the plumb line drawn from the ASIS and the center of patella.
    Intercondylar distance: Both the legs are rotated and held in such a way that both medial malleoli touch

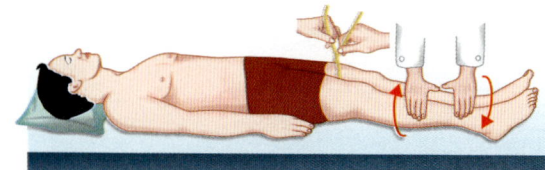

Fig. 6.15: Method of measuring the girth of a limb and checking the movements

Examination of Knee Joint

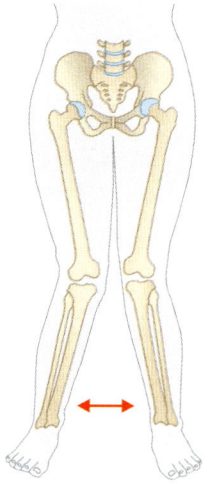

Fig. 6.16: Genu valgum or knock-knee deformity

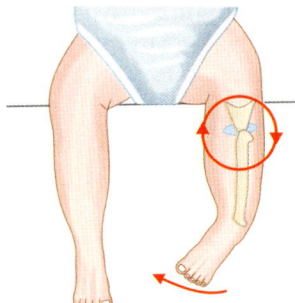

Fig. 6.18: Plumb line test to detect tibial torsion

or IV intermetatarsal space; and in external rotation deformity, the foot will lie outside the line (Fig. 6.18).

Quick Facts
Measurements
- Measure length of the thigh
- Measure length of the leg
- Measure breadth of the lower end of femur and upper end of tibia
- Measure the thigh and leg circumferences
- *Measurement of deformities*
  - Genu valgum deformity
    ◆ Intermalleolar gap
    ◆ Plumb line
  - *Genu varum deformity*
    ◆ Intercondylar distance
    ◆ Plumb line
  - *Rotational deformity*
    ◆ Plumb line

EXAMINATION OF THE POPLITEAL FOSSA

Examination of the popliteal fossae is done in standing and prone positions. The following are the important lesions in the popliteal fossa:
- *Baker's cyst:* It is prominently seen and felt during extension of the knee and disappears or becomes less prominent during flexion.
- *Aneurysm of the popliteal artery:* A pulsatile swelling is in the center of the popliteal fossa.
- *Enlarged popliteal lymph node:* This is enlarged in the early stages of TB arthritis.

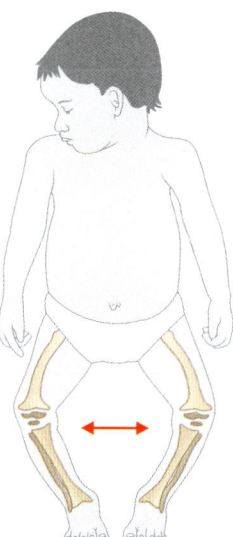

Fig. 6.17: Genu varum with increased intercondylar distance. Genu varum is said to exist if there is approximately 3 cm gap between the medial femoral condyles when the malleoli are together

each other. The intercondylar distance is measured (Fig. 6.17).

Note: X-ray of the limbs is the most accurate method of measuring the genu valgum and varum deformities in adults.

- *Rotational deformities* the patient is made to sit at the edge of the table with both the legs hanging down. Normally, a line drawn from the center of the patella and extended down cuts the I or II intermetatarsal space. In internal rotation deformity, this line cuts III

OTHER EXAMINATIONS

- *Systemic examination:* Useful in TB knee, rheumatoid arthritis, Charcot's joint (syphilis), etc.
- *Examination of other joints:* Especially hip joint as the pain in the knee may be a referred pain from the hip.

- *Examination of inguinal lymph nodes:* These are enlarged in later stages of TB arthritis.

> **Quick Facts**
> *Order of examination of knee*
> - History
> - Inspection
> - Palpation
> - Tests for stability
> - Movements
> - Measurements
> - Examination of popliteal fossa
> - Systemic examination
> - Examination of hip and other joints
> - Examination of inguinal and popliteal lymph nodes.

COMMON KNEE JOINT DISORDERS

- *Congenital:*
    - Genu recurvatum   (*see page 409)
- *Infective:*
    - Acute—septic arthritis   (*see page 556)
    - Chronic—TB knee   (*see page 550)
    - Charcot's knee   (*see page 559)
- *Inflammatory:*
    - Rheumatoid knee   (*see page 564)
- *Metabolic:*
    - Rickets (genu valgum)   (*see page 510)
- *Traumatic:*
    - Fracture patella   (*see page 242)
    - ACL tear   (*see page 232)
    - Menisci injuries   (*see page 238)
    - Collateral ligament injuries   (*see page 230)
    - Rupture of extensor apparatus   (*see page 246)
- *Degenerative:*
    - Genu varum (OA knee)   (*see page 408)
    - Chondromalacia patella   (*see page 413)
    - Cysts around the knee   (*see page 409)

---

*See *Textbook of Orthopedics,* John Ebnezar, 5th Edition.

7
CHAPTER

Examination of Sacroiliac Joint

The body weight is transferred from the single weightbearing axis of the trunk to the bipolar weightbearing of the lower extremities through the pelvis. The spine attaches to the pelvis through the sacroiliac (SI) joint. The SI joint is formed by the posterior and internal ilium and the lateral border of the sacrum. Although the SI joints can be affected by conditions involving any joint, the common ones are tuberculosis, ankylosing spondylitis and degenerative arthritis. The SI joint is supported by the thin anterior and thick posterior sacroiliac ligaments.

PHYSICAL EXAMINATION OF SACROILIAC JOINT

Inspection

The patient is examined in standing, sitting and recumbent positions and a look is made for any swelling, scar, sinuses, wasting, etc.

Palpation

Feel for the local rise of temperature. Tenderness is elicited by pressing with the thumb over the dimple which is situated just medial to the posterosuperior iliac spine.

Movements

Any movement which strains this joint like forward bending while standing or rotation causes pain. The following tests help to evaluate the SI joint movement and pain.

> **Remember**
> *Pain in SI Joint Involvement*
> - Felt locally over the joint
> - May be referred to groin, posterior thigh and down the leg on the same side
> - It increases by lying on the affected side

CLINICAL TESTS FOR SACROILIAC JOINT

Gapping Test (Sacroiliac Stretch Test)

Procedure

The patient is supine with the hips and knees extended. With crossed arms, place both the hands on the opposite anterosuperior iliac spines of each ilium and apply a downward and lateral pressure. Gluteal or posterior thigh sign suggests a positive test.

Inference

This test indicates sprain of the anterosacroiliac ligament.

Squish Test

Procedure

The patient is supine with the hips and knees extended. Place both the hands on the anterosuperior iliac spines and crests and push down at a 45° angle. Pain indicates a positive test.

Inference

The positive test indicates a sprain of the posterior sacroiliac ligaments.

Iliac Compression Test

Procedure

The patient is in a side-lying position on a hard surface. Place both the hands over the upper part of the superior iliac crest and exert a downward pressure. The test is positive, if the patient experiences pain (Fig. 7.1).

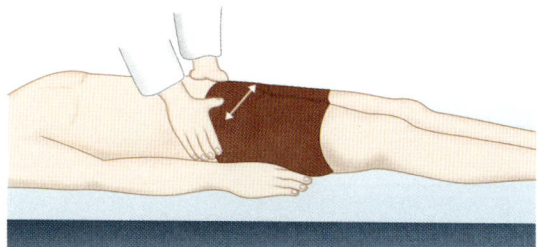

Fig. 7.1: Compression test for suspected sacoiliac joint involvement

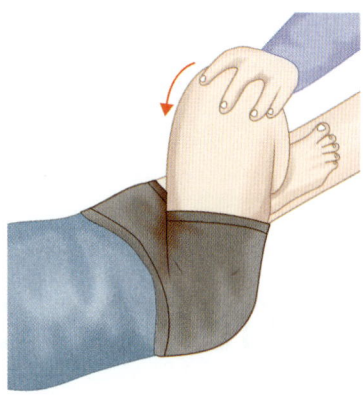

Fig. 7.2: Gaenselen's test

Inference

This test indicates sacroiliac sprain, fracture of the wing of the ilium, etc.

Gaenselen's Test

Procedure

The patient is supine with the affected side near the side of the table. Now flex the "unaffected" thigh over the abdomen pointing towards the opposite shoulder, while simultaneously hyperextending the affected SI joint by pressing on the thigh of the affected side. Pain indicates a positive test. The test is performed bilaterally (Fig. 7.2).

Inference

The test indicates a SI joint disease.

Knee-to-Shoulder Test

Procedure

The patient is supine. Flex the patient's knee and hip fully over the abdomen and then adduct the hip. Now move the knee towards the patient's opposite shoulder (Fig. 7.3). The test is positive if the patient complains of pain in the SI joint.

Inference

If the patient is afebrile, the positive test suggests mechanical dysfunction.

If the patient is febrile, it suggests pyogenic sacroiliitis.

Sacral Apex Test

Procedure

The patient is prone on a firm table. Pressure is applied with both the hands placed on the apex of the sacrum causing a shear stress of the sacrum on the ilium. Pain produced in the SI joint indicates a positive test.

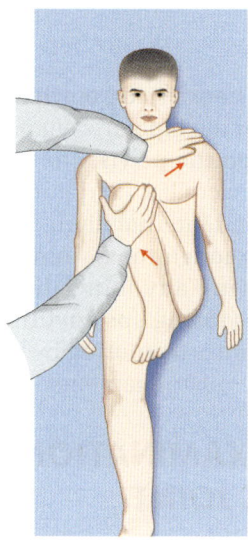

Fig. 7.3: Method of performing the knee-to-shoulder test

Inference

Positive test indicates SI joint arthritis.

TESTS TO DIFFERENTIATE PAIN DUE TO HIP JOINT AND SPINE

Erichsen's Test

Procedure

The patient is prone on a firm table. Place both the hands over the dorsum of the ilium and press down forcefully towards the midline. Pain over SI joint area suggests a positive test.

Inference

The test is positive in sacroiliac disease but not in hip joint disease.

Passive SLRT and Braggard's Sign

Procedure

Do a passive straight leg raising test (SLRT) till the point of pain and then dorsiflex the foot (Braggard's sign).

Inference

If sciatica is due to SI joint problems, there will be no increase in pain; but if it is due to nerve root compression by a prolapsed disk, pain increases.

Quick Facts
Tests for SI joints
- Test for tenderness—direct pressure over the SI joint
- Gapping test—for anterior sacroiliac ligament sprain
- Squish test—for posterior sacroiliac ligament sprain
- Iliac compression test—for fracture of the ilium
- Gaenslen's test—for SI joint disease
- Knee shoulder test—for mechanical dysfunction and pyogenic sacroiliitis
- Sacral apex test—for SI joint arthritis
- Erichsen's test—to differentiate from hip joint disease
- Passive SLRT and Braggard's sign—to differentiate from sciatica due to disk prolapse

CHAPTER 8

Examination of Spine

A normal spine is not straight. It is an S-shaped structure (Fig. 8.1). The cervical spine is more freely mobile while the thoracic spine is the least mobile, and the lumbar spine has a mobility lesser than the cervical.

Because of its mobility, cervical spine is more prone for injuries, while the thoracic spine is commonly involved in diseases like TB, etc. the lumbar spine is more vulnerable to degenerative diseases, particularly the disk diseases. The normal physiological spinal curves are mild lordosis of cervical spine, the thoracic kyphosis, lumbar lordosis and sacral kyphosis. If these curves are exaggerated due to disease or trauma, it is abnormal. Nevertheless, unlike the anteroposterior curves, the lateral curves (scoliosis) are always considered abnormal. These induce many compensatory changes in and around the spine and thereby pose one of the most difficult and challenging problems both in diagnosis and management.

Systematic examination of the spine will go a long way in making a good and proper diagnosis. The following protocol is helpful.

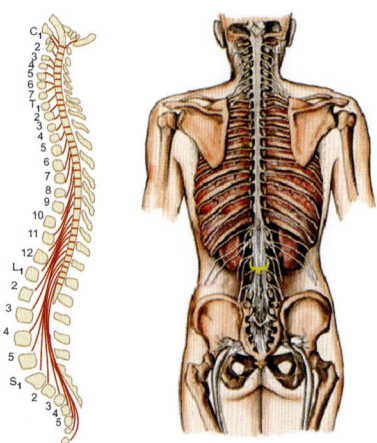

Fig. 8.1: Anatomical structure of spine

GENERAL EXAMINATION

General physical examination should be done before examining the spine to detect the role of systemic disease in the pathogenesis of back pain. After recording the vital signs, a search is made to detect any skin lesions like cafe-au-lait spots (neurofibromatosis), vesicles, petechial rashes, etc. as a number of spinal arthropathies are associated with skin disorders (e.g. psoriasis).

Other important general physical examinations include examination of the abdomen for diseases of liver, spleen, kidney, bladder, pancreas, uterus, aortic aneurysm, etc. Inguinal area is inspected for hernias and per rectal examination is carried out.

EXAMINATION OF THE SPINE

After the general examination, spine examination is carried out next.

Inspection

This is first carried out in standing position after the back is adequately exposed. Inspect the skin for cafe-au-lait spots (neurofibromatosis), lipoma and tuft of hair (meningocele), etc.

Posture

Does the patient have a normal posture or whether posture is altered due to deformities? The well-known postural deformities of spine are as follows (Figs 8.2A and B):

Kyphosis
Definition
This usually refers to the increased normal posterior convexity of the thoracic spine (Fig. 8.3).

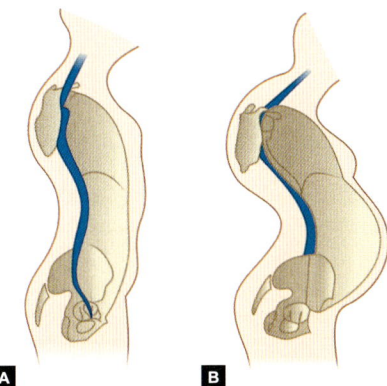

Figs 8.2A and B: Postures: (A) Normal posture; (B) Bad posture

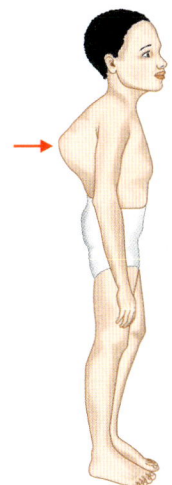

Fig. 8.3: Thoracic kyphosis arrow showing gibbus

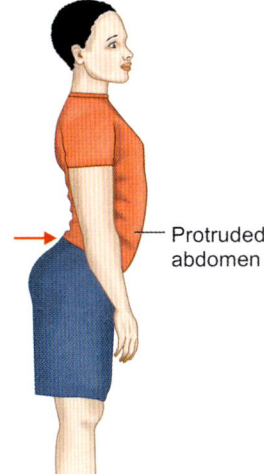

Fig. 8.4: Increased lumbar lordosis in spondylolisthesis

Causes

It could be due to localized injury, disease, generalized bone diseases, faulty growth, or postural habits.

Types

- Thoracolumbar or thoracic kyphosis (round back) with pelvic inclination of less than 20°.
- Gibbus or hump back this is a localized, sharp posterior angulation.
- Flat back or mobile spine with pelvic inclination less than 20°.
- Dowager's hump is seen in postmenopausal osteoporosis.

Thoracolumbar kyphosis is further classified into type I (postural kyphosis) or type II (structural kyphosis). Type I is mobile while type II is fixed.

Tests for Mobility

Instruct the patient to bend forwards in the standing position. If the deformity increases and decreases when the patient braces back the shoulder, the kyphosis is said to be mobile.

> **Note:**
> - Kyphosis is best examined from the back and sides.
> - *Gibbus:* This is a short, sharply angulated and acute kyphosis where only 2–3 vertebral elements are involved, e.g. tuberculosis spine.

Lordosis

Definition

Increase in the anterior convexity of the lumbar spine (Fig. 8.4).

Causes

The following are some of the important causes:
- *Compensatory:* This is the most common cause. Seen commonly in fixed flexion deformities of the hip, congenital dislocation of hip (CDH), Perthes' disease, etc.
- Pregnancy, large pendulous abdomen, uterine fibroid, etc. In these conditions, it attempts to correct the center of gravity.
- Spondylolisthesis.

Where there is a loss of normal lumbar lordosis, the following conditions are suspected:
- Prolapsed intervertebral disk.
- Infections of the spine.
- Ankylosing spondylitis.
- Osteoarthritis of spine, etc.

Lordosis of spine is best inspected from the sides.

Scoliosis

Definition

It is a lateral curvature of the spine and is always abnormal (Fig. 8.5).

Causes

It could be congenital, postural, paralytic compensatory (e.g. leg shortening), local bone diseases (e.g. TB, tumors, etc.) or idiopathic. The commonest cause of scoliosis is idiopathic.

Compensatory Changes

- Rotation of the affected vertebra (Figs 8.6A and B).
- Secondary compensatory curves above and below the primary curve (Fig. 8.5).
- Chest wall changes crowding of ribs (called as rib hump) occurs towards the side of scoliosis (Fig. 8.7).
- In the later stages, thoracic and abdominal viscera are affected, scapula becomes prominent, shoulder is pushed up and the opposite hip becomes prominent.

METHODS OF EXAMINATION

Standing Position

Scoliosis and the accompanying compensatory changes are noted and recorded.

Sitting Position

Next in the sitting position, if the scoliosis disappears, it is mobile and is secondary to leg shortening, etc.

Bending in Sitting Position

If the scoliosis persists in sitting position, ask the patient to bend forwards. If it disappears, it is mobile and is due to postural scoliosis. Nevertheless, if it persists, it is fixed. Presence of rib hump confirms the diagnosis of fixed scoliosis.

Adam's Positions

The patient is standing. The examiner notes any spinal asymmetry, scapular winging, chest asymmetry, etc.

Adam's Position—Posterior

This is to examine the thoracolumbar scoliosis.

Procedure

Here the examiner is positioned behind the patient. The patient flexes forward at the waist. The arms are allowed to hang towards the floor and the hands are placed in a prayer position. Now look for the thoracolumbar scoliosis, rib hump and muscle atrophy.

Adam's Position—Anterior

This is to examine the upper thoracic scoliosis.

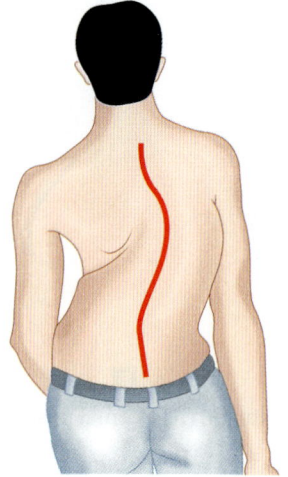

Fig. 8.5: Thoracic scoliosis

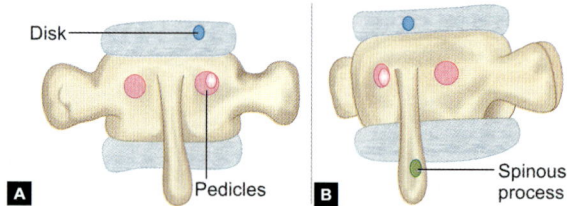

Figs 8.6A and B: (A) Normal PA view of the spine showing the normal positions of the pedicles and spinous processes; (B) The pedicles and spinous processes shadows are altered and indicate vertebral rotation in scoliosis

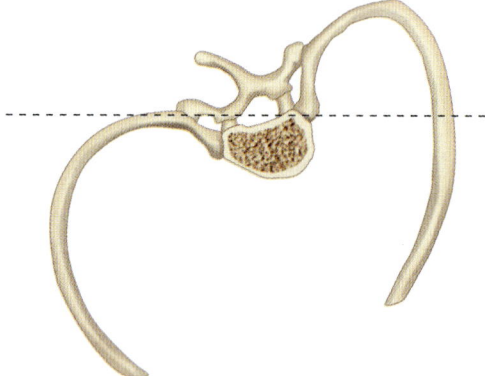

Fig. 8.7: Rib distortion due to vertebral rotation

Procedure

The examiner is standing in front. In addition to the above, the cervical spine is flexed. Look for the upper thoracic scoliosis.

Interpretation

Positive test: No changes in the scoliotic curve indicate structural scoliosis.

Negative test: Scoliosis disappears. Indicates functional scoliosis. Curves less than 25° indicate mild-to-moderate curves.

Spondylolisthesis

This is detected by the following clinical signs:
- A "step" at the upper angle of the sacrum.
- Increased lumbar lordosis.
- A transverse furrow encircles the body between the coastal margins and the iliac crest.

OTHER EXAMINATIONS

Examination of gait, evidence of swelling due to cold abscess. In spina bifida, it could be due to meningocele or myelomeningocele. In spina bifida occulta, there is no swelling but only a dimple, or dilated vessels or a tuft of hair.

Quick Facts
Inspection—spine deformities
- Kyphosis:
  - Four types
  - Sharp kyphosis is called gibbus
- Lordosis:
  - Commonest cause is compensatory
  - Loss in painful conditions of spine
- Scoliosis:
  - Commonest cause is idiopathic
  - Examined in standing, sitting and bending positions
  - Adam's position posterior is for thoracolumbar scoliosis
  - Adam's position anterior is for upper thoracic scoliosis
- Spondylolisthesis:
  - Transverse furrow
  - Increases lumbar lordosis
  - Step

RANGE OF MOVEMENTS

The normal movements taking place at the spine are forward flexion, extension, lateral bending and rotations. Most of the forward flexion and extension take place at the lumbar spine, whereas most of the lateral flexion and rotation takes place at the thoracic spine. The movements of the spine are best examined in standing position.

Flexion

Normal range is 105° (45° at the thoracic spine; 60° at the lumbar spine).

Thus, it is evident that the forward flexion takes place mainly in the lumbar spine. It is just possible that normal flexion takes place to the extent of obliteration of the normal convexity of the lumbar spine causing a smooth C-shaped configuration on bending. If the lumbar lordosis remains intact on bending forward, it suggests local lumbar disease.

Methods

- *Ask:* The patient to bend forward and note the distance between the fingers and the ground. Normally, the patient can touch the ground or reach within 7 cm off the ground. This test indicates the overall movements of the thoracic and lumbar segments ignoring the hip (Fig. 8.8).
- *Unequivocal method:* This method is more accurate than the one described above.

The spines of T_1 and S_1 are marked. With the patient fully erect and fully flexed, the distance between the two points is measured. Any increase in the distance indicates that the spine is flexing.

To assess the thoracic segment, mark T_1 and L_1 and repeat the procedure as mentioned above. Similarly, to measure the lumbar segment, repeat the above procedure between L_1 and S_1. If the increase in distance is 8 cm or more, it is considered as normal.

Extension

In the standing position, the patient is asked to arch his back while the examiner steadies the pelvis and a pull is exerted on the shoulder (Fig. 8.9). The angle between the long axis of the spine when erect and bent back is the angle of extension.

Alternatively, the distance between L_1 and S_1 is measured and is found to decrease in extension.

Normal range is 30° (thoracic—25°, lumbar—35°).

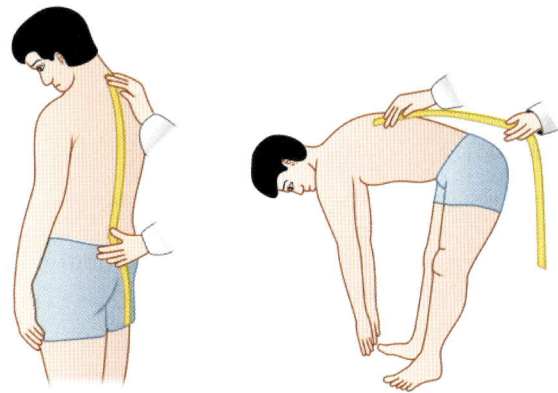

Fig. 8.8: Testing forward flexion movement of the spine

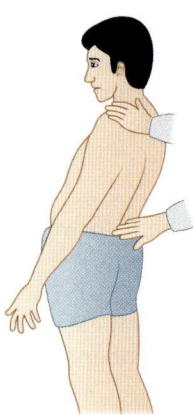

Fig. 8.9: Testing extension movement of the spine

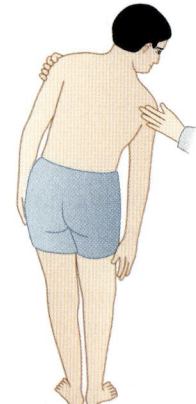

Fig. 8.10: Testing lateral flexion of the spine

Lateral Flexion

Normal range is 30° (thoracic and lumbar segments are equal).

Methods

Lateral flexion is best examined in standing position (Fig. 8.10).
- The patient is asked to slide down the hands on each side of the leg. The distance from the floor in cm or the position that the fingers reach in the legs is measured.
- The angle formed between the vertical and the line joining T_1 and S_1 on lateral flexion is measured.

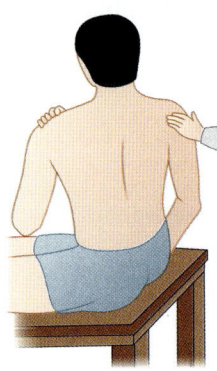

Fig. 8.11: Testing rotation movement of the spine

Rotations

Normal range is 40–45° (thoracic—40°, lumbar—5°).

Method

This is best examined in the sitting position. The patient sits at the edge of the table and holds it firmly to fix the pelvis. The patient is then asked to rotate on either side. The rotation is then measured between the plane of the shoulder and the pelvis (Fig. 8.11).

Palpation

Palpation is carried out with the patient in standing, sitting or prone positions (Fig. 8.12).

First, palpate both the groups of paraspinous muscles simultaneously for tenderness and firmness. Next, palpate the bony structures as follows for tenderness.

Percussion

In the standing position, ask the patient to bend forwards. From the root of the neck to the sacrum, the spine is lightly

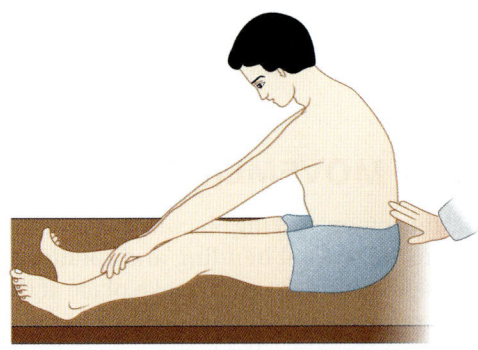

Fig. 8.12: Method of eliciting tenderness over the spine in the sitting position

percussed in an orderly fashion. The patient complains of marked pain in TB, infections, etc.

Rotation Method

This is the most accurate method. Here an attempt to rotate the vertebra by firmly pushing at the spinous process from the side elicits pain.

Rough Method

Gentle blows are given on either side of the spine. It is not advisable.

Anvil Method

Application of sudden jerk over the head. This is dangerous and is best avoided.

Other Sites

- *Facet joints:* Approximately 3 cm lateral to the midline facet joint tenderness can be elicited.
- In prolapsed intervertebral disks, tenderness is elicited in between the lumbar vertebrae.
- In mechanical back pain, tenderness is elicited over the lumbar muscles.
- Tenderness over sacroiliac (SI) joints is due to mechanical back pain or SI joint infection.

EXAMINATION OF SPINE FOR LOW BACK PAIN

Back pain is ubiquitous and one of the most common complaints all over the world. Exact diagnosis eludes most of the clinicians. In general, back pain can be put into three categories:
- *Referred pain:* Here the source of the problem is not in the back but elsewhere like intra-abdominal problems involving liver, spleen, gallbladder, pancreas, uterus, dissecting aortic aneurysms, renal calculi, etc. These form a large group of patients who should be excluded by appropriate examinations before examining the back proper.
- *True back pain:* This is the type of back pain, which will be discussed in this chapter at length.
- *Malingering:* This group causes the greatest confusion in diagnosis and one should be at guard in examining them. At the end of the chapter, guidelines are given as how to isolate this group of patients from the genuine patients.

TRUE BACK PAIN

True back pain can broadly be categorized into three groups:
- Back pain associated with spinal pathology (e.g. vertebral infections, tumors, ankylosing spnodylitis, etc.).
- Back pain due to nerve root compression. This is commonly due to prolapsed intervertebral disk causing compression of the nerve roots in the neural canals.
- Back pain due to alteration in the spine mechanics (Mechanical back pain). This forms the largest group of conditions that cause back pain, e.g. osteoarthritis, lumbar spondylosis, osteoporosis, etc.

NERVE ROOT PAIN

The most common cause of nerve root pain is intervertebral disk prolapse (IVDP). As explained in previous chapters, 95% of the disk prolapse takes place in the L_{4-5}, L_5S_1 region (low-disk prolapse) involving the L_4 and L_5 nerve roots and the remaining 5% involves the L_1 to L_3 levels (high-disk prolapse).

Tests to Detect Low-disk Prolapse (L_4-L_5)

Straight Leg Raising Test (SLRT)

It is a delicate accurate test to assess the presence or absence of nerve root irritation. Pain duplicating sciatica that is elicited by this test indicates a space-occupying lesion (SOL) such as lumbar disk herniation at the nerve root level.

Normally, the nerve roots are not stretched by the SLRT until 35–70° angulations has been reached. However, if there is a disk prolapse, the neural space is reduced, the nerve root is stretched, and the pain occurs early. In the dynamics of unilateral SLRT, during the first 0–35°, the slack sciatic nerve roots become taut and there is no dural movement. At 35°, tension is applied to the sciatic nerve roots. Between 35 and 70°, the sciatic nerve root stretches over the intervertebral disk. Above 70°, there is no further deformation of the root and the pain could originate in the joint. Thus, sciatica in the leg produced from 0–30° is due to nerve root compression due to SOL, from 30–60° is due to sacroiliac joint disease and above 90° is due to lumbosacral disease.

Procedure

It is a passive test (Fig. 8.13) and each leg is tested individually. The patient is supine with the legs extended. With one hand under the heel and the other over the knee, the examiner passively lifts the leg of the patient until the patient complains of pain or tightness. The test is positive if pain extends from the back, down the leg along the sciatic nerve distribution.

Now drop the leg slightly and the pain disappears. Instruct the patient to flex the neck or passively dorsiflex the foot (Braggard's sign). If the pain increases, it indicates dural stretch and traction on nerve roots. If pain does not increase, then it suggests hamstring tightness, lumbosacral or sacroiliac joint involvement and not disk prolapse (Fig. 8.14).

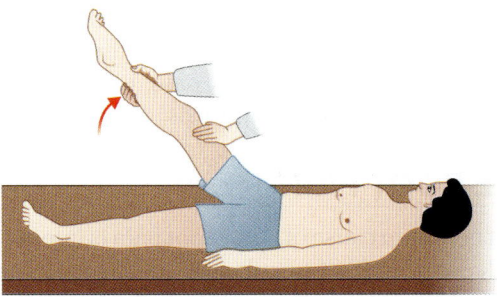

Fig. 8.13: Method of performing a passive SLRT

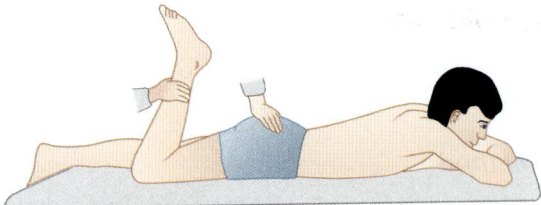

Fig. 8.15: Femoral nerve stretch test

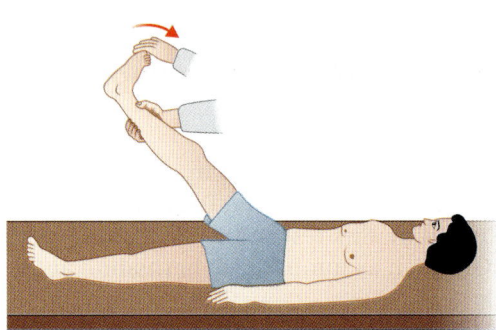

Fig. 8.14: Method of performing the Braggard's sign

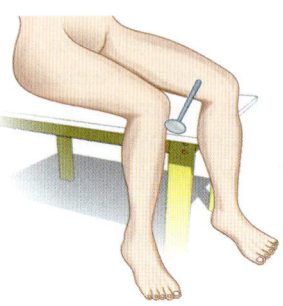

Fig. 8.16: Involvement of L_4 myotome (Patient is unable to extend the knee and loss of knee reflex)

Lasegue Test

The patient is supine. Flex the patient's hip and knee to 90°. The nerve roots are not under tension and no pain is elicited. Now extend the knee. If the patient complains of pain, the test is positive and it indicates nerve root compression or inflammation.

Tests to Detect High-disk Prolapse (L_1-L_2-L_3)

High-disk prolapse involves L_1, L_2 and L_3 nerve roots comprise only 5% of the cases of disk lesions. Since femoral nerve arises from L_1, L_2, L_3 and L_4, the tests are directed towards testing this nerve.

Femoral Nerve Traction Test

The patient lies on the side on the unaffected side with hip slightly flexed. Grasp the affected leg of the patient and gently extend the hip by 15° (Fig. 8.15). This stretches the femoral nerve. Now slowly flex the knee of the affected leg. This further stretches the femoral nerve. If pain radiates to the anterior thigh, it indicates a radiculopathy involving L_1, L_2, L_3 and L_4 nerve roots.

Interpretation

- If pain radiates to the groin and along the anterior medial thigh, it indicates L_3 nerve root radiculopathy.
- If pain radiates to midtibia—L_4 nerve root radiculopathy.

Neurological Signs

After having ascertained the nerve root compression due to disk prolapse, neurological examination of the lower limbs must be carried out to assess the damage caused to the neuromuscular system.

Motor Testing

Test the muscle strength of the following group of muscles and compare it with the normal side:
- The quadriceps group—test for the L_2, L_3 and L_4 roots (Fig. 8.16).
- Extensor hallucis longus—test for L_5 root (Fig. 8.17).
- The gastrocnemius—test for S_1 and S_2 (Fig. 8.18).
- The peroneus longus and brevis—test for S_1.

Quick Facts
Upper disc lesions
- Femoral nerve arises from L_1, L_2, L_3 and L_4 nerve roots. Hence, the traction tests for upper disk lesions are directed towards testing this nerve
- Features of upper disk lesions are:
  - Weakness of the quadriceps muscle
  - Diminished or absent patellar reflex
  - SLRT test and signs are negative
  - Hypo- or hyperesthesia at the L_4 dermatome

Interesting Facts
Sciatica versus herniated disk
- *Definition of Sciatica:* Radiating pain along the distribution of sciatic nerve along the posterior aspect of the buttocks, thigh, leg and foot

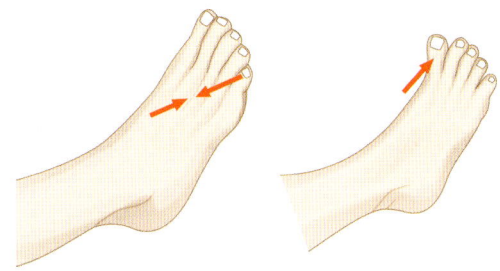

Fig. 8.17: Involvement of L_5 myotome, patient is unable to extend the toes

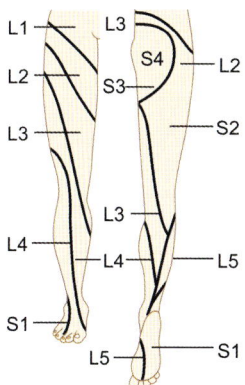

Fig. 8.19: Dermatomal pattern of lower limbs

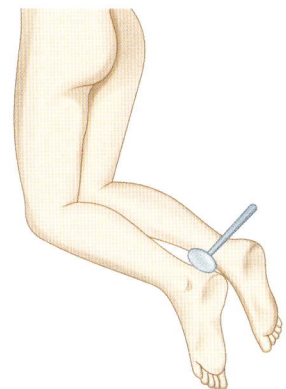

Fig. 8.18: S_1 myotome involvement loss of ankle jerk and plantar flexion

- *Causes:* There are plethora of causes for sciatica. The important ones being disk prolapse, tumors, lumbosacral disease, SI joint arthritis, etc.

There are five criteria to diagnose sciatica due to disk prolapse:
1. Leg pain > back pain
2. Paresthesia localized to a dermatome
3. SLRT is reduced to 50% of what is considered normal
4. Two of the four neurological signs are present (atrophy, motor weakness, and sensation ↓ reflexes ↑)
5. X-ray and imaging are positive

- The quadriceps group—test for the L_2, L_3 and L_4 roots.
- Extensor hallucis longus—test for L_5 root.
- The gastrocnemius—test for S_1 and S_2.
- The peroneus longus and brevis—test for S_1.

Interesting Facts
Quick screening tests for myotomes
Heel/toe walk test
Instruct the patient to walk on the toes and on the heel
Interpretation
- Inability to walk on the heel—L_5 myotome is affected (Weakness of anterior leg muscles)
- Inability to walk on the toes S_1 myotome is affected (Weakness of calf muscles)

Sensation

There is a considerable variation and overlap of the dermatomal patterns and hence it is difficult to chart the dermatomes precisely. In mapping out a sensory dermatome, it is advisable to go from zone of numbness to normal sensitivity.

General Guidelines
- L_4 dermatome affected—medial aspect of foot and leg.
- L_5 dermatome affected—dorsum of the foot and great toe.
- S_1 dermatome affected—lateral border of the foot.
- L_2, L_3, L_4 dermatome affected—anterior aspect of thigh.
- S_1, S_2, S_3, S_4 dermatome affected—perineum, and rectal tone (Fig. 8.19).

Reflexes
a. Knee reflex—to test the L_4 nerve root (Fig. 8.16).
b. Ankle reflex—to test the S_1 nerve root (Fig. 8.18).
No reliable reflex test is available for L_5 nerve roots.

Back Pain due to Spinal Pathology

In this group, ankylosing spondylitis is the common cause. Two important clinical tests help to diagnose this condition.

Chest Expansion

This is measured with the patient's arm held straight up over the head. In men, measurement is carried out at the level of fourth intercostals space and in women just below the breasts. Measurement is carried out in both inspiration and expiration. Normal expansion is more than 3 cm. It is decreased in ankylosing spondylitis.

> **Quick Recap**
> *Examination of spine*
> - General examination
> - Inspection
> - Palpation
> - Range of movements
> - Evaluation of the causes of low back pain
> - Tests for IVDP both high and low
> - Neurological examination
> - Tests to detect malingering
> - Tests for back pain, due to spinal pathology and mechanical back pain
> - Other examinations—for cold abscess, SI joint, systemic examination, examination of hip joint, etc.

IMPORTANT SPINE CONDITIONS

- Scoliosis (*see page 386)
- Spondylolisthesis (*see page 391)
- Low back pain and disk prolapse (*see page 447)
- TB spine (*see page 536)
- Injuries to the spine (*see page 300)

---

*See *Textbook of Orthopedics,* John Ebnezar, 5th Edition.

Index

Page numbers followed by *f* refer to figure, *fc* refer to flowchart and *t* refer to table

A

ABCDE's method 207
Abdomen 29
   muscle strain 788
Abduction
   limitation of 399*f*
   test 398
Abscess, psoas 540
Accident, scene of 49
Acetabular
   component 809*f*
   index 479
   labrum 806*f*
   preparation 806*f*
Acetabulum 288*f*, 478, 711*f*
   fracture of 291*f*
Achondroplasia 396, 499, 499*f*, 500
Acidosis 516
Ackermann's zone phenomenon 40
Acrocephalosyndactyly 506
Acromioclavicular joint 117
   injuries of 117, 118*f*
Acrylic bone cementation 611
Actinomycosis 522
Acupressure 580, 663
Adhesive skin traction 63
Adson's test 364, 364*f*
Adventitious bursa, inflammation of 374
Aerobic exercise 662
   program 662
Aeroplane splint 339*f*
Airway 49
   management 51
Albers-Schönberg disease 503
Albright's syndrome 505
Alfacalcidol 651

Alkaline phosphatase 569, 614
Allen's classification 301
Allen's test 364
Allis method 201, 207
Allograft 360
   fixation 72
American Academy of Orthopedic
      Surgeons 666
American College of Rheumatology 660
Aminoaciduria 511
Amniotic fluid examinations 594
Amphiarthrosis 11
Amputation 34, 381, 530, 612, 616, 773,
      773*f*, 774*f*
   level of 773, 775
   open 773, 775
   primary 156
   radical 598
Amyloidosis 530
Anal sphincter relaxation 317
Analgesic 357, 572
   anti-inflammatory drugs 92
Anderson and d'Olonzo's
      classification 307
Anderson's classification 22
Anemia, hypochromic 568
Anesthesia
   general 623, 741
   local 623
   spinal 708*f*
Aneurysmal bone cyst 608, 608*f*
Angulation osteotomy 357*f*, 641*f*
Angulatory malunion 41
Ankle 99, 587, 590, 768*f*
   amputation 774
   foot orthoses 781, 783, 784*f*
   fractures 74, 263*f*, 264*f*

   complications of 265
   nonunion of 265*f*
   injury 261, 262*f*, 266*f*, 788
      classification 262
      eversion mechanism of 262*f*
   inversion injury of 263*f*
   jerk 452*f*
   joint 40
      active movements of 95
      neuropathic 560*f*
   ligaments, anatomy of 261*f*
   plain X-ray of 562*f*
   radiograph of 266
   sprain 99, 265, 266*f*, 267*f*
      grading of 266
   strap 266*f*
   tuberculosis of 553, 553*f*
   units 780
Anorexia 516
Anoxia 523
Antalgic gait 398
Antibiotics 31, 47
   intravenous 525
   role of 25
   therapy 526
      principles of 524
Anticoagulant therapy 43
Antiepileptic drugs 510
Anti-inflammatory agents 357
Antinuclear antibody 569
Antiplatelets, role of 31
Antipyretic analgesics 92
Antitoxin 47
Apert's syndrome 506
Apical subungual infection 441
Apley's compression test 240
Apprehension test 128

Aquatic physical therapy 663
Arcuate line 288f
Arnold's classification 677
Arterial spasm 32
Arteriovenous malformation 439
Artery 522f
    lateral circumflex 634f
    medial circumflex 634f
Arthralgia 579
Arthritic hand 444
Arthritis 352, 549, 549fc, 552, 556, 558f, 574
    advanced 547, 549, 549fc
    crystal-induced 564
    gonococcal 558
    hemophilic 560, 561f
    hip 348
    infective 556
    metabolic 556
    post-traumatic 207, 295
    psoriatic 444, 575
    rheumatoid 571t
    septic 77, 396, 513, 519, 558f
    traumatic 564
Arthrodesis 34, 72, 174, 209, 324, 357, 358, 433, 549, 553, 574, 588, 631, 664
    extra-articular 358
    primary 260
    triple 492, 493, 493f
Arthrography 171, 400, 412
Arthrogryposis multiplex congenita 589
Arthroplasty 173, 358, 433, 549, 574, 611, 801
    amniotic 549
    bipolar 640
    excision 358, 359f
    hemireplacement 359f, 641, 707
    primary 209
    resurfacement 668
    types 358, 359f
Arthroscopic
    debridement 664
    examination 661
    meniscal repair 241f
    treatment 412
Arthroscopy 74, 171, 415, 415f, 791, 792
Arthrotomy 533, 549, 557
    closure of 825f
Articular facet
    inferior 299f
    superior 299f
Artificial respiration, technique of 50f
Aspiration 526, 541
Astro-sorb heel seat 784
Atelectasis 31
Atherosclerosis 580
Athletes 109
Atlantoaxial subluxation 569
Autologous chondrocyte grafting 664
Avascular necrosis 27, 38, 38f, 397, 640, 642
Axial skeleton 8
Axillary nerve injury 340
    treatment 340
Azathioprine 573

B

Backache 448, 461, 462f, 465, 467
    causes of 462, 578t
    epidemiology of 447
    low 447, 449, 451, 461, 788
Bado's classification 161t
Baker's cyst 411, 411t, 411f
Ball and socket joint 11f, 12
Balloon kyphoplasty 312
Bandaging techniques 776f
Bankart's lesion 127
Bankart's repair 129f
Barton's fracture 167, 168f
Baseball finger 182
Basket forceps 791
Baumann's angle 135
Bedsores
    formation of 315f
    management 315
Behçet's syndrome 575
Bence Jones protein 614
Benediction test 327, 328f
Bennett's fracture 174, 175, 175f, 190f
    K-wire fixation of 175f
Biceps
    muscle 303f
    tendon, rupture of 93f
Bigelow's method 201, 202f, 207
Bimalleolar ankle fracture 263f
Bioabsorbable fixation 74
Biochemical theory 30
Biopsy 597, 616
    types of 597fc
Biphosphonates 651
Bipolar prosthesis hip 642f
Birmingham hip 802
    resurfacing 668f
    arthroplasty 83
Bladder management 315f
Blade plate fixation 223, 224f
Blastomycosis 522
Bleeding gums 526
Blood
    tests 465
    transfusion 23, 525
    vessel 43, 44, 775
        injuries 44t
    volume 31

Blounts' disease 407
Blumensaat's line 413f
Body
    fracture of 172, 178, 286
Böhler's angle 280
Böhler's stirrup 64f
Böhler-Braun splint 61, 61f
Bologna cast 58
Bone 10, 24, 56, 478, 506, 775
    abscess 523
    affections of 108
    artificial 360
    cell types 7, 497
    clamps 731f
    cross-section 8f
    cyst 608
        unicameral 609f
    density of 37
    development 7, 497
    diseases 394
    disorders 352
    excision of 530
    extensive subperiosteal resorption of 518f
    flat 10
    formation 508
    fractures 23f, 29
    graft
        cortical 38, 38f
        method 84, 609
        role of 37, 360
    healing, primary 55, 87, 88
    homeostasis, dynamics of 509fc
    irregular thickening of 350, 527
    loss 15, 23f, 79
    metastatic tumors of 615
    mineral density 649f
    model 734f
    neoplasia 596
    organization of 8, 9f
    ossification methods 497
    parts of 8
    regeneration 86
    scan 110, 606, 616, 637
    structure of 8f, 508fc
    tumors 603
        classification of 598, 599t
        resorptive 608
    types of 10f
Bony
    anatomy of fibula 249f
    ankylosis 558f
        hip 558f
    procedures 492
    spicules, discharge of 527f
Boutonniere's deformity 18, 184, 566
Bow legs 407
Bowel program 316

Boxer's fracture 191, 191*f*
Boyd's classification 484*t*
Brachial plexus
　anatomy of 337*f*
　injury 337
　　causes 337
Brachial vessels 44*f*
Bracing, complications of 390
Brailsford's stages 559
Brain 583
Brand's operation 328
Brodies abscess 531, 531*f*
Brown tumor 518
Brucella bacillus 522
Bryant's traction 63
Buck's extension skin traction 63
Bucket handle tear 238*f*, 240*f*
Bückling's sign 453
Bulbocavernosus reflex 304
Bumper injuries 249*f*, 252*f*
Burkhalter splint 181
Bursa 97, 121
　around knee 99, 409, 410*f*
　enlargements 428
Bursitis 97
　infective 97
　painful 599
　prepatellar 410, 410*f*
Burst fracture 307, 307*f*
　stable 308*f*
　unstable 308*f*
Butcher's nail 70
Butterfly fractures 79
Buttress plate 68, 69, 69*f*, 223

C

Cafe-au-lait spots 506
Calcaneal
　fracture
　　displaced 283*f*
　　plating of 285*f*
　　reduction 283, 284*f*
　spurs 99, 430, 430*f*
　stress fracture 431
　traction 733*f*
Calcaneovalgus 485
Calcaneovarus 485
Calcaneum
　epiphysitis of 431
　fracture, intra-articular 283*f*
　intra-articular fractures of 281*f*
　stress fractures of 283*f*
Calcaneus deformity 584
Calcitonin 92, 651, 655*f*
Calcium 650
　hydroxyapatite 7
　metabolism 509
　pyrophosphate deposition
　　disease 580
　role of 509
Calipers, functions of 783
Campanacci's radiographic 610
Canal stenosis 677
Cancellous bone graft 38
Cancellous graft 753*f*
Cancellous screw 67, 67*f*
Canuati disease 504
Capital femoral epiphysis 397
Capitellum fracture 152, 152*f*
　types of 152*f*
Card test 327, 327*f*
Cardiovascular exercise 662
Carpal
　bones 530
　dislocations 19
　injury 170
　tunnel splint 383*f*
　tunnel syndrome 99, 381, 632
　　anatomy 381, 382*f*
　　causes 381
Carpenter's syndrome 506
Carpi ulnaris, flexor 324*f*
Carpometacarpal joint 671*f*
　injuries of 174
Cartilaginous, bone tumors of 598
Cast
　brace, functional 57-59, 61*f*, 79, 217*f*
　disease 59
　syndrome 59
Catterall classification 400
Cauda equina
　claudication 678
　lesion 317*f*
　syndrome 317
　　causes 317
　　symptoms 317
　　treatment 317
Causalgia 777
Cavendish's grading 473
Celiac disease 510
Cellulitis 526
Cemented total
　hip replacement 359*f*
　knee replacement 359*f*
Central intra-articular fragments 164
Central nervous system 347
　management 52
Central tumors 602
Ceramic 801
Cerebral palsy 583, 584*f*, 584*t*, 585, 595
　causes of 583*t*
　classification of 583*t*
　surgery in 585
Cervical
　collar 54, 306*f*, 354*f*, 675, 782, 783*f*
　coxa vara 396
　disk
　　herniation 673*f*
　　syndromes 365, 673, 675
　lordosis 298*f*
　nerve roots 303*f*
　orthosis 781, 783*f*
　plexus 319
　region 540
　rib 365
　　pathological anatomy 365
　　treatment 365
　　types 365
　　unilateral 365*f*
　spinal cord 314*f*
　　injury 304*t*
　spine 299, 675, 782
　　fractures 301
　　injuries 300, 301*f*, 302*f*
　spondylosis 671, 671*f*, 675, 675*f*
　　pain in 674*f*
　　treatment of 676*f*
　sprain syndrome 300
　traction 64, 355*f*
　vertebra fracture 305*f*
Cervico-thoraco-lumbo-sacral
　orthosis 781
Chance fracture 308*f*, 309
Charnley's compression
　arthrodesis 358*f*, 560*f*
　clamp 560*f*
Chauffeur's fracture 166
Chemonucleolysis 460
Chemotherapy 533-535, 598, 607, 614, 616
Chest 346*f*
　injuries 50
Chiari's osteotomy 483, 483*f*
Chlamydia 576
Chloroquine 572
Chondral resurfacing procedure 664
Chondroblastoma 601
Chondrocalcinosis 581
Chondroitin sulfate 663
Chondroma 599
Chondromalacia 414*f*
　hallmark of 414*f*
　patella 413, 414*f*
Chondromatosis, synovial 415, 562
Chondromyxoid fibroma 603, 603*f*
Chondro-osteodystrophy 396
Chondrosarcoma 601, 602, 602*f*
Chopart's operation 775
Chovstek's sign 511
Chromium 802
Cicatrix, excision of 34
Circular open amputation 773, 775
Citrovorum factor rescue 607

Clamps, types of 76
Classical claw hand 33
Claudication 678
    ischemic 678
    neurogenic 464, 678
    types of 678*t*
Clavicle
    aplasia of 474
    bone 114*f*
    bony anatomy of 113*f*
    fracture, pseudoparalysis in 114*f*
    functions of 113
    lateral end of 610*f*
Claw hand 325, 325*fc*
    causes 325
    deformity 328
    types 325
Claw toes 423, 434*f*, 435*f*, 584
Cleidocranial dysostosis 396, 474, 475*f*
Clergyman's knee 410*f*
Clostridium tetani 47
Clostridium welchii 47, 522
Clubfoot 485, 487, 490*f*, 495
    complex 487*fc*
    non-surgical treatment of 490*f*
    radiograph of 490
    recurrent 493
Cobalt 802
Cobb's method 388
Coccidioidomycosis 522
Coccyx 288*f*, 295
    fracture 295*f*, 296*f*
Cold abscess 538*f*, 545
    spread of 537*f*, 539*fc*
Coliforms 522
Collagen fibrils 565
Collateral ligament injury 99, 230
Colles' cast 624
Colles' fracture 16, 53, 164, 621, 621*f*-622*f*, 623, 624, 632*f*
Colton's classification 148
Compartmental syndrome 31, 32*f*, 33*f*, 59, 258*f*
Compression
    bandage 91, 94, 95, 267*f*
    fracture 15*f*
    injury 302*f*
    metatarsalgia 425
    plates, dynamic 69
Condylar
    fractures 249
    locking plates 223
    screw, dynamic 223
Condyle fracture 153*f*
    types of medial 154*f*
Conradi's disease 504
Conwell's classification 289
Cord injury, level of 314

Coronoid fractures, types of 151*f*
Cortical screw, placement of 704*f*
Corticosteroids 573
Corticotomy 38, 81
Costotransversectomy 543, 543*f*
Cotton fracture 265
Coxa plana 397
Coxa valga 396*f*, 397*f*
Coxa vara 396, 396*f*, 397*f*, 471
    congenital 396
    epiphyseal 396
Cozen's test 374, 375*f*
Crack fracture 15
Craniodiaphyseal dysplasia 504
Craniometaphyseal dysplasia 504
C-reactive protein 569
Crepitus 17, 18
Crescent sign 136
Crohn's disease 575
Cruciate ligament
    anterior 797, 798, 799*f*
    injury 99, 232
    posterior 238*f*
Crush
    injuries 32, 194, 195, 195*f*, 775, 776
    syndrome 45
Crutchfield tongs 306*f*
Cryotherapy 93, 94, 525
Crystalline arthropathies 580
Cubitus valgus 132*f*, 141
Cubitus varus 132*f*, 138, 140*f*, 141
    deformity 138*f*, 140*f*
Cuboid fractures 277, 278*f*
    classification 278
    treatment 278
Cuneiform injuries 278
    classification 278
    treatment 278
Cyanosis 30
Cyclophosphamide 573
Cylindrical cast 244*f*
Cyst 667
    formation 569
    popliteal 411, 411*f*
    subchondral 661
Cystic degeneration 238
Cytokine production 572
Cytotoxic drugs 357

D

Dancer tendinitis 432
Dapsone 572
Darrach's operation 706
Dashboard injury 198*f*
de Quervain's disease 98*f*, 99, 378, 378*f*
Dead tissues, excision of 767*f*
Death, causes of 4

Deep
    fascia, closure of 740*f*
    palmar abscess 442, 442*f*
    vein thrombosis 42, 43*f*
Deformity 17, 18, 158*f*, 215*f*, 253*f*, 402, 407, 505*f*, 528, 530, 545, 569, 683*f*, 697*f*, 708*f*, 730*f*, 757*f*, 760*f*
    abduction 545
    acquired 351, 476
    adduction 545, 546*f*
    classification 351
    correction of 356, 490
    flexion 545
    management 351
    since birth 351
    upper leg 729*f*, 730*f*
Dehydration 524
Delbet's classification 636*f*
Deltoid
    contracture 372, 372*f*
    muscle 303*f*
Denholm's method 269*f*
Denholm's repair 269
Denis Browne splint 494*f*
Denis Weber classification 263
Dermatitis, allergic 59
Destot's sign 291
Detsky quality index 836
Diaphyseal aclasia 502
Diaphysis 523
Diarthrosis 11
Diet therapy 579, 650*f*
Digestive system management 52
Digitorum profundus, flexor 324*f*
Dimeglio's classification 488
Dinner fork 622
    deformity 18, 18*f*, 622*f*, 625*f*
Disease-modifying antirheumatic drugs 572
Disk
    anatomy 449
    artificial 84*f*
    bulging 450
    functions of 299
    herniation 450
        posterolateral 455*f*
    physiology 449
    prolapse compressing nerve root 450*f*
    replacement, artificial 84
    slip 451*f*
Dislocation 13, 17, 26, 39, 62, 120, 802
    mechanism of 125
    subluxation of 547
    types of 26, 27
Displacement, stages of 153, 154
Distal radial
    epiphysis 476
    fracture, comminuted 164

Distal radioulnar ligament 630
Distal radius
   fracture 629f
      percutaneous fixation 624f
   resection of 611
Distal ulnar fracture 160
Distraction
   injury 309f
   test 292
Dorsal
   Barton's fracture 167f
   interosseous muscle 303f
   root ganglion 319f
   surface, comminuted 629
   trans-scaphoid perilunar
      dislocation 176
   ulnar split 164
Dorsiflexion
   loss of 631
   test 487, 488f
Double plate fixation 224
Draughtsman elbow 377
Drawer test
   anterior 233, 234f
   posterior 233
Drug
   anti-inflammatory 572
   antimalarial 572, 573
   anti-resorptive 650, 653, 653f
   therapy 31, 572, 585, 650
Duchenne muscular dystrophy 592
Duck waddle test 240
Dunlop's traction 63, 63f, 101, 106f
Duodenal biopsy 516
Duosoft insoles 784
Dupuytren's contracture 99, 380
   causes 380
   pathogenesis 380
   surgical methods 381
   treatment 381
Dynaplast pressure bandage 713f
Dyschondroplasia 502
Dysfunction, stage of 449
Dysplasia 8
   acetabular 478
   diaphyseal 504
   epiphyseal 503
   fibrous 108, 504
   hallmarks 498
   hemimelia, epiphyseal 504
   metaphyseal 504
   multiplexa, epiphyseal 503
   punctate, epiphyseal 504
   skeletal 396

E

Earle's sign 291
Edema, intramuscular 32

Egawa test 327, 327f
Elbow 375, 467, 589, 787
   amputation 775f
   arthroplasties, types of 146t
   disarticulation 773
   dislocation, reduction of 145f
   joint 40, 40f
      anatomy of 131f
      dislocation of 141
      posterior dislocation of 143f
   plaster slab 696f
   posterior dislocation of 142, 142f,
      142t, 143f, 147
   regional conditions of 373
   replacement, total 359f
   rheumatoid 568f
   X-ray of 134
Electrical stimulation, role of 38
Electrolyte balance 31
Elephant foot 35, 35f
Ellipsoid joint 11f
Ely's test 419, 419f
En bloc excision 611
Enchondroma 599, 601f
Endochondral ossification 497
Endocrine disorder 346
Endocrine
   abnormalities 646
   disorders 407
   system 456
Endoneurolysis 324
Endoprostheses 778
Engelmann's disease 504
Enneking's staging 597, 611
Epicondylitis 373
Epidural steroid injection, technique
   of 459f
Epiphyseal coxa vara 403
Epiphyseal stapling 408f
Epiphysis 8, 523
Episcleritis 566
Epithelioma 530
Epitrochleitis 376
Epstein's classification 199f, 205
Equinovalgus 485f
Equinovarus 485
Equinus 485, 492
   deformity 584
Erb's palsy 339, 339f
   management 339
Erysipelas 526
Erythema nodosum 526
Essex-Lopresti
   fracture 165
   method 283, 284f
Ewing's sarcoma 526, 612, 613, 612f
   femur 613f
Exacerbation, acute 530
Excision 598

Exercises
   active 91
   role of 457, 669
   therapeutic 662
   types of 669
Exoprostheses 778
Exostosis 598
   humerus 600f
Extensor
   digitorum longus 334f
   hallucis longus 334f
   lag 245, 421f
   pollicis tendon 631
   tendon
      injuries 194, 194f
      ruptured 183
      stretched 183
External fixation 55, 74, 176, 190, 223,
   624f, 766
External fixators 57, 57f, 76f, 493
   application of 766
   role of 256
   types of 76, 256
Extra-articular fractures 80, 281, 282
   classification 281
   treatment 282
   types of 281f
Extramedullary tibial alignment
   guide 817f

F

Fabre's test 577f
Facet joint 299f
   arthritis 449
   osteoarthritis 462
   sclerosis of 678
Facet syndromes 464
Facioscapulohumeral muscular
   dystrophy 593
Facture dislocation, posterior 199f, 204f
Fajersztajn's test 453
Falvo's classification 500
Faradic stimulation 323
Fascial tissues 475
Fasciectomy 381
Fasciitis 47
Fasciotomy, subcutaneous 381
Fat
   embolism 29, 802
      syndrome 30f
   pad
      atrophy of 431
      insufficiency 431
      sign 135
      syndrome 417
   source of 30
Fatal injuries 3
Fatigue fractures 15

Fatty white marrow 8
Femoral
   canal 811*f*
      plug 811*f*
      reaming of 809*f*
   condyles, flattening of 419
   cutaneous nerve, lateral 336*f*
   epiphysis, growth of capital 399
   fracture, proximal 26*f*
   functional braces 54
   head
      avascular necrosis of 39*f*, 637*f*
      blood supply of 634*fc*
      dislocation of 805*f*
      fracture of 199
      vascular anatomy of 634*f*
   instrument rotation 820*f*
   nails, proximal 643, 644
   neck
      fracture, complications of 640
      osteotomy 806*f*
      stress fracture of 110*f*
   nerve stretch test 454
   osteotomy, distal 664
   shaft fractures 46, 215*f*
   varus osteotomy 402*f*
Femur 528*f*, 612*f*
   compound fracture of 23*f*
   cut 819*f*
   delivering head of 710*f*
   fractures 26*f*, 72, 221*f*, 222*f*, 224
      classification of 215
      neck of 227
      proximal 211
      shaft of 228
   head of 478
   immobilize fracture 61
   interlocking 219*f*
      nail of 79*f*
   ipsilateral fracture of 226*f*
   malunion fracture 666*f*
   neck of 38*f*, 478
   nonunion fracture 220*f*
   proximal 633*f*
   pseudarthrosis of 485*f*
   sizing of 820*f*
   supracondylar fracture of 221, 222
   surgery of 719
   upper end of 602*f*
Fetal rickets 510
Fiberglass plasters 78
Fibroblastic tissue, zone of 40
Fibromyalgia 564, 579, 579*f*, 580*f*
Fibula 471
   congenital absence of 494
   fracture of 249, 253*f*
Fibular collateral ligament 238*f*
   injury 232
Fibular fractures 258

Fielding's classification 211, 211*f*
Figure of '8' 115
   bandaging 115*f*
Finger 467
   amputation of 195
   cot splint 182*f*
   extension splint 186*f*
   fracture 755
   trap traction 630*f*
Fingertip avulsions 194
Finkelstein's test 378*f*
Firearm injuries 5
Fish-tail sign 135
Fixation
   devices, complications of 220
   methods of 226
Fixed traction, method of 66*f*
Flail
   arm splint 338*f*
   upper limb 338*f*
Flatfoot 422*f*, 424*f*
   spasmodic 424
Flexion
   Deformity
      fixed 399
      minor 667*f*
   lateral 674*f*, 676
   loss of 674
Flexor tendon injuries 193
Fluid analysis, synovial 569
Fluoroscopy 171
Fluorosis 519, 677
Folic acid 572
Food supplementation 663
Foot 99, 270*f*, 584, 587, 589, 590, 788
   amputation 774
   arch 421, 422*f*
      deformities 422*f*
   cushion, ball of 784
   deformities 82, 485, 586
      classification of 590, 590*t*
   drop, causes of 334
   end elevation 94
   fracture of 271*fc*
   injuries of 270
   normal 422*f*, 424*f*, 487
   pain 425
      causes of 425*fc*
   radiograph of 591*f*
   regional disorders of 421
   rheumatoid 568*f*
   supports 784
Football injuries 270, 278
Footballer's ankle 40
Foot-drop 334, 335*f*, 591
   right 335*f*
   splint 336*f*
      dynamic 335*f*, 336*f*
   treatment algorithm of 335*fc*

Footwear 783, 784
Forearm 467
   bones of 157*f*, 159*f*
   fractures, distal 621
   greenstick fracture of 102*f*
   injuries of 157
   plain X-ray of 475
   volar compartment of 31*f*
Forefoot injuries classification 270
Fowler's operation 328
Fractures 13, 17-19, 29, 42, 51, 62, 78,
      100, 107, 158*f*, 264, 286, 352, 599,
      714*f*, 727*f*
   acetabulum 290, 292*f*
   acute 29, 273
   atypical 15, 15*f*
   avulsion 178, 183, 275*f*, 289*f*, 294
   bicondylar 250*f*
   birth 100
   calcaneal 282*f*, 284*f*
   calcaneum 279, 280, 281*f*
      classification 280
      functions 280
      structure 280
   capitellar 152
   clavicle 51, 113, 114*f*, 117
      classification of 113
      complications of 116
      internal fixation of 115
      plate fixation 116*f*
      treatment of 115
   comminuted 14, 79, 184*f*, 221*f*, 242*f*,
      281*f*
   complex 82
   complications of 29, 29*t*
   compound 13, 14*f*, 22, 36, 82
   compression 313*f*
   condylar 133, 184*f*, 730*f*
   coronoid 150, 151*f*
   diaphyseal 54
   disease 53, 57, 87
      eliminates 60
   dislocation 305*f*, 764*f*
   displaced 179, 244, 250, 254, 294
   displacement of 15
   distal 79
      femur 220
   examination 26
   exposure of 703*f*, 715*f*
   femur 60, 211, 214*f*, 215*f*, 217*f*
   flexion compression 310*f*
   fragments
      distraction of 36
      exposure of 684*f*
      reduction of 685*f*
      rotation of 79
   healing 86, 87*f*
      Hunter' stages of 86*f*
      methods of 86

immobilization 24, 53f
intercondylar 698f
intra-articular 80, 281f, 282, 415, 631
ipsilateral 224
lateral condyle 154f
line 14
linear 14
lunate 177
malleolus 72
management 20, 52
manipulation of 625f
medial calcaneal process 282
neck
   femur 19, 211, 633, 635f, 636f, 642, 644, 717
   radius 133, 162f
olecranon 72, 72f
open 13, 21, 24, 25, 54
operative treatment of 57
osteochondral 74, 146, 172
osteoporotic 656
patella 72, 243f
   surgical methods of 244fc
pathological 15, 16f, 79, 100, 107, 108, 528
pattern of 14, 101, 212, 621
pediatric 74
pelvic 29, 50, 289, 292, 294
pelvis 288
percutaneous fixation of 72
pertrochanteric 714f
phalangeal 187f
phalanx 56f, 181f
radial head 142f
reconstruction of 699f
reduction of 630f, 699f, 703f, 731f
segmental 14, 36, 720
shaft
   femur 66f, 214, 215f, 216fc
   humerus 70f, 88f, 683
simple 14f
sites of 79, 113
spine 677
spiral 79
stabilization of 21
straddle 290
subchondral 399, 399f
subtrochanteric 71f, 211
talus 284
temporary stabilization of 72
tibia 60, 253f
   technique of 254f
   treated 253f
tongue shaped 281f
treatment of 53, 56, 57, 57f, 76f, 101
   methods of 53, 78
trimalleolar 265
triquetral 177
tuberosity 172, 281f, 282
types of 13, 14f, 17t, 100
ulna 162f
undisplaced 149f, 153f, 179, 242f, 243, 250, 281f, 294
unicondylar 221f
unstable 172, 211, 311
waist 172
Fragility fractures 654
   management of 656f, 657f
Fragment, reduction of 728f
French osteotomy 140f
Froment's sign 326, 327f
Frostbite injury 194
Frozen
   biopsy 606
   hand shoulder syndrome 631, 632f
   shoulder 366, 367f, 368f
      arthrogram of 368f
      causes 366
      pain in 368f
      pathology 366
Fungal osteomyelitis 522

G

Galeazzi's fracture 164, 164f, 165f
   fixation 165f
   forces in 165f
   plating in 166f
Gallium scanning 541
Gallows' traction 63f, 101, 106f, 217f
Galvanic stimulation 323
Gamekeeper's thumb 189, 189f
Ganglion 99
   cyst 379
Garceaus method 493
   modified 493
Garden's classification 636f, 638
Garden's criteria 638
Gartland's classification 134
Gas gangrene 46, 47
Gastrointestinal system 456
Gaucher's disease 108
Genetic 416, 658
   theory 478
Genitourinary system 51
Genu recurvatum 405f, 409, 419, 584
   congenital 418f
Genu valgum 405, 405f, 406f, 511, 515f, 520f, 584
   causes of 405t
   complex 406, 406fc
   deformity 406, 406f, 515
   treatment of 406, 407t
Genu varum 405f, 407, 407f, 408f, 408t
   complex 408
   deformity 408f, 659f, 660f
Giant cell tumor 609, 610f
   benign 609
Gibson's approach 707
Girdle stone excision arthroplasty 550f
Gissane angle 280f
Glaucoma 566
Glenohumeral joint speaks 121
Glenoid cavity 127
Gliding joints 12
Glomerular failure 510
Glomerulonephritis 513
Glucosamine 663
Glutei bursitis 97, 99
Glutei muscles 478
Gluten-sensitive enteropathy 515
Golfer's elbow 99, 376, 376f
Gomphosis 11
Gout 444
Grafts
   fixation of 72
   placement of 753f
Granulation tissue 527
Granuloma 565f
Gray ramus communicans 319f
Great toe 97
   amputation of 774
   gangrene of 44f
Greenstick fracture 15, 100
Growth
   abnormal 397
   plate 8
Guinea pig test 533
Gunshot injuries 300
Gunstock
   deformity 138f
   elbow 138
Gustilo-Anderson and Tscherne classification 22
Gustilo-Anderson classification 22
Guyon's canal 326

H

Haemophilus influenzae 522
Hageland's disease 428
Hahn-Steinthal variety 152
Hairpin bend vessels 522f
Hallux
   rigidus 433
   valgus 432, 433f, 584
   varus 433
Halo body orthosis 783f
Hamate fractures 178
Hammer toe 434, 434f
Hamstrings strain 99
Hand 787
   deformities 592f
   disorders of 439

flexor zones of 193, 193f
infection of 440
injuries 180
intrinsic muscles of 324f
piece 780
sensory distribution of 326f
Hangman's fracture 308
Hard callus, stage of 87
Hardinge approach, modified 805f
Harris hormonal theory 403
Hawkin's types 286
Head
    injury 29, 50, 788
    traction 64
Headache 579
Heat therapy 356
Heel
    broadening of 281f
    compression test 283f
    pad 784
    pain, causes of 427f
    wedge 54
Heikel's classification 477
Helfet's sign 240
Hemarthropathy 562
Hemarthrosis 415
Hematoma 98, 777
    intermuscular 98, 99
    subungual 194
Hemilaminectomy 459, 459f
Hemipelvectomy 779f
Hemogram 226
Hemophilia 415, 561t, 666
    types of 560t
Hemopoiesis 7
Hemorrhage 4, 51f, 294
    external 46
    internal 46
    metaphyseal 522
    source of 46
Hereditary multiple exostosis 502
High density polyethylene 801
Hilgenreiner's line 479, 481f
Hill-Sachs lesion 127
Hindfoot
    injuries 279
    varus 492
Hinge joint 11, 11f
Hip 587, 589, 788
    advanced tuberculosis of 547f
    anterior dislocation of 18f, 205, 205f, 206f
    arthroplasties 668, 801
    central dislocation of 207, 209f
    congenital dislocation of 471, 477, 481, 496
    developmental dysplasia of 477, 478
    disarticulation 774, 779f
    dislocations 197, 199, 208t
        overall classification of 198
    flexion 670, 670f
    implants 21
    irritability, elimination of 401
    joint
        anatomy of 197f
        central fracture dislocation of 209f
        dislocation of 197
        posterior dislocation of 45f, 200f, 334f
        speaks 633
        tuberculosis of 544
    knee-ankle-foot orthoses 781, 783, 783f
    normal 714f
    osteoarthritis of 666, 668f, 669
    pointer 405
    posterior dislocation of 18f, 198f, 199, 205f
    primary osteoarthritis of 666
    radiograph of 547, 714
    reduction 812f
    regional conditions of 396
    replacement, total 359f
    rheumatoid 568f
    rotation 398f
    screw, dynamic 643, 714
    spastic contracture of 584
    stretch 458f
    surgery 707
        advances in 83
    X-ray of 226
Hippocrates method 124f
Hoffa's syndrome 417
Hohl and Moore's classification 250f
Homan's sign 42, 43f
Homocystinuria 506
Hondromyxoma 599
Hormonal theory 478
Hormone 357
    replacement therapy 651, 829
        process of 653f
    therapy 616
Horn cells, anterior 586f
Horner's syndrome 337, 338f
Hourglass constriction 478
Houser's method 413f
Hughston, jerk test of 233
Humeral line, anterior 135
Humeroscapular periarthritis 366
Humerus 72, 133, 612f
    atrophic nonunion of 37f
    displaced supracondylar fractures of 44f
    interlocking nail of 79f
    lateral condyle of 153
    medial condyle of 154
    pathological fracture 109f
    supracondylar fracture of 106f, 134f, 137f, 141
    surgeries of 683
    upper end of 608f
Hunter's disease 502
Hutchinson's fracture 166f
Hybrid fixation 74, 76, 260
Hydrocortisone injection 97, 98
Hydrotherapy 356, 662
Hydroxyapatite coated pins 75
Hyperbaric oxygen 47
    therapy 530
Hypercalcemia, treatment of 616
Hypercalciuria 518
Hyperextension
    brace, anterior 312f
    force 230
    injury 301f, 302f
Hyperflexion injury 301f
Hyperparathyroidism 108, 517, 518f, 666
    primary 517
    secondary 518, 518f
Hyperphosphaturia 518
Hyperplasia 518
Hyperpronation injury 161f
Hypertension 580
Hyperthermia 598
Hyperuricemia, role of 580
Hypoesthesia 678
Hypoplastic patella 419
Hypothenar, role of 324

I

Ice therapy 95
Idiopathic scoliosis, types of 387t
Iliac wing, fracture of 289f
Iliotibial band
    contractures 587
    syndrome 416
Iliotibial tract syndrome 99
Ilium 288f
Ilizarov's fixation 260
Ilizarov's frame 81f
Ilizarov's method 530
    principles of 81
Ilizarov's technique 80
    role of 38
Ilizarov's treatment 88f
Impingement syndrome 369, 371f, 372
    types of 370
Implants
    breakage of 802
    complications of 74
    loosening of 802
    types of 66
Incision 526

Infection 13, 74, 97, 666, 777, 802
Inflammation, stage of 87
Infraspinatus tendonitis 99
Inhibition test 569, 569*fc*
Injuries
  abdominal 50
    wall 295
  acceleration 300
  adduction 266*f*
  arterial 146, 295
  avulsion 39
  causes of 43
  common modes of 17
  compound 22
  epiphyseal 107, 107*f*
  mechanism of 4, 5, 17, 45, 89, 621, 635
  mode of 17*t*
  neurological 143
  prevention of 6
  traumatic 122
Intercondylar fracture humerus 696
Interlocking humerus 686
Interlocking nail 21, 70, 79, 79*f*, 218, 720
  technique 219
Intermittent claudication test 364
Internal fixation 24, 55, 101, 176, 182-184, 186, 190, 209, 244, 717
  complications of 639
  methods 71, 115
  primary 24
  technique of 55, 639
Internal rotation
  limitation of 398*f*
  test 398
Interphalangeal joint 442
  dislocations 272
    treatment 272
  injuries, distal 183
Interstitial nephritis, chronic 513
Intervertebral
  disk 448, 742
  foramina 675
  joints, posterior 448
Intra-articular arthrodesis 358
Intramedullary
  fixation 55, 73*f*, 159, 223
  nails 21, 70, 72, 79, 218
    types of 71*fc*
Intraosseous pressure, equalization of 65
Intrinsic minus hand 326
Iron deficiency anemia 516
Irradiation therapy 611
Ischemia 416
Ischium 288*f*
  stress fracture of 110*f*
Isometric exercises 94, 95, 97
Isotope scan 172, 637

J

Jaffe's criterion 609
Jaipur foot 780, 780*f*
Jefferson's fracture 307*f*
Jersey finger 18, 184
Jewett nail and plate 74
John Wein's
  classification 161*t*
  types 161*f*
Johnson's classification 494*t*
Joints 11, 92, 94, 95
  active movements of 94, 95
  biaxial 11
  bicondylar 11*f*
  cartilaginous 11
  condyloid 12
  contractures 82
  debridement 549
  diseases, treatment of 61
  dislocation 118*f*, 548*f*
  disorders of 556
  drainage 557
  examination 597
  fibrous 11
  function 92
  interference 599
  involvement 19, 523
  laxity 498
  line tenderness 240
  margins, erosion of 569
  mice 414
  mobilization 97
  movements 97, 349
    limitation of 348
    smooth 95
  multiaxial 12
  neuropathic 559, 802
  painful unstable 562
  patellofemoral 798*f*, 799*f*
  pathology 792
  reconstruction of 78
  saddle 11*f*
  space 569
    loss of 671*f*
  stiffness 27, 45, 59, 95, 220, 356
  swelling of 95
  synovial 11
  syphilis of 559
  tenderness, medial 239*f*
  types of 11*f*
  unaffected 91, 92, 97
  unstable 72
Jones fracture 275, 275*f*
  treatment 275
  screw fixation of 276*f*
Jumper's knee 415

Jupiter fracture 153
Juxtacortical tumors 602

K

Kanavel's sign 443*f*
Kaplan's lesion 188, 188*f*
Keinbock's disease 384, 385*f*
Kellegren and Lawrence radiological grading 661
King's osteotomy 141
Kirner's deformity 440
Kirschner's wire 57
Klumpke's paralysis 340
K-nail, complications of 219
Knee 40, 243*f*, 584, 587, 589
  acute dislocation of 247
  amputation 776, 776*f*, 779
  ankle-foot orthoses 781, 783, 783*f*
  arthroplasty 664, 801
  arthroscopy 792, 793*f*
  caliper 588*f*
  combined instabilities of 236
  congenital dislocation of 471, 483
  deformities 405*f*
  disarticulation 774, 776
  dislocation, congenital 484*f*
  extensor apparatus of 246
  flexion 670, 670*f*
    contracture 584
    deformity of 551*f*
    test 406
  gross swelling of 730*f*
  injuries of 229
  instability 236*t*
    classification of 237*t*
  joint 94*f*, 95*f*, 97*f*, 229, 581*f*, 661*f*, 788
    acute dislocation of 247*f*
    anatomy of 229*f*
    plain X-ray of 563*f*
    X-ray of 411
  ligament injuries 229, 230*f*, 233*t*, 236
  medial collateral ligament of 94*f*
  orthoses 781
  osteoarthritis of 658, 659*f*, 660*f*
  plain X-ray of 484, 666*f*
  radiograph of 234
  reflex, loss of 452*f*
  regional disorders of 405
  rheumatoid 568*f*
  septic arthritis of 557*f*
  splint 54
  stability depends upon 229
  swelling of 551*f*
  triple displacement of 551*f*
  tuberculosis of 550, 551*f*
Knock-knee deformity 405*f*

Kocher's method 124f, 125, 125f
Kullman and Leonart's surgery 409
Küntscher's nail 71f, 218
K-wire, fixation 756f, 764f
Kyphosis 394, 677
Kyphotic deformity 538f, 649f

L

Labrum 121
Lachman's test 233, 234, 234f
Lamellae 533
Laminectomy 394, 459, 544, 742, 751f, 752f
Lasègue's test 453
Laser 83f, 792
   treatment 83
Latex
   agglutination test 569fc
   fixation test 569
Lauge Hansen's classification 262, 263f
Lederham syndrome 432
Leg 788
   holder 792
   plaster casts 253
   stretch 669, 670f
Legg-Calvé-Perthes disease 397, 398fc
Leprosy 589, 590, 591f
   classification of 590t
   treatment in 590t
Less invasive stabilization system 80, 80f, 223
Leukocytopenia 566
Leukotriene synthesis 572
Levamisole 572
Lichtenstein's criteria 605
Lichtman classification 385
Ligament
   injury 93
   interspinous 299f
   intertransverse 238f
   medial collateral 238f
   tear, anterior cruciate 232
Ligamentum
   flavum 299f
   teres, artery of 634f
Limb
   elevation 51f, 91, 94, 95, 99
   girdle muscular dystrophy 593
   ischemic 776
   muscles 95, 789
   reflexes, upper 303f
   salvage 606
      surgery 617
Lisfranc's injuries 278, 279, 279f, 280f
Lisfranc's operation 775
Lobster claw hand 439

Low molecular weight dextran 31
Lower limb 27, 44, 323, 346f, 349, 584, 586, 774, 781, 788
   congenital disorders of 471, 477
   deformities 587f
   length 350f
   muscles 789
   orthosis 781, 783
   regional conditions of 396
   tractions 64
   trauma 44
Lumbar
   canal stenosis 395, 677f, 679f
   discectomy, endoscopic 83
   disk disease 449, 677
   lordosis 298f, 393f
   muscles 743f
   scoliosis 389f
   spine 299
      myelographic study of 455f
   spondylosis 449, 455f, 671, 671f
   traction 355f
Lunate
   anterior dislocation of 176
   burst fracture 177f
Lupus erythematosus 444
Luxatio erecta 129
Lymphangiectasia 411
Lymphangioma 439

M

Macnab classification 392
Madelung's deformity 440, 476, 476f
   radiograph of 476f
Mader's classification 529f
Maffucci's disease 502
Magerl classification, modified 309
Malgaigne's fracture 290
Malignant giant cell tumor 610
Malleolar
   fixation 265f, 736
   fractures 263
   screw 67, 67f
      placement of 738f
Malleolus, medial 737f
Mallet
   finger 18, 99, 182, 182f, 183, 183f
      injuries, mechanism of 788f
   fracture 183f
   splints 183
Malum coxae senilis 666
Malunion
   clavicle 116, 116f
   distal radius 42f
   femur, shortening in 42f
   fracture femur 220f

   olecranon fracture 151f
   proximal tibia fracture 252f
   subtrochanteric fracture 213f
Malunited Colles' fracture 630fc
Malunited supracondylar fracture
   femur 224f
   humerus 106f
Mantoux test 533
Marble bone disease 503
March fracture 276, 276f
Marfan's syndrome 505
Marie-Strumpell disease 576
Marrow
   biopsy 614
   cells 86
   fibrosis 518
   hypoplasia 566
Mason's classification 147
Matsen's mnemonic tubs 125
Maudsley's test 375
Mayo's operation 433
McAfee's classification 308
McFarland's bone grafting 485
McMurray's
   displacement osteotomy 641
   osteotomy 357f, 641f
   test 240
Meckel's cartilage 7
Medial malleolus
   fixation 740
   fracture 766f
      exposure of 737f
Medial meniscal
   injuries 241
   tear 799f
Medial parapatellar arthrotomy 814f
Medial scratch test 488
Median nerve 138, 382f
   compression test 383, 383f
   distribution 326f
   percussion test 383, 383f
Medulla 7
Medullary
   canal 761f
   cavity 523f
   fixation 149
   nails 485
   osteomyelitis 529
Megavoltage radiotherapy 606
Meningocele 594
Meniscal
   excision 814f
   injuries 99, 239fc, 415
      types of 238f
   pathology 792
   transplant 241
Meniscectomy 663

Meniscus injury, medial 239*f*, 240*f*
Mental
　amputation 632
　retardation 584*f*
Meralgia paresthetica 336
　treatment 336
　types 336
Metabolic bone disease 508
Metacarpal
　bones 189
　fracture 73, 189, 191, 275*f*, 760
　　K-wire fixation of 190*f*
　head fractures 191
Metacarpophalangeal joint 442
　dislocations 187
Metallic femoral component 813
Metaphyseal chondrodysplasia 504
Metaphysis 8, 523
Metatarsal
　arch 784
　bars 54, 427*f*
　bone 274*f*, 275*f*, 425, 774
　　stress fracture of III 109*f*
　fractures 274
　　classification 274
　　treatment 274
　injuries
　　classification 275
　　treatment 275
Metatarsophalangeal joint 272
　classification 273
　injuries 272
　treatment 273
Methotrexate 572
　drug 573
Meyer Ding's grading 393, 394*f*
Meyer's muscle pedicle graft 640
Middle volar space infection 442*f*
Midfoot
　fractures 277*fc*
　injuries 276
Midpatellar port 796
Migration 74
Mill's maneuver 375
Milwaukee brace 782, 782*f*
Miner's elbow 99, 377
Minerva jacket 782, 783*f*
Minimally invasive
　skeletal stabilization 80, 80*f*
　spinal surgery 83
　surgeries 224
Mobility
　abnormal 17
　loss of 138
Modern osteosynthesis, father of 55
Modules clamps 76
Monoarthritis, nonspecific 556
Monolateral fixator 260

Monosodium urate
　arthropathy 580
　crystals 580*f*
Monteggia's equivalents, types of 162*f*
Monteggia's fracture 19, 157, 133, 161, 161*f*-163*f*, 163*t*
Moore's approach 707, 709*f*
Morquio-Brailsford disease 501
Morton's neuroma 99, 426, 426*f*, 427*f*
Motor vehicle accidents 4
Movie sign 414*f*
Mucopolysaccharide disorders 501
Müller and Weber classification 35, 35*t*
Multiple
　bone cysts 518
　drill holes 526
　epiphyseal dysplasias 396
　fibrous septa 441*f*
　injuries 41
　metatarsal fractures 274*f*
　mycelia 108
　myeloma 613, 614*f*
　organ failure 4
　pins 639
　system injuries 57
Multisystem injuries 29, 41
Muscle 24, 40, 60, 65, 478, 709*f*, 775
　abdominal 458*f*
　atrophy 95
　closure of 739*f*
　complete tear of 92
　contraction 91*f*
　　active 92
　forces 14
　imbalance 352, 352*f*
　injury 90
　　types of 98
　ischemia 32
　normal 322
　re-education of 338
　relaxants 92, 93*f*, 357
　spasm 56, 62, 92, 398
　　severe 91
　strain 93*f*, 461
　　treatment of 92*t*
　　types of 90*f*
　strengthening 662
　　exercises 97
　supinator 475
　tethering 352*f*
　wasting of 335*f*, 545*f*
Muscular dystrophies 592, 593
　classification of 592*t*
Musculoskeletal system 456
Mycobacterium 522
　leprae 589
Myelocele 594, 594*f*
Myelography 465, 674

Myelomeningocele 594, 594*f*
Myodesis 775
Myoplasty 775
Myositis ossificans 28, 40, 40*f*, 138, 146, 204
　traumatic 39

N

Nade's indications 526
Nail 689*f*, 735*f*
　bed
　　injuries 195*f*
　　lacerations 194
　breakage 75*f*
　entry 734*f*
　fixed angle 639
　flexible medullary 70, 218
　interlocking 80*f*, 159*f*, 213*f*
　orientation of 722*f*
　patella syndrome 505
　plate 441
　types of 218
Narcotic analgesics 92
Nash and Moe's method 388
National Leprosy Eradication
　Program 589
Navicular bone fractures 277, 277*f*
　complications 277
　treatment 277
Neck 467
　bones 298*f*
　exercises 675
　extension 676
　femur, intracapsular fracture 637*f*
　flexion 300*f*, 676, 676*f*
　fracture, fixation of 227*f*
　ipsilateral fracture of 226*f*
　regional conditions of 362
　rheumatoid 569*f*
　rotation 676
Necrosis
　avascular 39, 205
　ischemic 31
Neer's classification 221, 221*f*
Neibauer and King technique 484
Nephritis 513
Nerve 44, 65, 448, 775
　degeneration 320
　　etiology 320
　　general causes 320
　　local causes 320
　　types 320
　grafting 324
　　interfascicular 323*f*
　injury 44*t*, 220, 321*t*802
　　classification of 320
　　principles of 320
　　types of 45

palsy, triple 592
pressure symptoms 365
regeneration 320
repair, types of 323, 323f
root 745f
  compression 451, 452t
  involvement 302
spinal 319
Nervous system 456, 585
Neural tube defects 593
Neurofibromas, locations of 506
Neurofibromatosis 391, 439
  congenital 506
Neurological system 452
Neurolysis 34
Neuromuscular disorders 583
Neuromyxofibroma 411
Neuron, part of 320
Neuropraxia 322
Neurorrhaphy 324
  epineural 323f
  epiperineural 323f
  partial 324, 726
  perineural 323f
Neurovascular injuries 18, 116, 134f
Neutralization plate 69
Newman classification 392
Nightstick fracture 160, 160f
Nonischemic limbs 776
Nonmetallic implants 66
Nonsteroidal anti-inflammatory
  drugs 20, 40, 92, 266, 336, 362, 413, 642
Nontraumatic orthopedic disorders 343

O

O' Donohue's unhappy triad 230
O'Brien's needle 268
Obesity 461, 580, 666, 802
Obturator foramen 288f
Odontoid process fracture 307, 308f
Olecranon 97
  bursitis 377, 377f
  fracture 74, 133, 148, 148f-150f
    comminuted 150f
    types of 149f
  osteotomy 700f
Ollier's disease 502
Omer's technique 333
Omoto technique 283, 284f
Onycho-osteodysplasia 505
Open reduction 101, 138, 176, 180, 182-184, 186, 190, 203, 207, 209, 244, 626, 643
  methods of 21
  principles of 21
  techniques of 203
Opioid analgesics 663

Opponens palsy 592
Optimum pressure 49
Orthopedic 53f, 589, 619
  deformities 566, 583, 587, 594f
    encountered 587t
  disease 345
  disorders 345, 345f
    treatment of 354
  emergency 31
  general 469
  goal 270, 276
  injury 16
  treatment, principles of 589
Orthosis 781, 782
  action of 781
Orthotic 778, 780
  treatment 389
Orthotrauma 19
Oschner's clasp test 327, 327f
Osgood-Schlatter disease 415
Ossification, types of 7
Osteitis fibrosa cystica 513, 517
Osteitis tuberculosa multiplex
  cystoides 554
Osteoarthritis 18, 415, 444, 556, 564, 571t, 658, 659, 668f, 802
  management of 669
  post-traumatic 46
  primary 658, 658f
  secondary 666, 667, 802
  spine 671
  traumatic 27, 205
  treatment of 665
Osteoarthrosis 658
Osteoblastic lesion 616f
Osteoblasts 86
Osteochondritis
  deformans juvenilis 397
  dissecans 415, 416, 417f
Osteochondroma 598, 600f
Osteoclastoma 360, 600f, 610f
  proximal tibia 600f
Osteoclasts 86
Osteodystrophy
  hepatic 510
  renal 510, 513, 519
Osteogenesis 60
  imperfecta 108, 500, 519
  tarda 500
Osteogenic sarcoma 604, 604f, 605, 605f-607f
Osteoid osteoma 603, 603f, 604f
Osteolysis 802
Osteoma 603
Osteomalacia 108, 516, 516f, 518, 519
Osteomyelitis 8, 45, 521, 522f, 523, 525t, 526, 529-531
  acute 513, 519, 521, 523f, 524, 524f, 525

chronic 65, 77, 522, 524, 524f, 525f, 527, 528f, 530f
  classification of 521t
  sclerotic 531
  subacute 527, 527f
  tibia 46f, 258f
Osteon 7
Osteopetrosis 109f, 503, 503f, 519
Osteophyte 661, 661f, 667
  anterior bridging 675f
  formation 675
Osteoporosis 15f, 109, 518, 646, 646f-651f, 653f-655f
  degree of 637
  juxta-articular 569
  management of 649, 654
  treatment of 652, 653f
  types of 647t
Osteosarcoma 605, 606
Osteosclerosis 519
Osteosynthesis 173
Osteotomy 42, 79, 101, 106f, 353, 357, 483f, 485, 549, 574, 640, 668f
  derotation 141
  displacement 549, 668
  innominate 403f, 482
  methods 140
  role of 482, 641
  types of 357f, 641f
Oxygen
  radical generation 572
  tension measurement 637

P

Paget's disease 108, 407, 507, 507f, 519, 677
Pain 17 19, 64, 56, 90, 91, 91f, 94, 95, 97, 464, 678
  abdominal 579
  arthritic 78
  chest 579
  chronic 356
  localized 90
  mild 95
  nature of 464
  sciatic 464
  subcalcaneal 428
Painful annular ligament 374
Paley's classification 35
Palmar
  flexion 631
  ganglion, compound 384, 384f
  rim dislocation 168
Paralysis 19, 591
Paraplegia 315f, 542
  causes of 542t
Parathyroid glands 518
Paresthesia 19, 678

Paronychia 440, 440f
Parrot beak tear 238f
Parson's radiological features 513
Passive rom exercises 94, 95
Patella 797
    acute dislocation of 247, 247f
    alta 584
    dislocation of 584
    displaced transverse fracture of 72f
    displacement of 419
    fracture of 242
    functions of 242
    high riding 419
    intercondylar notch of 243f
    nonunion 245f
    recurrent dislocation of 412
    surgery of 726
Patellar
    component 813
    fractures
        cause of 242f
        treatment of 246
    tendon bearing prosthesis 779
    tendonitis 99
    tracking 797, 800
Patellectomy 244, 664, 726
    disadvantages of 245
Paternalistic method 837
Pauwel's classification 636f
Pauwel's osteotomy 641f
Pectoralis major muscle, rupture of 93f
Pellegrini-Stieda disease 40
Pelvic
    compression test 577f
    fracture 289f, 290f, 292f
        operative fixation of 294f
        stable 290f
        types of 292f, 293, 293t
        unstable 288, 290f
    injuries 288
    osteotomies 482
    traction 679
Pelvis 478
    anatomy of 288f
    congenital disorders of 471
    deformity 511
    stability of 288
Pemberton's osteotomy 482, 483f
Pen test 327, 327f
Penicillamine 572
Percutaneous fixation 624, 626
    method of 691
Perilunar dislocation 177f
Periosteum 523, 533
    closure of 739f
Peripheral nerve
    injuries 59, 319
    root 320f
Peripheral tumors 602

Periprosthetic fractures 72, 75f, 802
Perkin's line 479, 481
Peroneal nerve 45
Persistent sinus, causes of 350
Perthes' disease 399f, 401, 401f, 401fc, 402f
Pertrochanteric fractures, fixation of 213
Pes cavus 422, 423, 424f
    classification of 422t
    degrees of 423t
Pes planus 423, 424t, 425f
Petechial rashes 30
Petrie cast 401, 402f
Phalangeal fractures 270, 272
    classification 271
    complications of 187
    nonoperative treatment 272
    operative treatment 272
Phalanges, multiple fractures of 271f
Phalanx 181
    Fracture
        proximal 185, 186f, 271f
        distal 181
Phalen's test 383, 383f
Phantom sensation 777
Phemister bone graft 38
Phosphorus metabolism 510t
Physeal fractures 152
Physiotherapy 34, 40, 580, 662, 668, 679
Physis 8
Pigeon chest 511
Pillar classification, lateral 400t
Pilon fracture 258, 259f, 260f
Pin 24, 75, 255
    breakage 77
    loosening 77
    migration 77
    number 76
    placement 76
    size 76
    tract infection 77
    types of 75
Pipkin's classification 199f
Pirani's classification 488
Piriformis syndrome 99
Pirogoff's amputation 774
Pisiform fractures 178, 178f
Pivot joint 11, 11f
Pivot shift test 233
Plague 3
Plantar
    fascia 428f
        fibromatosis of 432
    fasciitis 99, 428, 429f-431f
        types of 429fc
    fibromatosis 432
    flexion 452f
    ulcers 591, 591f, 592t
Plasmacytoma 613, 614f

Plaster
    allergy 59
    applications, types of 59f
    bandages 54
    cast 25
        application of 60f
    immobilization 87
Plaster of Paris 54, 55
    casts 25
    splint 58, 78
Plate 57, 68, 219
    breakage 75f
    fixation 733f
    osteosynthesis 80
    placement of 704f
    types of 68
Plica syndrome 99, 416
Plumb line test 406, 487, 488f
Pneumonia 31
    hypostatic 62
Podotech heel cushion 784
Pole fracture, proximal 172
Polio 3, 352f, 586
Poliomyelitis 586, 587f, 587t, 595
    acute anterior 526
    external appliances in 588t
Pollicis longus, flexor 193
Polyarthralgia 564
Polydactyly 439, 439f
Polydipsia 518
Polyethylene liner, insertion of 808f
Polyglycolic acid 74
Polylactic acid 74
Polymethylmethacrylate 66
Polytrauma 26f
Polyuria 518
Ponseti method 491
Ponseti technique 490, 490f
POP cast 98
    removal of 94
Popliteal artery, aneurysm of 411
Posterior segmental stabilization 72
Post-injection quadriceps contractures 418
Postpolio residual paralysis, stage of 588
Postreduction traction 203
Posture exercises 650
Pott's paraplegia, treatment of 543
Pressure
    abnormal external 97
    bandage 93, 94, 99
    intramuscular 32
    sores 59
Profunda femoris artery 634f
Progressive diaphyseal dysplasia 504
Pronation abduction 263f
    ankle fractures 264f
Pronation external rotation 263f

Prosthesis 779, 779f, 780
   choice of 801
   conventional type 779
   head of 710f
   metallic 801
   seating of 711f
   temporary 778, 778f
   types of 801
Prosthetic stem, breakage of 75f
Protrusio acetabuli 548f
Provocation tests 364, 426
Proximal
   femur
      breakage of 809f
      osteotomy of 207
   fragments, excision of 150, 174
   muscles, wasting of 516
   tibial fracture, classification of 250fc
Pseudarthrosis 485
   congenital 82, 471, 484, 495
   tibia 506f
Pseudogout 581f, 582
Pseudo-Jones fracture 275
Pseudoparalysis 526
Pseudorickets, renal 513
Psoriasis 444
Pubic symphysis 288f
Pubis 288f
Puller's technique 145f
Pulse rate 524
Pump handle test 577f
Punch forceps 791
Pusher's technique 145f
Pyelonephritis, chronic 513
Pyle's disease 504
Pyrexia 524
Pyrophosphate, inorganic 501

Q

Quadratus femoris 40, 478
Quadriceps
   contraction 242, 409
   drill 716f
   exercises 716f
   strain 99, 246
   strengthening of 662
Quicker fracture healing 80

R

Rachitis tarda 511
Radial
   club hand, radiograph of 477f
   column 164
   head 19
      excision 148f, 702
      fracture 74, 147, 147f
   nerve 138
      distribution 326f
      injury 45f, 329, 330, 332fc, 333
   styloid fracture 166
Radiocarpal
   dislocation 176
   injuries 176
Radioulnar
   joints, inferior 158f
   synostosis, congenital 440, 471, 475, 475f, 475t, 496
   translation, proximal 146
Radius 471
   congenital
      absence of 476
      dislocation of 477, 477f
   exposure of 703f
   fracture
      distal 163
      superior 292f
   greenstick fracture of 101f
   lower end of 611f
Randomized controlled trials 829, 831
Rectus femoris 409
Recurrent dislocation 27, 146, 205, 207
Reflex sympathetic dystrophy 45
Rehabilitation 20
   methods 429
   postoperative 421, 716f
Reisser's classification 388
Reisser's sign 388
Reiter's disease 575
Reiter's syndrome 444
Relaxation techniques 575
Relocation test 128
Respiratory distress syndrome, acute 29
Retinacular vessels, ascending 634f
Retrocalcaneal spur 430f, 431f
Rheumatic diseases 564
Rheumatoid 574
   arthritis 444, 556, 564-567, 569, 569f-571f, 574f, 575f, 802
   foot 567
   hand 566, 567f, 574f
   knee 570f
Ribs 19, 296f
   fractures 51, 296, 297f, 788
   treatment of fracture 297f
Richter's thermometer 323
Rickets 510, 512f, 512t, 515f, 516, 519
   infantile 511
   nutritional 108, 511
   renal 513t, 514fc, 515f
   types of 516t
Rigid
   fixation 57
   internal fixation 638
   spinal brace 782

Ring fixator 76, 81
   system 82
Riordan's operation 328
Road traffic accident 10, 13, 230, 242f, 289, 300, 521, 635
Rolando's fracture 175, 176f
Roll test 399, 399f
Romovac drain, placement of 732f
Root involvement 304t
Rotation injury, flexion 301f
Rotator cuff 121
   injuries 99
   lesions 368
   muscles of 369f
   repairs 73
   role of 368
   tear 370, 371f
      classification of 370
Roux's sign 291
Ruedi and Allgower classifications 259
Russel Taylor classification 212
Russell traction 217f

S

Sach foot 780, 780f
Sacroiliac joint
   involvement 577f
   sclerosis 579f
Sacrum, fracture of 289f
Sag sign 236f
Salter's extrusion angle 400, 401f
Salter's osteotomy 482
Salter-Harris classification 107f
Salter-Harris injury 108f
Salter-Thompson's classification 400
Sarcoidosis 518
Sarcoma, synovial 616
Sarmiento's amputation 774
Sarmiento's total contact below knee cast 254
Saturday night palsy 330, 330f
Saucerization 529
Scalene muscle insertion, abnormal 363f
Scaphoid 19
   blood supply of 172f
   bone 173f
   cast 173f
   fracture 19, 171, 172f, 173f, 174
      nonunion 173f
      treatment plan in 174fc
Scapula 129f
   congenital disorders of 471, 473, 496
   fracture 129, 130f
      lateral border 130f
   plain X-ray of 473
   winging of 340f
Scapular fractures, types of 130f

Scheuermann's disease 395
School bag syndrome 465, 466f
Sciatic nerve 333, 334f
    injury 205, 205f
Scleritis 566
Scleroderma 564
Scleromalacia perforans 566
Sclerosis
    loss of 671f
    subchondral 661f, 667
Scoliosis 386, 390, 391, 677
    congenital 386
    idiopathic 386
    neuromuscular 391
    nonstructural 386
    paralytic 386, 388f
    structural 386
    surgical treatment, methods of 391fc
    types of 387f
Scottish rite brace 401, 402f
Scottish terrier sign 394f
Scratch test 487
Screw 21, 57, 67
    outer diameter of 67
Scurvy 108, 519, 526
    infantile 513
Seatbelt injury 309
Seddon's carpectomy 34
Seddon's classification 320, 320t
Seinsheimer's classification 212
Semilunar cartilage injuries 237
Semi-tubular plate 69f
Senile osteoporosis 108
Sensory root 319f
Septic arthritis
    stages of 558f
    types of 557t
Sequestrectomy 529
Sequestrum 527, 528f
    forceps 529
Sesamoid bone 10
    fractures 274f
    function of 273
    injuries 273
        treatment 273
Sesamoidectomy 273
Sesamoiditis 435
Sever's disease 431, 432f
Sevitt's classification 30
Shaft femur, nonunion fracture 221f
Shanz angulation osteotomy 641, 641f
Sharrard classification 589
Shenton's line 200f, 479, 481, 637f
Shock 46
    spinal 304
    vasovagal 65
Shorbe's classification 155

Shoulder 467, 589
    anterior dislocation of 27f, 123, 124f, 125, 125f
    apprehension test 128f
    arthroscopy 793f
    complex 787
    disarticulation 773, 780
    dislocation 121, 123f
    drooping of 18
    flat 18
    joint 127f
        anatomy of 121f, 369f
        anterior dislocation of 123f, 124f
        dislocation 124f
        injuries of 121
        posterior dislocation of 129, 129f
    posterior dislocation of 122t, 124f
    recurrent anterior dislocation of 125
    replacement, total 359f
    rheumatoid 568f
    septic arthritis of 557f
    stabilization procedure 73
    tuberculosis of 552, 553f
Sicard's test 453
Sickle cell anemia 526
Simple fractures, management of 20
Sinding-Larsen-Johansson syndrome 415
Singh's index 637f
Sinus tract 350, 527
Sjögren's syndrome 566
Skeletal
    system 7
        bone of 512
    traction 24, 25, 63, 65, 209, 217, 306, 306t
        complications of 65
    trauma 44t
Skier's thumb 189
Skin
    changes 511f
    closure 704f, 728f, 745f, 813f, 826f
        final 686f, 732f
    exposure 727f
    flap 773, 775
    grafting 381
    incision 742f, 743f, 803f, 814f
    marking 802f
    resistance test 323
    tight cast 58
    traction 62, 63, 63f, 217
        method of 62f
        types of 63
Skull, base of 19
Small intervertebral muscles 448
Smallpox 3
Smillie's classification 238

Smillie's meniscus knife 241f
Smith's fracture 166, 167f
Smith's traction 17f, 106f
Sofield's method 501
Sofield's multiple osteotomies 485
Soft tissue 684f
    classification of 22
    contractures 77, 352f
    dissection 697f
    excision of 815f
    injuries 89, 89f, 194, 787f
        classification of 90
    neck injury 300
    procedures 491
    repair of 74
    swelling 19, 569
Solid action cushion heel 780
Soutter's release 588
Spasm 91f, 464
Spastic equinovalgus 585f
Spastic equinovarus 585f
Spica cast 56
Spina bifida 593, 594f, 595, 595f
    aperta 593, 594
    occulta 593, 594
    types of 594
Spinal
    canal 299f, 537f
    cord injuries 313, 318
    curves, normal 298f
    instrumentation, anterior 312
    muscles, retraction of 746f
    nerve 319
        mixed 319f
        root 320f
    orthoses 781, 782
        functions of 782
Spine 506, 584, 587
    implants 21
    injuries 51, 298, 308
        incidence of 300
    locking plate 306
    regional conditions of 386
    surgeries 72, 80f, 83, 742
    tuberculosis of 538f, 540f
Split skin graft 25
Spondylitis, ankylosing 575, 576, 577f, 578t, 579, 579f
Spondyloarthritis, seronegative 564
Spondylolisthesis 391, 393f, 393t, 471
Spondylosis, cervical 674, 675f
Sports injuries 5, 5f, 462f, 786, 787
    causes of 788f
    classification of 787
    treatment of 788
Sprain 13 28
    types of 93

Sprengel's shoulder 473, 474f
   deformity 473, 473f
   functions in 474f
Squamous cell carcinoma 530
Stabilization
   stage of 450
   temporary 21
Stable
   fracture 172, 211, 311
   injuries 264
   pelvic fracture 288
Staphylococcus aureus 440, 521, 527, 556
Starch test 322
Static
   encephalopathy 583
   foot-drop splint 335f
   metatarsalgia 425
   tension band 68
   wrist splint 332f
Steel's osteotomy 482, 483f
Steep learning curve 793
Steindler's release 588
Steinmann's pin 72, 64f, 768f
Steinmann's sign 240
Stenosis
   canal 678f
   spinal 462, 465
Sternoclavicular joint 118, 119f
   dislocation 119f
   injuries 118, 119f
Sternocleidomastoid muscle 471
Steroids 31, 92
   epidural 458, 679
   intra-articular 663, 668
   local 573
Stimson's classification 142, 142t
Stimson's gravity 203f
   method 124f, 207
Stompers gel heel pad 784
Straight leg raising test 453
Strain 13 28, 90
   first degree 90
   severity of 90
Streeter's dysplasia 439
Streptococcus 556
   haemolyticus 521
   pyogenes 440
Stress
   fractures 15, 109, 110
   injury 447, 466
   psychological 565
   tests 184, 231f
Student's elbow 99, 377
Stulberg classification 400
Stump neuroma 320
Styloid process test 622, 625f
Subclinical fat embolism syndrome 31

Subluxation 13 26f, 28, 120, 584
Subperiosteal abscess, formation of 523f
Subscapularis tendonitis 99
Subtalar dislocation 286f
Subtrochanteric fracture 211f, 213f
   femur 212f
   fixation of 213
Sudeck's osteodystrophy 631, 631f, 632f
Sulcus test 128
Sulfasalazine 572
Sultanpur technique 141
Sunderland's classification 320, 321t
Supracondylar fracture 32, 133, 138f, 221f, 222f, 691
   flexion type of 141
   management of 139fc
   type of 134f, 135f
Supracondylar pin traction 720f
Suprapatellar bursa 797
Supraspinatus tendinitis 99, 369
Supraspinous ligament 299f
   excision of 743f
Surgery, methods of 394
Swan neck deformity 18f, 566
Sweat test 322
Swelling 17, 94, 95, 97, 465
Syme's amputation 774, 776, 777f, 780
Syme's prosthesis 780f
Symphysis 11
Synarthrosis 11
Synchondroses 11
Syndesmosis 11
Synovectomy 549, 574
Synovial joints, types of 11
Synovioma 616
Synovitis 95, 549, 552, 558f, 565f
   acute 95
   chronic 95
   stage of 547, 547f
   traumatic 95f
Synovium 93, 94, 792
Syphilis, congenital 513
Syphilitic arthritis, classification of 559t
Syringomyelia 666
Syringomyelocele 594
Systemic lupus erythematosus 564

T

Tachycardia 30
Tachypnea 30
Tai chi 663
Talipes 485
   cavus 584
   equinovarus 584
      congenital 471, 485, 741
Talocalcaneal articulation 486

Talus 486
   blood supply of 284, 285f
   body of 286
   fracture 285f, 286f
      fixation of 287f
   neck of 284, 286f
   types 286
Tardy ulnar nerve palsy 329, 329f
Tarsal tunnel syndrome 99
Tarsometatarsal injuries 278, 279
   classification 279
   treatment 279
Tear drop sign 135, 135f
Technetium bone scan 171
Tendo-Achilles 97, 428, 588
   injuries 99, 267
   lengthening 491f
   repair 269
   rupture 268f
      injury of 268f
   trauma around region of 428
Tendon 65
   flexor 442
   grafting 193, 360, 361f
   injuries 192
      flexor 192
   origin 182
   surgeries 360
   transfer 34, 193, 324, 588
      operation 592
      techniques 333
Tennis elbow 99, 373, 373f, 375f, 376f
   medial 376
   tenderness in 375f
Tenosynovitis 98, 442, 443f, 564
Tenotomy, method of 491f
Tenovaginitis 98, 98f
Tensile trabeculae, primary 633f
Tension band
   dynamic 68
   principle 68, 69
   wiring 72f, 73f, 245, 245f, 726, 728f
Tension force, law of 81
Teratogenesis 471
Teriparatide, role of 654
Terminal flexion, loss of 660f
Tetanus 47
   immunoglobulin 48
Thermotherapy 94, 97
Thigh 776
   adductor muscles of 40
   hematoma of 98f
Thomas splint 54, 60
   parts of 61, 61f
   uses of 61
Thomas test 399, 419f, 545
Thompson and Epstein classification 199

Thompson's classification 129
Thompson's quadriceps plasty 409, 421
Thompson's test 268
Thoracic
  kyphosis 298
  nerve 340
  outlet syndrome 363
    complications 364
    tests 364
    treatment 364
  outlet, anatomy of 363*f*
  rib, anomalies of first 363
  spine 299
Thoracolumbar
  fractures 308*f*, 309*f*
  injuries
    stable 312*f*
    treatment plan for 311*fc*
  region 313
  spine 308
Thrombocytopenia 31
Thrombocytosis 566
Thumb metacarpophalangeal joint, dislocation of 189
Tibia 471, 486, 528*f*, 818*f*
  bony anatomy of 249*f*
  chronic osteomyelitis of 528*f*
  congenital absence of 494, 494*t*
  diaphyseal sequestrum of 524*f*
  fractures 57*f*, 72, 76*f*, 249, 252, 253, 253*f*, 255*fc*, 258
    cause of 249*f*
    complications of 256
    fixation 71*f*
    proximal 69*f*, 250*f*, 251*f*
  greenstick fracture of 15*f*
  hypertrophic nonunion of 37*f*
  interlocking nail of 79*f*, 733
  plafond fractures 258
  plating of 255*f*
  postsubluxation of 562
  shortening of 258*f*
  stress fracture of 110*f*
  surgery of 729
  vara 407
Tibial fractures
  distal 258
  open 260
  proximal 249
Tibial nerve
  anterior 333*f*
  posterior 333*f*
Tibial osteotomy
  high 357
  proximal 664
Tile's classification 291
Tinel's sign 322
Tip toe test 268

Toe
  fractures 763
  injuries 763
Torsion wedge nonunion 36*f*
Torticollis 362, 473*f*
  congenital 472*fc*
  management 362
Torus fracture 15, 15*f*, 16*f*, 101
Total hip replacement 549, 574*f*, 641, 802
Total knee
  arthroplasty 664
  replacement 574*f*, 664*f*, 813, 813*f*
Tourniquet palsy 330*f*
Toxic theory 30
Traction 54, 56, 62, 390, 668
  dynamic 184
  methods 62, 136, 207, 223
  points 64*t*
  skeletal 306*f*
  trabeculae 8
Traffic elbow 155*f*
Transfemoral amputations 779
Transiliac bone biopsy 649
Translational injuries 309, 310*f*
Transverse
  arch 422
  carpal ligament 384*f*
  costal facet 299*f*
  fracture 242*f*
Trapezius muscle 302*f*
Trauma 6, 39, 44, 97, 666
  care system, lack of 6
  mechanism of 4
  skeletal 44*t*
Trendelenburg's test 398, 547, 548*f*
Treponema pallidum 522, 559
Trethowan sign 404*f*
Trigen knee nail 224
Trochanteric fracture 55, 61, 642, 644, 644*f*
  fixation 644*f*
  nonunion 644*f*
  treatment of 643
Trochlea 797
Trunk
  congenital disorders of 471
  flex 458*f*
  muscle strains 788
  rotation 387
Tube defects 594
Tubercle bacillus 522
Tubercular
  abscess, treatment of 534
  arthritis 536
  dactylitis 554*f*
  osteomyelitis 531, 553
Tuberculosis 3, 535
  hip 549, 802
    stages of 546, 547*f*

knee, treatment of 552
musculoskeletal 535
skeletal 532, 533*f*, 534*t*, 536
spine 536
  complications of 542
Tuberosity, fracture of 172*f*
Tubular bones, tuberculosis of 554
Tumor 13
  endoprosthesis 606
  excision 82
  malignant 596*t*
Turco's procedure 491
Turn-o-plasty technique 611
Two-pin traction method 223
Tying external rotator muscles 709*f*
Typhoid 3
Typical Colles' cast 623*f*
Typical Colles' fracture 623

U

Ulcerative colitis 575
Ulna 705
  greenstick fracture of 101*f*
  reduplication of 440
Ulnar
  bursa 384*f*
  bursae 443*f*
  claw hand 325*f*, 325*fc*, 592
  nerve 45, 138, 324*f*
    distribution 326*f*
    injury 324-326, 327*f*, 328, 329
Unicondylar knee replacement 664*f*
Universal hand splint 181
Universal mini external fixator 83
Upper limb 27, 44, 99, 323, 349, 584, 587, 773, 787, 781
  amputations 780
  congenital disorders of 471
  deformities 586*f*
  dermatomal pattern of 674*f*
  muscles 789
  orthosis 781, 785
  regional conditions of 366
  tractions 64
  trauma 44
Upper tibial traction 223
Urinary tract, injuries of 294
Urogenital system 456

V

Vacuum mixing technique 811*f*
Valgus 485, 664*f*
  osteotomy 668
  pads 785
  stress test 231*f*, 233
Vanillylmandelic acid 613

Varus
  deformity 661f
  femoral osteotomy, technique of 403f
  stress test 231f
Vascular injury 138, 642, 802
Vasculitis 565f
Vastus lateralis 409
Vein 522f
Venography 637
Vertebra
  anatomy of 299f
  blood supply of 536f
Vertebral
  body 448
    excision, anterior 312
  column, normal appearance of 448f
  compression fractures 745
    treatment of 312
  injury 314
  reactions, types of 537t
Vertebroplasty 312, 313f
Vertical talus
  congenital 494
  radiograph of 495f
Viruses 586
Vital organs, protection of 7
Vitamin D 650
  intoxication 518
  resistant rickets 514, 515f
Volar Barton fracture 168f, 169f
  malunion of 169f
Volar trans-scaphoid perilunar
    dislocation 176
Volkmann's ischemia 31-33, 159
Volkmann's sign 33, 34
von Recklinghausen's disease 506, 517
von Rosen's line 479f, 482

W

Waist fracture 172f
Walking test 678
Wandering acetabulum 548
Watson-Jones method 202, 202f, 207
Web spaces, infection of 441
Well leg raising test 453
Wet method 58
Whiplash injury 300, 300f, 301f, 788
  signs 300
  symptoms 300
  treatment 301
Whipple's disease 575
Williams' classification 787, 787fc
Wound
  care 25
  closure of 732f, 745f
  exploration of 23
  exposure of 764f
  healing 775
  irrigation, after 767f
Wright's test 364, 364f
Wrist 99, 170, 467, 589, 622, 787
  bony anatomy of 170f
  cock-up splint 323f
  disarticulation 780
  drop 331f
    points, types of 332f
    splint 332f
    dynamic 332f
  extensors 303f
  flexors 192, 332
  hand orthoses 781
  joint 170
    palmar flexion of 355f
  regional conditions of 378
Wryneck 362f

X

Xenografting 360

Z

Zygoma 19